FOURTH
EDITION

EXERCISE PHYSIOLOGY

ENERGY, NUTRITION, AND HUMAN PERFORMANCE

WILLIAM D.
McARDLE

Professor, Department of Health and Physical Education
Queens College of the City University of New York
Flushing, New York

FRANK I.
KATCH

Professor, Department of Exercise Science
University of Massachusetts
Amherst, Massachusetts

VICTOR L.
KATCH

Professor, Department of Movement Science
Division of Kinesiology
Associate Professor, Pediatrics
School of Medicine
University of Michigan
Ann Arbor, Michigan

FOURTH EDITION

EXERCISE PHYSIOLOGY

ENERGY, NUTRITION, AND HUMAN PERFORMANCE

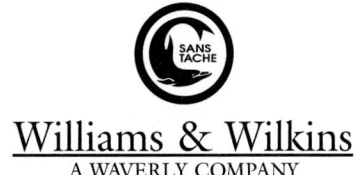

Williams & Wilkins
A WAVERLY COMPANY

BALTIMORE • PHILADELPHIA • LONDON • PARIS • BANGKOK
BUENOS AIRES • HONG KONG • MUNICH • SYDNEY • TOKYO • WROCLAW

Editor: Donna Balado
Managing Editor: Victoria M. Vaughn
Production Coordinator: Carol Eckhart
Copy Editors: Matthew Hauber, Thomas Lehr, Denise Wilson
Designer: Ashley Pound Design
Illustration Planner: Lorraine Wrzosek
Typesetter: Graphic World, Inc
Printer & Binder: Rand McNally

Copyright © 1996, Williams & Wilkins

351 West Camden Street
Baltimore, Maryland 21201-2436 USA

Rose Tree Corporate Center
1400 North Providence Road
Building II, Suite 5025
Media, Pennsylvania 19063-2043 USA

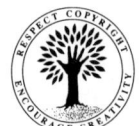

Accurate indications, adverse reactions and dosage schedules for drugs are provided in this book, but it is possible that they may change. The reader is urged to review the package information data of the manufacturers of the medications mentioned.

Printed in the United States of America

First Edition, 1981; Second Edition, 1986; Third Edition, 1991

Library of Congress Cataloging-in-Publication Data

McArdle, William D.
  Exercise physiology : energy, nutrition, and human performance /
William D. McArdle, Frank I. Katch, Victor L. Katch. — 4th ed.
      p. cm.
  Includes bibliographical references and index.
  ISBN 0-683-05731-6
  1. Exercise—Physiological aspects.   I. Katch, Frank I.
II. Katch, Victor L.   III. Title.
  [DNLM: 1. Exercise—physiology. 2. Nutrition. 3. Sports
Medicine. QT 260 M478e 1996]
  QP301.M375   1996
  612'.044—dc20
  DNLM/DLC
  for Library of Congress   95-38064
                                                                                          CIP

The publishers have made every effort to trace the copyright holders for borrowed material. If they have inadvertently overlooked any, they will be pleased to make the necessary arrangements at the first opportunity.

Call our customer service department at (800) 638-0672 for catalog information or fax orders to (800) 447-8438. For other book services, including chapter reprints and large quantity sales, ask for the Special Sales Department.

To purchase additional copies of this book or for information concerning American College of Sports Medicine certification and suggested preparatory materials, call (800) 486-5643.

Canadian customers should call (800) 268-4178, or fax (905) 470-6780. For all other calls originating outside of the United States, please call (410) 528-4223 or fax us at (410) 528-8550.

Visit Williams & Wilkins on the Internet: http://www.wwilkins.com or contact our customer service department at custserv@ wwilkins.com. Williams & Wilkins customer service representatives are available from 8:30 am to 6:00 pm, EST, Monday through Friday, for telephone access.

                                                                96 97 98 99 00
                                                        1 2 3 4 5 6 7 8 9 10

This edition is dedicated to our wives (Kathleen, Kerri, and Heather), our children (Theresa, Amy, Kevin, and Jennifer; David, Kevin, and Ellen; Erika, Leslie, and Jesse), and our parents (Harry and Claire; Roma and Kurt). All things considered, it is family that gives meaning to life.

We also dedicate this edition to that special group of former students who earned doctoral degrees in physical education and exercise science, and who have gone on to distinguish themselves as teachers and researchers in the related areas of exercise physiology. These include Doug Ballor, Dan Becque, George Brooks, Barbara Campaigne, Ken Cohen, Edward Coyle, Dan Delio, Julia Chase Delio, Chris Dunbar, Patti Freedson, Roger Glaser, Ellen Glickman, Nancy Greer, Everett Harmon, Tibor Hortobagyi, Betsy Keller, Jie Kang, George Lesmes, Steve Lichtman, Charles Marks, Karen Nau, Laurel Traeger-Mackinnon, Robert Mofatt, Steve Ostrove, James Rimmer, Stan Sady, Lapros Sidossis, Bob Spina, Mike Toner, Lorraine Turcotte, John Villanacci, Jonnis Vrabas, Nancy Wessinger, Stephen Westing, Art Weltman, Anthony Wilcox, and Linda Zwiren.

Finally, a sincere "thank you" to our former professors and cherished colleagues who had a profound influence on our personal and professional development: the late Albert Behnke and Franklin Henry, Jerry Ball, David Benson, John Faulkner, Don Fleming, Guido Foglia, Ernest Michael, Jr., Henry Montoye, George Q. Rich III, Bob Salmons, and Earl Wallis. Without the encouragement, stimulation, and example of these mentors, none of this would have been possible.

PREFACE

When we began to prepare the fourth edition of *Exercise Physiology, Energy, Nutrition, and Human Performance,* we knew we faced a huge undertaking, especially because so much new research had been published in fields related to exercise, health, and physical fitness. Our singular purpose was to provide the most up-to-date information in exercise physiology, particularly in the emerging areas of sport nutrition, exercise and immune function, body composition analysis, obesity and genetics, allometric scaling, and exercise and oxidative stress, without compromising coverage of the more established topics of exercise bioenergetics and environmental, neuromuscular, endocrine, cardiovascular, and pulmonary function. As the revision process unfolded, we added new and more complete information on neuromuscular physiology and adaptation with exercise (Chapters 18, 19, and 22) and expanded our presentations of bioenergetics (Chapters 5 and 6), exercise metabolism (Chapters 7 and 11), and the hormonal response to exercise and training (Chapter 20). We also added a new chapter (Chapter 31) that introduces the clinical aspects of exercise testing and rehabilitation in cancer and in cardiovascular and pulmonary disease.

A new feature at the beginning of each chapter is *Focus on Research,* a synopsis of an article selected for the pioneering aspects of the research, or the unique qualities of its methodology and design. We selected the articles not becaue they necessarily represented the "best" research available on a particular topic, although many of the lead authors are outstanding scientists. Our intention is that the *Focus On Research* provide the "flavor" of the research process, often in the early stages of inquiry on a particular topic in exercise physiology.

In this revision, we also wanted to pay tribute to the people and events that helped shape the field of exercise physiology. To accomplish this, we wrote a new introductory section that highlights many historical milestones, from the early Greek physicians to the European pioneers in anatomy, medicine, and physiology, to the American and Nordic physiologists, physicians, and physical educators who helped shape and define present-day exercise physiology. We hope you will gain a greater understanding about current themes in exercise physiology from this snapshot of the past. Never in our wildest dreams as graduate students or professors did we think we would become so fascinated with our professional history, let alone write about it! But it happened, and we are fortunate to have such esteemed colleagues and genuine friends as Charles Tipton, Roberta Park, and Per-Olaf Åstrand. They encouraged us to write the section and unselfishly provided keen insight and constructive suggestions on early drafts of our historical narrative (and also provided photographs of American and Nordic researchers). We also thank Tipton and Elsworth Buskirk for generously providing their original manuscripts (prior to publication) that present their views of the history of exercise physiology (references 9 and 53).

In preparing the revision of the text, we received significant input from undergraduate and graduate students regarding additional materials they would like to see accompany the main textbook. Students had benefited from the *Student Study Guide and Workbook* developed to accompany the *Essentials of Exercise Physiology* text, and requested that a similar workbook be developed for this text. This has been done in a manner that enables students to improve their assimilation of the material and at the same time "self test" their success. To enhance student understanding of key concepts and to keep pace with the rapidly expanding body of knowledge in exercise physiology, we modified many of our existing figures and added 113 new color graphics and 41 new tables. This brings the textbook's total to 377 color figures and 191 tables. We have also updated and expanded the appendixes to include the latest nutritional information on the composition of specialty and fast foods, coverage of SI units and terminology, and the American College of Sports Medicine's Position Stands on Osteoporosis and Exercise; Physical Activity, Physical Fitness, and Hypertension; and Exercise and Fluid Replacement. We are once again thankful to the Macintosh graphics wizards of ElectraGraphics, Inc., for their expertise and creative style in interpreting our ideas and making them come to life.

In addition to changes in the textbook and development of the accompanying workbook, we are introducing a new concept related to both the text material and the field itself. This project came about because of student requests for ancillary textbook information, as well as pertinent information about graduate school and employment opportunities in related areas after graduation. To meet these needs, we created a site on the World Wide Web of the Internet, called *The Exercise Physiology Club (EPC)*. The EPC provides the following:

- A comprehensive directory of allied health graduate programs in Exercise Science, Physical Therapy (undergraduate and graduate), Occupational Therapy, and Physician Assistant in the United States and Canada (including school listings by state, with information about entrance and degree requirements, deadlines, programs, number of students and faculty, accept/reject ratio, and contact person with addresses and phone numbers for correspondence).
- Practice questions for student use in preparation for exams.
- Crossword puzzles using exercise physiology terms and concepts to help students grasp material in a challenging and different way.
- An informational booklet about résumé writing, career planning, and job placement strategies that includes new and up-to-date materials for writing effective electronic resumes for job searching and finding internships, techniques of interviewing, and sites on the Internet that provide further information related to résumé writing, career planning, and job searching.
- A bulletin board to permit students and professors to correspond with us about exercise physiology–related topics.

- Up-to-date information about professional meetings, the American College of Sports Medicine, and topics related to exercise physiology.
- Information about sports nutrition, including sample low-fat, high-carbohydrate recipes for sport-specific meal planning.

It is our hope that the information provided by the EPC will catalyze and sustain interest in the diverse aspects of exercise physiology and its professional dimensions. You can assess the EPC using the following Internet URL:

HTTP://www.exer-phys-club.com

For further information about the EPC, write to Fitness Technologies at 1132 Lincoln, Ann Arbor, MI 48104 (fax [313] 662-8153).

We wish to acknowledge the following individuals who so kindly provided us with original data and/or photos: Bart Buxton, Edward Coyle, Michael Dechennes, Jim Dietz, Coop deRennie, Jay Graves, Hans Hoppeler, Richard Leiber, John-Eggs Magel, Bill Pearl, Jim Richardson, John Urbanchek, Art Weltman, and Judy Weltman. At Williams & Wilkins, we gladly acknowledge a group of dedicated professionals: editor Donna Balado; managing editor Victoria Vaughn; production coordinator Carol Eckhart; copy editors Matthew Hauber, Tom Lehr, and Denise Wilson; designer Ashley Pound; and marketing director Mary Finch. This fine team kept the project on track while orchestrating the numerous complexities involved in such an effort. Many thanks.

Special thanks to the American College of Sports Medicine for permission to use materials originally published in *Medicine and Science in Sports and Exercise*.

PUBLISHER'S NOTE

Williams & Wilkins is pleased to be one of the publishers leading the transition from traditional book printing to a new computer-to-plate technology. This process revolutionizes book manufacturing by enabling digital files to be sent directly from a computer system to a platesetter, which turns the digital input into full-size printing plates.

By eliminating photographic film from the prepress process, Williams & Wilkins and Rand McNally have made the book manufacturing process more environmentally friendly.

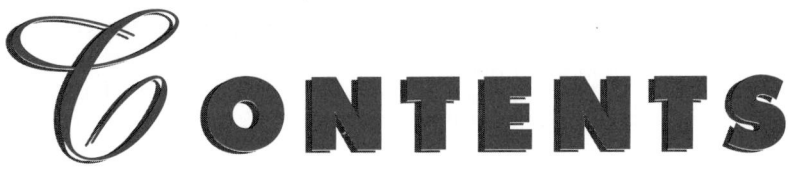ONTENTS

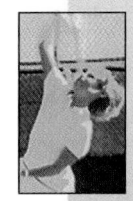

PART 1
EXERCISE PHYSIOLOGY

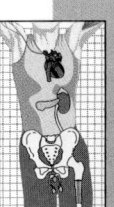

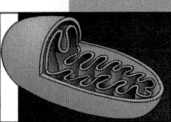

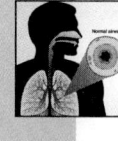

SECTION 3 • Systems of Energy Delivery and Utilization

PART 2
APPLIED EXERCISE PHYSIOLOGY

SECTION 4 • Enhancement of Energy Capacity

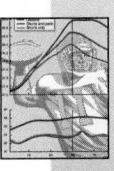
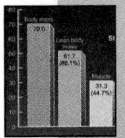

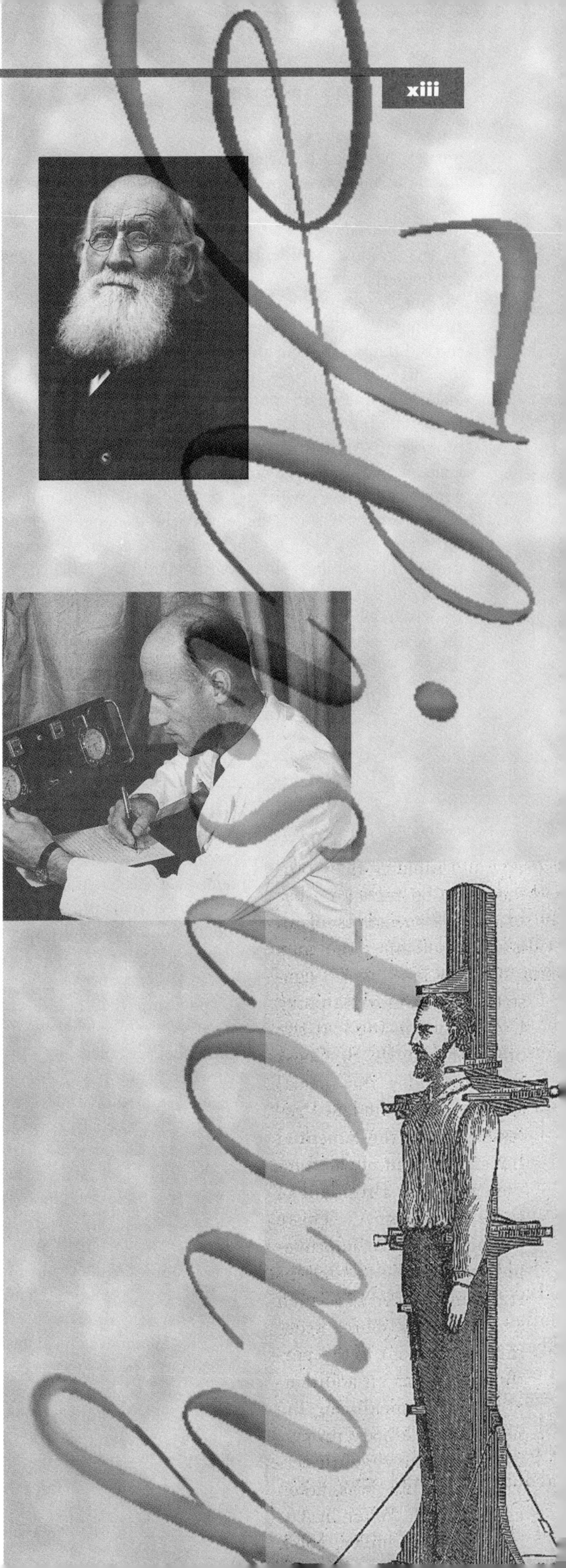

INTRODUCTION

Exercise Physiology: Roots and Historical Perspectives

The first edition of *Exercise Physiology: Energy, Nutrition, and Human Performance* appeared in 1981; since then, knowledge of the physiologic effects of exercise in general—and the body's unique and specific responses to training in particular—has exploded. Tipton's[53] search of the 1946 English literature for the terms *exercise* and *exertion* yielded 12 citations in five journals. Tipton also cited a 1962 study by Booth, who reported that in 1962 the number of citations of the term *exertion* increased to 128 in 51 journals, and that by 1981 there were 655 citations of *exercise* in 224 journals. A summary of our own computer search of the literature at 10-year intervals from 1966 to 1986 (and including 1994) is presented in the figure below; it shows the number of citations in *Index Medicus* (MEDLINE) in which *exercise* or *exertion* appears as a topic (illustrated in the top portion of each bar in the figure) and the number of times the word *exercise* appears in a journal title (bottom portion of each bar). In just 11 years, citations and topic headings increased almost sixfold to 3558! Interestingly, the

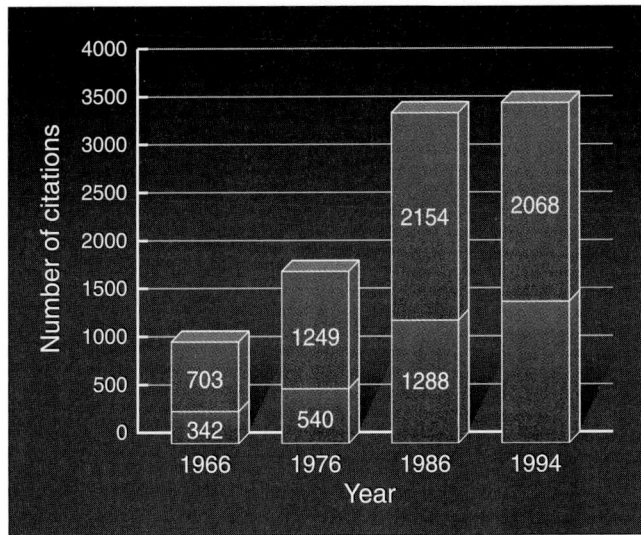

Exercise or *exertion* as a topic (*top bars*) and frequency of the word *exercise* appearing in a scientific journal title (*bottom bars*).

greatest increases occurred between 1976 and 1986; thereafter, the number of published articles about exercise or exertion and the occurrence of the word *exercise* in journal titles stabilized.

As graduate students in the late 1960s, we never dreamed that interest in exercise physiology would increase so quickly. A new generation of scholars committed to studying the scientific basis of exercise set to work. Some studied the physiologic mechanisms involved in the adaptations to regular exercise; others evaluated individual differences in exercise and sports performance. Both approaches contributed knowledge to the growing field of exercise physiology. At our first scientific conference (American College of Sports Medicine [ACSM] in Las Vegas, 1967), we rubbed elbows with the "giants" of the field, many of whom were themselves students of the leaders of their era. Sitting under an open tent in the Nevada desert with one of the world's leading physiologists, Dr. David Bruce Dill (then age 74), we listened to his researcher—a high school student—deliver a lecture about temperature regulation in the desert burro. Later, one of us (FK) sat next to a white-haired gentleman and chatted about a master's thesis pro-

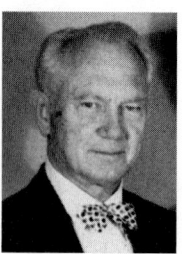

Albert R. Behnke (1899–1993).

ject. Only later did an embarrassed FK learn that this gentleman was Albert R. Behnke, M.D. (1898–1993; ACSM Honor Award, 1976), the modern-day "father" of human body composition analysis. His studies of underwater weighing in 1942, his development of a "reference man" and "reference woman" model, and his creation of the somatogram based on anthropometric measurements underlie much current work in body composition evaluation (refer to Chapter 27 and Focus on Research, p. 540). That meeting began a personal and professional friendship that lasted until Dr. Behnke's death in 1993.

Several hundred ACSM members listened attentively as the superstars of exercise physiology and physical fitness (such as Per-Olof Åstrand, Erling Asmussen, Bruno Balke, Elsworth Buskirk, Thomas Cureton, Lars Hermansen, Steven Horvath, Henry Montoye, Bengt Saltin, and Charles Tipton) presented their research and fielded tough questions from an audience of young graduate students eager to savor the latest scientific information.

Over the years, the three of us were fortunate to work with the very best in our field. William McArdle studied for the Ph.D. at Michigan with Dr. Henry Montoye (charter member of ACSM; President of ACSM, 1962–1963; Citation Award, 1973) and Dr. John Faulkner (President of ACSM, 1971–1972; Citation Award, 1973; and ACSM Honor Award, 1992). At the University of California, Berkeley, Victor Katch completed his M.S. thesis under the supervision of Dr. Jack Wilmore (President of ACSM, 1978–1979; Citation Award, 1984; and first editor of

Exercise and Sport Science Reviews, 1973–1974) and became a doctoral student of Dr. Franklin Henry (ACSM Honor Award, 1975; originator of the "Memory-Drum Concept" about the specificity of exercise; and author of the seminal paper "Physical Education—an Academic Discipline" [*JOHPER,* 35:32, 1964]) (see Focus on Research, p. 482). Frank Katch completed his M.S. degree at the University of California, Santa Barbara, under the supervision of Dr. Ernest Michael (a former student of pioneer exercise physiologist–physical fitness scientist Dr. Thomas Kirk Cureton, ACSM Honor Award recipient, 1969) and then also completed doctoral studies at the University of California, Berkeley, with Dr. Henry.

As the three of us examine those earlier times, we realize, like many of our colleagues, that our academic good fortunes occurred because our professors and mentors shared an unwavering commitment to study sport and exercise from a strong scientific and physiological perspective. These scholars demonstrated why it was crucial for physical educators to be well grounded in both the scientific basics and the underlying concepts and principles of exercise physiology.

We would be remiss if we did not acknowledge the pioneers who created exercise physiology. It is, of course, impossible in an introduction to present an adequate chronicle of the history of exercise physiology from its origins in ancient Asia to the present. Instead, our review presents historical information about topics not covered in prior exercise physiology textbooks or history texts. Our discussion begins with a brief acknowledgment of the ancient but tremendously influential Greek physicians; along the way, we highlight some milestones (and ingenious experiments), including the many contributions from Sweden, Denmark, Norway, and Finland that fostered the study of sport and exercise as a respectable field of scientific inquiry.

A treasure of information about the beginnings of exercise physiology in America was uncovered in the archives of Amherst College, Massachusetts: an anatomy and physiology textbook (incorporating a student study guide) written by the first American father-and-son writing team in exercise physiology. The father, Edward Hitchcock, was President of Amherst College; the son, Edward Hitchcock, Jr., an Amherst graduate and Harvard-trained physician, made detailed anthropometric and strength measurements of almost every student enrolled at Amherst College from 1861 to 1889. A few years later (1891–1892), much of what currently forms the college curriculum in exercise physiology, including evaluation of muscular strength and body size by anthropometry, began in the first physical education scientific laboratory at Harvard University's Lawrence Scientific School. Even before the creation of this laboratory, another less formal but still tremendously influential factor affected the development of exercise physiology: the publication during the 19th century of American textbooks on anatomy and physiology; physiology;

NORTHERN ATLANTIC OCEAN

Lugdunum

GAUL

Narbo

Aquileia

Corsica

Rome

Sardinia

Sicily

Syracuse

Carthage

ITALY

DALMATIA

THRACE

MACEDONIA

Thessalonica

BLACK SEA

MESOPOTAMIA

Pergamos

Ephesus

Athens

Sparta

Cos

Cnidus

Crete

Cyprus

Antioch

Damascus

PALESTINE

BABYLONIA

MEDITERRANEAN SEA

Alexandria

EGYPT

THE WORLD OF GALEN

lete, strongly advocated proper diet in physical training. His early writings and devoted followers influenced the famous physician Hippocrates ("father of preventive medicine"), who is credited with producing 87 treatises on medicine—including several on health and hygiene—during the Golden Age of Greece.[7] Today, physicians take the Hippocratic Oath, which is based on Hippocrates' *Corpus Hippocratum*.

Five centuries after Hippocrates, during the early decline of the Roman empire, Galen emerged as perhaps the most well-known and influential physician that ever lived. The son of a wealthy architect, Galen was born in the city of Pergamos[c] and was educated by scholars of the time. He began studying medicine at about age 16, and over the next 50 years he implemented and enhanced the current thinking about health and scientific hygiene, an area that some might consider applied exercise physiology. Throughout his life, Galen taught and practiced the "laws of health": breathe fresh air, eat proper foods, drink the right beverages, exercise, get adequate sleep, have a daily bowel movement, and control the emotions.[7] He was a prolific writer, producing at least 80 sophisticated treatises (and perhaps as many as 500 essays) on numerous topics, many of which were related to human anatomy and physiology, nutrition, growth and development, the beneficial effects of exercise and deleterious consequences of sedentary living, and a variety of diseases and their treatment. One of the first "bench physiologists," Galen made many observations in physiology, comparative anatomy, and medicine, including dissections on a variety of animals (for example, goats, pigs, cows, horses, and elephants—and other beasts from the gladiator games). Galen also was the physician to the gladiators of Pergamos, treating torn tendons and muscles by using many surgical procedures he invented. He developed numerous rehabilitation therapies and exercise regimens. Galen followed the Hippocratic school of medicine, which believed in logical science grounded in experimentation and observation. For example, Galen was first to prove that the arteries carried blood, not air, as previously believed, by tracing the main

physiology and hygiene; and anthropometry. Table 1 lists a sampling of 124 textbooks published between 1801 and 1899 containing information about the muscular, circulatory, respiratory, nervous, and digestive systems—including the influence of exercise and its effects—that eventually shaped the content area of exercise physiology during the next century. Additional textbooks from 1900 to 1947 deal with exercise, training, and exercise physiology.[a]

In the Beginning: Origins of Exercise Physiology from Ancient Greece to America in the 1850s

Exercise physiology arose mainly in early Greece and Asia Minor, although the topics of exercise, sports, games, and health concerned even earlier civilizations. These included the Minoan and Mycenaean cultures, the great biblical empires of David and Solomon, Assyria, Babylonia, Media, and Persia, as well as the Empires of Alexander. Other early references to sports, games, and health practices (personal hygiene, exercise, and training) were recorded in the ancient civilizations of Syria, Egypt, Macedonia, Arabia, Mesopotamia and Persia, India, and China. The greatest influence on Western civilization, however, came from the Greek physicians of antiquity—Herodicus (5th century B.C.); Hippocrates (460–377 B.C.), and Claudius Galenus or Galen (A.D. 131–201[b]). Herodicus, a physician and ath-

---

[a]Buskirk[10] provides a bibliography of books and review articles on exercise, fitness, and exercise physiology from 1920 to 1979. Berryman[7] lists many textbooks and essays from the time of Hippocrates through the Civil War period in the United States.

[b]According to Green, the dates for Galen's birth are estimates based on a notation Galen made when at age 38 he served as personal physician to the Roman emperors Marcus Aurelius and Lucius Verus.[21] Siegel's bibliography is an excellent source for references to Galen.[50]

[c]An important city on the Mediterranean coast of Asia Minor, Pergamos was influential in trade and commerce. Pergamos was renowned at the time for its library of 50,000 books (about one-fourth as many as in Alexandria, the greatest city for learning and education, where Galen studied from A.D. 152 to 156) and its famous medical center in the Temple of Asclepios.

Table 1

Sampling of textbooks on anatomy and physiology, anthropometry, exercise and training, and exercise physiology (1801–1947).

Year	Author and Text
1801	Willich, A.F.M. *Lectures on Diet and Regimen: Being a Systematic Inquiry Into the Most Rational Means of Preserving Health and Prolonging Life: Together With Physiological and Chemical Explanations, Calculated Chiefly for the Use of Families, in Order to Banish the Prevailing Abuses and Prejudices in Medicine.* New York, T and J Swords, 1801.
1831	Hitchcock, E. *Dyspepsy Forestalled and Resisted, or, Lectures on Diet, Regimen, and Employment.* 2nd ed., Northampton, J.S. & C. Adams. 1831.
1833	Beaumont, W. *Experiments and Observations on the Gastric Juice and the Physiology of Digestion.* Plattsburgh, F.P. Allen. 1833.
1839	Carpenter, W.B. *Principles of Physiology, General and Comparative.* London, John Churchill, 1839. 4th ed., 1854.
1842	Carpenter, W.B. *Principles of Human Physiology.* London, Churchill, 1842.
1843	Carpenter, W.B. *Principles of Human Physiology, with Their Chief Applications to Pathology, Hygiene, and Forensic Medicine. Especially Designed for the Use of Students.* Philadelphia, Lea & Blanchard, 1843. Numerous reprints and editions; 9th ed, 1881 (London); 4th American ed., 1890.
1843	Combe, A. *The Principles of Physiology Applied to the Preservation of Health, and to the Improvement of Physical and Mental Education.* New York, Harper & Brothers, 1843.
1844	Dunglison, R. *Human Health: The Influence of Atmosphere and Locality; Change of Air and Climate; Seasons; Food; Clothing; Bathing and Mineral Springs; Exercise; Sleep; Corporeal and Intellectual Pursuits, on Healthy Man; Constituting Elements of Hygiene.* Philadelphia, Lea & Blanchard, 1844.
1846	Warren, J.C. *Physical Education and the Preservation of Health.* Boston, William D. Ticknor, 1846.
1848	Cutter, C. *Anatomy and Physiology Designed for Academies and Families.* Boston, Benjamin B. Mussey and Co. 1848.
1852	Blackwell, E. *The Laws of Life, with Special Reference to the Physical Education of Girls.* New York, George P. Putnam, 1852.
1854	Stokes, W. *Diseases of the Heart and Aorta.* Philadelphia, Lindsay, 1854.
1855	Combe, A. *The Physiology of Digestion, Considered with the Relation to the Principles of Dietetics.* Philadelphia, Harper and Brothers, Publishers, 1855.
1856	Beecher, C. *Physiology and Calisthenics for Schools and Families.* New York, Harper and Brothers, 1856.
1859	Flint, A. *The Clinical Study of the Heart Sounds in Health and Disease.* Philadelphia, Collins, 1859.
1860	Hitchcock, E., and Hitchcock, E., Jr. *Elementary Anatomy and Physiology for Colleges, Academies, and Other Schools.* New York, Ivison, Phinney & Co., 1860.
1863	Ordronaux, J. *Manual of Instruction for Military Surgeons, on the Examination of Recruits and Discharge of Soldiers.* New York, D. Van Nostrand, 1863.
1866	Flint, A. *A Treatise on the Principles and Practice of Medicine; Designed for the use of Practitioners and Students of Medicine.* Philadelphia, H.C. Les, 1866 (fifth edition appeared 1884).
1866	Flint, A. *The Physiology of Man; Designed to Represent the Existing State of Physiological Science as Applied to the Functions of the Human Body.* Vol. I. Introduction; The Blood; Circulation; Respiration. New York, D. Appleton and Company. 1866. Vol. II. Digestion; Absorption; Lymph and Chyle (1867). Vol. III. Secretion; Excretion; Ductless Glands; Nutrition; Animal Heat; Movement; Voice and Speech (1870). Vol. IV. Nervous System (1873). Vol V. Special Senses; Generation (1874).
1866	Huxley, T.H. *Lessons in Elementary Physiology.* London, Macmillan and Co., 1866.
1866	Lewis, D. *Weak Lungs, and How to Make them Strong.* Boston, Ticknor and Fields, 1866.
1869	Dalton, J.C. *A Treatise on Physiology and Hygiene; for Schools, Families, and Colleges.* New York, Harper & Brothers, 1869.
1869	Gould, B.A. *Investigations in the Military and Anthropological Statistics of American Soldiers.* Published for the U.S. Sanitary Commission. New York, Hurd and Houghton, 1869.
1871	Flint, A. *On the Physiological Effects of Severe and Protracted Muscular Exercise; with Special Reference to its Influence Upon the Excretion of Nitrogen.* New York, D. Appleton & Co., 1871.
1873	Huxley, T.H., and Youmans, W.J. *The Elements of Physiology and Hygiene for Educational Institutions.* New York, D. Appleton & Co., 1873.
1873	Morgan, J.E. *University Oars.* London, MacMillan, 1873.
1875	Baxter, J.H. *Statistics, Medical and Anthropological, of the Provost-Marshal-General's Bureau, Derived from Records of the Examination for Military Service in the Armies of the United States During the Late War of the Rebellion, of Over a Million Recruits, Drafted Men, Substitutes, and Enrolled Men.* Vol. 1. Washington, D.C., U.S. Government Printing Office, 1875.
1876	Hitchcock, E. *A part of the course of instruction given in the Department of Physical Education and Hygiene in Amherst College. First issued by the class of 1877 while juniors.* Amherst, Mass., 1876.
1877	Flint, A. *A Text-Book of Human Physiology; Designed for the Use of Practitioners and Students of Medicine.* New York, D. Appleton, 1877. (2nd ed., rev. and cor. 1879; 3rd ed., rev. and cor. 1881, 1882, 1884, 1888; 4th ed., entirely rewritten, 1888 and published 1889, 1891, 1892, 1893, 1895, 1896, 1897, 1901)
1877	Flint, A. *The Source of Muscular Power, as Deduced from Observations Upon the Human Subject Under Conditions of Rest, and of Muscular Exercise.* London, 1877.
1878	Flint, A. *On the Sources of Muscular Power. Arguments and Conclusions Drawn from Observations Upon the Human Subject, Under Conditions of Rest and of Muscular Exercise.* New York, D. Appleton and Company, 1878.
1878	Foster, M. *A Text-Book of Physiology.* London, Macmillan and Co, 1878.

Year	Author and Text
1881	Huxley, T.H., and Youmans, W.J. *The Elements of Physiology and Hygiene: A Text-Book for Educational Institutions.* New York, Appleton and Co., 1881.
1884	Martin, H.N., and Martin, H.C. *The Human Body. A Beginners Text-book of Anatomy, Physiology and Hygiene.* New York, H. Holt and Company, 1884 (261 p), revised, 1885.
1885	Martin, H.N., and Martin, H.C. *The Human Body. A Beginners Text-book of Anatomy, Physiology and Hygiene, with Directions for Illustrating Important Facts of Man's Anatomy from that of the Lower Animals, and with Special References to the Effects of Alcoholic and other Stimulants, and of Narcotics.* New York, Henry Holt and Son, 1885.
1888	Huxley, T. H., and Martin. H. N. *A Course of Elementary Instruction In Practical Biology.* Rev. ed. London, Macmillan and Co., 1888.
1888	Lagrange, F. *Physiology of Bodily Exercise.* New York, D. Appleton and Company, 1890.
1889	Hitchcock, E, and Seelye, H.H. *An Anthropometric Manual, Giving the Average and Mean Physical Measurements and Tests of Male College Students and Method of Securing Them.* 2nd ed. Amherst, Mass., Williams, 1889.
1893	Kolb, G. *Physiology of Sport.* London, Krohne and Sesemann, 1893.
1895	Galbraith, A.M. *Hygiene and Physical Culture for Women.* New York, Dodd, Mead and Company, 1895.
1895	Galbraith, A.M. *Hygiene and Physical Culture for Women.* New York, Dodd, Mead and Company, 1895.
1896	Atkinson, E. *The Science of Nutrition.* Seventh edition. Boston, Damrell & Upham, 1896.
1896	Martin, H. N. *The Human Body. An Account of Its Structure and Activities and the Conditions of its Healthy Working.* New York, Holt & Co., 1881. 3rd ed. rev., 1884, 1885; 5th ed. rev., 1888, 1889 (621 p); 6th ed. rev., 1890, 1894 (621 p); 7th ed., 1896 (685 p); 8th ed., rev., 1896 (685 p).
1896	Seaver, J.W. *Anthropometry and Physical Examination. A Book for Practical Use in Connection with Gymnastic Work and Physical Education.* New Haven, Conn., Press of the O.A. Dorman Co., 1896.
1898	Martin, H.N. *The Human Body. A Text-book of Anatomy, Physiology and Hygiene; with practical exercises.* 5th ed., rev. by George Wells Fitz. New York, H. Holt and Company. 1898 (408 p), 1899 (408 p); 5th editions 1900, 1902, 1911, 1912, 1930.
1900	Atwater, W.O., and Bryant, A.P. *Dietary Studies of University Boat Crews.* U.S. Department of Agriculture, Office of Experiment Stations, Bulletin no. 25. Washington, D.C., U.S. Government Printing Office. 1900.
1900	Howell, W.H. (ed). *An American Text-Book of Physiology.* Vol. 1. Blood, Lymph, and Circulation; Secretion, Digestion, and Nutrition; Respiration and Animal Heat; Chemistry of the Body. 2nd. rev. Philadelphia, W.B. Saunders & Company, 1900.
1901	Howell, W.H. (ed). *An American Text-Book of Physiology.* Vol. 2. Muscle and Nerve; Central Nervous System; The Special Senses; Special Muscular Mechanisms; Reproduction. 2nd. rev. Philadelphia, W.B. Saunders & Company, 1901.
1902	Hastings, W.W. *A Manual for Physical Measurements for Use in Normal Schools, Public and Preparatory Schools, Boys Clubs, Girls Clubs, and Young Men's Christian Associations.* Springfield, Young Men's Christian Association Training School, 1902.
1903	Demeny, G. *Les Bases Scientifiques de l'Education Physique,* Paris, Felix Alcan, Editeur, 1903.
1903	Flint, A. *Collected Essays and Articles on Physiology and Medicine,* 2 volumes. New York, D. Appleton and Company. 1903.
1904	Butts, E.L. *Manual of Physical Drill.* United States Army. New York, D. Appleton and Company, 1904.
1904	Mosso, A. *Fatigue.* New York, G.P. Putnam's Sons, 1904.
1905	Atwater, W. O., and Benedict F.G. *A Respiration Calorimeter with Appliances for the Direct Determination of Oxygen.* Washington, D.C., Carnegie Institution of Washington, 1905.
1905	Flint, A. *Handbook of Physiology, for Students and Practitioners of Medicine.* New York, The Macmillan Company, 1905.
1906	Hough, T., and Sedgewick, W.T. *The Human Mechanism, Its Physiology and Hygiene and the Sanitation of Its Surroundings.* New York, Ginn and Company, 1906.
1906	Sargent, D.A. *Physical Education.* Boston, Ginn and Company, 1906.
1906	Sherrington, S.C. *The Integrative Action of the Nervous System.* New Haven, Conn., Yale University Press, 1906.
1906	Stevens, A.W., and Darling, E.D. *Practical Rowing and the Effects of Training.* Boston, Little, Brown and Company, 1906.
1908	Fisher, I. *The Effect of Diet on Endurance: Based on an Experiment with Nine Healthy Students at Yale University, January-June, 1906.* New Haven, Conn., Tuttle, Morehouse and Taylor Press, 1908.
1908	Fitz, G. W. *Principles of Physiology and Hygiene.* 2d ed., rev. New York, H. Holt and Company, 1908. 2nd ed., rev., 1909.
1909	McKenzie, R.T. *Exercise in Education and Medicine.* Philadelphia, W.B. Saunders Company, 1909.
1911	Cannon, W.B. *The Mechanical Factors of Digestion.* New York, Longmans, Green and Company, 1911
1914	Barcroft, J. *The Respiratory Function of the Blood.* Cambridge, University Press, 1914.
1914	Goodman, E.H. *Blood Pressure in Medicine and Surgery.* Philadelphia, Lea & Febiger, 1914.
1915	Benedict, F., and Murchhauser, J. *Energy Transformation During Horizontal Walking.* Carnegie Institute Publication. No. 231. Washington, D.C., Carnegie Institute of Washington, 1915.
1915	Cannon, W.B. *Bodily Changes in Pain, Hunger, Fear and Rage.* New York, D. Appleton Company, 1915.
1917	Haldane, J.S. *Organism and Environment as Illustrated by the Physiology of Breathing.* New Haven, Yale University Press, 1917.
1918	Fisher, I. *The Effect of Diet on Endurance.* New Haven, Yale University Press, 1918.
1918	Lewis, T. *The Soldier's Heart and the Effort Syndrome.* New York, P.B. Hoeber, 1918.
1918	Starling, E.H. *Linacare Lecture; The Law of the Heart.* London, Longmans, Green, and Company, 1918.
1918	Wilbur, W.C. *The Koehler Method of Physical Drill.* Philadelphia, J.B. Lippincott Company, 1918.
1919	Bainbridge, F.A. *Physiology of Muscular Exercises.* New York, Longmans, Green and Company, 1919.

Year	Author and Text	Year	Author and Text
1919	Love, A.G., and Davenport, C.B. *Physical Examination of the First Million Draft Recruits: Methods and Results.* Washington, D.C., U.S. Government Printing Office, 1919.	1931	Hill, A. V. *Adventures in Biophysics.* London, Oxford University Press, 1931.
1920	Amar, J. *The Human Motor.* New York, E.P. Dutton and Company, 1920.	1931	Schmidt, F.A., and Kohlrasch, W. *Physiology of Exercise.* (Translated by C.B. Sputh). Philadelphia, F.A. Davis and Company, 1931.
1920	Burton-Ovitz, R. *A Textbook of Physiology.* Philadelphia, W.B. Saunders Company, 1920.	1932	Boas, E.P. and E.F. Goldschmidt. *The Heart Rate.* Charles C. Thomas. Springfield, IL. 1932.
1920	Dreyer, G. *The Assessment of Physical Fitness.* New York, P.B. Hoeber, 1920.	1932	Creed, R.S., et al. *Reflex Activity of the Spinal Cord.* Oxford, Oxford University Press, 1932.
1920	Gaskell, W.H. *The Involuntary Nervous System.* New York, Longmans, Green and Company, 1920.	1932	Gould, A.G., and Dye, J.A. *Exercise and Its Physiology.* New York, A.S. Barnes and Company, 1932.
1920	Jansen, M. *On Bone Formation: Its Relation to Tension and Pressure.* New York, Longmans, Green and Company, 1920.	1932	Grollman, A. *The Cardiac Output of Man in Health and Disease.* Springfield, Ill., Charles C Thomas, Publisher, 1932.
1921	Martin, E.G. Tests of Muscular Efficiency. *Physiological Reviews.* 1: 454, 1921.	1932	McCloy, C.H. *The Measurement of Athletic Power.* New York, A.S. Barnes and Company, 1932.
1922	Haldane, J.S. *Respiration.* New Haven, Conn., Yale University Press, 1922.	1933	Haggard, H.W., and Greenberg, L.A. *Diet and Physical Efficiency.* New Haven, Conn., Yale University Press, 1933.
1922	Krogh, A. *The Anatomy and Physiology of Capillaries.* New Haven, Conn., Yale University Press, 1922.	1933	Schneider, E.C. *Physiology of Muscular Activity.* Philadelphia, W.B. Saunders, Co., 1933.
1923	MacKenzie, R.T. *Exercise in Education and Medicine.* Philadelphia, W.B. Saunders Company, 1923.	1934	Konradi, Slonim, D., and Farfel, V.S. *Work Physiology.* Moscow, Medgiz Publishing, 1934.
1924	Douglas, C.G., and Priestley, J.G. *Human Physiology.* Oxford, The Clarendon Press, 1924.	1935	Boorstein, S.W. *Orthopedics for the Teacher of Crippled Children.* New York, Aiden, 1935.
1926	Fulton, J.F. *Muscular Contraction and Reflex Control of Movement.* Baltimore, The Williams and Wilkins Company, 1926.	1935	Dawson, P.M. *The Physiology of Physical Education.* Baltimore, The Williams and Wilkins Company, 1935.
1926	Hill, A. V. *Muscular activity. Lectures on the Herter Foundation, sixteenth course;* "Muscles", 1924. Baltimore, Published for the Johns Hopkins University by Williams and Wilkins, 1926.	1935	Haggard, H.W., and Greenberg, L.A. *Diet and Physical Efficiency.* New Haven, Conn., Yale University Press, 1935.
1927	Deutsch, F., and Kauf, E. *Heart and Athletics.* Translation by L.M. Warfield. St. Louis, C.V. Mosby Company, 1927.	1935	Haldane, J.S., and Priestley, J.G. *Respiration.* New York, Oxford University Press, 1935.
1927	DuBois, E.F. Basal *Metabolism in Health and Disease.* Philadelphia, Lea and Febiger, 1927.	1937	Griffin, F.W.W. *The Scientific Basis of Physical Education.* London, Oxford University Press, 1937.
1927	Hill, A. V. *Living Machinery.* New York, Harcourt, Brace and Company, 1927.	1938	Benedict, F.G. *Vital Energetics. A Study in Comparative Basal Metabolism.* Washington, D.C., Carnegie Institute of Washington, 1938.
1927	Hill, A.V. *Muscular Movement in Man.* New York, McGraw-Hill Book Company, 1927.	1938	Dill, D.B. *Life, Heat, and Altitude. Physiological Effects of Hot Climates and Great Heights.* Cambridge, Harvard University Press, 1938.
1928	Henderson, L.J. *Blood. A Study in General Physiology.* New Haven, Conn., Yale University Press, 1928.	1939	Hrdlicka, A. *Practical Anthropometry.* Philadelphia, Wistar Institute of Anatomy and Biology, 1939.
1928	McCurdy, H.G., and McKenzie, R.T. *The Physiology of Exercise.* Philadelphia, Lea and Febiger, 1928.	1939	Krestovnikoff, A. *Fiziologia Sporta.* Moscow, Fizkultura and Sport, 1939.
1928	Schwartz, L., et al. *The Effect of Exercise on the Physical Condition and Development of Adolescent Boys.* U.S. Public Health Service Bulletin 179. Washington, D.C., U.S. Government Printing Office, 1928.	1939	McCurdy, J.H., and Larson, L.A. *The Physiology of Exercise.* Philadelphia, Lea and Febiger, 1939.
1929	Krogh, A. *The Anatomy and Physiology of Capillaries.* 2nd ed. New Haven, Conn., Yale University Press, 1929.	1939	Schneider, E.C. *Physiology of Muscular Activity.* 2nd ed. Philadelphia, W.B. Saunders, 1939.
1929	Macklin, C.C. The Musculature of the Bronchi and Lungs. *Physiological Reviews.* 9:1, 1929 (492 references).	1942	Cureton, T.K. *Physical Fitness Workbook.* Champaign, Ill., Stipes Publishing Company, 1942.
1930	Starling, E.H. *Human Physiology.* Philadelphia, Lea and Febiger, 1930.	1945	Cureton, T.K., et al. *Endurance of Young Men.* Washington, D.C., National Research Council, National Society for Research in Child Development, 1945.
1931	Bainbridge, F.A. *The Physiology of Muscular Exercise.* 3rd edition Rewritten by Bock, A.V., and Dill, D.B. London, Longmans Green and Company, 1931.	1947	Adolph, E.F., et al. *Physiology of Man in the Desert.* New York, Wiley, 1947.
		1947	Cureton, T.K., et al. *Physical Fitness Appraisal and Guidance.* St. Louis, The C.V. Mosby Company, 1947.

arteries accurately based on animal studies (human dissections were prohibited). However, Galen's ideas about the function of the heart and circulatory system were physiologically incorrect. He believed three kinds of spirits—natural, vital, and animal—ebbed and flowed throughout the body with the help of hollow nerve channels to sustain life. These beliefs about the inner workings of the body remained essentially unchallenged for almost 1500 years, until the experimental anatomists of the early 16th and 17th centuries discovered from post-mortem dissections how physiological function matched anatomical observation.

Galen wrote detailed descriptions about the forms, kinds, and varieties of "swift" and vigorous exercises, including their proper quantity and duration. The following definition of exercise is from the first complete English translation by Green[21] of *Hygiene* (*De Sanitate Tuenda;* pp. 53–54), Galen's insightful and detailed treatise on healthful living (the table of contents for the first two of the six sections or Books from *De Sanitate Tuenda* is presented as Table 2):

> To me it does not seem that all movement is exercise, but only when it is vigorous. But since vigor is relative, the same movement might be exercise for one and not for another. The criterion of vigorousness is change of respiration; those movements which do not alter the respiration are not called exercise. But if anyone is compelled by any movement to breathe more or less or faster, that movement becomes exercise for him. This therefore is what is commonly called exercise or gymnastics, from the gymnasium or public-place to which the inhabitants of a city come to anoint and rub themselves, to wrestle, throw the discus, or engage in some other sport.... The uses of exercise, I think are twofold, one for the evacuation of the excrements, the other for the production of good condition of the firm parts of the body. For since vigorous motion is exercise, it must needs be that only these three things result from it in the exercising body—hardness of the organs from mutual attrition, increase of the intrinsic warmth, and accelerated movement of respiration. These are followed by all the other individual benefits which accrue to the body from exercise; from hardness of the organs, both insensitivity and strength for function; from warmth, both strong attraction for things to be eliminated, readier metabolism, and better nutrition and diffusion of all substances, whereby it results that solids are softened, liquids diluted, and ducts dilated. And from the vigorous movement of respiration the ducts must be purged and the excrements evacuated.

The seeds of more "modern-day" exercise physiology include the periods of Renaissance, Enlightenment, and Scientific Discovery in Europe. It was then that Galen's ideas influenced the writings of the early physiologists, doctors, and teachers of hygiene and health.[41,44] For example, in Venice in 1539, the Italian physician Hieronymus Mercurialis (1530–1606) published *De arte Gymnastica apud ancientes* (*The Art of Gymnastics Among the Ancients*). This text, heavily influenced by Galen and other early Greek and Latin authors, profoundly affected subsequent writings about gymnastics (physical training and exer-

---

TABLE 2
TABLE OF CONTENTS FOR BOOK 1 AND BOOK 2[a]
OF GALEN'S *DE SANITATE TUENDA* (HYGIENE)

Book 1
The Art of Preserving Health

Chapter	
I	Introduction
II	The Nature and Sources of Growth and of Disease
III	Production and Elimination of Excrements
IV	Objectives and Hypothesis of Hygiene
V	Conditions and Constitutions
VI	Good Constitution a Mean Between Extremes
VII	Hygiene of the Newborn
VIII	The Use and Value of Exercise
IX	Hygiene of Breast-Feeding
X	Hygiene of Bathing and Massage
XI	Hygiene of Beverages and of Fresh Air
XII	Hygiene of the Second Seven Years
XIII	Causes and Prevention of Excrementary Retardation
XIV	Evacuation of Retained Excrements
XV	Summary of Book I

Book 2
Exercise and Massage

I	Standards of Hygiene Under Individual Conditions
II	Purposes, Time, and Methods of Exercise and Massage
III	Techniques and Varieties of Massage
IV	Theories of Theon and Hippocrates
V	Definitions of Various Terms
VI	Further Definitions About Massage
VII	Amount of Massage and Exercise
VIII	Forms, Kinds, and Varieties of Exercise
IX	Varieties of Vigorous Exercises
X	Varieties of Swift Exercises
XI	Effects, Exercises, Functions, and Movements
XII	Determination of Diet, Exercise, and Regime

[a]Book III. Apotherapy, Bathing, and Fatigue. Book IV. Forms and Treatment of Fatigue. Book V. Diagnosis, Treatment, and Prevention of Various Diseases. Book VI. Prophylaxis of Pathological Conditions.

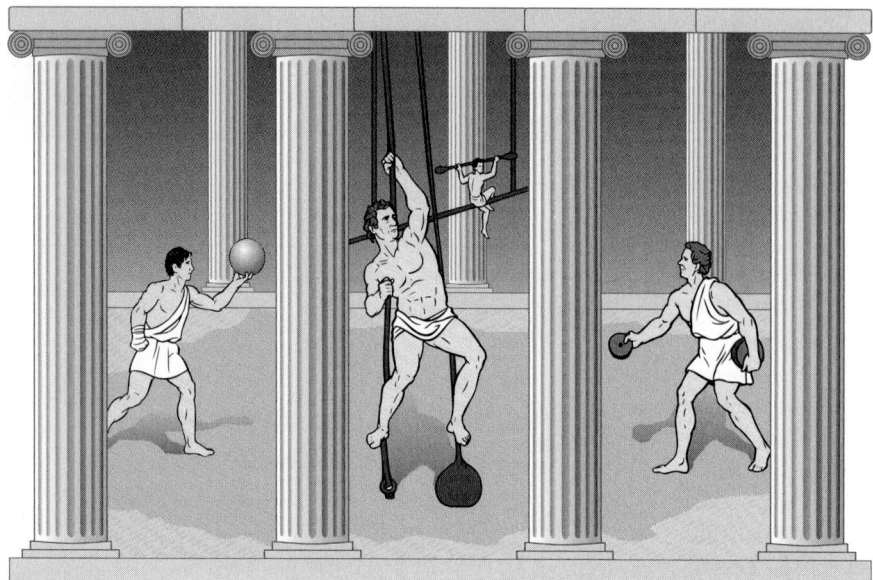

FIGURE 1

The early Greek influence of Galen's famous essay, *Exercise With the Small Ball*, as well as specific strengthening exercises (throwing the discus and rope climbing), appeared in Mercurialis' *De Arte Gymnastica*, a treatise about the many uses of exercise for preventive and therapeutic medical and health benefits. Mercurialis favored discus throwing to aid patients suffering from arthritis and to improve the strength of the trunk and arm muscles. He advocated rope climbing because it did not pose health problems, and he was a firm believer in walking (a mild pace was good for stimulating conversation, and a faster pace would stimulate appetite and help with digestion). He also believed that climbing mountains was good for those with leg problems, long jumping was desirable (but not for pregnant women), but tumbling and handsprings were not recommended because they would produce adverse effects from the intestines pushing against the diaphragm! The three panels represent the exercises as they might have been performed during the time of Galen.

cise) and health (hygiene), not only in Europe (influencing the Swedish and Danish gymnastic systems) but also in early America (the 19th-century gymnastic-hygiene movement). The panel in Figure 1, redrawn from *De Arte Gymnastica*, acknowledges the early Greek influence of one of Galen's famous essays, *Exercise with the Small Ball*, as well as his regimen of specific strengthening exercises (throwing the discus and rope climbing).

In the late 1700s in France, Antoine Lavoisier (the "Father of Chemistry") demonstrated that oxygen was the substance in the air responsible for combustion and thereby established the bases for modern conceptions of respiration. Research on metabolism was advanced by the physiologist Claude Bernard, the German chemist Justig von

Liebig, and others. By the 1840s, an understanding that foodstuffs were composed of carbohydrates, proteins, and lipids had been achieved. Events such as these led the way to the emergence of modern scientifically based medicine and physiology; by the mid-1800s, a small number of American physicians began to look to Europe for their ideas and training.[43]

Prior to 1800, only 39 first-edition American-authored medical books had been published, a few medical schools had been started (Harvard Medical School was founded in 1782), seven medical societies existed (the New Jersey State Medical Society being the first in 1766[8]), and only one medical journal was available (*Medical Repository*, which began publication in 1797). Outside of the United States there were 176 medical journals, but by 1850 the number in the United States had increased to 117.[51]

The steady growth in the number of scientific contributions from Europe, especially Germany, began to attract attention. Americans who desired the best medical training sought their education first in France and then in Germany until the late 1800s, when the Johns Hopkins Medical School opened and Harvard University reorganized its medical school curriculum. At the same time, there occurred an apparent "information explosion" that reached the American public through books, magazines, newspapers, and traveling "health salesmen," who sold an endless variety of tonics, elixirs, and other products for purposes of optimizing health and curing disease.[d] The "hot topics" of the early 19th century (as is also true today) included nutrition and dieting (slimming), general information about exercise, how best to develop overall fitness, training (or gymnastic) exercises for recreation and preparation for sport, and all matters relating to personal health and hygiene.

By the middle of the 19th century, fledgling medical schools in the United States began to graduate their own students, many of whom soon assumed positions of leader-

[d]According to Green,[20] many health reformers and physicians from 1800 to 1850 used "strange" procedures to treat disease and bodily discomforts. To a great extent, scientific knowledge was limited, quackery flourished, and primitive practices were often used to optimize health and treat disease. Except for three states, licensing laws for physicians has been repealed in 1845, thus enabling homeopathic and botanic medicine (bleeding, blistering, and purgation) to be promoted vigorously by many health reformers, dietary faddists, water-cure specialists, animal magnetizers, electromagnetizers, revivalist ministers, and evangelists. While these health faddists actually practiced medicine without a license, some enrolled in newly created medical schools (which did not have entrance requirements), obtaining the M.D. degree in as little as 16 weeks! Many of the newly trained physicians, however, contributed in significant ways to medical practice and to the development of exercise physiology. The contributions of two physicians, Austin Flint, Jr. and George Wells Fitz, are discussed in detail in subsequent sections.

ship in the academic world and allied medical sciences. Interestingly, physicians had the opportunity either to teach in medical school and conduct research (and write textbooks) or to become associated with departments of physical education and hygiene. Here they would oversee programs of physical training for students and athletes.

Within this framework, we begin our discussion of the early physiology and exercise physiology pioneers with Austin Flint, Jr., M.D., a respected physician, physiologist, and successful textbook author. His writings provided information for those wishing to place their beliefs about exercise on a scientific footing.

Austin Flint, Jr., M.D.: American Physician-Physiologist

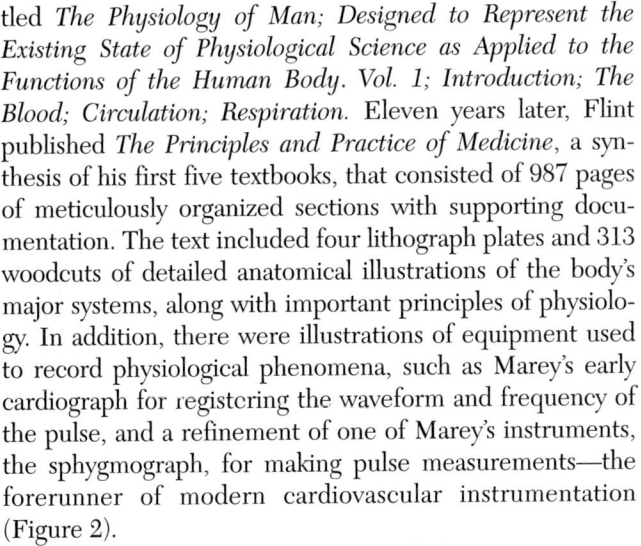

One of the first American pioneer physician-scientists whose writings contributed significantly to the burgeoning literature in physiology was Austin Flint, Jr., M.D., (1836–1915). He was a professor of physiology and physiological anatomy in the Bellevue Hospital Medical College of New York and was chair of the Department of Physiology and Microbiology from 1861 to 1897. In 1866, he published a series of five classic textbooks, the first entitled *The Physiology of Man; Designed to Represent the Existing State of Physiological Science as Applied to the Functions of the Human Body. Vol. 1; Introduction; The Blood; Circulation; Respiration.* Eleven years later, Flint published *The Principles and Practice of Medicine*, a synthesis of his first five textbooks, that consisted of 987 pages of meticulously organized sections with supporting documentation. The text included four lithograph plates and 313 woodcuts of detailed anatomical illustrations of the body's major systems, along with important principles of physiology. In addition, there were illustrations of equipment used to record physiological phenomena, such as Marey's early cardiograph for registering the waveform and frequency of the pulse, and a refinement of one of Marey's instruments, the sphygmograph, for making pulse measurements—the forerunner of modern cardiovascular instrumentation (Figure 2).

Dr. Flint, one of six generations of physicians spanning the years 1733 to 1955, was well trained in the scientific method (having studied under renowned physiologist Claude Bernard). In 1858, he received the American Medical Association's prize for basic research on the heart, and his medical school thesis, entitled "The phenomena of capillary circulation," was published in 1878 in the *American Journal of the Medical Sciences.* A characteristic of Flint's textbooks was his admiration for the work of other

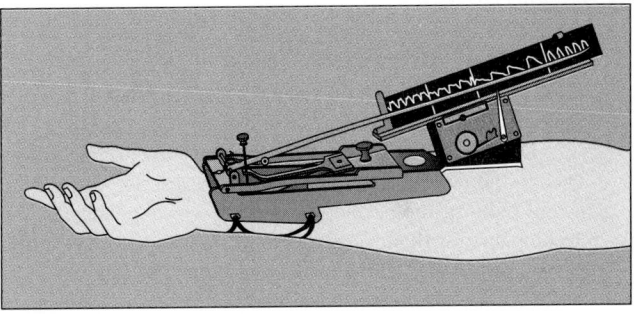

FIGURE 2

Marey's advanced sphygmograph, including actual portions of four tracings of the pulse under different conditions. It was not until the next century (in 1928) that Boas and Goldschmidt (cited in 1932 Boas and Goldschmidt text; see Table 1) reported on their human experiments with the first electronic cardiotachometer (Goldschmidt had invented the pulse resonator for recording pulse rate in 1927). The authors present a historical overview of pulse measuring devices, including the clepsydra (water clock) used by the Alexandrian physician Herophilus in the third century.

scholars. This included the pioneering work on liver physiology by the noted French physician Claude Bernard (1813–1878), who discovered that glycogen synthesis occurs in the liver regardless of what type of food is ingested; the celebrated observations of Dr. William Beaumont, an American physician, on his famous subject Alexis St. Martin (shot in the stomach at close range), which documented the digestive process; and William Harvey's momentous discovery in 1628 of the circulation of the blood, which revolutionized scientific research (Harvey's mentor, the Italian anatomist-surgeon Hieronymous Fabricius ab Aquapendente, had previously described the small semilunar valves in veins—providing Harvey with insight about the circulation).

Dr. Flint was a careful writer. This was a refreshing approach, particularly because so many "authorities" in physical training, exercise, and hygiene in the United States and abroad were uninformed and unscientific about exercise. In his 1877 textbook, Flint wrote about many topics related to exercise. The following sample passages are quoted from Flint's 1877 book to give the flavor of the emerging science of exercise physiology in the late 19th century.

1. Influence of posture and exercise on pulse rate (pp. 52–53)

> It has been observed that the position of the body has a very marked influence upon the rapidity of the pulse. Experiments of a very interesting character have been made by Dr. Guy and others, with a view to determine the difference in the pulse in different postures. In the male, there is a difference of about ten beats between standing and sitting, and fifteen beats between standing and the recumbent posture. In the female, the variations with position are not so great. The average given by Dr. Guy is, for the male standing, 81; sitting, 71; lying, 66;—for the female: standing, 91; sitting, 84; lying, 80.

This is given as the average of a large number of observations.

Influence of age and sex. In both the male and female, observers have constantly found a great difference in the rapidity of the heart's action at different periods of life.

During early life, there is no marked and constant difference in the rapidity of the pulse in the sexes; but, toward the age of puberty, the development of the sexual peculiarities is accompanied with an acceleration of the heart's action in the female, which continues even into old age. The differences at different ages are shown in the following table, compiled from the observations of Dr. Guy:

Ages	Males Average pulsations	Females Average pulsations
From 2 to 7 years	97	98
From 8 to 14 years	84	94
From 14 to 21 years	76	82
From 21 to 28 years	73	80
From 28 to 35 years	70	78
From 35 to 42 years	68	78
From 42 to 49 years	70	77
From 49 to 56 years	67	76
From 56 to 63 years	68	77
From 63 to 70 years	70	78
From 70 to 77 years	67	81
From 77 to 84 years	71	82

Influence of exercise, etc.—It is a fact generally admitted that muscular exertion increases the frequency of the pulsations of the heart; and the experiments just cited show that the difference in rapidity, which is by some attributed to change in posture (some positions, it is fancied, offering fewer obstacles to the current of blood than others), is mainly due to muscular exertion. Every one knows, indeed, that the action of the heart is much more rapid after violent exertion, such as running, lifting, etc. Experiments on this point date from quite a remote period. Bryan Robinson, who published a treatise on the "Animal Economy" in 1734, states, as the result of observation, that a man in the recumbent position has 64 pulsations per minute; sitting, 68; after a slow walk, 78; after walking four miles in one hour, 100; and 140 to 150 after running as fast as he could. This general statement, which has been repeatedly verified, shows the powerful influence of the muscular system on the heart. The fact is so familiar that it need not be farther dwelt upon.

2. Influence of muscular activity on respiration (pp. 150–151)

Nearly all observers are agreed that there is a considerable increase in the exhalation of carbonic acid during and imme-diately following muscular exercise. In insects, Mr. Newport has found that a greater quantity is sometimes exhaled in an hour of violent agitation than in twenty-four hours of repose. In a drone, the exhalation in twenty-four hours was 0.30 of a cubic inch, and during violent muscular exertion the exhalation in one hour was 0.34. Lavoisier recognized the great influence of muscular activity upon the respiratory changes. In treating of the consumption of oxygen, we have quoted his observations on the relative quantities of air vitiated in repose and activity.

The following results of the experiments of Dr. Edward Smith on the influence of exercise are very definite and satisfactory:

In walking at the rate of two miles an hour, the exhalation of carbonic acid during one hour was equal to the quantity produced during $1^4/_5$ hour of repose with food, and $2^1/_2$ hours with, and $3^1/_2$ hours without food.

One hour's labor at the tread-wheel, while actually working the wheel, was equal to $4^1/_2$ of rest with food, and 6 hours without food.

The various observers we have cited have remarked that, when muscular exertion is carried so far as to produce great fatigue and exhaustion, the exhalation of carbonic acid is notably diminished.

3. Influence of muscular exercise on nitrogen elimination (pp. 429–430)

We have had an opportunity of settling definitely the vexed question of the influence of muscular exercise upon elimination of nitrogen.[e] In 1871, we made an exceedingly elaborate series of observations upon Mr. Weston, the pedestrian. Of these we can only give here a brief summary. Mr. Weston walked for five consecutive days as follows: First day, 92 miles; second day, 80 miles; third day, 57 miles; fourth day, 48 miles; fifth day, 40.5 miles. The nitrogen of the food was compared with the nitrogen excreted for three periods; viz, five days before the walk, five days walking, and five days after the walk. A trusty assistant was with Mr. Weston day and night for the fifteen days; the food was weighed and analyzed; the excreta were collected; and other observations were made during the entire period. The analyses were made independently, under the direction of Prof. R.O. Doremus, who had no idea of the results until we had classified and tabulated them. The conclusions were most decided, and, as far as possible, all the physiological conditions were fulfilled. As regards the proportion of nitrogen eliminated to the nitrogen of the food, the general results were as follows:

For the five days before the walk, with an average exercise of about eight miles daily, the nitrogen eliminated was 92:82 parts for 100 parts of nitrogen ingested. For the five days of the walk, for every hundred parts of nitrogen ingested, there were discharged 153:99 parts. For the five days after the walk, when there was hardly any exercise, for every hundred parts of nitrogen ingested, there were discharged 84:63 parts. During the walk, the nitrogen excreted was in direct ratio to

---

[e]Flint, A., Jr.: On the physiological effects of severe and protracted muscular exercise, with special reference to its influence upon the excretion of nitrogen. *New York Medical Journal*, 1871, vol xiii., p. 609, et seq.

the amount of exercise; and, what was still more striking, the excess of nitrogen eliminated over the nitrogen of food almost exactly corresponded with a calculation of the nitrogen of the muscular tissue wasted, as estimated from the loss of weight of the body. Full details of the method of investigation, the processes employed, etc., are given in our original paper.

Austin Flint Jr., through his textbooks, influenced the first medically trained and scientifically oriented professor of physical education, Edward Hitchcock, Jr., M.D. Hitchcock quoted Flint about the muscular system in his syllabus of *Health Lectures* that was required reading for all students enrolled at Amherst College between 1861 and 1905.

The Amherst College Connection

Two physicians, father and son, pioneered the American sports science movement. Edward Hitchcock, D.D., LL.D. (1793–1864), was a professor of chemistry and natural history at Amherst College and also served as president of the college from 1845 to 1854. He convinced the college president in 1861 to allow his son Edward (1828–1911; Amherst undergraduate, 1849; Harvard medical degree, 1853) to assume the duties of his anatomy course. Subsequently, Edward Hitchcock Jr. was officially appointed on August 15, 1861, as Professor of Hygiene and Physical Education with full academic rank in the Department of Physical Culture at an annual salary of $1,000—a position he held almost continuously until 1911. This was the second such appointment in physical education to an American College in the United States.[f]

The Hitchcocks geared their textbook to college physical education (Hitchcock, E. and Hitchcock, E., Jr. *Elementary Anatomy and Physiology for Colleges, Academies, and Other Schools.* New York, Ivison, Phinney & Co., 1860); Edward Hitchcock Sr. had previously published a textbook on hygiene in 1831 that was more informed by contemporary science than most books then available. The Hitchcock and Hitchcock anatomy and physiology book (1860) predated Flint's anatomy and physiology text by 6 years. Topics covered were listed in numerical order by subject, and considerable attention was given to the physiology of species other than humans. The text included questions at the bottom of each page concerning the topics under consideration, making the textbook a "study guide" or "work-

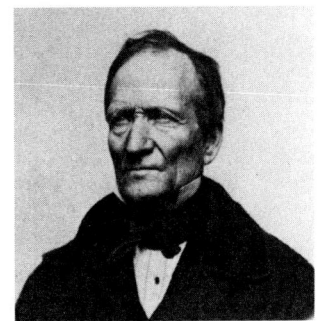 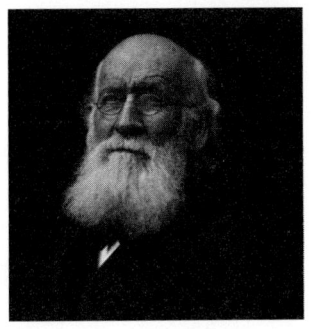

Dr. Edward Hitchcock (1793–1864).   Dr. Edward Hitchcock Jr., M.D. (1828–1911).

book," not an uncommon pedagogical feature (Cutter, 1848; see Table 1). Figure 3 shows sample pages on muscle structure and function from the Hitchcock and Hitchcock text.

From 1865 to about 1905, Professor Edward Hitchcock Jr.'s syllabus of *Health Lectures* (38-page pamphlet entitled *The Subjects and Statement of Facts Upon Personal Health Used for the Lectures Given to the Freshman Classes of Amherst College*) was part of the required curriculum. The topics included hygiene and physical education, with brief quotations about the topic, including a citation for the quote. In addition to quoting Austin Flint Jr. about care of the muscles, "The condition of the muscular system is an almost unfailing evidence of the general state of the body," other quotations peppered each section of the pamphlet, some from well-known physiologists such as Thomas Huxley and Henry Pickering Bowditch. For example, with regard to physical education and hygiene: "The successful men in life are those who have stored up such physical health in youth that they can in an emergency work sixteen hours in a day without suffering from it."—Professor Huxley. Concerning food and digestion: "A scientific or physiological diet for an adult, per day, is two pounds of bread, and three-quarters of a pound of lean meat." In regard to tobacco use: "Tobacco is nearly as dangerous and deadly as alcohol, and a man with tobacco heart is as badly off as a drunkard."—Dr. Bowditch. Other quotations were used for such tissues as skin: "Wear dark clothes in winter and light in summer. Have three changes of underclothing—heavy flannels for winter, light flannels for spring and fall, lisle thread, silk or open cotton for summer."—Dr. Dudley A. Sargent.

Anthropometric assessment of body build. During the years 1861 to 1888, Dr. Hitchcock Jr. obtained from almost

---

[f]Edward Hitchcock Jr. is often accorded the distinction of being the first professor of physical education in the United States, whereas in fact John D. Hooker was first appointed to this position at Amherst College in 1860. Because of poor health, Hooker resigned in 1861, and Hitchcock was appointed in his place. The original idea of a Department of Physical Education with a professorship had been proposed in 1854 by William Agustus Stearns, D.D., the fourth president of Amherst College, who considered physical education instruction essential for the health of the students and useful to prepare them physically, spiritually, and intellectually. Other institutions were slow to adopt this innovative concept; the next department of physical education in America was not created until 1879. In 1860, the Barrett Gymnasium at Amherst College was completed and served as the training facility where all students were required to perform systematic exercises for 30 minutes daily, 4 days a week. It is interesting to note that the gymnasium included a laboratory containing scientific equipment (e.g., spirometer, strength and anthropometric equipment) and also included a piano to provide rhythm during the exercises. Hitchcock reported to the Trustees that in his first year, he recorded the students vital statistics...including age, weight, height, size of chest and forearm, capacity of lungs, and some measure of muscular strength.

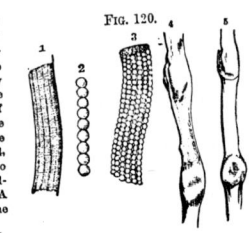
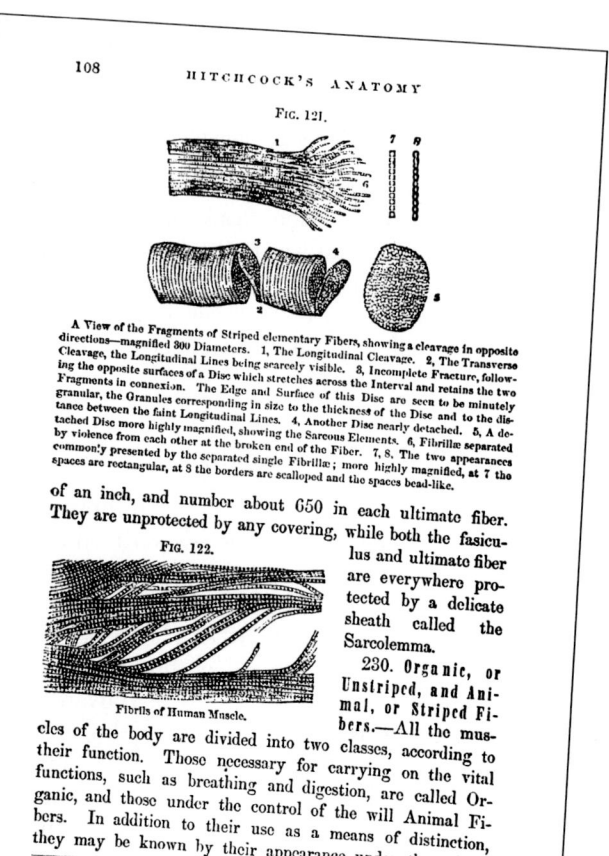

FIGURE 3

Examples from the Hitchcock text on structure and function of muscles. (Reproduced from Hitchcock, E., and Hitchcock, E., Jr.: *Elementary Anatomy and Physiology for Colleges, Academies, and Other Schools.* New York, Ivison, Phinney & Co., 1860, pp. 132 and 137. Materials courtesy of Amherst College Archives, and permission of the Trustees of Amherst College, 1995.)

every student who attended Amherst College six measurements of segmental height, 23 of girth, six of breadth, eight of length, eight of muscular strength, and measurements of lung capacity and pilosity (amount of hair on the body). From 1882 to 1888, according to Hitchcock, his standardization for measurement was improved based on suggestions of Dr. W.T. Brigham of Boston and Dr. Dudley A. Sargent (Yale medical degree, 1878; assistant professor of physical training and director of Harvard's Hemenway Gymnasium).

In 1889, Dr. Hitchcock and his colleague in the Department of Physical Education and Hygiene, Hiram H. Seelye, M.D. (who also served as college physician from 1884 to 1896), published a 37-page anthropometric manual that included five tables of anthropometric statistics of students from 1861 to 1891. This resource compendium provided detailed descriptions for taking measurements that also included eye testing and examining the lungs and heart before testing subjects for muscular strength. In the last section of the manual, Dr. Seelye wrote detailed instructions for using the various pieces of gymnasium apparatus for "enlarging and strengthening the neck, to remedy round or stooping shoulders, to increase the size of the chest and the capacity of the lungs, to strengthen and enlarge the arm, abdominal muscles, and weak back, and to enlarge and strengthen the thighs, calves, legs and ankles." The Hitchcock and Seelye manual, the first of its kind devoted to an analysis of anthropometric and strength data based on detailed measurements, influenced other departments of physical education in the United States (for example, Yale, Harvard, Wellesley, and Mt. Holyoke) to include anthropometric measurements as part of the physical education and hygiene curriculum.

Hitchcock's keen awareness of the history of anthropometry was succinctly stated in a speech entitled "The Need for Anthropometry," delivered as President of the American Association for the Advancement of Physical Education at the second annual meeting held in Brooklyn,

New York, November 26, 1886. Hitchcock's claim of the importance of anthropometry in the college curriculum as related to health and proper human development was not universally accepted; in fact, at the same conference, there was heated debate about the need for anthropometric assessment as part of training and exercise programs. Hitchcock was convinced that an important value of anthropometric assessment was its intrinsic relationship to human performance.[g] In fact, in his talk, he laid the groundwork for his rationale based on a historical perspective:

> The study of Anthropometry, or the proportions of the human body, is not modern, but reaches back to the remote civilization of India, when we find a treatise called Silpi Sastri, which investigated the outline of the body by dividing it into 480 parts. In later times the Greeks proposed a "Canon" or model in the shape of a statue called Doryphoros, which was claimed to be the pattern for the human figure. Still later the mathematical law was applied to the human body, an entirely artificial system; hence we obtain the terms cubit, handbreadth, ell and so on. An Italian sculptor, Alberti, proposed a module of one foot in height, which was divided into ten degrees and minutes, as a standard for the proportions of the human body. In 1854 a German, Carus, proposed an anatomical basis for determining human bodily proportions, assuming the hand length for the unit, and the adult vertebral column of 24 free vertebrae, to be the key to these proportions. But the father of anthropometry is Baron Quetelet of Belgium, who, in the middle part of the present century, offered the actual measurements of the body and the means and averages deduced from them as the true and scientific way of ascertaining human proportions; adopting the Baconian method of reasoning from the effect to the cause, from the concrete to the abstract.

One of the reasons for the early interest in anthropometric measurement was to demonstrate that engaging in daily, vigorous exercise produced desirable results, particularly in terms of muscular development. While none of the early physical education scientists used statistics to evaluate the outcomes of their exercise programs, it is instructive to apply modern methods of anthropometric analysis to the original data of Hitchcock on entering students at Amherst College in 1882 and upon their graduation in 1886. Figure

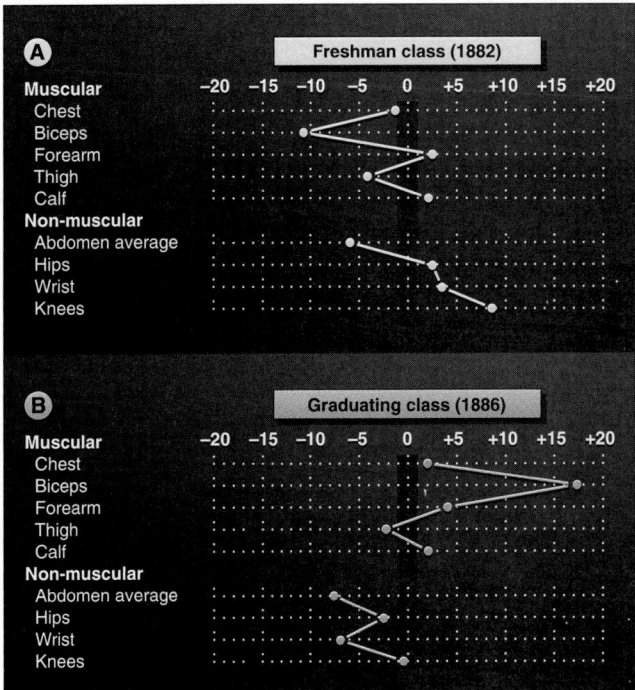

FIGURE 4

Changes in selected girth measurements of Amherst College men over 4 years of college using Behnke's reference man standards (presented in Chapter 27). **A,** The average body mass of the freshman class in 1882 was 59.1 kg (stature, 171.0 cm). **B,** Four years later, their body mass increased 5.5 kg (11.3 lb) and stature increased by 7.4 cm (2.9 in).

4 shows how the average student changed in anthropometric dimensions over 4 years of college in relation to Behnke's reference standards presented in Chapter 27. Note the dramatic increase in biceps girth and decreases in the nonmuscular abdomen and hip regions. Although data for a nonexercising "control" group of students were not available, these changes coincided with daily resistance training prescribed in the Hitchcock and Seelye *Anthropometric Manual*. This training used Indian club or barbell swinging exercises (see Figure 5) and other strengthening modalities (horizontal bar, rope and ring exercises, parallel-bar exer-

---

[g]Probably unknown to Hitchcock was the 1628 manuscript of the Flemish fencing instructor at the French Royal Court, Gerard Thibault, who studied optimal body proportions and success in fencing.[40a] This early text, *L'Académie de l'Espée*, appeared at a time when important discoveries were being made by European scientists, particularly anatomists and physiologists, whose contributions played such an important role in laboratory experimentation and scientific inquiry. Had Hitchcock known about this early attempt to link anthropometric assessment with success in sport, the acceptance of anthropometry in the college curriculum might have been easier. Nevertheless, just 67 years after Hitchcock began taking anthropometric measurements at Amherst, and 37 years following the creation of Harvard's scientifically based, exercise fitness–oriented B.S. degree program in 1892, anthropometric measurements were made of athletes at the 1928 Amsterdam Olympic Games. One of the athletes measured in Amsterdam, Ernst Jokl from South Africa, became a physician and then professor of physical education at the University of Kentucky, and was a charter member and founder of the American College of Sports Medicine. Thus, Hitchcock's visionary ideas about the importance of anthropometry finally caught on, and such assessment techniques are now used routinely in exercise physiology to assess physique status and the dynamics between physiology and performance. The more modern application of anthropometry is now known as kinanthropometry. This term, first defined at the International Congress of Physical Activity Sciences in conjunction with the 1976 Montreal Olympic Games,[47] was refined in 1980[48] as follows: "Kinanthropometry is the application of measurement to the study of human size, shape, proportion, composition, maturation, and gross function. Its purpose is to help us to understand human movement in the context of growth, exercise, performance, and nutrition. We see its essentially human-ennobling purpose being achieved through applications in medicine, education, and government."

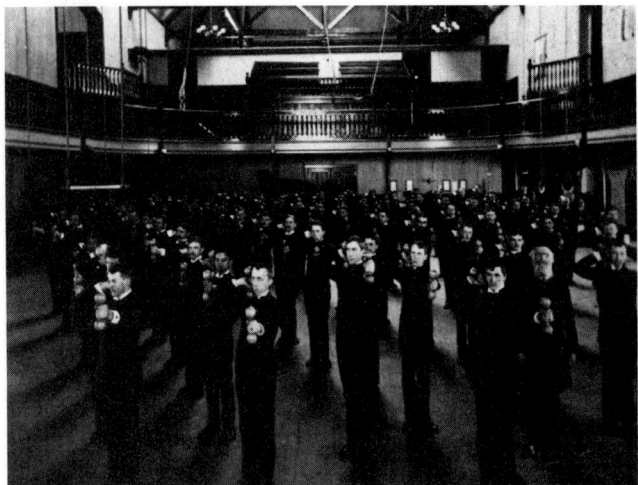

FIGURE 5

Dr. Edward Hitchcock, Jr. (second from right, with beard) observing the entire class of students perform barbell exercises in the Pratt Gymnasium of Amherst College. (Photo courtesy of Amherst College Archives, and by permission of the Trustees of Amherst College, 1995.)

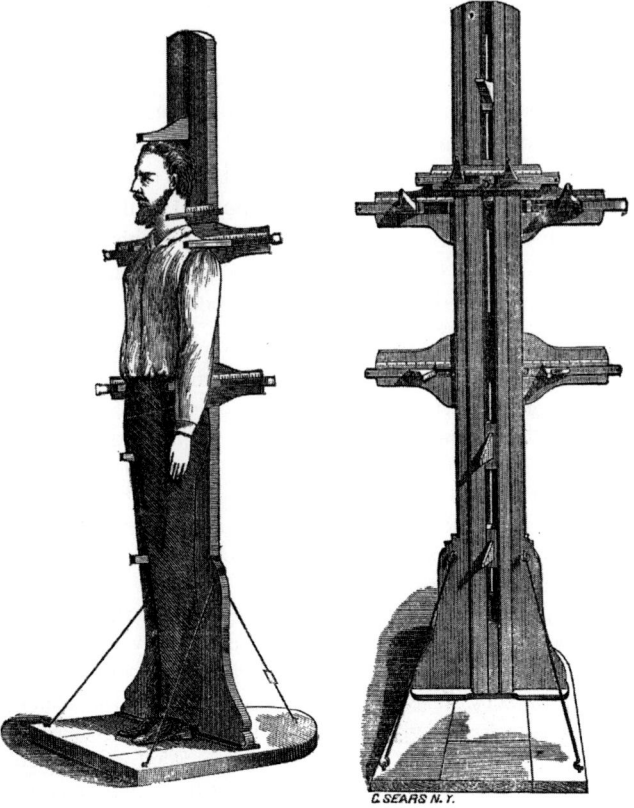

FIGURE 6

The andrometer was first used by the United States Sanitary Commission at numerous military installations along the Atlantic seaboard during the early 1860s to size soldiers for clothing.

cises, dipping machine, inclined presses with weights, pulley weights, and rowing machine workouts). "Old Doc" Hitchcock (as he was affectionately called) would have rejoiced to learn that his required physical education training program produced desirable results, something he fervently believed would occur. The Hitchcock data presentation, a first of its kind initially reported in the *Anthropometric Manual* in March 1892, used "bodily stature" as the basis of comparison "from measurements of 1322 students between 17 and 26 years of age. The strength tests are derived from 20,761 items." The Hitchcock studies were acknowledged in the first formal American textbook on anthropometry, published in 1896 by Jay W. Seaver, M.D. (1855–1915), physician and lecturer on personal hygiene at Yale University. Table 3 presents a sample of the average and "best" anthropometric values at Amherst College from 1861 to March 1900.

While Hitchcock was performing pioneering anthropometric studies at the college level, the military was making the first detailed anthropometric, spirometric, and muscular strength measurements on Civil War soldiers in the early 1860s; these were published in 1869 by Gould (cited in Table 1). The specially trained military anthropometrists used a unique device, the andrometer (Figure 6), to secure the physical dimensions of soldiers to the nearest tenth of an inch for purposes of fitting uniforms. The andrometer was originally devised in 1855 by a tailor in Edinburgh, Scotland, commissioned by the British government to determine the proper size for British soldiers' clothing. This device was set by special gauges to adjust "sliders" to measure total height; breadth of the neck, shoulders, and pelvis; length of the legs; and height to the knees and crotch. Each examiner

received 2 days of practice to perfect measurement technique before being assigned to different military installations (for example, Fort McHenry in Baltimore, Naval Rendezvous in New York City, Marine Barracks at the Brooklyn Navy Yard, and bases in South Carolina, Washington, D.C., Detroit, and New Orleans). Data were compiled on the actual and relative proportions of 15,781 men ("Whites, Blacks, Indians") between the ages of 16 and 45 years. One purpose of these military studies was to determine relationships among the anthropometric and other physical measurements as well as to gather demographic and anthropological statistics on enlisted and commissioned soldiers in the infantry, cavalry, and artillery. These early investigations into muscular strength and body dimensions were prototypical studies whose measurement techniques led the way to many later studies of muscular strength and human performance conducted in the military. Most laboratories in exercise physiology today include assessment procedures to evaluate aspects of muscular strength and body composition.

The top of Figure 7 shows two views of the instrument used to evaluate muscular strength in the military studies; the bottom of the figure shows the early spirometers used to

TABLE 3
THE AVERAGE AND THE BEST ANTHROPOMETRIC RECORDS OF AMHERST COLLEGE FROM 1861 TO 1900 INCLUSIVE

Items	Average		Maxima		Held By	Date of Record
	Metric	English	Metric	English		
Weight	61.2	134.9	113.7	250.6	K. R. Otis, '03	Oct. 2, '99
Height	1725	67.9	1947	76.6	B. Matthews '99	Oct. 28, '95
Girth, Head	572	22.5	630	24.8	W. H. Lewis '92	Feb. '92
Girth, Neck	349	13.7	420	16.5	D. R. Knight '91	Feb. '91
Girth, Chest, repose	880	34.6	1140	44.9	K. R. Otis '03	Oct. 2 '99
Girth, Belly	724	28.5	1017	40.1	G. H. Colman '99	May '97
Girth, Hips	893	35.1	1165	45.9	K. R. Otis '03	Oct. 2, '99
Girth, Right Thigh	517	20.3	745	29.3	K. R. Otis '03	Oct. 2, '99
Girth, Right Knee	361	14.2	460	18.1	K. R. Otis '03	Oct. 2, '99
Girth, Right Calf	359	14.1	452	17.8	K. R. Otis '03	Oct. 2, '99
Girth, Upper Right Arm	257	10.1	396	15.6	K. R. Otis '03	Oct. 2, '99
Girth, Right Forearm	267	10.5	327	12.8	K. R. Otis '03	Oct. 2, '99
Girth, Right Wrist	166	6.5	191	7.5	H. B. Haskell '94	April '92
Strength, Chest, Dip	6	—	45	—	H. W. Lane '95	March '95
Strength, Chest, Pull Up	9	—	65	—	H. W. Seelye '79	Oct. '75
Strength, Right Forearm	41	90	86	189.6	A. J. Wyman '98	April '96
Strength, Left Forearm	38	84	73	160.9	A. J. Wyman '98	April '96
Capacity of Lungs	377	230	6.66	406	E. D. Blodgett '87	June '87

From Hitchcock, E., Seelye, H.H., and Phillips, P.C.: *An Anthropometric Manual,* 4th ed. Amherst, MA, Carpenter and Morehouse, 1900.

evaluate pulmonary dimensions. The strength device predates the various strength-measuring instruments shown in Figure 8 used by Hitchcock (Amherst), Sargent (Harvard), and Seaver (Yale), as well as anthropometric measuring instruments used in their batteries of physical measurements. The inset shows the price list for some of the equipment from the 1889 and 1890 Hitchcock manuals on anthropometry. Note the progression in complexity of the early spirometers and strength devices used in the 1860 military studies (Fig. 7), and the more "modern" equipment of the 1889–1905 period displayed in Figure 8. Figure 9 includes three recently uncovered photographs (circa 1897–1901) of the strength testing equipment (Kellogg's Universal Dynamometer) acquired by Dr. Hitchcock in 1897 to assess the strength of the arms (A), anterior trunk and forearm supinators (B), and leg extensors, flexors, and thigh adductors (C).[h]

The First Exercise Physiology Laboratory and Associated Degree Program in the United States

The first formal exercise physiology laboratory in the United States was established in 1892 at Harvard University and was housed in a newly created Department of Anatomy,

---

[h]According to Hitchcock and Selye's *Anthropometric Manual* cited previously, the device consisted "of a lever acting by means of a piston and cylinder on a column of mercury in a closed glass tube. Water keeps the oil in the cylinder from contact with the mercury and various attachments enable the different groups of muscles to be brought to bear on the lever. By means of this apparatus, the strength of most of the large muscles may be tested fairly objectively."(p. 25). In the photographs, note the attachment of the tube to each device.

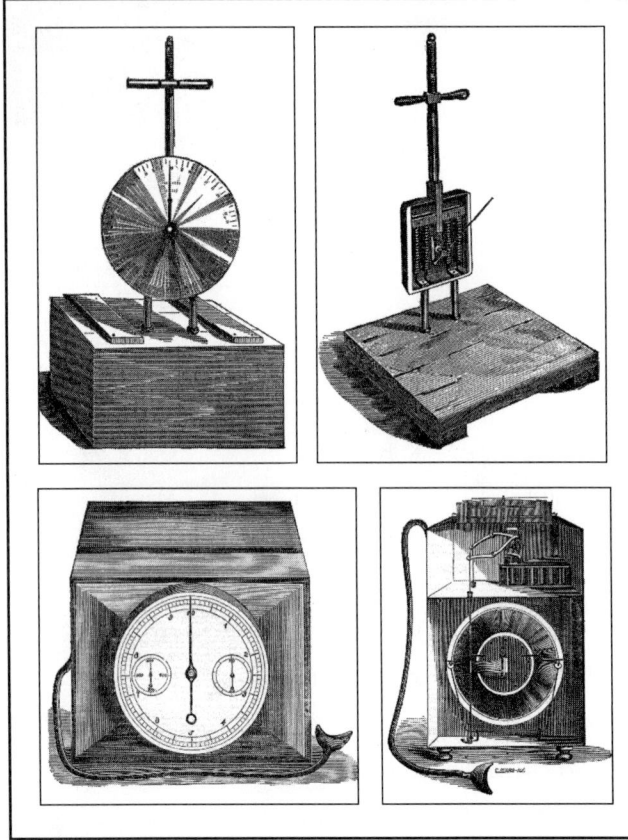

FIGURE 7

Top, Instrument used to evaluate muscular strength in the military studies of Gould in 1869. The illustration on the left shows the general look of the device, while the right side shows the internal arrangement without the face-plate. Gould (p. 458) described the procedure for measuring muscular strength as follows: "The man stands upon the movable lid of the wooden packing box, to which the apparatus is firmly attached, and grasps with both hands the rounded extremities of a wooden bar, of convenient shape and adjustable in height...The handle is conveniently shaped for firm and easy grasp, its height well suited for application of the full muscular power, and the mechanism such as to afford results which are to all appearance very trustworthy." This was not the first dynamometer; Gould cites Regnier (no date given), who published a description of a dynamometer to measure the strength of Parisians; and Péron, who carried a dynamometer on an expedition to Australia. Other researchers in Europe had also used dynamometers to compare the muscular strength of men of different races. Figure 22.1C shows the modern back-leg lift dynamometer still used for assessing muscular strength as part of physical fitness test procedures. *Bottom*, Spirometers, or dry gas meters, were used to measure vital capacity. These instruments were manufactured by the American Meter Company of Philadelphia. According to Gould (p. 469), the spirometers needed to be rugged "... to undergo the rough usage inseparable from transportation by army trains or on military railroads, which are in danger of being handled roughly at some unguarded moment by rude men..." The spirometers were graduated in cubic centimeters, and were "furnished with a mouthpiece of convenient form, connected with the instrument by flexible tubing."

Physiology, and Physical Training at the Lawrence Scientific School.[19,37] Several instructors in the initial undergraduate B.S. degree program in Anatomy, Physiology, and Physical Training started at the same time were Harvard-trained physicians; others—including Henry Pickering Bowditch, professor of physiology (who had discovered the all-or-none principle of cardiac contraction and treppe, the staircase phenomenon of skeletal muscle contraction), and William T. Porter, also a physiologist in the Harvard Medical School—were well known for their rigorous scientific and laboratory training.

George Wells Fitz, M.D.: A Major Influence. An important influence in creating the new departmental major and recruiting top scientists as faculty members in the Harvard program was George Wells Fitz, M.D. (1860–1934). Fitz vociferously supported a strong, science-based curriculum in preparing the new breed of physical educators. The archival records show that the newly formed major was grounded in the basic sciences, including formal coursework in exercise physiology, zoology, morphology (animal and human), anthropometry, applied anatomy and animal mechanics, medical chemistry, comparative anatomy, remedial exercises, physics, gymnastics and

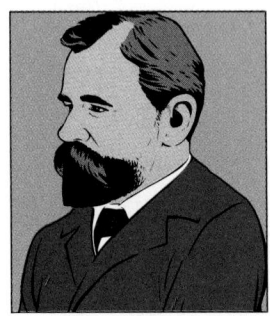

FIGURE 8

Anthropometric instruments used by Hitchcock, Seaver, and Sargent. Sargent, also an entrepreneur, constructed and sold specialized strength equipment used in his studies. **A**, Metric graduated scale. **B**, Height meter. **C**, Sliding anthropometer. **D**, Cloth tape measure, with an instrument made by the Narragansett Machine Co., at the suggestion of Dr. Gulick (head of the Department of Physical Training of the YMCA Training School, Springfield, MA), in 1887. The modern version of this tape, now sold as a "Gulick tape," was "for attachment to the end of a tape to indicate the proper tension, so that the pressure may be always alike." **E**, Calipers for taking depths. **F**, Several types of hand dynamometers, including push holder and pull holder instruments. **G**, Back and leg lift dynamometer, also used to measure the strength of the pectoral and "retractor" muscles of the shoulders. **H**, Vital capacity spirometer and Hutchinson's wet spirometer. **I**, Two stethoscopes. The soft rubber bell was used to "secure perfect coaptation to the surface of the chest." The Albion Stethoscope was preferred because it could be conveniently carried in the pocket. **J**, Parallel bars for testing arm extensors during push-ups, and testing of flexors in pull-ups. In special situations, physiological laboratories used Marey's cardiograph to record pulse, but the preferred instrument was a pneumatic kymograph (or sphygmograph; see Fig. 2). The inset figure shows a price comparison for the testing equipment from the 1889 and 1890 Hitchcock manuals. Note the yearly variation in prices. (Inset courtesy of Amherst College Archives, reproduced by permission of the Trustees of Amherst College, 1995.)

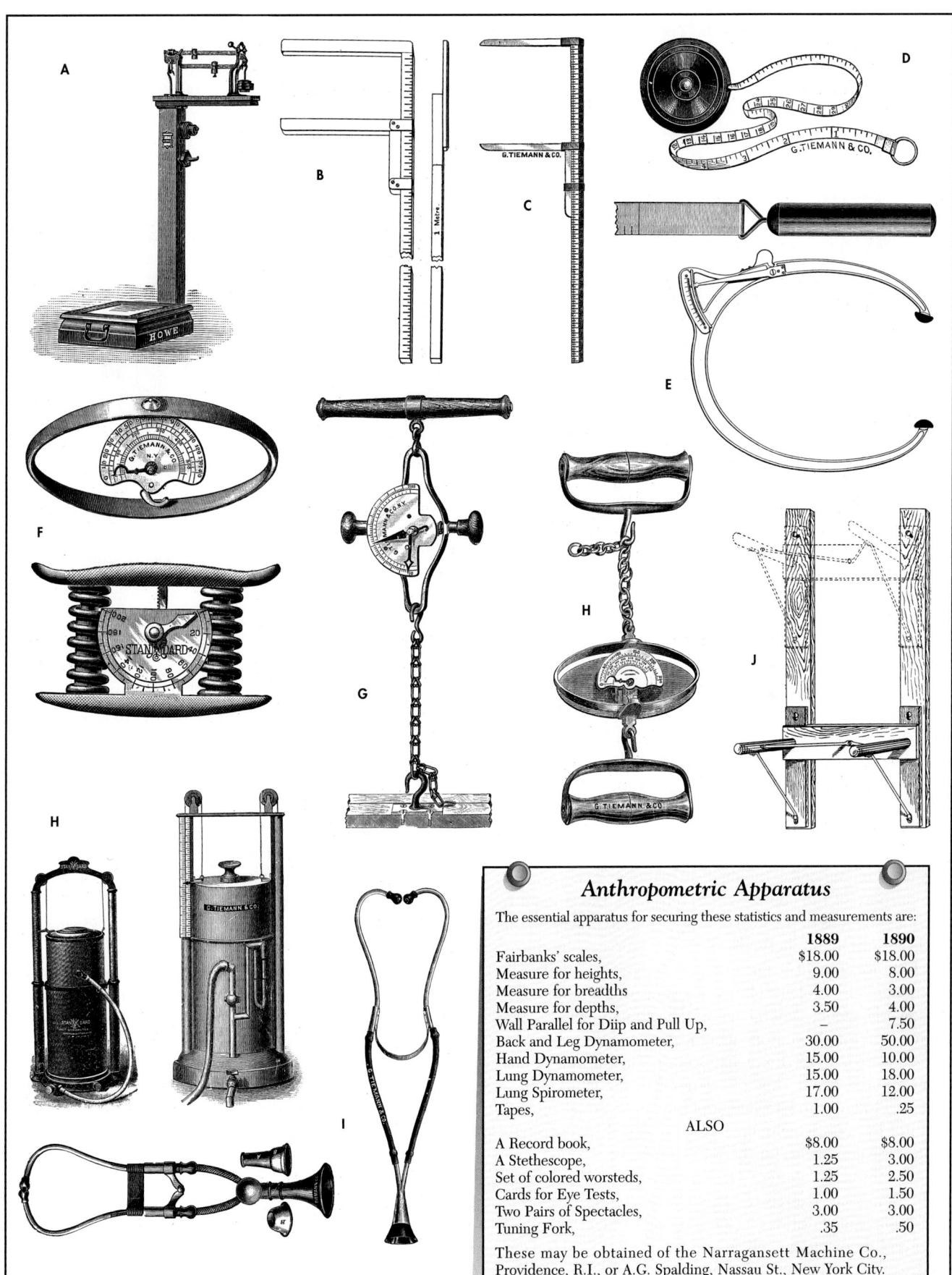

Anthropometric Apparatus

The essential apparatus for securing these statistics and measurements are:

	1889	1890
Fairbanks' scales,	$18.00	$18.00
Measure for heights,	9.00	8.00
Measure for breadths	4.00	3.00
Measure for depths,	3.50	4.00
Wall Parallel for Diip and Pull Up,	–	7.50
Back and Leg Dynamometer,	30.00	50.00
Hand Dynamometer,	15.00	10.00
Lung Dynamometer,	15.00	18.00
Lung Spirometer,	17.00	12.00
Tapes,	1.00	.25
ALSO		
A Record book,	$8.00	$8.00
A Stethescope,	1.25	3.00
Set of colored worsteds,	1.25	2.50
Cards for Eye Tests,	1.00	1.50
Two Pairs of Spectacles,	3.00	3.00
Tuning Fork,	.35	.50

These may be obtained of the Narragansett Machine Co.,
Providence, R.I., or A.G. Spalding, Nassau St., New York City.

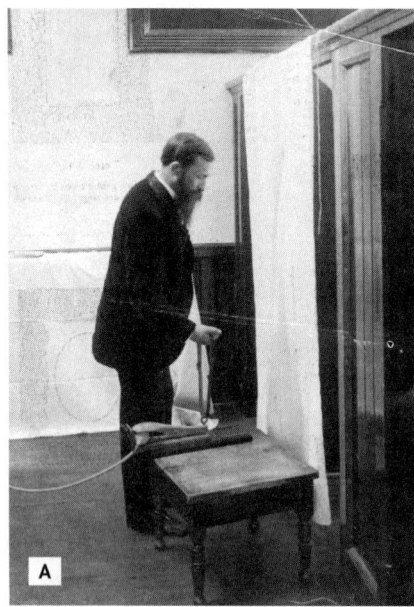 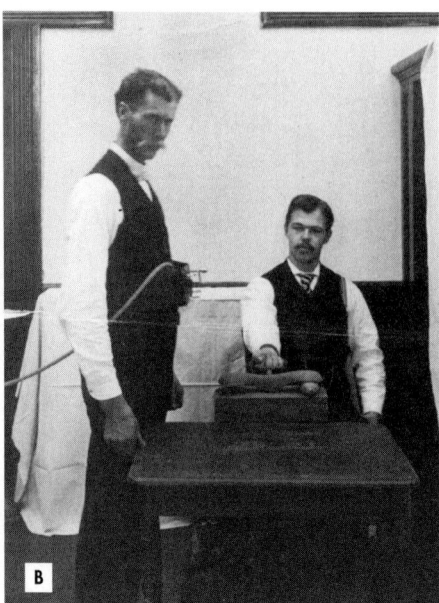 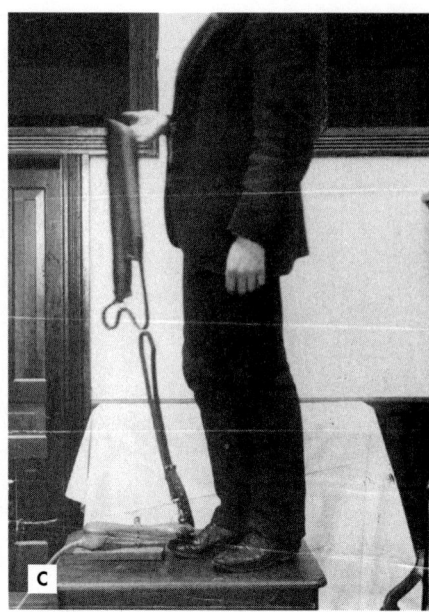

FIGURE 9

Kellogg's Universal Dynamometer acquired by Dr. Hitchcock to test the muscular strength of Amherst College students. From 1897 to 1900, strength measurements were taken on 328 freshmen, 111 sophomores, and 88 seniors, including retests on 58 individuals. Arm strength was measured bilaterally for the forearms and for the latissimus dorsi, deltoid, pectoral, and shoulder "retractor" muscles. Trunk measurements included the anterior trunk, and anterior and posterior neck. The leg measurements included the leg extensors and flexors and thigh adductors. **A**, "Arm pull." **B**, Anterior trunk (standing) and forearm supinators (sitting). **C**, Legs. (Photos courtesy of Amherst College Archives, and by permission of the Trustees of Amherst College, 1995.)

athletics, history of physical education, and English. Physical education students took general anatomy and physiology courses in the medical school; after 4 years of study, graduates could enroll as second-year medical students and graduate in 3 years with an M.D. degree. Dr. Fitz taught the physiology of exercise course; thus, we believe he was the first person to formally teach such a course. It included experimental investigation and original work and thesis, including 6 hours a week of laboratory study. The prerequisites for the Physiology of Exercise course included a course in general physiology at the medical school or its equivalent. The purpose of the course was to introduce the student to the fundamentals of physical education and to provide training in experimental methods related to exercise physiology. Dr. Fitz also taught a more general course entitled "The Elementary Physiology of the Hygiene of Common Life Personal Hygiene, Emergencies." The course included one lecture and one laboratory section per week for a year (or three times a week for a half year). The official course description stated, "This is a general introductory course intended to give the knowledge of human anatomy, physiology and hygiene which should be possessed by every student; it is suitable also for those not intending to study medicine or physical training." Dr. Fitz also gave a course entitled "Remedial Exercises. The Correction of Abnormal Conditions and Positions." Course content included observations of deformities such as spinal curvature (and the corrective effects of specialized exercises) and "the selection

and application of proper exercises, and in the diagnosis of cases when exercise is unsuitable." Several of Dr. Fitz's scientific publications dealt with spinal deformities. In addition to the remedial exercise course, students took a required course in "Applied Anatomy and Animal Mechanics. Action of Muscles in Different Exercises." This thrice weekly course, taught by Dr. Dudley Sargent, was the forerunner of modern biomechanics courses. Its prerequisite was general anatomy at the medical school or its equivalent.

Nine men graduated with B.S. degrees from the Department of Anatomy, Physiology, and Physical Training which had been discontinued in 1900. The aim of the major was to prepare students to become directors of gymnasia or instructors in physical training, to provide students with the necessary knowledge about the science of exercise, and to offer suitable training for entrance to the medical school. The stated purpose of the new exercise physiology research laboratory was as follows:

> A large and well-equipped laboratory has been organized for the experimental study of the physiology of exercise. The object of this work is to exemplify the hygiene of the muscles, the conditions under which they act, the relation of their action to the body as a whole affecting blood supply and general hygienic conditions, and the effects of various exercises upon muscular growth and general health.

With the activities of the department in full operation, its outspoken and critical director Dr. Fitz was not afraid to speak his mind about academic topics. For example, Fitz reviewed a new physiology text (*American Text-Book of Physiology,* edited by William H. Howell, Ph.D., M.D.) in the March 1897 issue of the *American Physical Education Review* (Vol. II, No. 1, p. 56). The review praised Dr. Howell's collection of contributions from outstanding physiologists (such as Bowditch, Lee, Lusk, and Sewall), and attacked an 1888 French book by Lagrange that some historians consider the first important text in exercise physiology.[i] The following is Fitz's review:

> No one who is interested in the deeper problems of the physiology of exercise can afford to be without this book [referring to Howell's Physiology text], and it is to be hoped it may be used as a text-book in the normal schools of physical training. These schools have been forced to depend largely on Lagrange's "physiology of exercise" for the discussion of specific problems, or at least for the basis of such discussions. The only value Lagrange has, to my mind, is that he seldom gives any hint of the truth, and the student is forced to work out his own problems. This does very well in well-taught classes, but, Alas! for those schools and readers who take his statements as final in matters physiological. We have a conspicuous example of the disastrous consequences in Treve's contribution of the "Cyclopaedia of Hygiene on Physical Education," in which he quotes freely from Lagrange and rivals him in the absurdity of his conclusions.
>
> The time has surely come for a thoroughly scientific investigation of the physiological problems involved in physical exercise and the promulgation of the exact and absolute. It is not too much to hope that the use of the American text-book of Physiology by training schools and teachers, may aid to bring about this much needed consummation.

Coinciding with Fitz's untimely departure from Harvard in 1899,[j] the department changed its curricular emphasis (the term physical training was dropped from the department title), thus terminating at least temporarily this unique experiment in higher education.

One of the legacies of the Fitz-directed "Harvard experience" between 1891 and 1899 was the training it provided to specialists who began their careers with a strong scientific basis in exercise and training and its relationship to health.

Unfortunately, it would take another six decades before the next generation of science-oriented physical educators (led by physiologists like A.V. Hill and D.B. Dill, not educators) who would once again exert strong influence on the physical education curriculum.

Exercise Studies in Research Journals. Another notable event in the growth of exercise physiology occurred in 1898 with the appearance of three articles dealing with physical activity in the first volume of the *American Journal of Physiology.*[k] This was followed in 1921 with the publication of the prestigious journal *Physiological Reviews.* Table 4 lists the articles in this journal (and two from the *Annual Review of Physiology*) from the first review of the mechanisms of muscular contraction by A.V. Hill in 1922, to Frances A. Hellebrandt's classic review of exercise in 1940. The German applied physiology publication *Internationale Zeitschrift fur angewandte Physiologie einschliesslich Arbeitsphysiologie* (1929–1973) was a significant journal for research in exercise physiology. The current title of this journal is *European Journal of Applied Physiology and Occupational Physiology.* The *Journal of Applied Physiology* was first published in 1948. Its first volume contained the now-classic paper on ratio expressions of physiological data with reference to body size and function by Tanner, a work that should be read by all exercise physiologists. The journal *Medicine and Science in Sports* first appeared in 1969. Its aim was to integrate both medical and physiological aspects of the emerging fields of sports medicine and exercise science. The official name of this journal was changed in 1980 (Volume 12) to *Medicine and Science in Sports and Exercise.*

The First Textbook In Exercise Physiology: The Debate Continues

What was the first textbook in exercise physiology? Several recent books give the distinction of being "first" to the English translation of Fernand Lagrange's book, *The Physiology of Bodily Exercise,* originally published in

---

[i] We disagree with Berryman's[6] assessment of the relative historical importance of the translation of the original Lagrange text. We give our reasons for this disagreement in a subsequent section, entitled "The First Textbook in Exercise Physiology: The Debate Continues."

[j] The reasons for Fitz's early departure from Harvard have been discussed in detail in Park's scholarly presentation of this topic.[44a] His leaving was certainly unfortunate for the next generation of students of exercise physiology. In his 1909 textbook *Principles of Physiology and Hygiene* (New York, Henry Holt and Company), the title page listed the following about Fitz's affiliation: *Sometime Assistant Professor Physiology and Hygiene and Medical Visitor, Harvard University.*

[k] The originator of the *American Journal of Physiology* was physiologist W.T. Porter of the St. Louis College of Medicine and Harvard Medical School, who remained editor until 1914.[9] Porter's research focused on cardiac physiology. The three articles in volume 1 concerned (*a*) spontaneous physical activity in rodents and the influence of diet (C.C. Stewart, Department of Physiology, Clark University), (*b*) neural control of muscular movement in dogs (R.H. Cunningham, College of Physicians and Surgeons, Columbia University), and (*c*) perception of muscular fatigue and physical activity (J.C. Welch, Hull Physiological Laboratory, University of Chicago). As pointed out by Buskirk,[9] the next four volumes of the *American Journal of Physiology* (1898–1901) contained six additional articles about exercise physiology from experimental research laboratories at Harvard Medical School, Massachusetts Institute of Technology, The University of Michigan, and The Johns Hopkins University.

TABLE 4
REVIEW ARTICLES ABOUT EXERCISE, 1922–1940

Year	Author and Article
1922	Hill, A.V. The mechnaism of muscular contraction *Physiol. Rev.* 2: 310, 1922.
1925	Cathcart, E.P. The influence of muscle work on protein metabolism. *Physiol. Rev.* 5: 225, 1925
1925	Cobb, S. Review on the tonus of skeletal muscle. *Physiol. Rev.* 5: 518, 1925.
1928	Vernon, H.M. Industrial fatigue in relation to atomspheric conditions. *Physiol. Rev.* 8: 1, 1921928.
1929	Eggleton, P. The position of phosphorus in the chemical mechansism of muscle contraction. *Physiol. Rev.* 9: 432, 1929.
1929	Richardson, H.B. The respiratory quotient (including: The source of energy used for muscular exertion). *Physiol. Rev.* 9: 61, 1929.
1930	Gasset, H.S. Contracture of skeletal muscle. *Physiol. Rev.* 10: 35, 1930
1931	Milroy, T.H. The present status of the chemistry of skeletal muscular contraction. *Physiol. Rev.* 11: 515, 1931.
1932	Baetzer, A.M. The effect of muscular fatigue upon resistance. *Physiol. Rev.* 12: 453, 1932.
1932	Hill, A.V. The revolution in muscle physiology. *Physiol. Rev.* 12: 56, 1932.
1933	Jordan, H.E. The structural changes in striped muscle during contraction. *Physiol. Rev.* 13: 301, 1933.
1933	Steinhaus, A.H. Chronic effects of exercise. *Physiol. Rev.* 13: 103, 1933.
1934	Hinsey, J.C. The innervation of skeletal muscle. *Physiol. Rev.* 14: 514, 1934.
1936	Dill, D.B. The economy of muscular exercise. *Physiol. Rev.* 16: 263, 1936.
1936	Fenn, W.O. Electrolytes in muscle. *Physiol. Rev.* 16: 450, 1936.
1937	Anderson, W.W. and Williams, H.H. Role of fat in diet. *Physiol. Rev.* 17: 335, 1937.
1939	Bozler, E. Muscle. *Annu. Rev. Physiol.* 1: 217, 1939
1939	Dill, D.B. Applied Physiology. *Annu. Rev. Physiol.* 1: 551, 1939
1939	Millikan, G.A. Muscle hemoglobin. *Physiol. Rev.* 19: 503, 1939.
1939	Tower, S.S. The reaction of muscle to denervation. *Physiol. Rev.* 19: 1, 1939.
1940	Hellebrandt, F.A. Exercise. *Annu. Rev. Physiol.* 2: 411, 1940.

French in 1888.[6,46,54] To deserve such historical recognition, we believe the work should meet the following three criteria:

1. Provide sound scientific rationale for major concepts.
2. Provide summary information (based on experimentation) about important prior research in a particular topic area (e.g., contain scientific references to research in the area).
3. Provide sufficient "factual" information about a topic area to give it academic legitimacy.

After reading the Lagrange book in its entirety, we came to the same conclusion as Fitz. Specifically, it was a popular book about health and exercise with a "scientific" title. It is our opinion that the book is not a legitimate scientific textbook of exercise physiology based on any reasonable criteria of the time. Despite Lagrange's assertion that the focus of his book is a study of physiology applied to exercise and not hygiene and exercise, it is informed by a 19th century hygienic perspective, not science. We believe Fitz and others would accept our evaluation.

There was much factual information available to Lagrange from existing European and American physiology textbooks on the digestive, muscular, circulatory, and respiratory systems, as well as limited information on physical training, hormones, basic nutrition, chemistry, and the biology of muscular contraction. Admittedly, this information was relatively scarce, but well-trained physiologists such as Flint, Howell, Martin, Huxley, Dalton, Carpenter, and Combe had already produced quality textbooks for their time that contained relatively detailed information about physiology in general, with some reference to muscular exercise. We now understand why Fitz was so troubled by the Lagrange book. By comparison, the two-volume text by Howell entitled *An American Text-Book of Physiology* was impressive; this edited volume contained articles from acknowledged American physiologists at the forefront of physiological research. This textbook was a high-level physiology text even by today's standards. Fitz, in his quest to provide the best possible science for his physical education students, could not tolerate a book that did not live up to his expectations for excellence. In fact, the Lagrange book contained fewer than 20 reference citations, and most of these were ascribed to French research reports or were based on observations of friends performing exercise. This plethora of anecdotal reports must have given Fitz "fits."

Lagrange was an accomplished writer who wrote extensively on exercise. Despite the titles of several of his books,[l] however, Lagrange was not a scientist. Bibliographic information about Lagrange is limited in the French and American archival records of the period—a further indication of his relative obscurity as a thinker of distinction. As far as we know, there have been no citations to his work in any physiology text or scientific article. For these reasons, we contend the Lagrange book does not qualify as the first exercise physiology textbook.[m]

Other Early Exercise Physiology Research Laboratories

Although the Nutrition Laboratory at the Carnegie Institute in Washington, D.C., had been created in 1904 to study nutrition and energy metabolism, the first research laboratories established in physical education in the United States to study exercise physiology were at George Williams College (1923), the University of Illinois (1925), and Springfield College (1927). However, the real impact of laboratory research in exercise physiology (along with many other research specialties) occurred in 1927 with the creation of the 800–square foot Harvard Fatigue Laboratory in the basement of Morgan Hall of Harvard University's Business School[30] (see below). The outstanding work of this laboratory over the next two decades established the legitimacy of exercise physiology on its own merits as an important area of research and study. Another exercise physiology

laboratory started prior to World War II was the Laboratory of Physiological Hygiene at the University of California, Berkeley, in 1934. The syllabus for the Physiological Hygiene course (taught by professor Frank Kleeberger), the precursor of contemporary exercise physiology courses, contained 12 laboratory experiments.[42] Several years later, Dr. Franklin M. Henry assumed responsibility for the laboratory. Henry began publishing the results of different experiments in various physiology-oriented journals, including the *Journal of Applied Physiology, Annals of Internal Medicine, Aviation Medicine, War Medicine,* and *Science.* Henry's first research project as a faculty member in the Department of Physical Education (published in 1938) concerned the validity and reliability of the pulse-ratio test of cardiac efficiency;[23] a later paper dealt with predicting aviator's bends (see Focus on Research, p. 482). Henry applied his training in experimental psychology to exercise physiology topics, including individual differences in the kinetics of the fast and slow components of the oxygen uptake and recovery curves during light- and moderate-cycle ergometer exercise; muscular strength; cardiorespiratory responses during steady-rate exercise; assessment of heavy-work fatigue; determinants of endurance performance; and neural control factors related to human motor performance (Fig. 10).

Contributions of the Harvard Fatigue Laboratory (1927–1946)

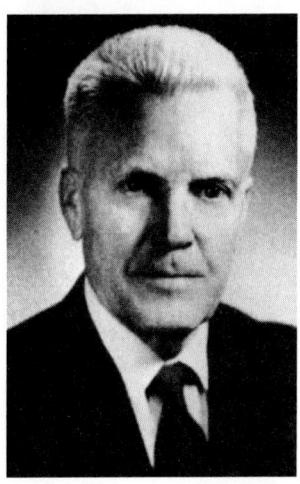

D.B. Dill (1891–1986).

Many of the great scientists of the 20th century with an interest in exercise were associated with the Harvard Fatigue Laboratory. This research facility was established by Lawrence J. Henderson, M.D. (1878–1942), a renowned chemist and professor of biochemistry at the Harvard Medical School. The first and only scientific director of the Fatigue Laboratory was David Bruce Dill (1891–1986), a Stanford Ph.D. in

---

[l]The following books (including translations, editions, and pages) were published by Lagrange beginning in 1888: *Physiologie des exercices du corps* (Paris, Alcan, 1888, 372 pp. [6th ed., 1892.]); *L'hygiene de l'exercice chez les enfants et les jeunes gens* (Paris, Alcan, 1890, 312 pp. [4th ed., 1893; 6th ed., 1896; 7th ed., 1901; 8th ed., 1905.]); *Physiology of Bodily Exercise* (New York, D. Appleton, 1890, 395 pp.); *De l'exercice chez les adultes* (Paris, Alcan, 1891, 367 pp. [2nd ed., 1892; 4th ed., 1900; Italian translation, *Fisiologia degli esercizj del corpo,* Milano, Dumolard, 1889; Hungarian translation, 1913.]); *La medication par l'exercice* (Paris, Alcan, 1894, 500 pp.).

[m]Possible pre-1900 candidates for "first" exercise physiology textbook listed in Table 1 also include Combe's 1843 text, *The Principles of Physiology Applied to the Preservation of Health, and to the Improvement of Physical and Mental Education;* Hitchcock and Hitchcock's *Elementary Anatomy and Physiology for Colleges, Academies, and Other Schools (1860);* Kolb's 1887 German monograph, translated into English in 1893 as *Physiology of Sport;* and the 1898 Martin text, *The Human Body. An Account of Its Structure and Activities and the Conditions of Its Healthy Working.*

FIGURE 10

A, Determining the velocity curve of 50-yard sprints (at 5-yard intervals) on the roof of Harmon Gymnasium. Henry's study[25] was prompted by A.V. Hill's 1927 observations concerning the "viscosity" factor of muscular contraction that at first helped to explain the large decline in metabolic efficiency at fast rates of movement, and that the oxygen requirement of running increased with the cube of speed. Henry verified that metabolic efficiency was uncorrelated to a muscle viscosity factor. **B,** Making limb and trunk anthropometric measurements on a sprinter during continuous studies of the force-time characteristics of the sprint start[26] to further evaluate A.V. Hill's theoretical equation for the velocity of sprint running. **C,** Recording the timing of the initial movements of blocking performance in football players.[40]

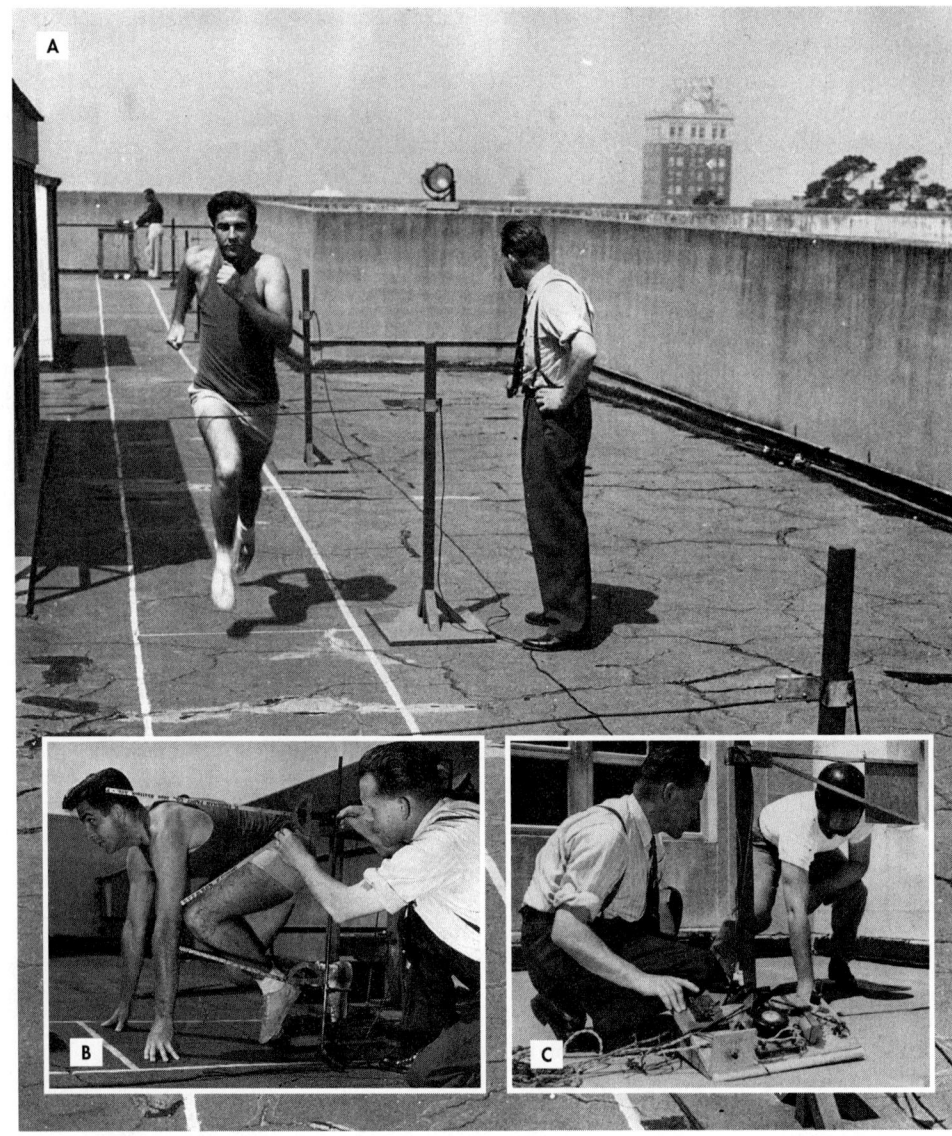

physical chemistry. Dill was transformed from a biochemist to an experimental physiologist while at the Fatigue Laboratory and was an important driving force behind the Laboratory's numerous scientific accomplishments. His early academic association with physician Arlie Bock (a student of famous high-altitude physiologist Dr. Barcroft in Cambridge, England,[5] and Dill's closest friend for 59 years), and contact with 1922 Nobel laureate Archibald Vivian Hill (for his discovery relating to the production of heat in the muscles) provided Dill with the confidence to successfully coordinate the research efforts of dozens of scholars from 15 different countries. A.V. Hill convinced Bock to write a third edition of Bainbridge's text *Physiology of Muscular Activity*. Bock, in turn, invited Dill to coauthor the book, which was republished in 1931.[15]

Over a 20-year period, at least 352 research papers and monographs and one book[16] were published in areas of basic and applied exercise physiology, including methodological refinements concerned with blood chemistry analysis and simplified methods for analyzing the fractional concentrations of expired air. Research at the Fatigue Laboratory included many aspects of acute responses and chronic physiologic adaptations to exercise under environmental stresses produced by exposure to altitude, heat, and cold. Most of the key exercise experiments were conducted with humans using treadmill and bicycle ergometer exercise, but several important studies were also conducted with animals. These studies formed the cornerstone for research in modern laboratories of exercise physiology, particularly in areas related to the assessment of physical working capacity and fitness, cardiovascular and hemodynamic responses during maximal exercise, kinetics of oxygen uptake and substrate utilization, metabolism during exercise and recovery, and maximal oxygen uptake. Detailed discussions of each of these topics can be found in various chapters of our textbook.

Similar to the legacy of the first exercise physiology laboratory established at Harvard's Lawrence Scientific School in 1892, the Harvard Fatigue Laboratory demanded excellence in research and scholarship. Particularly noteworthy was the cooperation among scientists from around the world that fostered lasting collaborations. Furthermore, many of the scientists who had contact with the Fatigue Laboratory profoundly influenced a new generation of exercise physiologists in the United States and abroad. Noteworthy were Ancel Keys, who established the Laboratory of Physiology and Physical Education (later renamed the Laboratory of Physiological Hygiene) at the University of Minnesota; Henry L. Taylor (Keys and Taylor were mentors to exercise physiologist Elsworth R. Buskirk, formerly at the National Institutes of Health and later the Noll Laboratory at Pennsylvania State University); Robert E. Johnson at the Human Environmental Unit at the University of Illinois; Sid Robinson at Indiana University; Robert C. Darling at the Department of Rehabilitation Medicine of Columbia University; Harwood S. Belding, who started the Environmental Physiology Laboratory at the University of Pittsburgh; C. Frank Consolazio of the U.S. Army Medical Research and Nutrition Laboratory in Denver; Lucien Brouha, who headed the Fitness Research Unit at the University of Montreal and then went to the Dupont Chemical Company in Delaware; and Steven M. Horvath, who established the Institute of Environmental Stress at the University of California, Santa Barbara, where he worked with visiting scientists and mentored graduate students in the Biology Department and Department of Ergonomics and Physical Education. After the Fatigue Laboratory was unfortunately forced to close in 1946, Dill continued as the deputy director of the U.S. Army Chemical Corps Medical Laboratory in Maryland for 13 years (1948 to 1961). Thereafter, he worked with Sid Robinson at Indiana University's physiology department before he started the Desert Research Institute (connected with the University of Nevada at Las Vegas), where he studied the physiological responses of men and animals to hot environments, a topic that culminated in a book on the subject.[18]

The group of scholars formerly associated with the Harvard Fatigue Laboratory mentored the next generation of students, who continue to make significant contributions to the field of exercise physiology. The monograph by Horvath and Horvath[30] and chronology by Dill[17] are the best sources of historical information about the Harvard Fatigue Laboratory. Exercise physiology continued to expand after the closing of the Fatigue Laboratory. Subsequent efforts probed the full range of physiologic functions in response to exercise, training, and environmental stress. The depth and breadth of this early investigation, summarized in Table 5, provided much of the current base for establishing exercise physiology as a respectable academic field of study.

TABLE 5
CURRENT AREAS OF INVESTIGATION THAT HELPED TO ESTABLISH EXERCISE PHYSIOLOGY AS AN ACADEMIC DISCIPLINE

1. Specificity of the exercise prescription
2. Genetic components of an exercise response
3. Selectivity of the adaptive responses by diseased populations
4. Differentiation between central and peripheral adaptations
5. The existence of cellular thresholds
6. Actions of transmitters and the regulation of receptors
7. Feed-forward and feedback mechanisms that influence cardiorespiratory and metabolic control
8. Matching mechanisms between oxygen delivery and oxygen demand
9. The substrate utilization profile with and without dietary manipulations
10. Adaptive responses of cellular and molecular units
11. Mechanisms responsible for signal transduction
12. The behavior of lactate in cells
13. The plasticity of muscle fiber types
14. Motor functions of the spinal cord
15. The ability of hormonally deficient animals to respond to conditions of acute exercise and chronic exercise
16. The hypoxemia of severe exercise

From Tipton C.M.: Personal communication to F. Katch, June 12, 1995. From a presentation made to the American Physiological Society Meetings, 1995.

Research Methodology Textbook Focusing on Physiological Research

In 1949, the Research Section and the Research Council of the Research Section of the American Association for Health, Physical Education, and Recreation or AAHPER (an outgrowth of the American Association for the Advancement of Physical Education, created in 1885), sponsored publication of the first textbook devoted to research methodology in physical education.[1] Thomas Cureton, Ph.D., a pioneer researcher in physical fitness evaluation and director of the exercise physiology research laboratory he established at the University of Illinois in 1944, appointed Dr. Henry to chair the committee to write the chapter on physiological research methods. The other committee members were respected scientists in their own right, and included Anna Espenshade (Ph.D. in psychology from Berkeley and a specialist in motor development and motor performance during growth); Pauline Hodgson (a Berkeley Ph.D. in physiology who did postdoctoral work at the Harvard Fatigue Laboratory); Peter V. Karpovich, M.D. (the originator of the Physiological Research Laboratory at Springfield College); Arthur H. Steinhaus, Ph.D. (director of the research laboratory at George Williams College, one of the 11 founders of the American College of Sports Medicine, and a research physiologist who authored an important review article [*Physiological Reviews*, 1933] about the chronic effects of exercise); and distinguished Berkeley physiologist Hardin Jones, Ph.D. (from the Donner Research Laboratory of Medical Physics).

The resulting book chapter by this distinguished committee stands as a hallmark of research methodology in exercise physiology. The 99 references, many of them key articles in this then-embryonic field, covered such exercise-related topics as the "heart and circulation, blood, urine and kidney function, work, lung ventilation, respiratory metabolism and energy exchange, and alveolar air."

Another masterful compendium of research methodologies published 14 years later, *Physiological Measurements of Metabolic Functions in Man*, provided complete details about specific measurements in exercise physiology.[14] Several sections in this book contained material previously published by the Harvard Fatigue Laboratory one year before its closing in 1946[31] and material from another book dealing with metabolic methods[13] published in 1951.

The Nordic Connection (Denmark, Sweden, Norway, and Finland)

Denmark and Sweden have had a significant historical impact on physical education as an academic field. In 1800, Denmark was the first European country to include physical training (military-style gymnastics) as a requirement in the school curriculum. Since that time, the Danish and Swedish approaches to physical training have influenced a large number of scientists who have made outstanding contributions to research in both traditional physiology and exercise physiology.

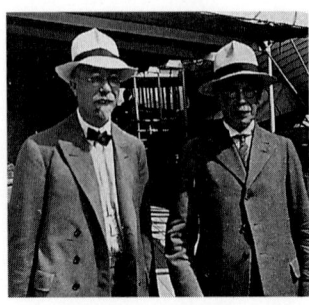

Danish Influence. In 1909, the University of Copenhagen endowed the equivalent of a Chair in Anatomy, Physiology, and Theory of

Professors August Krogh and Johannes Lindhard in the early 1930s.

Gymnastics.[38] The first Docent was Johannes Lindhard, M.D. (1870–1947). He later teamed with August Krogh, Ph.D. (1874–1949), an eminent scientist specializing in physiological chemistry and research instrument design and construction, to conduct many of the now classic experiments in exercise physiology. For example, Krogh and Lindhard investigated gas exchange in the lungs, pioneered studies of the relative contribution of lipid and carbohydrate oxidation during exercise (see Focus on Research, page 138), measured the redistribution of blood flow during different exercise intensities, and measured cardiorespiratory dynamics in exercise (including cardiac output using nitrous oxide gas, a method described by a German researcher in 1770).

By 1910, Krogh and his wife, Marie (a physician), had proven through a series of ingenious, decisive experiments[49]

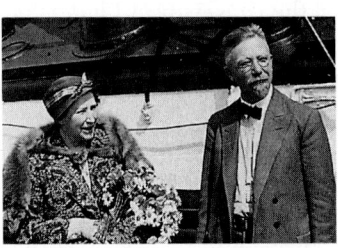

Marie and August Krogh

that diffusion was the mechanism by which pulmonary gas exchange occurred—not by the secretion of oxygen from lung tissue into the blood during exercise and exposure to altitude, as postulated by British physiologists Sir John Scott Haldane and James Priestley.[22] By 1919, Krogh had published reports of a series of experiments (with three appearing in the *Journal of Physiology* in 1919) concerning the mechanism of oxygen diffusion and transport in skeletal muscles. The details of these early experiments are included in Krogh's 1936 textbook,[33] but he also was quite prolific in many other areas of science.[32,34–36] In 1920, Krogh was awarded the Nobel Prize in physiology or medicine for discovering the mechanism of capillary control of blood flow in resting and exercising muscle (in frogs). To honor the achievements of this renowned scientist, an institute for physiological research in Copenhagen was named for him.

Three other Danish researcher-physiologists, Erling Asmussen (1907–1991; ACSM Citation Award, 1976; ACSM Honor Award, 1979), Erik Hohwü-Christensen (b. 1904; ACSM Honor Award, 1981), and Marius Nielsen (b. 1903) conducted pioneering studies in exercise physiology. These "three musketeers," as Krogh referred to them, published numerous research papers from the 1930s to the 1970s. Asmussen, initially an assistant in Lindhard's laboratory, became a prolific researcher specializing in muscle fiber architecture and mechanics. He also

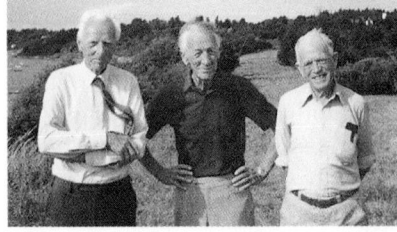

Drs. Erling Asmussen (*left*), Erik Hohwü-Christensen (*center*), and Marius Nielsen (*right*) (1988 photo).

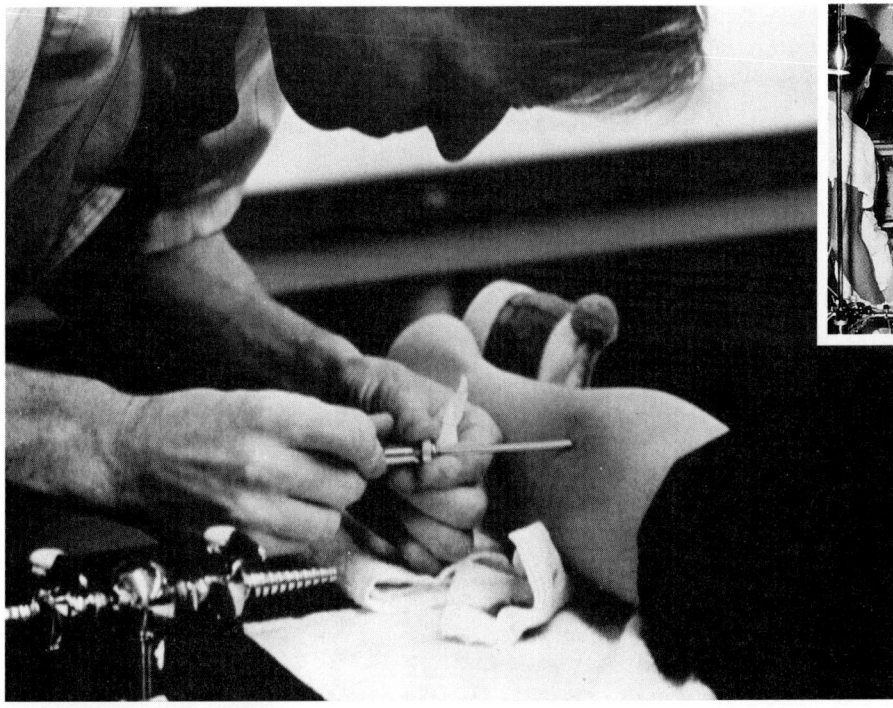

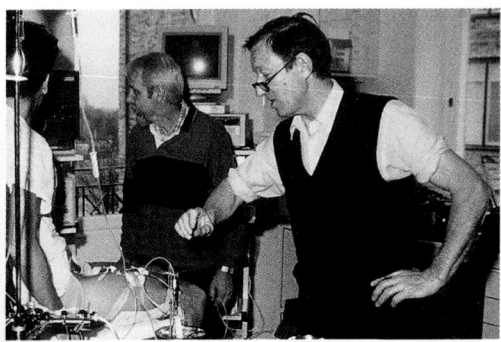

Bengt Saltin taking muscle biopsy of gastrocnemius muscle. (Photo courtesy Dr. David Costill.) Inset of Saltin (hand on hip) during an experiment at the August Krogh Institute, Copenhagen. (Photo courtesy Per-Olof Åstrand.)

published papers with Nielsen and Christensen as coauthors on many applied topics, including muscular strength and performance, ventilatory and cardiovascular response to changes in posture and exercise intensity, maximum working capacity during arm and leg exercise, changes in oxidative response of muscle during exercise, comparisons of positive and negative work, hormonal and core temperature response during different intensities of exercise, and respiratory function in response to decreases in oxygen partial pressure. In his classic review article[2] of muscular exercise that cites many of his own studies (plus 75 references from other Scandinavian researchers), Asmussen's grasp of the importance of the study of biologic functions during exercise is as relevant today as it was more than 30 years ago when this article was published. He clearly defines exercise physiology within the context of biological science:

> The physiology of muscular exercise can be considered a purely descriptive science: it measures the extent to which the human organism can adapt itself to the stresses and strains of the environment and thus provides useful knowledge for athletes, trainers, industrial human engineers, clinicians, and workers in rehabilitation on the working capacity of humans and its limitations. But the physiology of muscular exercise is also part of the general biological science, physiology, which attempts to explain how the living organism functions, by means of the chemical and physical laws that govern the inanimate world. Its important role in physiology lies in the fact that muscular exercise more than most other conditions, taxes the functions to their uttermost. Respiration, circulation, and heat regulation are only idling in the resting state. By following them through stages of increasing work intensities, a far better understanding of the resting condition is also achieved. Although the physiology of muscular exercise must be studied

primarily in healthy subjects, the accumulated knowledge of how the organism responds to the stresses of exercise adds immensely to the understanding of how the organism adapts itself to disease or attempts to eliminate its effects by mobilizing its regulatory mechanisms.

Christensen became Lindhard's student in Copenhagen in 1925. Together with Krogh and Lindhard, Christensen published an important review article in 1936 that described physiological dynamics during maximal exercise.[12] In his 1931 thesis, Christensen reported on studies of cardiac output using a modified Grollman acetylene method, measuring body temperature and blood sugar concentration during heavy exercise on a cycle ergometer, comparing arm exercise with leg exercise, and measuring the effects of training. Together with Ove Hansen, he used oxygen uptake and the respiratory quotient to describe how diet, state of training, and exercise intensity and duration affected carbohydrate and lipid utilization. (In fact, the concept of "carbohydrate loading" was first discovered in 1939!) Other notable studies included core temperature and blood glucose regulation during light to heavy fatiguing exercise at various ambient temperatures. A study by Christensen and Nielsen in 1942 used finger plethysmography to study regional blood flow (including skin temperature) during brief periods of constant-load cycle ergometer exercise.[11] Reports of experiments published in 1936 by physician Olé Bang, inspired by the work of his mentor Ejar Lundsgaard, described the fate of blood lactate during exercise of different intensities and durations.[4] The experiments of Christensen, Asmussen, Nielsen, and Hansen were conducted at the Laboratory for the Theory of Gymnastics at the University of Copenhagen. Today, the August Krogh Institute carries on the tradition of basic and applied research in exercise physiology. Since 1973, Swedish-trained scientist Bengt Saltin (the only Nordic researcher besides Erling Asmussen to receive both the ACSM Citation Award [1980] and the ACSM Honor Award [1990]; former student of Per-Olof Åstrand, discussed in the next section) has been a professor and continues his significant scientific studies at the Muscle Research Institute in Copenhagen.

Swedish Influence. Modern exercise physiology in Sweden can be traced to Per Henrik Ling (1776–1839), who

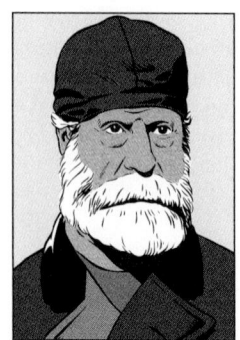

Hjalmar Ling.

in 1813 became the first director of Stockholm's Royal Central Institute of Gymnastics.[38] Ling, a specialist in fencing, developed a system of "medical gymnastics." This system, which became part of the school curriculum of Sweden in 1820, was based on Ling's studies of anatomy and physiology.

Ling's son, Hjalmar, also had a strong interest in medical gymnastics and physiology and anatomy, in part due to his attendance at lectures by physiologist Claude Bernard in Paris, in 1854. Hjalmar Ling published a book on the kinesiology of body movements in 1866.[38] As a result of the Lings' philosophy and influence, the physical educators who graduated from the Stockholm Central Institute were well schooled in the basic biological sciences, in addition to their high proficiency in sports and games. Currently, the College of Physical Education (Gymnastik-Och Idrottshögskolan) and the Department of Physiology in the Karolinska Institute Medical School in Stockholm continue to sponsor studies in exercise physiology.

Per-Olof Åstrand, M.D., Ph.D. (b. 1922) is the most famous graduate of the College of Physical Education (1946); in 1952 he presented his thesis to the Karolinska Institute Medical School. Åstrand taught in the Department of Physiology in the College of Physical Education from 1946 to 1977. When the College of Physical Education became a department of the Karolinska Institute, Åstrand served as professor and department head from 1977 to 1987. Christensen was Åstrand's mentor and supervised his doctoral dissertation, which included data on the physical

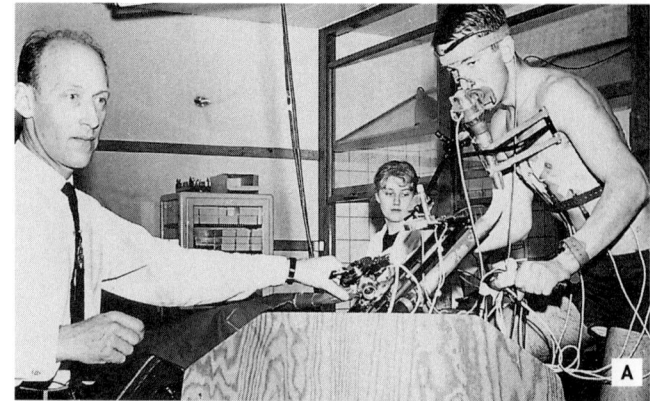

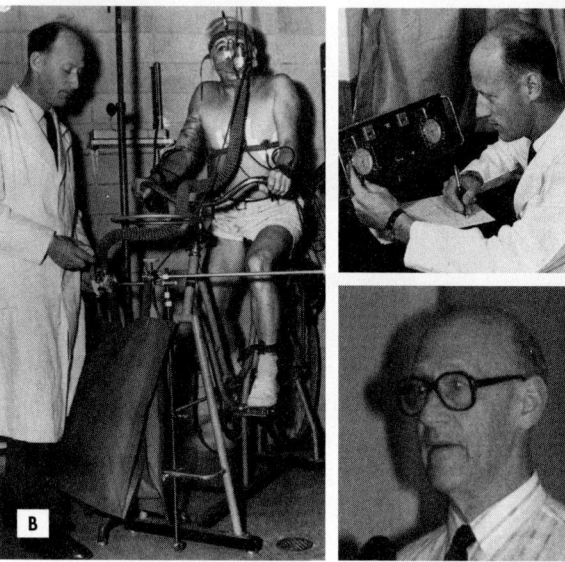

P.O. Åstrand, Department of Physiology. Karolinska Institute, Stockholm. **A,** Measuring maximal performance of Johnny Nilsson, Olympic Gold Medal speed skater, 1964. **B,** Maximal oxygen uptake measured during cycle ergometer exercise, 1958. **C,** Laboratory experiment, 1955. **D,** Invited lecture, 1992 International Conference on Physical Activity, Fitness and Health, Toronto.

working capacity of persons of both sexes aged 4 to 33 years. This important study—along with collaborative studies with his wife, Irma Ryhming—established a line of research that propelled Åstrand to the forefront of experimental exercise physiology, for which he achieved worldwide fame."[n] Four papers published by Åstrand in 1960, with Christensen as one of the authors, stimulated further studies on the

---

[n]Personal communication to F. Katch, June 13, 1995, from Dr. Åstrand regarding his professional background. Recipient of five honorary doctoral degrees (Université de Grenoble [1968], University of Jyväskylä [1971], Institut Superieur d'Education Physique, Université Libre de Bruxelles [1987], Loughborough University of Technology [1991], Aristoteles University of Thessaloniki [1992]), Åstrand is an honorary Fellow of nine international societies, is a Fellow of the American Association for the Advancement of Science (for "outstanding career contributions to understanding of the physiology of muscular work and applications of this understanding"), and has received many awards and prizes for his outstanding scientific achievements, including the ACSM Honor Award in 1973. Åstrand served on a committee for awarding the Nobel Prize in physiology or medicine from 1977 to 1988 and is coauthor with Kaare Rodahl of the third edition of *Textbook of Work Physiology* (1986) (translated into Chinese, French, Italian, Japanese, Korean, Portuguese, and Spanish). His English publications number about 200 (including book chapters, proceedings, a history of Scandinavian scientists in exercise physiology,[3] and monographs), and he has given invited lectures in approximately 50 countries and 150 different cities outside Sweden. His classic 1974 pamphlet *Health and Fitness* has an estimated distribution of 15 to 20 million copies (about 3 million copies in Sweden)—unfortunately, all without personal royalty!

TABLE 6
SELECTED CONTRIBUTIONS TO THE EXERCISE PHYSIOLOGY LITERATURE BY SWEDISH EXERCISE PHYSIOLOGISTS PER-OLOF ÅSTRAND AND BENGT SALTIN

Åstrand, P.-O.: Aerobic work capacity in men and women with special reference to age. *Acta Physiol. Scand.* (Suppl. 169), 1960.

Åstrand, P.-O.: *Experimental studies of physical working capacity in relation to sex and age.* Copenhagen: Munksgaard, 1952, 171 pp.

Åstrand, P.-O., and Grimby, G. (eds.): *Physical Activity in Health and Disease:* Proceedings of the Second Acta Medica Scandinavica International Symposium. Goteborg, Sweden, June 10–12, 1985.

Åstrand, P.-O., and Ryhming, I.: A nomogram for calculation of aerobic capacity (physical fitness) from pulse rate during sub maximal work. *J. Appl. Physiol.*, 7:218, 1954.

Åstrand, P.-O., and Rodahl, K.: *Textbook of Work Physiology*, 3rd ed. New York, McGraw-Hill, 1986.

Åstrand, P.-O., et al.: Girl swimmers. *Acta Paediatr.* (Suppl. 147), 1963.

Shephard, R.J., and Åstrand P.-O. (eds.): *Endurance in Sport.* Oxford, Blackwell Scientific Publications, 1992.

Saltin, B.: Aerobic work capacity and circulation of man. *Acta Physiol. Scand.* (Suppl. 230), 1964.

Saltin, B. (ed.): *International Symposium on Biochemistry of Exercise.* Champaign, IL, Human Kinetics, 1986.

Saltin, B., et al.: Physical training in sedentary middle-aged and older men. *Scand. J. Clin. Lab. Invest.*, 24:323, 1967.

Saltin, B., et al.: Response to submaximal and maximal exercise after bedrest and training. *Circulation*, 38 (Suppl. 7), 1968.

Pernow, B., and Saltin , B. (eds.): *Muscle Metabolism During Exercise.* Proceedings of a Karolinska Institutet symposium held in Stockholm, Sweden, September 6–9. New York, Plenum Press, 1971.

Viru, A., and Saltin , B. (eds.): *Adaptation in Sports Training.* Boca Raton, FL, CRC Press, 1995.

Saltin, B., and Åstrand, P.-O.: Maximal oxygen uptake in athletes. *J. Appl. Physiol.*, 23:353, 1967.

Hermansen, L., and Saltin, B.: Oxygen uptake during maximal treadmill and bicycle exercise. *J. Appl. Physiol.*, 26:31, 1969.

Saltin, B., and Hermansen, L.: Glycogen stores and prolonged severe exercise. In Blix, G. (ed.): *Nutrition and Physical Activity.* Symposia of the Swedish Nutrition Foundation. Stockholm, Almqvist & Wiksell, 1967.

Number of Citations in Scientific Literature						
Year	*1990*	*1991*	*1992*	*1993*	*1994*	*1995[a]*
Åstrand	183	192	217	190	223	115
Saltin	185	171	188	183	162	77

Source: *Science Citation Index.* Annual cumulations, 1990–1995 (CD-ROM). Philadelphia, Institute for Scientific Information. Numbers refer to citations in the published literature (including books).

[a]Through November 1995.

physiological responses to intermittent exercise. Åstrand has mentored an impressive group of exercise physiologists, including such "superstars" as Bengt Saltin and Björn Ekblom. Table 6 is a sampling of contributions to the exercise physiology literature by Åstrand and Saltin in books, book chapters, monographs, and research articles. As further evidence of their international influence, the bottom part of the table includes the number of times each

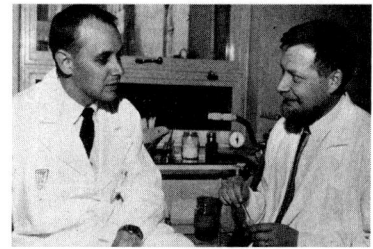

Drs. Jonas Bergstrom *(left)* and Eric Hultman, Karolinska Institute, mid 1960s.

was cited in the scientific literature from 1990 through November 1995.

Two Swedish scientists currently at the Karolinska Institute, Drs. Jonas Bergström and Erik Hultman, performed important experiments with the needle biopsy procedure that have provided a new vista from which to study exercise physiology. With this procedure, it became relatively easy to conduct invasive studies of muscle under various conditions of exercise, training, and nutritional status. Collaborative work with other Scandinavian researchers (Saltin and Hultman from Sweden and Lars Hermansen from Norway) and researchers in the United States (for example, Phillip Gollnick at Washington State University) contributed a whole new dimension to the study of muscular exercise.

Norwegian and Finnish Influence. The new generation of exercise physiologists trained in the late 1940s analyzed respiratory gases by means of a highly accurate sampling apparatus that measured minute quantities of carbon dioxide and oxygen in expired air. The method of analysis (and also the analyzer) was developed in 1947 by the Norwegian scientist Per Scholander (1905–1980). A diagram of Scholander's micrometer gas analyzer[50] is presented in Chapter 8, Figure 8.7 along with its larger counterpart, the Haldane analyzer.

Another prominent Norwegian researcher was Lars A. Hermansen (1933–1984; ACSM Citation Award, 1985) from the Institute of Work Physiology,

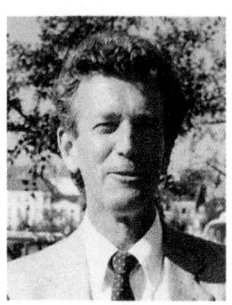 who died prematurely. Nevertheless, his many contributions include an impressive 1969 article entitled "Anaerobic Energy Release" that appeared in the first volume of *Medicine and Science in Sports.*[27] Other papers included work with fellow exercise physiologist K. Lange Andersen.[28]

Lars A. Hermansen (1933–1984). Institute of Work Physiology, Oslo.

In Finland, Martti Karvonen, M.D., Ph.D. (ACSM Honor Award, 1991) from the Physiology Department of the Institute of Occupational Health, Helsinki, is best known for a method to predict optimal exercise training heart rate, the so-called "Karvonen formula" (see Chapter 21, p. 403 and Focus on Research, p. 266). He also conducted studies dealing with exercise performance and the role of exercise in longevity. In 1952, Lauri Pikhala, a physiologist, suggested that obesity was the consequence and not the cause of physical "unfitness." Ilkka Vuori, starting in the early 1970s, reported on

hormone responses to exercise. Paavo Komi, from the Department of Biology of Physical Activity, University of Jyväskylä, has been Finland's most prolific researcher, with reports of numerous experiments published in the combined areas of exercise physiology and sport biomechanics. Table 7 lists the Nordic researchers who have received the prestigious ACSM Honor Award or ACSM Citation Award.

Other Contributors to the Knowledge Base in Exercise Physiology

In addition to the American and Nordic applied scientists who have achieved distinction in their own right, many other giants in the fields of physiology and experimental science[o] made monumental contributions that indirectly added to the knowledge base in exercise physiology. This list of scientists not mentioned previously includes Antoine Laurent Lavoisier (1743–1794; combustion[p]), Sir Joseph Barcroft (1872–1947; altitude), Christian Bohr (1855–1911; oxygen-hemoglobin dissociation curve), John Scott Haldane (1860–1936; respiration), Otto Myerhoff (1884–1951; Nobel Prize, cellular metabolic pathways), Nathan Zuntz (1847–1920; portable metabolism apparatus), Carl von Voit (1831–1908) and his student Max Rubner (1854–1932; direct and

TABLE 7 NORDIC RESEARCHERS[a] AWARDED THE ACSM HONOR AWARD AND ACSM CITATION AWARD	
ACSM Honor Award	*ACSM Citation Award*
Per-Olof Åstrand, 1973	Erling Asmussen, 1976
Erling Asmussen, 1979	Bengt Saltin, 1980
Erik Hohwü-Christensen, 1981	Lars A. Hermansen, 1985
Bengt Saltin, 1990	C. Gunnar Blomqvist, 1987
Martti J. Karvonen, 1991	

[a] Born and educated in a Nordic country.

---

[o]There are many excellent sources of information about the history of science and medicine, including the following: Bettman, O.: *A Pictorial History of Medicine* (Springfield, IL, Charles C Thomas, 1956); Clendening, L.: *Source Book of Medical History* (New York, Dover Publications/Henry Schuman, 1960); Coleman, W.: *Biology in the Nineteenth Century* (New York, Cambridge University Press, 1977); Franklin, K.: *A Short History of Physiology,* 2nd ed. (London, Staples Press, 1949); Fye, W.B.: *The Development of American Physiology. Scientific Medicine in the Nineteenth Century* (Baltimore, Johns Hopkins University Press, 1987); Guthrie, D.: *A History of Medicine* (London, T. Nelson & Sons, 1945); Haskins, T.: *Science and Enlightenment* (New York, Cambridge University Press, 1985); Holmes, F.L.: *Lavoisier and the Chemistry of Life* (Madison, WI, University of Wisconsin Press, 1985); Knight, B.: *Discovering the Human Body* (London, Bloomsbury Books, 1992); Lesch, J.E.: *Science and Medicine in France. The Emergence of Experimental Physiology,* 1790-1855 (Cambridge, MA, Harvard University Press, 1984); Vertinsky, P.A.: *The Eternally Wounded Woman: Women, Exercise and Doctors in the Late Nineteenth Century* (Urbana, IL, University of Illinois Press, 1994); Walker, K.: *The Story of Medicine* (London, Arrow Books, 1954).

[p]Lavoisier was the first person to conduct experiments on human respiration (about 1770). According to Lusk,[39] Lavoisier told of his experiments in a letter to a friend dated November 19, 1790, as follows: "(1) The quantity of oxygen absorbed by a resting man at a temperature of 26°C is 1200 *pouces de France* [1 cubic *pouce* = 0.0198 liters] hourly. (2) The quantity of oxygen required at a temperature of 12°C rises to 1400 *pouces.* (3) During the digestion of food the quantity of oxygen amounts to from 1800 to 1900 *pouces.* (4) During exercise 4000 *pouces* and over may be the quantity of oxygen absorbed." Lusk's excellent 1909 textbook provides a detailed summary of the early history of energy research in metabolism in Europe and the United States.

indirect calorimetry, and specific dynamic action of food), Max von Pettenkofer (1818–1901; nutrient metabolism), and Eduard F.W. Pflüger (1829–1910; tissue oxidation).

■ SUMMARY ■

This introductory section on the historical development of exercise physiology illustrates that interest in exercise and health had its roots with the ancients. Over the next 2000 years, the field we now call exercise physiology evolved from a symbiotic (albeit sometimes rocky) relationship between the classically trained physicians, the academically based anatomists and physiologists, and a small cadre of physical educators who struggled to achieve their identity and academic credibility through research and experimentation in the basic and applied sciences. While the physiologists used exercise to study the dynamics of human physiology, the early physical educators often used the methodology and knowledge of physiology to study exercise.

Beginning in the early 1860s in America, there was a small but slowly growing effort to raise standards for the scientific training of physical education and hygiene specialists who were primarily involved in teaching at the college and university level. The creation of the first exercise physiology laboratory at Harvard University in 1892 contributed to an already burgeoning knowledge base in basic physiology. Originally, medically trained physiologists made the significant scientific advances in most of the subspecialties that are now included in the exercise physiology course curriculum. They studied oxygen metabolism, muscle structure and function, gas transport and exchange, mechanisms of circulatory dynamics, and neural control of voluntary and involuntary muscular activity.

The field of exercise physiology also owes a debt of gratitude to the pioneers of the physical fitness movement in the United States, notably Thomas K. Cureton (1901–1993; ACSM charter member; ACSM Honor Award, 1969) at the University of Illinois, Champaign—a prolific, insightful exercise physiology–fitness researcher who trained four generations of physical educators beginning in 1941. Many of these pioneers assumed leadership positions as professors with teaching and research responsibilities in exercise physiology at numerous colleges and universities in the United States and throughout the world.

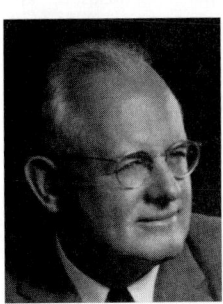

Dr. Thomas Kirk Cureton (1901–1993).

While we have focused on the contributions of selected early American scientists and physical educators and their counterparts from the Nordic countries to the development of modern-day exercise physiology, we would be neglectful not to acknowledge the numerous contributions from many scholars in other countries. The group of foreign contributors, many still active, includes but certainly is not limited to the following individuals: Roy Shephard, School of Physical and Health Education, University of Toronto (ACSM Citation Award, 1991); Claude Bouchard, Laval University, Québec City (ACSM Citation Award, 1992); Oded Bar-Or, McMaster University, Hamilton, Ontario, Canada; Rodolfo Margaria, P.E. di Prampero, P. Cerretelli, and Giovanni Cavagna, Institute of Human Physiology, Medical School of the University of Milan; Michio Ikai, School of Education, University of Japan; Wildor Holloman, Director of the Institute for Circulation, Research and Sports Medicine, and L. Brauer and H.W. Knipping, Institute of Medicine, University of Cologne, Germany (in 1929, they described the "vita maxima," now called the maximal oxygen uptake); L.G.C.E. Pugh, Medical Research Council Laboratories, London; Z.I. Barbashova, Sechenov Institute of Evolutionary Physiology, Leningrad; Sir Cedric Stanton Hicks, Human Physiology Department, University of Adelaide, Australia; Otto Gustaf Edholm, National Institute for Medical Research, London; John Valentine George Andrew Durnin, Department of Physiology, Glasgow University; Reginald Passmore, Department of Physiology, University of Edinburgh; Ernst F. Jokl (ACSM Founder and charter member), Witwatersrand Technical College, Johannesburg, and later the University of Kentucky; and C.H. Wyndham and N.B. Strydom, University of the Witwatersrand, Johannesburg. There were also many early German scientific contributions to exercise physiology and sports medicine.[29]

■ CONCLUDING COMMENT ■

One theme unites the history of exercise physiology: the value of mentoring by those visionaries who spent an extraordinary amount of their careers "infecting" students with love for hard science. These demanding but inspiring relationships developed researchers who in turn nurtured the next generation of productive scholars. This applies not only to the current group of exercise physiologists, but also to scholars of previous generations. Siegel[52] cites Payne,[45] who in 1896 wrote the following about Harvey's 1628 discovery of the mechanism of the circulation, acknowledging the discoveries of the past:

> No kind of knowledge has ever sprung into being without an antecedent, but is inseparably connected with what was known before.... We are led back to Aristotle and Galen as the real predecessors of Harvey in his work concerning the heart. It was the labors of the great school of Greek anatomists...that the problem though unsolved, was put in such a shape that the genius of Harvey was enabled to solve it.... The moral is, I think, that the influence of the past on the present is even more potent than we commonly suppose. In common and trivial things, we may ignore this connection; in what is of enduring worth we cannot.

We end our overview of the history of exercise physiology with a passage from an American physiology and hygiene textbook written over 130 years ago by J.C. Dalton, M.D., a professor of physiology in the College of Physicians and Surgeons in New York City. It shows how current themes in exercise physiology share a common bond with what was known and advocated at that time (the benefits of moderate exercise, walking as an excellent exercise, the appropriate exercise intensity, the specificity of training, the importance of mental well-being). Even the "new" thoughts and ideas of Dalton penned in 1869 had their roots in antiquity—reinforcing to us the importance of maintaining a healthy respect for the past.

Exercise. The natural force of the muscular system requires to be maintained by constant and regular Exercise. If all of the muscles, or those of any particular part, be allowed to remain for a long time unused they diminish in size, grow softer, and finally become sluggish and debilitated. By use and exercise, on the contrary, they maintain their vigor, continue plump and firm to the touch, and retain all the characters of their healthy organization. It is very important, therefore, that the muscles should be trained and exercised by sufficient daily use. Too much confinement by sedentary occupation, in study, or by simple indulgence in indolent habits, will certainly impair the strength of the body and injuriously affect the health. Every one who is in a healthy condition should provide for the free use of the muscles by at least two hour's exercise each day; and this exercise can not be neglected with impunity, any more than the due provision of clothing and food.

The muscular exercise of the body, in order to produce its proper effect, should be regular and moderate in degree. It will not do for any person to remain inactive during the greater part of the week, and then take an excessive amount of exercise on a single day. An unnatural deficiency of this kind can not be compensated by an occasional excess. It is only a uniform and healthy action of the parts which stimulates the muscles, and provides for their nourishment and growth. Exercise which is so violent and long-continued as to produce exhaustion or unnatural fatigue is an injury instead of an advantage, and creates a waste and expenditure of the muscular force instead of its healthy increase.

Walking is therefore one of the most useful kinds of exercise, since it calls into easy and moderate action nearly all the muscles of the body, and may be continued for a long time without fatigue. Riding on horseback is also exceedingly efficacious, particularly as it is accompanied by a certain amount of excitement and interest which acts as an agreeable and healthy stimulus to the nervous system. Running and leaping, being more violent should be used more sparingly. For children, the rapid and continuous exercise which they spontaneously take in their various games and amusements in the open air is the best. The exact quantity of exercise to be taken is not precisely the same for different persons, but should be measured by its effect. It is always beneficial when it has fully employed the muscular powers without producing any sense of excessive fatigue or exhaustion.

It should be remembered, also, that the object of exercise is not the mere acquisition or increase of muscular strength, but the proper maintenance of the general health. A special increase of strength may be produced to a very great extent by the constant practice or training of particular muscles. Thus the arms of the blacksmith and the legs of the dancer become developed in excessive proportions; and by the continued practice, in a gymnasium, of raising weights, or carrying loads, the muscular system generally may be greatly increased in force. But this unusual muscular development is not necessary to health, and is not even particularly beneficial about it. The best condition is that in which all the different organs and systems of the body have their full and complete development, no one of them preponderating excessively over the others. The most useful kind of exercise, accordingly, is that which employs equally all the limbs, and cultivates agility and freedom of movement, as well as simple muscular strength.

In all cases, also, the exercise which is taken should be regular and uniform in degree, and should be repeated as nearly as possible for the same time every day.

As a student in an Exercise Physiology course, you are about to embark on an exciting journey into the world of human physiological response and adaptation to physical activity. We hope our tour of the beginnings of exercise physiology inspires you in your studies to begin your own journey to new discoveries.

Photograph of Dr. Austin Flint, Jr., M.D. from the Library of the College of Physicians of Philadelphia. Photographs of Dr. Edward Hitchcock and Dr. Edward Hitchcock, Jr., from the Amherst College Archives and by permission of the Trustees of Amherst College.

■ REFERENCES ■

1. American Association for Health, Physical Education, and Recreation: Physiological Laboratory Research. In *Research Methods Applied to Health, Physical Education, and Recreation*, Chapter 11. Washington, DC, American Association for Health, Physical Education, and Recreation, 1949, pp. 254–274.

2. Asmussen, E: Muscular exercise. In *Handbook of Respiration, vol. 2, section 3, Respiration.* Fenn, W.O. and Rahn, H. (Eds.). Washington, DC, American Physiological Society, 1965, pp. 939–978.

3. Åstrand, P.-O.: Influence of Scandinavian scientists in exercise physiology. *Scand. J. Med. Sci. Sports*, 1:3–9, 1991.

4. Bang, O., et al.: Contributions to the physiology of severe muscular work. *Skand. Arch. Physiol.* 74 (Suppl.): 1, 1936.

5. Barcroft, J.: *The Respiratory Function of the Blood. Part 1. Lessons from High Altitude.* Cambridge, Cambridge University Press, 1925.

6. Berryman, J.W.: *Out of Many, One. A History of the American College of Sports Medicine.* Champaign, IL, Human Kinetics, 1995.

7. Berryman, J.W.: The tradition of the "six things non-natural": Exercise and medicine from Hippocrates through Ante-Bellum America. *Exerc. Sport Sci. Rev.*, 17: 515, 1989.

8. Billings, J.S.: Literature and institutions. In *A Century of American Medicine*, Clarke, E.H., et al. (Eds.). Philadelphia, Henry C. Lea, 1876, p. 294.

9. Buskirk, E.R.: Early History of Exercise Physiology in the United States. Part 1. A contemporary historical perspective. In *History of*

Exercise and Sport Science. Messengale, J.D., and Swanson, R.A. (Eds.). Champaign, IL, Human Kinetics, in press, 1996.

10. Buskirk, E.R.: The emergence of exercise physiology in physical education. In *Perspectives on the Academic Discipline of Physical Education*, Brooks, G.A. (Ed.). Champaign, IL, Human Kinetics, 1981, pp. 55–74.

11. Christensen, E.H., and Nielsen, M.: Investigations of the circulation in the skin at the beginning of muscular work. *Acta Physiol. Scand.*, 4:162, 1942.

12. Christensen, E.H., et al.: Contributions to the physiology of heavy muscular work. *Skan. Arch. Physiol.*, Suppl. 10, 1936.

13. Consolazio, C.F.: *Metabolic Methods.* St. Louis, C.V. Mosby, 1951.

14. Consolazio, C.F.: *Physiological Measurements of Metabolic Functions in Man.* New York, McGraw-Hill, 1961.

15. Dill, D.B.: Arlie V. Bock, pioneer in sports medicine. December 30, 1888–August 11, 1984. *Med. Sci. Sports Exerc.*, 17:401, 1985.

16. Dill, D.B.: *Life, Heat, and Altitude; Physiological Effects of Hot Climates and Great Heights.* Cambridge, MA, Harvard University Press, 1938.

17. Dill, D.B.: The Harvard Fatigue Laboratory: Its development, contributions, and demise. *Circ. Res.*, 20 & 21 (Suppl. 1): 161, 1967.

18. Dill, D.B.: *The Hot Life of Man and Beast.* Springfield, IL, Charles C. Thomas, 1985.

19. Gerber, E.W.: *Innovators and Institutions in Physical Education.* Philadelphia, Lea & Febiger, 1971.

20. Green, H.: *Fit For America. Health, Fitness, Sport, and American Society.* New York, Pantheon, 1986.

21. Green, R.M.: *A Translation of Galen's Hygiene.* Springfield, IL, Charles C. Thomas, 1951.

22. Haldane, J.S., and Priestley, J.G.: *Respiration.* New York, Oxford University Press, 1935.

23. Henry, F.M., and Farmer, D.: Functional Tests: II. The reliability of the pulse-ratio test. *Res. Q.*, 4:81, 1938.

24. Henry, F.M., and Kleeberger, F.L.: Functional Tests: I. The validity of the pulse-ratio test of cardiac efficiency. *Res. Q.*, 4:32, 1938.

25. Henry, F.M., and Trafton, I.R.: The velocity curve of sprint running with some observations on the muscle viscosity factor. *Res. Q.*, 22: 409, 1951.

26. Henry, F.M.: Force-time characteristics of the sprint start. *Res. Q.*, 23:301, 1952.

27. Hermansen, L.: Anaerobic energy release. *Med. Sci. Sports*, 1:32, 1969.

28. Hermansen, L., and Andersen, K.L.: Aerobic work capacity in young Norwegian men and women. *J. Appl. Physiol.*, 20:425, 1965.

29. Hoberman, J.M. The early development of sports medicine in Germany. In *Sport and Exercise Science*, Berryman, J.W., and Park, R.J. (Eds.). Urbana, IL, University of Illinois Press, 1992, pp. 233–282.

30. Horvath, S.M., and Horvath, E.C.: *The Harvard Fatigue Laboratory: Its History and Contributors.* Englewood Cliffs, NJ, Prentice-Hall, 1973.

31. Johnson, R.E., et al.: *Laboratory Manual of Field Methods for the Biochemical Assessment of Metabolic and Nutrition Conditions.* Boston, Harvard Fatigue Laboratory, 1946.

32. Krogh, A.: *Osmotic Regulation in Aquatic Animals.* New York, Dover Publications, 1939.

33. Krogh, A.: *The Anatomy and Physiology of Capillaries.* New Haven, CT, Yale University Press, 1936.

34. Krogh, A.: *The Comparative Physiology of Respiratory Mechanisms.* Philadelphia, University of Pennsylvania Press, 1941.

35. Krogh, A.: *The Composition of the Atmosphere; An Account of Preliminary Investigations and a Programme.* Copenhagen, A.F. Host, 1919. (19-p. monograph)

36. Krogh, A.: *The Respiratory Exchange of Animals and Man.* New York, Longmans, Green, 1916. (includes 17-page reference list)

37. Kroll, W.: *Perspectives in Physical Education.* New York, Academic Press, 1971.

38. Leonard, F.G.: *A Guide to the History of Physical Education.* Philadelphia, Lea & Febiger, 1923.

39. Lusk, G.: *The Elements of the Science of Nutrition*, 2nd ed. Philadelphia, W.B. Saunders, 1909.

40. Manolis, G.G.: Relation of charging time to blocking performance in football. *Res. Q.*, 26:170, 1955.

40a. Ostyn, M.: Preface. In *Kinanthropometry II.* Ostyn, M., et al. (Eds.). Baltimore, University Park Press, 1980, p. xvii.

41. Park, R.J.: Concern for health and exercise as expressed in the writings of 18th century physicians and informed laymen (England, France, Switzerland). *Res. Q.*, 47:756, 1976.

42. Park, R.J.: Franklin M. Henry—Scientist, mentor, pioneer. *Res. Q. Exerc. Sports.*, 65:295–307, 1994.

43. Park, R.J.: Physiologists, physicians, and physical educators: nineteenth century biology and exercise, hygienic and educative. *J. Sport Hist.*, 14:28, 1987.

44. Park, R.J.: The emergence of the academic discipline of physical education in the United States. In *Perspectives on the Academic Discipline of Physical Education.* Brooks, G.A. (Ed.). Champaign, IL, Human Kinetics, 1981, pp. 20–45.

44a. Park, R.J.: The rise and demise of Harvard's B.S. program in anatomy, physiology, and physical training: a case of conflicts of interest and scarce resources. *Res. Q. Exerc. Sport.* 63:1, 1992.

45. Payne, J.F.: *Harvey and Galen.* The Harveyan Oration. Oct. 19, 1896. London, Frowde, 1897.

46. Powers, S.K., and Howley, E.T.: *Exercise Physiology.* Dubuque, IA, Wm. C. Brown Publishers, 1994.

47. Ross, W.D.: Kinanthropometry: an emerging scientific technology. In *Biomechanics of Sports and Kinanthropometry.* Book 6. Landry, F., and Orban, W.A.R. (Eds.). Miami, Symposia Specialists, Inc. 1978, pp. 269–282.

48. Ross, W.D., et al.: Kinanthropometry: traditions and new perspectives. In *Kinanthropometry II.* Ostyn, M., et al. (Eds.). Baltimore, University Park Press, 1980, pp. 3–27.

49. Schmidt-Nielsen, B.: August and Marie Krogh and respiratory physiology. *J. Appl. Physiol.*, 57:293, 1984.

50. Scholander, P.F.: Analyzer for accurate estimation of respiratory gases in one-half cubic centimeter samples. *J. Biol. Chem.*, 167:235, 1947.

51. Shaffel, N.: The evaluation of American medical literature. In *History of American Medicine.* Marti-Ibanez, F. (Ed.). New York, MD Publications, 1958.

52. Siegel, R.: *Galen's System of Physiology and Medicine.* New York, S. Karger, 1968.

53. Tipton, C.M.: A history of exercise physiology in the United States. Part II. A contemporary historical perspective. In *History of Exercise and Sport Science.* Messengale, J.D., and Swanson, R.A. (Eds.). Champaign, IL, Human Kinetics, in press, 1996.

54. Wilmore, J.H., and Costill, D.L.: *Physiology of Sport and Exercise.* Champaign, IL, Human Kinetics, 1994.

PART 1

EXERCISE
PHYSIOLOGY

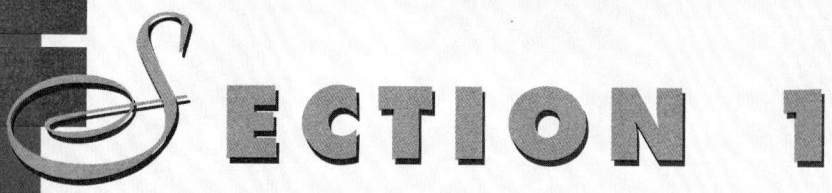

SECTION 1

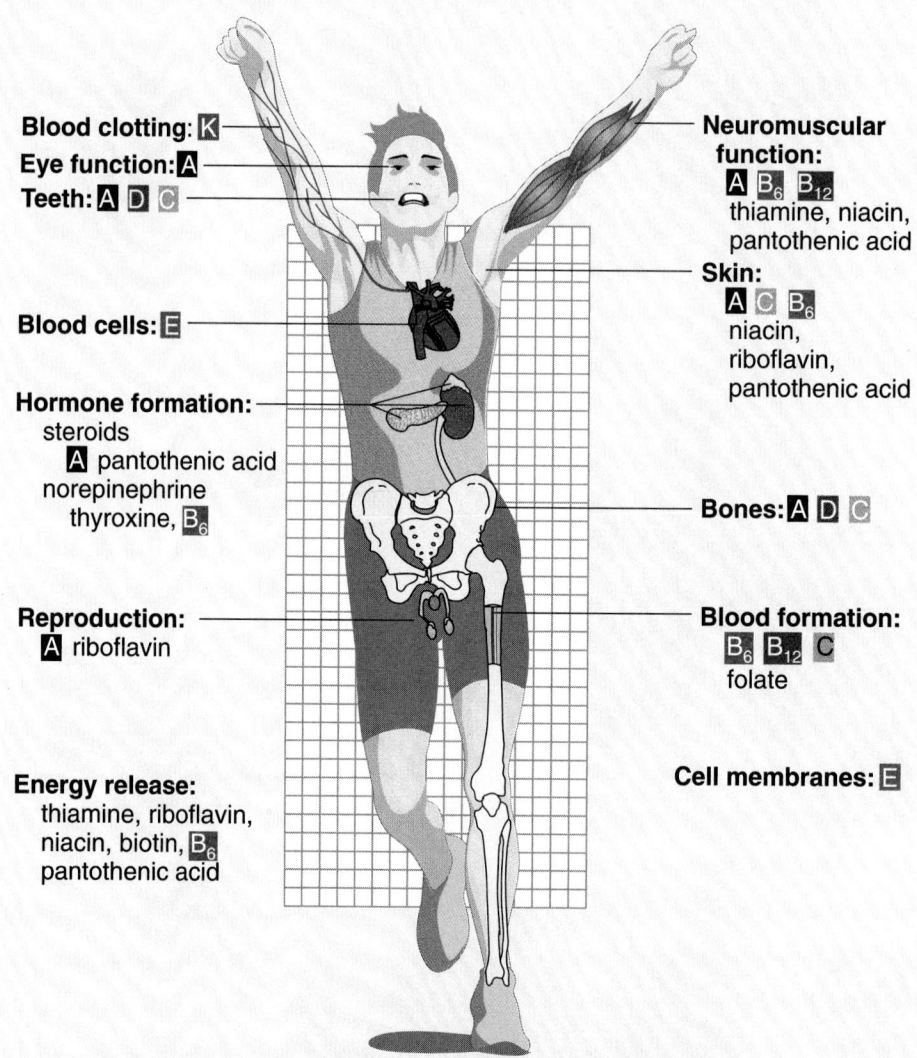

Blood clotting: K

Eye function: A

Teeth: A D C

Blood cells: E

Hormone formation:
steroids
A pantothenic acid
norepinephrine
thyroxine, B6

Reproduction:
A riboflavin

Energy release:
thiamine, riboflavin,
niacin, biotin, B6
pantothenic acid

Neuromuscular
function:
A B6 B12
thiamine, niacin,
pantothenic acid

Skin:
A C B6
niacin,
riboflavin,
pantothenic acid

Bones: A D C

Blood formation:
B6 B12 C
folate

Cell membranes: E

"THE CONSENSUS IS THAT

PHYSICALLY ACTIVE PEOPLE

DO NOT REQUIRE ADDITIONAL

NUTRIENTS BEYOND THOSE

OBTAINED IN A BALANCED DIET."

Nutrition: The Base for Human Performance

There is a natural linkage between nutrition and exercise physiology. Proper nutrition forms the foundation for physical performance; it provides the fuel for biologic work and the chemicals for extracting and using the potential energy contained within this fuel. In addition, food nutrients provide the essential elements for synthesizing new tissue and repairing existing cells.

Some may argue that adequate nutrition for exercise is readily obtained with a well-balanced diet, and thus a knowledge of nutrition has little value in studying exercise. We maintain, however, that the study of exercise, when viewed within the framework of energy capacities and human performance, must begin with a good understanding of the sources of food energy and the role of nutrients in the process of energy release. With this perspective, the exercise specialist appreciates the importance of "adequate" nutrition and critically evaluates the validity of claims concerning nutrient supplements and special dietary modifications to enhance physical performance. Because various food nutrients provide energy and regulate physiologic processes associated with exercise, it is tempting to link dietary modification to improved athletic performance. Too often individuals spend considerable time and "energy" striving for optimum exercise performance, only to fall short due to inadequate, counterproductive, and sometimes harmful nutritional practices. Finally, sound nutritional practices ameliorate many disease conditions; these conditions are also positively affected by a lifestyle that includes regular physical activity.

In the chapters that follow, we look at the six broad categories of nutrients: carbohydrates, lipids, proteins, vitamins, minerals, and water. We explore the following questions: What are they? Where are they found? What are their functions? What is their specific role in physical activity?

Tarnopolsky, M.A., et al.: Influence of protein intake and training status on nitrogen balance and lean body mass. *J. Appl. Physiol.* 64:187, 1988.

There is controversy concerning the protein needs of athletes during training. Numerous factors influence protein utilization; these include fitness level, type and volume of training, nutritional status, different types of athletes have different protein requirements.

This study determined whether either endurance exercise or heavy resistance training increased urea excretion and altered nitrogen balance during two different levels of protein intake (LP, low protein; HP, high protein). Three groups of six men served as subjects: a sedentary control group (S), a group of elite endurance athletes (EA), and a group of competitive bodybuilders (BB). Measurement over 10 days included total nitrogen balance (N-BAL) during LP and HP conditions. For the EA group, the protein intake at LP was 1.70 $g \cdot kg^{-1} \cdot d^{-1}$, compared with 2.65 $g \cdot kg^{-1} \cdot d^{-1}$ for HP. For the BB group, protein intake averaged 1.05 $g \cdot kg^{-1} \cdot d^{-1}$ (LP) and 2.77 $g \cdot kg^{-1} \cdot d^{-1}$ (HP), and for the S group, average protein intake levels were 1.05 $g \cdot kg^{-1} \cdot d^{-1}$ (LP) and 1.90 $g \cdot kg^{-1} \cdot d^{-1}$ (HP). To determine total nitrogen excretion (TNF), there were three sequential 24-hour urine collections, 72-hour fecal collections, and representative sampling of resting and exercise sweat secretion. Determination of N-BAL required assessment of TNF and protein intake.

The figure presents the N-BAL (grams N per day) plotted with different protein intake levels for each group. The zero N-BAL horizontal line represents the point where nitrogen intake equals the body's nitrogen requirement. The point where the regression line intersects (daily protein intake) theoretically represents the protein requirement at nitrogen balance. The calculated protein intake necessary for N-BAL was 0.73 $g \cdot kg^{-1}d^{-1}$ for the S group; for the BB group, it was 0.82 $g \cdot kg^{-1}d^{-1}$; and for the EA group, 1.37 $g \cdot kg^{-1} \cdot d^{-1}$. These calculated protein intakes for the different groups probably represent an overestimation of true levels.

The researchers argued that determining the minimal protein intake required several N-BAL studies at protein intakes just below and above the levels required to attain N-BAL. This overestimation was used to calculate safe levels of protein intake for the BB (1.2 $g \cdot kg^{-1} \cdot d^{-1}$) and EA groups (1.6 $g \cdot kg^{-1} \cdot d^{-1}$). The projected protein requirements consider the high-energy and high-carbohydrate diet usually maintained by competitive athletes. Endurance exercise apparently increased net protein catabolism and resulted in an increased protein requirement not evident for the BB group. The protein supplements so commonly used among bodybuilders are expensive, cause strain on the kidneys, and are probably unnecessary. The researchers recommended that bodybuilders reduce protein intake, while endurance athletes could possibly benefit from increased protein intake.

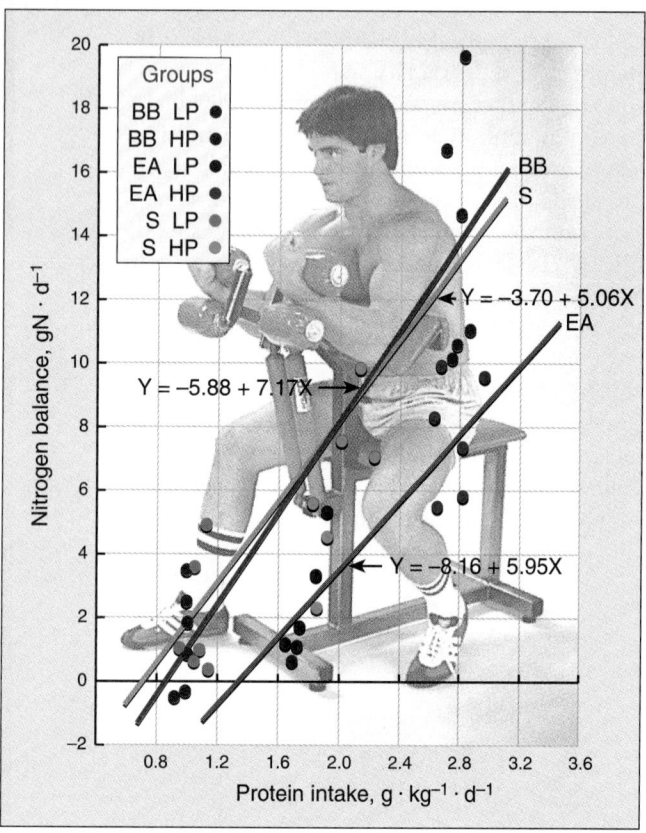

Nitrogen balance plotted in relation to the different protein intake levels for each of the three groups. The zero horizontal line represents the point of nitrogen balance where nitrogen intake equals the body's nitrogen requirement. The point where the regression line intersects this horizontal axis theoretically represents the protein requirement for nitrogen balance.

and the energy density and carbohydrate content of the diet. The current recommendation in the United States for daily protein intake is 0.82 g of mixed protein per kilogram of body mass. This recommendation does not consider individuals undergoing exercise training. Because endurance and resistance exercise increases net protein utilization (evidenced by increased protein oxidation and urea excretion during exercise), the authors argued that

Carbohydrates, Lipids, and Proteins

The carbohydrate, lipid, and protein nutrients provide the necessary energy to maintain body functions at rest and during various forms of physical activity. Aside from their role as biologic fuel, these nutrients, called **macronutrients,** play important roles in maintaining the structural and functional integrity of the organism. In this chapter, we discuss each macronutrient for its general structure, function, source in specific foods in the diet, and importance in optimizing physiologic function during varied physical activities differing in intensity.

ATOMS: NATURE'S BUILDING BLOCKS

Of the 103 different atoms or elements identified in nature, the mass of the human organism is composed of about 3% nitrogen, 10% hydrogen, 18% carbon, and 65% oxygen. These atoms play the major role in the chemical composition of nutrients and make up the structural units for the body's biologically active substances.

The union of two or more atoms forms molecules. The specific atoms as well as their arrangement give the molecule its particular properties. Glucose is glucose because of the arrangement of three different kinds of 24 atoms within its molecule. Chemical bonding involves a common sharing of electrons between atoms, as when atoms of hydrogen and oxygen join to form the water molecule. The force of attraction between the positive and negative charges of atoms forms the basis for bonding and provides the "chemical cement" that keeps the atoms and molecules within a substance from readily coming apart. A larger aggregate of matter (a substance) is formed when two or more molecules bind chemically. This substance may take the form of a gas, a liquid, or a solid, depending on the force of interaction between molecules. When these forces are altered due to the removal, transfer, or exchange of certain electrons, energy is released, some of which is used to power cellular functions.

CARBON: THE VERSATILE ELEMENT

All of the nutrients except water and minerals contain carbon. Almost all of the substances within the body are composed of carbon-containing (organic) compounds. Carbon atoms can easily share their chemical bonds with other carbon atoms, as well as with atoms of other elements, to form large carbon-chain molecules.

Lipids and carbohydrates are formed from specific linkages of carbon atoms with atoms of hydrogen and oxygen. A protein molecule is formed when nitrogen is added with certain mineral substances. Atoms of carbon, hydrogen, oxygen, and nitrogen are the atomic building blocks from which the nutrients are made.

PART 1
CARBOHYDRATES

THE NATURE OF CARBOHYDRATES

Carbohydrates, as the name implies, are composed of carbon and water. Atoms of carbon, hydrogen, and oxygen combine to form a carbohydrate or sugar molecule in the general formula $(CH_2O)_n$, where n can be from three to seven carbon atoms with the hydrogen and oxygen atoms attached by single bonds. The most typical sugar, **glucose,** is illustrated in Figure 1.1, along with the different carbohydrates formed during photosynthesis. This molecule consists of 6 carbon, 12 hydrogen, and 6 oxygen atoms with the chemical formula $C_6H_{12}O_6$. Each of the carbon atoms has four bonding sites that can link to other atoms, including carbon atoms. Carbon bonds not linked to other carbon atoms are "free" to hold hydrogen (which has only one bond site), oxygen (with two bond sites), or an oxygen-hydrogen combination (OH), termed a hydroxyl. **Fructose** and **galactose** are two other simple sugars that have the same chemical formula as glucose, but with a slightly different carbon-to-hydrogen-to-oxygen linkage. This alteration in the arrangement of atoms makes fructose, galactose, and glucose different substances with different biochemical characteristics. The structural characteristics of the simple sugars were uncovered at the beginning of the 20th century by the German chemist Emil Fischer.

KINDS AND SOURCES OF CARBOHYDRATES

Carbohydrates are classified as either **monosaccharides, oligosaccharides,** or **polysaccharides.** Each of these carbohydrate types is distinguished by the number of simple sugars linked within the molecule. Table 1.1 provides the general classification of carbohydrates.

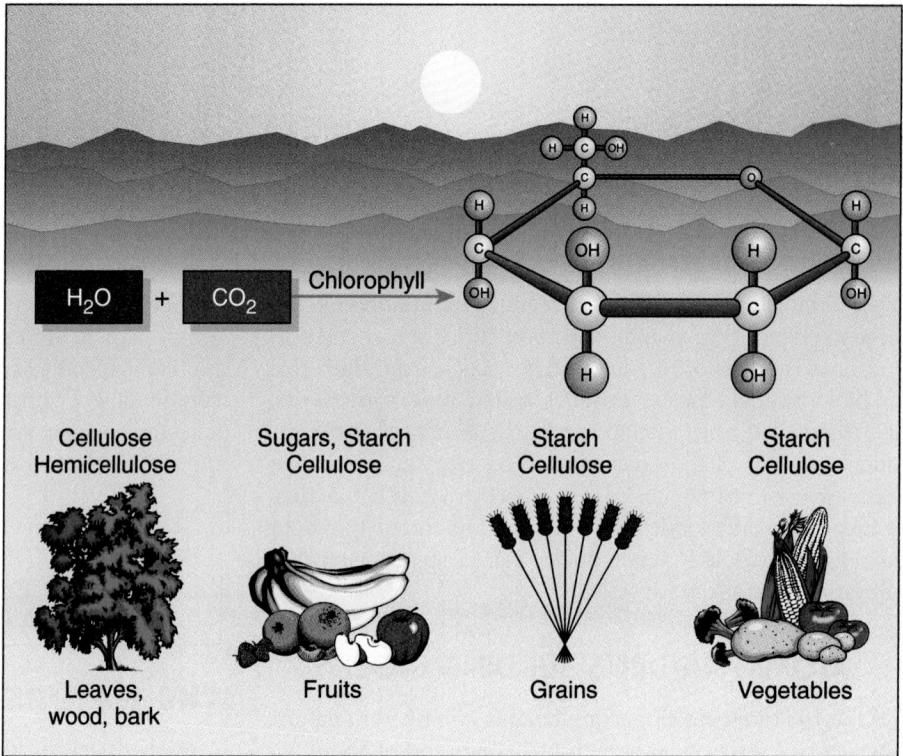

FIGURE 1.1

Three-dimensional ring structure of the simple sugar molecule glucose formed during photosynthesis when the energy from sunlight interacts with water, carbon dioxide, and the green pigment chlorophyll. The molecule resembles a hexagonal plate for attachment of H and O atoms. About 75% of the dry matter of plants consists of carbohydrate, and photosynthesis forms approximately 100 billion tons of carbohydrates yearly.

MONOSACCHARIDES

The basic unit of carbohydrates is the sugar molecule or monosaccharide. More than 200 monosaccharides have been found in nature.[77] They are categorized by the number of carbon atoms in their ring, using the Greek name for this number and ending with "ose" to indicate that they are sugars. For example, three-carbon monosaccharides are known as trioses, four-carbon sugars are tetroses, five-carbon sugars are pentoses, six-carbon sugars are hexoses, and the seven-carbon sugars are heptoses. The nutritionally important monosaccharides are the hexose sugars glucose, fructose, and galactose. Glucose, also called dextrose or blood sugar, is a natural sugar in food or is produced in the body through the digestion of more complex carbohydrates. It can also be produced by the process of **gluconeogenesis,** whereby it is synthesized primarily in the liver from the carbon skeletons of other compounds (amino acids, glycerol, pyruvate, lactate). After absorption by the small intestine, glucose can be used directly by the cell for energy, stored as glycogen in the muscles and liver, or converted to lipids for energy storage.

Fructose, or fruit sugar, the sweetest of the simple sugars, is present in large amounts in fruits and honey. Although some fructose is absorbed directly into the blood from the digestive tract, it is all converted to glucose in the liver.[39] Galactose is not found freely in nature; rather, it is combined in milk sugar in the mammary glands of lactating animals. In the body, galactose is converted to glucose for energy metabolism.

OLIGOSACCHARIDES

Oligosaccharides are formed from the joining together of a few (*oligo* in Greek) monosaccharides. The major oligosaccharides are the **disaccharides** or double sugars, formed from the combination of two monosaccharide molecules.

The monosaccharides and disaccharides collectively make up what are commonly called **simple sugars.** These sugars are packaged under a variety of guises—brown sugar, corn syrup, invert sugar, honey, and "natural sweeteners."

In the structure of each of the disaccharides, glucose is one of the simple sugars. The three principal disaccharides are:

- **Sucrose,** composed of glucose plus fructose, is the most common dietary disaccharide; it constitutes up to 25% of the total caloric intake in the United States. It occurs naturally in most foods that contain carbohydrates, particularly in beet and cane sugar, brown sugar, sorghum, maple syrup, and honey. (Honey, while sweeter than table sugar because of its higher fructose content, is not superior either nutritionally or as an energy source.)

- **Lactose,** composed of glucose plus galactose, is found in natural form only in milk and is called milk sugar. Lactose is the least sweet of the disaccharides; it can be artificially

TABLE 1.1
GENERAL CLASSIFICATION OF CARBOHYDRATES

Monosaccharides		*Oligosaccharides*	*Polysaccharides*		
Trioses	*Tetroses*				
Pentoses $C_5H_{10}O_5$	**Hexoses** $C_6H_{12}O_6$	**Disaccharides** $C_{12}H_{22}O_{11}$	**Pentosans** $(C_5H_8O_4)n^2$	**Hexosans** $(C_6H_{10}O_5)n^2$	**Mixed Polysaccharides**
Arabinose	Fructose	Lactose	Araban	Cellulose	Agar
Ribose	Galactose	Maltose	Xylan	Glycogen	Pectin
Xylose	Glucose	Sucrose		Inulin	Chitin
Deoxyribose	Mannose	Trehalose		Mannan	Hemicelluloses
				Starch (amylose and amylopectin)	Carrageenan
					Vegetable gums

Derivatives of Monosaccharides

Sugar alcohols: glycerol, inositol, mannitol, sorbitol

Amino sugars: galactosamine (formed from galactose—present in cartilage, tendons, and aorta); glucosamine (formed from glucose—present in connective tissues)

Sugar acids: ascorbic acid (vitamin C, not formed in the body); gluconic acid (formed from glucose); glucuronic acid (formed from glucose, aids in detoxification and excretion of other compounds, and is present in connective tissue)

processed and is often present in carbohydrate-rich, high-calorie liquid meals. A substantial number of people around the world are lactose intolerant; that is, they lack adequate quantities of the enzyme lactase, which splits lactose to glucose and galactose during the digestive process.

• **Maltose,** composed of glucose plus glucose, is present in beer, cereals, and germinating seeds. Also called malt sugar, maltose is a negligible component of the carbohydrate content of the average person's diet.

POLYSACCHARIDES

The term polysaccharide is used when from three to thousands of sugar molecules are linked together. There are two classifications of polysaccharides, plant and animal.

Plant Polysaccharides

Two common forms of plant polysaccharides are **starch** and **fiber.**

Starch. Starch, the storage form of carbohydrate in plants, is the most familiar form of plant polysaccharide. It is found in seeds, corn, and the various grains from which bread, cereal, spaghetti, and pastries are made. Large amounts are also present in peas, beans, potatoes, and roots, where it serves as an energy store for future use by plants. Plant starch is still the most important dietary source of carbohydrate in the American diet, accounting for approximately 50% of the total carbohydrate intake. The daily intake of starch, however, has decreased about 30% since the turn of the century, whereas the consumption of simple sugars such as sucrose has correspondingly increased from 30% to about 50% of total carbohydrate intake. Dietary starch is commonly referred to as **complex carbohydrates.**

Fiber. Fiber is classified as a nonstarch polysaccharide, of which cellulose is the most abundant organic molecule on earth. Nonstarch fibrous materials are resistant to human digestive enzymes, although a portion are fermented by intestinal bacteria and ultimately used in metabolic reactions following their intestinal absorption. Fibers are found exclusively in plants and make up the structure of leaves, stems, roots, seeds, and fruit coverings. The various fibers differ widely in physical and chemical characteristics and in physiologic action; they are found mostly within the cell wall as cellulose, hemicellulose, pectin, and the noncarbohydrate

TABLE 1.2
FIBER CONTENT OF SOME COMMON FOODS LISTED FOR OVERALL FIBER CONTENT

	Serving Size	Total Fiber (g)	Soluble Fiber (g)	Insoluble Fiber (g)
100% bran cereal	½ cup	10.0	0.3	9.7
Peas	½ cup	5.2	2.0	3.2
Kidney beans	½ cup	4.5	0.5	4.0
Apple	1 small	3.9	2.3	1.6
Potato	1 small	3.8	2.2	1.6
Broccoli	½ cup	2.5	1.1	1.4
Strawberries	¾ cup	2.4	0.9	1.5
Oats, whole	½ cup	1.6	0.5	1.1
Banana	1 small	1.3	0.6	0.7
Spaghetti	½ cup	1.0	0.2	0.8
Lettuce	½ cup	0.5	0.2	0.3
White rice	½ cup	0.5	0	0.5

lignin, whereas other fibers such as mucilage and gums are found within the plant cell itself.

Health Implications.   Although technically not a nutrient, dietary fiber has received considerable attention by researchers and the mainstream press. Much of this interest originated from studies that linked high fiber intake with a lower occurrence of obesity, diabetes, intestinal disorders, and heart disease.[50] Because the Western diet is high in fiber-free animal foods and loses much of its natural fiber through processing, it is speculated that this accounts for the prevalence of intestinal disorders in these countries compared to countries where people consume a more primitive kind of diet high in unrefined, complex carbohydrates. For example, the typical American diet contains a daily fiber intake of about 12 g,[a] whereas diets in Africa and India range between 40 and 150 g per day.[43, 52] Fibers hold considerable water and thus give "bulk" to the food residues in the small intestine, often increasing stool weight and volume by 40 to 100%. This bulking action may aid gastrointestinal functioning by exerting a scraping action on the cells of the gut wall, by binding or diluting harmful chemicals or inhibiting their activity, and by shortening the transit time for the passage of food residues (and possibly carcinogenic materials) through the digestive tract. This may reduce the chances of contracting colon cancer and various other gastrointestinal diseases later in life.[8]

Fiber intake also may cause modest reductions in serum cholesterol in humans, especially the **water-soluble** mucilaginous fibers such as pectin and guar gum present in oats, beans, brown rice, peas, carrots, and a variety of fruits.[17, 30, 41]

For men with elevated blood lipids, for example, adding 100 g of oat bran to the daily diet caused a 13% reduction in serum cholesterol and favorably affected the ratio of the blood's lipoproteins.[45] Also, increasing the daily intake of guar gum fiber reduced cholesterol, specifically by lowering the low-density lipoprotein component of the cholesterol profile.[30, 84] In contrast, the **water-insoluble** fibers, such as cellulose, hemicellulose, and lignin, and cellulose-rich products like wheat bran showed no cholesterol-lowering effect.[43, 90] The precise mechanism by which dietary fibers favorably affect serum cholesterol is unclear. It may be that the addition of fiber simply replaces cholesterol-laden items in the diet. On the other hand, some types of fiber may actually hinder cholesterol absorption, while others may reduce cholesterol metabolism in the gut. These actions would depress the synthesis of cholesterol while at the same time facilitating the excretion of existing cholesterol bound to the fiber in the feces. Dietary fiber also slows the rate of digestion of carbohydrate so it is absorbed into the bloodstream more slowly by the intestine. Fiber decreases the total number of calories that will be consumed in subsequent meals. Consuming a fiber-rich breakfast, for example, decreased the caloric intake both during breakfast and during a buffet-type lunch consumed 3.5 hours later.[55]

Present nutritional wisdom maintains that a dietary fiber intake of about 20 to 35 g per day (ratio of 3:1 for water-insoluble to soluble fiber) is an important part of a well-structured diet. Table 1.2 gives the fiber content of some common foods, and Table 1.3 presents a sample daily 2200-kcal menu that includes 31 g of fiber (21 g insoluble

---

[a]Scientific measurement is generally presented in terms of the metric system. Appendix A shows the relationship between metric units and English units relevant to exercise physiology. Also presented are some common expressions of work, energy, and power.

fiber). In this particular diet, total lipid calories are 30% (saturated fat, 32%), protein is 19%, and carbohydrate is 54% of the total calories ingested. Perhaps as research progresses and the specific fiber content of various foods is clarified, a recommended daily requirement for specific fibers will be established. Excessive fiber intake, however, is not prudent for persons with marginal levels of nutrition. This is because an increase in fiber intake can decrease the absorption of calcium, iron, magnesium, phosphorus, and certain trace minerals.

Animal Polysaccharides

Glycogen is the storage carbohydrate peculiar to mammalian muscle and liver. It is a large polysaccharide polymer synthesized from glucose in the process of **glucogenesis** and stored in the tissues of animals. This irregularly shaped macromolecule's size ranges from a few hundred to thousands of glucose molecules linked together, much like the links in a chain of sausages, with some branch points for additional glucose linkage. As shown in Figure 1.2, the synthesis of glycogen from glucose occurs by the addition of individual glucose units to an already existing glycogen polymer.

In well-nourished humans, approximately 375 to 475 g of carbohydrate is stored in the body. Of this, approximately 325 g is muscle glycogen (largest reserve), 90 to 110 g is liver glycogen (highest concentration that represents between 3 to 7% of the liver's weight), and only about 5 g is present as blood glucose.[29] As each gram of glycogen contains 4 calories of energy, the average person stores between 1500 and 2000 calories as carbohydrate. This is approximately enough energy to power a 20-mile run.

Several factors determine the rate and quantity of both the breakdown and synthesis of glycogen. During exercise, muscle glycogen is the **major** source of carbohydrate energy for the active muscles in which it is stored. In the liver, in contrast, glycogen is reconverted to glucose (under the control of a specific **phosphatase** enzyme) and transported in the blood for use by the working muscles. The term **glycogenolysis** describes this reconversion process, which provides a rapid extramuscular supply of glucose for muscular action. When liver and muscle glycogen is depleted through dietary restriction or heavy exercise, glucose synthesis from the structural components of the other nutrients, principally proteins, increases through the gluconeogenic metabolic pathways.

Hormones play an important role in regulating liver and muscle glycogen stores by controlling the level of circulating blood sugar. When blood sugar level is elevated, the beta cells of the pancreas secrete additional insulin and the excess circulating glucose is taken up by the cells, which inhibits further insulin secretion. This feedback regulation maintains blood glucose at an appropriate physiologic concentration. In contrast, if blood sugar falls below normal, insulin's opposing hormone, glucagon, is immediately secreted by the alpha cells of the pancreas to normalize the blood sugar level. This "insulin antagonist" hormone raises the blood glucose level by stimulating both glycogenolysis and gluconeogenesis in the liver. More will be said in Chapter 19 concerning the role of hormones in exercise.

Because comparatively little glycogen is stored in the body, its quantity can be modified considerably through the diet. For example, a 24-hour fast or a low-carbohydrate, normal-calorie diet results in a large reduction in glycogen reserves.[36] On the other hand, maintaining a carbohydrate-rich diet for several days enhances the body's carbohydrate stores to a level almost twice that obtained with a normal, well-balanced diet.[5] The upper limit for glycogen storage in the body is about 15 g per kilogram of body mass. This is a capacity of 1150 g for an average-sized man who weighs 70 kg. The effect of enhanced carbohydrate storage on exercise performance is discussed in a later section of this chapter.

TABLE 1.3
SAMPLE DAILY MENU FOR BREAKFAST, LUNCH, AND DINNER (2200 KCAL) CONTAINING 31 G OF DIETARY FIBER. THE DIET'S TOTAL CHOLESTEROL CONTENT IS LESS THAN 200 MG, AND TOTAL CALCIUM IS 1242 MG

Breakfast	*Lunch*	*Dinner*
Whole grain cereal (0.75 cup)	Bran muffin (1)	Green salad (3.5 oz)
Whole wheat toast (2 slices)	Milk, 2% (1 cup)	Broccoli, steamed (0.5 cup)
Margarine (2 tsp)	Hamburger on bun, lean beef patty (3 oz)	Roll, whole wheat (1)
Jelly, strawberry (1 Tbsp)	with 2 slices tomato and lettuce, catsup	Margarine (2 tsp)
Milk, 2% (1 cup)	(1 Tbsp) and mustard (1 Tbsp)	Brown rice (0.5 cup)
Raisins (2 Tbsp)	Whole wheat crackers (4 small)	Chicken breast, skinless, broiled (3 oz)
Orange juice (0.5 cup)	Split-pea soup (1 cup)	Salad dressing, vinegar and oil (1 Tbsp)
Coffee (or tea)	Coffee (or tea)	Pear, medium (1)
		Yogurt, vanilla, lowfat (0.5 cup)

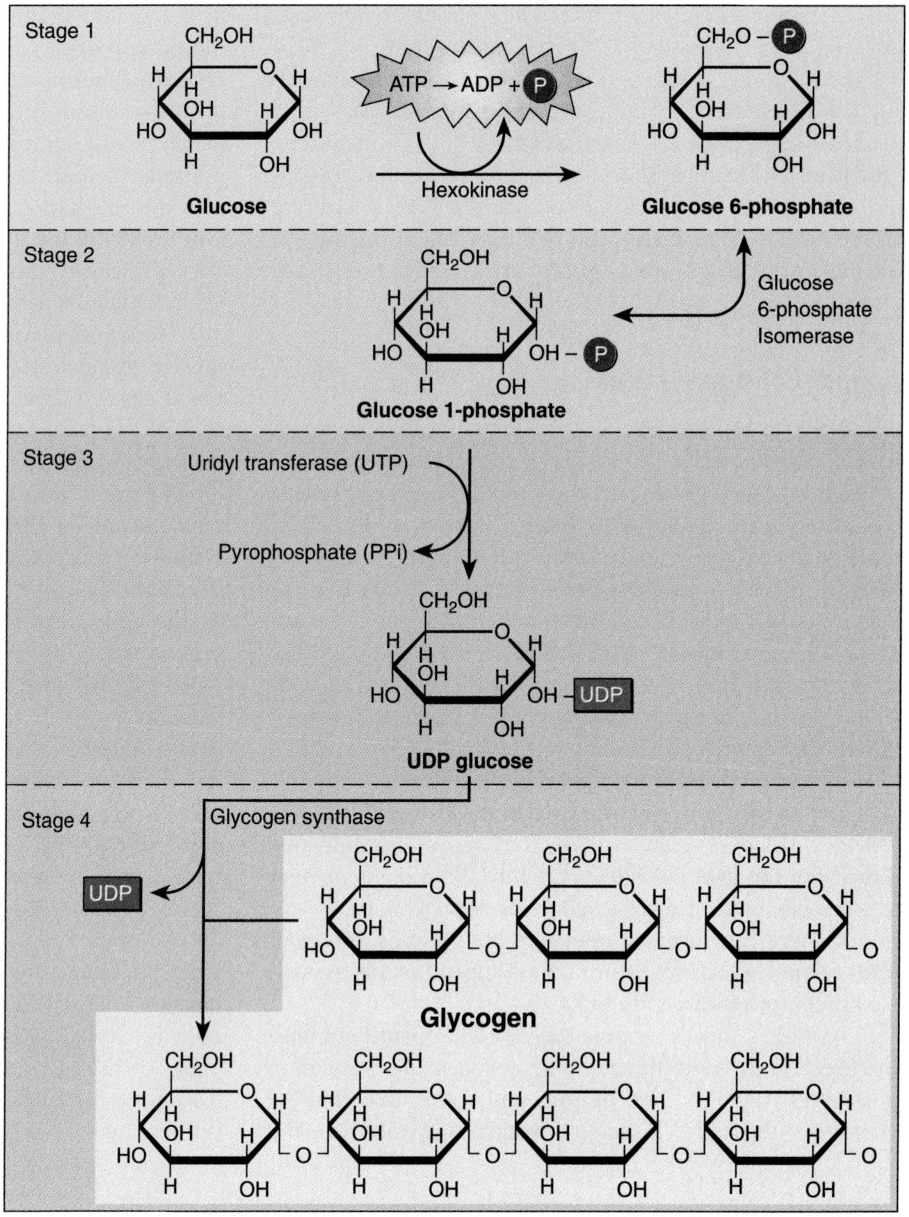

FIGURE 1.2

The synthesis of glycogen is a four-step process. *Step 1,* ATP donates a phosphate to glucose to form glucose 6-phosphate. This reaction involves the enzyme hexokinase. *Step 2,* Glucose 6-phosphate is isomerized to glucose 1-phosphate by the enzyme glucose 6-phosphate isomerase. *Step 3,* The enzyme uridyl transferase (UTP) reacts with glucose 1-phosphate to form UDP-glucose (a phosphate is released as UTP → UDP). *Step 4,* UDP-glucose attaches to one end of an already existing glycogen polymer chain. This forms a new bond (known as a glycoside bond) between the adjacent glucose units, with the concomitant release of UDP. For each glucose unit added, there is conversion of 2 moles of ATP to ADP and phosphate.

RECOMMENDED DIETARY CARBOHYDRATE INTAKE

Figure 1.3 illustrates the carbohydrate content of selected foods. Cereals, cookies, candies, breads, and cakes are rich carbohydrate sources. Because the values are based on carbohydrate percentage in relation to the food's total weight, including water content, fruits and vegetables appear to be less valuable sources of carbohydrates. The dry portions of these foods, however, are almost pure carbohydrate.

The typical American diet includes between 40 and 50% of its total calories as carbohydrate. For a sedentary 70-kg person, this amounts to a daily intake of about 300 g of carbohydrate. For more physically active people and those in-volved in exercise training, about 60% of daily calories (400 to 600 g) should be carbohydrates, predominantly of the un-refined, fiber-rich complex variety in fruits and vegetables. This quantity will be sufficient to replenish the carbohydrate used to power the increased level of physical activity.

Important dietary carbohydrate sources are generally fruits and vegetables, although this is not true for all people. The average American consumes about 50% of carbohydrate as simple sugars, predominantly as sucrose and high-fructose corn syrup (formed by enzyme action on corn-starch that emphasizes fructose formation). This amount represents more than 16 teaspoons a day or 60 lb of table sugar and 46 lb of corn syrup each year, as contrasted to a 4 lb per person intake of table sugar 100 years ago!

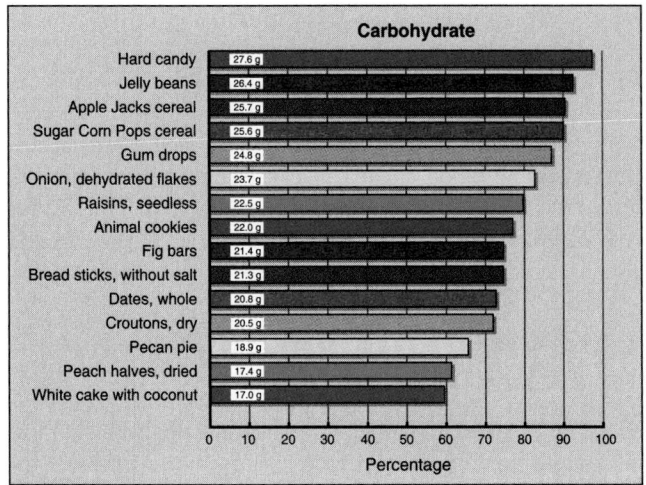

FIGURE 1.3
Percentage of carbohydrates in commonly served foods. The insert box displays the number of grams of carbohydrate per ounce (28.3 g) of the food.

Excessive fermentable carbohydrate (principally sucrose) in the diet is a main cause of tooth decay.[23] The precise role, if any, that excessive dietary sugar plays in diseases such as diabetes, obesity, and coronary heart disease has not been established. One way to reduce sucrose intake is to substitute fructose, a monosaccharide that is about twice as sweet as table sugar. This provides equal sweetness with fewer calories. In addition, fructose does not stimulate pancreatic insulin secretion and may be taken up by the muscle without the assistance of insulin. As a result, the blood-glucose level remains fairly stable following fructose ingestion.[64]

ROLE OF CARBOHYDRATES IN THE BODY

Carbohydrates serve four important functions related to energy metabolism and exercise performance.

ENERGY SOURCE

The main function of carbohydrate is to serve as an energy fuel, particularly during exercise. The energy derived from the breakdown of blood-borne glucose and liver and muscle glycogen is ultimately used to power the contractile elements of muscle as well as other forms of biologic work.[75]

Daily carbohydrate intake must be adequate to maintain the body's relatively limited glycogen stores. On the other hand, once the capacity of the cell for glycogen storage is reached, excess sugars are converted to and stored as lipid. This action helps to explain how the body's fat content can increase when excess carbohydrates are consumed, even if the diet is low in lipid.

PROTEIN SPARING

Adequate carbohydrate intake helps to preserve tissue proteins. Normally, protein serves a vital role in tissue maintenance, repair, and growth and, to a considerably lesser degree, as a nutrient source of energy. Glycogen reserves, however, can readily become reduced in starvation or in diets with reduced calorie and/or carbohydrate content and through strenuous exercise. The effect of reduced energy intake (40-hour fast) and total food deprivation (7-day starvation) on levels of plasma glucose and lipid breakdown components is readily seen in Table 1.4. After almost 2 days of fasting, blood glucose becomes reduced by 35% but does not decrease to a lower level during a further prolonged abstinence from food. At the same time, circulating fatty acid and ketone (byproducts of incomplete lipid breakdown) levels increase rapidly, with plasma ketones rising dramatically after 7 days of starvation.

When glycogen reserves are reduced and plasma glucose level falls, metabolic pathways exist for the synthesis of glucose from both protein and the glycerol portion of the lipid molecule. This process of gluconeogenesis provides a metabolic option for augmenting carbohydrate availability (and maintaining plasma glucose levels) in the face of depleted glycogen stores, as occurs in dietary restriction or prolonged exercise. The price paid, however, is a temporary reduction in the body's protein "stores," particularly muscle protein. In extreme conditions, this causes a significant reduction in the lean tissue mass and an accompanying solute load on the kidneys, which must increase their workload to excrete the nitrogen-containing byproducts of protein breakdown.

METABOLIC PRIMER

Carbohydrates serve as a "primer" for lipid metabolism. Certain products from carbohydrate breakdown must be

TABLE 1.4
CHANGES IN THE PLASMA CONCENTRATIONS OF GLUCOSE, FATTY ACIDS, AND KETONES FOLLOWING 40 HOURS OF FASTING AND SUBSEQUENT 7 DAYS OF STARVATION

Nutrient $(mmol \cdot L^{-1})$	Normal	40 hours Fasting	7 days Starvation
Glucose	5.5	3.6	3.5
Fatty acids	0.3	1.15	1.19
Ketones	0.01	2.9	4.5

Adapted from Bender, D.A.: *Introduction to Nutrition and Metabolism.* London, UCL Press, 1993.

available to facilitate the metabolism of lipid. If carbohydrate metabolism is insufficient—either through limitation in the transport of glucose into the cell, as occurs in diabetes, or through depletion of glycogen through improper diet or prolonged exercise—the body will mobilize a greater amount of lipid than it can metabolize. The result is incomplete lipid breakdown and the accumulation of acetone-like byproducts (chiefly acetoacetate and hydroxybutyrate) called **ketone bodies**.[49] This situation may lead to a harmful increase in the acidity of body fluids, a condition called acidosis or, more specifically with regard to lipid breakdown, **ketosis**. More is said in Chapter 6 of the role of carbohydrate as a primer for lipid metabolism.

FUEL FOR THE CENTRAL NERVOUS SYSTEM

Carbohydrate is essential for the proper functioning of the central nervous system. Under normal conditions and in short-term starvation, the brain uses blood glucose almost exclusively as its fuel and essentially has no stored supply of this nutrient. In poorly regulated diabetes, however, or during starvation or with a low carbohydrate intake, metabolic adaptations occur so that after about 8 days the brain uses relatively large amounts of lipid in the form of acetoacetate for its fuel requirement.[12] There is even indication that adaptations take place in skeletal muscle that increase its ability to burn lipids for energy during exercise and concurrently spare muscle glycogen.[63]

At rest and during exercise, liver glycogenolysis is the primary means for maintaining normal blood glucose levels, usually at an average of 100 mg · dL^{-1} or 5.5 mM. With the depletion of liver glycogen and a continued large use of blood glucose by active muscle, blood glucose eventually falls below normal levels. The symptoms of a modest reduction in blood glucose (**hypoglycemia**) include feelings of weakness, hunger, and dizziness. This condition impairs exercise performance and may partially explain the "central" fatigue associated with prolonged exercise. Sustained and profound low blood sugar can cause loss of consciousness and irreversible brain damage. Because of the important role of glucose in nerve tissue metabolism, blood sugar is usually regulated within narrow limits.

CARBOHYDRATE BALANCE IN EXERCISE

The fuel mixture in exercise depends on the intensity and duration of effort, as well as the fitness and nutritional status of the exerciser.[20, 20a, 40] The energy contribution of intramuscular and extramuscular nutrients during physical activity can be studied with the use of biochemical and biopsy techniques and labeled nutrient tracers. For example, the needle biopsy technique permits the serial sampling of specific muscles with little interruption during exercise for purposes of assessing the kinetics of intramuscular nutrient use throughout exercise. Under most conditions, exercise brings about a marked increase in the release of glucose by the liver and its subsequent use by active muscle.[46, 99] At the same time, the predominant carbohydrate energy source during exercise is the glycogen stored within this muscle.[73]

INTENSE EXERCISE

With strenuous exercise, neural-humoral factors increase the hormonal output of epinephrine, norepinephrine, and glucagon, and decrease insulin release. These actions have a

FIGURE 1.4
Exercise duration and intensity affect blood glucose uptake by the leg muscles. Exercise intensity is expressed as a percentage of one's V̇o₂max. (From Felig, P., and Wahren, J.: Fuel homeostasis in exercise. *N. Engl. J. Med.*, 293: 1078, 1975.)

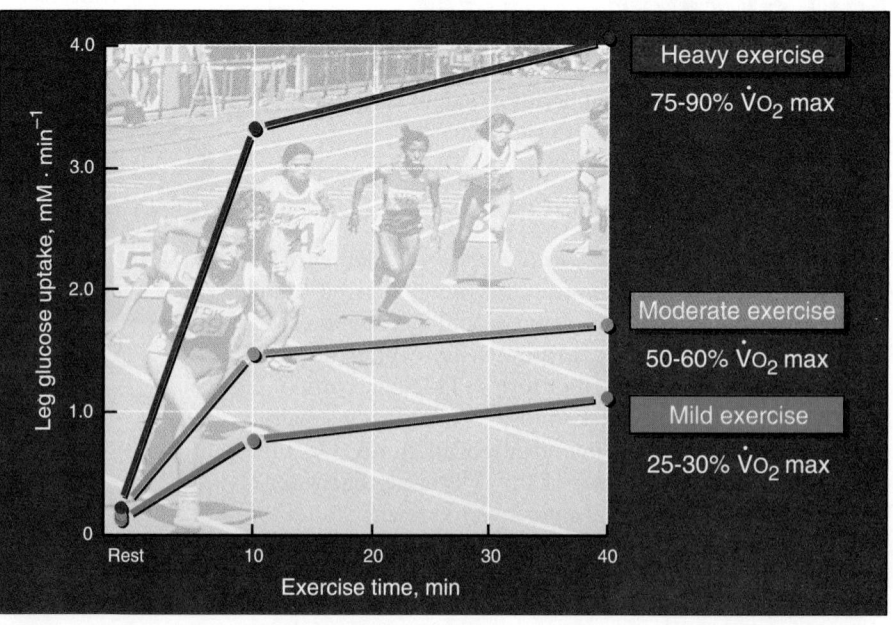

stimulating effect on the enzyme **glycogen phosphorylase** that facilitates glycogenolysis in the liver and active muscle. Because of its ability to provide energy without oxygen, stored muscle glycogen is the prime contributor of energy in the early minutes of exercise when oxygen utilization does not meet the metabolic demands. As exercise progresses, blood-borne glucose increases its contribution as a metabolic fuel. Blood glucose, for example, may supply 30% of the total energy required by vigorously active muscles, with the remaining **majority** of carbohydrate energy supplied by muscle glycogen.[29, 67, 73] An hour of high-intensity exercise can decrease liver glycogen by about 55%; a 2-hour strenuous workout can just about deplete the glycogen in the liver and specifically exercised muscles. As illustrated in Figure 1.4, the uptake of circulating blood glucose by the muscles increases sharply during the initial stage of exercise and continues to increase as exercise progresses. By the 40th minute of exercise, glucose uptake has risen to between 7 and 20 times the uptake at rest, depending on the exercise intensity.

The increased contribution of carbohydrate in intense anaerobic exercise occurs because it is the **only** macronutrient to provide energy rapidly when the oxygen supply and/or utilization do not meet a muscle's oxygen needs. During heavy, fatiguing aerobic exercise, the advantage of a selective dependence on carbohydrate metabolism lies in its rapidity for energy transfer compared to lipids (about twice as fast) and proteins. Also, the energy generated per unit oxygen consumed is about 6% greater for carbohydrate than for lipid. The specifics of the role of carbohydrate in energy release under anaerobic and aerobic conditions are explained in Chapter 6.

MODERATE AND PROLONGED EXERCISE

Almost all the energy in the transition from rest to submaximal exercise is supplied from glycogen stored in the active muscles, as was the case in intense exercise. During the next 20 minutes or so, liver and muscle glycogen supply between 40 and 50% of the energy requirement, with the remainder provided by lipid breakdown, including a small utilization of protein. (This nutrient energy mixture depends on the relative intensity of exercise. If the exercise is light to moderate, the main energy substrate throughout exercise is lipid; refer to Figure 1.12). As exercise continues and glycogen stores become reduced, blood glucose becomes the major source of carbohydrate energy, and an increasingly greater percentage of the total energy is supplied through lipid breakdown. Eventually, glucose output by the liver fails to keep pace with its use by muscle and plasma glucose concentration decreases.[1] The level of circulating blood glucose may actually fall to hypoglycemic levels (less than 45 mg glucose per 100 mL blood) during 90 minutes of strenuous exercise.[27]

Figure 1.5 depicts the metabolic profile during prolonged exercise in both the glycogen-depleted and the

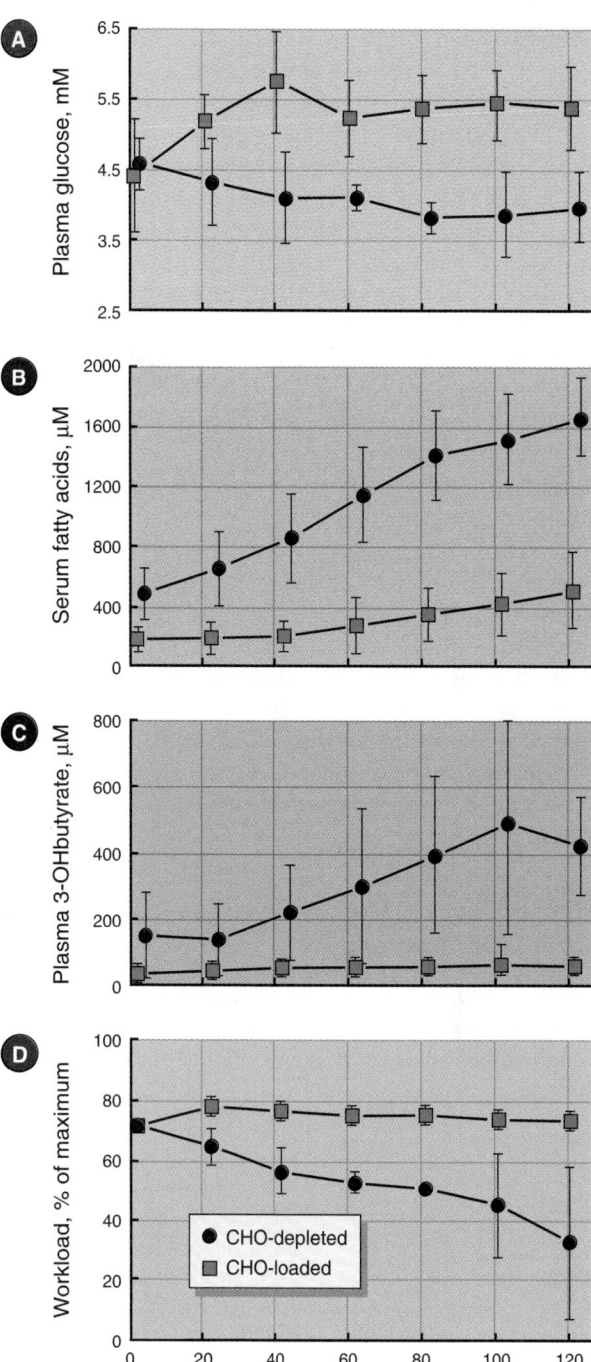

FIGURE 1.5

Dynamics of nutrient metabolism in the glycogen-loaded and glycogen-depleted states. During exercise with limited carbohydrate availability, blood glucose levels (A) progressively decrease and lipid metabolism (B) progressively increases compared to similar exercise when glycogen loaded. In addition, protein utilization for energy (C), reflected by plasma levels of 3-OH butyrate, is considerably higher with glycogen depletion. After 2 hours, exercise capacity (D) reduces to about 50% of maximum in exercise begun in the glycogen-depleted state. (From Wagenmakers, A.J.M., et al.: Carbohydrate supplementation, glycogen depletion, and amino acid metabolism. *Am. J. Physiol.*, 260: E883, 1991.)

glycogen-loaded state.[91] As submaximal exercise progresses in the glycogen-depleted state, blood glucose levels fall and the level of circulating lipid increases dramatically compared to exercise in the glycogen-loaded state. Concurrently, there is an increased contribution of protein to the energy pool. Under such conditions of carbohydrate depletion, work capacity (expressed as a percentage of maximum) progressively decreases so that at 2 hours, only about 50% of maximum capacity can be sustained due to the relatively slow rate of aerobic energy release from lipid breakdown.

Fatigue occurs if exercise continues to the point where liver and muscle glycogen become severely lowered, even though sufficient oxygen is available to the muscles and the potential energy from stored lipid is almost unlimited. Endurance athletes commonly refer to this sensation of fatigue as "bonking" or "hitting the wall." Because of the absence in muscle of the phosphatase enzyme that would allow for glucose exchange between muscles, the relatively inactive muscles maintain their full glycogen content. It is unclear in prolonged exercise why the depletion of muscle glycogen coincides with the point of fatigue. Part of the answer may be related to the functions of blood glucose as energy for the central nervous system and muscle glycogen as a "primer" in lipid metabolism. In addition, there is a slower rate of energy release from lipid compared to carbohydrate breakdown.

Effect of Diet on Muscle Glycogen Stores and Endurance

Ingested carbohydrate is a readily available energy nutrient for active muscles.[38] Diet composition, however, can profoundly affect glycogen reserves. Figure 1.6 shows the re-

sults of one experiment in which muscle glycogen was varied in six subjects through dietary manipulation.[5] In one condition, the normal caloric intake was maintained for 3 days but the major quantity of calories was supplied as lipid with less than 5% as carbohydrate. In the second condition, the 3-day diet was normal and contained the recommended daily percentages of carbohydrate, lipid, and protein. With the third diet, 82% of the calories were provided as carbohydrates. The glycogen content of the quadriceps femoris muscle, determined by needle biopsy, averaged 0.63 g of glycogen per 100 g wet muscle with the high-fat diet, 1.75 g for the normal diet, and 3.75 g for the high-carbohydrate diet.

Endurance capacity during cycling exercise varied considerably depending on the diet each person consumed during the 3 days prior to the exercise test. With the normal diet, exercise could be tolerated for an average of 114 minutes, whereas endurance averaged only 57 minutes with the high-fat diet. The endurance capacity of subjects who were fed the high-carbohydrate diet was more than three times greater than when the same subjects consumed the high-fat diet. In all instances, the point of fatigue was associated with the same low level of muscle glycogen. These results clearly demonstrate the importance of muscle glycogen for high-intensity exercise lasting more than an hour. Such data also emphasize the important role nutrition can have in establishing the appropriate energy reserves for both long-term exercise and strenuous training.

A diet deficient in carbohydrates rapidly depletes muscle and liver glycogen and subsequently affects performance in intense short-term exercise as well as in prolonged submaximal endurance activities. These observations are important for athletes and physically active individuals who have modified their diet by reducing the recommended

FIGURE 1.6

Effects of a low-carbohydrate diet, mixed diet, and high-carbohydrate diet on the glycogen content of the quadriceps femoris muscle and the duration of endurance exercise on a bicycle ergometer. With a high-carbohydrate diet, endurance time increases 3 times compared to a diet low in carbohydrate. (Adapted from Bergstrom, J., et al.: Diet, muscle glycogen and physical performance. *Acta Physiol. Scand.*, 71: 140, 1967.)

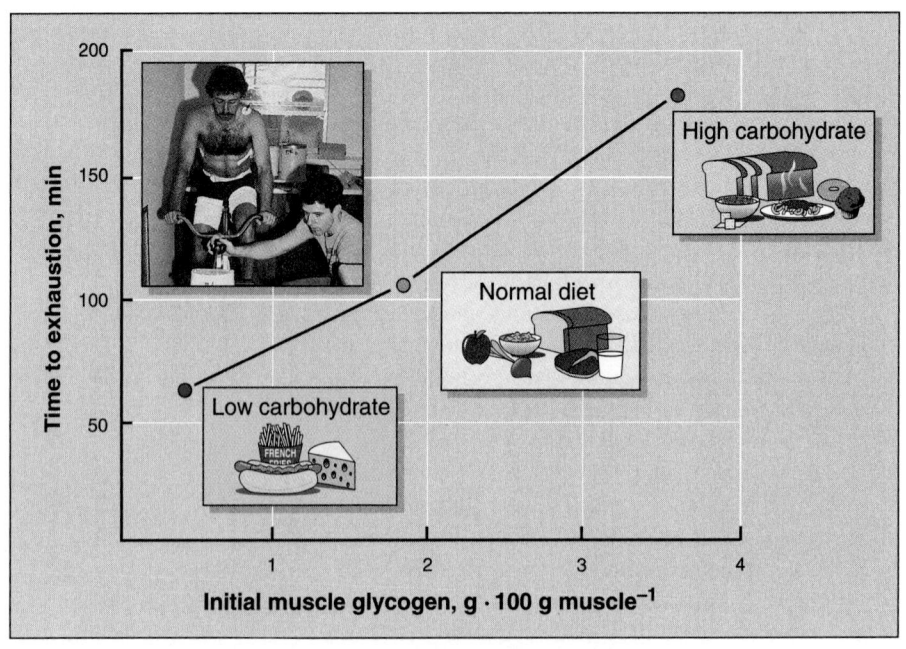

percentage of carbohydrate intake. Reliance on starvation diets or on other potentially harmful diets such as high-fat, low-carbohydrate diets, "liquid-protein" diets, or water diets, is counterproductive for weight control, exercise performance, optimal nutrition, and good health. Such low-carbohydrate diets make it extremely difficult from the standpoint of energy supply to participate in vigorous physical activity or training.[22] More will be said in Chapter 3 concerning optimal provision for carbohydrate needs prior to, during, and in recovery from different intensities of exercise.

■ SUMMARY ■

1. Atoms are the basic building blocks of all matter and play the major role in the composition of food nutrients and biologically active substances.

2. Carbon, hydrogen, oxygen, and nitrogen are the primary structural units for most of the biologically active substances in the body. Specific combinations of carbon with oxygen and hydrogen form carbohydrates and lipids, whereas proteins are composed of combinations of carbon, oxygen, and hydrogen with the addition of nitrogen and minerals.

3. Simple sugars consist of chains of from three to seven carbon atoms with hydrogen and oxygen in the ratio of 2 to 1. Glucose, the most common simple sugar, contains a six-carbon chain as $C_6H_{12}O_6$.

4. There are three kinds of carbohydrates: monosaccharides (sugars such as glucose and fructose); oligosaccharides (disaccharides such as sucrose, lactose, and maltose), and polysaccharides that contain three or more simple sugars to form starch, fiber, and the large glucose polymer glycogen.

5. Glycogenolysis is the process of reconverting glycogen to glucose, whereas gluconeogenesis refers to the process of glucose synthesis, especially from protein sources.

6. Americans typically consume 40 to 50% of their total calories as carbohydrates. This is generally in the form of fruits, grains, and vegetables, although greater sugar intake in the form of sweets (simple sugars) is common and possibly harmful.

7. Carbohydrates, which are stored in limited quantity in liver and muscle, serve (*a*) as a major source of energy, (*b*) to spare the breakdown of proteins, (*c*) as a metabolic primer for lipid metabolism, and (*d*) as fuel for the central nervous system.

8. Muscle glycogen and blood glucose are the primary fuels during intense exercise. The body's glycogen stores also serve an important role in energy metabolism in sustained high levels of aerobic exercise such as marathon running, distance cycling, and swimming.

9. A carbohydrate-deficient diet rapidly depletes muscle and liver glycogen and can profoundly affect both high-intensity anaerobic and long-duration aerobic ex-

ercise capacity. Individuals involved in heavy training should consume about 60% of their daily calories (400 to 600 g) as carbohydrates, predominantly in unrefined complex form.

PART 2
LIPIDS

THE NATURE OF LIPIDS

A lipid (from the Greek *lipos*, meaning fat) molecule possesses the same structural elements as a carbohydrate except that it differs markedly in the linking of the specific atoms. Specifically, the ratio of hydrogen to oxygen is considerably higher in the lipid. For example, the common lipid stearin has the formula $C_{57}H_{110}O_6$. Whereas the H-to-O ratio for carbohydrate is $2:1$, for stearin it $18.3:1$. Lipid is a general term that includes oils, fats, and waxes. Oils are liquid at room temperature, while fats remain solid. Approximately 98% of dietary fat is in the form of triglycerides (see below), and about 90% of fat in the body is stored in the adipose tissue depots, mostly in the subcutaneous tissues.

KINDS AND SOURCES OF LIPIDS

Lipids are long hydrocarbon chains found in both plants and animals. They are generally greasy to the touch and are insoluble in water but soluble in organic solvents such as ether, chloroform, and benzene. According to common classification, lipids can be placed into one of three main groups: **simple lipids, compound lipids,** and **derived lipids.** Table 1.5 lists the general classification for lipids with specific examples of each form.

SIMPLE LIPIDS

The simple lipids or "neutral fats" consist primarily of **triglycerides,** also called triacylglycerols. These are the most plentiful lipids in the body. They constitute the major storage form of lipid in adipose (fat) cells, in that more than 95% of the body fat is in the form of triglycerides. The triglyceride molecule consists of two different clusters of atoms. One cluster is **glycerol,** a three-carbon molecule that itself is not a lipid because it is readily soluble in water. Attached to the glycerol molecule are three clusters of carbon-chained atoms, usually an even number, termed **fatty acids.**

When glycerol and fatty acids are joined in the synthesis of the triglyceride molecule during the chemical process of condensation, three molecules of water are formed. Conversely, during hydrolysis, when the lipid molecule is cleaved into its constituents by the action of **lipase** enzymes, three molecules of water are added at the point

TABLE 1.5
GENERAL CLASSIFICATION OF LIPIDS

Type of Lipid	Example
I. Simple lipids	
Neutral fats	Triglycerides (triacylglycerols)
Waxes	Beeswax
II. Compound lipids	
Phospholipids	Lecithins, cephalins, lipositols
Glycolipids	Cerebrosides, gangliosides
Lipoproteins	Chylomicrons, very low-density lipoproteins (VLDLs), low-density lipoproteins (LDLs), high-density lipoproteins (HDLs)
III. Derived lipids	
Fatty acids	Palmitic acid, oleic acid, stearic acid, linoleic acid
Steroids	Cholesterol, ergosterol, cortisol, bile acids, vitamin D, estrogens, progesterone, androgens
Hydrocarbons	Terpenes

where the lipid molecule is split. The basic structures of the two kinds of fatty acid molecules, **saturated** and **unsaturated,** are shown in Figure 1.7. All lipid-containing foods consist of a mixture of different proportions of saturated and unsaturated fatty acids. The reason these substances are called fatty acids is because of the organic acid (COOH) molecule that is part of their chemical structure.

Saturated Fatty Acids

A saturated fatty acid contains no double bonds between carbon atoms; the remaining bonds attach to hydrogen. The fatty acid molecule is said to be saturated because it holds as many hydrogen atoms as is chemically possible.

Saturated fatty acids are found primarily in animal products such as beef, lamb, pork, and chicken. Saturated fatty acids are also present in egg yolk and in the dairy fats of cream, milk, butter, and cheese. Coconut and palm oil, vegetable shortening, and hydrogenated margarine are sources of saturated fatty acids from the plant kingdom and are present to a relatively high degree in commercially prepared cakes, pies, and cookies.

Unsaturated Fatty Acids

Fatty acids containing one or more double bonds along the main carbon chain are classified as unsaturated. In this case, each double bond in the carbon chain reduces the number of potential hydrogen-binding sites; therefore the molecule is said to be unsaturated with respect to hydrogen. If only one double bond is present along the main carbon chain, as in canola, olive, and peanut oil, the fatty acid is said to be **monounsaturated.** If there are two or more double bonds along the main carbon chain, as in safflower, sunflower, soybean, and corn oil, the fatty acid is **polyunsaturated.**

Fatty acids from plant sources are generally unsaturated and tend to liquefy at room temperature. Generally, the less firm the lipid the greater the degree of unsaturation. Unsaturated fats that are present as liquids are called oils. Unsaturated oils can be changed to semisolid compounds by the chemical process of **hydrogenation.** This process, utilizing hydrogen gas and a nickel catalyst, reduces a double bond in the unsaturated fatty acid to a single bond to allow more hydrogen atoms to attach to the carbon atoms along the chain. This creates a firmer fat because the addition of hydrogen increases the lipid's melting temperature. Consequently, the hydrogenated oil behaves as a saturated fat. The most common hydrogenated fats include lard substitutes and margarine.

Butter versus Margarine: A Health Risk in Trans Fatty Acids?

The distinguishing characteristic between margarine and butter is not the caloric content, as they are about equal, but the composition of their fatty acids. About 62% of the fatty acids in butter are saturated compared with 20% in margarine. During the manufacture of margarine and some other vegetable shortenings, unsaturated corn, soybean, or sunflower oil is partially hydrogenated. This rearranges the chemical structure of the original polyunsaturated oil to a lipid not found in nature that is more hardened (saturated), but not as hard as butter. When one of the hydrogen atoms

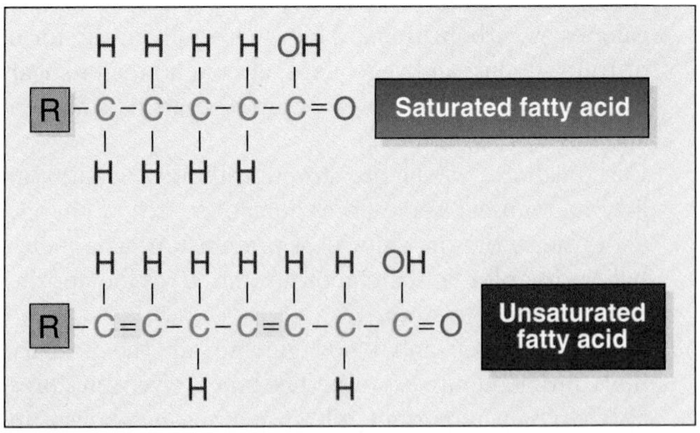

FIGURE 1.7
The presence or absence of double bonds between the carbon atoms constitues the major structural difference between saturated and unsaturated fatty acids. **R** represents the glycerol portion of the triglyceride molecule.

along the carbon chain moves from its naturally occurring position (*cis* position) to the opposite side of the double bond that separates two carbon atoms (*trans* position), the restructured fatty acid is referred to as a ***trans* unsaturated fatty acid.** From 17 to 25% of the fatty acids in margarine are *trans* unsaturated fatty acids, compared with only 7% in butter fat. Because margarine is made from vegetable oil, it contains no cholesterol; butter, on the other hand, is made from a dairy source and contains between 11 and 15 mg of cholesterol per teaspoon.

The current controversy over margarine versus butter centers on the possible detrimental health effects of *trans* unsaturated fatty acids.[37, 88] A diet high in margarine and other foods containing partially hydrogenated vegetable oils increases LDL cholesterol concentration to about the same degree as a diet high in saturated fat. Unlike saturated fats, however, they also decrease the concentration of the beneficial HDL cholesterol. Scientists estimate that dietary *trans* fatty acids cause 30,000 deaths annually from heart disease.[95] If it is discovered that *trans* unsaturated fatty acids do contribute to increased risk for heart disease, then it is to be hoped that the manufacturers of many foods containing hydrogenated vegetable oils will change their methods of production.

Lipids in The Diet

Figure 1.8 shows the approximate percentage contribution of some common food groups to the total lipid content of the typical American diet. Vegetables generally contribute about 34% to the daily lipid intake, whereas the remaining 66% is from lipids of animal origin.

The average person in the United States now consumes about 15% of total calories as saturated fats (or over 50 lb of saturated fats per year), and most of this fat is of animal origin. This is in contrast to groups like the Tarahumara Indians of Mexico, whose diet high in complex, unrefined carbohydrates contains only 2% of the total calories as saturated fat.[19] The relationship between intake of saturated fatty acids and risk of coronary heart disease has led many nutritionists and medical personnel to suggest replacing at least a portion of the saturated fat in one's diet with lipids that are unsaturated.[32] At present, it is probably prudent to recommend that no more than 10% of total energy intake be in the form of saturated fatty acids.

Fish Oils May Be Healthful. Attention has focused on the possible health benefits of ingesting two long-chain polyunsaturated fatty acids, eicosapentaenoic acid and docosahexenoic acid. These oils belong to an **omega-3** family of fatty acids found primarily in the oils of cold-water fish such as tuna, herring, sardines, and mackerel. It is now apparent that regular intake of fish and fish oil has a beneficial effect on the various aspects of one's lipid profile,[34, 93] overall heart disease risk,[6, 79] and (for smokers) risk of contracting chronic obstructive pulmonary disease.[76] One proposed

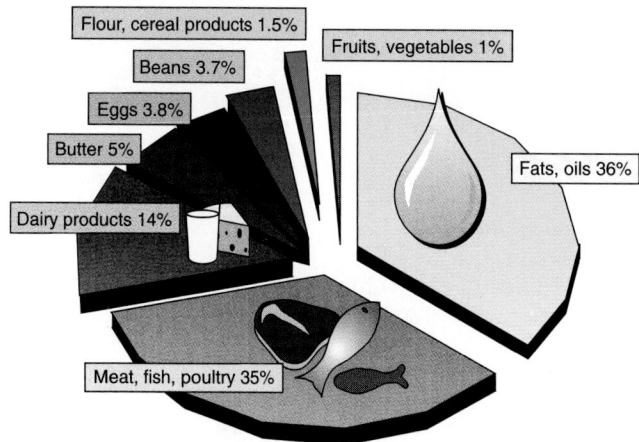

FIGURE 1.8
Contribution from the major food groups to the lipid content of the typical American diet.

protective mechanism from heart attack is that fish oil helps prevent blood clots from forming on arterial walls.

In the quest for good health, it has become common practice to cook with and ingest lipids derived primarily from vegetable sources, such as corn oil. This approach, however, may be too simplistic, because the total intake of lipids—both saturated and unsaturated fatty acids—may constitute a risk for both diabetes and heart disease; if so, then the intake of all lipids should be reduced. Concern has also been expressed concerning the association of high-fat diets with ovarian, breast, and colon cancer, as well as the possibility that such diets promote the growth of other cancers as well. Reducing the lipid content of the diet also may provide benefits for weight control. Due to the energy requirements of various metabolic pathways, the body is particularly efficient in converting excess calories of dietary fat to stored lipid.[80] Consequently, greater increases in body fat can occur when the diet is high in lipid content compared to an equivalent caloric excess of carbohydrate.

The saturated and unsaturated fatty acid content of various sources of dietary lipid are listed in Table 1.6. Several polyunsaturated fatty acids, most prominently **linoleic acid,** a fatty acid present in cooking and salad oils, must be consumed in the diet because it is a precursor of other fatty acids and cannot be synthesized by the body. This is an **essential fatty acid** required for ensuring the integrity of plasma membranes and for growth, reproduction, skin maintenance, and general body functioning.

COMPOUND LIPIDS

Compound lipids consist of a triglyceride in combination with other chemicals. One such group, the **phospholipids,** contains one or more fatty acid molecules combined with a phosphate group and a nitrogenous base. These lipids are formed in all cells, though most are synthesized in the liver.

TABLE 1.6
COMMON DIETARY SOURCES OF LIPIDS

Food	Percent Fat	Percent Saturated	Percent Unsaturated
Animal Sources			
Beef heart	6	50	50
Veal cutlet	10	50	50
Chicken	10-17	30	70
Beef	16-42	52	48
Lamb	19-29	60	40
Ham, sliced	23	45	55
Pork	32	45	55
Butter	81	55	36
Plant Sources			
Carrots	0	0	0
Potato chips	35	25	75
Cashew nuts	48	18	82
Peanut butter	50	25	75
Margarine	81	26	66
Corn oil	100	7	78
Cottonseed oil	100	21.5	71.5
Olive oil	100	14	86
Soybean oil	100	14	71.5

The phospholipid in the plasma membrane is important because the phosphorous part of the molecule is hydrophilic (attracts water) and the lipid portion is hydrophobic (repels water). Thus, phospholipids, as an integral part of the plasma membrane bilayer, can interact with both water and lipid to control fluid movement across the cell membrane. Phospholipids also help to maintain the structural integrity of the cell and are important in blood clotting and in the structure of the insulating sheath around nerve fibers.

Other compound lipids are the **glycolipids,** which are fatty acids bound with carbohydrate and nitrogen, and the water-soluble **lipoproteins,** formed primarily in the liver from the union of protein with either triglycerides or phospholipids. *The lipoproteins are important because they constitute the main form for lipid transport in the blood.* If blood lipids were not bound to protein, they would literally float to the top like cream in nonhomogenized milk.

High- and Low-Density Lipoproteins

Figure 1.9 illustrates the general scheme and interaction between dietary cholesterol and the lipoproteins, and their transport between the intestine, the liver, and the peripheral tissues. There are basically four types of lipoproteins, categorized according to their gravitational density. **Chylomicrons** are formed after emulsified lipid droplets (including triglyceride, phospholipids, and free fatty acids) leave the intestine and enter the lymphatic vasculature. Under normal conditions, the chylomicrons are then taken up by the liver, metabolized, and delivered to be stored in adipose tissue. The chylomicrons also serve as the transporter of the lipid-soluble vitamins A, D, E, and K.

High-density lipoproteins (HDLs) are produced in the liver and small intestine. Of all the lipoproteins, they contain the greatest percentage of protein (about 50%), the least total lipid (about 20%), and the least cholesterol (about 20%). A **low-density lipoprotein (LDL)** is a remnant of a **very low-density lipoprotein (VLDL).** The VLDL contains the greatest percentage of lipid (95%), of which about 60% is in the form of triglyceride. This lipoprotein transports to muscle and adipose tissue the triglycerides formed in the liver from lipids, carbohydrates, alcohol, and cholesterol. Once the VLDL is acted on by the enzyme **lipoprotein lipase,** it becomes a denser LDL molecule because it now contains less lipid. The LDL and the VLDL fractions contain the greatest lipid and the least protein components.

"Bad" Cholesterol. Among the lipoproteins, the LDLs that normally carry between 60 and 80% of the total serum cholesterol have the greatest affinity for the cells of the arterial wall. They help to deliver cholesterol to arterial tissue, where it may become oxidized and ultimately participate in the proliferation of smooth muscle cells and further unfavorable changes that damage and narrow the artery.[82] LDL concentration is influenced by exercise, visceral fat accumulation, and diet.

"Good" Cholesterol. Unlike LDL, HDL operates as so-called good cholesterol to protect against heart disease.[65] HDL acts as a scavenger in the **reverse transport of cholesterol** by removing it from the arterial wall and transporting it to the liver, where it is incorporated into bile and excreted via the intestinal tract.

The quantities of LDL and HDL cholesterol, as well as the specific ratios of these lipoproteins (e.g., HDL:total cholesterol) and subfractions, provide more meaningful indicators of coronary artery disease risk than total cholesterol per se.[44, 59] Regular aerobic exercise and abstinence from cigarette smoking increase the HDL level and can favorably affect the LDL:HDL ratio.[26] This is discussed more fully in Chapter 30.

DERIVED LIPIDS

Derived lipids include substances derived from the simple and compound lipids. The most widely known derived lipid is **cholesterol,** a sterol found **only** in animal tissue. The chemical structure of cholesterol provides the backbone for synthesizing other steroid compounds. Cholesterol does not contain fatty acids but does share some of the physical and chemical characteristics of lipid. Thus, from a dietary viewpoint it can be considered a lipid. Cholesterol is widespread in the plasma membrane of all cells and is either obtained through the diet (exogenous cholesterol) or synthesized within the cells (endogenous cholesterol). Even when an individual maintains a "cholesterol-free" diet, the rate of endogenous cholesterol synthesis varies from 0.5 to 2.0 g per day. More can be produced, especially if the diet is high in saturated fat, to facilitate cholesterol synthesis by the liver. While the liver is the major organ for cholesterol synthesis (about 70%), other tissues—including the walls of the arteries and intestines—can synthesize this compound. The rate of endogenous synthesis is usually sufficient for the body's needs; hence, a severe reduction in cholesterol intake, except in infants, is probably not harmful.

Functions of Cholesterol

Cholesterol is normally required in many complex bodily functions, including the building of plasma membranes, and as a precursor in the synthesis of vitamin D and the adrenal gland hormones as well as estrogen, androgen, and progesterone, the hormones responsible for secondary sex characteristics. Cholesterol also plays a crucial role in the formation of the bile that emulsifies lipids during digestion.

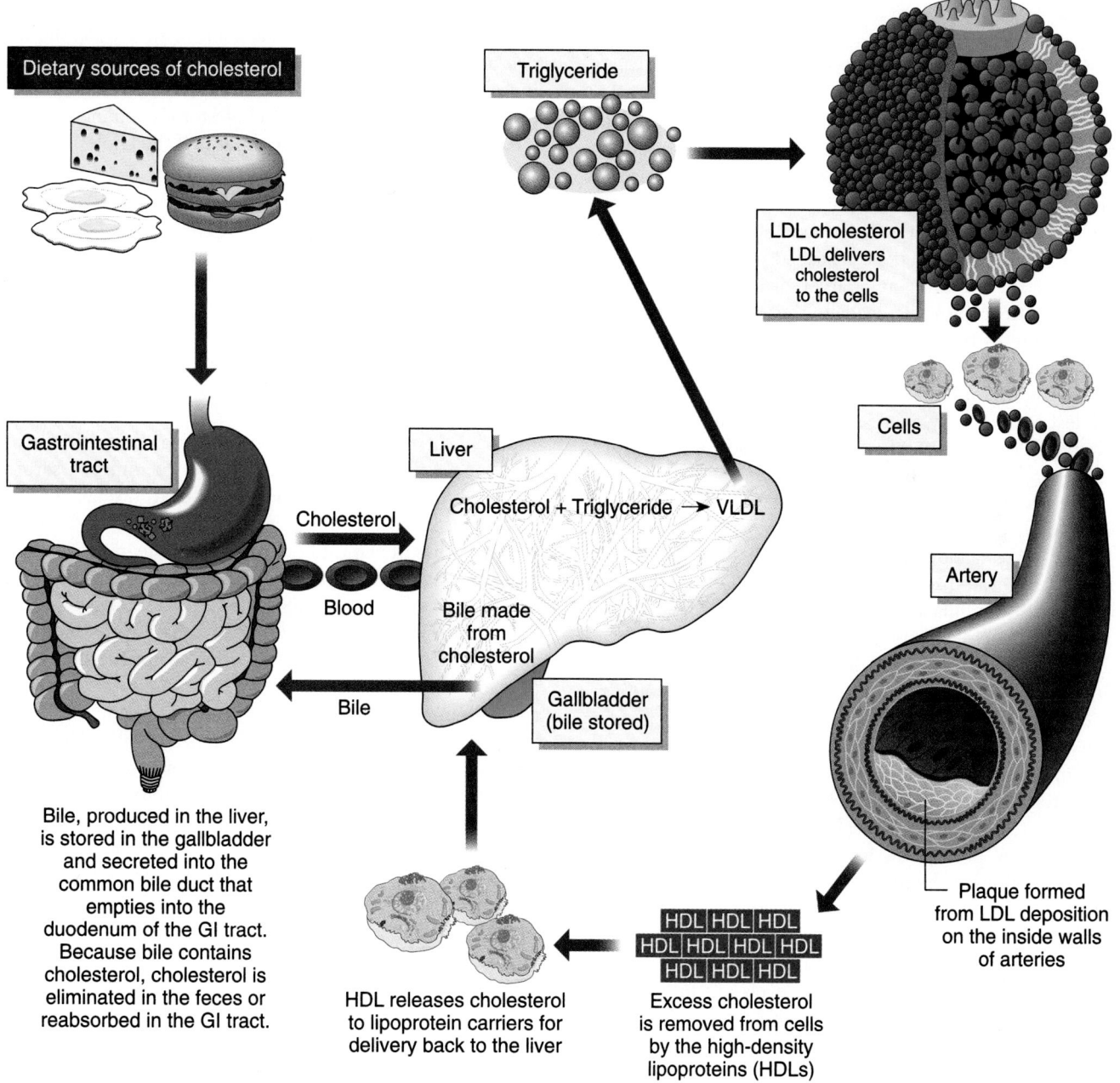

FIGURE 1.9
General scheme and interaction between dietary cholesterol and the lipoproteins, and their transport between the intestine, liver, and peripheral tissues.

The richest dietary source of cholesterol is egg yolk. Cholesterol is also plentiful in red meats and organ meats such as liver, kidney, and brains. It is also abundant in shellfish, especially shrimp, and in dairy products such as ice cream, cream cheese, butter, and whole milk. *Cholesterol is not present in any foods of plant origin.*

Cholesterol-Heart Disease Controversy

High levels of both serum cholesterol and the cholesterol-rich LDL molecule are powerful predictors of coronary artery disease,[47, 60] particularly in the presence of other risk factors such as smoking and untreated hypertension.[37a] The relationship between serum cholesterol and death from coronary artery disease is not linked to some threshold level, but instead is continuous and graded; therefore any lowering of cholesterol offers protection from heart disease.[56, 83] Numerous animal studies indicate that diets high in cholesterol and saturated fat raise serum cholesterol in "susceptible" animals. This eventually produces a degenerative process characterized by the formation of cholesterol-rich deposits called **plaque** on the inner lining of the medium and larger arteries. This process, termed **atherosclerosis,** leads to the narrowing and eventual closure of these vessels. In humans, a reduced intake of saturated fatty acids and cholesterol generally lowers serum cholesterol, although for most people the effect is modest.[3, 11] Similarly, increased dietary intake of monounsaturated and polyunsaturated fatty acids also exerts a cholesterol-lowering effect.

A cause-and-effect relationship between serum cholesterol and heart disease has been shown in a controlled 7- to 10-year investigation of nearly 4000 healthy middle-aged men with elevated serum cholesterol.[57, 58] Lowering cholesterol by 25% significantly reduced the risk of heart attack, and the chances for survival were improved if an attack did occur. With the aid of diet and a cholesterol-lowering drug, the reduction in serum cholesterol caused a 50% reduction in the rate of heart disease. The improvement in one's coronary heart disease risk is closely linked to the cholesterol decrease by the factor of 1:2—a 1% reduction in cholesterol caused a 2% reduction in risk! These findings, corroborated in other clinical trials,[13, 31] are encouraging because they provide an important "missing link" in the diet-heart disease theory and support the effort of health professionals to encourage people to reduce serum lipids through diet, exercise, and weight control. Specific recommended values for "desirable," "borderline," and "undesirable" plasma lipid and lipoprotein levels are presented in Chapter 30.

Even the Young Benefit. Research with children aged 10 to 15 years indicates that lifestyle habits such as regular exercise, good cardiovascular fitness, and a prudent nutritional profile are related to favorable lipid profiles similar to the effects of exercise seen with adults.[85]

RECOMMENDED DIETARY LIPID INTAKE

Dietary lipid represents about 38% of total caloric intake in the United States, or about 50 kg of lipid consumed per person each year. Although standards for optimal lipid intake have not been firmly established, it is believed that to promote better health, lipid intake should not exceed 30% of the total energy content of the diet, and less may be even more desirable. Of this intake, at least 70% and preferably 80% should be in the form of unsaturated fatty acids, equally distributed between the polyunsaturates and the monounsaturates.

The American Heart Association recommends the intake of no more than 300 mg (0.01 oz) of cholesterol daily, limiting intake to 100 mg per 1000 calories of food ingested. This is almost the amount of cholesterol contained in the yolk of one large egg and just about half the cholesterol ingested daily by the average American male. A reduction in daily cholesterol intake toward 150 to 200 mg may be even more desirable.[96] The main sources of dietary cholesterol are the same animal food sources rich in saturated fatty acids. Thus, reducing the intake of these foods will not only reduce the intake of preformed cholesterol but, more importantly, reduce the intake of the fatty acids known to stimulate endogenous cholesterol synthesis. The cholesterol and saturated fat content of one serving of some common foods is presented in Table 1.7.

While it is prudent to apply appropriate methods of nutrition, exercise, and weight control to improve serum lipids and lipoproteins, the cholesterol-heart disease controversy is far from resolved. For one thing, there are no controlled studies of cholesterol lowering and heart disease risk in women, and it is doubtful whether cholesterol lowering is necessary or effective for the elderly. The standard indices of dyslipidemia are unrelated to heart disease morbidity or mortality or all-cause mortality in persons older than 70 years.[51]

Recommendations to the general population are based on inferences from studies of middle-aged men with high cholesterol levels. It is disturbing to note that in clinical trials of such men who were administered powerful cholesterol-lowering drugs, the significant reduction in heart disease was not accompanied by an increased longevity. This was because, for reasons unknown, the group receiving treatment had an increased incidence of violent and accidental deaths as well as an excess of gastrointestinal disorders.

ROLE OF LIPID IN THE BODY

The important functions of lipids in the body include (*a*) providing the body's largest store of potential energy, (*b*) serving as a cushion for the protection of vital organs, and (*c*) providing insulation from the thermal stress of a cold environment.

TABLE 1.7
CHOLESTEROL AND SATURATED FATTY ACID CONTENT OF SOME COMMON FOODS

Food	Saturated Fat (mg)	Cholesterol (mg)
Butter	50.7	219
Peanut butter	8.5	0
Chocolate fudge	7.3	4
French fries, McDonald's	6.8	13
Ice cream, vanilla	6.2	44
Taco, beef	6.2	57
Doritos, taco flavor	4.8	0
Kentucky Fried Chicken	4.2	76
Hamburger, Big Mac	3.6	36
Pizza, cheese	3.4	47
Egg, raw	3.0	410
Beef liver, fried	2.8	482
Chicken breast, fried with skin	2.5	90
Chocolate milkshake	2.3	13
Milk, whole	2.1	14
Swordfish, broiled	1.4	50
Chicken breast, fried without skin	1.3	91
Milk, lowfat 2%	1.2	9
Yogurt, plain lowfat	1.0	6
Shrimp, raw	0.3	152

ENERGY SOURCE AND RESERVE

Lipid constitutes the ideal cellular fuel because each molecule carries large quantities of energy per unit weight, is easily transported and stored, and is readily used for energy. At rest in well-nourished individuals, lipid may provide as much as 80 to 90% of the body's energy requirement. One gram of lipid contains about 9 calories of energy, more than **twice** the energy in an equal quantity of carbohydrate or protein. This is due to the greater quantity of hydrogen in the lipid molecule compared to carbohydrate or protein. As discussed in Chapters 6 and 7, it is the oxidation of these hydrogen atoms that provides the energy for bodily functions at rest and during exercise. Recall that three molecules of water are produced from the union of glycerol and three fatty acid molecules in the synthesis of a lipid molecule. In contrast, when glycogen is formed from glucose, 2.7 g of water is stored with each gram of glycogen. *Thus, lipid is a relatively water-free, concentrated fuel, whereas glycogen is hydrated and heavy relative to its energy content.*

The body's lipid content is approximately 15% of the body mass for males and 25% for females. Consequently, the potential energy stored in the lipid molecules of an average 70-kg college-aged male is about 94,500 kcal (10,500 g body fat $\times$ 9.0 kcal $\cdot$ g^{-1}). Most of this energy is available for exercise and could fuel a run from New York City to Madison, Wisconsin, assuming an energy expenditure of about 100 calories per mile. Contrast this to the limited 2000-calorie reserve of stored carbohydrate that could provide energy for a 20-mile run! Viewed from a different perspective, the body's energy reserves from carbohydrate could power marathon running for only about 1.6 hours, but the lipid reserves could fuel about 120 hours! As was the case with carbohydrates, the use of lipid as a fuel "spares" protein to carry out its important functions of tissue synthesis and repair.

PROTECTION AND INSULATION

Up to 4% of the body's fat protects against trauma to the vital organs such as the heart, liver, kidneys, spleen, brain, and spinal cord. Lipids in storage depots just below the skin (subcutaneous fat) serve an important insulating function, determining one's ability to tolerate extremes of cold exposure.[61] Swimmers who excelled in swimming the English Channel showed only a slight decrease in body temperature while resting in cold water and essentially no lowering effect while swimming.[70] In contrast, the body temperature of leaner, non-Channel swimmers decreased considerably under both conditions. The insulatory layer of fat, which usually assumes a greater proportion of total body weight with increasing age, probably contributes little except for those engaged in cold-related activities such as deep-sea divers, ocean or channel swimmers, or Arctic inhabitants. In most instances, excess body fat is a liability in terms of temperature regulation. This is apparent during sustained exercise in air, when the body's heat production can increase 20 times above the resting level. In this situation, heat flow from the body is greatly retarded by the shield of insulation from subcutaneous fat.

For some larger-sized athletes such as football linemen, excess lipid storage provides an additional cushion that may protect from the sport's normal hazards. This possible protective benefit, however, must be evaluated against the liability imposed by the excess "dead weight" in terms of energy expenditure, thermal regulation, and the possible detrimental effects on exercise performance.

VITAMIN CARRIER AND HUNGER DEPRESSOR

Dietary lipid serves as a carrier and transport medium for the fat-soluble vitamins—vitamins A, D, E, and K—and ingesting about 20 g a day can serve this purpose. Thus, a significant reduction in dietary lipid can lead to a reduced level of these vitamins that could ultimately lead to vitamin deficiency. Dietary lipid is also believed to be necessary for the absorption of vitamin A precursors from nonlipid plant sources such as carrots. Because the movement of lipid from the stomach takes about 3.5 hours after ingestion, some lipid in the diet helps delay the onset of "hunger pangs" and contributes to the feeling of satiety after eating. This is one reason why reducing diets that contain moderate amounts of lipid are sometimes considered more successful in blunting the urge to eat than the more extreme low-fat diets.

LIPID BALANCE IN EXERCISE

The energy requirements of light to moderate exercise are largely provided by fatty acids released from triglyceride storage sites and delivered to muscle as free fatty acids (FFA) bound to blood albumin, as well as triglycerides in muscle itself. As exercise begins, there is a transient initial drop in plasma FFA concentration due to their increased uptake by active muscles. This is followed by an increased FFA release from adipose tissue via hormonal stimulation by the sympathetic nervous system and a decrease in insulin levels. During brief periods of moderate exercise, energy is derived in approximately equal amounts from carbohydrate and lipid. There is a gradual increase in the utilization of lipid for energy as exercise continues for an hour or more and carbohydrates become depleted. Toward the end of prolonged exercise, lipid (mainly as circulating FFA) may supply nearly 80% of the total energy required. Figure 1.10 shows this phenomenon for a subject who exercised continuously for 6 hours. There was a steady decline in the combustion of carbohydrate for energy (as reflected by the RQ; refer to Chapter 8) during the exercise period with a concomitant increase in lipid utilization. Toward the end of exercise, an estimated 84% of the total energy for exercise was provided from the breakdown of lipid! This experiment, conducted over 60 years ago, clearly illustrates the important contribution of lipid oxidation in prolonged exercise.

The large lipid metabolism in prolonged exercise is probably brought about by a small drop in blood sugar as exercise progresses, accompanied by a subsequent decrease in insulin and increase in glucagon output by the pancreas. This ultimately reduces glucose metabolism and further stimulates the liberation of FFA for energy. The data in Figure 1.11 show that the uptake of FFA by working muscles rises during 1 to 4 hours of moderate exercise. In the first hour of exercise, about 50% of the energy was supplied by lipid; at the third hour, lipid contributed up to 70% of the total energy requirement.

The metabolic mixture is somewhat different during exercise of varying intensities. This is illustrated in Figure 1.12 for trained men cycling at 25 to 85% of their maximum level for aerobic metabolism.[73] With light to mild exercise (40% or less) the main energy source is lipid, predominantly as plasma FFA delivered from the adipose tissue depots. As exercise intensity increases, there is an eventual **crossover** in the balance of fuel utilization—that is, the total energy from lipid breakdown remains essentially unchanged while the added energy for the more intense exercise is provided almost exclusively by blood glucose and muscle glycogen. The

total energy derived from lipids during exercise at 85% of maximum is **no different** than during 25%. *Such data highlight the important role of carbohydrate, especially muscle glycogen, as the major energy source during high-intensity aerobic exercise.*[67]

EXERCISE TRAINING AND LIPID UTILIZATION

Exercise training has a profound effect on the metabolism of lipid during exercise.[74, 89] This is shown in Figure 1.13, which displays the contribution of various energy substrates to the exercise metabolism of trained and untrained limb muscles. The important point is the greater uptake of plasma free fatty acids by the trained limb during moderate exercise. This augmented lipid mobilization and utilization with training helps to conserve the relatively limited glycogen reserves in the active muscles. Such adaptations in skeletal muscle with exercise training may be the result of:

- Increased quantity of enzymes involved in β-oxidation, Krebs cycle metabolism, and the electron-transport chain.
- Improved transport of fatty acids through the plasma membrane (sarcolemma) of the muscle fiber.
- Augmented transport of fatty acids within the muscle cell by the action of carnitine and carnitine transferase.

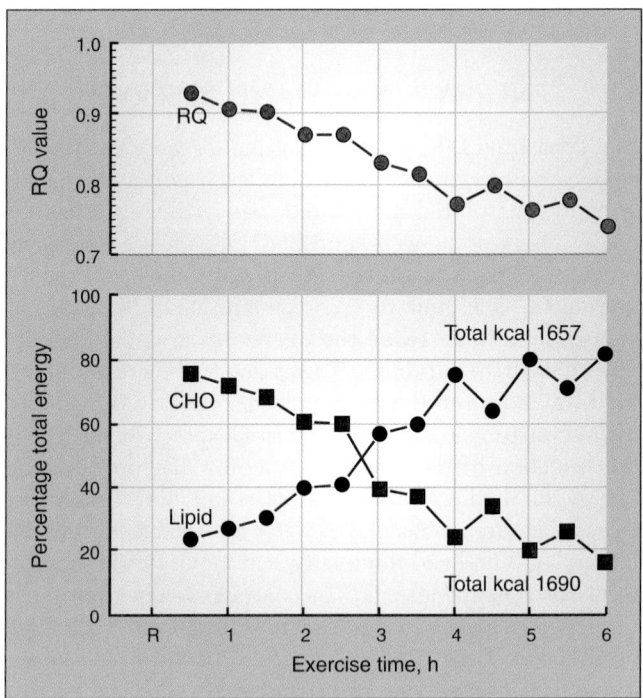

FIGURE 1.10

Top, Reduction in respiratory quotient (*RQ*) at an oxygen uptake of 2.36 L · min⁻¹ during 6 hours of continuous exercise. *Bottom,* Percentage of energy derived from carbohydrate and fat (1 kcal = 4.2 kJ). (Modified from Edwards, H.T., et al.: Metabolic rate, blood sugar and utilization of carbohydrate. *Am. J. Physiol.,* 108: 203, 1934.)

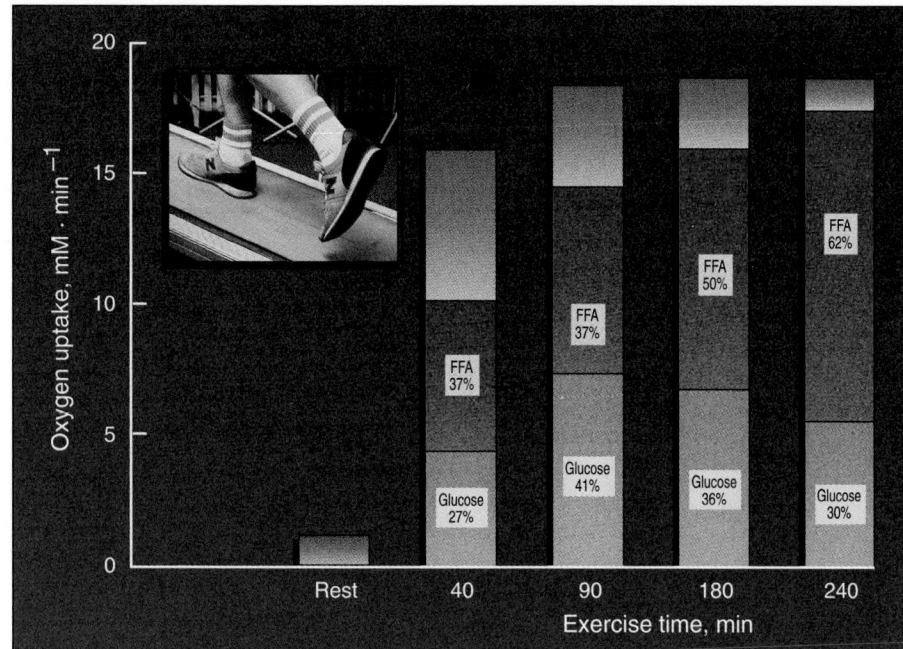

FIGURE 1.11
Uptake of oxygen and nutrients by the legs during prolonged exercise. (*Red* and *orange areas* represent the proportion of the total oxygen uptake caused by the oxidation of free fatty acids (FFA) and blood glucose. *Purple areas* indicate the oxidation of non-blood-borne fuels (muscle glycogen and intramuscular lipids and proteins). (From Ahlborg, G., et al.: Substrate turnover during prolonged exercise in man. *J. Clin. Invest.*, 53: 1080, 1974.)

• Proliferation of capillaries in trained muscle as reflected by both a greater total number and greater density of these microvessels.

Improvement in the aerobic production of ATP from lipids with aerobic training may aid in maintaining cellular integrity and a high level of function that would contribute to enhanced endurance independent of glycogen reserves. More is said on this important topic in Chapters 6 and 7, which deal with energy transfer and exercise metabolism.

■ SUMMARY ■

1. Like carbohydrates, lipids contain carbon, hydrogen, and oxygen atoms, but the ratio of hydrogen to oxygen is much higher. For example, the lipid stearin has the formula $C_{57}H_{110}O_6$. Lipid molecules are composed of one glycerol molecule and three fatty acid molecules.
2. Lipids are synthesized by plants and animals. They can be classified into three groups: simple lipids (glycerol plus 3 fatty acids), compound lipids (phospholipids, glycolipids, and lipoproteins) composed of simple lipids in combination with other chemicals, and derived lipids like cholesterol, which are synthesized from simple and compound lipids.
3. Saturated fatty acids contain as many hydrogen atoms as is chemically possible; thus, the molecule is said to be saturated with respect to hydrogen. Saturated fatty acids are present primarily in animal meat, egg yolk, dairy fats, and cheese. High intakes of saturated fatty acids have been linked to elevated blood cholesterol and the development of coronary heart disease.

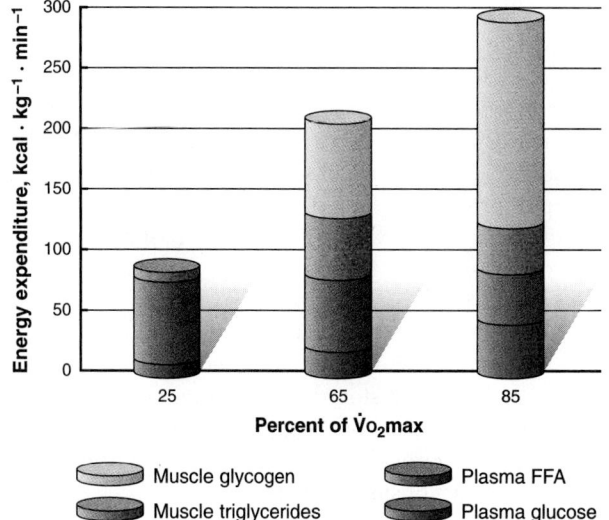

FIGURE 1.12
Steady-state substrate utilization calculated using three isotopes and indirect calorimetry in trained men performing cycle ergometer exercise at 25, 65, and 85% of $\dot{V}O_2$max. As exercise intensity increases, absolute use of glucose and muscle glycogen increases, while use of muscle triglycerides and plasma free fatty acids (FFA) decreases. (From Romijn, J.A., et al.: Regulation of endogenous fat and carbohydrate metabolism in relation to exercise intensity and duration. *Am. J. Physiol.*, 265: E380, 1993.)

4. Unsaturated fatty acids contain fewer hydrogen atoms attached to the carbon chain. Instead, the carbon atoms are joined by double bonds, and they are said to be either monounsaturated or polyunsaturated with respect to hydrogen. Increasing the proportion of these lipids in the diet may offer protection against heart disease.

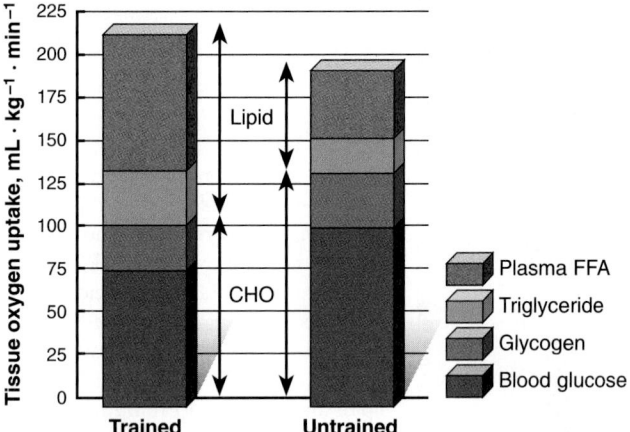

FIGURE 1.13

Estimated contribution of various substrates to energy metabolism in trained and untrained limb muscles. (From Saltin, B., and Åstrand, P.O.: Free fatty acids and exercise. *Am. J. Clin. Nutr.*, 57[Suppl]: 752S, 1993.)

5. Lowering blood cholesterol, especially that carried by the LDLs, provides significant protection against coronary heart disease.

6. Dietary lipid currently represents about 38% of the total caloric intake. Prudent recommendations suggest that a 30% level or lower is desirable. Of this, 70 to 80% should be in the form of unsaturated fatty acids.

7. Lipids provide the largest nutrient store of potential energy for biologic work. They protect vital organs and provide insulation from the cold. Lipid also acts as the carrier of the fat-soluble vitamins, A, D, E, and K.

8. During light and moderate exercise, lipid contributes about 50% of the energy requirement. As exercise continues, the role of stored lipid becomes even more important, and during prolonged work, the fatty acid molecules may provide more than 80% of the energy requirements of such exercise.

PART 3
PROTEINS

THE NATURE OF PROTEINS

Proteins (from the Greek word meaning "of prime importance") are similar to carbohydrates and lipids because they contain atoms of carbon, oxygen, and hydrogen. Proteins also contain nitrogen that makes up approximately 16% of the molecule, along with sulfur, phosphorus, and iron. Just as glycogen forms from the linkage of many simple glucose subunits, so also is the protein molecule polymerized from its "building-block" constituents, the **amino acids.** These amino acids are linked by peptide bonds in long chains in

various forms and chemical combinations. There are thousands of different protein molecules in a single cell, and approximately 50,000 different protein-containing compounds in the human body. It is the specific amino acids as well as their sequencing that determine the properties and biochemical function of all types of proteins.

Of the 20 different amino acids required by the body, each contains a positively charged amino radical at one end and a negatively charged radical called an organic acid at the other end. The amino radical is composed of two hydrogen atoms attached to nitrogen (NH_2), whereas the organic acid radical (technically termed a carboxylic acid group) is made up of one carbon atom, two oxygen atoms, and one hydrogen atom (COOH). The remainder of the amino acid molecule may take on several different forms and often is referred to as the **side chain** of the amino acid. The amino acid **alanine** is shown in Figure 1.14. This contains the basic amino and organic acid group with its unique structural side chain. *It is the specific structure of this side chain that gives an amino acid its particular characteristics.*

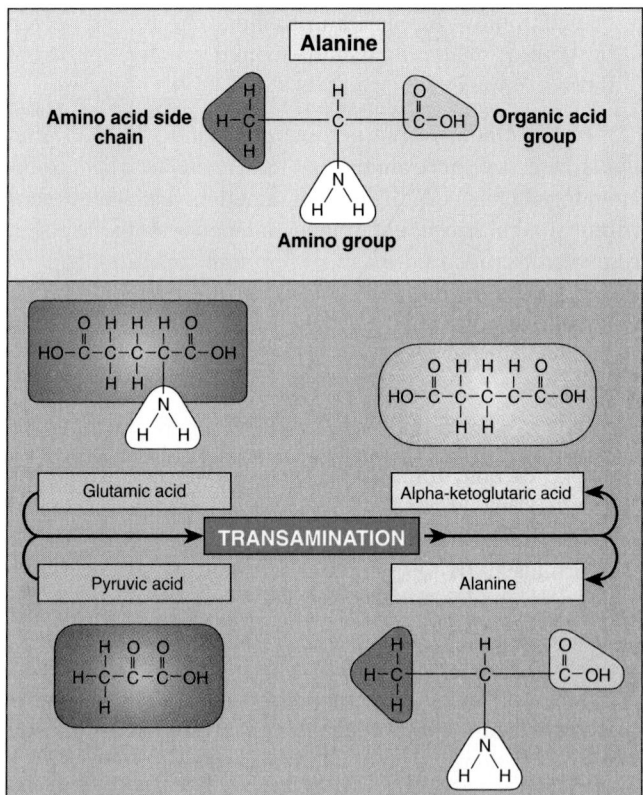

FIGURE 1.14

Chemical structure of alanine and the process of transamination where an amino group from a donor amino acid transfers to an acceptor acid forming a new amino acid. A specific transferase enzyme accelerates the transamino reaction. In the muscle, transamination uses branched-chain amino acids (BCAAs) that generate branched-chain ketoacids (mediated by BCAA aminotransferase).

Because there are so many ways the 20 amino acids can combine, there is an almost infinite number of possible proteins depending on the combination of amino acids. For example, if we consider only proteins formed from the linkage of three different amino acids, there could be 20^3 or 8000 different proteins! With few exceptions, the proteins in the body are composed of numerous combinations of linkages of amino acids.

KINDS OF PROTEIN

Eight amino acids (nine in children and certain older adults) cannot be synthesized by the body and therefore must be provided preformed in foods. These are called **essential amino acids.** They are isoleucine, leucine, lysine, methionine, phenylalanine, threonine, tryptophan, and valine; in addition, the body synthesizes cystine from methionine and tyrosine from phenylalanine. Furthermore, infants cannot synthesize histidine, and children have a reduced capability to synthesize arginine. The remaining nine amino acids that can be manufactured in the body are termed **nonessential.** This does not mean that they are unimportant, but simply that they can be synthesized from compounds ordinarily available in the body and at a rate that meets the demands for normal growth.

Proteins that contain the essential amino acids can be found in both animals and plants. There is nothing "better" about a specific amino acid from an animal compared to the same amino acid of vegetable origin. Plants make their protein by incorporating nitrogen contained in the soil to synthesize amino acids. Carbon, oxygen, and hydrogen are available from the air and water. In contrast, animals do not have a broad capability for protein synthesis and thus must derive much of their protein from ingested sources.

For a specific protein to be constructed, the appropriate amino acids must be available at the time of protein synthesis. Foods that contain all of the essential amino acids in the quantity and correct ratio to maintain nitrogen balance and allow for tissue growth and repair are known as **complete proteins,** or higher quality proteins. An **incomplete protein,** or lower quality protein, lacks one or more essential amino acid. Diets containing predominantly incomplete protein eventually result in protein malnutrition, even though they are adequate in caloric value and protein quantity.

Protein Sources

Sources of complete protein include eggs, milk, meat, fish, and poultry. The mixture of essential amino acids in eggs has been judged to be the best among food sources; hence, eggs are given the highest quality rating of 100 for comparison with other foods. Some common sources of protein in the diet are rated in Table 1.8. Presently, almost two-thirds of dietary protein comes from animal sources, whereas 80 years ago protein was ingested equally from both the plant

TABLE 1.8
RATING OF COMMON SOURCES OF DIETARY PROTEIN

Food	Protein Rating
Eggs	100
Fish	70
Lean beef	69
Cow's milk	60
Brown rice	57
White rice	56
Soybeans	47
Brewer's hash	45
Whole-grain wheat	44
Peanuts	43
Dry beans	34
White potato	34

and animal kingdom. This present-day reliance on animal protein is largely responsible for the relatively high intake of cholesterol and saturated fatty acids.

The "biologic value" of food refers to the completeness with which it supplies essential amino acids. High-quality protein foods are of animal origin whereas vegetables (lentils, dried beans and peas, nuts, and cereals) are incomplete in terms of one or more essential amino acids and thus have a relatively lower biologic value. However, **all** of the essential amino acids can be obtained by consuming a **variety** of plant foods (grains, fruits, and vegetables), each with a different quality and quantity of amino acids.

The Vegetarian Approach

Grains and legumes are excellent protein sources, but neither provides the full complement of essential amino acids. Grains lack the essential amino acid lysine, while legumes contain lysine but lack the sulfur-containing essential amino acid methionine for which grains are rich sources. Consequently, tortillas and beans, rice and beans, rice and lentils, rice and peas, and peanuts and wheat (bread) are staples in various cultures that provide **complementary** sources of all essential amino acids from the plant kingdom.

True vegetarians or **vegans** obtain all of their nutrients from the plant kingdom and in the form of dietary supplements. Vegans make up less than 1% of the US population. There are, however, an increasing number of competitive and champion athletes whose diet consists predominately of nutrients from varied plant sources as well as some dairy products.[66, 81] Two-thirds of the world's population are adequately nourished on largely vegetarian diets using only small amounts of animal protein. In contrast to diets that rely heavily on animal sources for protein, well-balanced vegetarian and vegetarian-type diets provide relatively large

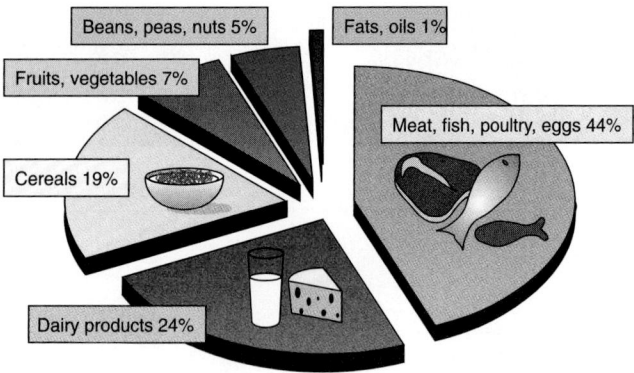

FIGURE 1.15

Contribution from the major food sources to the protein of the typical American diet.

amounts of carbohydrate that are crucial to the endurance athlete and others involved in heavy training. These diets are usually low or devoid of cholesterol, high in fiber, and rich in fruit and vegetable sources of antioxidant vitamins. In fact, a recent meta-analysis of 38 controlled clinical trials concluded that substituting the animal protein in one's diet with soy protein significantly decreases plasma triglycerides, total cholesterol, and the harmful LDL cholesterol without reducing the beneficial HDL cholesterol.[4] Except for the nutrients calcium, phosphorus, iron and vitamin B_{12} (produced by bacteria in the digestive tract of animals), a strict vegetarian's nutritional problem is one of getting ample high-quality protein. This is easily resolved with a **lactovegetarian** diet that allows the addition of milk and related products such as ice cream, cheese, and yogurt. The lactovegetarian approach minimizes the problem of getting sufficient high quality protein and increases the intake of calcium, phosphorus, and vitamin B_{12}. An intake of high-quality protein is assured by adding an egg to the diet (**ovolactovegetarian diet**).

The contribution of various food groups to the protein content of the American diet is shown in Figure 1.15. By far, the greatest intake of protein comes from animal sources, with only about 30% coming from plants.

RECOMMENDED DIETARY PROTEIN INTAKE

Despite the beliefs of many coaches, trainers, and athletes, there is probably no benefit from eating excessive amounts of protein. Increasing the protein intake by more than three times the recommended level does not enhance work capacity during intensive training.[21] For athletes, muscle mass is **not** increased simply by eating high-protein foods. If all of the extra protein intake of the typical athlete were used exclusively for lean tissue synthesis, then the muscle mass would increase tremendously. For example, consuming an extra 100 g (400 calories) of protein daily would translate

into a 500-g daily increase in muscle mass. This obviously does not happen. Additional calories in the form of protein are, after deamination (nitrogen removal), used directly for energy or recycled as components of other molecules including lipids that are stored in the subcutaneous depots. Excessive dietary protein can be harmful because the breakdown of large quantities of this nutrient produces undesirable quantities of urea and other compounds that may strain liver and kidney function.

Many Americans consume more than twice the protein requirement. On a population basis, for example, the actual intake of protein in relation to the total energy consumed is 12% (US), 11% (Germany), 14.4% (Japan), 12% (Sweden), and 12.6% (Italy). For both endurance-trained and resistance-trained athletes, many of whom consume considerable quantities of food, the diet may contain more than three times the required protein.[78]

The RDA: A Liberal Standard

The **Recommended Dietary Allowance** or **RDA** for protein, as well as for the various vitamins and minerals required by the body, are standards for nutrient intake expressed as a daily average developed by the Food and Nutrition Board of the National Research Council/National Academy of Science and revised ten times since 1943. RDA levels are believed to represent a liberal yet safe excess to meet the nutritional needs of practically all **healthy** people. It is important to emphasize that the RDA reflects nutritional needs of a population over a long time period. Malnutrition is the cumulative result of weeks, months, and even years of inadequate nutrient intake. Also, an individual who regularly consumes a diet that contains certain nutrients below the RDA standards may not necessarily be or become malnourished. The RDA is best viewed as a probability statement for adequate nutrition: as nutrient intake falls below the RDA the statistical probability for malnourishment for that person is increased, and this probability becomes progressively greater as the nutrient intake becomes lower.

Table 1.9 shows the protein RDAs for adolescent and adult men and women. On average, a daily intake of 0.83 g of protein per kg body mass is recommended.[68] (To determine the protein requirement for men and women ages 18 to 65, multiply the body mass in kg by 0.83. Thus, for a 90-kg man, total daily protein requirement would be 90×0.83 or 75 g.) This recommendation holds even for people who are overweight, and includes a reserve of about 25% to account for individual differences in protein requirement for about 98% of the population. Generally, the protein requirement as well as the quantity of the required essential amino acids decreases with age. On the other hand, for infants and growing children, the daily recommended protein intake is 2.0 to 4.0 g per kilogram body mass, whereas pregnant women should increase their daily protein intake by 20 g, and nursing mothers should increase their intake by 10 g. Likewise, stress, disease, and injury increase the protein requirement.

It is currently debated whether there is a larger protein requirement for adolescent athletes who are still growing, athletes involved in strength development programs that enhance muscle growth and endurance programs that increase protein breakdown, and athletes subjected to recurring trauma.[14, 35, 62, 86, 87] If an additional requirement exists, it is more than likely met by the generally increased food intake of these athletes to compensate for the increased energy expenditure associated with training. A more complete discussion of protein balance in training is presented on page 28.

Preparations of Simple Amino Acids

Male and female weight lifters, body builders, and other power athletes commonly consume between 0.5 and 4.0 times the RDA for protein each day.[48] Much of this excess is in the form of liquids, powders, or pills of "purified" protein at a cost in excess of $50 per pound of actual protein. These preparations often contain proteins that are "predigested" to simple amino acids through chemical action in the laboratory. The belief is that the simple amino-acid molecule is absorbed more readily and rapidly by the body to optimize the expected muscle growth brought on by training, or to acutely improve strength, power, or "vigor" for a heavy workout. This, however, is not the case. Amino acids are absorbed rapidly in the healthy intestine when they are part of the more complex di- and tripeptide molecules as well as in simple amino acid form. The intestinal tract is quite efficient at handling protein in its more complex form, whereas a concentrated amino-acid

solution draws water into the intestine. This process can cause irritation, cramping, and diarrhea. *Simply stated, amino acid supplementation in any form above the RDA has not been shown by adequate experimental design and methodology to increase muscle mass or significantly improve muscular strength, power, or endurance.*

ROLE OF PROTEIN IN THE BODY

The three major sources of body protein are blood plasma, visceral tissue, and muscle. There are, however, no body stores or "reservoirs" of this macronutrient because all protein is part of tissue structures or exists as important constituents of metabolic, transport, and hormonal systems. Protein makes up between 12 to 15% of the body mass, but there is considerable variability in the protein content of different cells. A brain cell is only about 10% protein; red blood cells and muscle cells, on the other hand, contain as much as 20% of their total weight as protein. The protein content of skeletal muscle, which represents about 65% of the body's total protein, increases with the systematic application of resistance training.

Amino acids provide the major building blocks for the synthesis of tissue. They also provide a means to incorporate nitrogen into compounds such as RNA and DNA, the coenzyme electron carriers NAD^+ and FAD, the heme components of the oxygen-binding hemoglobin and myoglobin, as well as the catecholamines epinephrine and norepinephrine and the neurotransmitter serotonin. Amino acids are needed to activate vitamins that play a key role in metabolic and physiologic regulation. The process of building tissue is termed **anabolism,** and the amino acid requirement for anabolic processes can vary considerably. During periods of rapid growth in infancy and childhood, over one-third of the protein intake is retained for tissue anabolism. As the growth rate declines, so does the percentage of protein retained for growth-related processes. Once an optimal body size is attained and growth stabilizes, there is still a continuous turnover of tissue protein.

Proteins are present in all cells and are the primary constituents that make up plasma membranes as well as internal cellular material. The proteins found in the nuclei of the cell (nucleoproteins) transmit hereditary characteristics and are responsible for continued protein synthesis within the cell. The hair, skin, nails, bones, tendons, and ligaments are comprised of special forms of collagen **structural** proteins. The **globular** proteins make up the nearly 2000 different enzymes that speed up chemical reactions. These compounds are critical in helping to regulate the breakdown of lipids, carbohydrates, and proteins for energy release. Blood plasma also contains the specialized proteins thrombin, fibrin, and fibrinogen that are required for blood clotting. Within the red blood cell, the oxygen-carrying compound hemoglobin contains the large protein molecule globin.

TABLE 1.9
RECOMMENDED DIETARY ALLOWANCES (RDAS) OF PROTEIN FOR ADOLESCENT AND ADULT MEN AND WOMEN

Recommended Amount	Men		Women	
	Adolescent	Adult	Adolescent	Adult
Grams of protein per kg body weight	0.9	0.8	0.9	0.8
Grams per day based on average weight[a]	59.0	56.0	50.0	44.0

[a]Average weight is based on a "reference" man and woman. For adolescents (ages 14–18), average weight is approximately 65.8 kg (145 lb) for males and 55.7 kg (123 lb) for females. For adult men, average weight is 70 kg (154 lb); for adult women, average weight is 56.8 kg (125 lb).

Proteins play a role in regulating the acid-base quality of the body fluids. This buffering function is important when large quantities of acid metabolites are formed during vigorous exercise. Proteins also are essential for muscle action; actin and myosin are the structural proteins that slide past each other as muscles shorten and lengthen during movement. Even for adults, the protein-containing structures in the body are actually "turned over" or replaced on a regular basis; this places a special importance on regular and adequate protein intake simply to replace the amino acids that are continually degraded in the turnover process.

DYNAMICS OF PROTEIN METABOLISM

Although the main function of dietary protein is its contribution of amino acids to various anabolic processes, protein is also catabolized for energy. In well-nourished individuals at rest, the protein breakdown contributes between 2 to 5% of the body's total energy requirement. During this **catabolism,** protein must first be degraded into its amino acid components. Nitrogen is then stripped from the amino acid molecule in the process of **deamination** in the liver and is excreted from the body as **urea** (H_2NCONH_2). Deamination involves the removal of the amino group from the amino acid molecule. A new amino acid can then be synthesized from the deaminated amino acid, or the remaining deaminated carbon compound can be synthesized into a carbohydrate or lipid, or it can be metabolized directly for energy. The urea formed in deamination (including some ammonia) leaves the body in solution as urine. Because urea must be excreted dissolved in water, excessive protein catabolism augments the body's fluid requirements.

In muscle, enzymes are available that facilitate nitrogen removal from certain amino acids and subsequently pass this nitrogen to other compounds in the biochemical reactions of **transamination** (see Fig. 1.14). This process involves the shifting of an amino group from a donor amino acid to an acceptor acid (keto acid), the acceptor thus becoming a new amino acid. This allows certain amino acids to be constructed from non nitrogen-carrying organic compounds formed in metabolism. In both deamination and transamination, the resulting carbon skeleton of the non-nitrogenous amino acid residue can then be further degraded during energy metabolism.

A **nitrogen balance** exists, when nitrogen intake (protein) equals nitrogen excretion. If the body is in **positive nitrogen balance,** where nitrogen intake is greater than nitrogen excretion, then protein is retained as new tissue is being synthesized. This is often observed in children, during pregnancy, in recovery from illness, and during resistance exercise training where protein synthesis occurs in muscle cells. It is unlikely that the body can develop a protein reserve, as is the case with lipid in adipose tissue and to some extent carbohydrate. Nevertheless, individuals fed a diet with adequate protein have a higher content of muscle and liver protein than individuals fed a low-protein diet. Also, by use of radioactive protein (injecting protein that has one or several of its carbon atoms "tagged"), it has been shown that certain proteins are more easily recruited for energy metabolism, whereas other proteins in nervous and connective tissues are relatively "fixed" as cellular constituents and cannot be used without tissue damage.[28]

A greater output of nitrogen relative to its intake indicates protein use for energy and a possible encroachment on the body's available amino acids, primarily those in skeletal muscle. If this occurs, a **negative nitrogen balance** can exist even at levels of protein intake above the standards established as the minimum requirement. This could happen if the body catabolizes protein because of a lack of other energy nutrients. For example, an individual may consume adequate or even excess protein but too little carbohydrate or lipid. Consequently, protein becomes used as a primary energy fuel, the result being a negative protein (nitrogen) balance. The protein sparing role of dietary lipid and carbohydrate discussed previously is important during periods of growth and high-energy output in intensive training. Also, the greatest negative nitrogen balance is observed in starvation. *For these reasons, starvation diets or diets with reduced carbohydrate and/or energy result not only in the depletion of glycogen reserves, but also in a possible protein deficiency and accompanying loss of lean tissue.*

PROTEIN BALANCE IN EXERCISE AND TRAINING: IS THE RDA REALLY ADEQUATE?

Nutritionists and exercise physiologists have long maintained that the RDA for protein represents a liberal "margin of safety" to provide for any amino acids catabolized for energy during exercise or required for the augmented protein synthesis following exercise.[14, 54] Over the past 100 years, the contention that protein is used only to a limited extent as an energy fuel has generally been based on two observations: (*a*) protein's primary role is to provide the amino-acid building blocks for tissue synthesis, and (*b*) the findings of early studies that there was only minimal protein breakdown during endurance exercise as reflected by urinary nitrogen in the immediate 24-hour recovery period. In addition, theoretical computations of the protein required for muscle tissue synthesis with resistance training, as well as some experimental evidence, support the position that the protein RDA is adequate for both anabolic and catabolic requirements of exercise and training.[9, 25, 35]

Recent research on protein balance in exercise, however, presents a compelling argument that protein is used as an energy fuel to a much greater extent than previously thought,[16, 72, 87] and that such protein utilization varies with energy expenditure and nutritional status.[91] *This is particularly true for the branched-chain (for the way the side chain branches from the molecule's amino core) amino acids leucine, valine, and isoleucine that are oxidized in muscle rather than the liver.* As was shown in Figure 1.5, exercise in a carbohydrate-depleted state caused a significantly greater utilization of protein than when there were ample carbohydrate reserves, particularly for extended durations of exercise. Also, if energy intake is not equal to energy expenditure during heavy training, even an augmented protein intake of two times the RDA may be insufficient to maintain nitrogen balance.[10] In this regard, dieting could negatively affect training regimens geared to increase muscle mass or maintain a high level of strength and power.[92]

While protein breakdown generally increases only modestly with exercise, muscle protein synthesis rises markedly following both endurance and resistance-type exercise. The data illustrated in Figure 1.16 for aerobic exercise indicate that the rate of muscle protein synthesis (determined from the rate of incorporation of labeled leucine into muscle) increased between 10 and 80% within 4 hours after exercise. It then remained elevated for at least 24 hours.[14] Thus, the two factors of (1) an increased protein breakdown during exercise, and (2) a somewhat larger increased protein synthesis in recovery would justify a reexamination of the recommendations for protein intake for those involved in heavy training.

Much of the current belief concerning protein dynamics and exercise is based on studies that expanded the classic method of determining protein breakdown through urea excretion. For example, the output of "labeled" CO_2 from amino acids either injected or ingested increased during exercise in a manner proportional to the metabolic rate.[94] It is now also apparent that as exercise progresses there is an increase in the concentration of plasma urea. This increase is coupled with a dramatic rise in nitrogen

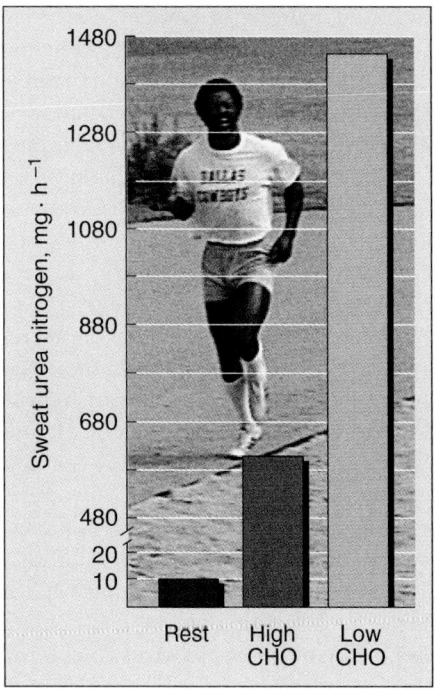

FIGURE 1.17

Excretion of urea in sweat at rest, and during exercise after carbohydrate loading (*High CHO*) and carbohydrate depletion (*Low CHO*). The largest utilization of protein (as reflected by sweat urea) occurs when glycogen reserves are low. (From Lemon, P.W.R., and Nagel, F.: Effects of exercise on protein and amino acid metabolism. *Med. Sci. Sports Exerc.*, 13: 141, 1981.)

excretion in sweat, often without any change in urinary-nitrogen excretion.[33, 71] These observations account for earlier conclusions of minimal protein breakdown during endurance exercise because the early studies only measured nitrogen in the urine. Figure 1.17 illustrates that the sweat mechanism is an important means for excreting the nitrogen from protein breakdown during exercise. Furthermore, urea production may not reflect all aspects of protein breakdown.[15] This is because the oxidation of both plasma and intracellular leucine, a branched chain essential amino acid, can increase significantly during moderate exercise regardless of changes in urea production.[98]

Figure 1.17 also shows that protein use for energy in exercise was greatest when subjects exercised in the glycogen-depleted state. This emphasizes the important role of carbohydrate as a protein sparer and suggests that the demand on protein "reserves" in exercise is linked to carbohydrate availability.[91] Certainly protein breakdown and accompanying gluconeogenesis would become important factors in endurance exercise or in frequent heavy training where glycogen reserves become greatly reduced.[86, 97] Chemically blocking the process for gluconeogenesis produces hypoglycemia, which greatly impairs endurance performance.[42]

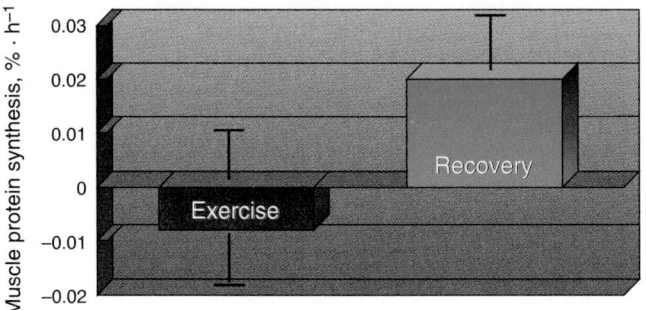

FIGURE 1.16

Stimulation of human protein synthesis during the recovery period from aerobic exercise. Values shown are differences between an exercise group and a control group that received the same diet for each time interval. (From Carraro, F., et al.: Whole body and plasma protein synthesis in exercise and recovery in human subjects. *Am. J. Physiol.*, 258: E821, 1990.)

The increased pattern of protein catabolism during endurance exercise and heavy training often mirrors the metabolic mixture during short-term starvation. With depleted glycogen reserves, the liver's glucose output is maintained largely by the process of gluconeogenesis. More than likely this augmented protein breakdown reflects the body's attempt to provide glucose for central nervous system functioning. *These observations certainly support the importance of a high-carbohydrate diet as a means to conserve muscle protein for athletes who engage in protracted and hard training.* The potential for an increased use of protein for energy (and the depression of protein synthesis during heavy exercise) may explain why individuals who participate in resistance training to augment muscle size generally refrain from glycogen-depleting, endurance-type exercise.

The beginning phase of an exercise training program also places a transient but increased demand on body protein, due perhaps to both muscle injury and metabolic requirements.[53, 69] A continuing area of controversy is whether this effect contributes to a true long-term increase in the protein requirement above that provided by the RDA.[72, 86]

The Alanine-Glucose Cycle

Some proteins in the body can not readily be utilized for energy. Proteins in muscle, however, are more labile, and when the demand arises as in exercise, can enter the process of energy metabolism.[16, 18, 29] Figure 1.18 shows that the increased release of the amino acid alanine (and possibly glutamine) from active leg muscles is related to the severity of exercise; as exercise intensity increases, alanine

output correspondingly increases in proportion to exercise intensity.

A model has been proposed that alanine **indirectly** serves the energy requirements of exercise.[28] Alanine is synthesized in active skeletal muscle during transamination from pyruvate (with nitrogen derived in part form the amino acid leucine). It then leaves the muscle and is transported to the liver where it is deaminated. The resulting carbon skeleton is converted to glucose (gluconeogenesis) which is released into the blood and delivered to the working muscles. The remaining carbon fragments from the amino acid used to form alanine can be oxidized for energy within the specific muscle cell. Figure 1.19 summarizes the sequence of the **alanine-glucose cycle.** After 4 hours of continuous light exercise, the liver's output of alanine-derived glucose can account for 45% of the total glucose released from the liver. *As much as 10 to 15% of the total exercise energy requirement can be generated from the alanine-glucose cycle.*

In summary, protein breakdown above the resting level occurs during both endurance and resistance training exercise to a degree greater than previously thought.[24, 53, 62] This is most apparent when carbohydrate and/or energy reserves are low. Such observations support the importance of supplying adequate carbohydrate and sufficient calories during training. Unfortunately, little is known concerning the actual protein requirements for individuals who train 4 to 6 hours a day by resistive-type exercise. Some evidence suggests that their requirement for protein may be only slightly greater than for sedentary individuals.[86] It also is possible that despite an increased utilization of protein for energy during heavy training, adaptations occur to augment the body's efficiency to utilize dietary protein and thus enhance amino

FIGURE 1.18

Influence of 40 minutes of exercise at various intensities on estimated alanine release from the leg muscles. As the severity of exercise increases, corresponding increases occur in alanine release. (From Felig, P., and Wahren, J.: Amino acid metabolism in exercising man. *J. Clin. Invest.*, 50: 2703, 1971.)

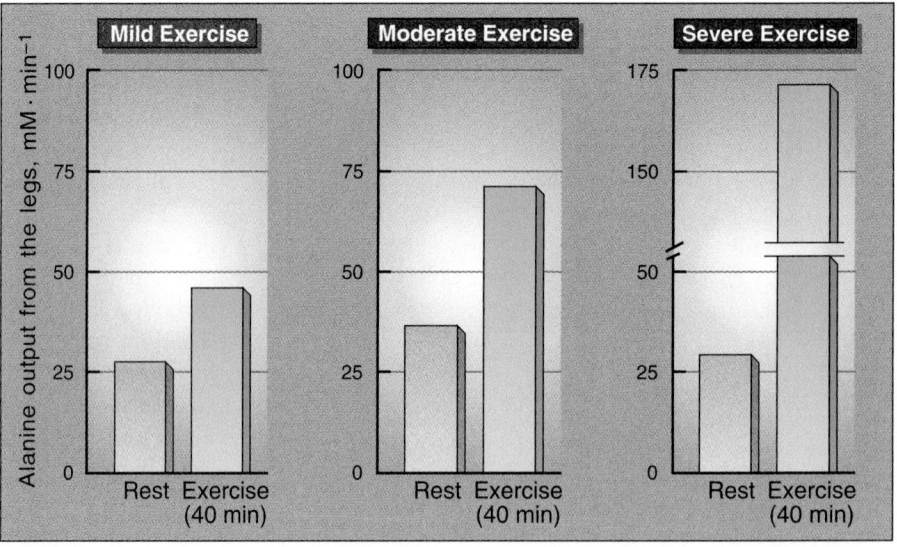

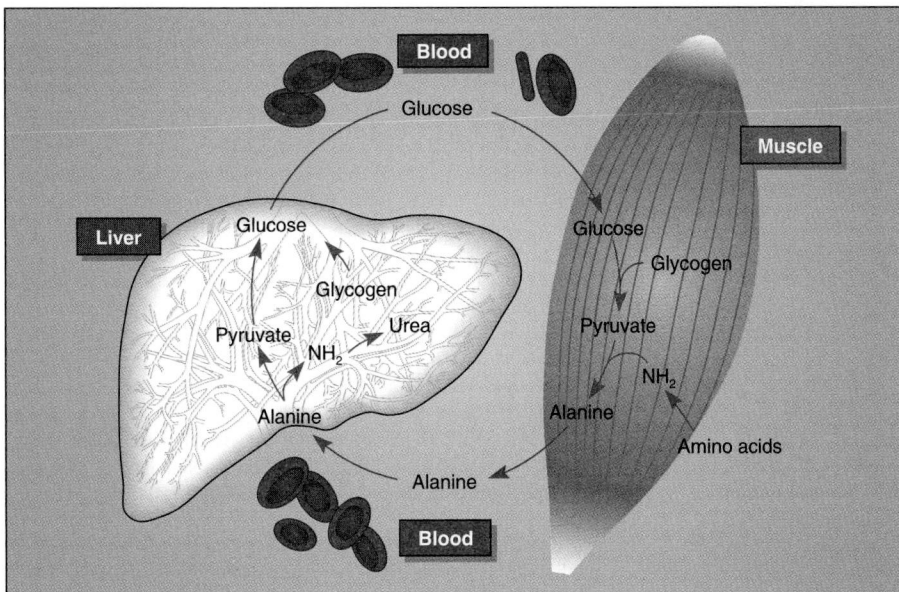

FIGURE 1.19

The alanine-glucose cycle. Alanine, synthesized in muscle from glucose-derived pyruvic acid via transamination, releases into the blood and converts to glucose and urea in the liver. Glucose released into the blood coincides with delivery to the muscle for energy. During exercise, the increased production and output of alanine from muscle helps to maintain blood glucose for the needs of the nervous system and active muscles. (From Felig, P., and Wahren, J.: Amino acid metabolism in exercising man. *J. Clin. Invest.*, 50: 2703, 1971.)

acid balance.[2, 7] Further research hopefully will determine whether there will be a modification of the current protein RDA for specific athletic groups such as body builders, weight lifters, and others who typically use resistance exercise to increase muscle size, strength, and power, as well as those involved in prolonged endurance competitions and heavy training. Until such data become available, it seems reasonable to acknowledge the heretofore unrecognized significant role of protein as a potential energy fuel for exercise.

■ SUMMARY ■

1. Proteins differ chemically from lipids and carbohydrates because they contain nitrogen in addition to other elements such as sulfur, phosphorus, and iron.

2. Proteins are formed from subunits called amino acids. The body requires 20 different amino acids, each containing an amino radical (NH_2) and an organic acid radical called a carboxyl group (COOH). In addition to NH_2 and COOH, amino acids contain a side-chain that gives the amino acid molecule its particular chemical characteristics.

3. There is almost an infinite number of possible protein structures because of the almost infinite number of combinations for the 20 different amino acids.

4. Eight of the 20 amino acids cannot be synthesized in the body. These are known as essential amino acids and they must be consumed in the diet.

5. Proteins are found in the cells of all animals and plants.

Proteins containing all the essential amino acids are called complete (higher-quality) proteins; the others are called incomplete (lower-quality) proteins. Animal proteins found in eggs, milk, cheese, meat, fish, and poultry are examples of higher-quality, complete proteins.

6. All of the essential amino acids can be obtained by consuming a variety of plant foods because each food source has a different quality and quantity of amino acids.

7. Proteins provide the building blocks for the synthesis of cellular material during anabolic processes. Under certain conditions, the amino acids also contribute their "carbon skeletons" for the catabolic process of energy metabolism.

8. The RDA is the recommended quantity for nutrient intake. It represents a liberal, yet safe level of excess to meet the nutritional needs of practically all healthy people. For adults, the protein RDA is 0.83 g per kg of body mass.

9. Certain proteins, particularly those in nervous and connective tissue, are generally not sacrificed in energy metabolism. The amino acids such as alanine, however, play a key role in providing carbohydrate fuel, especially in prolonged exercise. This is achieved through the process of gluconeogenesis. During strenuous exercise of long duration, the alanine-glucose cycle may account for up to 40 to 50% of the total glucose released by the liver.

10. Protein catabolism during exercise becomes most apparent when the body's carbohydrate reserves are low. Such findings further support the wisdom of main-

taining optimal levels of glycogen during strenuous training.

11. Future research must determine whether the increased demand on body protein with training is sufficient to increase the protein requirement above that specified by the RDA for individuals in energy balance.

■ REFERENCES ■

1. Ahlborg, G., and Felig, P.: Lactate and glucose exchange across the forearms, legs, and splanchnic bed during and after prolonged leg exercise. *J. Clin. Invest.*, 69:45, 1982.

2. Albert, J.K., et al.: Exercise-mediated tissue and whole body amino acid metabolism during intravenous feedings in normal men. *Clin. Sci.*, 77:113, 1989.

3. American Heart Association Steering Committee for Medical and Community Programs: Risk Factors and Coronary Disease. *Circulation*, 62:449A, 1980.

4. Anderson, J.W., et al.: Meta-analysis of the effects of soy protein intake on serum lipids. *N. Engl. J. Med.*, 333:276, 1995.

5. Bergstrom, J., et al.: Diet, muscle glycogen and physical performance. *Acta Physiol. Scand.*, 71:140, 1967.

6. Bónaa, K.H., et al.: Effect of eicosapentaenoic and docosahexaenoic acids on blood pressure in hypertension. *N. Engl. J. Med.*, 322:795, 1990.

7. Brooks, G.A.: Amino acid and protein metabolism during exercise and recovery. *Med. Sci. Sports Exerc.*, 19:S150, 1987.

8. Burkitt, D.: Dietary Fiber. In *Medical Applications of Clinical Nutrition*. New Canaan, CT, Keats, 1983.

9. Butterfield-Hodgen, G., and Calloway, D.H.: Protein utilization in men under two conditions of energy balance and work. *Fed. Proc.*, 39:377, 1977.

10. Butterfield, G.E.: Whole body protein utilization in humans. *Med. Sci. Sports, Exerc.*, 19:S157, 1987.

11. Caggiula, A.W., et al.: The multiple risk factor intervention trial (Mr. Fit): IV. Intervention on blood lipids. *Prev. Med.*, 10:443, 1981.

12. Cahill, G.E., Jr., and Aoki, T.T.: Partial and total starvation. In *Assessment of Energy Metabolism in Health and Disease*. Columbus, OH, Ross Laboratories, 1980.

13. Canner, P.L., et al.: Fifteen year mortality in Coronary Drug Project patients: long-term benefit with niacin. *J. Am. Coll. Cardiol.*, 8:1245, 1986.

14. Carraro, F., et al.: Effect of exercise and recovery on muscle protein synthesis in human subjects. *Am. J. Physiol.*, 259:E470, 1990.

15. Carraro, F., et al.: Urea kinetics in humans at two levels of exercise intensity. *J. Appl. Physiol.*, 75: 1180, 1993.

16. Carraro, F., et al.: Alanine kinetics in humans during low-intensity exercise. *Med. Sci. Sports Exerc.*, 26: 48, 1994.

17. Cassidy, M., et al.: Morphological aspects of dietary fibers in the intestines. In *Advances in Lipid Research*. Edited by R. Paoletti and D. Kaitchevsky. New York, Academic Press, 1982.

18. Christensen, H.N.: Role of amino acid transport and counter transport in nutrition and metabolism. *Physiol. Rev.*, 70:43, 1990.

19. Conner, W.E., et al.: The plasma lipids, lipoproteins, and diet of the Tarahumara Indians of Mexico. *Am. J. Clin. Nutr.*, 31:1131, 1978.

20. Coggan, A.R., et al.: Plasma glucose kinetics in subjects with high and low lactate thresholds. *J. Appl. Physiol.*, 73:1873, 1992.

20a. Coggan, A.R., et al.: Glucose kinetics during high-intensity exercise in endurance-trained and untrained humans. *J. Appl. Physiol.*, 78:1203, 1995.

21. Consolazio, C.F., et al.: Protein metabolism during intensive physical training in the young adult. *Am. J. Clin. Nutr.*, 28:29, 1975.

22. Costill, D.L., et al.: Effects of repeated days of intensified training on muscle glycogen and swimming performance. *Med. Sci. Sports Exerc.*, 20:249, 1988.

23. Crapo, P.A.: Sugar and sugar alcohols. *Contemp. Nutr.*, 7 (12):1981.

24. Dohm, G.L., et al.: Time course of changes in gluconeogenic enzyme activities during exercise and recovery. *Am. J. Physiol.*, 249:E6, 1985.

25. Durnin, J.V.G.A.: Protein requirements and physical activity. In *Nutrition, Physical Fitness and Health*. Edited by J. Parizkova and V.A. Rogozkin. Baltimore, MD, University Park Press, 1978.

26. Durstine, J.L., and Haskell, W.L.: Effects of exercise training on plasma lipids and lipoproteins. *Exerc. Sport Sci. Rev.*, 22:477, 1994.

27. Felig, P., et al.: Hypoglycemia during prolonged exercise in normal men. *N. Engl. J. Med.*, 306:895, 1982.

28. Felig, P., and Wahren, J.: Amino acid metabolism in exercising man. *J. Clin. Invest.*, 50:2703, 1971.

29. Felig, P., and Wahren, J.: Fuel homeostasis in exercise. *N. Engl. J. Med.*, 293:1078, 1975.

30. Fernandez, M.L., et al.: Guar gum effects on plasma low-density lipoprotein and hepatic cholesterol metabolism in guinea pigs fed low- and high-cholesterol diets: a dose-response study. *Am. J. Clin. Nutr.*, 61:127, 1995.

31. Frick, M.H., et al.: Helsinki Heart Study: primary-prevention trial with gemfibrozil in middle-aged men with dyslipidemia. Safety of treatment, changes in risk factors, and incidence of coronary heart disease. *N. Engl. J. Med.*, 317:3217, 1987.

32. Ginsberg, H.N.: Reduction of plasma cholesterol levels in normal men on an American Heart Association Step 1 diet or a Step 2 diet with added monounsaturated fat. *N. Engl. J. Med.*, 322:574, 1990.

33. Harlambie, G., and Sensor, L.: Metabolic Changes in man during long-distance swimming. *Eur. J. Appl. Physiol.*, 43:115, 1980.

34. Harris, W.S., et al.: Fish oils in hypertriglyceridemia: a dose response study. *Am. J. Clin. Nutr.*, 51:399, 1990.

35. Hickson, J.F., et al.: Repeated days of body building exercise do not enhance urinary nitrogen excretions from untrained young males. *Nutr. Res.*, 10:723, 1990.

36. Hultman, E.: Liver as a glucose supplying source during rest and exercise, with special reference to diet. In *Nutrition, Physical Fitness, and Health*. Edited by J. Parizkova and V.A. Rogozkin. Baltimore, MD, University Park Press, 1978.

37. Hunter, J.E., and Applewhite, T.H.: Reassessment of trans fatty acid availability in the U.S. *Am. J. Clin. Nutr.*, 54:363, 1991.

37a. Iribarren, C., et al.: Serum total cholesterol and mortality: compound factors and risk modification in Japanese-American men. *JAMA*, 273:1926, 1995.

38. Jandrain, B.J., et al.: Metabolic availability of glucose ingested three hours before prolonged exercise in humans. *J. Appl. Physiol.*, 56:1314, 1984.

39. Jandrain, B.J., et al.: Fructose utilization during exercise in men: rapid conversion of ingested fructose to circulating glucose. *J. Appl. Physiol.*, 74:2146, 1993.

40. Jansson, E., and Kaijser, L.: Effect of diet on the utilization of blood-borne and intramuscular substrates during exercise in man. *Acta Physiol. Scand.*, 115:19, 1982.

41. Jenkins, D.J.A., et al.: Effect on blood lipids of very high intakes of fiber in diets low in saturated fat and cholesterol. *N. Engl. J. Med.*, 329: 21, 1993.

42. John-Adler, H.B., et al.: Reduced running endurance in gluconeogenesis-inhibited rats. *Am. J. Physiol.*, 251, 1986.

43. Kay, R.M.: Dietary fiber. *J. Lipid Res.*, 23:221, 1982.

44. Kinosian, B., et al.: Cholesterol and coronary heart disease: predicting risk by levels and ratios. *Ann. Intern. Med.*, 121:641, 1994.

45. Kirby, R.W., et al.: Oat-bran intake selectively lowers serum low-density lipoprotein cholesterol concentrations of hypercholesterolemic men. *Am. J. Clin. Nutr.*, 34:824, 1981.

46. Kjaer, M., et al.: Increased epinephrine response and inaccurate glucoregulation in exercising athletes. *J. Appl. Physiol.*, 61:1693, 1986.

47. Klag, M.J., et al.: Serum cholesterol in young men and subsequent cardiovascular disease. *N. Engl. J. Med.*, 328:313, 1993.

48. Kleiner, S.M., et al.: Metabolic profiles, diet and health practices of championship male and femal body builders. *J. Am. Diet. Assoc.* 90:962, 1990.

49. Koeslag, J.H.: Post-exercise ketosis and the hormone response to exercise: a review. *Med. Sci. Sports Exerc.*, 4:327, 1982.

50. Kromhout, D., et al.: Dietary fiber and 10 year mortality from coronary heart disease, cancer, and all causes. *Lancet*, 2:518, 1982.

51. Krumholz, H.M., et al.: Lack of association between cholesterol and coronary heart disease mortality and morbidity and all-cause mortality in persons older than 70 years. *JAMA*, 272:1335, 1994.

52. Lanza, E., et al.: Dietary fiber intake in the U.S. population. *Am. J. Clin. Nutr.*, 46:790, 1987.

53. Lemon, P.W.R.: Protein and exercise: Update 1987. *Med. Sci. Sports Exerc.*, 19:S179, 1987.

54. Lemon, P.W.R., and Mullin, J.P.: The effect of initial muscle glycogen levels on protein catabolism during exercise. *J. Appl. Physiol.*, 48:624, 1980.

55. Levine, A.S., et al.: Effect of breakfast cereals on short-term food intake. *Am. J. Clin. Nutr.*, 50:1303, 1989.

56. Levy, D., et al.: Stratifying the patient at risk for coronary disease: new insights from the Framingham Heart Study. *Am. Heart J.*, 119:712, 1990.

57. Lipid Research Clinics Program: The Lipid Research Clinics coronary primary prevention trial results. I. Reduction in incidence of coronary heart disease. *JAMA*, 251:351, 1984.

58. Lipid Research Clinics Program: The Lipid Research Clinics coronary primary prevention trial results. II. The relationship of reduction in incidence of coronary heart disease to cholesterol lowering. *JAMA*, 251:365, 1984.

59. Manninen, V., et al.: Lipid alternations and decline in the incidence of coronary heart disease in the Helsinki Heart Study. *JAMA*, 260:641, 1988.

60. Martin, M.J., et al.: Serum cholesterol, blood pressure, and mortality: implications from a cohort of 361,662 men. *Lancet*, 2:933 1986.

61. McArdle, W.D., et al.: Thermal adjustment to cold-water exposure in resting men and women. *J. Appl. Physiol.*, 56:1565, 1984.

62. Meridith, C.N., et al.: Dietary protein requirements and body protein metabolism in endurance-trained men. *J. Appl. Physiol.*, 66:2850, 1989.

63. Miller, V.C., et al.: Adaptations to high-fat diet that increase exercise endurance in male rats. *J. Appl. Physiol.*, 56:78, 1984.

64. Murray, R., et al.: The effects of glucose, fructose, and sucrose ingestion during exercise. *Med. Sci. Sports Exerc.*, 21:275, 1989.

65. NIH Consensus Congerence. Triglyceride, high-density lipoprotein, and coronary heart disease. *JAMA*, 269:505, 1993.

66. Nieman, D.: Vegetarian dietary practices and endurance performance. *Am. J. Clin. Nutr.*, 48:754, 1988.

67. O'Brien, M.J., et al.: Carbohydrate dependence during marathon running. *Med. Sci. Sports Exerc.*, 25:1009, 1993.

68. Pellet, P.L.: Protein requirements in humans. *Am. J. Clin. Nutr.*, 51:723, 1990.

69. Pivarnik, J.M., et al.: Urinary 3-methylhistidine excretion increases with repeated weight training exercise. *Med. Sci. Sports Exerc.*, 21:283, 1989.

70. Pugh, L.G.C.E., and Edholm, O.G.: The physiology of channel swimmers. *Lancet*, 2:761, 1955.

71. Refsum, H.E., et al.: Changes in plasma amino acid distribution and urinary amino acid excretion during prolonged heavy exercise. *Scand. J. Clin. Invest.*, 39:407, 1979.

72. Rennie, M.J., et al.: Physical activity and protein metabolism. In *Physical Activity, Fitness, and Health.* Edited by C. Bouchard, et al., Champaign, IL, Human Kinetics, 1994.

73. Romijn, J.A., et al.: Regulations of endogenous fat and carbohydrate metabolism in relation to exercise intensity and duration. *Am. J. Physiol.*, 265:E380, 1993.

74. Saltin, B., and Åstrand, P -O.: Free fatty acids and exercise. *Am. J. Clin. Nutr.*, 57 (Suppl):752S, 1993.

75. Saltin, B., and Gollnick, P.D.: Fuel for muscular exercise: role of carbohydrate. In *Exercise, Nutrition, and Energy Metabolism.* Edited by E.S. Horton, and R.L. Terjung. New York, Macmillan, 1988.

76. Shahar, E., et al.: Dietary n-3 polyunsaturated fatty acids and smoking-related chronic obstructive pulmonary disease. *N. Engl. J. Med.*, 331:228, 1994.

77. Sharon, N.: Carbohydrates. *Sci. Am.*, 243:90, 1980.

78. Short, S.H., and Short, W.R.: Four-year study of university athletes' dietary intake. *J. Am. Diet. Assoc.*, 82:632, 1983.

79. Simopolous, A.P.: Omega-3 fatty acids in health and disease and in growth and development. *Am. J. Clin. Nutr.*, 54:438, 1991.

80. Sims, E.A.H., and Danforth, Jr., E.: Expenditure and storage of energy in man (perspective). *J. Clin. Invest.*, 79:1019, 1987.

81. Slavin, J.L. et al.: Nutritional practices of women cyclists including recreational riders and elite racers. In *Sport, Health, and Nutrition.* Edited by F.I. Katch. Champaign, IL, Human Kinetic Publishers, 1986.

82. Slyper, A.H., et al.: Low-density lipoprotein and atherosclerosis. *JAMA*, 272:305, 1994.

83. Stamler, J., et al.: Is relationship between serum cholesterol and risk of premature death from coronary heart disease continuous or graded? Findings in 356,222 primary screenees of the Multiple Risk Factor Intervention Trial (Mr Fit). *JAMA*, 256:2823, 1986.

84. Superko, H.R., et al.: The effect of solid and liquid gum on the reduction of plasma cholesterol in patients with moderate hypercholesterolemia. *Am. J. Cardiol.*, 62:51, 1988.

85. Suter, E., and Hawes, M.R.: Relationship of physical activity, body fat, diet, and blood lipid profile in youths 10-15 yr. *Med. Sci. Sports Exerc.*, 25:748, 1993.

86. Tarnopolosky, M.A., et al.: Influence of protein intake and training status on nitrogen balance and lean body mass. *J. Appl. Physiol.*, 64:187, 1988.

87. Tarnopolosky, M.A., et al.: Effect of bodybuilding exercise on protein requirements. *Can. J. Sport Sci.*, 15:225, 1990.

88. Troisi, R., et al: Trans-fatty acid intake in relation to serum lipid concentrations in adult men. *Am. J. Clin. Nutr.*, 56:1019, 1992.

89. Turcotte, L.P., et al.: Increased plasma FFA uptake and oxidation during prolonged exercise in trained versus untrained humans. *Am. J. Physiol.*, 262:E791, 1992.

90. Vahouny, G.V.: Dietary fiber, lipid metabolism, and atherosclerosis. *Fed. Proc.*, 41:2801, 1982.

91. Wagenmakers, A.J.M., et al.: Carbohydrate supplementation, glycogen depletion, and amino acid metabolism. *Am. J. Physiol.*, 260:E883, 1991.

92. Walberg, J.L., et al.: Macronutrient content of a hypoenergy diet affects nitrogen retention and muscle function in weight lifters. *Int. J. Sports Med.*, 9:261, 1988.

93. Warner, J.G., Jr., et al.: Combined effect of aerobic exercise and omega-3 fatty acids in hyperlipidemic persons. *Med. Sci. Sports Exerc.*, 21:498, 1989.

94. White, T.P., and Brooks, G.A.: [u-^{14}C] glucose-alanine and leucine oxidation in rats at rest and two intensities of running. *Am. J. Physiol.*, 240:E155, 1981.

95. Willett, W.C., and Ascherio, A.: Trans fatty acids: are the effects only marginal? *Am. J. Public Health.*, 84:722, 1994.

96. Williams, O.D., et al.: Common methods, different populations: The Lipid Research Clinics program prevalence study. *Circulation*, 62(Suppl. 4):18, 1980.

97. Wolfe, R.R., et al.: Glucose metabolism in man: response to intravenous glucose infusion. *Metabolism*, 28:210, 1979.

98. Wolfe, R.R., et al.: Isotopic analysis of leucine and urea metabolism in exercising humans. *J. Appl. Physiol.*, 52:458, 1982.

99. Wolfe, R.R., et al.: Role of changes in insulin and glucagon in glucose homeostasis in exercise. *J. Clin. Invest.*, 77:900, 1986.

Smith, E.L., et al.: Physical activity and calcium modalities for bone mineral increase in aged women. *Med. Sci. Sports Exerc.* **13:60, 1981.**

In normal, well-nourished males and females the rate of bone formation balances bone resorption to maintain a constancy in bone mass and density. In females older than 35 years of age, however, bone mineral content decreases at a rate of about

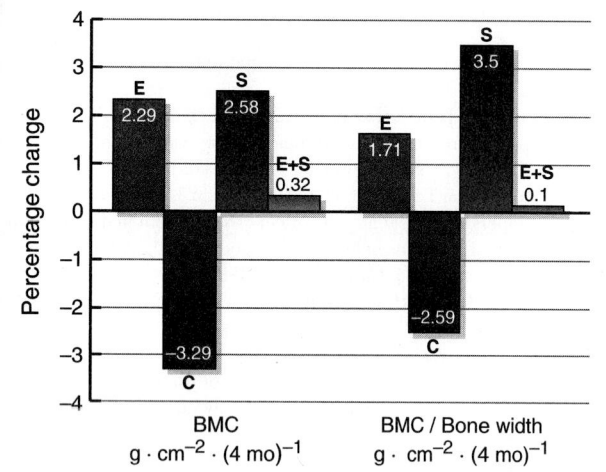

Percent change after 4 months in bone mineral content and bone mineral content/bone width for exercise (E), diet supplement (S), control (C), and exercise plus diet supplement (E + S) groups. The experiment lasted 36 months.

1% per year. Qualitatively, bone remains the same but it is less dense. The causes for decreased bone density and bone mass loss in middle-aged women include a sedentary lifestyle and an inadequate intake of dietary calcium. In this study of the role of exercise and diet, Smith and colleagues made in vivo bone mineral content (BMC) and bone width measurements by photon absorptiometry of the nondominant arm in 80 Caucasian women ranging in age from 69 to 95 years. Following pretesting, which included a Balke treadmill stress test, subjects were placed randomly into one of four groups: control (C), exercise (E), diet supplement (S), and exercise plus diet supplement (E + S). The groups were matched for age, body mass, and degree of ambulation. The supplement group (N = 17) consumed calcium carbonate tablets containing 750 mg of elemental calcium and 400 IU of vitamin D each day. The controls (N = 26) received a placebo tablet containing 360 mg of lactose, 5 mg of magnesium stearate, and 80 mg of microcrystalline cellulose. The exercise group (N = 19) par-

ticipated in group exercise sessions consisting of light to mild aerobics at about 3 METs intensity 3 days a week for 30 minutes per session. The exercise plus supplement group (N = 18) received both the exercise and the supplement throughout the 36-month study.

As shown in the figure, BMC declined significantly by about 3.3% for the control group. On the other hand, BMC increased by 0.32% for the exercise plus supplement group, 2.29% for the exercise group, and 2.58% for the supplement-only group. The changes in BMC for the exercise and supplement groups were significantly different than that of the control group, while the BMC change in the exercise plus supplement group was marginally significant. The figure also presents the changes in the bone width measurements. The differences are in the same direction as the BMC changes, although they are not statistically significant.

The results showed that the groups that exercised and added calcium to their food intake (E and S groups) showed slight increases in bone mineral content over the 36-month study. However, the combined treatments were no more effective in maintaining bone mineral content or bone width than each treatment alone. This indicated that the treatments were not additive, as one might have expected. The authors suggested that perhaps the individuals in the E + S group had a higher rate of overall decline in physical and mental function that prevented a positive bone mass response to exercise plus calcium supplementation.

The authors hypothesized a different mechanism to explain the similar positive results in bone mineral content and bone width data for the supplement-only and exercise-only groups. They suggested that the supplemented group had increased bone mass because of increased calcium availability and absorption, which contributed to the maintenance of a positive calcium balance in the intestinal tract. In contrast, the increased BMC in the exercise group could not be attributed to increased calcium availability because they received no supplement, and their diet was not different from that of the control group, which continued to lose bone density. The only plausible explanation for the increased BMC in the exercise group was their increased level of physical activity.

This was one of the early studies to clearly indicate reversal of bone loss in middle-aged women through the use of increased levels of mild to moderate physical activity or calcium and vitamin D supplementation.

Vitamins, Minerals, and Water

The effective regulation of all metabolic processes requires a delicate blending of food nutrients in the watery medium of the cell. Of special significance in the metabolic mixture are the **micronutrients**—the small quantities of vitamins and minerals that play highly specific roles in facilitating energy transfer and tissue synthesis. For example, the average adult requires only about 350 g (12 oz) of vitamins from the 820 kg (1820 lb) of food consumed each year. These nutrients are readily obtained from the foods consumed in well-balanced meals. With proper nutrition from a variety of food sources, there is little need to consume vitamin and mineral supplements; such practices often are physiologically and economically wasteful.

PART 1
VITAMINS

THE NATURE OF VITAMINS

Centuries before scientists isolated and classified vitamins, their importance was known. For example, the Greek physician Hippocrates advocated the ingestion of liver to cure night blindness. Although the reason for the cure was unknown at the time, we now know that vitamin A, which helps prevent night blindness, is plentiful in this organ meat. In 1897, scientists observed that a regular diet of polished rice caused beriberi, but supplementing the diet with thiamine-rich rice polishings cured this disease. In the early 19th century, the disease scurvy was eliminated by adding lemons (then known as limes) to the diet of British sailors, many of whom would have perished from lack of the then unknown vitamin C. It was not until 1932, however, that ascorbic acid or vitamin C was isolated from lemon juice.

Vitamins were formally discovered as organic substances needed by the body in minute amounts. Vitamins have no particular chemical structure in common and often are considered accessory nutrients because they neither supply energy nor contribute substantially to body mass. With the exception of vitamin D, the body cannot manufacture vitamins; hence, they must be supplied through diet or supplementation.

Some foods contain an abundant quantity of vitamins. For example, vitamins are manufactured in green leaves and roots of plants during photosynthesis. Animals obtain vitamins from the plants, seeds, grains, and fruits they eat or from the meat of other animals that have previously consumed these foods. Several vitamins, most notably vitamins A and D, niacin, and folic acid, are activated from their inactive precursor or **provitamin** form. The best known of the provitamins are the **carotenes,** the yellow and yellow-orange pigment precursors of vitamin A that give color to vegetables and fruits such as carrots, squash, corn, pumpkins, apricots, and peaches.

KINDS OF VITAMINS

Thirteen different vitamins have been isolated, analyzed, classified, and synthesized, and recommended dietary allowance (RDA) levels have been established. These vitamins are classified as either **lipid soluble** or **water soluble.** The lipid-soluble vitamins are vitamins A, D, E, and K; the water-soluble vitamins are vitamin C (ascorbic acid) and the B-complex vitamins: vitamin B_6 (pyridoxine), thiamine (B_1), riboflavin (B_2), niacin (nicotinic acid), pantothenic acid, biotin, folic acid (folate), and cobalamin (B_{12}).

LIPID-SOLUBLE VITAMINS

Daily ingestion of lipid-soluble vitamins is not absolutely necessary, because these substances are dissolved and stored in the fatty tissues of the body. In fact, it may take years for symptoms of a lipid-soluble vitamin insufficiency to become evident. Vitamins A and D are stored predominantly in the liver, whereas vitamin E is distributed throughout the body's fatty tissues. Vitamin K is stored only in small amounts, mainly in the liver. Lipid-soluble vitamins are often obtained from dietary lipids, and consuming a "fat-free" diet could certainly accelerate the development of an insufficiency.

At the other extreme, consuming an excessive amount of lipid-soluble vitamins can have harmful effects. For example, daily ingestion of a moderate to large amount of vitamins A and D eventually can have serious toxic effects. Women who consume excess vitamin A early in pregnancy increase the risk of birth defects in their unborn children. In young children, excessive vitamin A intake (called hypervitaminosis A) causes irritability, swelling of the bones, weight loss, and dry, itchy skin. In adults, symptoms can include nausea, headache, drowsiness, loss of hair, diarrhea, and loss of calcium from bones, causing brittleness. Discontinuing high intakes of vitamin A reverses these symptoms. Kidney damage can result from a regular excess of vitamin D.

Lipid-soluble vitamins should not be consumed in excess without proper medical supervision. Although an "overdose" of vitamins E and K is rare, intakes above the recommended level are believed to yield no health benefits.

WATER-SOLUBLE VITAMINS

Water-soluble vitamins function largely as **coenzymes,** which are small molecules that combine with larger protein compounds (apoenzymes) to form active enzymes that accelerate the interconversion of chemical compounds. Coenzymes participate directly in chemical reactions, but when the reaction is completed, they remain intact to be used again. Water-soluble vitamins are similar to their lipid-soluble counterparts because they are composed of atoms of carbon, hydrogen, and oxygen. They also contain nitrogen and metal ions such as iron, molybdenum, copper, sulfur, and cobalt.

Because of their water solubility, these vitamins are dispersed in the body fluids and are not stored to an appreciable extent. Generally, any excess intake is eventually voided in the urine. Water-soluble vitamins probably exert their influence for as long as 8 to 14 hours after ingestion; thereafter, their potency in the body begins to decrease. For maximum benefit, for example, vitamin C should be consumed at least every 12 hours. In most cases, the loss of water-soluble vitamins in perspiration, even during extreme physical activity, is probably negligible.[47]

ROLE OF VITAMINS IN THE BODY

Many of the biologic functions of vitamins in the body are summarized in Figure 2.1. Whereas vitamins contain no useful energy for the body, they do serve as essential links and regulators in metabolic reactions that release energy from food; vitamins also control the process of tissue synthesis. For example, vitamin B_1 facilitates the conversion of pyruvate to acetyl-CoA in carbohydrate breakdown, while niacin and vitamin B_2 regulate mitochondrial energy metabolism. Vitamins B_6 and B_{12} act as catalysts in protein synthesis, and pantothenic acid is a constituent of coenzyme-A that plays a

FIGURE 2.1.
Biologic functions of vitamins in the body.

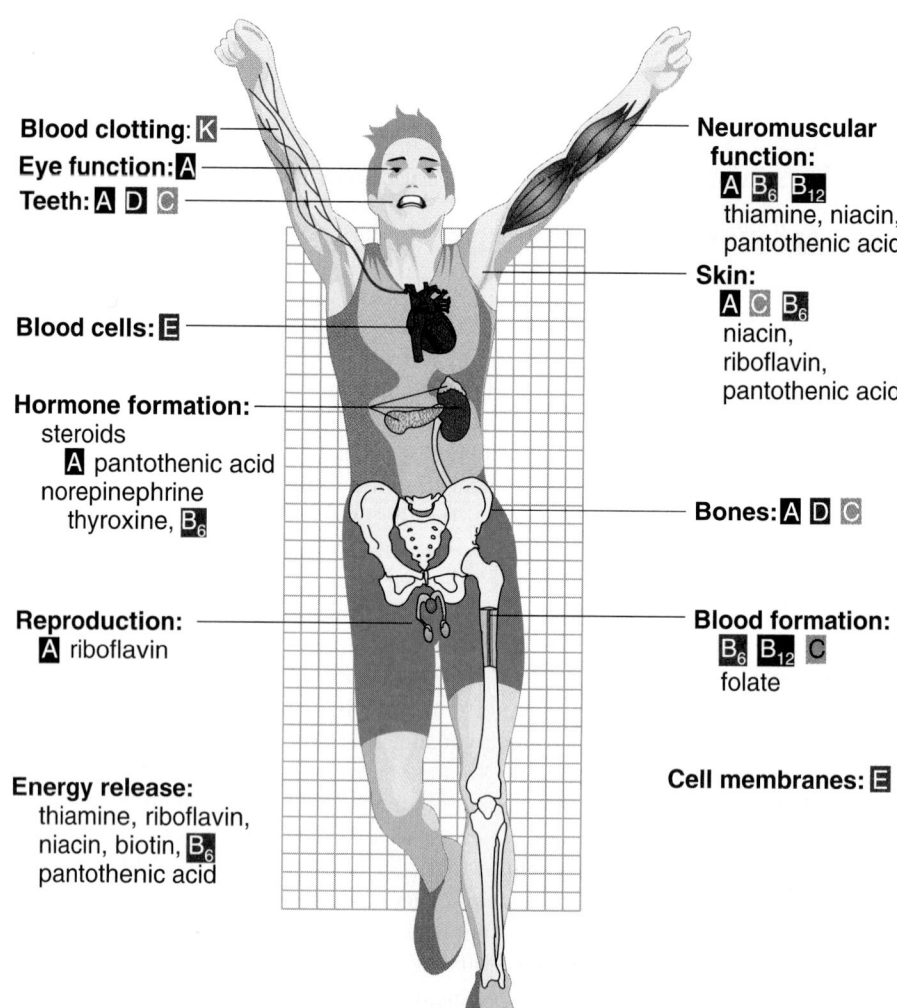

Blood clotting: K
Eye function: A
Teeth: A D C

Blood cells: E

Hormone formation:
steroids
A pantothenic acid
norepinephrine
thyroxine, B_6

Reproduction:
A riboflavin

Energy release:
thiamine, riboflavin,
niacin, biotin, B_6
pantothenic acid

Neuromuscular
function:
A B_6 B_{12}
thiamine, niacin,
pantothenic acid

Skin:
A C B_6
niacin,
riboflavin,
pantothenic acid

Bones: A D C

Blood formation:
B_6 B_{12} C
folate

Cell membranes: E

TABLE 2.1
THE MAJOR COENZYMES, THEIR VITAMIN SOURCE, AND THEIR FUNCTION[a]

Name	Abbreviation	Vitamin Source	Function
Coenzyme A	CoA	Panthothenic acid	Acyl transfer reactions
Flavin adenine dinucleotide	FAD	B_2 (riboflavin)	Oxidation reactions
Nicotinamide adenine dinucleotide	NAD^+	Niacin	Oxidation and reduction reactions
Pyridoxal phosphate	PLP	B_6	Amino acid metabolism

[a]Many of the vitamins function as coenzymes in metabolic reactions. For example, vitamin B_1 (thiamine) is involved in carbohydrate metabolism and in the citric acid cycle (Krebs cycle). The active coenzyme of thiamine is thiaminediphosphate. Vitamin C is a cofactor in some hydroxylation reactions (e.g., dopamine to noradrenalin), and pantothenic acid is involved in fatty acid synthesis.

crucial role in the aerobic breakdown of macronutrients. *Because vitamins can be used repeatedly in metabolic reactions, the vitamin requirements of athletes are generally no greater than those of sedentary people.* The major coenzymes, along with their derivations and principal functions, are listed in Table 2.1. These compounds are not synthesized by the body and thus must be derived from dietary sources.

The bodily functions, dietary requirements, and major dietary sources of water-soluble and lipid-soluble vitamins are listed in Table 2.2. An adequate quantity of all vitamins is available in well-balanced meals. This is true for all individuals, regardless of age and level of physical activity. Indeed, there is no need for individuals who expend considerable energy exercising to consume extra vitamins in the form of special foods or supplements. Also, at high levels of daily physical activity, food intake is generally increased to sustain the added energy requirements of exercise. If this additional food is obtained through a variety of well-balanced meals, a proportionate increase in vitamin and mineral intake is ensured.

Several possible exceptions to this rule should be noted. Vitamin C and the B-vitamin folic acid are contained in foods that usually comprise only a minimal amount of the caloric content of the diet of most Americans; the availability of these foods varies by season. Also, intake of vitamins B_1 and B_6 has been reported to be insufficient in some athletic groups.[32] Adequate intake of these vitamins can be ensured, however, if the daily diet contains fresh fruit, grains, and uncooked or steamed vegetables. For individuals on meatless diets, a small amount of milk, milk products, or eggs should be consumed because vitamin B_{12} is available only in foods of animal origin.

ANTIOXIDANT ROLE OF SPECIFIC VITAMINS

Most of the oxygen consumed during energy metabolism in the mitochondria combines with hydrogen to produce water. Normally, however, approximately 2 to 5% of this oxygen will form oxygen-containing free radicals such as superoxide (O_2^-), hydrogen peroxide (H_2O_2), and hydroxyl (OH^-) rad-

icals due to electron "leakage" at various steps in the electron transport chain.[113] *A free radical is a highly chemically reactive molecule or molecular fragment that contains at least one unpaired electron in its outer orbital or valence shell.* These are the same free radicals produced by external factors such as heat and ionizing radiation and carried in cigarette smoke, environmental pollutants, and even some medications. Once formed, free radicals can interact with other compounds to create new free radical molecules.

When superoxide forms, for example, it dismutates to hydrogen peroxide. Normally, superoxide is rapidly converted to O_2 and H_2O by the enzyme **superoxide dismutase.** An accumulation of free radicals increases the potential for cellular damage, or **oxidative stress,** to many biologically important substances. These include the genetic material of DNA, proteins, and lipid-containing structures, particularly the polyunsaturated fatty acid-rich bilayer membrane that helps to isolate the cell against noxious agents such as toxins and carcinogens.[45] In fact, the major effect of oxygen radicals is their affinity to the polyunsaturated fatty acids that make up the lipid bilayer of the cell membrane. During unchecked oxidative stress, there is a deterioration of the fatty acids in the plasma membrane, which becomes damaged through a chain-reaction series of events termed **lipid peroxidation.** These reactions increase the vulnerability of the cell and its constituents.[44] Free radicals also can facilitate the oxidation of low density lipoprotein (LDL) cholesterol, which accelerates the process of atherosclerosis.[70] Oxidative stress ultimately increases the likelihood of cellular deterioration associated with advanced aging as well as cancer, diabetes, and coronary artery disease.

Although there is no way to stop oxygen reduction and the production of free radicals, an elaborate natural defense against their damaging effects exists within the cytosol and mitochondria of the cell and its surrounding extracellular space. This defense includes the antioxidant scavenger enzymes such as catalase, glutathione peroxidase, superoxide dismutase, and metal-binding proteins.[58, 123] In addition, nutritive-reducing agents such as vitamins A, C, and E

TABLE 2.2
RECOMMENDED DIETARY ALLOWANCE, FOOD SOURCES, MAJOR BODILY FUNCTIONS, AND SYMPTOMS OF DEFICIENCY OR EXCESS OF THE LIPID-SOLUBLE AND WATER-SOLUBLE VITAMINS FOR HEALTHY ADULTS (19 TO 50 YEARS OF AGE)[a]

Vitamin	RDA (mg) Males	RDA (mg) Females	Dietary Sources	Major Body Functions	Deficiency	Excess
Lipid Soluble						
Vitamin A (retinol)	1.0	0.8	Provitamin A (β-carotene) widely distributed in green vegetables. Retinol present in milk, butter, cheese, fortified margarine	Constituent of rhodopsin (visual pigment). Maintenance of epithelial tissues. Role in mucopolysaccharide synthesis	Xerophthalmia (keratinization) of ocular tissue), night blindness, permanent blindness	Headache, vomiting, peeling of skin, anorexia, swelling of long bones
Vitamin D	0.01[a]	0.01	Cod-liver oil, eggs, dairy products, fortified milk, and margarine	Promotes growth and mineralization of bones. Increases absorption of calcium	Rickets (bone deformities) in children. Osteomalacia in adults	Vomiting, diarrhea, loss of weight, kidney damage
Vitamin E (tocopherol)	10.0	8.0	Seeds, green leafy vegetables, margarines, shortenings	Functions as an antioxidant to prevent cell damage	Possibly anemia	Relatively nontoxic
Vitamin K (phylloquinone)	0.08	0.06	Green leafy vegetables. Small amount in cereals, fruits, and meats	Important in blood clotting (involved in formation of active prothrombin)	Conditioned deficiencies associated with severe bleeding; internal hemorrhages	Relatively nontoxic. Synthetic forms at high doses may cause jaundice
Water Soluble						
Vitamin B$_1$ (thiamin)	1.5	1.1	Pork, organ meats, whole grains, legumes	Coenzyme (thiamin prophosphate) in reactions involving the removal of carbon dioxide	Beriberi (peripheral nerve changes, edema, heart failure)	None reported
Vitamin B$_2$	1.7	1.3	Widely distributed in foods	Constituent of two flavin nucleotide coenzymes involved in energy metabolism (FAD and FMN)	Reddened lips, cracks at mouth corner (cheilosis), eye lesions	None reported
Niacin	19	15	Liver, lean meats, grains, legumes (can be formed from tryptophan)	Constituent of two coenzymes in oxidation-reduction reactions (NAD$^+$ and NADP)	Pellagra (skin and gastrointestinal lesions, nervous, mental disorders)	Flushing, burning and tingling around neck, face, and hands
Vitamin B$_6$ (pyridoxine)	2.0	1.6	Meats, vegetables, whole-grain cereals	Coenzyme (pyridoxal phosphate) involved in amino acid and glycogen metabolism)	Irritability, convulsions, muscular twitching, dermatitis, kidney stones	None reported

TABLE 2.2—continued

Vitamin	RDA (mg) Males	RDA (mg) Females	Dietary Sources	Major Body Functions	Deficiency	Excess
Water Soluble—cont'd						
Pantothenic acid	4–7[b]	4–7[b]	Widely distributed in foods	Constituent of coenzyme A, which plays a central role in energy metabolism	Fatigue, sleep disturbances, impaired coordination, nausea	None reported
Folacin	0.2	0.2	Legumes, green vegetables, whole-wheat products	Coenzyme (reduced form) involved in transfer of single-carbon units in nucleic acid and amino acid metabolism	Anemia, gastrointestinal disturbances, diarrhea, red tongue	None reported
Vitamin B$_{12}$	0.002	0.002	Muscle meats, eggs, dairy products, (absent in plant foods)	Coenzyme involved in transfer of single-carbon units in nucleic acid metabolism	Pernicious anemia, neurologic disorders	None reported
Biotin	0.03	0.10	Legumes, vegetables, meats	Coenzymes required for fat synthesis, amino acid metabolism, and glycogen (animal starch) formation	Fatigue, depression, nausea, dermatitis, muscular pains	None reported
Vitamin C (ascorbic acid)	60[c]	60	Citrus fruits, tomatoes, green peppers, salad greens	Maintains intercellular matrix of cartilage, bone, and dentine. Important in collagen synthesis.	Scurvy (degeneration of skin, teeth, blood vessels, epithelial hemorrhages)	Relatively nontoxic. Possibility of kidney stones

Recommended Dietary Allowances. Revised 1989. Food & Nutrition Board, National Academy of Sciences-National Research Council, Washington, D.C.

[a]0.005 mg for adults 25 and older.

[b]Because there is less information on which to base allowances, these figures are given in the form of ranges.

[c]100 for adults who smoke.

and the vitamin A-precursor, β-carotene, serve important protective functions. These antioxidant vitamins protect the plasma membrane by reacting with and removing the free radicals, thus quenching the chain reaction. Maintaining a diet that provides appropriate levels of the antioxidant vitamins, especially vitamin C and β-carotene, is linked to a reduced risk of several types of cancers,[31, 118] whereas a normal to above-normal intake of vitamin E and β-carotene and/or serum levels of carotenoids may blunt the progression of coronary artery narrowing and reduce heart attack risk.[54a, 59, 76, 98, 119] One proposed mechanism for heart disease protection is that the ingestion of antioxidant vitamins prevents oxidation of LDL cholesterol and its subsequent uptake into the foam cells embedded in the arterial wall. It is the oxidation of LDL cholesterol—a process similar to butter turning rancid—that contributes to the plaque-forming, artery-clogging process of atherosclerosis.

In fact, recent research shows that the reduction of heart disease risk in menopausal women who receive estrogen supplements may lie in this hormone's antioxidant properties for blunting the oxidation of LDL cholesterol.[104] An additional benefit of vitamin E is that it may protect against heart disease and stroke by preventing the formation of blood clots via the anticoagulant properties of a natural by-product of vitamin E's metabolism.

Exercise, Free Radicals, and Antioxidants. Although the beneficial effects of physical activity are well known, the potential for possible negative effects is currently being reviewed in the literature.[62] This potential is based on the reasoning that the elevated aerobic metabolism in exercise increases the production of free radicals. (In humans, free radical production and tissue damage are not directly measured but rather inferred via markers of free radical by-products.) This possibly could overwhelm the body's natural defenses and pose a health risk due to an increased level of oxidative stress.[58, 63, 120] The opposing position is that while free radical production may increase during exercise, the body's normal antioxidant defenses are either adequate[126] or are concomitantly improved as natural enzymatic defenses are "upregulated" through training adaptations.[1, 23] This latter position is supported by research showing the beneficial effects of regular exercise on the incidence of various forms of cancer and heart disease, the occurrence of which has been linked to oxidative stress.

Reactive oxygen or free radicals can be produced during exercise in at least two ways. The first is via an electron leak in the mitochondria, probably at the cytochrome level where superoxide radicals are produced. The second is during alterations in blood flow and oxygen supply—underperfusion often occurs during intense exercise and is then followed by reperfusion in the recovery period. Some argue that the potential for free radical damage may be increased during trauma, stress, muscle damage, and exercise and by environmental pollutants such as smog. With exercise, the risk seems to depend on intensity and the individual's state of training, because exhaustive exercise by untrained individ-uals is more likely to produce oxidative damage in the active muscles. The questions that arise are (*a*) whether physically active individuals are more prone to free-radical damage and (*b*) whether protective agents with antioxidant properties are required in increased quantities in physically active individuals.

In answer to the first question, recent research suggests that for well-nourished humans, the natural defenses of the body are adequate for its protection.[126] Although a single bout of submaximal exercise increased oxidant production, the natural antioxidant defenses coped effectively. Even when repeated bouts of exercise were performed on consecutive days, various indices of oxidative stress indicated that the body's antioxidant system was not depleted. The answer to the second question is equivocal. *Limited research suggests that vitamin E may be the most important antioxidant related to exercise.*[39, 90]

Research revealed that vitamin E-deficient animals began an exercise program with plasma membrane function compromised from oxidative damage and thus reached exhaustion earlier than animals with normal levels of vitamin E. In animals who received a normal diet, vitamin E supplements appeared to diminish oxidative damage caused by exercise in certain muscle fiber types.[39] Limited evidence in humans suggests a possible benefit from vitamin E supplementation.[90, 102] The effects of 3 weeks of a daily 200-mg vitamin E supplement on pentane elimination are listed in Figure 2.2 (pentane is a primary marker of free radical production). As can be seen, free radical production was dramatically reduced in the vitamin E-supplemented trials. In humans who received a daily antioxidant vitamin mixture of β-carotene, ascorbic acid, and α-tocopherol, serum and breath markers of lipid peroxidation were lower at rest and following exercise than in those who did not receive supple-

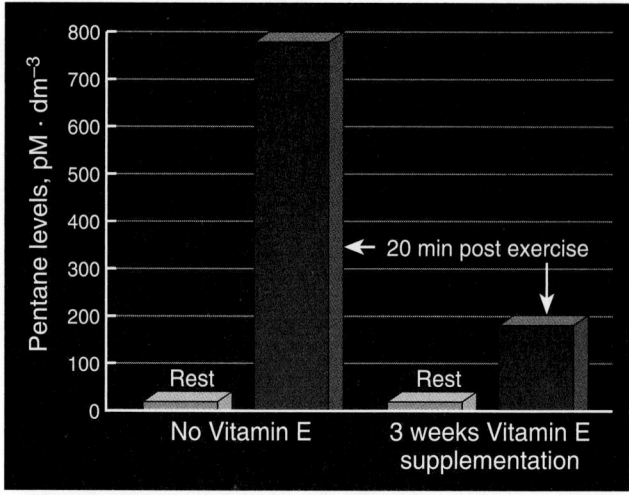

FIGURE 2.2

Pentane levels before and after 20 minutes of exercise at 100% $\dot{V}O_2$max; with and without vitamin E supplementation. (Adapted from Pincemail, J., et al.: Pentane measurement in man as an index of lipoperoxidation. *Bioelectronchem. Bioenerg.*, 18:117, 1987.)

ments.[63] Five months of α-tocopherol supplementation in racing cyclists had a protective effect on markers of oxidative stress induced by extreme endurance exercise.

Research on the antioxidant effects of selenium and coenzyme-Q_{10} is not well defined. Selenium (and other minerals such as copper, manganese, and zinc) may possess antioxidant properties due to its incorporation within the structure of glutathione peroxidase and other enzymes.[123] However, the occurrence of a selenium deficiency in humans is quite rare. Coenzyme-Q_{10} is believed to act as an antioxidant either by itself within the respiratory chain or as a recycler of vitamin E. There is little evidence that this substance has the same direct antioxidant effect as vitamin E. Whereas vitamin C is known as a strong antioxidant, its effect in exercise is less well known. Although there is some evidence that supplements of various antioxidant compounds can blunt exercise-induced free radical formation or augment the body's natural defense system, more research will be forthcoming in this important area.[31, 38, 58, 63] A prudent recommendation is consumption of a well-balanced diet that contains fruits, grains, and vegetables. Rich dietary sources of antioxidants include the following:

- **β-Carotene** (best known of the pigmented compounds, or carotenoids, that give color to yellow and green leafy vegetables): carrots; dark-green leafy vegetables such as spinach, broccoli, turnips, beet and collard greens; sweet potatoes; winter squash; apricots; cantaloupe; mangos; papaya.
- **Vitamin C:** citrus fruits and juices, cabbage, broccoli, turnip greens, cantaloupe.
- **Vitamin E:** vegetable oils, wheat germ, whole-grain bread and cereals, dried beans, green leafy vegetables.

VITAMIN SUPPLEMENTS: THE COMPETITIVE EDGE?

Vitamins synthesized in the laboratory are no less effective for bodily functions than vitamins from natural sources. Although vitamin supplements can reverse the symptoms of vitamin deficiency, once a deficiency is cured, supplements do not further improve a normal status. In addition, more than 40 years of research has not supported the use of vitamin supplements to improve exercise performance or the ability to participate in arduous training in nutritionally adequate healthy people.[8, 9, 73, 124] When vitamin intake is at recommended levels, supplements neither improve exercise performance nor necessarily increase the blood levels of these nutrients.[127] The facts have become clouded by the "testimonials" of coaches and elite athletes who profess that their successes were because of a particular dietary modification, which usually included specific vitamin supplements.

VITAMINS AND EXERCISE PERFORMANCE

As noted previously, many vitamins serve as coenzyme components or precursors of coenzymes that regulate energy metabolism. Figure 2.3 illustrates that the B-complex vitamins play key roles as coenzymes in important energy-yielding reactions during carbohydrate, lipid, and protein catabolism. They also contribute to hemoglobin synthesis and red blood cell production. It is tempting to speculate that an increased intake of these vitamins would enhance energy release and lead to improved physical performance. The belief that "if a little is good, more must be better" has led many coaches, athletes, fitness enthusiasts, and even some scientists to advocate the use of vitamin supplements. This approach is simply not supported by research findings or by the overwhelming majority of professional nutritionists.[91]

Supplementing the diet with vitamin B_6, an essential cofactor in glycogen and amino acid metabolism, was of no benefit to the mixture metabolized by women during intense aerobic exercise.[73] No exercise benefit has been shown for vitamins other than the B-complex group such as vitamins C and E. Vitamin C, for example, is a factor in the synthesis of collagen and the stress-related adrenal hormone norepinephrine. Supplements of vitamin C had negligible effects on endurance performance and on the rate, severity, and duration of injuries compared with placebo treatment.[37] However, runners who received a 600-mg daily supplement before and for 3 weeks after a 90-km ultramarathon competition experi-

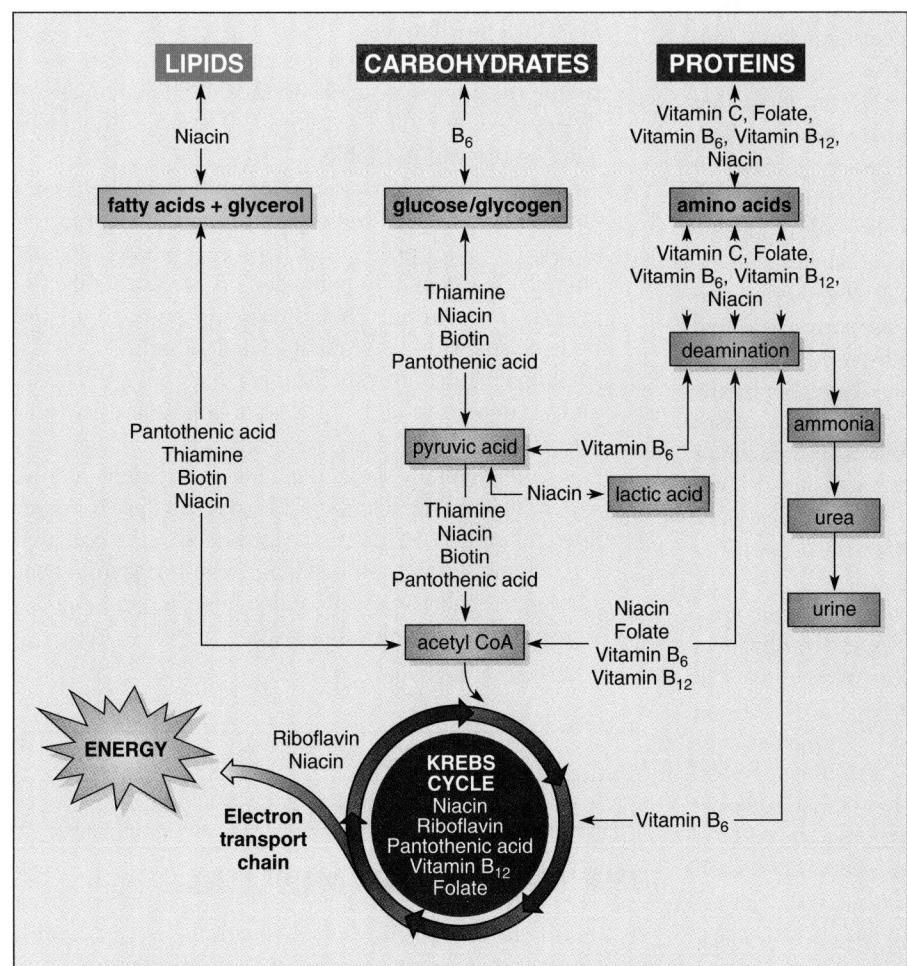

FIGURE 2.3.

General schema for the role of water-soluble vitamins in the metabolism of carbohydrates, lipids, and proteins.

enced significantly fewer symptoms of upper respiratory tract infection (running nose, sneezing, sore throat, coughing, fever) than runners who received a placebo.[89] In addition, the duration and severity of the symptoms were less in a nonrunning control group who took vitamin supplements. Interestingly, the risk of infection was inversely related to race performance, in that those who performed best suffered more symptoms. Infection was greatest in runners whose training regimens were the most strenuous.

It has never been firmly established that a deficiency state for vitamin E exists for normal individuals or that vitamin E supplements above the RDA level are beneficial to stamina, circulatory function, or energy metabolism. Chronic high-potency multivitamin-mineral supplementation for well-nourished healthy individuals was of no benefit on measures of aerobic fitness, muscular strength, and athletic performance.[112]

MEGAVITAMINS

Although physically active individuals who eat a well-balanced diet do not need to take additional vitamins, most nutritionists believe that there is little harm in taking a multivitamin capsule containing the recommended allowance of each vitamin. For some people, the psychological effects may even be beneficial. It is of great concern, however, that some athletes resort to taking **megavitamins,** or doses of at least **tenfold** and up to 1000 times the RDA, in hopes that "supercharging" with vitamins will improve exercise performance. Such a practice can be harmful, except in cases of specific serious medical illness.

Once the enzyme systems that are catalyzed by specific vitamins are saturated, the excess vitamins taken in megadose function as chemicals in the body. A megadose of water-soluble vitamin C, for example, can raise serum uric acid levels and precipitate gout in people predisposed to this disease. Also, some American blacks, Asians, and Sephardic Jews have a genetic metabolic deficiency in which excesses of vitamin C can lead to hemolytic anemia.[19] In individuals who are iron-deficient, megadoses of vitamin C may destroy significant amounts of vitamin B_{12}.[53] In healthy individuals, vitamin C supplements frequently irritate the bowel and cause diarrhea.

It is currently believed that excess vitamin B_6 may produce liver disease and nerve damage.[106] Excessive riboflavin (B_2) can impair vision, whereas a megadose of nicotinic acid inhibits the uptake of fatty acids by cardiac muscle during exercise. Possible side effects of vitamin E megadose include headache, fatigue, blurred vision, gastrointestinal disturbances, muscular weakness, and low blood sugar.[51] Because vitamin E is usually found with unsaturated fatty acids, it is difficult to "construct" a vitamin E-deficient diet. The toxicity to the nervous system of megadoses of vitamin A and the damaging effects to the kidneys of excess vitamin D have been well demonstrated.[108]

It is indeed troublesome that data from the U.S. National Health Interview Survey indicate that more than 30% of American adults use vitamin and/or mineral supplements, often at potentially toxic dosages.[125] If vitamin supplementation plays a role in physically active individuals, it may be only in those who have marginal vitamin stores. Well-controlled research is needed to fully determine whether and under what circumstances such supplementation would be beneficial. Perhaps the misuse and abuse of vitamins by individuals hoping to improve athletic performance can be put in proper perspective by the following quotation from nearly 20 years ago:[88] "The sale of vitamins is probably the biggest ripoff in our society today. Their only effect would appear to be a highly enriched sewage around athletic training or competition sites."

■ S U M M A R Y ■

1. Vitamins are organic substances that neither supply energy nor contribute to body mass. Vitamins serve crucial functions in almost all bodily processes. Vitamins must be obtained from food or dietary supplementation.
2. Vitamins are synthesized by plants and also are found in animals that produce them from precursor substances known as provitamins.
3. There are 13 known vitamins classified as either water soluble or lipid soluble. The lipid-soluble vitamins are vitamins A, D, E, and K; vitamin C and the B-complex vitamins are water soluble.
4. Excess lipid-soluble vitamins accumulate in the tissues and can increase to toxic concentrations. Except in relatively rare and specific instances, excess water-soluble vitamins are generally nontoxic and are eventually excreted in the urine. Their maximum potency for the body occurs within an 8- to 14-hour period.
5. Vitamins regulate metabolism, facilitate energy release, and are important in the process of bone and tissue synthesis.
6. Research generally shows that vitamin supplementation (above that obtained in the well-balanced diet) is not related to improved exercise performance or the potential for training. In fact, serious illness can result from consuming a regular excess of lipid-soluble and, in some instances, water-soluble vitamins.

PART 2
MINERALS

THE NATURE OF MINERALS

In addition to the organic elements carbon, oxygen, hydrogen, and nitrogen, approximately 4% of the body's mass (about 2 kg for a 50-kg woman), is composed of a group of 22 mostly metallic elements collectively called **minerals.** Most of these minerals are found in living cells although not all are essential for life. Minerals are constituents of enzymes, hormones, and vitamins; they are combined with other chemicals (for example, calcium phosphate in bone and iron in the heme of hemoglobin) or exist singularly (such as free calcium in body fluids).

In the body, minerals are classified as **major minerals** (required in amounts of more than 100 mg daily) and minor or **trace minerals** (required in amounts of less than 100 mg daily). The total quantity of the body's trace minerals is less than 15 g (or approximately 0.5 oz). Any excess minerals are useless to the body and even may be toxic. RDAs have been established for many minerals; it is believed that if the re-

quirements are met for these and other nutrients, then the remaining minerals can be obtained in adequate amounts.

Most minerals, major or trace, occur freely in nature—mainly in the waters of rivers, lakes, and oceans, in topsoil, and beneath the earth's surface. Minerals can be found in the root systems of plants and in the body structure of animals that consume plants and water containing minerals. Absorption of minerals takes place in the small intestine.

KINDS AND SOURCES OF MINERALS

The important minerals and their functions, food sources, and daily requirements are listed in Table 2.3. As with vita-

---

TABLE 2.3
THE IMPORTANT MAJOR AND MINOR (TRACE) MINERALS FOR HEALTHY ADULTS (19 TO 50 YEARS OF AGE) AND THEIR DIETARY REQUIREMENTS, FOOD SOURCES, FUNCTIONS, AND THE EFFECTS OF DEFICIENCIES AND EXCESSES

Mineral	RDA Males and Females[a] (mg)	Dietary Sources	Major Body Functions	Deficiency	Excess
Major					
Calcium	1200[b] 1200	Milk, cheese dark green vegetables, dried legumes	Bone and tooth formation Blood clotting Nerve transmission	Stunted growth Rickets, osteoporosis Convulsions	Not reported in humans
Phosphorus	1200[b] 1200	Milk, cheese, yogurt, meat, poultry, grains, fish	Bone and tooth formation Acid-base balance	Weakness, demineralization of bone Loss of calcium	Erosion of jaw (phossy jaw)
Potassium	2000	Leafy vegetables, cantelope, lima beans, potatoes, bananas, milk, meats, coffee, tea	Fluid balance Nerve transmission Acid-base balance	Muscle cramps Irregular cardiac rhythm Mental confusion Loss of appetite Can be life-threatening	None if kidneys function normally Poor kidney function causes potassium buildup and cardiac arrythmias
Sulfur	Unknown	Obtained as part of dietary protein and is present in food preservatives	Acid-base balance Liver function	Unlikely to occur if dietary intake is adequate	Unknown
Sodium	1100–3300	Common salt	Acid-base balance Body water balance Nerve function	Muscle cramps Mental apathy Reduced appetite	High blood pressure
Chlorine (chloride)	700	Chloride is part of salt-containing food Some vegetables and fruits	Important part of extracellular fluids	Unlikely to occur if dietary intake is adequate	Along with sodium, contributes to high blood pressure
Magnesium	350 280	Whole grains, green leafy vegetables	Activates enzymes Involved in protein synthesis	Growth failure Behavioral disturbances	Diarrhea

TABLE 2.3—continued

Mineral	RDA Males and Females[a] (mg)	Dietary Sources	Major Body Functions	Deficiency	Excess
Minor					
Iron	10 / 15	Eggs, lean meats, legumes, whole grains, green leafy vegetables	Constituent of hemoglobin and enzymes involved in energy metabolism	Iron deficiency anemia (weakness; reduced resistance to infection)	Siderosis Cirrhosis of liver
Fluorine	1.5–4.0	Drinking water, tea, seafood	May be important in maintenance of bone structure	Higher frequency of tooth decay	Mottling of teeth, increased bone density Neurologic disturbances
Zinc	15 / 12	Widely distributed in foods	Constituent of enzymes involved in digestion	Growth failure Small sex glands	Fever, nausea, vomiting, diarrhea
Copper	1.5–3.0[c] / 1.5–3.0	Meats, drinking water	Constituent of enzymes associated with iron metabolism	Anemia, bone changes (rare in humans)	Rare metabolic condition (Wilson's disease)
Selenium	0.070 / 0.055	Seafood, meat, grains	Functions in close association with vitamin E	Anemia (rare)	Gastrointestinal disorders, lung irritation
Iodine (Iodide)	150	Marine fish and shellfish, dairy products, vegetables, iodized salt	Constituent of thyroid hormones	Goiter (enlarged thyroid)	Very high intakes depress thyroid activity
Chromium	0.075–0.25[c] / 0.05–0.25[c]	Legumes, cereals, organ meats	Constituent of some enzymes	Not reported in humans	Inhibition of enzymes
		Fats, vegetable oils, meats, whole grains	Involved in glucose and energy metabolism	Impaired ability to metabolize glucose	Occupational exposures: skin and kidney damage

Recommended Dietary Allowances, Revised 1989. Food and Nutrition Board, National Academy of Sciences-National Research Council, Washington, D.C.

[a]First values are for males; second values are for females.

[b]800 mg for adults 25 and older.

[c]Because there is less information on which to base allowances, these figures are given in the form of ranges.

mins, mineral supplements generally are not needed, because most minerals are readily available in the foods we eat and the water we drink. Some supplementation may be necessary, however, in geographic regions where the soil or water supply is lacking a particular mineral. For example, in certain regions of the United States, particularly the basin of the Great Lakes and Pacific Northwest, as well as in central Brazil and the Himalayan mountain region, sources of the mineral **iodine** are relatively poor. Iodine is required by the thyroid gland to synthesize the hormones **thyroxine** and triiodothyronine, which exert an accelerating influence on the cells' resting metabolism. An iodine deficiency can easily be prevented by adding iodine to the water supply or to table salt (iodized salt).

A common mineral deficiency in this country results from a lack of iron in the diet. Between 30 and 50% of American women of childbearing age suffer some form of dietary iron insufficiency. There are two sources of iron in food: the first is the heme source in meat and animal products, particularly red meat, liver, kidney, and heart; the second is from the inorganic iron salts found in foods of plant origin such as beans, peas, dried uncooked fruits, and leafy green vegetables.

ROLE OF MINERALS IN THE BODY

Whereas vitamins activate chemical processes without becoming part of the products of the reactions they catalyze, minerals often become incorporated within the structures and existing chemicals of the body. Minerals serve three broad roles in the body:

- They provide **structure** in the formation of bones and teeth.
- In terms of **function,** they are intimately involved in maintaining normal heart rhythm, muscular contractility, neural conductivity, and the acid-base balance of the body.
- They play crucial roles in the **regulation** of cellular metabolism by serving as important parts of enzymes and hormones that modulate cellular activity.

Various minerals that participate in catabolic and anabolic cellular processes are shown in Figure 2.4. Minerals are important in activating the numerous reactions that release energy during the breakdown of carbohydrates, lipids, and proteins. In addition to these processes of catabolism, minerals are essential for the synthesis of biologic nutrients—glycogen from glucose, lipids from fatty acids and glycerol, and proteins from amino acids. Without the essential minerals, the fine balance between catabolism and anabolism would be disrupted. Minerals also form important constituents of hormones. For example, an inadequate thyroxine production due to iodine deficiency significantly slows the body's resting metabolism. In extreme cases, this reduced level of energy output could predispose a person to develop obesity. The synthesis of insulin, the hormone that facilitates glucose uptake by the cells, requires the mineral zinc (as do about 100 other enzymes), whereas the digestive acid hydrochloric acid is formed from the mineral chlorine. In the subsequent sections, specific functions are described for several of the more important minerals that relate to physical activity.

CALCIUM

Calcium is the most abundant mineral in the body. Calcium combines with phosphorus to form the bones and teeth. These two minerals represent approximately 75% of the body's total mineral content (about 2.5% of body mass). In its ionized form (about 1% of the body's 1200 mg of calcium), calcium is crucial for muscle action and the transmission of nerve impulses. It also activates several enzymes, is part of calcitrol, the active form of vitamin D, and is essential for blood clotting and the transport of fluids across cell membranes.

Osteoporosis: Calcium, Estrogen, and Exercise. Bone is a dynamic tissue formed from collagen and minerals and composed of about 50% water. It is in a continual state of **remodeling** in which specific bone cells (osteoclasts) cause the breakdown (resorption) of bone while bone-forming osteoblast cells cause bone synthesis. Calcium availability greatly affects the dynamics of bone remodeling. The plasma calcium level, which is regulated by hormonal action, is maintained by either calcium derived from food or from resorption of the bone mass. The two broad categories of bone are as follows:

- **Cortical bone:** dense, hard outer layer of bone, such as the shafts of the long bones of the arms and legs.
- **Trabecular bone:** spongy, less dense, and relatively weaker bone most prevalent in the vertebrae and the ball of the femur.

Although it is true that growing children need more calcium per unit body mass on a daily basis than adults, it also is clear that many adults are deficient in their intake of this mineral. As a general guideline, adolescents and young adults require 1200 mg of calcium daily (800 to 1000 mg for adults over age 24) or about as much calcium as in five 8-oz glasses of milk. In reality, however, calcium is one of the most frequently lacking nutrients in the diet. For example, more than 75% of adults consume less than the RDA, and approximately 25% of females in the United States consume less than 300 mg of calcium daily.[50] As a result of inadequate calcium intake, the body draws upon its calcium "reserve" in bone to restore the deficit. If this imbalance is prolonged, the condition of **osteoporosis** (literally meaning "porous bones") develops progressively as bone loses its mineral mass and progressively becomes porous and brittle (Fig. 2.5); bone may eventually break under the stresses of normal living.

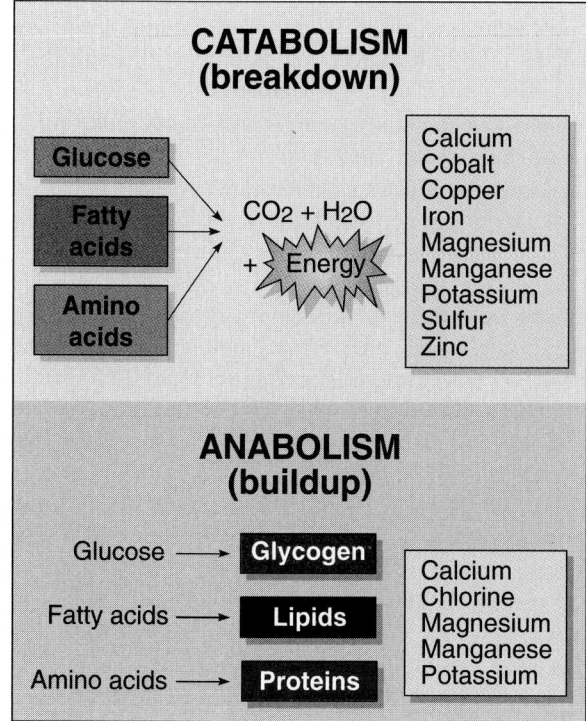

FIGURE 2.4.
Minerals are involved in the catabolism and anabolism of macronutrients.

Currently, osteoporosis afflicts about 25 million Americans; 90% of individuals with osteoporosis are women. Among older individuals, especially women over age 60, this disease has reached near-epidemic proportions. For example, osteoporosis accounts for more than 1.5 million fractures (the clinical manifestation of the disease) yearly, including about 500,000 to 600,000 spinal fractures and 250,000 hip fractures. The increased susceptibility to osteoporosis among older women is closely associated with the marked decrease in estrogen secretion that accompanies menopause.[85, 94] Exactly how estrogen exerts its protective effect on bone is not known; however, estrogen is believed to enhance calcium absorption and limit its withdrawal from bone. The major reason for the significantly lower prevalence of osteoporosis among men is that men normally produce a significant amount of estrogen. In addition, some circulating testosterone is converted into estrogen, which also promotes positive calcium balance—the overwhelming majority of men have adequate testosterone levels throughout life.

A Progressive Disease. With proper nutrition and increased levels of physical activity, women normally continue to show gains in bone mass throughout the third decade of life, although the prime bone-building years are the early teens.[93] In reality, osteoporosis begins early in life for many women because the average teenager consumes suboptimal calcium to support growing bones. This imbalance worsens into adulthood, and by middle age, adult women consume only about one-third of the calcium they require for optimal bone maintenance. Beginning around age 50, the average man experiences bone loss of about 0.4% each year, whereas the female begins to lose twice this amount at age 35. For men, the normal rate of bone mineral loss does not usually pose a problem until the eighth decade

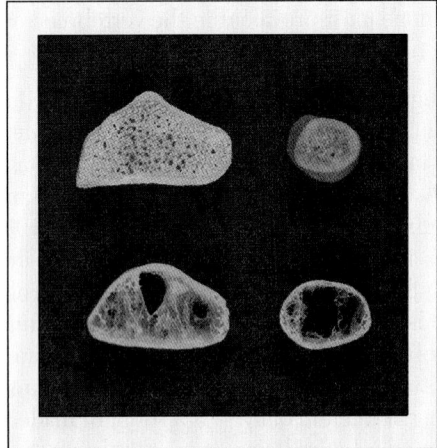

FIGURE 2.5.
Normal radius and ulna (*top*), and radius and ulna in a patient with bone loss due to osteoporosis (*bottom*). (Photos courtesy of Dr. Lisbeth Nilas, Department of Clinical Chemistry, Glostrup Hospital, Glostrup, Denmark.)

of life. Women, however, become highly susceptible to osteoporosis at menopause. At this time, there is little or no release of estrogen from the ovaries, although some estrogen continues to be produced by muscle, adipose tissue, and connective tissue. The dramatic fall in estrogen production at menopause coincides with reduced intestinal calcium absorption, decreased production of calcitonin (a hormone that inhibits bone demineralization), and an increase in bone resorption. Under these conditions, bone loss accelerates to 3 to 6% per year in the 5 years after menopause; the rate then drops to approximately 1% yearly. At this rate, the typical woman will lose about 15% of her bone mass in the first decade after menopause; for some women, a loss of as much as 30% of bone mineral mass is observed by age 70.[114]

Certain characteristics or risk factors can indicate a predisposition to osteoporosis. These include white or Asian heritage, female sex, slight build or a tendency to be underweight, sedentary lifestyle, early menopause, cigarette and alcohol abuse, poor or calcium-deficient diet in the years before and after menopause, and family history of osteoporosis.

Prevention. *A prime defense against bone loss with age is adequate calcium intake throughout life.*[61, 93, 97] Increasing the calcium intake of adolescent girls from the current 80% of the RDA level to the 110% level through supplementation significantly increased total body calcium and spinal bone density.[69] Many experts recommend an increase in calcium intake for middle-aged women to between 1200 and 1500 mg per day, especially for estrogen-deprived women after menopause to ensure a positive calcium balance later in life.[49, 95, 117] This added calcium seems to be beneficial in slowing the rate of bone loss despite the absence of adequate estrogen.[95]

Good calcium sources include milk and milk products, sardines and canned salmon, kidney beans, and dark green leafy vegetables. Calcium supplements also can help to correct dietary deficiencies regardless of whether the extra calcium comes from supplements (calcium citrate is readily absorbed) or food products. Adequate availability of vitamin D facilitates calcium uptake, whereas excessive consumption of meat, salt, coffee, and alcohol inhibits its absorption. In postmenopausal women, estrogen supplements or low-dose, slow-release fluoride-plus-calcium supplements serve as a treatment for severe osteoporosis. Estrogen therapy must be continued for prolonged periods, thus increasing the risk for cancers of the uterus, breast, and other organs. Therefore, hormone treatment for osteoporosis is often viewed as a more dramatic approach.

Exercise Is Helpful. *Regular exercise helps slow the rate of aging of the skeleton.* Regardless of age, children and adults who maintain an active lifestyle have significantly greater bone mass compared with their sedentary counterparts,[42, 43, 54, 80, 109] and this benefit is maintained into the seventh and even eighth decade of life![115, 121] In fact, the decline in vigorous exercise with the sedentary lifestyle associated with advancing age closely parallels the age-related loss of

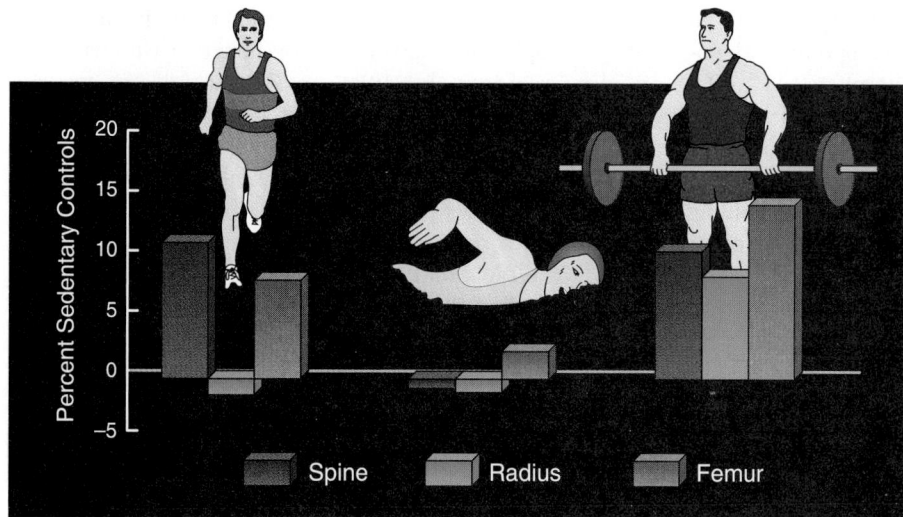

FIGURE 2.6
Bone mineral density as a percentage of sedentary control values at three skeletal sites for runners, swimmers, and weight lifters. (Adapted from Drinkwater, B.L.: Physical activity, fitness, and osteoporosis. In *Physical Activity, Fitness, and Health.* Edited by C. Bouchard, et al. Champaign, IL, Human Kinetics, 1994.)

bone mass. Exercise provides a safe and potent stimulus to maintain and even increase bone mass in adults, although it is not as effective as hormone replacement therapy in preventing bone loss in the early postmenopausal period.[2] As illustrated in Figure 2.6, exercise of a weight-bearing nature is especially beneficial, including walking, running, dancing, skipping rope, or activities such as heavy-resistance exercises and circuit-resistance training, in which significant muscle force is generated against the long bones of the body.[29, 46, 121a, 129] Even walking as little as 1 mile per day is beneficial for women in maintaining bone mass during and after menopause. Men and women participating in muscular strength and power activities have equal or higher bone mass than endurance-type athletes.[101a] In fact, bone mineral density is related to measures of muscular strength and regional lean tissue mass;[81] the lumbar spine and proximal femur bone mass of elite teenage weight lifters is greater than representative values for fully mature bone of reference adults.[20]

In a normal hormonal milieu, muscle forces (mechanical loading) acting on specific bones during physical activity modify bone metabolism at the point of stress.[25, 34, 42, 55a, 68a] For example, the lower limb bones of older cross-country runners have greater bone mineral content compared with the bones of their less active counterparts. Likewise, the playing arm of tennis players and the throwing arm of baseball players show greater bone thickness compared with the less-used, nondominant arm. The prevailing theory considers bone to behave as a piezoelectric crystal that converts mechanical stress into electrical energy. The electrical changes created when bone is mechanically stressed stimulate the activity of osteoblasts that leads to calcium buildup. The quantity of bone buildup depends on both the magnitude of the force as well as its frequency of application. Chemicals produced in bone itself may also contribute to bone formation.

Five Principles for Planning Exercise to Promote Bone Health[21, 29]

- **Specificity:** exercise provides a local osteogenic effect.
- **Overload:** there must be a progressive increase in the intensity of the exercise for continued improvement.
- **Initial values:** individuals with the smallest total bone mass have the greatest potential for improvement.
- **Diminishing returns:** as the biologic ceiling for bone density is approached, greater effort is required to obtain further gain.
- **Reversibility:** the positive osteogenic effects of exercise on bone are lost by discontinuing the exercise program (overload).

Is Too Much Training Harmful?   An apparent paradox between exercise and bone dynamics has been noted for premenopausal women who train intensely and reduce body mass and body fat to a point at which the menstrual cycle actually ceases, a condition termed **secondary amenorrhea.**[24] The cessation of menstruation may remove estrogen's protective effect on bone and makes young women more vulnerable to calcium loss with concomitant decrease in bone mass.[14, 40, 54, 74a] Concurrently, nutritional factors (e.g., low protein, lipid, and energy intake) magnify the problem. If amenorrhea persists, then the benefits of exercise on bone mass would be negated and the risk of musculoskeletal injuries during exercise would increase as osteoporosis sets in at an early age.[78] A disturbing factor is that if the normal menses is reestablished, some bone mass is regained but does not appear to reach levels attained by those women who have maintained normal menses.[30]

PHOSPHORUS

Besides its important function in combining with calcium to form hydroxyapatite and calcium phosphate—compounds that give rigidity to bones and teeth—phosphorus is an essential component of the high-energy compounds adenosine triphosphate (ATP) and creatine phosphate (CP). ATP is crucial in supplying the energy for all forms of biologic work. Phosphorus combines with lipids to form phospholipid compounds, which are integral to the bilayer of the cell's plasma membrane. The phosphorus-containing phosphatase enzymes help regulate cellular metabolism; phosphorus also participates in the buffering of the acid end products of energy metabolism. For this latter reason, some coaches and trainers recommend the consumption of special "phosphate drinks" to reduce the effects of acid production in heavy exercise and perhaps to enhance oxygen release from red blood cells.[16a] In Chapter 23, the usefulness of buffering drinks for augmenting exercise performance is discussed in more detail.

MAGNESIUM

Magnesium is present in about 300 enzymes that regulate metabolic processes. It plays a vital role in glucose metabolism by facilitating the formation of muscle and liver glycogen from blood-borne glucose. Magnesium also participates as a cofactor in the breakdown of glucose, fatty acids, and amino acids during energy metabolism. Furthermore, magnesium is important in the synthesis of lipids and proteins and in stabilizing the neuromuscular system in terms of nerve conduction and muscle action.

IRON

Between 3 and 5 g (about ⅙ oz) of iron is normally contained in the body. Of this iron, approximately 80% is in functionally active compounds, predominantly combined with **hemoglobin** in the red blood cells.[11] This iron-protein compound increases the oxygen-carrying capacity of blood approximately 65 times. Iron serves other important exercise-related functions aside from its role in oxygen transport by red blood cells. It is a structural component of **myoglobin** (about 5% of total iron), a compound similar to hemoglobin that aids in the storage and transport of oxygen within the muscle cell. Small amounts of iron are also present in specialized substances called **cytochromes,** which facilitate energy transfer within the cell. About 20% of the body's iron is not combined in functionally active compounds; this constitutes the iron stores located in the liver, spleen, and bone marrow as **hemosiderin** and **ferritin.** It is these stores that replenish iron lost from the functional compounds and provide the iron reserve during periods of insufficient dietary intake. Another plasma protein **(transferrin)** transports iron from ingested food and damaged red blood cells and delivers it to tissues in need. Plasma levels of this compound tend to reflect the adequacy of the current iron intake.

Athletes should include iron-rich foods in their daily diets. People with inadequate iron intake or who have limited rates of iron absorption or high rates of iron loss can develop a condition in which there is a reduced concentration of hemoglobin in red blood cells. This extreme condition of iron insufficiency, commonly called **iron-deficiency anemia,** is characterized by general sluggishness, loss of appetite, and a reduced capacity to sustain even mild exercise.[36, 107] With "iron therapy," both the hemoglobin content of the blood and the exercise response can be returned to normal levels.[67] The recommendations for iron intake for children and adults are listed in Table 2.4.

Females: A Population at Risk. Inadequate iron intake frequently occurs among young children, teenagers, and females of childbearing age, including physically active women.[16a, 17, 92a] Moderate iron-deficiency anemia is common during pregnancy, when there is an increased demand for iron for both mother and fetus. In addition, females usually lose between 5 and 45 mg of iron during menstruation.

The additional 5 mg of iron required daily for premenopausal females compared to males increases the average monthly iron intake by approximately 150 mg. Because between 10 and 15% of the ingested iron is absorbed (depending on iron status, form of iron, and composition of the meal), an additional 20 to 25 mg of iron would be available in females each month for the synthesis of red blood cells lost during menstruation. When this added iron requirement for the female is combined with the fact that the normal American diet contains only about 6 mg of iron in each 1000 calories of food ingested, it is not surprising that 30 to 50% of American women have significant dietary iron insufficiencies.

TABLE 2.4
RECOMMENDED DIETARY ALLOWANCES FOR IRON

	Age	Iron (mg)
Children	1–10	10
Males	11–18	12
	19	10
Females	11–50	15
	51	10
	Pregnant	30[a]
	Lactating	15[a]

Recommended Dietary Allowances, Revised 1989, Food and Nutrition Board, National Academy of Sciences-National Research Council, Washington, D.C.
[a]Generally, this increased requirement cannot be met by ordinary diets; therefore, the use of 30 to 60 mg of supplemental iron is recommended.

Source of Iron is Important. Whereas intestinal absorption of iron varies closely with iron need, considerable variation in absorption occurs in relation to the diet's composition. For example, usually only between 2 and 10% of iron from plants (ferric or nonheme iron) is absorbed, whereas 10 to 35% of animal (ferrous or heme) iron is absorbed. The presence of heme iron also increases the absorption or bioavailability of iron from nonheme sources. In fact, meat supplements are more effective in maintaining iron status in exercising women than commercially prepared iron supplements.[72]

The relatively low bioavailability of nonheme iron places women on vegetarian diets at risk for developing iron insufficiency. This is supported by data from vegetarian female runners who had a poorer iron status than their counterparts who consumed the same quantity of iron from predominantly animal sources.[116] This problem can be alleviated somewhat by including foods rich in vitamin C in the diet, because ascorbic acid increases the solubility of nonheme iron and makes it available for absorption at the alkaline pH of the intestine. The ascorbic acid in one glass of orange juice, for example, stimulates a threefold increase in nonheme iron absorption from a breakfast meal.[103] Heme sources of iron include beef, beef liver, pork, tuna, and clams; nonheme sources are oatmeal, dried figs, spinach, beans, and lentils.

Exercise-Induced Anemia: Fact or Fiction? Because of the great interest in endurance sports combined with the increased participation of women in such activities, research has focused on the influence of hard training on the body's iron status.[82, 86] The term "sports anemia" is frequently used to describe reductions in hemoglobin to levels approaching **clinical anemia** (12 g in women and 13 to 14 g in men per 100 mL of blood) that are believed to be due to intense training. Some researchers maintain that exercise training creates an added demand for iron that outstrips its intake.[17] As a result, iron reserves are taxed, which eventually leads to a fall in hemoglobin levels and/or a reduction in iron-containing compounds within the cell's energy transfer system.[10, 26] Of concern is the possibility that individuals susceptible to "iron drain" may ultimately experience a reduced capacity for exercise due to the crucial role of iron in both oxygen transport and use.

It is postulated that heavy training creates an augmented iron demand because of a loss of iron in sweat[67] or because of the loss of hemoglobin in urine due to the actual destruction of red blood cells with increased temperature, spleen activity, and circulation rates, as well as from mechanical trauma caused by pounding of the feet on the running surface.[33, 84] In addition, gastrointestinal bleeding that is unrelated to age, sex, or performance time may occur after long-distance running.[13, 74, 100] Any such iron loss would certainly stress the body's iron reserves for the daily synthesis of more than 260 billion new red blood cells in the bone

marrow of the skull, upper arm, sternum, ribs, spine, pelvis, and upper leg.[77] This loss would be particularly significant to women, who have the greatest requirement and lowest intake of iron.

To support the possibility of exercise-induced anemia, some data indicate that suboptimal hemoglobin concentration and hematocrit are more prevalent among endurance athletes.[55] On closer scrutiny, it appears that reductions in hemoglobin concentration are transient, occurring in the early phase of training and then returning toward pretraining values.[35] This general response for hematologic variables is illustrated in Figure 2.7 for high-school female cross-country runners during a competitive season.[92] It is noteworthy that the decrease in hemoglobin concentration generally parallels the disproportionately large expansion in plasma volume in relation to total hemoglobin with training. For example, just 4 days of exercise training increased plasma volume by 20%, whereas the total volume of red blood cells remained unchanged.[41] Consequently, whereas **total** hemoglobin (an important factor in endurance performance) may remain the same or increase somewhat with training, its concentration decreases in the plasma. Despite this apparent dilution of hemoglobin, aerobic capacity and exercise performance consistently increase during training.

Although there may be some mechanical destruction of red blood cells with vigorous exercise and some loss of iron in sweat (probably minimal[12]), it has yet to be verified whether these factors are sufficient to strain an athlete's iron reserves and precipitate anemia if iron intake is normal.[7, 71] In fact, using stringent criteria for both anemia

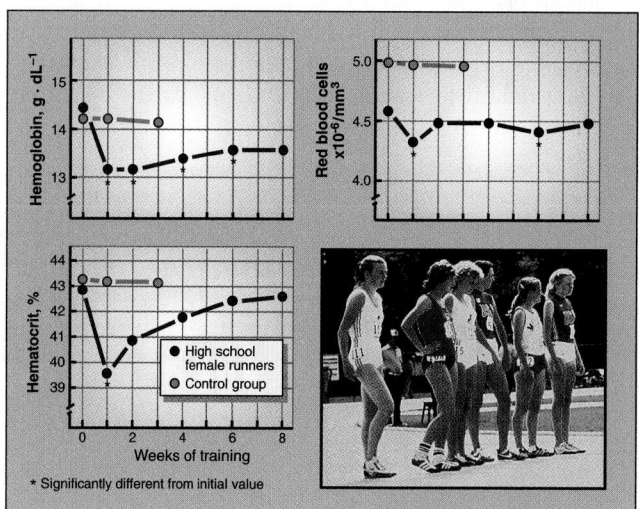

FIGURE 2.7

Hemoglobin, red blood cell count, and hematocrit in high school female cross-country runners and a comparison group during the competitive season. (Adapted from Puhl, J.L., et al.: Erythrocyte changes during training in high school women cross-country runners. *Res. Q. Exerc. Sport*, 52:484, 1981.)

and insufficiency of iron reserves, the condition of sports anemia is much less prevalent among athletes than generally believed.[128] Data from a relatively large number of female athletes indicated that the prevalence of iron-deficiency anemia did not differ in comparisons among specific athletic groups or with a nonathletic control group.[99] Because adolescent and premenopausal women have a relatively high iron requirement and because many women consume inadequate dietary iron, any increase in iron loss with training could strain an already limited iron reserve. This does not mean that all athletes in training should take supplementary iron or that all indications of sports anemia are the result of an iron intake deficiency or iron loss. It does suggest, however, that the iron status of athletes should at least be monitored. This is best achieved by periodic evaluation of both hematological characteristics as well as iron reserves. These reserves are indirectly indicated by measuring serum ferritin concentration;[18] values below $20 \ \mu g \cdot L^{-1}$ for females and $30 \ \mu g \cdot L^{-1}$ for males indicate depleted iron reserves.

In an individual whose diet contains the recommended iron intake, iron supplementation does not cause an increase in hemoglobin or hematocrit or other measures of iron status.[48, 87] Even in instances of mild iron insufficiency without anemia, iron supplementation and improved iron reserve status may not enhance exercise capacity or aerobic performance.[64, 79] When supplements are administered, they should not be used indiscriminately, because excessive iron can accumulate to toxic levels in the body and contribute significantly to diabetes, liver disease, and heart and joint damage. Additionally, there is current controversy regarding whether men with high levels of body iron stores are at higher risk for coronary heart disease than men with iron levels in the low normal range.[105, 110] If this risk exists, the possible explanation is that high serum iron may catalyze free radical formation, which augments the oxidation of LDL cholesterol, thus promoting the process of atherosclerosis.

SODIUM, POTASSIUM, AND CHLORINE

The minerals sodium, potassium, and chlorine are collectively termed **electrolytes** because they are dissolved in the body as electrically charged particles called ions. Sodium and chlorine are the chief minerals in blood plasma and extracellular fluid. A major function of these electrolytes is to modulate fluid exchange within the body's various fluid compartments. This allows for a constant, well-regulated exchange of nutrients and waste products between the cell and its external fluid environment. Potassium is the chief intracellular mineral.

Perhaps the most important function of sodium and potassium is their role in establishing the proper electrical gradient across cell membranes. This electrical difference between the interior and exterior of the cell is required for the transmission of nerve impulses, for the stimulation and action of muscle, and for the proper functioning of glands. Electrolytes are also important in maintaining the permeability of the plasma membrane and regulating the acid and base qualities of body fluids, especially blood. Values considered normal for electrolyte concentrations in blood serum and sweat, as well as the electrolyte and carbohydrate concentrations of some common oral rehydration beverages, are presented in Table 2.5.

Sodium: How Much is Enough? Normally, if sodium intake is low, the hormone **aldosterone** acts on the kidneys to conserve sodium. With high sodium intake, the excess is excreted in the urine. Consequently, salt balance is maintained at normal levels throughout a wide range of intakes. This is not the case for certain susceptible individuals, and excessive sodium intake is inadequately regulated. This intake contributes to an increase fluid volume and elevates

TABLE 2.5
ELECTROLYTE CONCENTRATIONS IN BLOOD SERUM AND SWEAT, AND CARBOHYDRATE AND ELECTROLYTE CONCENTRATIONS OF SOME COMMON BEVERAGES

Substance	Na^+ $(mEq \cdot L^{-1})$	K^+ $(mEq \cdot L^{-1})$	Ca^{2+} $(mEq \cdot L^{-1})$	Mg^{2+} $(mEq \cdot L^{-1})$	Cl^- $(mEq \cdot L^{-1})$	Osmolality $(mOsm \cdot L^{-1})$	CHO $(g \cdot L^{-1})$
Blood serum	140	4.5	2.5	1.5–2.1	110	300	—
Sweat	60–80	4.5	1.5	3.3	40–90	170–220	—
Coca-Cola	3.0	—	—	—	1.0	650	107
Gatorade	23.0	3.0	—	—	14.0	280	62
Fruit juice	0.5	58.0	—	—	—	690	118
Pepsi-Cola	1.7	Trace	—	—	Trace	568	81
Water	Trace	Trace	—	—	Trace	10–20	—

blood pressure to levels that may pose a health risk. Sodium-induced hypertension occurs in about one-third of individuals with hypertension. In the United States, sodium intake regularly exceeds the recommended level for adults of between 1100 and 3300 mg per day, or the amount of sodium in 0.5 to 1.5 teaspoons of salt (approximately 40% of table salt is sodium). In fact, for the person consuming the typical Western diet, approximately 4500 mg of sodium or 8 to 12 g of salt is ingested daily. This value is 10 times the 500 mg of sodium that the body actually needs. This high sodium intake is primarily due to the heavy reliance on table salt in processing, curing, cooking, seasoning, and storing foods. Aside from table salt, common sodium-rich dietary sources are monosodium glutamate (MSG), soy sauce, condiments, canned foods, baking soda, and baking powder.

For decades, one low-risk, first-line defense in treating high blood pressure was to eliminate excess sodium from the diet. Sodium is so widely distributed naturally in foods that it is easy to obtain the daily requirement without adding salt. By reducing sodium intake, it is believed that sodium and fluid in the body will be reduced, thereby lowering blood pressure. If dietary constraints are ineffective, drugs that induce a water loss (diuretics) are the next line of defense. In addition to reducing sodium and fluid in the body, however, diuretics also cause a loss in other minerals, particularly potassium. For a patient using diuretics, a potassium-rich diet is a necessity. Although the effectiveness of sodium restriction for controlling hypertension in the general population is presently debated among medical specialists, it does seem that certain individuals are "salt sensitive;" when dietary sodium is reduced, they respond favorably in terms of lowering blood pressure.

MINERALS AND EXERCISE PERFORMANCE

There is no evidence that supplementation benefits exercise performance for normal individuals receiving the RDA of minerals. An important consequence of prolonged exercise, especially in hot weather, is the loss of water and mineral salts, primarily sodium and some potassium chloride, in sweating. Excessive water and electrolyte losses impair heat tolerance and exercise performance and can lead to severe dysfunction in the form of heat cramps, heat exhaustion, or heat stroke. The yearly number of heat-related deaths during spring and summer football practice provides a tragic illustration of the importance of fluid and electrolyte replacement. It is not uncommon during practice or a game for an athlete to lose between 1 and 5 kg of water due to sweating. This fluid loss corresponds to a depletion of 1.5 to 8.0 g of salt, because each kilogram (1 L) of sweat generally contains about 1.5 g of salt. The crucial and immediate need in these situations is replacement of the water lost through sweating.

Chronic mineral supplementation does not enhance physical performance in well-nourished, active individuals.[122]

Vigorous exercise triggers a rapid and coordinated release of the hormones vasopressin, renin, and aldosterone, which reduce sodium and water loss through the kidneys.[27] Sodium conservation by the kidneys is increased, even under extreme conditions such as marathon running in warm weather, during which sweat output may be as much as 2 L per hour. Any electrolytes that are lost usually can be replenished by adding a slight amount of salt to the fluid ingested or to the normal daily food intake. In one study of runners during a 20-day road race in Hawaii, plasma minerals were maintained at normal levels when the athletes consumed an unrestricted diet without mineral supplements.[28] This and other findings indicate that ingesting so-called athletic drinks is of no special benefit in replacing the minerals lost through sweating compared with ingesting a well-balanced diet.[60] In fact, research shows that most individuals unconsciously consume more salt when the need exists. For fluid losses in excess of 4 or 5 kg and for prolonged activity in the heat, salt supplements may be necessary and can be achieved with a 0.1 to 0.2% salt solution by adding approximately 0.3 tsp of table salt per liter of water.[3] Although a potassium deficiency may occur with intense exercise during heat stress, an adequate potassium level with most exercise and training is generally ensured by consuming a diet containing normal amounts of this mineral.[22, 68] A glass of orange or tomato juice replaces almost all of the calcium, potassium, and magnesium lost in 3 L (7 lb) of sweat.

Trace Elements. Strenuous exercise may place a drain on the body's content of the trace elements chromium (necessary for carbohydrate and lipid catabolism and proper insulin function and protein synthesis), copper (required for red blood cell formation), manganese (part of superoxide dismutase in the body's antioxidant defense system), and zinc (proper enzyme function in numerous different reactions, many related to energy metabolism). In one study, urinary losses of zinc and chromium were between 1.5- and 2.0-fold higher on the day of a 6-mile run compared to a rest day.[4] In addition, sweat loss of copper and zinc can be relatively high. While such trace mineral losses do not necessarily mean that athletes should supplement these micronutrients, it is possible that for men and women with marginal micronutrient intakes any further loss with strenuous exercise needs to be replaced to prevent an overt deficiency. Because iron, zinc, and copper are highly interactive with each other and compete for the same carrier during intestinal absorption, an excessive intake of one mineral may cause a deficiency in the other. However, in one study in which collegiate football players received supplements of 200 mg of chromium picolinate for 9 weeks, no benefit was seen for augmenting changes in body composition and muscular strength during a program of intense weight lifting training compared to a control group that received a placebo.[15]

There is recent evidence that the body's stores of several of the trace minerals, particularly copper and zinc,

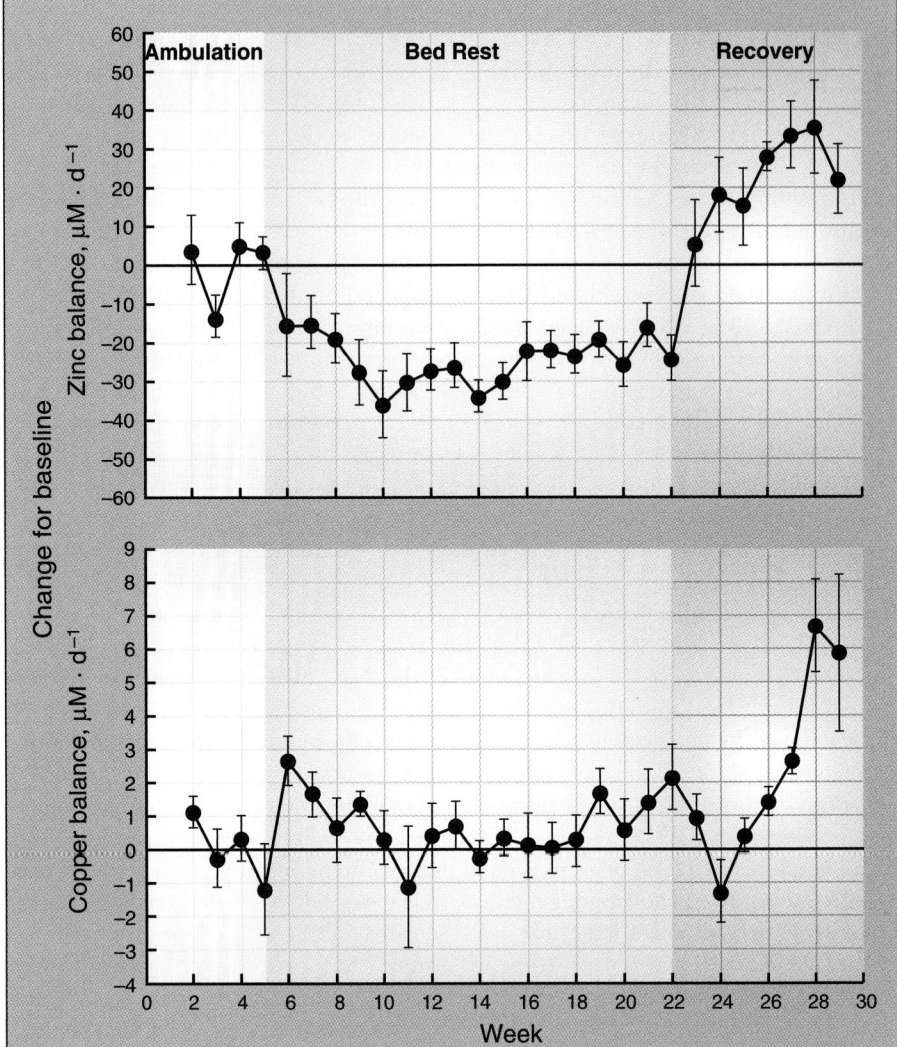

FIGURE 2.8

Changes in weekly zinc (*top*) and copper (*bottom*) balance during a 5-week control period, a 17-week period of bed rest, and a 7-week recovery period. (From Krebs, J.M., et al.: Zinc and copper balances in healthy adult males during and after 17 wk of bed rest. *Am. J. Clin. Nutr.*, 58:897, 1993.)

become depleted during a continuous period of bed rest.[66] Because about one-half of the body's copper and zinc are constituents of the muscle and bone mass,[57] excessive bed rest (and perhaps physical inactivity) could possibly cause a drain of these minerals from the body. In this regard, it becomes important to determine the dynamics of trace mineral balance during abnormal situations such as prolonged inactivity to better understand potential variations in the requirements of these elements. The time course for zinc and copper balance during a 30-week period is shown in Figure 2.8; the course included a 5-week control period in which ambulation was permitted, 17 weeks of continuous bed rest, and a 7-week period of recovery in which ambulation was again permitted.[66] Dietary intake remained constant at approximately 2,688 kcal (11,115 kJ) throughout the observation period. The results were clear; bed rest caused a marked decrease in the body's copper and zinc stores. During the recovery period with modest physical activity, these trace minerals were retained to a greater extent compared with the bed rest condition. Although

this study represented an extreme and prolonged condition of physical inactivity, it does indicate that trace mineral dynamics in the body can be affected by physical inactivity. We are hopeful for an increase in research in the area of trace mineral metabolism in general and the effects of exercise and training on their requirements in particular.[5, 16, 71]

■ SUMMARY ■

1. Approximately 4% of body mass is composed of 22 elements called minerals. Minerals are a part of enzymes, hormones, and vitamins; they are found in muscles, connective tissues, and all body fluids.

2. Minerals occur freely in nature, in the waters of rivers, lakes, and oceans, and in soil. They are absorbed into the root system of plants and eventually incorporated into the tissues of animals that consume plants.

3. A primary function of minerals is in metabolism, in which they serve as important parts of enzymes.

Minerals provide structure in the formation of bones and teeth and are also important for the synthesis of the biologic macronutrients, glycogen, lipids, and protein.

4. A balanced diet provides generally adequate mineral intake, except perhaps in geographic locations in which there is a lack of certain minerals such as iodine.

5. Among older individuals, particularly women, the disease of osteoporosis has reached almost epidemic proportions. Adequate calcium intake and regular exercise provide an effective defense against bone loss at any age.

6. Paradoxically, women who train intensely and reduce body weight to the point at which menstruation is adversely affected often show advanced bone loss at an early age.

7. There is some evidence that about 40% of American women of childbearing age suffer from iron insufficiency. This could lead to iron-deficiency anemia, which would negatively affect exercise performance.

8. It is not clear whether regular physical activity creates a significant drain on the body's iron reserves. If this does occur, females, who have the greatest iron requirement and lowest intake, could be at risk for developing anemia. Assessment of the body's iron status should include an evaluation of both hematological characteristics and iron reserves.

9. As a result of excessive sweating during exercise, significant losses of body water and related minerals can occur. These should be replaced during and following exercise. Specific mineral supplementation is not required in most instances.

PART 3
WATER

WATER IN THE BODY

Water makes up from 40 to 60% of an individual's body mass and constitutes 65 to 75% of the weight of muscle and approximately 50% of the weight of body fat. Consequently, differences in total body water between individuals largely are due to variations in body composition (that is, differences in lean versus fat tissue).

Figure 2.9 depicts the fluid compartments of the body, the normal variability, and specific terminology describing the various states of human hydration. The body has two main water "compartments:" **intracellular,** referring to inside the cell, and **extracellular,** referring to fluids surrounding the cells. Extracellular fluid includes the blood plasma and lymph, saliva, fluid in the eyes, fluid secreted by glands and the digestive tract, fluid that bathes the nerves of the spinal cord, and fluid excreted from the skin and kidneys. Blood plasma accounts for 20% of the extracellular

fluid (between 3 and 4 L). Much of the fluid lost through sweating is extracellular fluid, predominantly from the blood plasma. Of total body water, an average of 62% is intracellular and 38% is extracellular.

FUNCTIONS OF BODY WATER

Water is a remarkable nutrient. Without water, death occurs within days. It serves as the body's transport and reactive medium; diffusion of gases always takes place across surfaces moistened by water. Nutrients and gases are transported in aqueous solution; waste products leave the body through the water in urine and feces. Water has tremendous heat-stabilizing qualities because it can absorb considerable

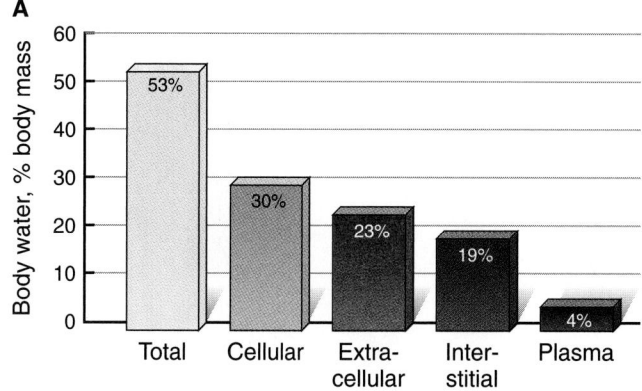

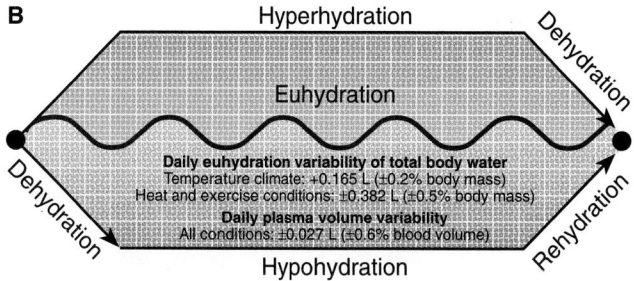

Hydration Terminology
- Euhydration: Sinusoidal line indicating normal daily water variation
- Hyperhydration: New steady-state condition of increased water content
- Hypohydration: New steady state condition of decreased water content
- Dehydration: Process of losing water either from the hyperhydrated state to euhydration, or from euhydration downward to dehydration
- Rehydration: Process of gaining water from a hypohydrated state toward euhydration

FIGURE 2.9

Fluid compartments, average volumes and variability, and hydration terminology. Volumes are for an 80-kg man. Approximately 60% of the body mass is composed of water in striated muscle (80% water), skeleton (32% water), and adipose tissue (50% water). For a man and woman of similar body mass, the woman contains less total water because of her larger ratio of adipose tissue to lean body mass (striated muscle + skeleton). (Adapted from Greenleaf, J. E.: Problem: thirst, drinking behavior, and involuntary dehydration. *Med. Sci. Sports Exerc.*, 24:645, 1992.)

heat with only a small change in temperature. Water lubricates joints. Because it is essentially noncompressible, water helps give structure and form to the body through the turgor it provides for body tissues.

WATER BALANCE: INTAKE VERSUS OUTPUT

The body's water content remains relatively stable over time. Although water output may frequently exceed water intake,

this imbalance is quickly adjusted with appropriate fluid intake to restore the body's fluid level balance. The sources of water intake and output are shown in Figure 2.10.

WATER INTAKE

Normally, approximately 2.5 L of water is required each day for a fairly sedentary adult in a normal environment. This water is supplied from three sources: (*a*) from liquids, (*b*) in foods, and (*c*) during metabolism.

FIGURE 2.10
Water balance in the body. *Top*, Little or no exercise in normal ambient temperature and humidity. *Bottom*, Moderate to heavy exercise in a hot, humid environment.

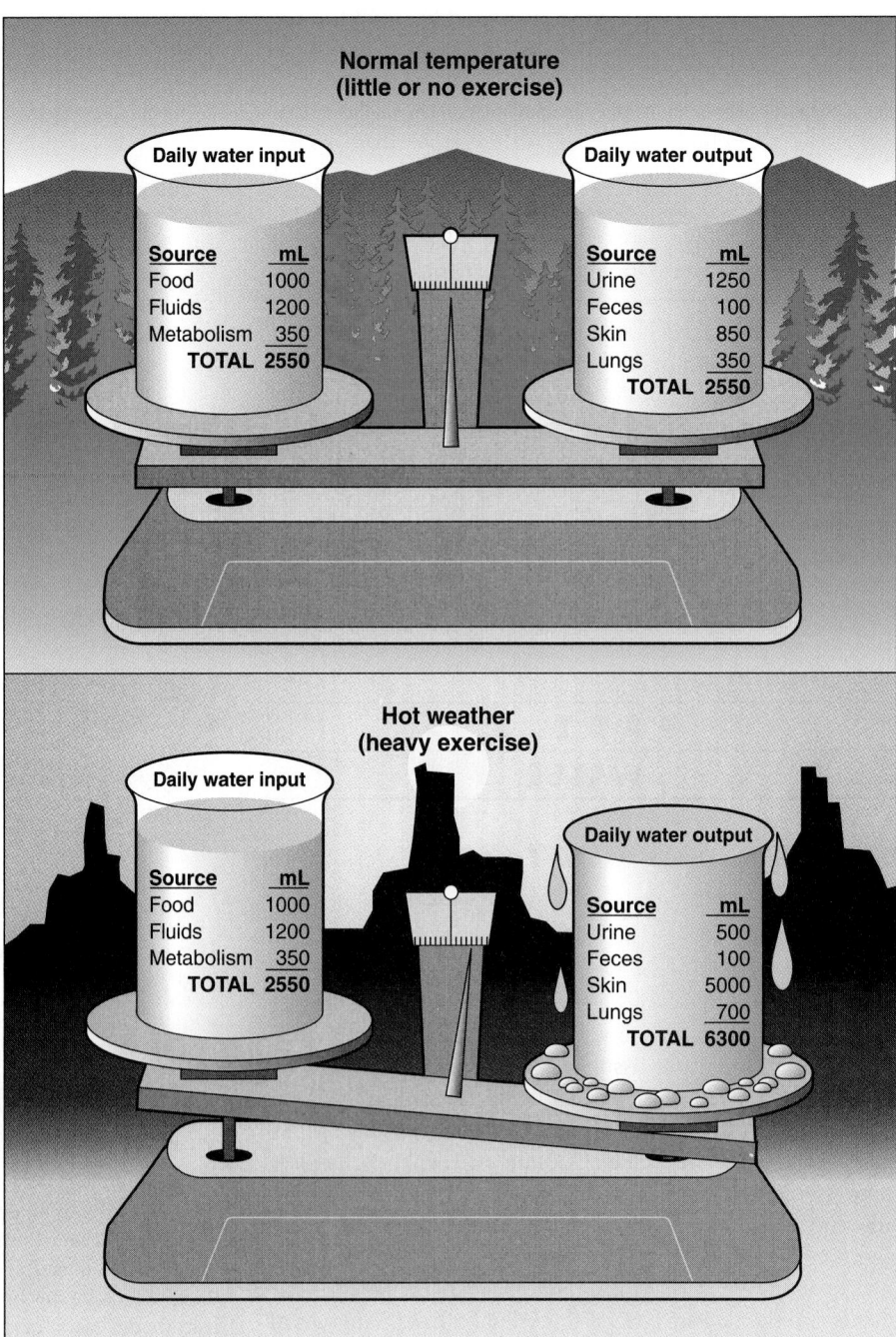

Water from Liquids. The average individual normally consumes 1200 mL or 41 oz of water each day. Of course, during exercise and thermal stress, fluid intake can increase five or six times above normal. There are reports of an individual losing 13.6 kg (30 lb) of water weight during a 2-day, 17-hour, 55-mile run across Death Valley, California.[101] With proper fluid ingestion, however, including salt supplements, the actual body weight loss was only 1.4 kg. In this example, fluid loss and replenishment amounted to between 3.5 and 4 gallons of liquid!

Water in Foods. Most foods, especially fruits and vegetables, contain large amounts of water. Such foods as lettuce, watermelon and cantaloupe, pickles, green beans, and broccoli are examples of foods that have a high water content, whereas the water content is relatively low in butter, oils, dried meats, chocolate, cookies, and cakes.

Metabolic Water. Carbon dioxide and water are formed when food molecules are degraded for energy. This water is termed **metabolic water** and accounts for about 25% of the daily water requirement of a sedentary person. The complete breakdown of 100 g of carbohydrate, protein, and lipid produces 55, 100, and 107 g of metabolic water, respectively. As mentioned in Chapter 1, each gram of glycogen is hydrated with 2.7 g of water. Consequently, this water also becomes available when glycogen is used for energy.

WATER OUTPUT

Water is lost from the body in urine, through the skin, as water vapor in the expired air, and in feces.

Water Loss in Urine. Under normal conditions, the kidneys reabsorb approximately 99% of the 140 to 160 L of filtrate formed each day; consequently, the volume of urine excreted by the kidneys ranges from 1000 to 1500 mL or about 1.5 quarts per day.

Approximately 15 mL of water is required to eliminate 1 g of solute. Thus, a portion of water in urine is "obligated" to rid the body of metabolic by-products such as urea, an end product of protein breakdown. In this way, the use of large quantities of protein for energy (as would occur with a high-protein diet) can actually accelerate the body's dehydration during exercise.

Water Loss Through the Skin. A small quantity of water, perhaps 350 mL, seeps from the deeper tissues through the skin to the body's surface. This continuous loss of water is termed **insensible perspiration.**

Water is also lost through the skin in the form of sweat produced by specialized sweat glands located beneath the skin. Evaporation of sweat provides the refrigeration mechanism to cool the body. Under normal conditions, 500 to 700 mL of sweat is secreted each day. This by no means reflects sweating capacity, because a well-acclimatized person can produce up to 12 L of sweat (about 12 kg at a rate of 1 L per hour) during prolonged exercise in a hot environment.

Water Loss as Water Vapor. The amount of insensible water loss through small water droplets in exhaled air is 250 to 350 mL per day. Exercise also affects this source of water loss. For physically active persons, 2 to 5 mL of water is lost from the respiratory passages each minute during strenuous exercise.[75] This amount varies considerably with climate; water loss is lowest in hot, humid weather and highest in cold temperatures, in which the inspired air contains little moisture, or at altitudes at which ventilatory volumes are significantly elevated at rest and during exercise.

Water Loss in Feces. Between 100 and 200 mL of water is lost through intestinal elimination, because water constitutes about 70% of fecal matter. The remainder is composed of nondigestible material, including bacteria from the digestive process and the residues of digestive juices from the intestine, stomach, and pancreas. With diarrhea or vomiting, water loss can increase to between 1500 and 5000 mL.

WATER REQUIREMENT IN EXERCISE

The most serious consequence of profuse sweating is the loss of body water. The amount of water lost through sweating depends on the severity of physical activity and environmental temperature. The **relative humidity** (water content of the ambient air) is also an important factor affecting the efficiency of the sweating mechanism in temperature regulation. During conditions of 100% relative humidity, the air is completely saturated with water vapor. Thus, evaporation of fluid from the skin to the air is impossible and this important avenue for body cooling is closed. Under such conditions, sweat beads on the skin and eventually rolls off. On a dry day, the air can hold considerable moisture, and fluid rapidly evaporates from the skin. Thus, the sweat mechanism functions at optimal efficiency and body temperature is more easily regulated. A more detailed discussion of fluid replacement with exercise is presented in Chapter 3. It is noteworthy, however, that plasma volume becomes reduced when sweating causes a fluid loss of 2 or 3% of body mass. This loss of fluid places a significant strain on circulatory function, which ultimately impairs the capacity for both exercise and thermoregulation. A convenient method for assessing fluid loss is through changes in body weight during exercise and/or heat stress. Each 1 lb of body weight loss corresponds to 450 mL (15 oz) of dehydration.

HYPONATREMIA: SWEATING + WATER INTAKE = TOO MUCH OF TWO GOOD THINGS

Major concerns in hot-weather exercise are dehydration, decreased plasma volume and resulting hemoconcentration, impaired physical performance and thermoregulatory capacity, and the increased risk of heat injury (especially heat stroke). As a result, the physiological literature is replete with warnings for the need to consume fluid before, during, and after exercise. In many instances, the beverage recommended is plain, hypotonic water. It now is apparent that under certain exercise conditions, excessive fluid intake may actually be counterproductive and may result in the condition of **hyponatremia** or "water intoxication." This potentially significant medical complication is characterized by symptoms ranging from mild—headache, confusion, malaise, nausea, cramping—to severe—seizures, coma, pulmonary edema, and even death.

Hyponatremia is considered to exist when the concentration of serum sodium falls below 136 mEq · L^{-1}; severe symptoms are often observed with serum sodium below 130 mEq · L^{-1}. The condition most conducive to hyponatremia is high-intensity, ultramarathon-type, continuous exercise lasting 6 to 8 hours, although it may occur with exercise lasting only 4 hours.[6] Hyponatremia in ultraendurance athletes competing in hot weather is not rare. For example, nearly 30% of the athletes competing in the 1984 Ironman Triathlon had symptoms of hyponatremia, most frequently observed late in the race or in the recovery period.

Development of hyponatremia requires a large loss of sodium through prolonged sweating coupled with the dilution of existing extracellular sodium (and accompanying reduced osmolality) through fluid ingestion, especially fluids containing low or no sodium. Because exercise in hot, humid weather often produces a sweat rate of more than 1 L per hour (with a sweat-sodium concentration ranging between 20 and 100 mEq · L^{-1}), a significant sodium loss can occur after several hours of exercise. The occurrence of hyponatremia becomes a distinct possibility when this sodium loss is combined with the diluting effects on extracellular fluid of large volumes of ingested water. It is also possible that frequently ingesting large volumes of plain water causes sodium from the extracellular fluid compartment to be drawn into the unabsorbed intestinal water. This further dilutes the serum sodium concentration.[56]

Factors That Predispose to Hyponatremia

- Prolonged high-intensity exercise in hot weather.
- Relatively poor fitness level associated with sweat production containing high sodium concentration, thus augmenting sodium loss.
- Beginning physical activity in a sodium-depleted state due to "salt-free" or "low-sodium" diet or use of diuretic medication for hypertension.
- Frequent and prolonged ingestion of sodium-free fluid.

To reduce the risk of hyponatremia in prolonged exercise, it is recommended to refrain from overhydration—that is, not to consume extreme amounts of plain water (more than 1000 mL · hr^{-1}) either before, during, or after exercise—and to include some sodium (approximately 25 mEq · L^{-1}) in the ingested fluid. Also, the inclusion of some glucose in the rehydration drink facilitates intestinal water uptake via the glucose-sodium transport mechanism (see Chapters 3 and 25).[83]

■ SUMMARY ■

1. Water makes up 40 to 60% of the total body mass. Muscle is 72% water by weight, whereas water represents only about 50% of the weight of body fat.

2. Of the total body water, roughly 62% is intracellular (inside the cells) and 38% is extracellular (in the plasma, lymph, and other fluids outside the cell).

3. The normal average daily water intake of 2.5 L is supplied from (a) liquid intake (1.2 L), (b) food (1.0 L), and (c) metabolic water produced during energy-yielding reactions (0.3 L).

4. Water is lost from the body each day in the urine (1 to 1.5 L), through the skin as insensible perspiration (0.50 to 0.70 L), as water vapor in expired air (0.25 to 0.30 L), and in feces (0.10 L).

5. Food and oxygen are always supplied in the body in aqueous solution and waste products always exit via watery medium. Water also helps give structure and form to the body and plays a vital role in temperature regulation.

6. Exercise in hot weather greatly increases the body's water requirement. In extreme conditions, the fluid needs can increase to five or six times above normal.

7. Excessive sweating combined with the ingestion of large volumes of plain water during prolonged exercise sets the stage for hyponatremia or water intoxication. This potentially dangerous condition is related to a decrease in the concentration of extracellular sodium.

■ REFERENCES ■

1. Alessio, H.M.: Exercise-induced oxidative stress. *Med. Sci. Sports Exerc.*, 25:218, 1993.
2. Aloia, J.F., et al.: Calcium supplementation with and without hormone replacement therapy to prevent postmenopausal bone loss. *Ann. Intern. Med.*, 120:97, 1994.
3. American College of Sports Medicine: Position statement on prevention of heat injuries during distance running. *Med. Sci. Sports Exerc.*, 16:ix, 1984.
4. Anderson, R.A., et al.: Strenuous running: acute effects on chromium, copper, zinc, and selected variables in urine and serum of male runners. *Biol. Trace Elem. Res.*, 6:327, 1984.
5. Anderson, R.A., and Guttman, H.N.: Trace minerals and exercise. In *Exercise, Nutrition, and Energy Metabolism*. Edited by E.S. Horton and R.L. Terjung. New York, Macmillan, 1988.
6. Armstrong, L.E., et al.: Symptomatic hyponatremia during prolonged exercise in heat. *Med. Sci. Sports Exerc.*, 25:543, 1993.
7. Balban, E.P., et al.: The frequency of anemia and iron deficiency in the runner. *Med. Sci. Sports Exerc.*, 21:643, 1989.
8. van der Beek, E.J.: Vitamin supplementation and physical exercise performance. In *Foods, Nutrition and Sports Performance*. Edited by C. Williams and J.T. Devlin. London, E. and F.N. Spon, 1992.

9. Belko, A.Z.: Vitamins and exercise: an update. *Med. Sci. Sports Exerc.*, 19:S191, 1987.

10. Blum, S.M., et al.: The effects of fitness-type exercise on iron status in adult women. *Am. J. Clin. Nutr.*, 43:456, 1986.

11. Bothwell, T.H., et al.: *Iron Metabolism in Man.* Boston, Blackwell, 1979.

12. Brune, M., et al.: Iron loss in sweat. *Am. J. Clin. Nutr.*, 43:438, 1986.

13. Buckman, M.T.: Gastrointestinal bleeding in long distance runners. *Ann. Intern. Med.*, 101:127, 1984.

14. Cann, E.C.: Decreased spinal mineral content in amenorrheic women. *JAMA*, 251:626, 1984.

15. Clancy, S.P., et al.: Effects of chromium picolinate supplementation on body composition, strength, and urinary chromium loss in football players. *Int. J. Sport Nutr.*, 4:142, 1994.

16. Clarkson, P.M.: Minerals: exercise performance and supplementation in athletes. *J. Sports Sci.*, 9:91, 1991.

16a. Clarkson, P.M., and Haymes, E.M.: Exercise and mineral status of athletes: calcium, magnesium, phosphorus, and iron. *Med. Sci. Sports Exerc.*, 27:831, 1995.

17. Clement, D.B., and Asmundson, R.C.: Nutritional intake and hematological parameters in endurance runners. *Phys. Sportsmed.*, 10:37, 1982.

18. Clement, D.B., and Sawchuk, L.L.: Iron status and sports performance. *Sports Med.*, 1:65, 1984.

19. Clinical nutrition: vitamin C toxicity. *Nutr. Rev.*, 34:236, 1977.

20. Conroy, B.P., et al.: Bone mineral density in elite junior Olympic weight lifters. *Med. Sci. Sports Exerc.*, 25:1103, 1993.

21. Consensus Statement. *Physical Activity, Fitness, and Health.* Edited by C. Bouchard, et al. Champaign, IL, Human Kinetics, 1994.

22. Costill, D.L., et al.: Dietary potassium and heavy exercise: effects on muscle water and electrolytes. *Am. J. Clin. Nutr.*, 36:266, 1982.

23. Criswell, D., et al.: High intensity training-induced changes in skeletal muscle antioxidant enzyme activity. *Med. Sci. Sports Exerc.*, 25:1135, 1993.

24. Dalsky, G.P., et al.: Effect of exercise on bone: permissive influence of estrogen and calcium. *Med. Sci. Sports Exerc.*, 22:281, 1990.

25. Davee, A.M., et al.: Exercise patterns and trabecular bone density in college women. *J. Bone Miner. Res.*, 5:245, 1990

26. Davies, K.J.A., et al.: Muscle mitochondrial bioenergetics, oxygen supply, and work capacity during dietary iron deficiency and repletion. *Am. J. Physiol.*, 242:E418, 1982.

27. De Souza, M.J., et al.: Menstrual status and plasma vasopressin, renin activity, and aldosterone exercise responses. *J. Appl. Physiol.*, 67:736, 1989.

28. Dressendorfer, R.H., et al.: Plasma mineral levels in marathon runners during a 20-day road race. *Phys. Sportsmed.*, 10:113, 1982.

29. Drinkwater, B.L.: C.H. McCloy Research Lecture: Does physical activity play a role in preventing osteoporosis? *Res. Q. Exerc. Sport.*, 65:197, 1994.

30. Drinkwater, B.L., et al.: Menstrual history as a determinant of current bone density in young athletes. *JAMA*, 263:545, 1990.

31. Eichner, E.R.: Physical activity and free radicals. In *Physical Activity, Fitness, and Health.* Edited by C. Bouchard, et al. Champaign, IL, Human Kinetics, 1994.

32. van Erp-Bart, A.M.J., et al.: Nationwide survey on nutritional habits in elite athletes. Part 1. Energy, carbohydrate, protein and fat intake. *Int. J. Sports Med.*, 10(Suppl. 1):S3, 1989.

33. Falsetti, H.L., et al.: Hematological variations after endurance running with hard- and soft-soled running shoes. *Phys. Sportsmed.*, 11:118, 1983.

34. Faulkner, R.A., et al.: Comparison of bone mineral content and bone mineral density between dominant and nondominant limbs in children 8-16 years of age. *Am. J. Hum. Biol.*, 5:491, 1993.

35. Frederickson, L.A., et al.: Effects of training on indices of iron status of young female cross-country runners. *Med. Sci. Sports Exerc.*, 15:271, 1983.

36. Gardner, G.W., et al.: Cardiorespiratory, hematological and physical performance responses of anemic subjects to iron treatment. *Am. J. Clin. Nutr.*, 28:982, 1975.

37. Gey, G.O., et al.: Effects of ascorbic acid on endurance performance and athletic injury. *JAMA*, 211:105, 1970.

38. Goldfarb, A.H.: Antioxidants: role of supplementation to prevent exercise-induced oxidative stress. *Med. Sci. Sports Exerc.*, 25:232, 1993.

39. Goldfarb, A.H., et al.: Vitamin E effects on indexes of lipid peroxidation in muscle from DHEA-treated and exercised rats. *J. Appl. Physiol.*, 76:1630, 1994.

40. Gonzalez, E.R.: Premature bone loss found in some nonmenstruating sports-women. *JAMA*, 248:513, 1982.

41. Green, H.J., et al.: Training induced hypervolemia: lack of an effect on oxygen utilization during exercise. *Med. Sci. Sports Exerc.*, 19:202, 1987.

42. Grimston, S.K., et al.: Mechanical loading regimen and its relation to bone mineral density. *Med. Sci. Sports Exerc.*, 25:1203, 1993.

43. Haliova, L., and Anderson, J.J.B.: Lifetime calcium intake and physical activity habits: independent and combined effects on the radial bone of healthy premenopausal Caucasian women. *Am. J. Clin. Nutr.*, 49:534, 1989.

44. Halliwell, B., and Chirico, S.: Lipid peroxidation: its mechanism, measurement and significance. *Am. J. Clin. Nutr.*, 57(Suppl.):715S, 1993.

45. Halliwell, B., and Gutteridge, J.M.C.: *Free Radicals in Biology and Medicine.* Oxford, Clarendon Press, 1989.

46. Hamdy, R.C., et al.: Regional differences in bone density of young men involved in different exercises. *Med. Sci. Sports Exerc.*, 26:884, 1994.

47. Haymes, E.M.: Vitamin and mineral supplementation to athletes. *Int. J. Sport Nutr.*, 1:146, 1991.

48. Haymes, E.M., et al.: Training for cross-country skiing and iron status. *Med. Sci. Sports Exerc.*, 18:162, 1986.

49. Heaney, R.: Bone mass, nutrition and other life style factors. *Am. J. Med.*, 95(Suppl. 5A):29, 1993.

50. Heaney, R.P., et al.: Calcium nutrition and bone health in the elderly. *Am. J. Clin. Nutr.*, 36:986, 1982.

51. Herbert, V.: Toxicity of vitamin E. *Nutr. Rev.*, 35:158, 1977.

52. Herbert, V.: Megavitamin therapy. *Contemp. Nutr.*, 2:10, 1977.

53. Herbert, V., et al.: Destruction of vitamin B by vitamin C. *Am. J. Clin. Nutr.*, 30:297, 1977.

54. Hetland, M.L., et al.: Running induces menstrual disturbances but bone mass is unaffected, except in amenorrheic women. *Am. J. Med.*, 95:53, 1993.

54a. Hodis, H.N., et al.: Serial coronary angiographic evidence that antioxidant vitamin intake reduces progression of coronary artery disease. *JAMA*, 273:1849, 1995.

55. Hundig, A., et al.: Runner's anemia and iron deficiency. *Acta Med. Scand.*, 209:315, 1981.

55a. Hutchinson, T.M., et al.: Factors in daily physical activity related to calcaneal mineral density in men. *Med. Sci. Sports Exerc.*, 27:745, 1995.

56. Irving, R.A., et al.: Evaluation of renal function and fluid homeostasis during recovery from exercise induced hyponatremia. *J. Appl. Physiol.*, 70:342, 1991.

57. Jackson, M.J.: Physiology of zinc: general aspects. In *Zinc in Human Biology.* Edited by C.F. Mills. London, Springer-Verlag, 1989.

58. Ji, L.L.: Exercise and oxidative stress: role of the cellular antioxidant systems. *Exerc. Sport Sci. Rev.*, 23:135, 1995.

59. Jialal, I., and Grundy, S.M.: Effect of combined supplementation with alpha-tocopherol, ascorbate, and beta carotene on low-density lipoprotein oxidation. *Circulation*, 88:2780, 1993.

60. Johnson, H.L., et al.: Effects of electrolyte and nutrient solutions on performance and metabolic balance. *Med. Sci. Sports Exerc.*, 20:26, 1988.

61. Johnston, C.C., Jr., et al.: Calcium supplementation and increases in bone mineral density in children. *N. Engl. J. Med.,* 327:82, 1992.

62. Kanter, M.M.: Free radicals and exercise: effects of nutritional antioxidant supplementation. *Exerc. Sport Sci. Rev.,* 23:375, 1995.

63. Kanter, M.M., et al.: Effects of an antioxidant vitamin mixture on lipid peroxidation at rest and postexercise. *J. Appl. Physiol.,* 74:965, 1993.

64. Klingshirn, L.A., et al.: Effect of iron supplementation on endurance capacity in iron-depleted female runners. *Med. Sci. Sports Exerc.,* 24:819, 1992.

65. Krebs, P., et al.: The acute and prolonged effects of marathon running on 20 blood parameters. *Phys. Sportsmed.,* 10:58, 1982.

66. Krebs, J.M., et al.: Zinc and copper balances in healthy adult males during and after 17 wk of bed rest. *Am. J. Clin. Nutr.,* 58:897, 1993.

67. Lamanca, J.J., et al.: Sweat iron loss of male and female runners during exercise. *Int. J. Sports Med.,* 9:52, 1988.

68. Lane, H.W., et al.: Effect of physical activity on human potassium metabolism in a hot and humid environment. *Am. J. Clin. Nutr.,* 31:838, 1978.

68a. Lee, E.J., et al.: Variations in bone status of contralateral and regional sites in young athletic women. *Med. Sci. Sports Exerc.,* 27:1354, 1995.

69. Lloyd, T., et al.: Calcium supplementation and bone mineral density in adolescent girls. *JAMA,* 270:841, 1993.

70. Luc, G., et al.: Oxidation of lipiproteins and atherosclerosis. *Am. J. Clin. Nutr.,* 55:265S, 1991.

71. Lukaski, H.C., et al.: Physical training and copper, iron, and zinc status of swimmers. *Am. J. Clin. Nutr.,* 51:1093, 1990.

72. Lyle, R.M., et al.: Iron status in exercising women: the effect of oral iron therapy vs increased consumption of muscle foods. *Am. J. Clin. Nutr.,* 56:1099, 1992.

73. Manore, M.M., and Leklem, J.E.: Effect of carbohydrate and vitamin B_6 on fuel substrates during exercise in women. *Med. Sci. Sports Exerc.,* 20:233, 1988.

74. McCabe, M.E., et al.: Gastrointestinal blood loss associated with running a marathon. *Dig. Dis. Sci.,* 31:1229, 1986.

74a. Micklesfield, L.K., et al.: Bone mineral density in mature, premenopausal ultramarathon runners. *Med. Sci. Sports Exerc.,* 27:688, 1995.

75. Mitchel, J., et al.: Respiratory weight loss during exercise. *J. Appl. Physiol.,* 32:474, 1972.

76. Morris, D.L., et al.: Serum carotenoids and coronary heart disease: the Lipid Research Clinics Coronary Prevention Trial and Follow-up Study. *JAMA,* 272:439, 1994.

77. Moses, F.M.: Physical activity and digestive processes. In *Physical Activity, Fitness, and Health.* Edited by C. Bouchard, et al. Champaign, IL, Human Kinetics, 1994.

78. Myburgh, K.H., et al.: Low bone mineral density at axial and appendicular sites in amenorrheic athletes. *Med. Sci. Sports Exerc.,* 25:1197, 1993.

79. Newhouse, I.J., et al.: The effects of prelatent/latent iron deficiency on physical work capacity. *Med. Sci. Sports Exerc.,* 21:263, 1987.

80. Nichols, D.L., et al.: The effects of gymnastics training on bone mineral density. *Med. Sci. Sports Exerc.,* 26:1220, 1994.

81. Nichols, D.L., et al.: Relationship of regional body composition to bone mineral density in college females. *Med. Sci. Sports Exerc.,* 27:178, 1995.

82. Nickerson, H.J., and Tripp, H.J.: Iron deficiency in adolescent cross-country runners. *Phys. Sportsmed.,* 11:60, 1983.

83. Nose, H., et al.: Role of osmolality and plasma volume in rehydration of humans. *J. Appl. Physiol.,* 65:325, 1988.

84. O'Toole, M.L., et al.: Hemolysis during triathlon races: its relation to race distance. *Med. Sci. Sports Exerc.,* 20:172, 1988.

85. Owen, R.A., et al.: The national cost of acute care of hip fractures associated with osteoporosis. *Clin. Orthop.,* 150:172, 1980.

86. Pate, R.: Sports anemia: a review of the current literature. *Phys. Sportsmed.,* 11:115, 1983.

87. Pate, R., et al.: Dietary iron supplementation in women athletes. *Phys. Sportsmed.,* 7:16, 1979.

88. Percey, E.C.: Ergogenic aids in athletics. *Med. Sci. Sports Exerc.,* 10:298, 1978.

89. Peters, E.M., et al.: Vitamin C supplementation reduces the incidence of postrace symptoms of upper-respiratory-tract infection in ultramarathon runners. *Am. J. Clin. Nutr.,* 57:170, 1993.

90. Pincemail, J., et al.: Pentane measurement in man as an index of lipoperoxidation. *Bioelectronchem. Bioenerg.,* 18:117, 1987.

91. Position of the American Dietetic Association: Nutrition for physical fitness and athletic performance for adults. *ADA Reports,* 87:933, 1987.

92. Puhl, J.L., et al.: Erythrocyte changes during training in high school women cross-country runners. *Res. Q. Exerc. Sport,* 52:484, 1981.

92a. Rajaram S., et al.: Effects of long-term moderate exercise on iron status in young women. *Med. Sci. Sports Exerc.,* 27:1105, 1995.

93. Recker, R.R., et al.: Bone gain in young adult women. *JAMA,* 268:2403, 1992.

94. Regelson, W., and Sines, F.: *Intervention in the Aging Process.* New York, Alan R. Liss, 1983.

95. Reid, I.R., et al.: Effect of calcium supplementation on bone loss in postmenopausal women. *N. Engl. J. Med.,* 328:460, 1993.

96. Report of the Council on Scientific Affairs: Diet and cancer: where do matters stand? *Arch. Intern. Med.,* 153:50, 1993.

97. Riis, B., et al.: Does calcium supplementation prevent postmenopausal bone loss? A double-blind controlled clinical study. *N. Engl. J. Med.,* 36:173, 1987.

98. Rimm, E.B., et al.: Vitamin E consumption and the risk of coronary heart disease in men. *N. Engl. J. Med.,* 328:1450, 1993.

99. Risser, W.L., et al.: Iron deficiency in female athletes: its prevalence and impact on performance. *Med. Sci. Sports Exerc.,* 20:116, 1988.

100. Robertson, J.O., et al: Fecal blood loss in response to exercise. *BMJ,* 205:303, 1987.

101. Robinson, S.: Cardiovascular and respiratory reactions to heat. In *Physiological Adaptations.* Edited by M.K. Yousef, et al. New York, Academic Press, 1972.

101a. Robinson, T.L., et al.: Gymnasts exhibit higher bone mass than runners despite similar prevalence of amenorrhea and oligomenorrhea. *J. Bone Mineral Res.,* 10:26, 1995.

102. Rokitzki, L., et al.: α-tocopherol supplementation in racing cyclists during extreme endurance training. *Int. J. Sport Nutr.,* 4:255, 1994.

103. Rossander, L., et al.: Absorption of iron from breakfast meals. *Am. J. Clin. Nutr.,* 32:2484, 1979.

104. Sack, M.N., et al.: Oestrogen and inhibition of oxidation of low-density lipoproteins in postmenopausal women. *Lancet,* 343:269, 1994.

105. Salonen, J.T., et al.: High stored iron levels are associated with excess risk of myocardial infarction in Eastern Finnish men. *Circulation,* 86:803, 1992.

106. Schawmberg, H., et al.: Sensory neuropathy from pyridoxine abuse: a new megavitamin syndrome. *N. Engl. J. Med.,* 309:445, 1983.

107. Schoene, R.B., et al.: Iron repletion decreases maximal exercise lactate concentrations in female athletes with minimal iron-deficiency anemia. *J. Lab. Clin. Med.,* 102:306, 1983.

108. Schrimshaw, N.S., and Young, V.R.: The requirements of human nutrition. *Sci. Am.,* 235:50, 1976.

109. Selemenda, C.W., et al.: Role of physical activity in the development of skeletal mass in children. *J. Bone Miner. Res.,* 6:1227, 1991.

110. Sempos, C.T., et al.: Body iron stores and risk of coronary heart disease. *N. Engl. J. Med.,* 330:1119, 1994.

111. Serfass, W.C.: Nutrition for the athlete. *Contemp. Nutr.,* 2:1977.

112. Singh, A., et al.: Chronic multivitamin-mineral supplementation does not enhance physical performance. *Med. Sci. Sports Exerc.,* 24:726, 1992.

113. Sjodin, B., et al.: Biochemical mechanisms for oxygen free radical formation during exercise. *Sports Med.,* 10:233, 1990.

114. Smith, E.L.: Exercise for prevention of osteoporosis: a review. *Phys. Sportsmed.*, 10:72, 1982.

115. Smith, E.L., et al.: Physical activity and calcium modalities for bone mineral increase in aged women. *Med. Sci. Sports Exerc.*, 13:60, 1981.

116. Snyder, A.C., et al.: Importance of dietary iron source on measures of iron status among female runners. *Med. Sci. Sports Exerc.*, 21:7, 1989.

117. Spencer, H., and Kramer, L.: NIH Consensus Conference: osteoporosis. *J. Nutr.*, 116:316, 1986.

118. Stahelin, H.B., et al.: Beta carotene and cancer prevention: the Basel study. *Am. J. Clin. Nutr.*, 53:265S, 1991.

119. Stampfer, M.J., et al.: Vitamin E consumption and the risk of coronary heart disease in women. *N. Engl. J. Med.*, 328:1444, 1993.

120. Starnes, J., et al.: Skeletal muscle lipid peroxidation in exercised and food restricted rats. *J. Appl. Physiol.*, 67:69, 1989.

121. Suominen, H., and Rahkila, P.: Bone mineral density of the calcaneus in 70- to 81-yr-old males athletes and a population sample. *Med. Sci. Sports Exerc.*, 23:1227, 1991.

121a. Taaffle, D.R., et al.: Differential effects of swim versus weight bearing activity on bone mineral status of eumenorrheic athletes. *J. Bone Mineral Res.*, 10:586, 1995.

122. Telford, R., et al.: The effect of 7 to 8 months of vitamin/mineral supplementation on athletic performance. *Int. J. Sport Nutr.*, 2:135, 1992.

123. Tessier, F., et al.: Selenium and training effects on the glutathione system and aerobic performance. *Med. Sci. Sports Exerc.*, 27:390, 1995.

124. Trembly, A., et al.: The effects of riboflavin supplementation on the nutritional status and performance of elite swimmers. *Nutr. Res.*, 4:201, 1984.

125. Use of vitamin and mineral supplements in the United States. *Nutr. Rev.*, 70:43, 1990.

126. Viquie, C.A., et al.: Antioxidant status and indexes of oxidative stress during consecutive days of exercise. *J. Appl. Physiol.*, 75:566, 1993.

127. Weight, L.M., et al.: Vitamin and mineral supplementation: effect on running performance of trained athletes. *Am. J. Clin. Nutr.*, 47:192, 1988.

128. Weight, L.M., et al.: Sports anemia: a real or apparent phenomenon in endurance-trained athletes. *Int. J. Sports Med.*, 13:344, 1992.

129. Williams, J.A.: The effect of long-distance running upon appendicular bone mineral content. *Med. Sci. Sports Exerc.*, 16:223, 1984.

Connor, W.E., et al.: The plasma lipoproteins, and diet of the Tarahumara Indians of Mexico. *Am. J. Clin Nutr.* 31:1131, 1978.

The Tarahumara Indians are a group of about 50,000 relatively unacculturated farmers who inhabit the rugged Sierra Madre Occidental Mountains in the north-central state of Chihuahua, Mexico. These individuals, renowned for their en-

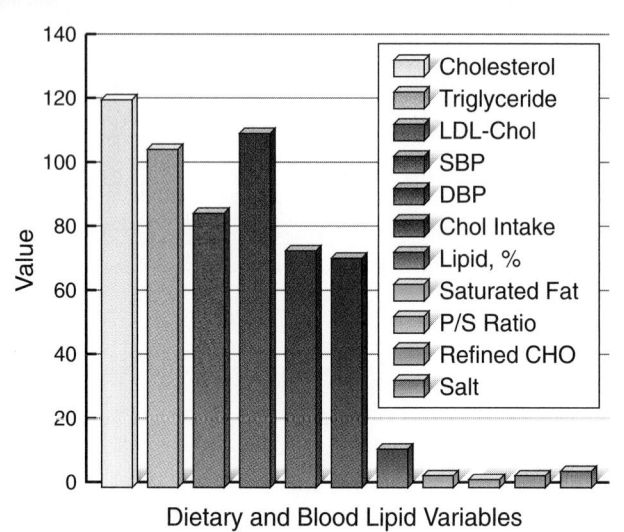

Different dietary and blood lipid variables for the Tarahumara Indians of Mexico. Plasma cholesterol, triglycerides, and LDL cholesterol are in milligrams per deciliter. *Chol intake* is cholesterol intake in grams per day. Lipid intake (*Lipid %*) and saturated fat intake (*Saturated Fat*) are expressed as percentage of total caloric intake; *P/S ratio* is the ratio of polyunsaturated to saturated fatty acid intake; *Refined CHO* is the percentage of the total kcal of refined sugar; *Salt* is salt intake in grams per day; *SBP* and *DBP* represent systolic and diastolic blood pressure in millimeters of mercury.

durance capacity, reportedly run distances of up to 200 miles in the competitive sport of "kickball" that lasts 1 to 2 days. This research investigated the diet, blood lipid status, and blood pressure of these 20th-century "Spartans." Measurements of 523 Tarahumaras over a 3-year period included plasma cholesterol and triglycerides, lipoprotein fractions, body stature and mass, triceps skinfold, resting blood pressure, and nutrient intake by dietary history and observation of food intake. The most striking findings included extremely low values for blood cholesterol, blood lipoproteins (VLDL and LDL), blood pressure, fatfold thickness, and dietary fat. The average blood cholesterol levels (below 136 mg · dL^{-1} for men, 117 mg · dL^{-1} for women, and 116 mg · dL^{-1} for children) contrast sharply with typical American values of more than 200 mg · dL^{-1}.

The low plasma cholesterol of the Tarahumaras is largely related to their unique dietary patterns. Their diet, extremely low in cholesterol, averaged 71 mg · d^{-1} (the typical U.S. cholesterol intake is 500 to 750 mg · d^{-1}). Additionally, fat intake averaged only 11% of total caloric intake compared to nearly 40% for the U.S. diet. Corn and beans accounted for 95% of total lipid consumption, mainly from polyunsaturated and monounsaturated fatty acid sources. Saturated fat constituted only 2% of total calories, compared to 15% in the United States. Thus, the polyunsaturated/saturated fat ratio exceeded 2.0, compared to only 0.35 for the U.S. diet.

Simple sugars provided only 5% of total energy intake compared to 25% for the typical North American diet. No occurrence of obesity or hypertension occurred in the Tarahumaras. Vegetable sources provided more than 96% of dietary protein, while protein intake averaged 79 to 96 g · d^{-1} and accounted for 236 to 1221% of the total essential amino acid requirements based on the U.S. RDA. The Tarahumaras' high level of physical activity coincided with a favorable blood lipid and blood pressure profile and other low coronary risk factors. Overall, the results illustrated that favorable dietary factors and increased physical activity contributed to the group's relatively good health status.

Optimal Nutrition for Exercise

An optimal diet is one in which the supply of required nutrients is adequate for tissue maintenance, repair, and growth without excess energy intake. It is now possible to make reasonable estimates of nutritional needs for men and women that account for normal variation in daily energy expenditure. Dietary recommendations for athletes, however, must also consider the specific energy requirements of a particular sport as well as by the athlete's dietary preferences. Although there is no one diet for optimal exercise performance, careful planning and evaluation of food intake should follow sound nutritional guidelines.

At the extreme negative end of the nutrition continuum, reliance on low-calorie "semi-starvation" diets or other potentially harmful practices such as high-fat, low-carbohydrate diets, "liquid-protein" diets, or single-food diets are counterproductive to good health, exercise performance, and the maintenance of optimum body composition. Reliance on low-carbohydrate diets compromises energy reserves for vigorous physical activity or regular training. Athletes who do not include sufficient carbohydrate energy in their diets will eventually train in a state of relative glycogen depletion, which may eventually result in "staleness" that hinders the ability to train and compete.

NUTRIENT REQUIREMENTS

Many coaches make dietary recommendations based on their own "feelings" and past experiences rather than on available evidence. This problem is compounded because athletes often have either inadequate or incorrect information concerning prudent dietary practices. Although research in the area of **sports nutrition** is far from complete, the general consensus is that physically active people do not require additional nutrients beyond those obtained in a balanced diet. This is important because a large number of adults exercise regularly to keep fit. In terms of nutrition, active Americans, including those involved in exceptional endurance activities, consume typical diets that are remarkably similar in composition to those consumed by their more sedentary counterparts.[6, 34, 39] As shown in Table 3.1, the main difference is that athletes eat more of the same foods, which results in a larger total **quantity** of food consumed to support the extra energy for training. *In essence, sound nutrition for athletes is sound human nutrition.* For endurance athletes and others who engage regularly in heavy training, special consideration should focus on maintaining adequate, regular carbohydrate intake and fluid intake.

RECOMMENDED NUTRIENT INTAKE

The recommended intakes for proteins, lipids, and carbohydrates, as well as the food sources of these macronutrients for active men and women, are listed in Figure 3.1. These guidelines provide the necessary vitamin, mineral, and protein requirements even though the energy content of the food intake amounts to only about 1200 calories daily. (A calorie or kcal is a unit of heat used to express the energy value of food.) In terms of average values for young adults, the total daily energy requirement is approximately 2100 kcal for women and 2700 kcal for men. *After the basic nutrient requirements are met (as recommended in Figure 3.1), extra energy needs can be supplied from a variety of food sources based on individual preference.*

Proteins. As discussed in Chapter 1, the recommended dietary allowance (RDA) for protein intake is 0.8 g per kilogram of body mass (0.128 oz per pound of body weight). A person who weighs 77 kg (170 lb) would therefore require approximately 62 g or 2.2 oz of protein daily. Assuming that even during exercise there is relatively little protein loss through energy metabolism (an assumption that may not be entirely correct), the protein recommendation is probably adequate for most active men and women. Also, the protein intake in the average American diet significantly exceeds the RDA for protein, and the athlete's diet is usually two to five times more than this protein recommendation!

Lipids. Standards for optimal lipid intake have not been firmly established because relatively little is known concerning the human requirement for this nutrient. The amount of dietary lipid varies widely according to personal taste, money spent on food, and the availability of lipid-rich foods. For example, only about 10% of the energy in the average diet of people living in Asia is furnished by lipids, whereas in many Western countries, lipids account for 40 to 45% of the caloric intake. To promote good health, lipid intake probably should not exceed 30% of the energy content of the diet. Of this, at least 70% should be in the form of unsaturated fatty acids. To attempt to eliminate all lipids from the diet, however, is unwise and may be detrimental

TABLE 3.1
COMPARISON OF CARBOHYDRATE, LIPID, PROTEIN, AND CALORIC INTAKE OF MIDDLE-AGED MALE AND FEMALE RUNNERS AND SEDENTARY CONTROLS[a]

	Runners	Sedentary Controls
Males		
Calories (kcal · day^{-1})	2959.0[b]	2361.0
Protein (g · day^{-1})	102.1	93.6
Protein (%)	13.8[b]	15.8
Lipid (g · day^{-1})	134.4[b]	109.0
Lipid (%)	40.8	41.5
Carbohydrate (g · day^{-1})	294.6[b]	225.7
Carbohydrate (%)	39.8	38.6
Cholesterol (mg · 1000 kcal^{-1})	175.0	190.0
Saturated fat (g · 1000 kcal^{-1})	16.2	16.0
Polyunsaturated fat (g · 1000 kcal^{-1})	9.0	9.3
Females		
Calories (kcal · day^{-1})	2386.0[b]	1871.0
Protein (g · day^{-1})	82.2	76.7
Protein (%)	14.2[b]	17.4
Lipid (g · day^{-1})	110.7	83.0
Lipid (%)	41.1	40.3
Carbohydrate (g · day^{-1})	234.3[b]	174.7
Carbohydrate (%)	39.5	39.1
Cholesterol (mg · 1000 kcal^{-1})	190.0	205.0
Saturated fat (g · 1000 kcal^{-1})	16.8	16.5
Polyunsaturated fat (g · 1000 kcal^{-1})	8.5	7.9

From Blair, S.N., et al.: Comparisons of nutrient intake in middle-aged men and women runners and controls. *Med. Sci. Sports. Exerc.*, 13:310, 1981.

[a]% calories do not total 100% because alcohol calories constitute the difference.

[b]Values for runners are significantly different from controls.

to exercise performance. With low-fat diets, it is difficult to increase carbohydrate and protein intake during strenuous training to furnish sufficient energy to maintain body weight and muscle mass. Also, because essential fatty acids such as linoleic acid and many vitamins are ingested through dietary lipids, a low-fat diet could eventually result in a relative state of malnutrition.

Carbohydrates. The prominence of dietary carbohydrates varies widely throughout the world, depending on factors such as the availability and relative cost of lipid-rich and protein-rich foods. Carbohydrate-rich foods such as grains, starchy roots, and dried peas and beans are usually cheapest in relation to their energy value. In the Far East, carbohydrates (rice) contribute 80% of the total caloric intake, whereas in the United States, only about 40 to 50% of energy intake comes from carbohydrates. Most evidence

suggests that there is little health hazard in subsisting chiefly on a variety of fiber-rich complex carbohydrates, provided that the essential amino acids and fatty acids, minerals, and vitamins are also consumed in adequate amounts. In fact, the diet of the Tarahumara Indians of Mexico is high in fiber and complex carbohydrates (75% of calories) and correspondingly low in cholesterol (71 mg/day), lipids (12% of calories), and saturated fat (2% of calories).[16] These people are noted for their remarkable physical endurance; they reportedly run distances of up to 200 miles in competitive soccer-type sports events that often last several days. This type of diet may confer health benefits. Particularly notable among the Tarahumaras is the virtual absence of hypertension, obesity, and death from cardiac and circulatory complications.

Adequate carbohydrate intake is crucial for an active person.[15] When the oxygen supply to active muscles is inadequate, stored muscle glycogen and blood-borne glucose are prime energy contributors. In addition to this anaerobic role of carbohydrates, stored glycogen provides substantial energy during more intense levels of aerobic exercise. Consequently, dietary carbohydrates are of utmost importance to men and women who maintain a physically active lifestyle. *Their diet should contain at least 50 to 60% of calories in the form of carbohydrates, predominantly starches, derived from fiber-rich, unprocessed grains, fruits, and vegetables.* During more strenuous training for specific sports and before competition, the carbohydrate intake may even be increased further to ensure adequate glycogen reserves. A general recommendation for athletes in heavy endurance training is maintenance of a daily carbohydrate intake of 10 g per kilogram of body mass. Thus, the daily carbohydrate intake for a 46-kg (100-lb) athlete who expends about 2800 kcal each day should be approximately 450 g or 1800 kcal. The athlete weighing 68 kg (150 lb) should take in approximately 675 g of carbohydrates (2700 kcal) as part of a daily energy requirement of 4200 kcal. In both examples, carbohydrates represent approximately 65% of the total energy intake. Specific diet and exercise techniques for facilitating glycogen storage in the days before endurance competition are presented in Chapter 23.

Carbohydrate Needs in Intense Training. Athletes training for endurance activities such as distance running, swimming, cross-country skiing, or cycling frequently experience a state of chronic fatigue in which successive days of hard training become progressively more difficult. This "staleness" can be related to a gradual depletion of the body's carbohydrate reserves with repeated strenuous training, even though the athlete's diet contains the typical percentage of carbohydrates. As shown in Figure 3.2, after 3 successive days of running 16.1 km (10 miles), the glycogen in the thigh muscle was nearly depleted.[18] This occurred even though the diets of the runners contained 40 to 60% carbohydrates. In addition, the amount of glyco-

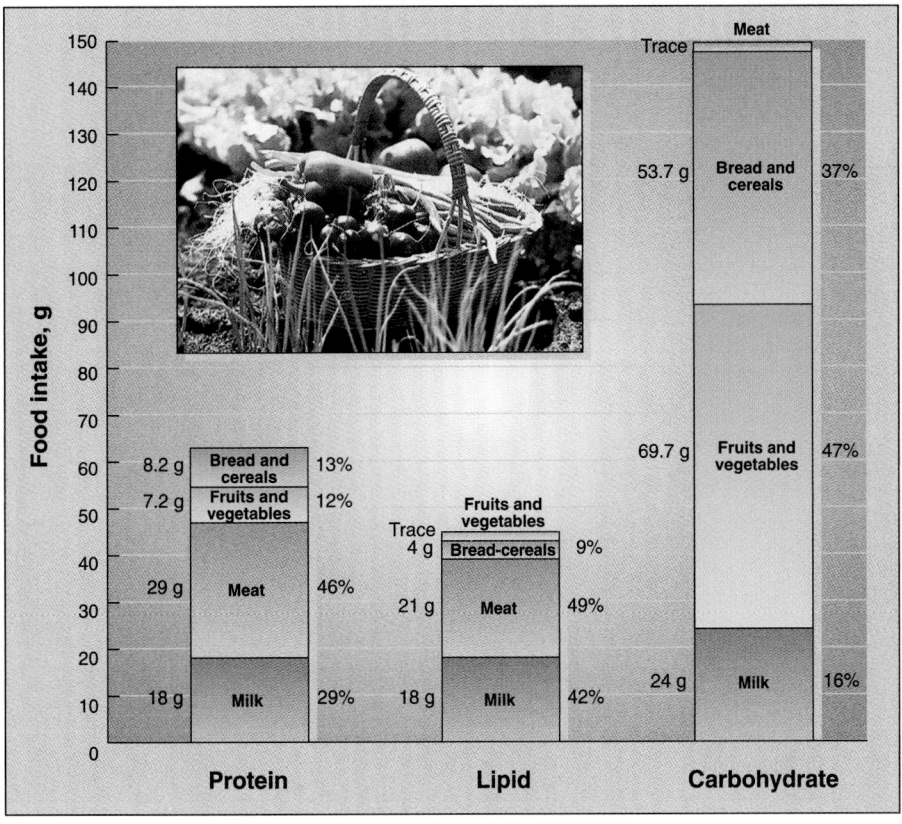

Food intake, g

	Protein		Lipid		Carbohydrate	
					Trace Meat	
					53.7 g Bread and cereals	37%
	8.2 g Bread and cereals	13%			69.7 g Fruits and vegetables	47%
	7.2 g Fruits and vegetables	12%	Trace 4 g Fruits and vegetables Bread-cereals	9%		
	29 g Meat	46%	21 g Meat	49%		
	18 g Milk	29%	18 g Milk	42%	24 g Milk	16%

FIGURE 3.1
Basic recommendations for carbohydrate, lipid, and protein components and the general categories of food sources in a balanced diet.

gen used on the third day of the run was much less than the amount used on the first day. Presumably, the energy for exercise was supplied predominantly by the body's lipid reserves. Because glycogen synthesis is related to carbohydrate intake, researchers now recommend increasing the daily carbohydrate intake to 70% of total calories (612 g for 3500 calories) or higher to prevent the depletion of glycogen stores and to induce protein sparing with successive days of hard training.[8, 9, 17] With more moderate training, a minimum of 400 to 500 g of carbohydrates should be ingested (usually equivalent to between 50 and 60% of caloric intake). Even if the diet is high in carbohydrates, muscle glycogen is not rapidly restored to the pre-exercise level. Although liver glycogen is restored at a faster rate, it takes at least 24 hours to replenish muscle glycogen levels after prolonged, exhaustive exercise.[22]

Unmistakably, if a person performs unduly heavy exercise on successive days, daily allowances must be adjusted to permit optimal glycogen resynthesis and the maintenance of high-quality training. *In addition, after exhaustive training and competition, at least 1 to 2 days of rest or lighter exercise combined with a high carbohydrate intake must be provided to reestablish the pre-exercise muscle glycogen levels.* This certainly provides a nutritional justification for the recommendation of many coaches and trainers to gradually re-

duce or taper the intensity of workouts several days before a competition.

THE EATING-RIGHT PYRAMID: THE ESSENTIALS OF GOOD NUTRITION

Variety and moderation are the key principles of good eating. Earlier approaches to formulating recommendations for sound nutrition, such as the Four-Food-Group Plan developed by the U.S. Department of Agriculture (USDA), were greatly influenced by lobbyists for the beef and dairy industries. Findings from research in nutrition, cancer, and heart disease during the past 35 years have revealed the shortcomings of the "basic four," with its overemphasis on meat and milk products, as a guide to healthful eating. To reflect the current state of nutritional knowledge more clearly, the USDA has developed a new model for good nutrition—the "Eating-Right Pyramid" (Fig. 3.3). This practical approach to sound nutrition maintains the concept of the four food groups and categorizes foods that make similar nutrient contributions; a recommended number of servings from each category is then provided. Emphasis, however, is focused on grains, vegetables, and fruits as the basis of the diet; food sources high in animal protein, lipids, and dairy products are downplayed. Serving size and number

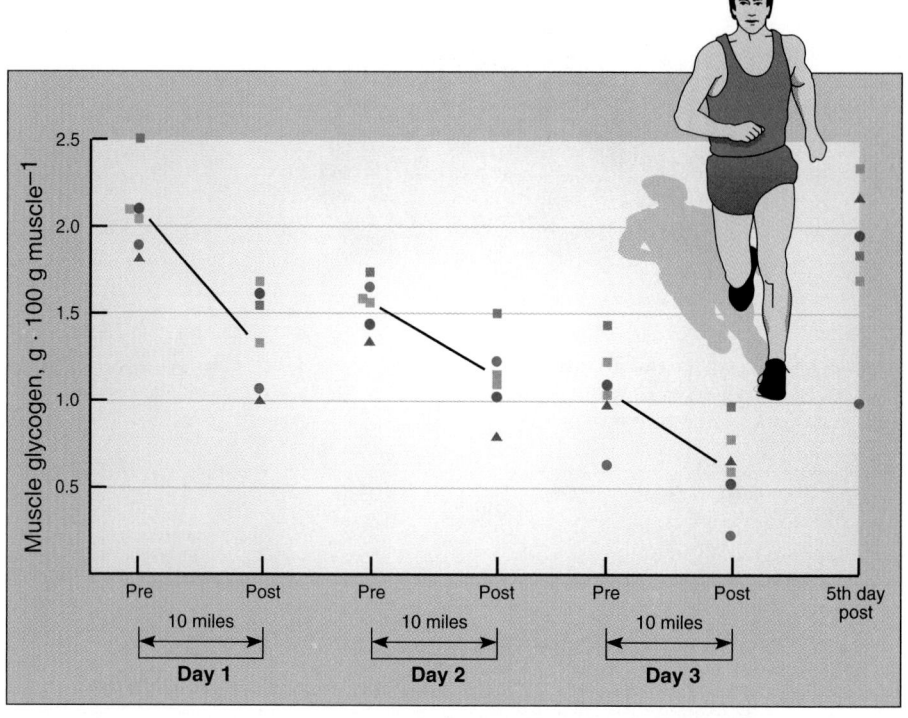

FIGURE 3.2

Changes in muscle glycogen concentration for six male subjects before and after 16.1-km runs performed on 3 successive days. Muscle glycogen was also measured 5 days after the last run (referred to as "5th day post"). (Modified from Costill, D.L., et al.: Muscle glycogen utilization during prolonged exercise on successive days. *J. Appl. Physiol.*, 31:834, 1971.)

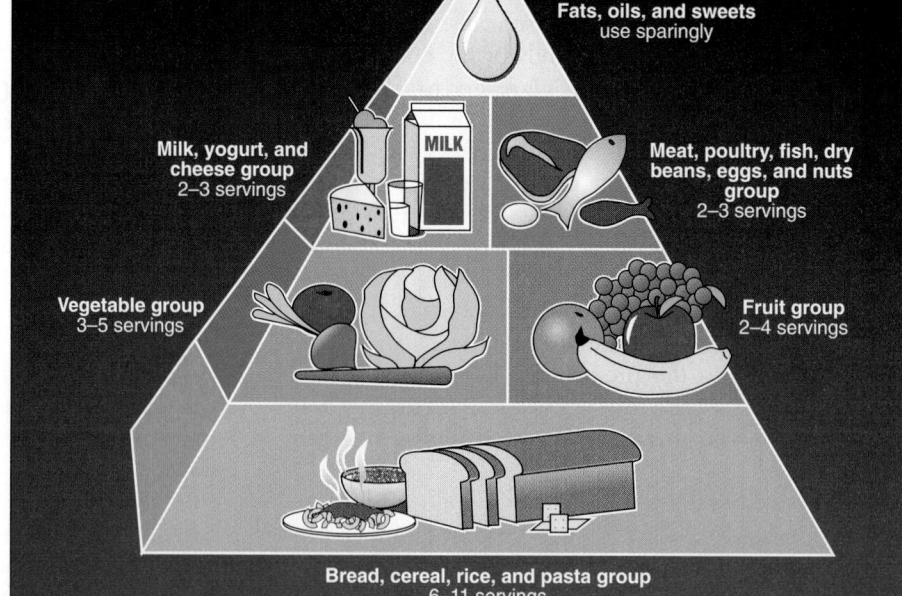

FIGURE 3.3

The Eating-Right Pyramid emphasizes grains, vegetables, and fruits as important sources of nutrients.

of servings are then regulated as needed for growth, level of physical activity, and the maintenance of a desirable body weight.

EXERCISE AND FOOD INTAKE

For individuals who engage regularly in moderate to intense physical activity, it is relatively easy to match food intake with the daily level of energy expenditure. Lumber workers, for example, who expend approximately 4500 calories daily, unconsciously adjust their caloric intake to closely balance their energy output. Consequently, body mass remains stable despite an extremely large food intake. When balancing food intake to meet a new level of energy output, the body requires 1 or 2 days to attain a new energy equilibrium. This fine balance between energy expenditure and food intake often is not maintained in sedentary people, and caloric intake generally exceeds the daily energy expenditure. The lack of precision in regulating food intake at the low end of the physical activity spectrum probably accounts for the "creeping obesity" commonly observed in highly mechanized and technically advanced societies.

The daily food intake of athletes in the 1936 Olympics reportedly averaged more than 7000 calories or roughly three times the average daily intake of nonathletic counterparts.[1] These caloric values often are quoted to justify what seems to be an enormous food requirement for athletes in training. However, these figures are only estimates, because objective dietary data were not presented in the original report. It is likely that the figures were inflated estimates of the energy expended (and required) by the athletes.[34] For example, distance runners who train upwards of 100 miles per week (6 minutes per mile at approximately 15 kcal per minute) probably do not expend more than 800 to 1300 "extra" calories each day above their normal energy requirement. For these endurance athletes, the daily food intake should supply approximately 4000 kcal to balance the increased energy expenditure. Data on energy intake from a large sample of elite male and female endurance, strength, and team sport athletes in the Netherlands are presented in Figure 3.4.[27] For the men, daily energy intake ranged between 2900 and 5900 kcal, whereas the intake of female competitors ranged between 1600 and 3200 kcal. With the exception of the high energy intake of athletes at extremes of

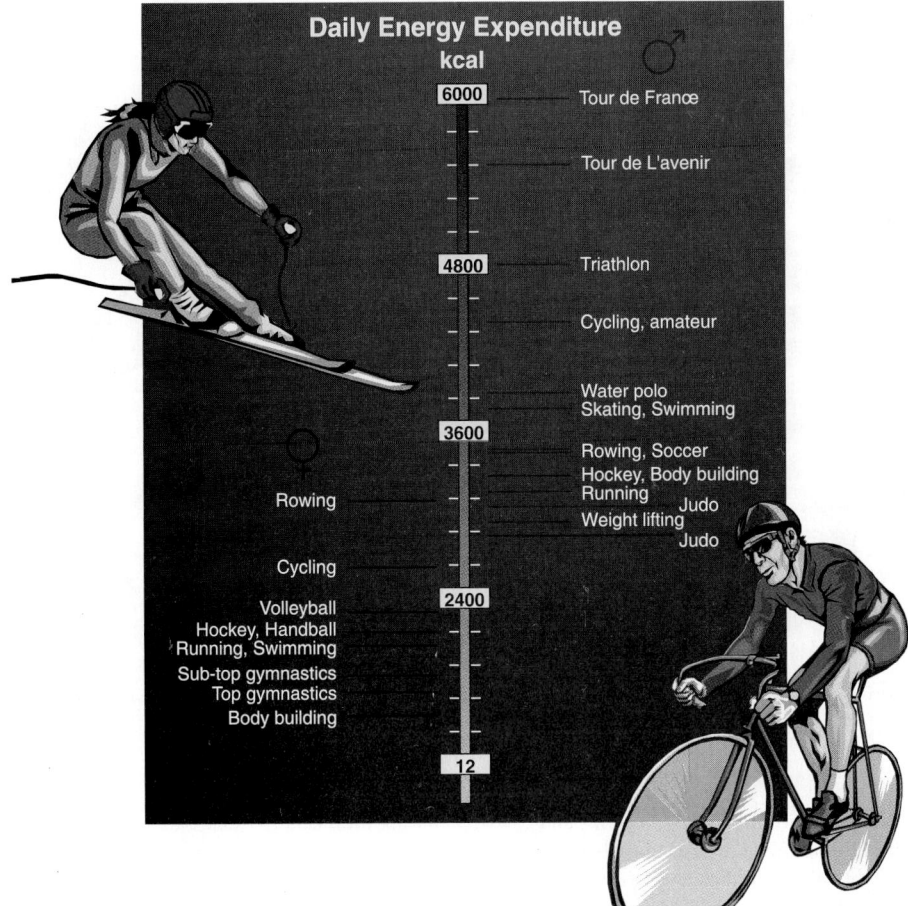

FIGURE 3.4

Daily energy intake (in kcal) of elite male and female endurance, strength, and team sport athletes. (Modified from van Erp-Baart, A.M.J., et al.: Nationwide survey on nutritional habits in elite athletes. *Int. J. Sports Med.*, 10:53, 1989.)

performance and training, daily caloric intake generally did not exceed 4000 kcal for the men and 3000 kcal for the women. Additional nutritional data for eight groups of male and female athletes, including four separate groups of male athletes, are summarized in Figure 3.5. The data are presented as percentage of total calories consumed as carbohydrates, proteins, and lipids, including total kcal per kg body mass. Not surprisingly, male triathletes and cyclists have the largest energy requirement in relation to body mass, whereas female dancers and football lineman have the lowest caloric intake in relation to body mass. Protein intake ranged from 13.4% (male lightweight rowers) to 20% (male weight lifters); carbohydrate percentage ranged from 66.2% (female triathletes) to 38.4% (male dancers); and lipid percentage ranged from a surprisingly high 45.1% (male dancers) to a low of 23.7% (male lightweight rowers).

Tour de France. Certain physical activities require an unusually large caloric output and have a correspondingly high energy intake requirement during competition or periods of high-intensity training. For example, the daily energy requirements of elite cross-country skiers during 1 week of training averaged from 3740 to 4860 calories for women and from 6120 to 8570 for men.[58] The variation in daily energy expenditure for a male competitor in the Tour de France professional cycling race is outlined in Figure 3.6.[9] During this event, the energy expenditure averaged approximately 6500 calories daily for nearly 3 weeks. Large daily variation was noted, however, depending on the level of activity for a particular day; the daily energy expenditure fell to approximately 3000 calories on a "rest" day and increased to approximately 9000 calories when cycling over a mountain pass. By combining liquid nutrition with normal meals, it

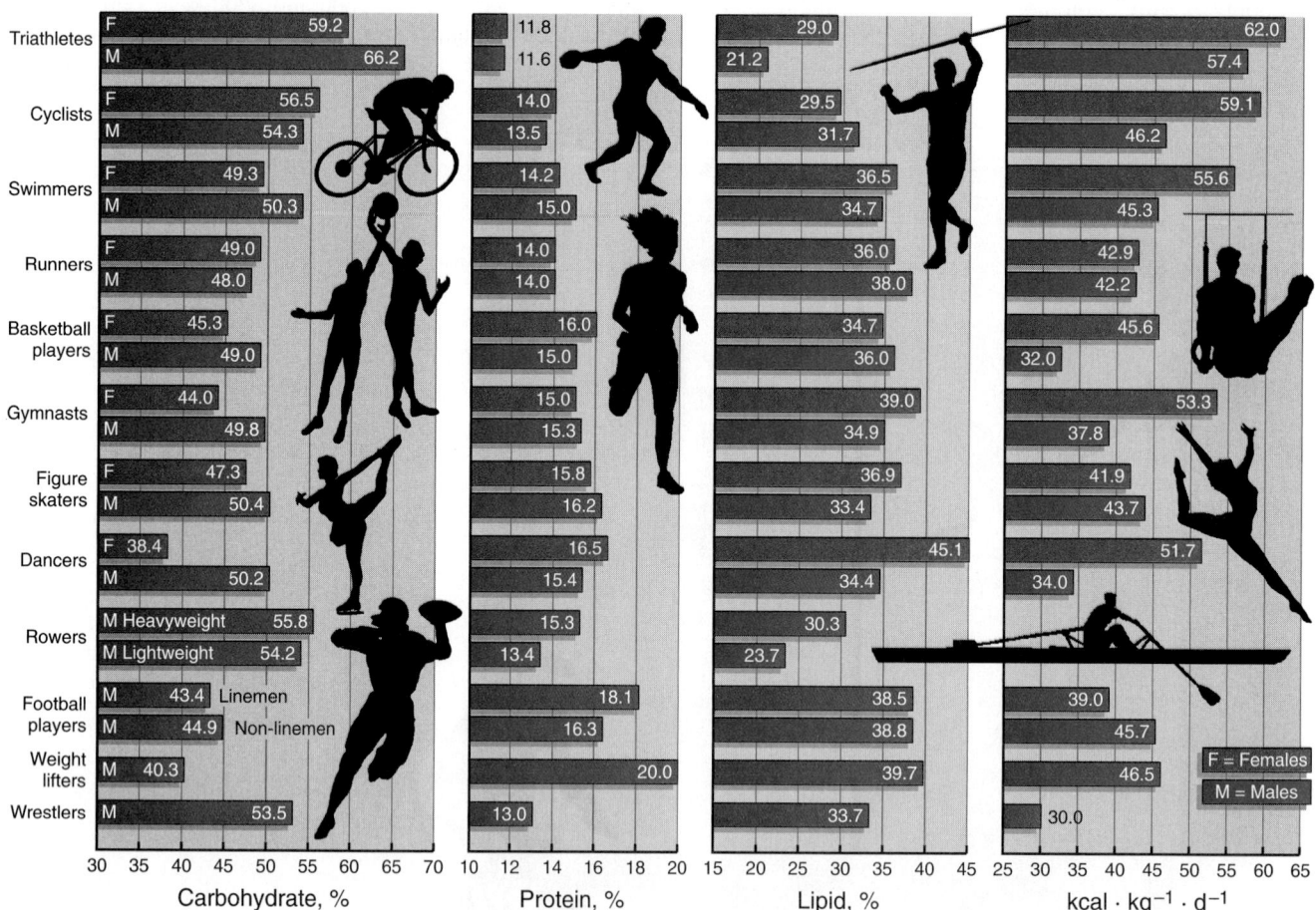

FIGURE 3.5

Percentage of total calories consumed in the form of carbohydrates, proteins, and lipids, including total kcal per kilogram body mass, for eight groups of male and female athletes and four additional groups of male athletes. The data represent averages for each group of athletes based on the world literature. (Data for lightweight and heavyweight male rowers courtesy of Likomitrou, M. Comparison of physical performance, nutritional and calorie intake, and body composition among heavyweight and lightweight oarsmen. Unpublished Master's thesis. University of Massachusetts, Amherst, MA, 1995.)

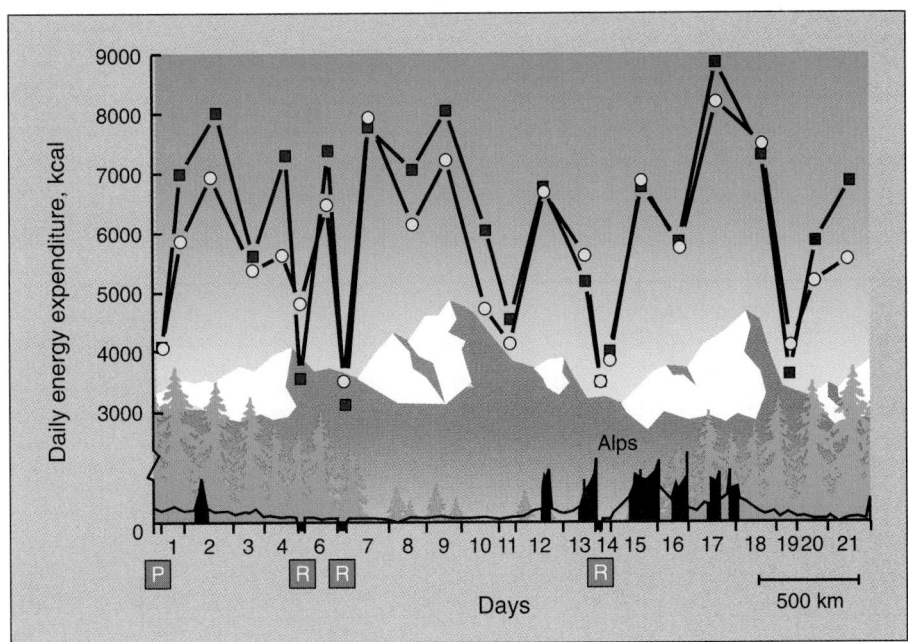

FIGURE 3.6

Daily energy expenditure (*purple squares*) and energy intake (*yellow circles*) for a cyclist during the Tour de France competition. Of note are the extremely high energy expenditure and the ability to achieve energy balance with the use of liquid nutrition in addition to normal meals. P, stage; R, rest day. (Modified from Saris, W.H.M., et al.: Adequacy of vitamin supply under maximal sustained workloads: the Tour de France. In *Elevated Dosages of Vitamins*. Edited by P. Walter, et al. Toronto, Huber Publishers, 1989.)

was possible for this athlete to match fairly closely the daily energy expenditure with energy intake.

Ultraendurance Running Competition. The energy balance (caloric intake and energy expenditure) has been studied during a 1000-km (approximately 600-mile) race from Sidney to Melbourne, Australia.[53] The Greek ultra-marathon champion Kouras completed this race in 5 days, 5 hours, and 7 minutes, finishing 24 hours and 40 minutes ahead of the next competitor. The relevant features of race conditions, distance covered, average daily speed, and rest and sleep patterns are listed in Table 3.2 (*top*). One striking feature is that Kouras did not sleep during the first 2 days of competition. He covered 463 km (287.8 miles) at an average speed of 11.4 km · h^{-1} during day 1 and 8.3 km · h^{-1} on day 2. During the remaining days, he took frequent rest periods, including periodic breaks for short "naps." Weather ranged from spring to winter conditions (8 to 30°C), and terrain was variable. The pertinent details of food and water intake are listed in Table 3.2 (*bottom*).

The remarkable part of this performance was the near equivalence between estimated total energy intake (55,970 kcal) and energy expenditure (59,079 kcal). Of the total energy intake, 95.3% was carbohydrates, 3% was lipids, and the remaining 1.7% was proteins. The latter averaged considerably below the generally recommended (RDA) level. The unusually large daily energy intake, which ranged between 8,600 and 13,770 kcal, was provided from Greek sweets (baklava, cookies, doughnuts), some chocolate, dried fruit and nuts, various fruit juices, and fresh fruits. Every 30 minutes after the first 6 hours of running, Kouras replaced sweets and fruit with a small biscuit soaked

in honey or jam. He consumed a small amount of roasted chicken on day 4 and drank coffee every morning. He took a 500-mg vitamin C supplement every 12 hours and a protein tablet twice daily.

The remarkable achievement by the champion Kouras exemplifies a highly conditioned athlete's exquisite regulatory control for energy balance during strenuous exercise. Not only did this runner perform at a pace that required a continuous supply of energy averaging 49% of aerobic capacity during the first 2 days of competition (and 38% for days 3 through 5), but he accomplished this without compromising overall health (no muscular injuries or thermoregulatory problems; body mass remained unchanged), except for a severe bout of constipation during the run and frequent urination that persisted for several days after the race.

Other Athletic Groups. At another extreme, training for some groups of athletes (gymnasts, ballet dancers, ice dancers, and weight class athletes in boxing, wrestling, and judo) is arduous; however, due to the nature of their sport, they continually strive to maintain a lean, light body mass. In these situations, energy intake often intentionally falls short of energy expenditure and a relative state of malnutrition develops. For these athletes, nutritional supplementation might be beneficial. This point is illustrated by the daily nutrient intake data (% of RDA) in Figure 3.7 for 97 competitive female gymnasts (11 to 14 years of age). Twenty-three percent of these adolescent girls consumed less than 1500 calories daily, and more than 40% consumed less than two-thirds of the RDA for vitamin E and folate and the minerals iron, magnesium, calcium, and zinc. Clearly, many of these gymnasts need to upgrade the

TABLE 3.2
FEATURES OF RACE CONDITIONS, DISTANCE COVERED, AVERAGE DAILY SPEED, REST AND SLEEP PATTERNS, AND NUTRIENT BALANCE DURING AN ELITE ULTRAENDURANCE PERFORMANCE (TOP). DAILY AND TOTAL ENERGY BALANCE, NUTRIENT DISTRIBUTIONS IN FOOD, AND WATER INTAKE DURING THE RACE (BOTTOM). THE RUNNER KOURAS WEIGHED 65 KG, STATURE WAS 171 CM, PERCENT BODY FAT WAS 8%, AND Vo$_2$MAX WAS 62.5 ML · KG^{-1} · MIN^{-1}

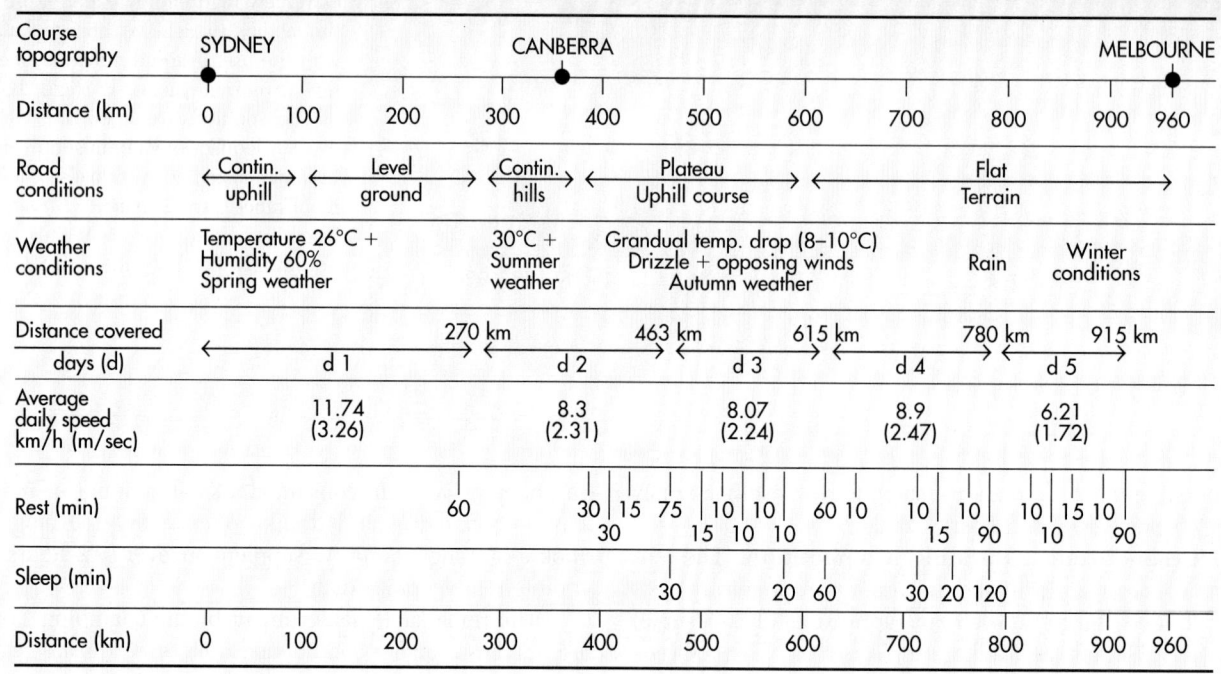

Day of the race	Distance covered	Estimated energy expenditure	Estimated energy intake	Carbohydrates			Lipids			Proteins			H$_2$O
	km	**kcal**	**kcal**	**g**	**%**	**kcal**	**g**	**%**	**kcal**	**g**	**%**	**kcal**	**L**
1	270	15367	13770	3375	98.0	13502	20	1.3	180	22	0.7	88	22.0
2	193	10741	8600	1981	92.2	7923	53	5.5	477	50	2.3	200	19.2
3	152	8919	12700	3074	96.8	12297	27	1.9	243	40	1.3	160	22.7
4	165	9780	7800	1758	90.1	7032	56	6.5	504	66	3.4	264	14.3
5	135	7736	12500	3014	96.4	12058	30	2.2	270	43	1.4	172	18.3
5 h	45	2536	550	138	100.0	550	—	—	—	—	—	—	3.2
Total	960	55079	55970	13340		53362	186		1674	221		734	99.7

nutritional quality of their food intake or consider supplementation.

Eat More, Weigh Less. As shown in Table 3.1, the caloric intake of 61 middle-aged men and women who ran an average of 60 km per week amounted to about 40 to 60% more calories per kg body mass compared to sedentary controls. The larger caloric intake for the runners was accounted for by the extra energy required to run between 8 and 10 km daily. Paradoxically, the most active men and women who ate considerably more on a daily basis weighed considerably less than subjects who were less physically active. Such data generally are consistent with other studies of physically active people and add further evidence to the strong argument that regular exercise provides an effective means by which a person actually can "eat more yet weigh less" and maintain a lower percentage of body fat.[10, 64] Active people maintain a lighter and leaner body and a healthier heart disease risk profile despite an increased intake of the typical American diet. A general model for food intake for active athletes as well as an example of a 2500-kcal menu containing 350 g of carbohydrates are presented in Table 3.3. The important role of

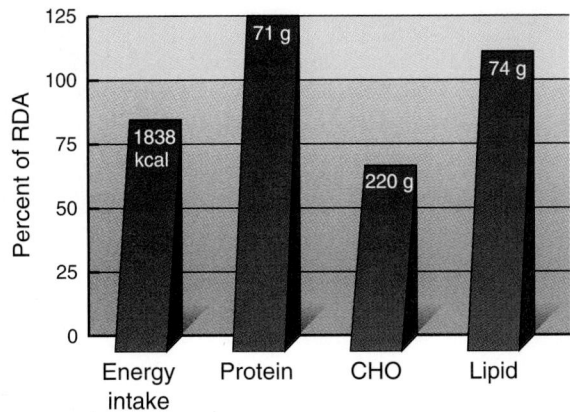

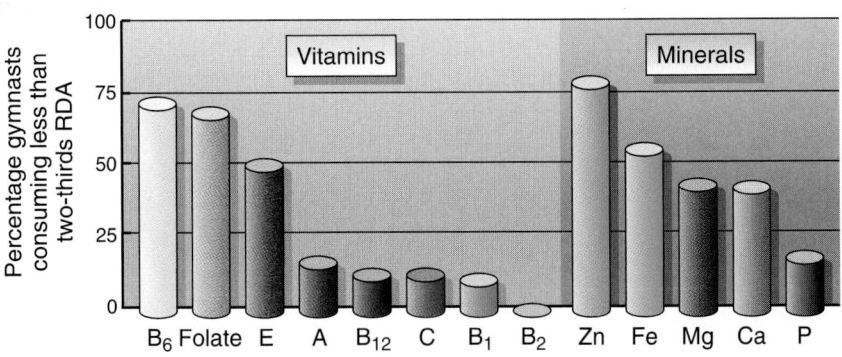

FIGURE 3.7
Average daily nutrient intake for 97 adolescent female gymnasts (11 to 14 years of age) in relation to recommended values. The RDA on the y axis reflects only protein, while energy, CHO, and lipid reflect "recommended" values (*top*). Percentage of gymnasts consuming less than two-thirds of the RDA (*bottom*). Mean age was 13.1 years, mean stature was 152.4 cm (60 in.), and mean body mass was 43.1 kg (94.8 lb). (Modified from Loosli, A.R., and Benson, J.: Nutritional intake in adolescent athletes. *Sports Med.*, 37:1143, 1990.)

exercise for weight control is discussed more fully in Chapter 29.

THE PRECOMPETITION MEAL

The main purpose of the precompetition meal is to provide the athlete with adequate carbohydrate energy and to ensure optimal hydration. Within this framework, fasting before competition or training makes no sense physiologically because it rapidly leads to a depletion of liver and muscle glycogen. The food preference of the athlete, the "psychological set" of the competition, and the digestibility of the foods should be considered in individualizing the meal plan. As a rule, foods high in lipid and protein content should be eliminated from the diet on the day of competition. This is because these foods are digested slowly and remain in the digestive tract longer than foods containing a similar amount of energy in the form of carbohydrates. Consideration should be given to the timing of the precompetition meal. With the increased stress and tension that usually accompany competition, there may be a significant decrease in blood flow to the digestive tract and an accompanying decrease in intestinal absorption.

PROTEIN OR CARBOHYDRATE?

Many athletes are psychologically accustomed to and even dependent on the classic "steak and eggs" pregame meal.

Although this meal may be satisfying to the athlete, coach, and restaurateur, its benefits in terms of exercise performance have yet to be demonstrated. In fact, such a meal, with its low carbohydrate content, actually may be detrimental to optimal performance.

There are several reasons for modifying or even abolishing the high-protein pregame meal in favor of one high in carbohydrates. One reason is that the normal overnight fast results in a significant depletion of carbohydrates in the liver and muscle that must be replenished by dietary carbohydrates. Carbohydrates also are digested and absorbed more rapidly than either proteins or lipids. Therefore, they are available for energy faster and reduce the feeling of fullness following a meal. Furthermore, the digestion, absorption, and assimilation of a high-protein meal elevates the resting metabolic rate considerably more than a high-carbohydrate meal. This metabolic heat adds additional strain to the body's heat-dissipating mechanisms, which could be detrimental to exercise performance in hot weather. Concurrently, the breakdown of protein for energy facilitates dehydration during exercise, because the by-products of amino acid breakdown demand water for urinary excretion. More specifically, approximately 50 mL of water "accompanies" the excretion of each gram of urea in the urine. Carbohydrate intake should be favored because it is the main energy nutrient for both short-term anaerobic activity as well as high-intensity endurance exercise.

TABLE 3.3
AN ACTIVE ATHLETE REQUIRES APPROXIMATELY 50 CALORIES OF FOOD PER KILOGRAM (23 CALORIES PER POUND) OF BODY MASS EACH DAY TO PROVIDE ENOUGH CALORIES FOR "OPTIMAL" ATHLETIC PERFORMANCE. A SAMPLE TRAINING DIET WOULD IDEALLY CONSIST OF APPROXIMATELY 60% CARBOHYDRATES, 15 TO 20% PROTEIN, AND LESS THAN 25% LIPIDS

Body Weight	110 lb (50 kg)	132 lb (60 kg)	154 lb (70 kg)	176 lb (80 kg)
Total kcal	**2500**	**3000**	**3500**	**4000**
Milk group (90 kcal) Skim milk, 1 cup Plain, low-fat yogurt, 1 cup	4[a]	4	4	4
Meat group (55–75 kcal) Cooked, lean meat (fish, poultry), 1 oz Egg, 1 Peanut butter, 1 tbsp Low-fat cheese, 1 oz Cottage cheese, 1/4 cup	5	5	6	6
Fruits	7	9	10	12
Vegetables	3	5	6	7
Grains	16	18	20	24
Lipid	5	6	8	10

Sample high-carbohydrate 2500-kcal menu (350 g)

Breakfast	Lunch	Dinner	Snack #1	Snack #2

1 cup bran cereal
8 oz low-fat milk
1 english muffin
1 tsp margarine
4 oz orange juice
	3 oz lean roast beef
	1 hard roll
	2 tsp mayonnaise or
	  mustard, lettuce
	  and tomato
	1/2 cup cole slaw
	2 fresh plums
	2 oatmeal cookies
	8 oz seltzer water
	  with lemon
		Chicken stir-fry:
		3 oz chicken
		1 cup diced vegetables
		2 tsp oil
		2 cup rice
		1 cup orange and
		  grapefruit sections
		1 cup vanilla yogurt
		Iced tea with lemon
			3 cups popcorn	8 oz apple cider

Modified from Carbohydrates and Athletic Performance. *Sports Science Exchange.* Vol. 7. Gatorade Sports Science Institute, Chicago, 1988.

[a]Unbolded numbers below total kcal values are recommended number of daily servings.

A precompetition meal containing 150 to 300 g of carbohydrates consumed 3 to 4 hours before exercising has the potential to improve performance by maximizing muscle and liver glycogen storage as well as by providing glucose for intestinal absorption during exercise. The precompetition meal is only of real significance if the athlete has maintained a nutritionally sound diet throughout training. This meal cannot correct nutritional deficiencies or inadequate nutrient intake during the weeks before competition. For endurance athletes, precompetition glycogen storage can be augmented in conjunction with specific exercise/diet modifications for "carbohydrate loading" (see Chapter 23).

LIQUID AND PREPACKAGED MEALS

Commercially prepared liquid meals offer an alternative approach to the precompetition meal. These foods are generally well balanced in nutritive value. They are high in carbohydrates but contain enough lipids and proteins to contribute to a feeling of satiety. Because they are in liquid form, they contribute to the athlete's fluid requirements. The liquid meal also is advantageous because it is digested rapidly, leaving essentially no residue in the intestinal tract. Liquid meals are particularly effective during day-long meets such as in swimming and track or in some tennis and basketball tournaments. In these situations, an athlete may have relatively little time for (or interest in) food. Liquid meals serve as a practical approach to supplementing caloric intake during the high energy output phase of training. They also can be used by athletes who have difficulty maintaining body weight or who desire to increase body mass.

Application in the Military. Although commercially prepared meals have been fairly well accepted by the athletic community, various military groups have long relied on prepackaged meals to optimize nutrition of personnel in a variety of work situations.[60] For example, soldiers during peacetime and military maneuvers are often required to work under diverse environmental conditions, including extremes of temperature, humidity, terrain, and terrestrial elevations. The Military Recommended Daily Allowances (MRDA) for food rations under operational conditions (and restricted rations) in relation to the RDA for men aged 19 to 22 years are listed in Table 3.4. These rations must have a useful storage life of up to 3 years at an ambient temperature of 27°C. Restricted rations are in certain operations, such as long-range patrol, assault, and reconnaissance, during which troops are required to subsist for up to 10 days on an energy-restricted ration. Whereas the RDAs do not provide recommendations for carbohydrate and lipid intake, the MRDA specifies the minimum intake of carbohydrates

(440 g or 48% of total kcal), lipids (160 g or 40% of total kcal), and protein (100 g or 11.1% of total kcal). The generally higher absolute protein intake is recommended under the assumption that the additional amino acids may be beneficial during stressful working conditions.[26]

A new development in creating palatable and nutritious rations for the military is the self-heating individual meal module (SHIMM).[60] This prepackaged ration contains a chemically activated, flameless heating system that brings food to the proper temperature within 10 minutes. Another development is the concept of a tailored system in which rations are optimized to environmental conditions that might modify nutritional requirements. In this system, a core module of food contains 1500 calories, with supplementary modules for hot (desert) and cold (Arctic) weather as well as high altitudes. Total caloric content is 3000 for the standard ration, which would be increased to 4500 for the Arctic ration. The 1500-calorie core module might contain dehydrated pork and rice, bread, a meat stick, two compressed cereal bars, two maltodextrin packets, and a dairy bar that could be made into a pudding.

Although military operations are not often thought of as athletic contests, soldiers often are required to perform pro-

TABLE 3.4
NUTRITIONAL STANDARDS FOR OPERATIONAL AND RESTRICTED RATIONS FOR MALES AGED 19 TO 22 YEARS AND COMPARISON TO THE UNITED STATES RDA

Nutrient	Unit	Operational Rations	Restricted Rations	RDA
Energy	kcal	3600	100–1500	2900 ± 400
Protein	g	100	50–70	56
Carbohydrate	g	440	100–200	—
Lipid	g	160 (maximum)	50–70	—
Vitamin A	μg	1000	500	1000
Vitamin D	μg	10	5	300
Vitamin E	mg	10	5	10
Ascorbic acid	mg	60	30	60
Thiamin	mg	1.8	1.0	1.5
Riboflavin	mg	2.2	1.2	1.7
Niacin	mg	24	13	19
Vitamin B_6	mg	2.2	1.2	2.2
Folacin	μg	400	200	400
Vitamin B_{12}	μg	3	1.5	3
Calcium	mg	800	400	800
Phosphorus	mg	800	400	800
Magnesium	mg	800	400	350
Iron	mg	18	9	10
Zinc	mg	15	7.5	15
Sodium	mg	5000–7000	2500–3500	1100–3300
Potassium	mg	1875–5625	950–2800	1880–5620

Data from Dunne, P.C.: Biochemical strategies for ration design: concerns of bioavailability. In *Food Components to Enhance Performance.* Edited by B.M. Marriot. Washington, D.C., National Academy Press, 1994.

longed arduous work that can be compared to a sporting event. It is not uncommon for some specialized military groups to endure environmental extremes for months at a time, often performing heavy exercise for up to 19 hours daily. Such metabolic demands pose a significant challenge to the scientists who collaborate to optimize military rations. These scientists must not only create prepackaged, compact, nutritious meals, but the meals also must be palatable, be resistant to contamination, and retain their nutritional potency for years.

CARBOHYDRATE FEEDINGS BEFORE, DURING, AND IN RECOVERY FROM EXERCISE

High-intensity aerobic exercise for 1 hour can decrease liver glycogen by about 55%, whereas a 2-hour strenuous workout can almost deplete the glycogen content of the liver and specifically exercised muscles. Even supermaximal, repetitive 1- to 5-minute bouts of exercise interspersed with brief rest (as in soccer and ice hockey) can dramatically lower liver and muscle glycogen reserves in a relatively short time period.[40, 57] This "vulnerability" of the body's glycogen stores during heavy exercise has caused a significant amount of research to focus on the potential beneficial role of carbohydrate feedings immediately before and during exercise. Scientists are also researching ways of optimizing carbohydrate replenishment during the postexercise recovery period.

DURING EXERCISE

Carbohydrates in either liquid or solid form that are consumed during exercise benefit performance in relatively high-intensity, long-term aerobic exercise and repetitive short bouts of near-maximal effort.[3, 25, 40, 42, 43, 46, 54, 67] In low-intensity exercise, the beneficial effect is negligible for carbohydrate feeding, because such exercise is fueled mainly by the oxidation of lipids with relatively small demand on carbohydrate breakdown.[2] Glucose feedings provide supplementary carbohydrate when the demand on glycogen is great, as in high-intensity exercise. This may either spare muscle glycogen, because the ingested glucose is used as fuel to power exercise, or help maintain a more optimal level of blood glucose, which prevents headache, lightheadedness, nausea, and other symptoms of central nervous system distress.[24, 41, 67] This maintenance of blood glucose also supplies muscles when glycogen reserves become depleted later in prolonged exercise.[14, 35, 50, 51]

Fatigue is postponed by 15 to 30 minutes with carbohydrate feeding during exercise at an intensity of 60 to 80% of aerobic capacity.[21] This effect is potentially significant in endurance competition because, for well-nourished athletes, fatigue usually occurs within 2 hours during intense aerobic exercise (performed at about 70% of maximum). The effect of a single concentrated carbohydrate feeding approximately

30 minutes before anticipated fatigue (usually 2 to 3 hours into exercise, when blood glucose and glycogen reserves are low) is as effective as periodic carbohydrate ingestion during exercise. This later feeding restores the blood glucose level, as shown in Figure 3.8. The result is an increase in carbohydrate availability and a delay in fatigue as blood glucose provides the energy needs of the active muscles.[21]

The endurance benefits of carbohydrate feedings are most effective during exercise at about 75% of aerobic capacity. With exercise that starts out above 75% of maximum, subjects were forced to reduce exercise intensity to about 75% during the final stages so they could maintain the benefits from the carbohydrate feedings.[14] With light to moderate exercise at or below 50% of maximum, the primary energy fuel is lipid, so the glycogen reserves are probably not taxed to a degree that would limit endurance. Research also shows that repeated feedings of carbohydrates in solid form (43 g sucrose with 400 mL water) at the beginning and at 1, 2, and 3 hours during exercise maintains blood glucose and reduces glycogen depletion during 4 hours of cycling; there also were enhancements for sprint performance to exhaustion at the end of the activity.[3, 3a, 5, 28, 36] *These findings illustrate that carbohydrate feedings during high-intensity aerobic exercise contribute to metabolism in a way that conserves the muscle's glycogen content for later use and/or maintains blood glucose for use later as exercise progresses and muscle glycogen becomes depleted.* The result is improved endurance at a high, steady pace or in prolonged high-intensity intermittent exercise, as well as a greater sprint capacity toward the end of prolonged physical effort. In a marathon run, the biochemical ability to sustain effort and sprint to the finish often determines the winner.

BEFORE EXERCISE

Feedings of high-glycemic carbohydrates in the 1-hour period before exercise have the potential to negatively affect exercise performance by:

- Rapidly raising blood sugar, causing an excess release of insulin to produce a relative hypoglycemia.
- Facilitating glucose influx into muscle to increase the substrate's availability for metabolism. At the same time, high insulin levels inhibit lipid mobilization from adipose tissue. Both factors cause an inordinately large carbohydrate metabolism and rapid depletion.

Research in the late 1970s indicated that drinking a highly concentrated sugar solution during the 30 minutes before exercise often caused early fatigue in endurance activities. For example, the riding time of young men and women on a bicycle ergometer was reduced 19% when they consumed a 300-mL solution containing 75 g of glucose 30 minutes before exercise, compared to similar trials preceded by the same volume of plain water or a liquid meal of protein, lipids, and carbohydrates.[29] Paradoxically, the muscle

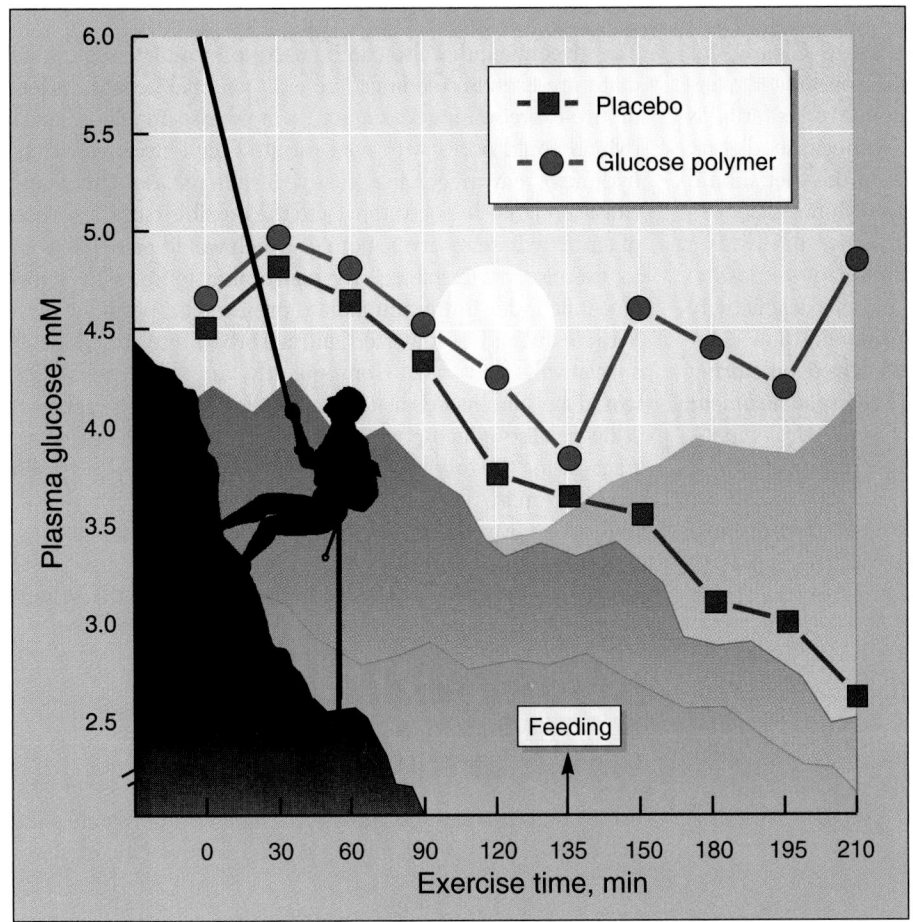

FIGURE 3.8
Average plasma glucose concentration during prolonged high-intensity aerobic exercise when subjects were fed a placebo (■) or glucose polymer (O) (3 g per kg body weight in a 50% solution). (Modified from Coggan, A.R., and Coyle, E.F.: Metabolism and performance following carbohydrate ingestion late in exercise. *Med. Sci. Sports Exerc.*, 21:59, 1989.)

glycogen reserves became prematurely depleted when using concentrated pre-event sugar drinks in contrast with drinking plain water. The explanation was that a pre-exercise challenge of simple carbohydrate causes a dramatic rise in blood sugar 5 to 10 minutes after ingestion. This rise leads to an overshoot in insulin release from the pancreas, which actually produces a decline in blood sugar (hypoglycemia) as glucose moves rapidly into the muscle.[37, 65] At the same time, insulin inhibits the mobilization and utilization of lipid for energy. Consequently, when exercise begins, intramuscular carbohydrate is used to a much greater degree than under normal conditions, causing premature glycogen depletion and fatigue. If more than 60 minutes are allowed after initiating pre-exercise glucose feedings, endurance performance would not be impaired because hormonal balance would be reestablished before exercise begins.[29, 33] Although these earlier research findings and explanations were impressive, the negative effects of concentrated pre-exercise sugar feedings observed in prior studies have **not** been duplicated in subsequent investigations.[19] No clear explanation for this discrepancy has been presented.

Fructose is absorbed more slowly from the gut than either glucose or sucrose, and causes only a minimal insulin response with essentially no decline in blood glucose. This has stimulated debate as to whether fructose would be beneficial as an immediate pre-exercise carbohydrate feeding.[47, 49] Although the theoretical rationale for the use of fructose appears strong, the ergogenic benefits are inconclusive concerning such feedings. What is important, however, is that the consumption of a high-fructose beverage is often accompanied by significant gastrointestinal distress, which in itself can negatively affect exercise performance.

IN RECOVERY

Not all carbohydrates are digested and absorbed by the body at the same rate. The **glycemic index** is a relative measure of the extent to which blood glucose increases after ingesting a food containing 50 g of carbohydrates. This increase is evaluated in relation to the increase observed when eating a "standard" for carbohydrate such as white bread or glucose, which is given the value of 100. Some common foods are classified in Figure 3.9 based on their glycemic index. It is noteworthy that the index is not formulated simply on the complexity of the ingested carbohydrate, because the plant starch in white rice and potatoes rates higher than the availability of the simple sugars in apples and peaches. Because of fiber content, which slows the rate of digestion, many fruits and vegetables, especially peas and beans (legumes), have a low glycemic index. Clearly, for rapid replenishment of carbohydrates after prolonged exercise, a food with a moderate to high glycemic index rating is more desirable than one rated low.[11, 19] Because dietary lipids delay gastric emptying, fatty foods in the diet should be limited to optimize carbohydrate replenishment.

The need for glycogen in previously active muscle is a primary factor affecting glycogen resynthesis in the postexercise period.[68] When food is available and physical activity is low, the hormonal milieu (elevated insulin and low catecholamines) increases the activity of the glycogen-storing enzyme **glycogen synthetase.** *To speed the replenishment of carbohydrates after a hard period of training or competition, it is wise to begin consuming carbohydrate-rich foods as soon as possible after exercising.* It is a good idea to eat about 50 to 75 g high- to moderate-glycemic carbohydrates every 2 hours until 500 g are consumed or until a large high-carbohydrate meal is eaten. Legumes, fructose, and milk products should be avoided because of their slow rates of intestinal absorption. More rapid resynthesis takes place if the person remains inactive during the recovery period.[13] With optimal carbohydrate intake, glycogen stores are replenished at a rate of about 5 to 7% per hour. Therefore, under the best of circumstances, it still will take at least 20 hours to reestablish glycogen stores after a glycogen-depleting bout of exercise.[22]

The Glycemic Index and Pre-Exercise Feedings. The glycemic index also can be used to formulate the immediate pre-exercise feeding. The one potential negative effect of pre-exercise simple sugars, a rapid rise in blood sugar (which could occur with concentrated high-glycemic carbohydrates), may trigger an excessive insulin release. This would cause a relative hypoglycemia and the possible early depletion of carbohydrate reserves, both of which would be deleterious to exercise performance. By consuming foods with a low glycemic index in the immediate pre-exercise period, carbohydrates would be digested and absorbed into the blood at a relatively slow rate. Consequently, any surge of insulin would be eliminated; at the same time, a steady supply of "slow-release" glucose would be available from the digestive tract during the exercise period. The wisdom of this approach to pre-exercise feeding has been supported by a study of trained cyclists performing high-intensity aerobic exercise. For equivalent carbohydrate content, a low-glycemic meal of lentils significantly extended endurance compared to feedings of glucose or a high-glycemic meal of potatoes.[61]

GLUCOSE FEEDINGS, ELECTROLYTES, AND WATER UPTAKE

Fluid ingestion before and during exercise attenuates the detrimental effects of dehydration on cardiovascular dynam-

FIGURE 3.9
Categorization for glycemic index of common food sources of carbohydrates.

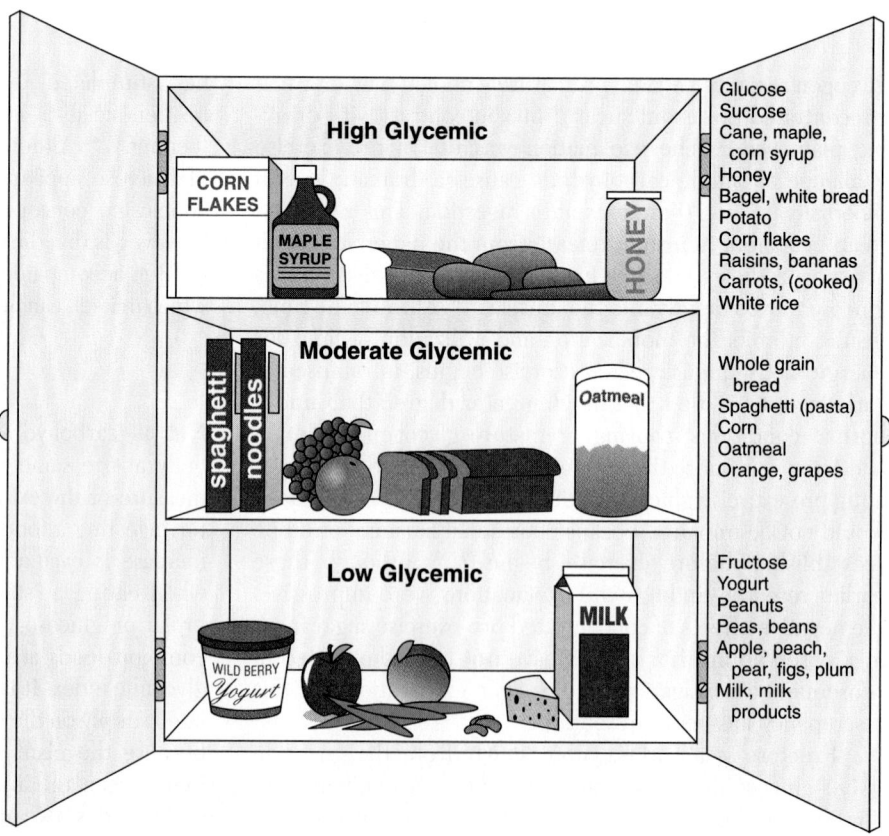

ics, temperature regulation, and exercise performance. By adding carbohydrates to the **oral rehydration solution**, additional energy for exercise is provided as the endogenous carbohydrate becomes depleted. To reduce fatigue and prevent dehydration, it is important to determine the optimal fluid/carbohydrate mixture and volume for an endurance activity. These combinations are important because the intake of a large fluid volume may impair carbohydrate uptake, and a concentrated sugar solution may impair fluid replacement. When sugars are consumed during exercise, there is no augmented reaction in insulin response (and resulting hypoglycemia) that could occur in the pre-exercise condition. During exercise, insulin release is inhibited because of the release of sympathetic nervous system hormones. Concurrently, exercise augments a muscle's ability to absorb glucose so the added exogenous glucose moves into the cells with a lower insulin requirement.

IMPORTANT CONSIDERATIONS

The absorption of fluid and nutrients is greatly affected by the rate at which they are emptied from the stomach into the small intestine. The important factors that influence gastric emptying are illustrated in Figure 3.10. There generally is little negative effect of exercise on gastric emptying up to an intensity of about 75% of maximum, at which point the stomach's emptying rate becomes somewhat reduced.[55]

Gastric emptying, however, is greatly influenced by gastric volume, and the rate of emptying decreases exponentially as fluid volume decreases. *Consequently, keeping fluid volume in the stomach at a relatively high level is a major factor to speed gastric emptying and may actually compensate for any inhibitory effects of the beverage's carbohydrate content.*[4, 55] This beneficial effect of an increased stomach volume on the passage of fluid and nutrients into the intestine is optimized by consuming 400 to 600 mL of fluid immediately before exercise. Then, regularly ingesting 150 to 250 mL of fluid (at 15-minute intervals) throughout exercise continually replenishes the fluid passed into the intestine and maintains a large gastric volume during exercise.[48] Although earlier research indicated that colder fluid was emptied from the stomach at a faster rate than fluid at room temperature, this is probably not a major factor during exercise.[44]

Of considerable concern regarding sugar drinks is their potential negative effect on water absorption from the digestive tract. Gastric emptying is slowed by an increased concentration of particles in solution (**osmolality**) as well as by the caloric density of the ingested fluid.[7, 14, 63] This could be deleterious during prolonged exercise in hot weather, when adequate intake **and** absorption of fluid are of prime importance to the athlete's health and safety. In this regard, the negative effects of sugar molecules on gastric emptying can be reduced and plasma volume can be maintained if a glucose polymer (**maltodextrin**) solution is

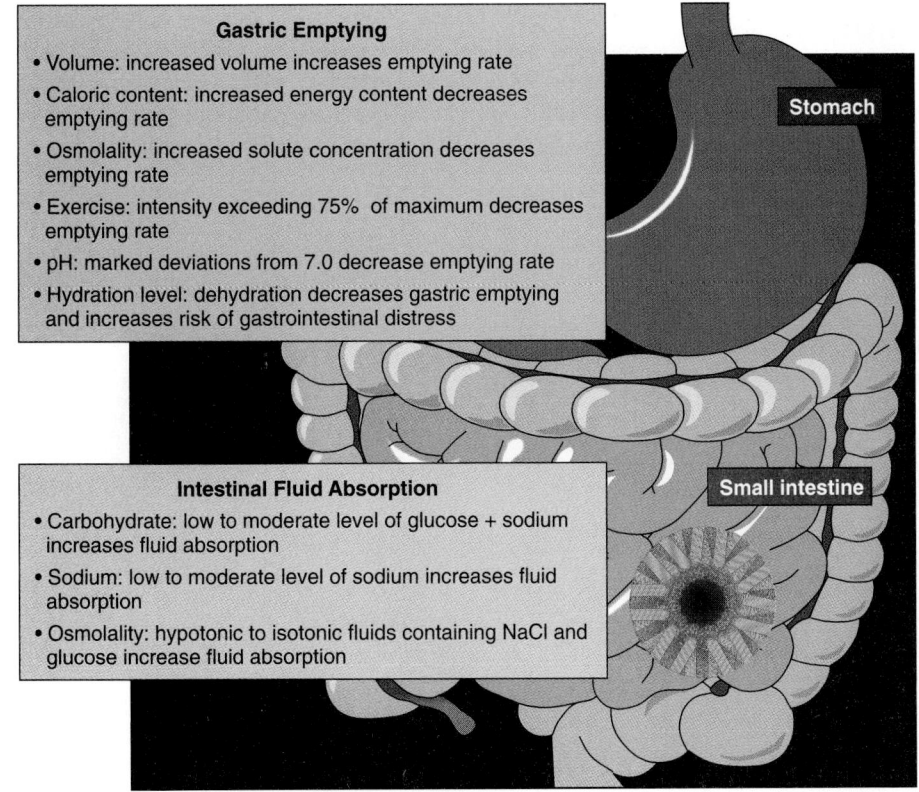

Gastric Emptying
- Volume: increased volume increases emptying rate
- Caloric content: increased energy content decreases emptying rate
- Osmolality: increased solute concentration decreases emptying rate
- Exercise: intensity exceeding 75% of maximum decreases emptying rate
- pH: marked deviations from 7.0 decrease emptying rate
- Hydration level: dehydration decreases gastric emptying and increases risk of gastrointestinal distress

Stomach

Intestinal Fluid Absorption
- Carbohydrate: low to moderate level of glucose + sodium increases fluid absorption
- Sodium: low to moderate level of sodium increases fluid absorption
- Osmolality: hypotonic to isotonic fluids containing NaCl and glucose increase fluid absorption

Small intestine

FIGURE 3.10
Major factors that affect gastric emptying (stomach) and fluid absorption (small intestine).

used in formulating the drink.[54, 56, 59] The use of short-chain polymers (3 to 20 glucose units) derived from corn starch breakdown reduces the number of particles in solution; this facilitates the movement of water from the stomach to the intestine for absorption. Furthermore, the addition of a small amount of glucose and sodium (glucose being the more important factor) to the oral rehydration solution has only a small negative effect on gastric emptying and may actually facilitate a fluid's uptake once in the intestinal lumen.[31, 32, 32a] The reason for this is that the active coupled or cotransport of glucose-sodium across the intestinal mucosa is rapid, thus stimulating the passive uptake of water by osmotic action.[55] Consequently, not only is water replenished effectively, but the additional glucose uptake can contribute to the maintenance of blood glucose. This might then spare muscle and liver glycogen and/or provide glucose if glycogen reserves fall during the later stage of exercise.

The addition of small amounts of sodium to the ingested fluid probably has little effect on glucose and water absorption.[32a, 38] This extra sodium may, however, contribute to maintaining plasma sodium concentrations. This would benefit the ultraendurance athlete, who is at risk for hyponatremia because of a potentially large sweat-sodium loss coupled with a large water intake (see Chapter 2). More than likely, the intake of sodium and water aids in maintaining an elevated plasma osmolality. This sustains the osmotic drive to drink and thus promotes continued fluid intake during the postexercise period.

RECOMMENDED ORAL REHYDRATION SOLUTION

The ideal oral rehydration solution contains a carbohydrate concentration of between 5 and 8%.[12, 45, 52, 62, 66] To determine the percentage of carbohydrate in a drink,

divide the carbohydrate content (in grams) by the fluid volume (in milliliters) and multiply by 100. Oral rehydration solutions within this range generally permit carbohydrate replenishment without hindering water uptake, fluid homeostasis, and temperature regulation compared to ingesting plain water during prolonged exercise in the heat. Of course, various environmental and exercise conditions interact to influence the optimal composition of the rehydration solution. If the duration of the intense aerobic effort is relatively short (less than 1 hour) and the thermal stress is high, fluid replenishment is of utmost importance to health and safety, and it is advisable to consume a diluted carbohydrate-electrolyte solution (less than 5% carbohydrates). A more concentrated beverage of approximately 15% carbohydrates may be appropriate in cooler weather, in which dehydration is not a major factor. There is little difference between liquid glucose, sucrose, or starch as the ingested carbohydrate fuel source during exercise.[30] Fructose is not desirable because its absorption by the gut does not involve the active cotransport process required for glucose-sodium. Therefore, fructose absorption is relatively slow and promotes less fluid uptake than an equivalent amount of glucose. The optimal carbohydrate replacement rate is between 30 and 60 g (about 1 to 2 oz) per hour ingested at least 30 minutes before the time when fatigue would normally occur without a carbohydrate supplement.

A general guideline for fluid intake during each hour of exercise for a given amount of carbohydrate replenishment is presented in Figure 3.11.[23] Although there is a tradeoff between carbohydrate ingestion and gastric emptying, it is possible to empty up to 1700 mL of water per hour from the stomach, even when drinking an 8% carbohydrate solution. However, 1000 mL (about 1 quart) of fluid ingestion per hour is probably optimal to offset dehydration, because larger amounts of fluid often result in gastrointestinal discomfort.

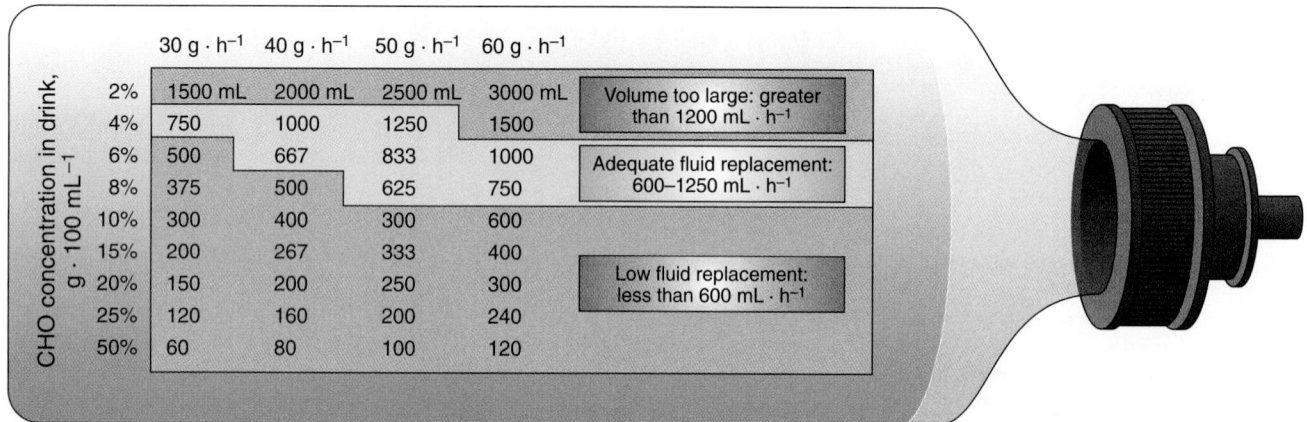

FIGURE 3.11
Volume of fluid to ingest each hour to obtain the noted amount of carbohydrates. (Modified from Coyle, E.F., and Montain, S.J.: Benefits of fluid replacement. *Med. Sci. Sports Exerc.*, 24:S324, 1992.)

Practical Recommendations for Fluid and Carbohydrate Replacement[23]

- Monitor the rate of dehydration by changes in body weight. Each pound of weight loss corresponds to 450 mL (15 fluid oz) of dehydration.
- Drink fluids at the same rate that they are being depleted (or at least drink at a rate that is close to 80% of the sweating rate) during prolonged exercise in which there is cardiovascular stress, excessive heat, and dehydration.
- The endurance athlete can meet both carbohydrate (30 to 60 g per hour) and fluid requirements by drinking between 625 to 1250 mL of a beverage containing 4 to 8% carbohydrates each hour.

■ SUMMARY ■

1. Within rather broad limits, the nutrient requirements of athletes and other individuals engaged in training programs can be achieved with a balanced diet. With well-planned menus, the vitamin, mineral, and protein requirements can be met with a food intake of about 1200 calories a day. Additional food then can be consumed to meet energy needs depending on the daily level of physical activity.

2. The recommended protein intake of 0.8 g per kilogram body mass is a liberal requirement believed to be adequate for all people, regardless of physical activity level. Athletes generally consume two to five times the protein RDA because their greater caloric intake usually provides proportionately more protein.

3. Precise recommendations have not been established for lipid and carbohydrate intake. A prudent recommendation is that no more than 30% of the daily calories should be obtained from lipids; of this amount, most should be in the form of unsaturated fatty acids. For people who are physically active, 60% or more of the calories should come from carbohydrates, particularly unrefined polysaccharides. This generally represents between 400 and 600 g on a daily basis.

4. Successive days of hard training can gradually deplete the body's carbohydrate reserves, even when maintaining the recommended carbohydrate intake. This could lead to a training "staleness" in which continued training becomes exceedingly more difficult.

6. The Eating-Right Pyramid provides broad recommendations for healthful nutrition. Emphasis is placed on fruits, grains, and vegetables; deemphasized are foods high in animal protein, lipids, and dairy products. This approach to nutrition is ideal for the physically active man and woman.

7. The most important factor determining the daily caloric requirement is the level of physical activity. It is likely that the daily caloric requirements of athletes in strenuous sports do not exceed 4000 calories unless body mass is excessive or the training level or competition is extreme. Such a high caloric intake usually exceeds the RDA requirements for protein, vitamins, and minerals.

8. The precompetition meal should include foods that are readily digested and contribute to the energy and fluid requirements of exercise. For this reason, the meal should be high in carbohydrates and relatively low in lipids and proteins. Clearly, the typical low-carbohydrate "steak-and-eggs diet" does not meet the requirements for optimal pre-event nutrition.

9. Three hours should be sufficient to permit digestion and absorption of the precompetition meal.

10. Commercially prepared liquid meals offer a practical approach to precompetition nutrition and caloric supplementation. These "meals" are well balanced in nutritive value, contribute to fluid needs, and are absorbed rapidly, leaving practically no residue in the digestive tract.

11. Carbohydrate-containing rehydration solutions consumed during exercise can enhance high-intensity endurance performance by maintaining blood sugar concentration. This can then be used by the active muscles to either spare muscle glycogen or serve as reserve glucose for later use if muscle glycogen becomes depleted.

12. The glycemic index is a relative measure of the extent to which blood glucose increases after ingesting a specific carbohydrate. For rapid carbohydrate replenishment after exercise, individuals should consume carbohydrate-containing foods (50 to 75 g each hour) with a moderate to high glycemic index.

13. Maintaining a relatively large fluid volume in the stomach throughout exercise greatly enhances gastric emptying. This is achieved by consuming 400 to 600 mL of fluid immediately before exercise followed by regular fluid ingestion during exercise (approximately 200 mL every 15 minutes).

14. Concentrated sugar drinks slow the rate of gastric emptying, which could ultimately upset the body's fluid balance. The ideal oral rehydration solution should probably contain between 5 and 8% carbohydrates. This would permit carbohydrate replenishment without adversely affecting fluid balance and thermoregulation.

■ REFERENCES ■

1. Abrahams, A.: The nutrition of athletes. Br. J. Nutr., 2:266, 1948.
2. Ahlborg, G., and Felig, P.: Influence of glucose ingestion on the fuel-hormone response during prolonged exercise. J. Appl. Physiol., 41:683, 1976.
3. Bacharrach, D.W., et al.: Carbohydrate drinks and cycling performance. J. Sports Med. Phys. Fitness, 34:161, 1994.
3a. Ball, T.C., et al.: Periodic carbohydrate replacement during 50 min of high-intensity cycling improves subsequent sprint performance. Int. J. Sports Nutr., 5:151, 1995.
4. Beckers, E.J., et al.: Comparison of aspiration and scintigraphic techniques for the measurement of gastric emptying rates in man. Gut, 33:115, 1992.

5. Below, P.R., et al.: Fluid and carbohydrate ingestion independently improve performance during 1 h of intense exercise. *Med. Sci. Sports Exerc.*, 27:200, 1995.

6. Blair, S.N., et al.: Comparison of nutrient intake in middle-aged men and women runners and controls. *Med. Sci. Sports Exerc.*, 13:310, 1981.

7. Brouns, F., and Beckers, E.: Is the gut an athletic organ? *Sports Med.*, 15:242, 1993.

8. Brouns, F., et al.: Eating, drinking, and cycling. A controlled Tour de France simulation study, Part I. *Int. J. Sports Med.*, 10:532, 1989.

9. Brouns, F., et al.: Eating, drinking, and cycling. A controlled Tour de France simulation study, Part II. Effect of diet manipulation. *Int. J. Sports Med.*, 10:541, 1989.

10. Brownell, K.D., and Stunkard, A.J.: Physical activity in the development and control of obesity. In *Obesity*. Edited by A.J. Stunkard. Philadelphia, W.B. Saunders, 1980.

11. Burke, L.M., et al.: Muscle glycogen storage after prolonged exercise: effect of the glycemic index on carbohydrate feedings. *J. Appl. Physiol.*, 75:1019, 1993.

12. Burstein, R., et al: Glucose polymer ingestion—effect on fluid balance and glycemic state during a 4-d march. *Med. Sci. Sports Exerc.*, 26:360, 1994.

13. Choi, D., et al.: Effect of passive and active recovery on the resynthesis of muscle glycogen. *Med. Sci. Sports Exerc.*, 26:992, 1994.

14. Coggan, A.R., and Coyle, E.F.: Metabolism and performance following carbohydrate ingestion late in exercise. *Med. Sci. Sports Exerc.*, 21:59, 1989.

15. Coggan, A.R., and Coyle, E.F.: Carbohydrate ingestion during prolonged exercise: effects on metabolism and performance. *Exerc. Sport Sci. Rev.*, 19:1, 1991.

16. Connor, W.E., et al.: The plasma lipids, lipoproteins, and diet of the Tarahumara Indians of Mexico. *Am. J. Clin. Nutr.*, 31:1131, 1978.

17. Costill, D.L., and Miller, J.: Nutrition for endurance sports: carbohydrate and fluid balance. *Int. J. Sports Med.*, 1:2, 1980.

18. Costill, D.L., et al.: Muscle glycogen utilization during prolonged exercise on successive days. *J. Appl. Physiol.*, 31:834, 1971.

19. Coyle, E.F.: Timing and method of increased carbohydrate intake to cope with heavy training, competition and recovery. *J. Sports Sci.*, 9:29, 1991.

20. Coyle, E.F.: Substrate utilization during exercise in active people. *Am. J. Clin. Nutr.*, 61:968S, 1995.

21. Coyle, E.F., and Coggan, A.R.: Effectiveness of carbohydrate feeding in delaying fatigue during prolonged exercise. *Sports Med.*, 1:446, 1984.

22. Coyle, E.F., and Coyle, E.: Carbohydrates that speed recovery from training. *Phys. Sportsmed.*, 21:111, 1993.

23. Coyle, E.F., and Montain, S.J.: Benefits of fluid replacement with carbohydrate during exercise. *Med. Sci. Sports Exerc.*, 24:S324, 1992.

24. Coyle, E.F., et al.: Carbohydrate feeding during prolonged strenuous exercise can delay fatigue. *J. Appl. Physiol.*, 55:230, 1983.

25. Coyle, E.F., et al.: Muscle glycogen utilization during prolonged strenuous exercise when fed carbohydrate. *J. Appl. Physiol.*, 61:165, 1986.

26. Dunne, P.C.: Biochemical strategies for ration design: concerns of bioavailability. In *Food Components to Enhance Performance*. Edited by B.M. Marriot. Washington, D.C., National Academy Press, 1994.

27. van Erp-Baart, A.M.J., et al.: Nationwide survey on nutritional habits in elite athletes. Part I. Energy, carbohydrate, protein, and fat intake. *Int. J. Sports Med.*, 10:53, 1989.

28. Fielding, R.A., et al.: Effect of carbohydrate feeding frequencies and dosage on muscle glycogen use during exercise. *Med. Sci. Sports Exerc.*, 17:472, 1985.

29. Foster, C., et al.: Effects of pre-exercise feedings on endurance performance. *Med. Sci. Sports Exerc.*, 11:1, 1979.

30. Fujisawa, T., et al.: The effects of exercise on fructose absorption. *Am. J. Clin. Nutr.*, 58:75, 1993.

31. Gisolfi, C.V., et al.: Human intestinal water absorption: direct vs. indirect measurements. *Am. J. Physiol.*, 258:G216, 1990.

32. Gisolfi, C.V., et al.: Intestinal water absorption from select carbohydrate solutions in humans. *J. Appl. Physiol.*, 7:2142, 1992.

32a. Gisolfi, C.V., et al.: Effect of sodium concentration in a carbohydrate-electrolyte solution on intestinal absorption. *Med. Sci. Sports Exerc.*, 27:1414, 1995.

33. Gleeson, M., et al.: Comparison of the effects of pre-exercise feedings of glucose, glycerol, and placebo on endurance and fuel homeostasis in man. *Eur. J. Appl. Physiol.*, 55:645, 1986.

34. Grandjean, A.C.: Macronutrient intakes of U.S. athletes compared with the general population and recommendations made for athletes. *Am. J. Clin. Nutr.*, 49:1070, 1989.

35. Hargreaves, M., and Briggs, C.A.: Effect of carbohydrate ingestion on exercise metabolism. *J. Appl. Physiol.*, 65:1553, 1988.

36. Hargreaves, M., et al.: Effect of carbohydrate feedings on muscle glycogen utilization and exercise performance. *Med. Sci. Sports Exerc.*, 16:219, 1984.

37. Hargreaves, M., et al.: Effect of fructose ingestion on muscle glycogen usage during exercise. *Med. Sci. Sports Exerc.*, 17:360, 1985.

38. Hargreaves, M., et al.: Influence of sodium on glucose bioavailability during exercise. *Med. Sci. Sports Exerc.*, 26:365, 1994.

39. Hartung, G.H., et al.: Effects of marathon running, jogging, and diet on coronary risk factors in middle-aged men. *Prev. Med.*, 10:316, 1981.

40. Hawley, J.A., et al.: Carbohydrate, fluid, and electrolyte requirements of the soccer player: a review. *Int. J. Sports Med.*, 4:221, 1994.

41. Krzentowski, B., et al.: Availability of glucose given orally during exercise. *J. Appl. Physiol.*, 56:315, 1984.

42. Lugo, M., et al.: Metabolic responses when different form of carbohydrate energy are consumed during cycling. *Int. J. Sports Nutr.*, 3:398, 1993.

43. Mason, W.L., et al. Carbohydrate ingestion during exercise: liquid vs. solid feeding. *Med. Sci. Sports Exerc.*, 25:966, 1993.

44. Maughan, R.J.: Effects of CHO-electrolyte solution on prolonged exercise. In *Perspectives in Exercise Science and Sports Medicine*. Edited by D.R. Lamb and M.H. Williams. Carmel, Benchmark Press, 1991.

45. Millard-Stafford, M.L., et al.: Carbohydrate-electrolyte replacement improves distance running performance in the heat. *Med. Sci. Sports Exerc.*, 24:934, 1992.

46. Mitchell, J.B., et al.: Effects of carbohydrate ingestion on gastric emptying and exercise performance. *Med. Sci. Sports Exerc.*, 20:110, 1988.

47. Murray, R., et al.: The effects of glucose, fructose, and sucrose ingestion during exercise. *Med. Sci. Sports Exerc.*, 21:275, 1989.

48. Noakes, T.D., et al.: The importance of volume in regulating gastric emptying. *Med. Sci. Sports Exerc.*, 23:307, 1991.

49. Okano, G., et al.: Effect of pre-exercise fructose ingestion on endurance performance in fed man. *Med. Sci. Sports Exerc.*, 20:105, 1988.

50. Pallikarikas, N., et al.: Remarkable metabolic activity of oral glucose during long-duration exercise in humans. *J. Appl. Physiol.*, 60:1035, 1986.

51. Pirnay, F., et al.: Fate of exogenous glucose during exercise of different intensities in man. *J. Appl. Physiol.*, 53:1620, 1982.

52. Rehrer, N.J., et al.: Gastric emptying, absorption, and carbohydrate oxidation during prolonged exercise. *J. Appl. Physiol.*, 72:468, 1992.

53. Rontoyannis, G.P., et al.: Energy balance in ultramarathon running. *Am. J. Clin. Nutr.*, 49:976, 1989.

54. Ryan, A.J., et al.: Gastric emptying during prolonged exercise in the heat. *Med. Sci. Sports Exerc.*, 21:51, 1989.

55. Schedl, H.P., et al.: Intestinal absorption during rest and exercise: implications for formulating an oral rehydration solution (ORS). *Med. Sci. Sports Exerc.*, 26:267, 1994.

56. Seiple, R.S., et al.: Gastric-emptying characteristics of two glucose polymer-electrolyte solutions. *Med. Sci. Sports Exerc.*, 15:366, 1983.

57. Simard, C., et al.: Effect of carbohydrate intake before and during an ice hockey match on blood and muscle energy substrates. *Res. Q. Exerc. Sport.*, 59:144, 1988.

58. Sjödin, A.M., et al.: Energy balance in cross-country skiers: a study using doubly labeled water. *Med. Sci. Sports Exerc.*, 26:720, 1994.

59. Sole, C.C., and Noakes, T.D.: Faster emptying for glucose-polymer and fructose solutions than for glucose in humans. *Eur. J. Appl. Physiol.*, 58:605, 1989.

60. Taub, I.A.: Optimizing the design of combat rations. In *Food Components to Enhanced Performance*. Edited by B.M. Marriot. Washington, D.C., National Academy Press, 1994.

61. Thomas, D.E., et al.: Carbohydrate feeding before exercise: effect of glycemic index. *Int. J. Sports Med.*, 12:180, 1991.

62. Vist, G.E., and Maughn, R.J.: Gastric emptying of dilute glucose solutions in man. *Med. Sci. Sports Exerc.*, 22:S70, 1992.

63. Vist, G.E., and Maughan, R.J.: Gastric emptying of ingested solutions in man: effect of beverage glucose concentration. *Med. Sci. Sports Exerc.*, 26:1269, 1994.

64. Wood, P.D., et al.: Exercise and plasma lipoproteins: a one-year randomized, controlled trial. *Council on Epidemiology Newsletter*, 30:20, 1981.

65. Yannick, C., et al.: Oxidation of corn starch, glucose, and fructose ingested before exercise. *Med. Sci. Sports Exerc.*, 21:45, 1989.

66. Yaspelkis, B.B. III, and Ivy, J.L.: Effects of carbohydrate supplements and water on exercise metabolism in the heat. *J. Appl. Physiol.*, 71:680, 1991.

67. Yaspelkis, B.B. III, et al.: Carbohydrate supplementation spares muscle glycogen during variable intensity exercise. *J. Appl. Physiol.*, 75:1477, 1993.

68. Zachwieja, J.J., et al.: Influence of muscle glycogen depletion on the rate of resynthesis. *Med. Sci. Sports Exerc.*, 23:44, 1991.

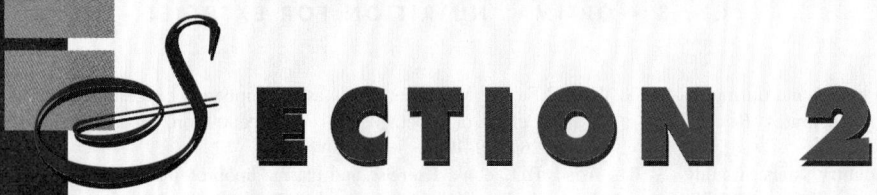

SECTION 2

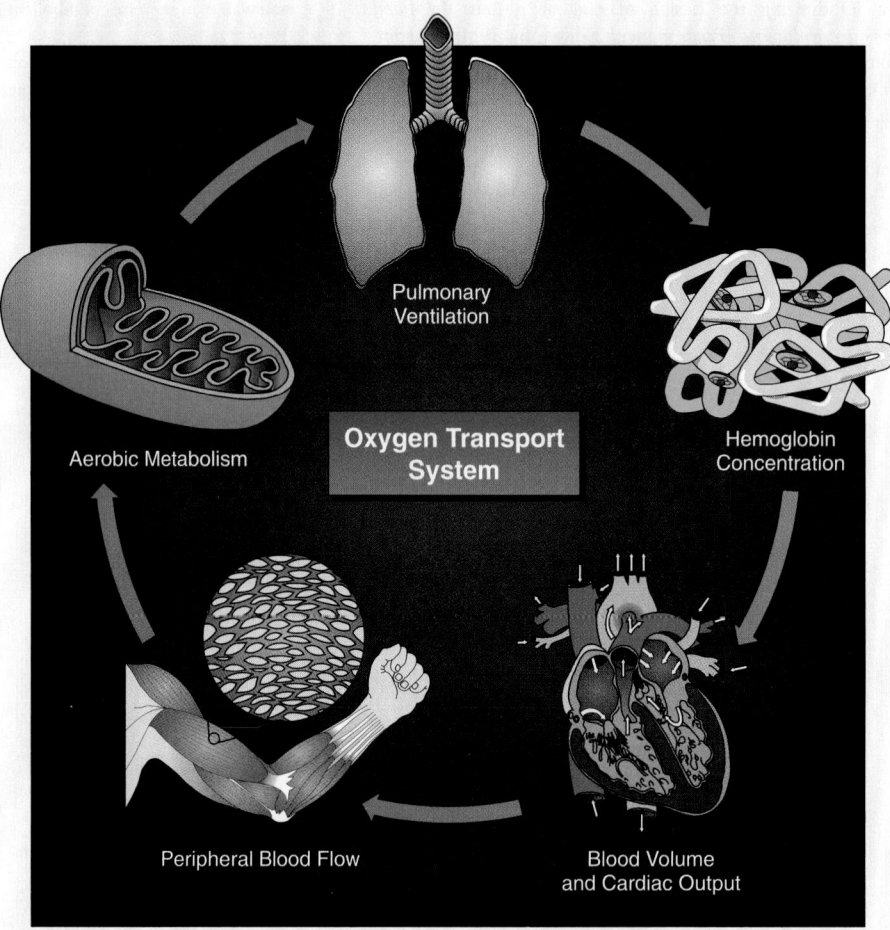

Oxygen Transport System

- Pulmonary Ventilation
- Hemoglobin Concentration
- Blood Volume and Cardiac Output
- Peripheral Blood Flow
- Aerobic Metabolism

"PHYSICAL ACTIVITY BY FAR PROVIDES THE GREATEST DEMAND ON HUMAN ENERGY EXPENDITURE."

Energy for Physical Activity

Biochemical reactions that do not consume oxygen generate considerable amounts of energy for short durations. This rapid generation of anaerobic energy is crucial in maintaining a high standard of performance during sprint activities and other all-out bursts of exercise. In comparison, during longer duration aerobic exercises, energy is extracted more slowly from food through reactions that require oxygen. The effective training of the various physiologic systems begins with an understanding of how energy is generated to sustain exercise, of the sources that provide that energy, and of the energy requirements of particular activities.

This section presents a broad overview of how cells extract the chemical energy bound within the food molecule and use it to power biologic work. Emphasis is placed on the importance of the food nutrients and the processes of energy transfer in sustaining physiologic function during light, moderate, and strenuous exercise.

Segal, K.R., and Gutin, B.: Thermic effects of food and exercise in lean and obese women. *Metabolism* **32:581, 1983.**

Considerable research concerns the association between obesity and impaired thermogenesis (a diminished capacity to increase metabolism in response to different stimuli). A number of studies had concluded that the rise in metabolic rate after ingestion of a meal, exposure to cold, infusion of noradrenaline, or the combination of a meal plus exercise occurred less often in obese than in lean persons. A blunted thermogenic response probably played an important role in total energy conservation, contributing to the onset or persistence of human obesity.

77.9 kg) and ten lean (percent fat, 18.8; body mass, 53.2 kg) women measured under six different conditions: (*a*) resting metabolic rate ($\dot{V}o_2$) for 4 hours; (*b*) $\dot{V}o_2$ for 4 hours following consumption of a 910-kcal meal (14% protein, 46% carbohydrate, 40% lipid); (*c*) $\dot{V}o_2$ during exercise at a constant submaximal work rate of 300 kg · m · min⁻¹ (cycling for 5 minutes every 0.5 hour for 4 hours); (*d*) $\dot{V}o_2$ during exercise at a relative work rate equal to the subject's lactate threshold (cycling for 5 minutes every 0.5 hour for 4 hours); (*e* and *f*) same as protocols *c* and *d*, except the subjects consumed the test meals before exercising.

The figure presents the effects of exercise and the 910-kcal meal on the metabolic rates of lean and obese subjects. Eating increased the $\dot{V}o_2$ during exercise more for the lean than the obese subjects. Stated somewhat differently, there was a greater difference between the fed and fasting conditions for the lean group at both exercise intensities. The postprandial exercise $\dot{V}o_2$ for the lean group also remained elevated above the corresponding fasting value at the end of the 4 hours, while for the obese group, the postprandial value at 4 hours equaled their fasting exercise metabolism. Thus, using a 4-hour measurement period underestimated the total amount that eating augmented energy expenditure during exercise for the lean group. For the lean subjects, a larger thermic effect of food occurred during exercise compared to rest. For obese subjects, on the other hand, similar effects of food intake occurred during exercise and rest, with no added thermogenic benefit of exercise after eating.

The researchers concluded that exercise significantly potentiated the thermic effect of food for lean but not for obese females. The large differences in the thermogenic response to the combination of food and subsequent exercise occurred despite similar thermogenic responses of the lean and obese women to food alone and exercise alone. In obesity, therefore, the cumulative effect of a reduced metabolic rate during exercise following food ingestion favored energy conservation rather than energy dissipation.

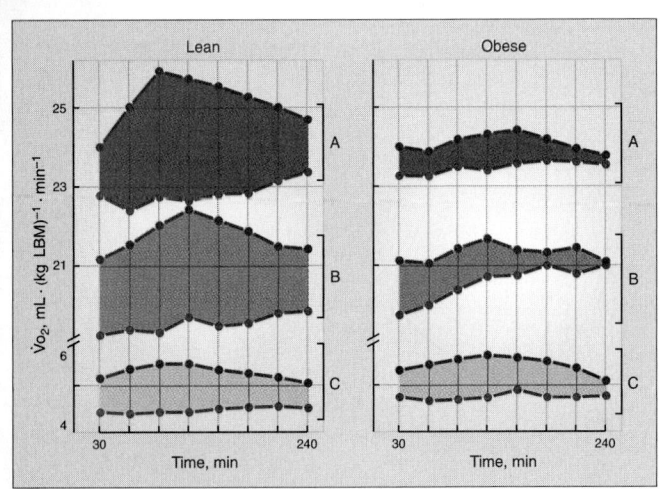

Effects of exercise and a 910-kcal meal on metabolic rates of lean and obese women. *A*, exercise at lactate threshold; *B*, exercise at 300 kg · m · min⁻¹; and *C*, rest condition. The *purple circles* represent postprandial (after the meal) data; *red circles* represent postabsorptive (after fasting) data. The *shaded areas* indicate the thermic effect of food under each condition.

This study evaluated the difference in thermogenesis between obese and lean women in response to food intake, two levels of exercise, and the possible potentiation of the thermic effect of food intake with physical activity. Subjects included ten obese (percent fat, 37; body mass,

Energy Value of Food

All biologic functions require energy. Because carbohydrate, lipid, and protein macronutrients contain the energy that ultimately powers biologic work, it is possible to classify both food and physical activity in terms of this common factor: energy. The discussion in this chapter concerns the quantification of food energy.

THE CALORIE AS A UNIT OF ENERGY MEASUREMENT

One calorie is defined as the quantity of heat necessary to raise the temperature of 1 kg (1 L) of water 1°C (for example, from 14.5 to 15.5°C). Thus, a calorie is more accurately termed a **kilogram calorie** or kilocalorie, abbreviated **kcal**. If 300 kcal is the caloric content of a particular food, then the energy trapped within the chemical bonds of this food, if released, would increase the temperature of 300 L of water 1°C. Different foods contain different amounts of energy. One-half cup of apricot nectar, for example, has a caloric value of 70 kcal, or the equivalent of the heat energy needed to increase the temperature of 70 L of water 1°C.

The standard international unit for expressing energy is the **joule**, or **kilojoule** (kJ). To convert kilocalories to kilojoules, multiply the kilocalorie value by 4.2. The kilojoule value of one-half cup of apricot nectar, for example, would be 70 kcal × 4.2, or 294 kJ.

GROSS ENERGY VALUE OF FOODS

Laboratories use **bomb calorimeters** similar to the one illustrated in Figure 4.1 to measure the total, or **gross**, energy value of various food nutrients. Bomb calorimeters operate on the principle of **direct calorimetry**: food is burned completely and a measurement is taken of the heat liberated.

As shown in Figure 4.1, food is placed inside a sealed chamber and oxygen is added. An electrical current moving through the fuse at the top ignites the food-oxygen mixture. As the food burns, the heat (energy) liberated is absorbed by a water jacket that surrounds the bomb. Because the calorimeter is fully insulated from the outside environment, a measured increase in water temperature directly reflects the amount of heat liberated during oxidation of the specific food nutrient.

The heat liberated by the oxidation, or burning, of a specific food is referred to as its **heat of combustion** and represents the total energy value of the food. For example, a teaspoon of margarine releases 100 kcal of heat energy when burned completely in a bomb calorimeter, enough energy to raise 1.0 kg (2.2 lb) of ice water to its boiling point. Although the oxidation pathways of the intact organism and the bomb calorimeter differ, the quantity of energy liberated in the complete breakdown of a food is the same and is independent of the pathways by which combustion occurs.

HEAT OF COMBUSTION

Lipid

The heat of combustion for lipid varies depending on the structural composition of the fatty acids that make up the triglyceride. For example, 1 g of either beef or pork fat yields 9.50 kcal, whereas the oxidation of 1 g of butterfat liberates 9.27 kcal. The average caloric value for 1 g of lipid in meat, fish, and eggs is 9.50 kcal. In dairy products, it is 9.25 kcal per gram, and in vegetables and fruits, 9.30 kcal. *The average heat of combustion for lipid is generally considered to be 9.4 kcal per gram of lipid oxidized in the bomb calorimeter.*

Carbohydrate

The heat of combustion for a carbohydrate also varies depending on the arrangement of atoms in the particular carbohydrate molecule. For glucose, the heat of combustion is 3.74 kcal per gram, which is less than the value for glycogen (4.19 kcal) and starch (4.20 kcal). *The value of 4.2 kcal generally represents the average heat of combustion for a gram of carbohydrate.*

Protein

Energy released from the combustion of the protein portion of food also varies depending on two factors: (*a*) the type of protein in the food, and (*b*) the relative nitrogen content of the particular protein. Many common proteins, such as those found in eggs, meat, corn (maize), and beans (jack, lima, navy, soy), contain approximately 16% nitrogen and have corresponding heats of combustion that average 5.75 kcal per gram. Proteins in other food items contain a higher nitrogen content, such as most nuts and seeds (18.9%) and whole-kernel wheat, rye, millets, and barley

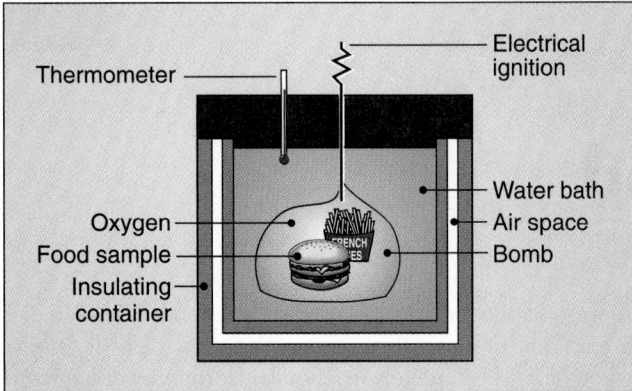

FIGURE 4.1

A bomb calorimeter is used to directly measure the energy value of food.

(17.2%). Other food proteins contain slightly lower percentages of nitrogen, for example, whole milk (15.7%) and bran (15.8%). *An average value for the heat of combustion of protein is 5.65 kcal per gram.*

COMPARING THE ENERGY VALUE OF NUTRIENTS

A comparison of the average heats of combustion for the three nutrients (carbohydrate, 4.2 kcal · g^{-1}; lipid, 9.4 kcal · g^{-1}; protein, 5.65 kcal · g^{-1}) demonstrates that the complete oxidation of lipid in the bomb calorimeter liberates about 65% more energy per gram than the oxidation of protein and 120% more energy per gram than the oxidation of carbohydrate. Recall from Chapter 1 that a lipid molecule contains more hydrogen atoms than either a carbohydrate or protein molecule. The common fatty acid palmitic acid, for example, has the structural formula $C_{16}H_{32}O_2$. In palmitic acid and other lipids, the ratio of hydrogen atoms to oxygen atoms is always considerably greater than the 2 : 1 ratio in carbohydrates. Simply stated, lipid molecules have more hydrogen atoms that can be cleaved away and oxidized to generate energy for the body's needs than do carbohydrates or protein.

One can conclude from this discussion that lipid-rich foods contain a higher energy content than relatively fat-free foods. One cup of whole milk, for example, contains 160 kcal, whereas the same quantity of skimmed milk contains only 90 kcal. If a person who normally consumes one quart of whole milk each day should switch to skimmed milk, the total calories ingested each year would be reduced by an amount equivalent to 25 lb of body fat. In 5 years, this would amount to approximately 125 lb in body fat—indeed a large quantity of "extra" fat. This comparison warrants serious consideration, because the nutritional values of whole and skim milk are basically identical. Switching to skimmed milk also greatly reduces the saturated fatty acids and cholesterol normally consumed.

NET ENERGY VALUE OF FOODS

The energy value of a particular food changes when its heat of combustion (gross energy value) as determined by direct calorimetry is compared with the **net** energy actually made available to the body. This is particularly true for proteins, because the body cannot oxidize the nitrogen component of these nutrients. In the body, nitrogen atoms combine with hydrogen to form urea, which is excreted in the urine. The elimination of hydrogen in this manner represents a loss of approximately 19% of the protein molecule's potential energy. This loss reduces the heat of combustion of protein in the body to approximately 4.6 kcal per gram instead of the 5.65 kcal per gram released during complete oxidation in the bomb calorimeter. In contrast, the physiologic fuel values for carbohydrates and lipids (that contain no nitrogen) are **identical** to their heats of combustion determined by bomb calorimetry.

COEFFICIENT OF DIGESTIBILITY

Another consideration in determining the ultimate caloric yield of food nutrients is the efficiency of the digestive process, numerically defined as the **coefficient of digestibility.** The coefficient of digestibility indicates the proportion of ingested food actually digested and absorbed to serve the metabolic needs of the body. The quantity of food exceeding this coefficient remains unabsorbed in the intestinal tract and is voided in the feces. Dietary fiber is one of the factors that reduces the coefficient of digestibility: Total energy absorbed is less from a high-fiber meal than from a fiber-free meal of equivalent caloric content. This variance may result from the ability of fiber to move food more rapidly through the intestine, reducing the time for absorption. Fiber may also cause mechanical erosion of the intestinal mucosa, which must be resynthesized through energy-requiring processes.

Table 4.1 presents digestibility coefficients as well as heat of combustion and net energy values for nutrients in the various food groups. As can be seen, different food categories exhibit different coefficients of digestibility. The relative percentages of macronutrients completely digested and absorbed are 97% for carbohydrate; 95% for lipid; and 92% for protein. There is little difference in digestive efficiency between obese and lean individuals. It is noteworthy that these values only are averages, and some variability can be expected in efficiency percentages for any food within a particular category. With proteins in particular, digestive efficiencies range from a low of about 78% for legumes to a high of 97% for protein from animal sources. The relatively low coefficient of digestibility from plant protein is used by some to argue for the use of vegetables in weight-loss diets. Those who do choose a vegetarian diet should take great care to maintain adequate protein intake, in terms of both quantity and quality, to obtain all the essential amino acids.

From the data in Table 4.1, *the average net energy values can be rounded to simple whole numbers: 4 kcal per gram for dietary carbohydrate, 9 kcal per gram for lipid, and 4 kcal per gram for protein.* These values, referred to as the **Atwater general factors,** have been used by nutritionists for the past 100 years to represent the energy available to the body from ingested food nutrients. Except when exact energy values are desired, as for preparing experimental or therapeutic diets, the Atwater general factors can be used to estimate the net metabolizable energy value of typical foods consumed in a diet. For the consumption of alcohol, a

value of 7 kcal (29.4 kJ) is given for each gram (milliliter) of pure (200 proof) alcohol ingested.

CALORIC VALUE OF A MEAL

If the composition and weight of a food are known, the caloric content of any portion of food or an entire meal can be determined using the Atwater factors. Table 4.2 illustrates the method for calculating the kilocalorie value of 100 g (3.5 oz) of vanilla ice cream. Based on laboratory analysis, vanilla ice cream contains approximately 4% protein, 13% lipid, and 21% carbohydrate, with the remaining 62% essentially water. Thus, each gram of ice cream contains 0.04 g protein, 0.13 g lipid, and 0.21 g carbohydrate. Using these compositional values and the Atwater factors,

TABLE 4.1
FACTORS FOR DIGESTIBILITY, HEATS OF COMBUSTION, AND NET PHYSIOLOGIC ENERGY VALUES[a] OF PROTEIN, LIPID, AND CARBOHYDRATE

Food Group	Digestibility (%)	Heat of Combustion (kcal $\cdot$ g^{-1})	Net Energy (kcal $\cdot$ g^{-1})
Protein			
Meats, fish	97	5.65	4.27
Eggs	97	5.75	4.37
Dairy products	97	5.65	4.27
Animal food	97	5.65	4.27
Cereals	85	5.80	3.87
Legumes	78	5.70	3.47
Vegetables	83	5.00	3.11
Fruits	85	5.20	3.36
Vegetable food	85	5.65	3.74
Total Food	92	5.65	4.05
Lipid			
Meat and eggs	95	9.50	9.03
Dairy products	95	9.25	8.79
Animal food	95	9.40	8.93
Vegetable food	90	9.30	8.37
Total Food	95	9.40	8.93
Carbohydrate			
Animal food	98	3.90	3.82
Cereals	98	4.20	4.11
Legumes	97	4.20	4.07
Vegetables	95	4.20	3.99
Fruits	90	4.00	3.60
Sugars	98	3.95	3.87
Vegetable food	97	4.15	4.03
Total Food	97	4.15	4.03

From Merrill, A.L., and Watt, B.K., Energy values of foods . . . basis and derivation. Agricultural Handbook No. 74, Washington, D.C., U.S. Department of Agriculture, 1973.

[a]Net physiologic energy values are computed as the coefficient of digestibility × heat of combustion adjusted for energy loss in urine.

the kilocalorie value per gram of ice cream is determined as follows: The net kilocalorie values indicate that 0.04 g of protein contains 0.16 kcal (0.04 × 4.0 kcal · g^{-1}), 0.13 g of lipid contains 1.17 kcal (0.13 × 9 kcal · g^{-1}), and 0.21 g of carbohydrate contains 0.84 kcal (0.21 × 4.0 kcal · g^{-1}). Combining the separate values for the nutrients yields a total energy value for each gram of vanilla ice cream equal to 2.17 kcal (0.16 + 1.17 + 0.84). A 100-g serving yields a caloric value 100 times as large, or 217 kcal. This computation can produce an estimate of the kilocalorie value for any food serving. Of course, increasing or decreasing portion sizes or adding rich sauces or candies, or, conversely, adding fruits or calorie-free substitutes will affect the caloric content accordingly.

The procedure for computing the kilocalories in foods is time consuming and laborious. Various government agencies in the United States and elsewhere have evaluated and compiled nutritive values of thousands of foods. The most comprehensive data bank resources available are the U.S. Nutrient Data Bank (USNDB) maintained by the U.S. Department of Agriculture's Consumer Nutrition Center[7a] and a computerized data bank maintained by the Bureau of Nutritional Sciences of Health and Welfare Canada.

Large differences exist between the energy values of various foods. Consuming an equal number of calories from different foods often requires increasing the intake of a particular food. For example, to consume 100 kcal from each of six common foods—carrots, celery, green peppers, grapefruit, medium-sized eggs, and mayonnaise—one must eat 5 carrots, 20 stalks of celery, 6 green peppers, 1 large grapefruit, and 1¼ eggs, but only 1 tablespoon of mayonnaise. Consequently, for an average sedentary adult female to meet her daily energy needs (2100 kcal), she would need

to consume about 420 celery stalks, 105 carrots, 136 green peppers, or 26 eggs, yet only 1 cup of mayonnaise or 8 oz of salad oil. These examples illustrate dramatically that foods high in lipid content contain considerably more calories than foods low in lipid and correspondingly high in water content.

Another important consideration is that a calorie is a measure of food energy regardless of its source. Thus, from an energy standpoint, 100 calories from mayonnaise is no more fattening than the same 100 calories contained in 20 stalks of celery. The more one eats of any given food, the more calories one consumes. The difference is that a small quantity of fatty foods represents a considerable number of calories; thus, these foods are considered "fattening." An individual's caloric intake, however, equals the sum of **all** energy consumed, be it from a small or large quantity of food.

■ SUMMARY ■

1. A calorie or kilocalorie (kcal) is a measure of heat that expresses the energy value of food. To obtain a kilocalorie value, food is literally burned and the released energy is measured directly in a bomb calorimeter.

2. The heat of combustion measurement represents the amount of heat liberated by the complete oxidation of a given food. Average gross energy values are 4.2 kcal per gram for carbohydrate, 9.4 kcal per gram for lipid, and 5.65 kcal per gram for protein.

3. The coefficient of digestibility is the proportion of ingested food actually digested and absorbed by the body. Coefficients of digestibility average approximately 97% for carbohydrates, 95% for lipids, and 92% for proteins. Thus, the net energy values are 4 kcal per gram of carbohydrate, 9 kcal per gram of lipid, and 4 kcal per gram of protein. These values, referred to as the Atwater general factors, are used to estimate the net energy value of typical foods in a diet.

4. Knowing the Atwater calorific values allows one to compute the caloric content of any meal—as long as the carbohydrate, lipid, and protein compositions are known.

5. From an energy standpoint, the calorie as a unit of heat energy remains constant regardless of the food source. It is incorrect to consider 500 kcal of chocolate ice cream topped with whipped cream and nuts any more fattening than 500 kcal of watermelon, 500 kcal of cheese and pepperoni pizza, or 500 kcal of a bagel with salmon, onions, and sour cream.

TABLE 4.2
METHOD OF CALCULATING THE CALORIC VALUE OF A FOOD FROM ITS COMPOSITION OF MACRONUTRIENTS

Food: ice cream (vanilla)
Weight: three-fourths cup = 100 grams

	Composition		
	Protein	Lipid	Carbohydrate
Percentage	4%	13%	21%
Total grams	4	13	21
In one gram	0.04 g	0.13 g	0.21 g
Calories per gram	0.16	1.17	0.84

(.04 × 4.0 kcal) + (.13 × 9.0 kcal) + (.21 × 4.0 kcal)

Total calories per gram: .16 + 1.17 + .84 = 2.17 kcal
Total calories per 100 grams: 2.17 × 100 = 217 kcal

■ REFERENCES ■

1. Atwater, W.O., and Woods, C.D.: *The Chemical Composition of American Food Materials.* USDA Bulletin No. 28, Washington, DC, U.S. Department of Agriculture, 1896.

2. Brooks, G.A., et al.: *Exercise Physiology, Human Bioenergetics and Its Applications.* 2nd ed., Mountain View, CA, Mayfield, 1996.

3. Gibson, R.S.: *Principles of Nutritional Assessment.* New York, Oxford University Press, 1990.

4. Guthrie, H.A. (Ed.): *Introductory Nutrition.* 7th ed., St. Louis, C.V. Mosby, 1988.

5. Guyton, A.C.: *Textbook of Medical Physiology.* 8th ed., Philadelphia, W.B. Saunders, 1990.

6. Hamilton, E.M., et al.: *Nutrition: Concepts and Controversies.* 5th ed, St. Paul, MN, West, 1991.

7. Health and Welfare Canada: *Nutrient Value of Some Common Foods.* Ottawa, Canada, Health Services and Promotion Branch, Health and Welfare Canada, 1988.

7a. Katch, F.I. U.S. government raises serious questions about reliability of U.S. Department of Agriculture's Food Composition Tables. *Int. J. Sports Nutr.,* 5:62, 1995.

8. McCance, R.A., and Widdowson, E.M.: *The Composition of Foods.* 5th ed., London, Royal Society of Chemistry, Ministry of Agriculture, Fisheries and Food, 1991.

9. Miles, C.W., et al.: Effect of dietary fiber on the metabolizable energy of human diets. *J. Nutr.,* 118:1075, 1988.

10. Pennington, J.A.T., and Church, H.N.: *Bowes and Church's Food Values of Portions Commonly Used.* 15th ed, Philadelphia, J.B. Lippincott, 1989.

11. Rand, W.M., et al. (Eds.): *Food Composition Data: A User's Perspective.* Tokyo, The United Nations University, 1987.

12. Shils, M.E., et al.: *Modern Nutrition in Health and Disease,* 8th ed., Philadelphia, Lea & Febiger, 1993.

13. U.S. Department of Agriculture. *Composition of Foods—Raw, Processed, and Prepared.* USDA Bulletin No. 8, Washington, DC, U.S. Department of Agriculture, 1963–1987.

Wilmore, J.H., and Costill, D.L.: Adequacy of the Haldane transformation in the computation of exercise V̇o₂ in man. *J. Appl. Physiol.* 35:85, 1973.

A fundamental measurement in exercise physiology is oxygen uptake using open-circuit spirometry. A primary assumption of this methodology requires no nitrogen production or retention by the body, so the nitrogen volume remains exactly equal in the inspired and expired air. Because of this intrinsic relationship, no need exists to collect and

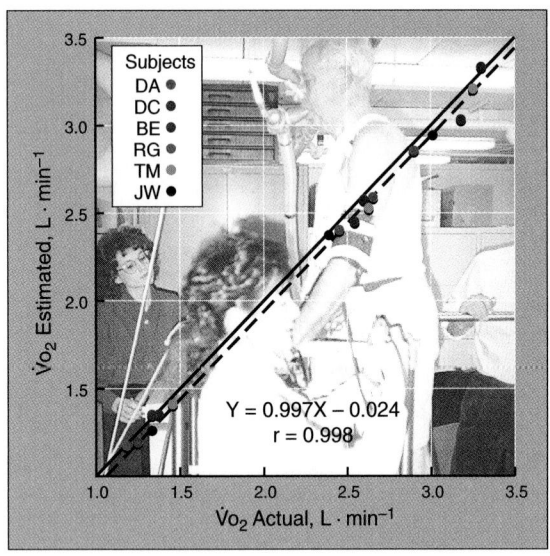

Actual versus estimated exercise oxygen uptake for six subjects. The *solid line* represents the line of identity, and the *dashed line* represents the regression line for predicting the oxygen uptake estimated from the Haldane transformation (y axis) from the actual oxygen uptake values (x axis). Note that the slope is nearly 1.0 and the intercept is zero.

analyze both inspired and expired air volumes during measurement of oxygen uptake and carbon dioxide production. The following mathematical relationship, known as the Haldane transformation, exists between inspired and expired air volumes:

$$\dot{V}_I = \dot{V}_E \times F_{EN_2} \div F_{IN_2}$$

where $\dot{V}_I$ equals air volume inspired, $\dot{V}_E$ equals air volume expired, and F_{EN_2} and F_{IN_2} equal the fractional concentrations of nitrogen in the expired and inspired air. Because the fractional concentrations for inspired oxygen, carbon dioxide, and nitrogen are known, only $\dot{V}_E$ (or $\dot{V}_I$) and the concentrations in expired air of CO_2 (F_{ECO_2}) and O_2 (F_{EO_2}) are required to calculate $\dot{V}_{O_2}$:

$$\dot{V}_{O_2} = \dot{V}_E \times F_{EN_2}/F_{IN_2} \times F_{IO_2} - \dot{V}_E \times F_{EO_2}.$$

In this formula, F_{EN_2} usually equals

$$1.00 - (F_{EO_2} + F_{ECO_2}).$$

This study determined any nitrogen retention or production, and how it influenced the accuracy of the calculations of oxygen uptake using the traditional Haldane transformation during light to heavy exercise. Six subjects completed treadmill exercise by walking on the level at 4 mph; a 5-minute jog followed at 6.0 mph, followed again by a 5-minute run at 7.5 mph. Oxygen uptake, continuously monitored using open-circuit spirometry, included measurement of inspired and expired pulmonary ventilation. Measurements also included barometric pressure, inspired and expired gas temperatures, relative humidity, and F_{EO_2}, F_{ECO_2}, F_{IO_2}, and F_{ICO_2}.

The figure presents the $\dot{V}_{O_2}$ calculated from the inspired and expired air volumes for all subjects compared to the values estimated from the Haldane transformation. The slope of the regression line deviated only 0.003 unit from unity (the intercept was almost zero), demonstrating the closeness between the actual oxygen uptake and that predicted by the Haldane transformation. The largest difference between the 68 actual and estimated $\dot{V}_{O_2}$ values was 230 mL, an error of 7.3%. The average difference of 0.8% for all subjects was within the measurement error of the instruments. For the nitrogen data, a difference of 1.6% occurred between the minute volume of nitrogen inspired and expired for any subject at any work rate; 11 of 17 subject-work rates exhibited less than a 1% difference. The largest difference, 1099 mL $N_2 \cdot min^{-1}$, occurred during heavy exercise (2.1% difference).

The researchers calculated that the major sources of variation in assessing $\dot{V}_{O_2}$ included the measurement of ventilation volume, gas meter calibration, and determination of the water vapor pressure (P_{H_2O}) of inspired air. The measurement of ventilation volume presented a problem, because accuracy depended on the subject being "switched in" and "switched out" at the same phase of the tidal volume at the beginning and end of the collection period. Because this remains difficult (if not impossible) to achieve, an inspired–to–expired volume differential nearly always occurs. Also, a 10 percentage point difference in inspired P_{H_2O} (for example, from 50 to 60% relative humidity) results in more than a 100-mL change between the inspired and expired N_2 volumes.

The results from this study supported the continued use of the Haldane transformation to calculate $\dot{V}_{O_2}$ during exercise. While production and/or retention of N_2 can occur during exercise, it had little or no effect on the $\dot{V}_{O_2}$ computation.

Introduction to Energy Transfer

The ability to swim, run, or ski long distances is framed largely by a person's capacity to extract energy from food nutrients and transfer it to the contractile elements of skeletal muscle. Likewise, specific energy-transferring capacities also determine one's level of success in weight lifting, sprinting, jumping, and football line play. Although most of the discussion in this textbook concerns muscular activity, the direct transfer of chemical energy is required to power **all** forms of biologic work.

The sections that follow introduce general concepts dealing with bioenergetics. These sections provide the basis for understanding energy metabolism during physical activities of varying intensity.

ENERGY: THE CAPACITY TO WORK

Unlike matter and its physical properties, energy eludes a concrete definition in terms of size, shape, or mass. Rather, the term *energy* implies a dynamic state—a condition of change—because the presence of energy is revealed only when a change takes place. It is impossible to assign absolute values to energy: values can only be assigned to the **changes** in energy that occur during a process. Within this context, *energy is related to the ability to perform work*. As work increases, the transfer of energy also increases such that a change occurs.

The **first law of thermodynamics** states that energy is neither created nor destroyed, but is transformed from one form to another. In essence, this defines the immutable principle of the **conservation of energy** that applies to both living and nonliving systems. The large amount of chemical energy in fuel oil, for example, is readily converted to heat energy in a home oil burner. In the body, however, not all of the chemical energy trapped within the bonds of the food nutrients is immediately lost as heat; rather, a considerable portion is conserved as chemical energy and then changed into mechanical energy (and, ultimately, heat energy) by the action of the musculoskeletal system. The key point related to the first law of thermodynamics is that energy is not produced, consumed, or used up in the body; it merely changes from one form to another as the various bodily functions undergo transformations.

POTENTIAL AND KINETIC ENERGY

The total energy of any system consists of two components—**potential energy** and **kinetic energy.** Potential energy can mean energy of position, such as that possessed by a car parked on a steep hill. It also can mean light energy, electric energy, or bound energy, such as that contained within the internal molecular structure of a lump of coal before it burns. *When potential energy is released (as when the car's brake is released and the car rolls down the hill), it is transformed into kinetic energy, or energy of motion.* The conversion from potential to kinetic energy can take many forms. For example, this conversion occurs with the rearrangement of the chemical structure of a substance when the bonds between its atoms are broken. This results in a release of potential energy with a concomitant increase in kinetic energy. In some instances, the bound energy in one substance can be directly transferred to other substances to increase the potential energy of the recipient molecules. Energy transfers of this type are required for the chemical work of biosynthesis in the body. During biosynthesis, specific building-block molecules are activated and join other molecules to synthesize important biologic compounds. Some of these compounds serve structural needs, while others can then serve the energy needs of the cell.

Figure 5.1 depicts the relationship between potential and kinetic energy as related to position. Calm water at sea level possesses little potential energy and cannot drive the water wheel. However, water from a mountain stream flows downhill and picks up speed as it cascades over the fall, its potential energy rapidly transforming into kinetic energy of motion. Some of this energy is harnessed to turn the water wheel. The amount of kinetic energy generated increases with the distance the water falls. Water at the brink of the fall possesses more potential and less kinetic energy than water at the bottom, and vice versa. Hence, the potential energy stored in the water at the top of the fall changes into kinetic energy as it drops from a higher to a lower level.

ENERGY-RELEASING AND ENERGY-CONSERVING PROCESSES

Any physical or chemical process that releases (frees) energy to its surroundings is termed **exergonic.** Exergonic reactions can be viewed as "downhill" processes: they result in a decline in **free energy,** the "useful" energy needed for the life-sustaining processes of biologic work in the cell. Chemical processes that store or absorb energy are termed **endergonic.** Endergonic reactions represent "uphill" processes and result in an increase in free energy for biologic

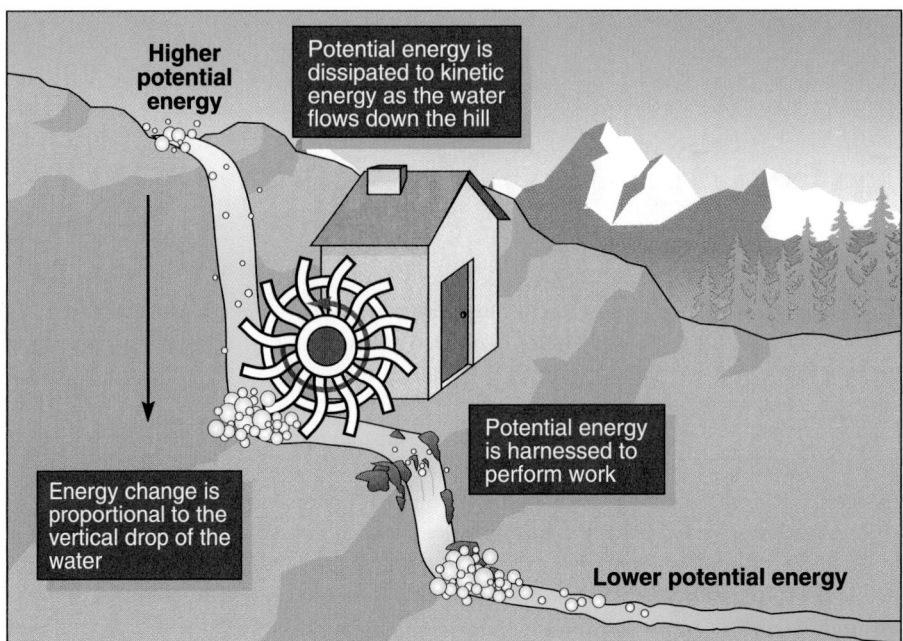

FIGURE 5.1
High-grade potential energy capable of performing work is degraded to a useless form of kinetic energy.

work. In some instances, exergonic processes are linked, or **coupled,** with endergonic reactions, enabling the transfer of some of the energy to the endergonic process. In the next chapter, we emphasize that coupled reactions are important because they serve as the means to link exergonic and endergonic processes. *In the body, coupled reactions conserve a large portion of the chemical energy in food nutrients in a usable form.*

During exergonic chemical reactions, potential energy stored within the chemical structure of a compound is released. This liberated energy is equal to the difference between the potential energy of the reactant and the potential energy of the products. For example, the union of hydrogen and oxygen to form water releases 68 kcal of free energy, as shown in the following reaction:

$$H_2 + O \rightarrow H_2O - 68 \text{ kcal} \cdot \text{mol}^{-1}$$

The negative sign indicates that heat is lost from the system as the reaction proceeds. One mole represents the molecular weight of a substance in grams. A mole of glucose, for example, weighs 180 g. The process shown above is reversible. During the reverse endergonic reaction, the chemical bonds of the water molecule split apart, freeing the original hydrogen and oxygen atoms by supplying 68 kcal of energy to each mole of water. This "uphill" energy-transfer process, depicted below, provides the hydrogen and oxygen atoms with their original energy contents, satisfying the principle of the conservation of energy.

$$H_2 + O \leftarrow H_2O + 68 \text{ kcal} \cdot \text{mol}^{-1}$$

The process of energy transfer in cells follows the same principles outlined in the waterfall/water wheel example:

the carbohydrate, lipid, and protein nutrients possess considerable potential energy. The formation of product substances causes a progressive loss of potential energy from the nutrient molecule and a corresponding increase in kinetic energy. Aided by appropriate enzyme-regulated transfer systems, a portion of this chemical energy is harnessed or conserved in the new compounds, which are then used for biologic work. Generally speaking, all living cells rely primarily on chemical energy; they perform work by utilizing the potential energy in the chemical bonds of their energy sources. In essence, living cells are transducers with the capacity to extract and utilize the energy stored in a compound's atomic structure. Conversely, and of equal importance, living cells can bond atoms and molecules together, raising the level of potential energy.

The transfer of potential energy in any spontaneous process is unidirectional: it always proceeds such that the capacity of the total energy to perform work decreases. The tendency of potential energy to degrade to kinetic energy with a lower capacity for work (that is, an increase in **entropy** occurs) mirrors the **second law of thermodynamics.** A good example of this law is a car battery: the electrochemical energy stored within its cells is slowly released even if the battery is not in use. The energy from sunlight is also degraded continually to heat energy when sunlight strikes and is absorbed by a surface. Foods and other chemicals store potential energy quite effectively. This energy, however, is gradually released as the compounds decompose through normal oxidative processes. Energy, similar to water, always runs downhill and, thus, potential energy continually decreases. *Ultimately, all of the potential energy in a system is degraded to the nonusable form of kinetic energy or heat.*

INTERCONVERSIONS OF ENERGY

Because the total energy in an isolated system remains constant, a decrease in one form of energy is matched by an equivalent increase in another form. In the process of energy conversion, a loss of potential energy from one source can produce a temporary increase in the potential energy of another source. Using this principle, vast quantities of potential energy can be harnessed in nature for useful purposes. However, even under such favorable conditions, the tendency toward entropy dominates, and the net flow of energy in the biologic world ultimately results in the degradation of potential energy.

Entropy was discovered by the chemist Ludwig Boltzmann in the late 1800s, and the equation that describes the disorder of the universe was later carved on his tombstone. Entropy is a measure of the continual process of energy change. All chemical and physical processes proceed in such a direction that total randomness or disorder increases and the energy available to do work decreases. In coupled reactions that occur during biosynthesis, part of a system may show a decrease in entropy while another shows an increase. Nevertheless, there is no circumventing the second law: the entire system always shows a net increase in entropy. In a more global sense, the biochemical reactions within the body's trillions of cells (as within the universe as a whole) "tilt" in the direction of spontaneity, disorder, and randomness.

FORMS OF ENERGY

Figure 5.2 shows that energy can be categorized as one of six forms: chemical, mechanical, heat, light, electric, or nuclear.

Examples of Energy Conversions

The conversion of energy from one form to another occurs readily in both the inanimate and animate worlds. The most fundamental processes of energy conversion in living cells are **photosynthesis** and **respiration.**

Photosynthesis. The sun, with a temperature of fifteen million degrees Fahrenheit, releases part of its potential energy stored in the nuclei of hydrogen atoms through the process of nuclear fusion. This energy in the form of gamma radiation is converted to radiant energy that ultimately represents the sole source of energy for green plants.

As shown in Figure 5.3, the pigment chlorophyll in the chloroplasts of green plants, through the reactions of photosynthesis, absorbs solar (radiant) energy and transforms it into the chemical potential energy of carbohydrates. This endergonic process driven by light energy involves the synthesis of glucose from carbon dioxide and water and the release of oxygen to the atmosphere (subsequently used by animals in the process of cellular respiration). Photosynthesis requires an input of 689 kcal of energy per mole of glucose synthesized. Because only a change in free energy that occurs during a process can be measured, the value of that

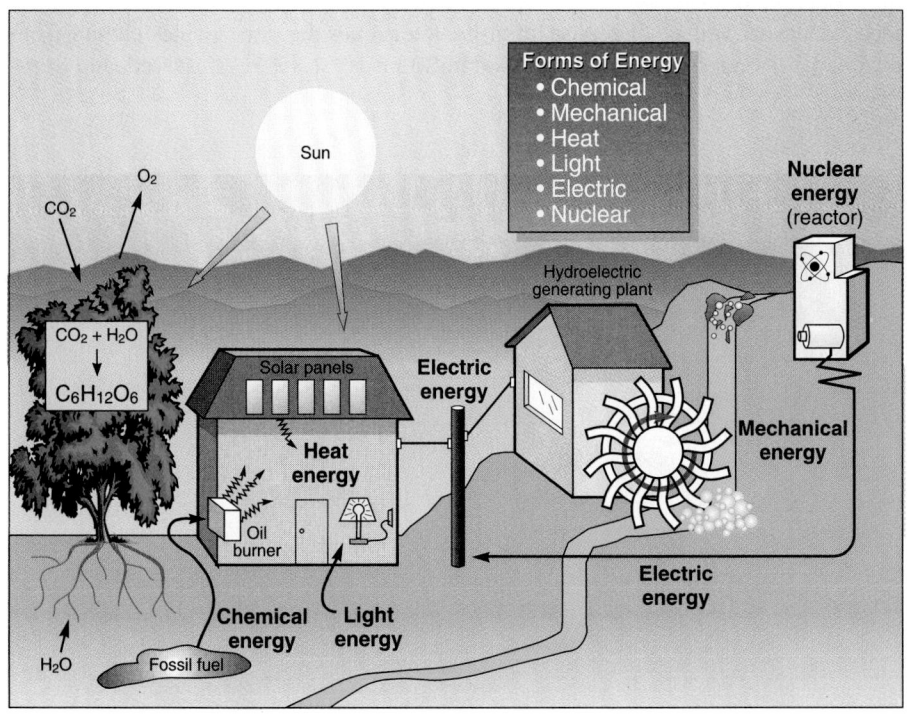

FIGURE 5.2
Interconversions of six forms of energy.

change is indicated by the symbol ΔG. (Interestingly, the letter G was chosen to honor the chemist J. Willard Gibbs (1839–1903), whose research provided the foundation of biochemical thermodynamics.) Carbohydrates can be converted to lipids and proteins for storage in the plant as a reserve of potential energy. Animals ingest the plant nutrients to serve their own energy needs. *In essence, solar energy, coupled with the process of photosynthesis, powers the animal world with food and oxygen.*

Cellular Respiration.   The process of respiration, diagrammed in Figure 5.4, is the reverse of photosynthesis: the stored energy in plants is recovered for use in biologic work. During these exergonic reactions, the chemical energy stored in the glucose, lipid, and protein molecules is extracted in the presence of oxygen. For glucose, this results in the release of 689 kcal per mole oxidized. *A portion of the energy released during cellular respiration can be conserved in other chemical compounds and converted to mechanical work in the body by muscle action; the remaining energy flows to the environment as heat.*

Biologic Work in Humans

The energy released during cellular respiration in humans sustains biologic work. This work can take one of three familiar forms:

- **Mechanical work** of muscle action.
- **Chemical work** involving the synthesis of cellular molecules.
- **Transport work** that concentrates various substances in the intracellular and extracellular fluids.

Mechanical Work.   The most obvious example of energy transformation in the body is the mechanical work generated by muscle action. The protein filaments of muscle fibers directly convert chemical energy into mechanical energy. This is not the only form of mechanical work performed in the body. In the cell nucleus, for example, contractile elements similar to those found in muscle literally tug at the chromosomes to facilitate the process of cell division. Mechanical work also is performed by specialized structures, such as cilia, that are part of many cells.

Chemical Work.   Chemical work is performed by all cells for growth and maintenance. Cellular components undergo continual synthesis as other components are destroyed. This biosynthesis opposes the tendency toward entropy and requires a substantial input of energy to rebond different cellular elements.

Transport Work.   Much less conspicuous than mechanical or chemical work is the work of transporting or concentrating substances in the body. Cellular materials normally flow from an area of high concentration to one of low concentration. This passive process, called **diffusion,** requires no energy. For proper physiologic functioning, however, certain chemicals also must be transported "uphill" against their normal concentration gradients, that is, from an area of lower to one of higher concentration. The term **active transport** is usually associated with this process. Secretion and reabsorption in the kidney tubules require active transport, as does the establishment of proper electrochemical gradients around the plasma membrane. Stored chemical energy must be continually expended to accomplish these "quiet" forms of biologic work.

FACTORS THAT AFFECT THE RATE OF BIOENERGETICS

Exercise intensity determines the rate at which chemical energy in the food nutrients is extracted, conserved, and trans-

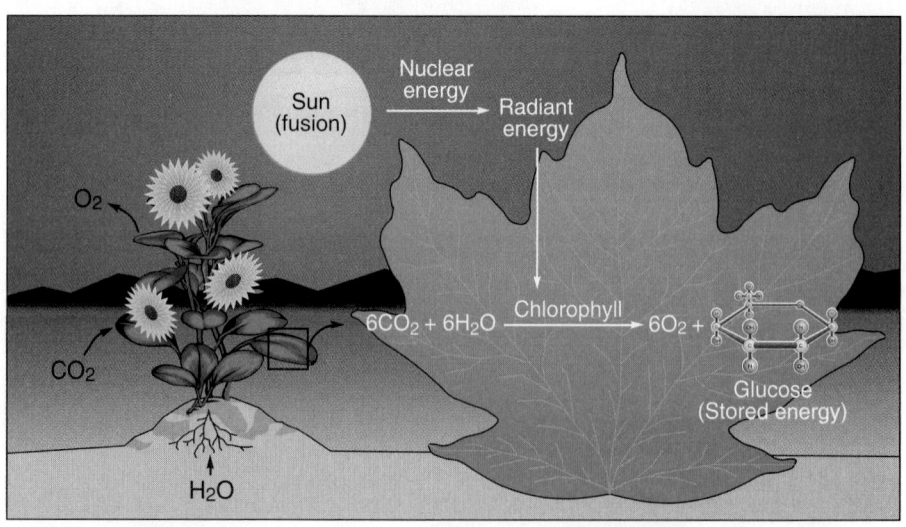

FIGURE 5.3
The endergonic process of photosynthesis. These reactions requiring an input of energy, such as the synthesis of glucose in green plants, undergo a positive standard free energy (useful energy) change ($+\Delta G$).

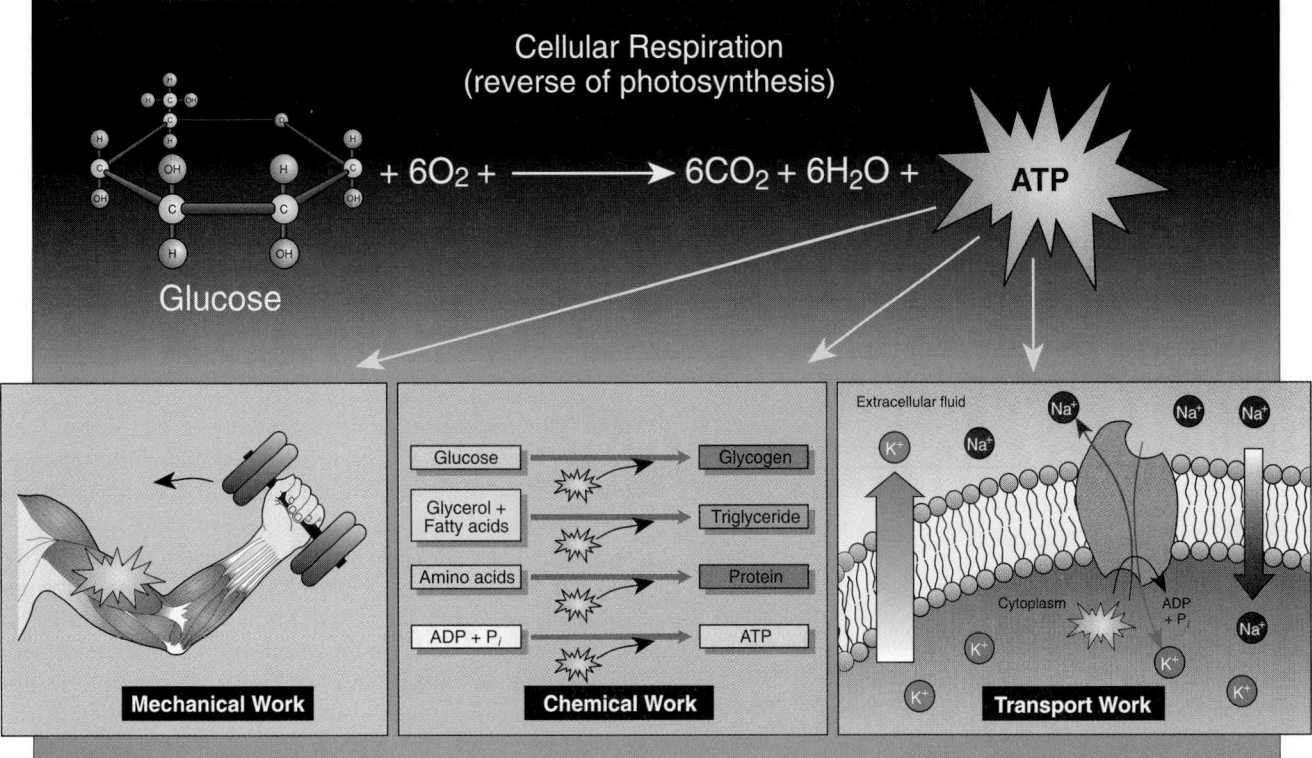

FIGURE 5.4

The exergonic process of cellular respiration. These reactions releasing potential energy, such as the burning of gasoline or oxidation of glucose, undergo a negative standard free energy change (that is, a reduction in total energy available for work; $-\Delta G$). In this illustration, the potential energy in the glucose molecule is harvested to form ATP during cellular respiration. Subsequently, the energy in ATP is used to power all forms of biologic work.

ferred to the contractile filaments of skeletal muscle. *The sustained pace of the marathon runner at close to 80% of aerobic capacity, or the rapid speed of the sprinter, is a direct expression of the body's capacity to transfer chemical energy to mechanical work.* Enzymes and coenzymes are two important substances that affect the rate of energy release during chemical reactions.

ENZYMES: BIOLOGIC CATALYSTS

An enzyme is a highly specific protein catalyst that accelerates the forward and reverse rates of chemical reactions within the body without being consumed or changed in the reaction. Enzymes do not induce reactions that could not otherwise occur under proper conditions. Rather, they facilitate the interaction of substances that normally would occur at a much slower rate. In a way, enzymes reduce the required **activation energy,** that is, the energy input to initiate a reaction, so that the reaction rate changes. This change occurs even though the equilibrium constants and total energy released (free energy change) per reaction remain unaltered. Figure 5.5 illustrates the effectiveness of a catalyst in initiat-

ing a chemical reaction compared to the uncatalyzed state. The X-axis represents the progress of the reaction, while the Y-axis compares the energy requirements for the activation of catalyzed and uncatalyzed reactions. Clearly, the initiation of an uncatalyzed reaction (activation energy) requires much more energy than the initiation of a catalyzed reaction. Biochemists estimate that without proper enzyme action, full digestion of a breakfast might take 50 years!

Enzymes possess the unique property of not being readily altered by the reactions in which they participate. Consequently, the turnover of enzymes in the body is relatively slow and specific enzymes are continually reused.

A typical mitochondrion may contain as many as 10 billion enzyme molecules, each carrying out millions of operations within a short time period. During exercise, the rate of enzyme activity within the cell increases tremendously. The increased rate of a catalyzed reaction can be 10^6 to 10^{20} times faster than an uncatalyzed reaction under similar conditions. The fluids of a single cell can contain as many as four thousand different enzymes, each performing a specific function. Almost every chemical reaction within a cell

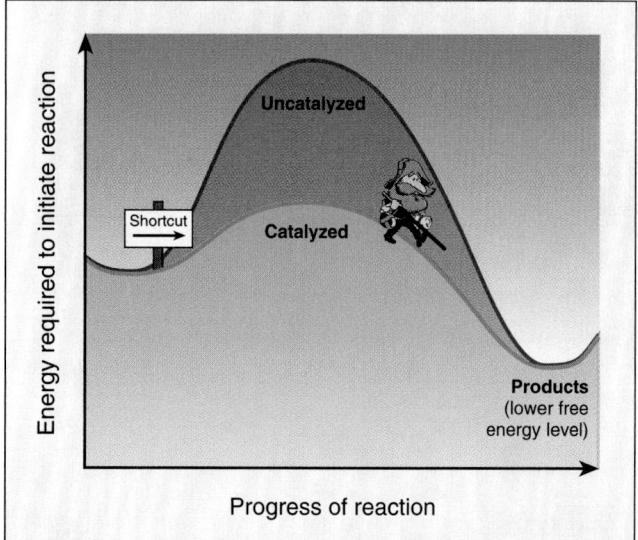

FIGURE 5.5
The presence of a catalyst greatly reduces the activation energy required to initiate a chemical reaction compared to the energy required for an uncatalyzed reaction. For the reaction to occur at all, however, the reactant must have a higher free-energy level than that of the product.

is catalyzed by a specific enzyme. For example, the breakdown of glucose to carbon dioxide and water requires 19 different chemical reactions, each catalyzed by a specific enzyme. Enzymes make contact at precise locations on the surfaces of cell structures; they can also work within the structure itself. Many enzymes can operate outside the cell, such as in the bloodstream, digestive mixture, or fluids of the small intestine.

Enzymes usually take their names from the functions they perform. The suffix *-ase* often is appended to the specific molecule on which the enzyme operates. For example, hydrol*ase* adds water during hydrolysis reactions, prote*ase* interacts with protein, oxid*ase* adds oxygen to a substance, and ribonucle*ase* splits apart ribonucleic acid (RNA). Remarkably, enzymes do not all operate at the same rate: some operate slowly, others quite rapidly.

Enzymes often work cooperatively among their binding sites. While one substance is "turned on" at a particular site, its neighbor is "turned off" until the job is completed. The operation then can be reversed, with one enzyme becoming inactive and the other active. Enzymes can also act along small regions of a **substrate** (any substance acted upon by an enzyme), each time working at a different rate than previously! Some enzymes delay the beginning of their work. A good example is the precursor enzyme trypsinogen, which is manufactured by the pancreas. After a delay, trypsinogen is secreted into the small intestine where it functions as the active enzyme trypsin, digesting complex proteins into simple amino acids. This process is referred to

as proteolytic action. Without this delay in activity, trypsinogen would literally digest the pancreatic tissue that produced it.

The temperature and the hydrogen ion concentration of the reactive medium dramatically affect enzyme activity. Each enzyme performs its maximum activity at a specific pH. For some enzymes, optimal activity requires a relatively high level of acidity; for others, the optimal pH is on the alkaline side of neutrality. Increases in temperature generally accelerate enzyme reactivity. As the temperature rises above 40 to 50°C, the protein enzyme becomes permanently denatured and its activity ceases.

A unique characteristic of an enzyme's three-dimensional globular protein structure is interaction with its specific substrate. Interaction works similarly to a key fitting a lock. As illustrated in Figure 5.6, the enzyme turns on when its **active site,** usually a groove, cleft, or cavity on the protein's surface, is joined in a "perfect fit" with the active site on the substrate. Upon formation of the enzyme-substrate complex, the newly formed product is released when chemical bonds are broken and new bonds are formed. The enzyme is once again available to act upon more substrate. Figure 5.6 depicts the interaction sequence of the enzyme maltase as it disassembles its substrate maltose into its component glucose building blocks in the intestinal wall during digestion:

Step 1: The active sites of the enzyme and substrate line up to achieve a perfect fit, forming an enzyme-substrate complex.
Step 2: The enzyme catalyzes (greatly speeds up) the chemical reaction with the substrate. Note that a water molecule is liberated during this hydrolysis process.
Step 3: An end product is produced. In the example, the end product is two glucose molecules.

Because the enzyme-substrate interaction resembles a key fitting into a lock, it is known as the **lock and key mechanism.** This interactive process ensures that the correct enzyme "mates" with its specific substrate to carry out a particular function. Once the enzyme and substrate join, the enzyme conformationally changes shape as it molds to the substrate. Even if an enzyme happens to link with a substrate, unless the specific conformational change in the shape of the enzyme occurs, the enzyme will not interact chemically with the substrate.

The lock and key mechanism is essentially protective in that only the correct substrate becomes activated by the correct enzyme. A typical example involves the enzyme hexokinase, which accelerates a chemical reaction when it links with a glucose molecule. When this occurs, a phosphate molecule is transferred from ATP to a specific binding site on one of glucose's carbon atoms. Once the two binding sites join to form a glucose-hexokinase complex, the substrate undergoes a stepwise degradation to less complex molecules in the process of energy metabolism. This process

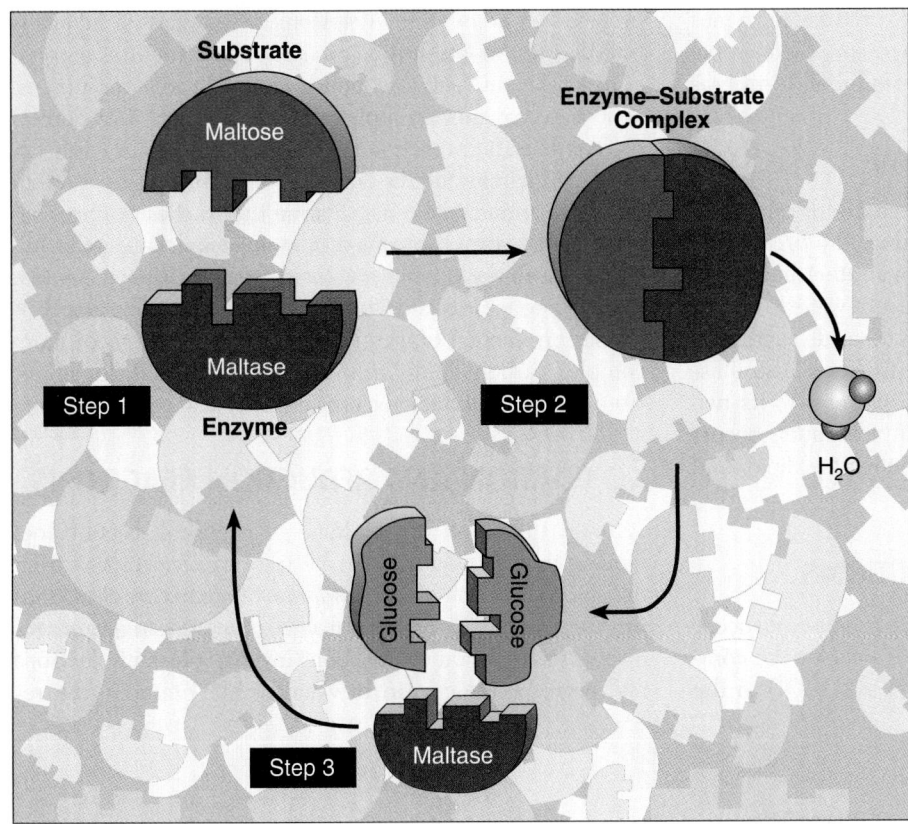

FIGURE 5.6
Sequence of steps in the "lock and key" mechanism of an enzyme with its substrate. The example shows how two molecules of the monosaccharide glucose are formed through the interaction of the enzyme maltase with its disaccharide substrate maltose.

is discussed in Chapter 6 as it applies to energy extracted from carbohydrate, lipid, and protein molecules for use by the body.

COENZYMES

Some enzymes are totally inactive in the absence of additional substances termed coenzymes. These complex, nonprotein, organic substances facilitate enzyme action by helping to bind the substrate with its specific enzyme. Coenzymes then regenerate to assist in further similar reactions. Metallic ions such as iron and zinc also often play coenzyme roles, as do vitamins, particularly the B-vitamins or their derivatives. B-vitamins such as riboflavin and niacin are involved in oxidation-reduction reactions, while others serve as transfer agents for groups of compounds in metabolic processes. Some advertisements for vitamins imply that taking vitamin supplements provides immediate usable energy for exercise. Although vitamins "make the reactions go," they contain no chemical energy that is available for biologic work.

The action of a coenzyme is less specific than that of an enzyme because the coenzyme can act in a number of different reactions. It can act as a "cobinder," or it can serve as a temporary carrier of intermediary products in the reaction. For example, the hydrogen atoms and electrons that split from food fragments during energy metabolism are transported by the coenzyme **nicotinamide adenine dinucleotide (NAD$^+$)** to form NADH. The electrons are then passed to other special transporter molecules in another series of chemical reactions that ultimately deliver them to molecular oxygen.

HYDROLYSIS AND CONDENSATION: THE BASES FOR DIGESTION AND SYNTHESIS

HYDROLYSIS REACTIONS

Hydrolysis is a basic process by which complex organic molecules such as carbohydrates, lipids, and proteins are degraded (catabolized) to simpler forms that the body can easily assimilate. During the decomposition process of hydrolysis, energy is released when chemical bonds are split apart by the addition of the constituents of water (H$^+$ and OH$^-$) to the by-products of the reaction. Examples of hydrolytic reactions include the digestion of food nutrients: starches and disaccharides to monosaccharides, proteins to amino acids, and lipids to glycerol and fatty acids. The hydrolysis of each nutrient is catalyzed by a specific enzyme. For disaccharides, the specific enzymes are lactase (lactose), sucrase (sucrose), and maltase (maltose). The lipid enzymes, lipases, degrade lipid molecules when water is added, causing the fatty acids to be cleaved from their glycerol backbone.

During the digestion of proteins, the protease enzymes need water to degrade the peptide linkages into their simple constituent amino acids. The general form for all hydrolysis reactions is:

$$AB + HOH \rightarrow A\text{-}H + B\text{-}OH$$

When water is added to the substance AB, the chemical bond that joins AB decomposes to produce the breakdown products A-H (H is a hydrogen atom from water) and B-OH (OH is the remaining hydroxyl group from water). Figure 5.7A illustrates the hydrolysis of the disaccharide sucrose to its end product molecules glucose and fructose. Also illustrated is the hydrolysis of a dipeptide (protein) to its two constituent amino acid units. Intestinal absorption occurs quickly following hydrolysis of the carbohydrate, lipid, and protein nutrients.

CONDENSATION REACTIONS

Because the reactions illustrated for hydrolysis also can occur in the opposite direction, that is, are reversible, the compound AB can be synthesized from A-H and B-OH in the process of condensation. A molecule of water is formed in this building up, or **anabolic,** process. The structural components of the nutrients are bound together in condensation reactions to form more complex molecules. Figure 5.7B depicts the condensation reaction for the synthesis of maltose from two glucose units and the creation of a more complex protein from two amino acid units. During the synthesis of protein, note that a hydroxyl removed from one amino acid and a hydrogen from the other amino acid create a water molecule. For the protein, the new bond is called a **peptide bond.** A similar production of water occurs in the synthesis of more complex carbohydrates from simple sugars and, for lipids, from the union of their glycerol and fatty acid components.

OXIDATION AND REDUCTION REACTIONS

Literally thousands of simultaneous chemical reactions occurring in the body involve the transfer of electrons from one substance to another. *Oxidation reactions are those that involve the transfer of either oxygen atoms, hydrogen atoms, or electrons.* Oxidation reactions involve a **loss** of electrons and corresponding **gain** in valence. For example, the re-

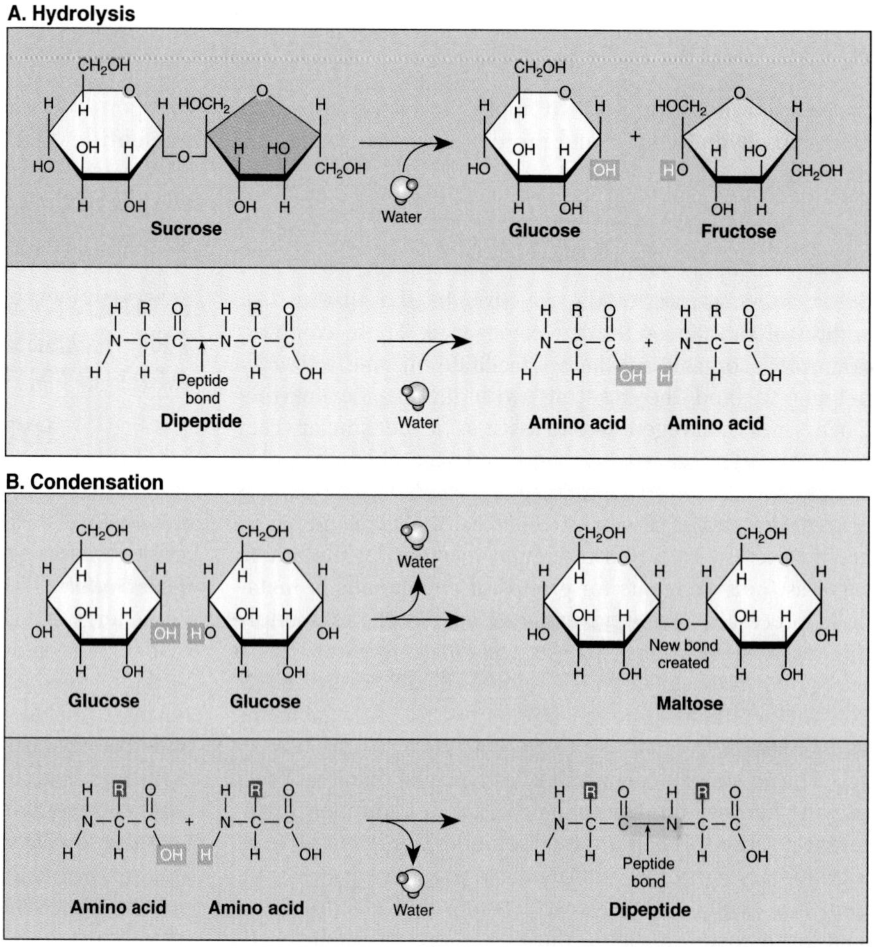

FIGURE 5.7

A, A *hydrolysis* chemical reaction of the disaccharide sucrose to the end-product molecules glucose and fructose and a hydrolysis reaction of a dipeptide (protein) into two amino acid constituents. **B,** A *condensation* chemical reaction to synthesize maltose from two glucose units and the creation of a protein dipeptide from two amino acid units. The latter reaction is the reverse of the hydrolysis reaction for the dipeptide. The symbol R represents the remainder of the amino acid molecule.

moval of hydrogen from a substance corresponds with a net gain of valence electrons. In contrast, reduction reactions involve a gain of electrons from a substance and net loss of valence electrons from another substance. *Reduction involves any process by which either electrons, oxygen atoms, or hydrogen atoms are gained with a corresponding decrease in valence.*

The substance that donates or loses electrons as it is oxidized is called a **reducing agent,** while the substance reduced or gaining electrons is called the electron acceptor, or **oxidizing agent.** For a transfer of electrons to take place, both the oxidizing agent and reducing agent must be present. Oxidation and reduction reactions are characteristically coupled: whenever oxidation occurs, the reverse reaction of reduction also takes place, and the electrons lost from one substance are gained by the other. An oxidation-reduction reaction is also known as a **redox** reaction.

An excellent example of a redox reaction is the transfer of electrons in the mitochondria. Here, hydrogen atoms are oxidized and the removed electrons passed by special carriers to be delivered ultimately to oxygen (they are reduced). The sources of hydrogen are the carbohydrate, lipid, and protein macronutrient substrates. The enzymes that speed up the redox reactions are called dehydrogenases or oxidases. Two of the hydrogen-accepting coenzymes are the vitamin-B-containing nicotinamide adenine dinucleotide (NAD^+) and flavin adenine dinucleotide (FAD). Energy in the form of ATP is harnessed during the transfer of electrons from NADH and $FADH_2$.

Figure 5.8 illustrates a redox reaction during vigorous physical activity. This coupled process constitutes the oxidation of hydrogen and subsequent reduction of oxygen. Much of the energy generated in cellular oxidation-reduction reactions is conserved as chemical energy to power the cell's various forms of biologic work. As exercise intensifies, more hydrogen atoms are stripped from the carbohydrate substrate than can be oxidized in reactions that utilize oxygen. For energy metabolism to continue, these nonoxidized excess hydrogens must be "accepted" by a chemical other than oxygen. This is exactly what takes place as a molecule of pyruvic acid, an intermediate compound formed in the initial phase of carbohydrate metabolism, temporarily accepts a pair of hydrogens (electrons). This reduction of pyruvic acid through the

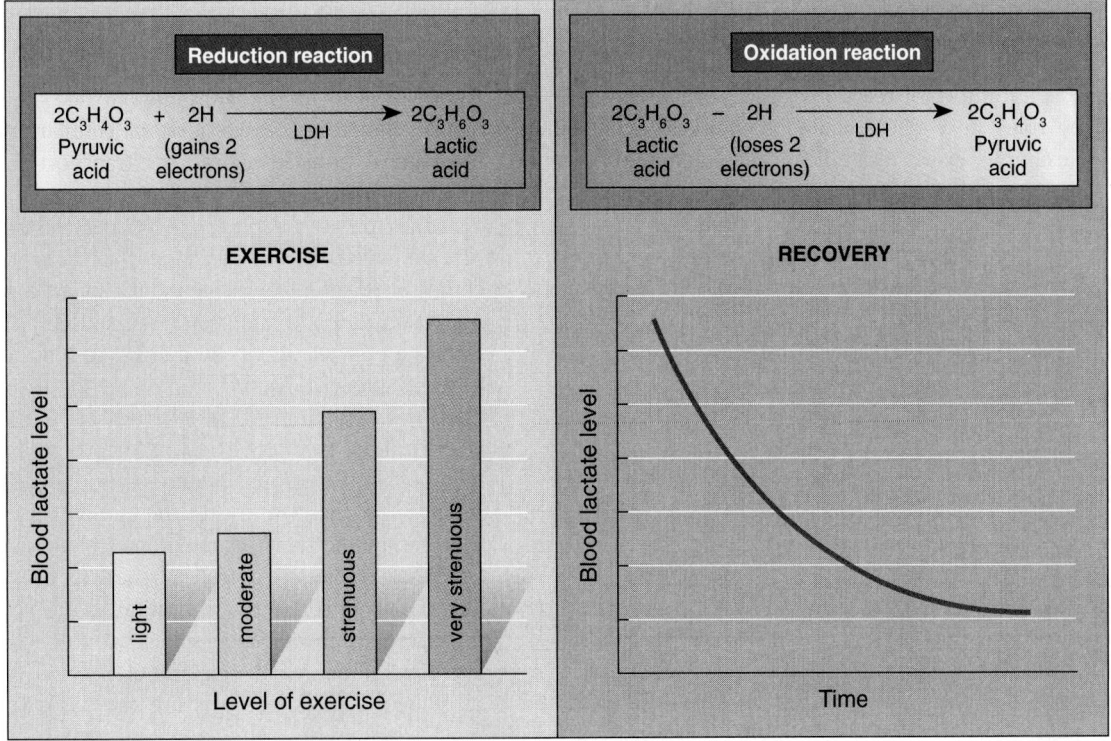

FIGURE 5.8

Example of a redox (oxidation-reduction) reaction. During progressively strenuous exercise when either oxygen supply or its metabolism becomes inadequate, some pyruvic acid formed during energy metabolism gains two hydrogens (gains two electrons) and is *reduced* to a new compound, lactic acid. During recovery, when oxygen supply is adequate, lactic acid gives up two hydrogens (loses two electrons) and is *oxidized* back to pyruvic acid. This example illustrates how a redox reaction enables energy metabolism to progress despite the limited availability of oxygen in relation to its demands during exercise.

acceptance of two hydrogens forms a new compound called **lactic acid;** the more intense the exercise, the greater the flow of excess hydrogens to pyruvic acid, with a rapid increase in lactic acid. During recovery, the excess hydrogens used to form lactic acid can then be oxidized (that is, electrons removed and passed to NAD^+) with the reformation of the oxidized pyruvic acid molecule. The enzyme that mediates this reaction is **lactate dehydrogenase** or **LDH.** Oxidation-reduction reactions in energy metabolism are discussed further in Chapter 6.

THE MASS ACTION EFFECT

The effect of the concentration of chemicals on the occurrence of a particular chemical reaction represents the **law of mass action** and is called the **mass action effect.** In essence, a chemical reaction will progress to the right when reactants are added and move to the left with the addition of by-products. The formation of a product in a simple chemical reaction increases linearly with the concentration of chemicals available to undergo the reaction. During an enzyme-mediated reaction, however, the rate of product formation is curvilinear, with a small change in substrate concentration having a relatively large effect on product formation. It is not uncommon to find certain substances in the body tied to several reactions; thus, the products of one reaction can become reactant substances for other reactions. Simply changing the concentration of one substance profoundly affects a number of reactions. Also, certain chemicals play key roles in a whole chain of chemical events. Oxygen, for example, exerts a significant mass action effect on reactions required for energy transfer. If the oxygen supply to the tissues is diminished (known as tissue hypoxia), several chemical processes cease and the net energy available for biologic work reduces dramatically.

MEASURING ENERGY RELEASE IN HUMANS

The gain or loss of heat in a biological system offers a simple means for determining the energy change of any chemical process. During the breakdown of foods, for example, the energy change can be determined **directly** as the amount of heat (kilocalories) liberated in a bomb calorimeter.

Because the complete combustion of food is achieved at the expense of molecular oxygen, the heat generated in these exergonic reactions can be conveniently and accurately estimated by measuring oxygen uptake. This type of measurement forms the basis of **indirect calorimetry** and enables one to infer the energy metabolism of humans both at rest and during many forms of physical activity by measuring the amount of oxygen consumed. The use of direct and indirect calorimetry for determining heat production (energy metabolism) in humans is discussed in Chapter 8.

■ SUMMARY ■

1. Energy is defined as the ability to perform work and, therefore, is revealed only when change takes place.
2. Energy exists in either potential or kinetic form. Potential energy is the energy associated with a substance's structure or position, whereas kinetic energy is the energy of motion. Potential energy can be measured when it is transformed into kinetic energy.
3. The six forms of energy are chemical, mechanical, heat, light, electric, and nuclear. Each form of energy can be converted or transformed into another form.
4. Exergonic energy reactions result in a transfer of energy to the surroundings. Endergonic energy reactions result in the storage or conservation of, or increase in, free energy. All potential energy is ultimately degraded to kinetic or heat energy. In living organisms, however, a portion of this energy is conserved within the structure of new compounds, which are then used for biologic work.
5. Entropy is an expression of the tendency of potential energy to degrade to kinetic or heat energy having a lower capacity for work.
6. Photosynthesis is the endergonic process by which plants transfer the energy of light to the potential energy of carbohydrates, lipids, and proteins. Respiration is the exergonic process by which the stored energy in plants is released and coupled to other chemical compounds for use in biologic work.
7. Energy transfer in humans generally takes one of three forms: chemical (biosynthesis of cellular molecules), mechanical (muscle action), or transport (transfer of substances between cells).
8. Enzymes are highly specific protein catalysts that facilitate the interaction of substances so that the rate of a chemical reaction accelerates greatly. In a supportive role, coenzymes are nonprotein, organic substances that facilitate enzyme action by helping to bind a substrate to its specific enzyme.
9. Hydrolysis (catabolism) of complex organic molecules is critical in the processes of digestion and energy metabolism. Reactions of condensation (anabolism) are required for the synthesis of the complex biomolecules required by the body for maintenance and growth.
10. Oxidation-reduction or redox reactions are intimately linked or coupled so that oxidation, or the loss of electrons from a substance, coincides with the reverse reaction of reduction, or the gaining of electrons by another substance. Redox reactions are the bases for energy-transfer processes in the body.

■ REFERENCES ■

1. Åstrand, P.O., and Rodahl, K.: *Textbook of Work Physiology.* 3rd ed., New York, McGraw-Hill, 1986.
2. Atkins, P.W.: *The Second Law.* San Francisco, W.H. Freeman, 1984.

3. Brooks, G.A., et al.: *Exercise Physiology: Human Bioenergetics and Its Applications.* 2nd ed., Mountain View, CA, Mayfield, 1996.

4. Campbell, M.K.: *Biochemistry.* Philadelphia, W.B. Saunders, 1991.

5. Kraut, J.: How do enzymes work? *Science*, 242:533, 1988.

6. Lehninger, A.L.: *Bioenergetics: The Molecular Bases of Biological Energy Transformations.* Menlo Park, CA, W.A. Benjamin, 1971.

7. Lehnigner, A.L., et al.: *Principles of Biochemistry.* 2nd ed., New York, Worth Publishers, 1993.

8. Stryer, L.: *Biochemistry.* 2nd ed., San Francisco, Freeman, 1988.

9. Szent Györgi, A.: *Chemistry of Muscular Contraction.* New York, Academic Press, 1951.

10. Vander, A.J., et al.: *Human Physiology: The Mechanisms of Body Function.* 6th ed., New York, McGraw-Hill, 1993.

Hill, A.V., and Lupton, H.: Muscular exercise, lactic acid and the supply and utilization of oxygen. Q. J. Med. 16:135, 1923.

Perhaps no scientist has contributed more to the field of exercise physiology than A.V. Hill. Although he won the Nobel prize for studies of energy metabolism using mostly frog muscle, he also pioneered studies of the physiology of running. His careful experiments on oxygen uptake during exercise and recovery led to an understanding of the dynamics of energy metabolism and work efficiency. Hill and Lupton's 1923 article dealt with interrelationships among exercise intensity, oxygen uptake, and lactic acid production and recovery oxygen uptake. This lengthy article reported the results of many experiments on several individuals (including the authors) performing different "athletic" events such as running, continuous jumping, and "violent" gymnastics of 10 to 40 minutes' duration. Measurements included oxygen uptake and blood lactic acid during exercise and recovery using what currently seem like crude techniques.

"The subject finished the exercise in front of a stand carrying a wide pipe with nine projecting tubes. To one of these tubes the valves and mouth piece were fixed: to the others were attached rubber bags through single-way stopcocks. The subject on cessation of exercise adopted the standard resting position adjusted the valves, and nose clip, and commenced to expire into the first bag. At the end of about one-half minute (end of nearest expiration) the first bag was turned off, and the second one turned on for a like interval. This process was continued, the intervals of collection being gradually increased."

The topics covered in this article included the following: the role of lactic acid in muscle; heat production; the efficiency and speed of the recovery process; the production of lactic acid in humans; lactic acid and oxygen debt; the maximal lactic acid production in muscular exertion; the rate of oxidative processes in recovery from exercise; the steady state during exercise; the maximal oxygen uptake; the relation between speed and oxygen uptake during running; the importance of tissue buffers in muscular effort; and the oxidative factor in exercise.

A salient feature of this pioneering article is the inclusion of a detailed description of the recovery oxygen uptake following different exercise intensities. The figure shows the oxygen uptake during recovery from moderate (*Exp. 1*) and severe (*Exp. 3*) exercise. The time course of the recovery oxygen uptake was related to the intensity of the previous exercise and the supposed amount of lactic acid production. Sixty years of research has confirmed most of Hill's astute observations.

Another interesting finding concerned maximal (peak) oxygen uptake. Prior to 1923, few data existed on the aerobic capacity of highly skilled individuals "of athletic disposition." Hill reported $\dot{V}O_2$ peak on five individuals during running (see last row of inset table). Also presented were other $\dot{V}O_2$ peak data collected between 1913 and 1934. Of interest are comparisons of the Hill and Lupton data with more recent $\dot{V}O_2$max data presented in Figure 11.9. Can you speculate on possible reasons for these differences?

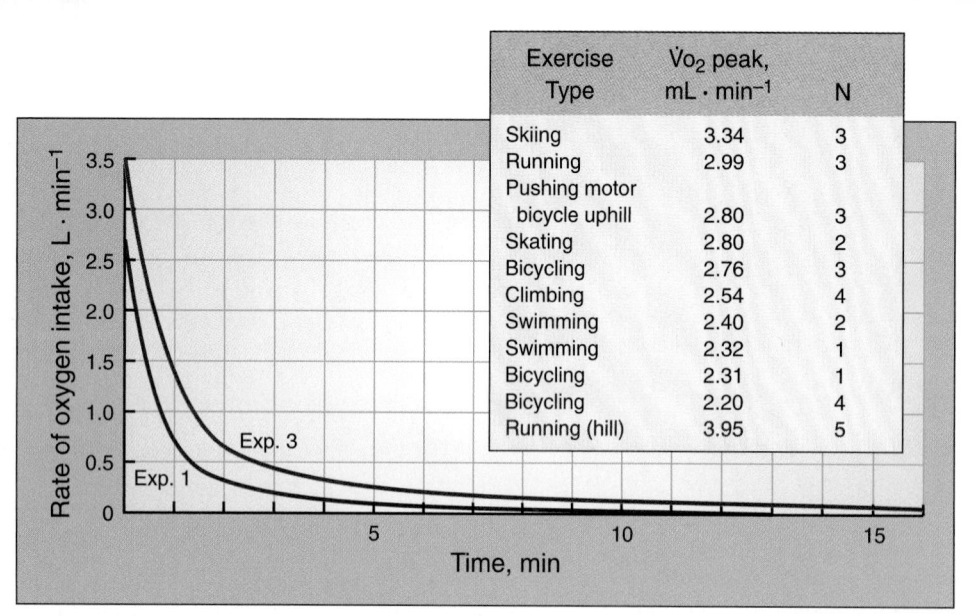

Exercise Type	$\dot{V}O_2$ peak, mL · min⁻¹	N
Skiing	3.34	3
Running	2.99	3
Pushing motor bicycle uphill	2.80	3
Skating	2.80	2
Bicycling	2.76	3
Climbing	2.54	4
Swimming	2.40	2
Swimming	2.32	1
Bicycling	2.31	1
Bicycling	2.20	4
Running (hill)	3.95	5

Plot of postexercise oxygen uptake during recovery from moderate (*Exp. 1*) and severe (*Exp. 3*) exercise. Note the elevated and more prolonged period of recovery from the strenuous exercise. The postexercise oxygen uptake curve represented a quantitative function of exercise intensity. The inset table presents values for $\dot{V}O_2$ peak obtained by Hill (*last row*) and others between 1913 and 1934.

Energy Transfer in the Body

The human body must receive a continuous supply of chemical energy to perform its many complex functions. Energy derived from the oxidation of food is not released suddenly at some kindling temperature because the body's cells, unlike a combustion engine, cannot use heat energy. If they could, our fluids would actually boil and our tissues burst into flames. Rather, the chemical energy trapped within the bonds of the carbohydrate, lipid, and protein molecules is extracted in small amounts during enzymatically controlled reactions, which occur in the relatively cool, watery medium of the cell. This slow extraction process reduces the loss of energy as heat and provides for much greater efficiency in energy transformations. These transformations enable the body to make direct use of **chemical energy** for biologic work. In a sense, energy is supplied to the cells as it is needed. The story of how the body maintains its continuous energy supply begins with adenosine triphosphate, or ATP, the special carrier for free energy.

PART 1
PHOSPHATE BOND ENERGY

ADENOSINE TRIPHOSPHATE: THE ENERGY CURRENCY

The energy in food is not transferred directly to the cells for biologic work. Rather, this "nutrient energy" released through oxidation is harvested and funneled as an accessible form of chemical energy through the energy-rich compound **ATP.** The potential energy within the ATP molecule is utilized for **all** of the energy-requiring processes of the cell. This energy receiver–energy donor cycle, in essence, represents the two major energy-transforming activities of the cell: (a) the formation of energy-rich ATP from the potential energy in food, and (b) the use of the chemical energy in ATP for biologic work.

Although the cell contains other high-energy compounds, ATP is the most important. Figure 6.1 shows the ATP molecule (one of a group of compounds called nucleotides) formed from a molecule of adenine and ribose, called adenosine, linked to three phosphates, each consist-

ing of phosphorus and oxygen atoms. The bonds that link the two outermost phosphates, symbolized as ~, are termed high-energy bonds because upon hydrolysis, they release a considerable quantity of useful energy.

When ATP joins with water, a chemical reaction catalyzed by the enzyme **adenosine triphosphatase** (**ATPase**), the outermost phosphate bond is cleaved to release a phosphate ion (also called inorganic phosphate) and forms a new compound called **adenosine diphosphate,** or **ADP.** This reaction liberates approximately 7.3 kcal of free energy per mole of ATP degraded to ADP.

$$ATP + H_2O \xrightarrow{ATPase} ADP + P_i - 7.3 \text{ kcal} \cdot \text{mol}^{-1}$$

The free energy of hydrolysis liberated in the breakdown of ATP equals the difference between the energy of the reactant and of the end products. ATP is often referred to as a **high-energy phosphate** because considerable energy is generated in its breakdown. Additional energy is released (albeit infrequently) when the second phosphate splits from ADP. During some reactions of biosynthesis, the two terminal phosphates from ATP are simultaneously donated in the construction of new cellular material. The remaining molecule with a single phosphate group is adenosine monophosphate, or **AMP.**

The energy liberated during ATP breakdown directly transfers to or couples with other energy-requiring molecules. In muscle, for example, this chemical energy activates specific sites along the contractile elements, causing the muscle fiber to shorten. Because the energy harnessed from ATP powers all forms of biologic work, ATP is considered the cell's "energy currency." Figure 6.2 illustrates the role of ATP as energy currency for biologic work and its subsequent recycling from ADP and a phosphate ion via the oxidation of stored macronutrients.

The splitting of ATP takes place whether oxygen is available or not. This reaction is rapid, **anaerobic** (not dependent on oxygen), and energy-liberating. The cell's capacity for ATP breakdown enables it to generate energy for immediate use; this would not occur if oxygen were required. Thus, exercise such as sprinting for a bus, spiking a volleyball, doing a double back flip, smashing a nail with a hammer, or lifting a heavy barbell can begin immediately without oxygen.

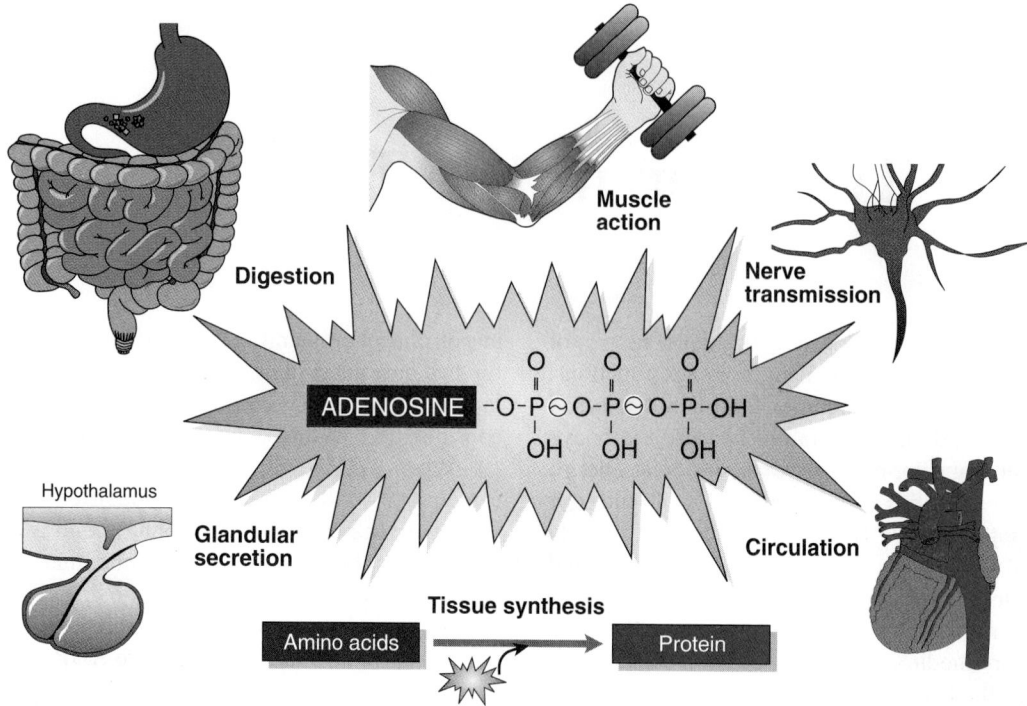

FIGURE 6.1

Simplified illustration of the structure of ATP, the energy currency that powers all forms of biologic work. The symbol ~ represents the high-energy bonds.

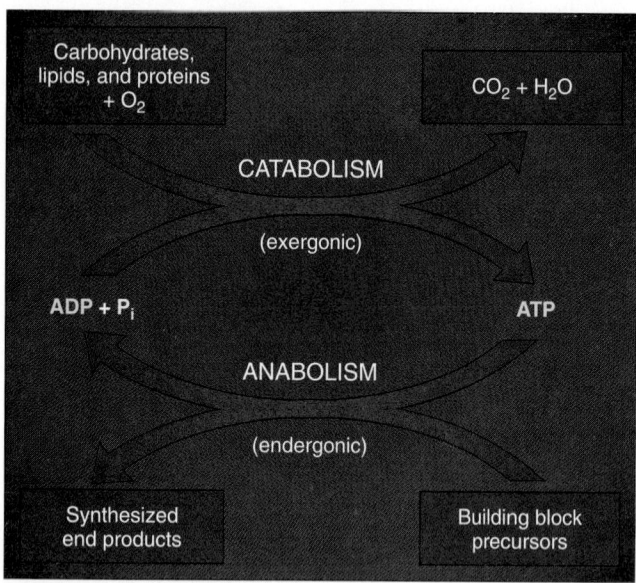

FIGURE 6.2

The role of ATP as energy currency. This compound, which is relatively heavy in relation to its energy content, is continually recycled from the energy generated during oxidation of the stored macronutrients.

CREATINE PHOSPHATE: THE ENERGY RESERVOIR

Because only a small quantity of ATP is actually stored in the cell and cannot be supplied through the blood or from other tissues, it must be continually resynthesized at its rate of usage. This situation provides a sensitive mechanism for regulating energy metabolism. Because ATP is maintained only in small amounts, its relative concentration (and the corresponding concentration of ADP) changes rapidly with an increase in energy metabolism. This change immediately stimulates the breakdown of stored nutrients to provide energy for ATP resynthesis. In this way, energy metabolism increases rapidly in the early stage of exercise.

The total quantity of ATP in the body is limited to about 80 to 100 g (3.5 oz), only enough energy to perform at a maximum exercise level for several seconds. One advantage of having a limited quantity of this "stored" fuel is that the ATP molecule is quite heavy. Biochemists estimate that sedentary persons each day use an amount of ATP approximately equal to 75% of their body mass. For an endurance athlete running a marathon race and generating about 20 times the resting energy expenditure over the course of the 2 + hour run, ATP usage could amount to about 80 kg!

Although the major sources of chemical energy for ATP resynthesis are lipids and carbohydrates, some of the energy for ATP resynthesis is generated rapidly and without oxygen

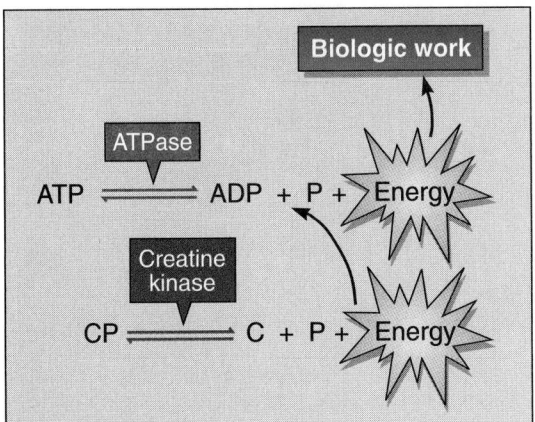

FIGURE 6.3

ATP and CP are nonaerobic sources of phosphate-bond energy. The energy liberated from the hydrolysis (splitting) of CP is used to rebond ADP and P to form ATP.

from another high-energy phosphate compound called **creatine phosphate,** or **CP.** Energy transfer from CP, depicted in Figure 6.3, is crucial during transitions from low to high energy demand, such as at the beginning of an exercise, when energy requirements exceed the energy provided from the breakdown of the stored macronutrients. The concentration of CP in the cell is about four to six times greater than that of ATP. Thus, CP is considered the high-energy phosphate "reservoir."

The CP molecule resembles ATP in that a large amount of free energy is released when the bond is cleaved between the creatine and phosphate molecules. Because CP yields more free energy during hydrolysis than ATP, CP hydrolysis (catalyzed by the enzyme **creatine kinase**) drives the phosphorylation of ADP. The arrows pointing in opposite directions in Figure 6.3 indicate that the reactions are reversible. If sufficient energy is available, creatine (C) and phosphate (P) can join to re-form CP. The same is true for ATP: the top reaction illustrates the union of ADP and phosphate to re-form ATP.

It should now be apparent that human energy dynamics involve the transfer of energy via chemical bonds. Potential energy released by the splitting of bonds is conserved by means of coupled reactions that cause the formation of new bonds. Some energy lost by one molecule can be transferred to the chemical structure of another molecule without being lost as heat. Compounds relatively low in potential energy are "juiced-up" for biologic work by energy transfer via phosphate bonds. This means of energy transfer is termed **phosphorylation.** Adenosine triphosphate serves as the ideal energy-transfer agent; in one respect, it "traps" in its phosphate bonds a large portion of the potential energy from the original food molecule, yet it readily transfers this energy to other compounds to raise them to a higher energy level.

The oxidation of the macronutrients consumed in the diet ultimately generates the energy for phosphorylation.

CELLULAR OXIDATION

During energy metabolism, hydrogen atoms are continually stripped from the carbohydrate, lipid, and protein nutrient substrates. Carrier molecules within the **mitochondria,** the cell's "chemical factories," then remove electrons from these hydrogen atoms and pass them to molecular oxygen. To complete the process, oxygen also accepts hydrogen to form water. Much of the energy generated in cellular oxidation (that is, the transfer of electrons from hydrogen to oxygen) is trapped or conserved as chemical energy in the form of ATP.

ELECTRON TRANSPORT

Energy is extracted from food in a series of small steps involving the transfer of electrons from donor to acceptor molecules. This process, known as oxidation-reduction, is fundamental to cellular energy dynamics. Figure 6.4 illustrates the general scheme for the oxidation of hydrogen and the accompanying exergonic transport of electrons to oxygen. During cellular oxidation, hydrogen atoms are not merely turned loose in the cell fluid. Rather, hydrogen release from the nutrient substrate is catalyzed along the inner surface of the mitochondrion by highly specific **dehydrogenase** enzymes. The electrons (energy) from hydrogen are picked up in pairs by the coenzyme part of the dehydroge-

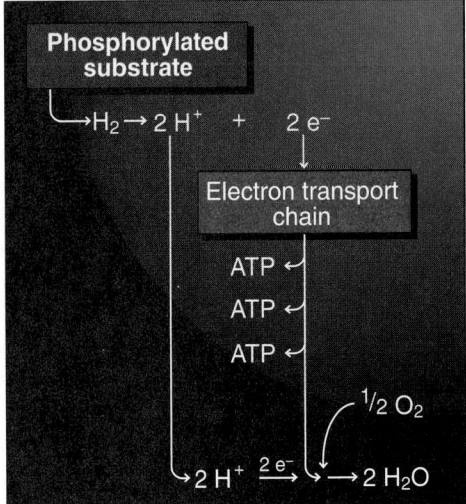

FIGURE 6.4

A general scheme for the oxidation (loss of electrons) of hydrogen and accompanying electron transport. During this process, oxygen is reduced (gain of electrons) and water is formed.

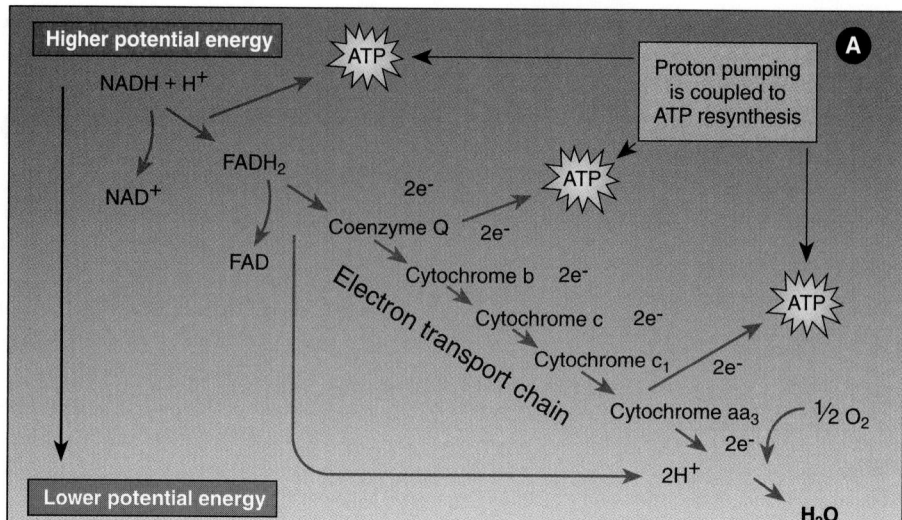

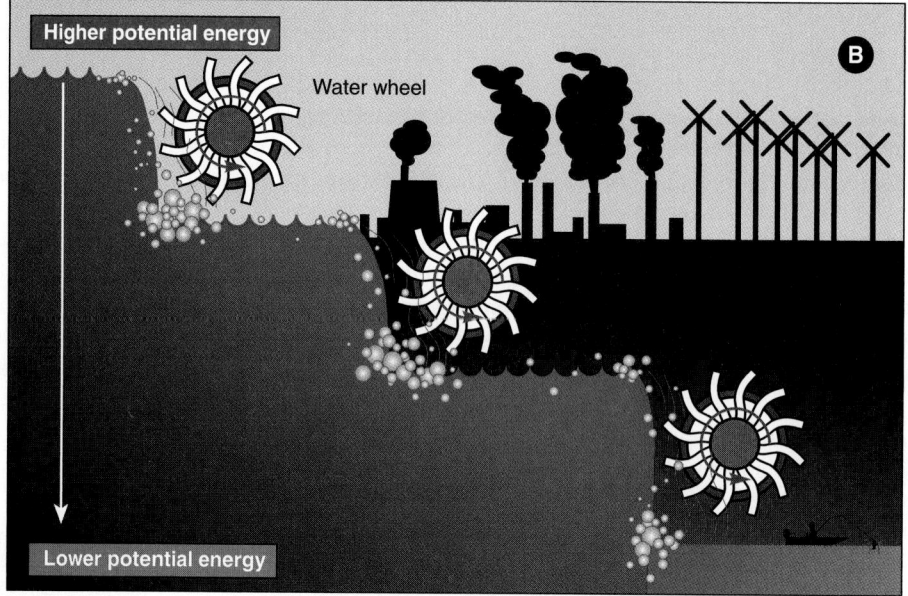

FIGURE 6.5

Examples of harnessing potential energy. **A,** *In the body:* the electron-transport chain involves the removal of electrons from hydrogens and their ultimate delivery to oxygen. During this oxidation-reduction process, a portion of the chemical energy within the hydrogen atom, rather than being dissipated to kinetic energy, is conserved in forming ATP. **B,** *In industry:* energy from falling water is harnessed to turn a water wheel used for mechanical work.

nase, usually the vitamin B (niacin)-containing coenzyme **nicotinamide adenine dinucleotide,** or **NAD$^+$.** While the substrate is being oxidized and losing hydrogen (electrons), NAD$^+$ is gaining a hydrogen and two electrons and being reduced to NADH; the remaining hydrogen appears in the cell fluid as H$^+$. The other important coenzyme electron acceptor in the oxidation of food, **flavin adenine dinucleotide,** or **FAD,** is derived from the B-vitamin riboflavin. Unlike NAD$^+$, FAD accepts both hydrogens to become FADH$_2$.

The NADH and FADH$_2$ generated in the catabolism of food are energy-rich molecules because they carry electrons that have a high energy-transfer potential. Along the inner membrane of the mitochondrion, the electrons carried by NADH and FADH$_2$ are passed in "bucket brigade" fashion

to coenzyme Q and then to a series of iron-protein electron carriers called **cytochromes.** Unlike the iron (heme) portion of the blood's hemoglobin, which remains in its reduced form as Fe^{2+} during oxygen transport, the heme portion of each cytochrome can exist in the oxidized state as ferric ion (Fe^{3+}) or in the reduced state as ferrous ion (Fe^{2+}). By accepting an electron, the ferric portion of a specific cytochrome is reduced to its ferrous form; in turn, the electron is donated to the next cytochrome, and so on down the line. By shuttling between these two iron forms, the cytochromes transfer electrons to their ultimate destination, where they reduce oxygen to form water. The NAD$^+$ and FAD are then recycled for subsequent use in energy metabolism.

The transport of electrons from hydrogen to oxygen by specific intermediate carrier molecules constitutes the **res-**

piratory chain. Of the five specific cytochromes, only the last, **cytochrome oxidase** (cytochrome aa$_3$), which has an extremely strong affinity for oxygen, can discharge its electron directly to an oxygen atom. Oxidation is complete when two electrons and two protons (H$^+$) join with oxygen to form water. Figure 6.5A illustrates the route for the oxidation of hydrogen and the accompanying electron transport and energy transfer in the respiratory chain. *Free energy is released in relatively small amounts, and in several of the electron transfers, energy is conserved by the formation of high-energy phosphate bonds during the phosphorylation of ADP.*

OXIDATIVE PHOSPHORYLATION

In the oxidative phosphorylation process, ATP is synthesized during the transfer of electrons from NADH and FADH$_2$ to molecular oxygen. This process is separate from, yet dependent on, electron transport. Figure 6.6 illustrates how the energy generated during the reactions of electron transport pumps protons across the inner mitochondrial membrane into the intermembranous space. The electrochemical gradient generated by this reverse flow of protons represents stored potential energy, which provides the coupling mechanism that binds ADP and a phosphate ion to synthesize ATP. Biochemists refer to this process as **chemosmotic coupling.** This important endergonic process occurring in the inner wall of the mitochondrion represents the cell's primary means of extracting and trapping chemical energy in the form of high-energy phosphates. More than 90% of ATP synthesis is accomplished in the respiratory chain of the mitochondrial proteins by oxidative reactions coupled with phosphorylation.

In a way, the process of oxidative phosphorylation resembles a waterfall divided into several separate cascades by the intervention of water wheels spaced at different heights. As depicted in Figure 6.5B, the water wheels harness the energy of the falling water. Similarly, the electrochemical energy generated in electron transport from one respiratory chain component to the next is harnessed and transferred or coupled to ADP. The energy in NADH is transferred to ADP to drive the reformation of ATP at three distinct coupling sites during electron transport (Figure 6.5A). This oxidation of hydrogen and subsequent phosphorylation can be summarized as follows:

$$NADH + H^+ + 3\,ADP + 3\,P + \tfrac{1}{2}\,O_2 \longrightarrow NAD^+ + H_2O + 3\,ATP$$

The **P/O ratio** quantitatively reflects the coupling of ATP production to electron transport. The P/O ratio equals 3 when NADH is the substrate oxidized. If, however, hydrogen is originally donated by FADH$_2$, then only two molecules of ATP are formed for each hydrogen pair oxidized (P/O ratio = 2). This occurs because FADH$_2$ enters the respiratory chain at a lower energy level and at a point beyond the site of the first ATP synthesis.

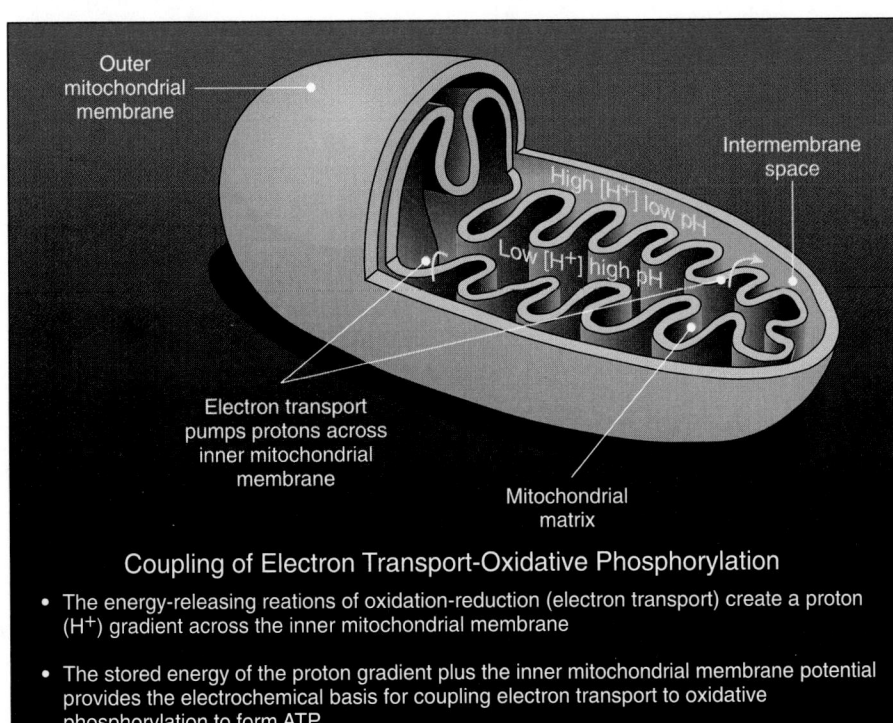

Outer mitochondrial membrane

Intermembrane space

High [H$^+$] low pH

Low [H$^+$] high pH

Electron transport pumps protons across inner mitochondrial membrane

Mitochondrial matrix

Coupling of Electron Transport-Oxidative Phosphorylation

- The energy-releasing reations of oxidation-reduction (electron transport) create a proton (H$^+$) gradient across the inner mitochondrial membrane

- The stored energy of the proton gradient plus the inner mitochondrial membrane potential provides the electrochemical basis for coupling electron transport to oxidative phosphorylation to form ATP

FIGURE 6.6

The mitochondrion is the site of aerobic energy metabolism. Electron transport causes a proton (H$^+$) gradient across the inner mitochondrial membrane. This leads to a net flow of protons that provides the coupling mechanism to drive ATP resynthesis. The number of molecules of ATP resynthesized in relation to oxygen consumed is termed the P/O ratio. When NADH is oxidized, the P/O ratio = 3; when FADH$_2$ donates its hydrogens, the P/O ratio = 2.

EFFICIENCY OF ELECTRON TRANSPORT AND OXIDATIVE PHOSPHORYLATION

The synthesis of each mole of ATP requires approximately 7 kcal of energy. Because 3 moles of ATP result from the oxidation of 1 mole of NADH, the chemical energy conserved amounts to about 21 kcal. In total, the oxidation of a mole of NADH liberates 52 kcal. Thus, the relative efficiency of electron transport-oxidative phosphorylation for harnessing chemical energy is approximately 40% (21 kcal ÷ 52 kcal × 100). The remaining 60% of the energy is lost to the body as heat. Considering that a steam engine transforms fuel into useful energy at an efficiency of only about 30%, the value of 40% for the human body represents a high efficiency rating.

ROLE OF OXYGEN IN ENERGY METABOLISM

Three prerequisites must be met for the continual resynthesis of ATP:

- A donor of electrons (reducing agent) must be available in the form of NADH (or FADH$_2$)
- Although many intermediate electron acceptors take part in the metabolic process, adequate oxygen must be present as the final electron and hydrogen acceptor (oxidizing agent)
- Enzymes and associated "metabolic machinery" must be present in sufficient concentrations to move the energy transfer reactions to completion

When these three conditions are satisfied, hydrogen and electrons are continually shuttled down the respiratory chain to molecular oxygen during the catabolism of food substrate.

Strenuous exercise, during which the rate of oxygen delivery (second prerequisite) or utilization (third prerequisite) often is inadequate, creates a relative imbalance between the release of hydrogen and its final acceptance by oxygen. In a sense, electron flow down the respiratory chain begins to "back up" and hydrogen atoms bound to NAD$^+$ accumulate. As discussed in a subsequent section, pyruvate temporarily accepts these excess hydrogens (electrons) to form lactic acid, permitting energy metabolism to continue at relatively high levels for an additional time period.

During energy metabolism, oxygen serves as the final electron acceptor in the respiratory chain and combines with hydrogen to form water. The process of electron transport and oxidative phosphorylation in the respiratory chain is referred to as **aerobic metabolism.** In one sense, this term is misleading because oxygen does not participate directly in the synthesis of ATP. In reality, however, the availability of oxygen as the oxidizing agent at the "end of the line" largely determines one's capability for sustained aerobic energy release during exercise.

■ SUMMARY ■

1. The energy contained within the chemical structure of carbohydrates, lipids, and proteins is not released in the body suddenly at some kindling temperature. Rather, it is released slowly in small amounts during complex, enzymatically controlled reactions, enabling more efficient energy transfer.
2. About 40% of the potential energy in food nutrients is transferred to the high-energy compound ATP. When the terminal phosphate bond of ATP is broken, the free energy liberated powers all forms of biologic work. Thus, ATP is considered the body's energy currency, although its quantity in the body amounts to only about 3.5 ounces.
3. Creatine phosphate interacts with ADP to form ATP and thus serves as a nonaerobic, high-energy reservoir to replenish ATP rapidly.
4. Phosphorylation is the process by which energy is transferred in the form of phosphate bonds. In this process, ADP and creatine are continually recycled into ATP and CP.
5. Cellular oxidation occurs on the inner lining of the membranes of the mitochondria and involves the transfer of electrons from NADH and FADH$_2$ to molecular oxygen. This transfer results in the release and coupled transfer of chemical energy to form ATP from ADP plus phosphate ion.
6. During the aerobic resynthesis of ATP, oxygen serves primarily as the final electron acceptor in the respiratory chain and combines with hydrogen to form water.

PART 2
ENERGY RELEASE FROM FOOD

The energy generated in the breakdown of food macronutrients serves one purpose: to phosphorylate ADP and reform the energy-rich compound ATP. Although food catabolism is geared toward generating phosphate-bond energy, the specific pathways of degradation differ depending on the nutrients metabolized. In the sections that follow, we will look at how the potential energy in food is extracted and utilized to synthesize ATP.

Figure 6.7 outlines the basic macronutrient fuel sources that supply substrates for oxidation to form ATP. These are the triglyceride and glycogen molecules stored within the muscle cells themselves, as well as glucose derived from liver glycogen and free fatty acids (from both the liver and adipocytes) that enter the bloodstream and are delivered to active muscle. A small amount of ATP is also generated from anaerobic reactions that take place in the cytosol in the initial phase of glucose or glycogen breakdown and rephos-

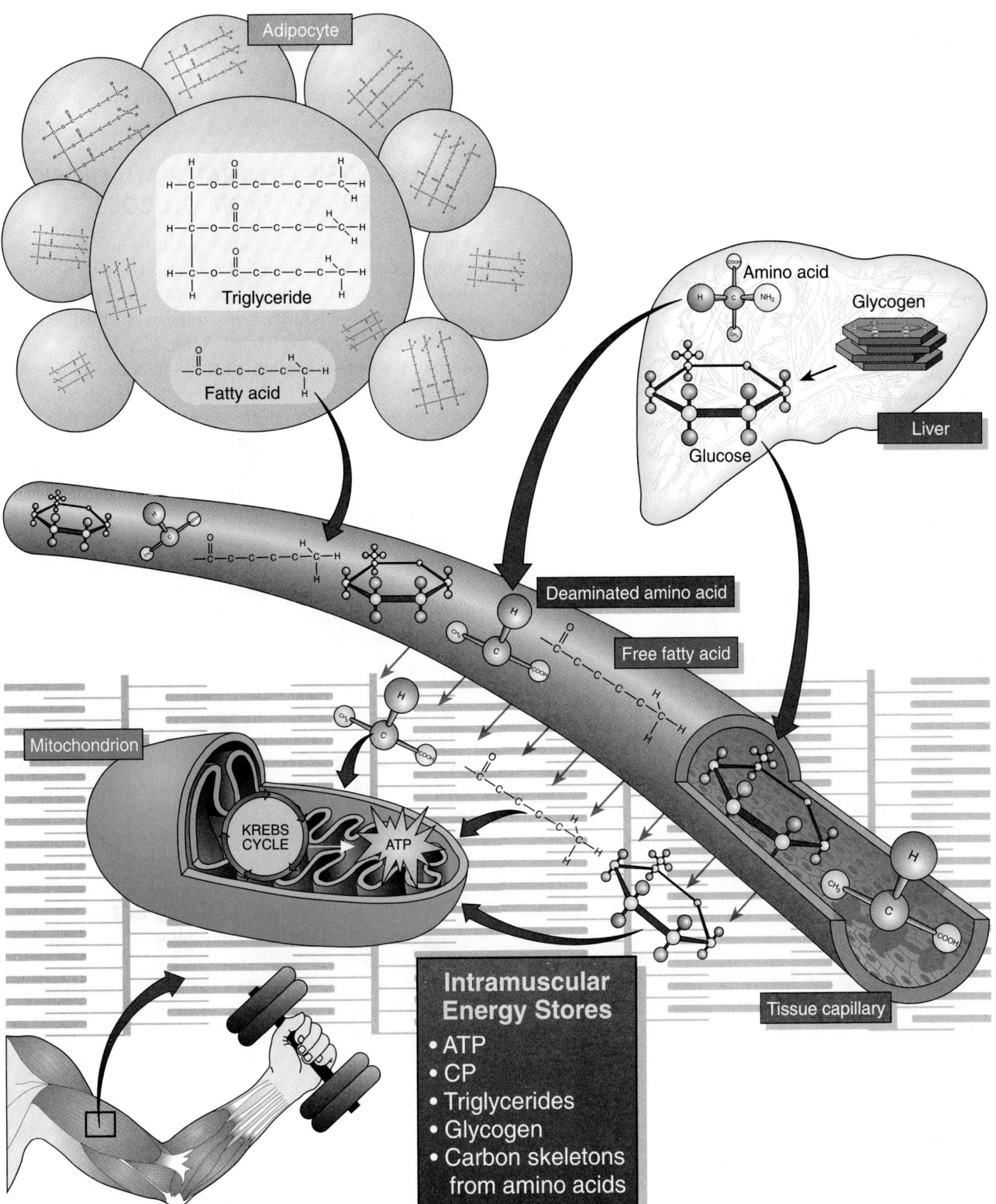

FIGURE 6.7

Basic macronutrient fuel sources that supply substrates for the regeneration of ATP. The liver is a rich source of amino acid and glucose release, while the adipocytes generate large quantities of the energy-rich fatty acid molecules. Once released, these compounds are delivered to the muscle cell via the bloodstream. Most of the cells' energy production takes place within the mitochondria. The mitochondrial proteins carry out their roles of oxidative phosphorylation in the inner membranous walls of this architecturally elegant mitochondrial complex. The intramuscular energy sources consist of the high-energy phosphates, ATP and CP, and triglycerides, glycogen and amino acids.

phorylation of ADP from CP under enzymatic control of creatine kinase.

ENERGY RELEASE FROM CARBOHYDRATES

The primary function of carbohydrates is to supply energy for cellular work. Our discussion of nutrient energy metabolism begins with carbohydrates for several reasons:

- Carbohydrates are the only macronutrients whose stored energy can be used to generate ATP anaerobically. This ability is important during vigorous exercise requiring a rapid energy release above levels supplied by aerobic metabolism. In such a case, stored glycogen and blood-borne glucose must supply the main portion of energy for ATP resynthesis.
- During light and moderate exercise, carbohydrates supply about one-half of the body's energy requirement.
- Some carbohydrates must continually be degraded so that lipid nutrients can be processed through the metabolic mill and used for energy. During prolonged, high-intensity aerobic exercise such as marathon running, participants commonly experience "nutrient fatigue"—a state associated with glycogen depletion in the muscles and liver.

The complete breakdown of one mole of glucose to carbon dioxide and water yields a maximum of 689 kcal of chemical free energy (that is, energy available for work) as follows:

$$C_6H_{12}O_6 + 6O_2 \longrightarrow 6CO_2 + 6H_2O - \Delta G\ 689\ kcal \cdot mol^{-1}$$

In the cell, the breakdown of glucose to its simple, stable end-products is accompanied by the conservation of some energy in the form of ATP. Because 7.3 kcal is required to synthesize each mole of ATP from ADP and phosphate ion, coupling all of the energy in glucose oxidation to phosphorylation could theoretically form 94 moles of ATP per mole of glucose (689 kcal ÷ 7.3 = 94). In the muscle, however, only about 38%, or 263 kcal, of energy is actually conserved in phosphate bonds, with the remainder dissipated as heat. Consequently, 36 moles of ATP is regenerated in glucose breakdown (263 kcal ÷ 7.3 = 36), with an accompanying gain of 263 kcal of free energy.

Anaerobic versus Aerobic Metabolism

There are two stages for glucose degradation in the body. The first stage involves the rapid 10-step breakdown (fermentation) of a glucose molecule in the cell's cytosol to two molecules of pyruvate. *These reactions involve energy transfers that do not require oxygen and are termed anaerobic.* Without this anaerobic production of ATP, all of the energy liberated in the degradation of glucose to pyruvate or lactic acid would be lost to the body and dissipated as heat. In the

second phase of glucose catabolism, the pyruvate molecules are further degraded in the mitochondrion to carbon dioxide and water. *Energy transfers from these reactions involve electron transport and accompanying oxidative phosphorylation and are termed aerobic.*

GLYCOLYSIS GENERATES ANAEROBIC ENERGY FROM GLUCOSE

When a glucose molecule enters a cell for use as energy, it undergoes a series of chemical reactions collectively termed **glycolysis,** also called the Embden-Myerhoff pathway after the pioneering chemists who uncovered this sequence of reactions.[3] These reactions, summarized in Figure 6.8, occur in the watery medium of the cell outside of the mitochondrion. In terms of evolutionary sequence, glycolysis represents a more primitive form of energy transfer that is well developed in amphibians, reptiles, fish, and diving mammals.

In the first reaction, ATP acts as a phosphate donor to phosphorylate glucose to glucose 6-phosphate. This reaction "traps" the glucose molecule in most cells. Liver cells (and, to a small extent, kidney cells) contain the enzyme **phosphatase,** which splits phosphate from glucose 6-phosphate, enabling glucose to leave the cell for transport throughout the body. The phosphorylated glucose molecule can then be converted to uridine diphosphate glucose and linked together or polymerized with other glucose molecules (under the control of the enzyme glycogen synthetase) to form glycogen, the storage form of glucose (refer to Fig. 1.2).

During energy metabolism, however, glucose 6-phosphate is changed to the isomer fructose 6-phosphate. At this stage, no useful energy has been extracted, but energy has been incorporated into the original glucose molecule at the expense of one molecule of ATP (see reaction 1 in Fig. 6.8). In a sense, this phosphorylation has "primed the pump" so that energy metabolism can proceed. Controlled by the enzyme **phosphofructokinase (PFK),** the fructose 6-phosphate molecule is then phosphorylated and changed in a highly exergonic and irreversible reaction to fructose 1,6-diphosphate. The **regulatory control** of PFK limits the rate of glycolysis during maximum exercise. Fructose 1,6-diphosphate then splits into two phosphorylated, three-carbon molecules, which are further degraded to pyruvate in five successive reactions.

Glycogen Catabolism

When glycogen serves as the source of glucose for energy, a process termed **glycogenolysis,** one glucose component at a time is cleaved from the glycogen molecule. This process is regulated by the action of the enzyme **glycogen phosphorylase,** the activity of which is greatly influenced by the action of epinephrine, a hormone of the sympathetic nervous system.[6] The glucose residue then reacts with a phosphate ion to produce glucose 6-phosphate, thus bypass-

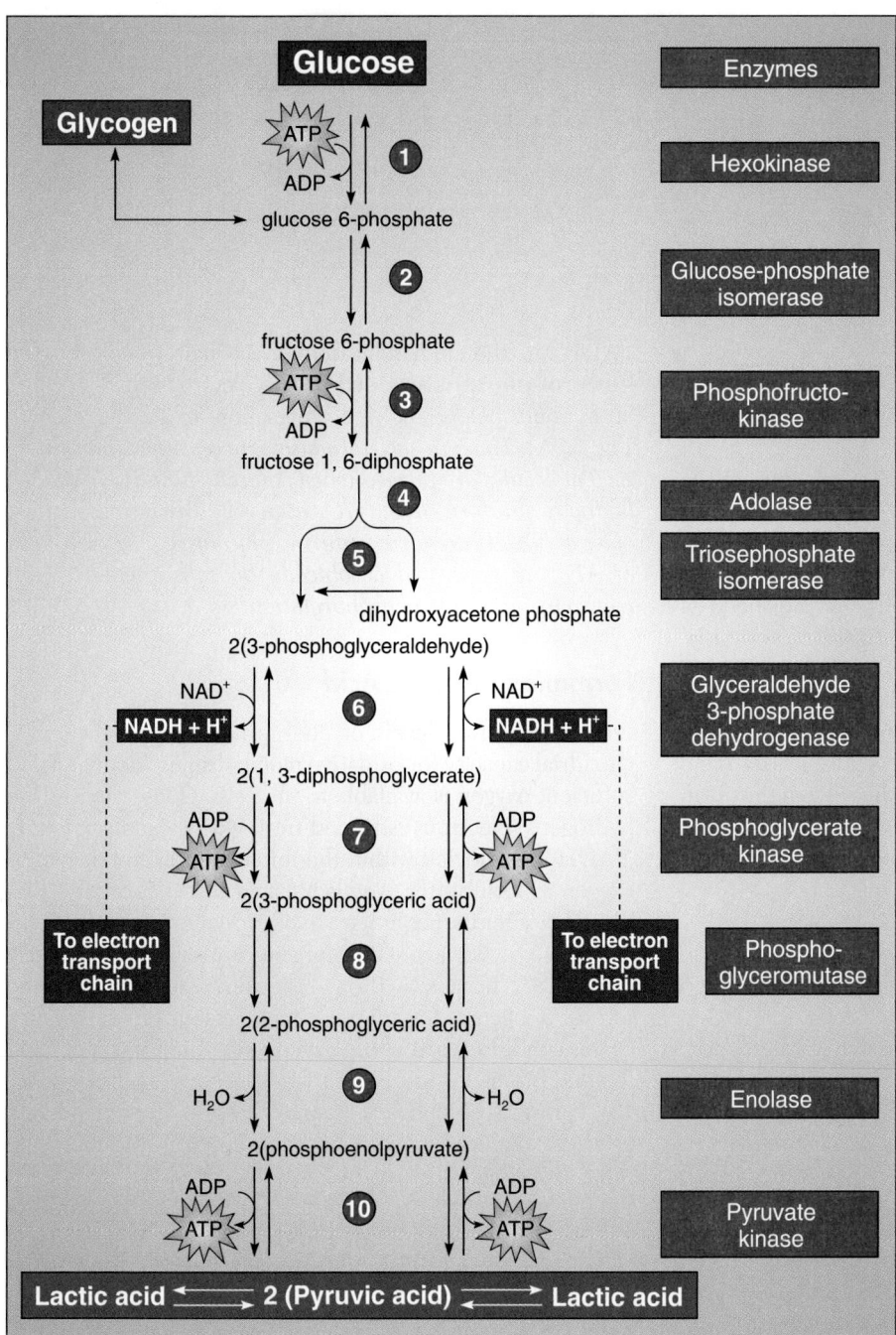

FIGURE 6.8

Glycolysis is a series of 10 enzymatically controlled chemical reactions that occur during the anaerobic breakdown of glucose to two molecules of pyruvate. Lactic acid is formed by the process of anaerobic glycolysis when the oxidation of NADH does not keep pace with its formation in glycolysis.

ing the first step of the glycolytic pathway. When glycolysis begins with a glucose molecule derived from glycogen, there is a net gain of 3 ATP rather than 2 ATP as occurs when glycolysis begins with glucose itself (see below).

Substrate-Level Phosphorylation in Glycolysis

Most of the energy generated in the exergonic reactions of glycolysis (44 kcal · mol⁻¹) is not sufficient to resynthesize ATP and is lost to the body as heat. In reactions 7 and 10,

however, the energy released from the glucose intermediates is sufficient to stimulate the direct transfer of a phosphate ion to ADP, with the generation of a total of four molecules of ATP. *Because two molecules of ATP are lost in the initial phosphorylation of glucose, the net energy transfer from glycolysis results in a gain of two molecules of ATP (endergonic conservation of 14.6 kcal · mol⁻¹).* These specific energy transfers from substrate to ADP through phosphorylation do not require oxygen or ATP. Rather, the source of the phosphate group is the phosphate ion itself. This

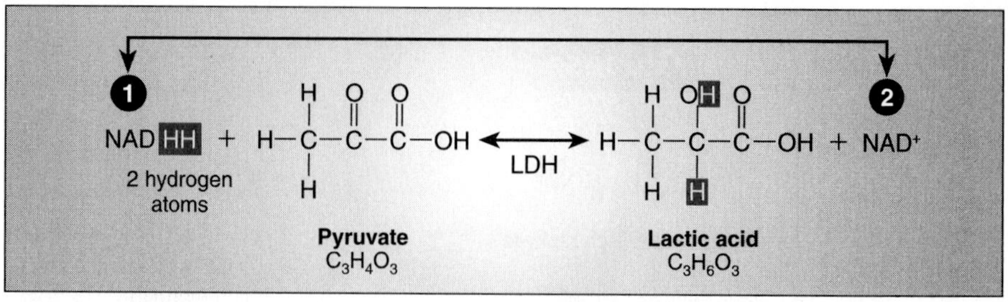

FIGURE 6.9
The formation of lactic acid occurs when excess hydrogens from NADH combine temporarily with pyruvate (**1**). This frees up NAD⁺ to accept additional hydrogens generated in glycolysis (**2**).

method of phosphate bond energy transfer via glycolysis is called **substrate-level phosphorylation**—an anaerobic process of energy conservation that operates at an efficiency of about 33%.

Only about 5% of the total ATP generated in the complete breakdown of a glucose molecule is formed during glycolysis. However, significant energy for muscle action can be provided **rapidly** through glycolysis because of the high concentration of glycolytic enzymes and the speed of these reactions. In fact, the rate of energy release from glycolysis is about three times as fast as the aerobic energy release from stored lipids. The cells' capacity for glycolysis is crucial during physical activity requiring all-out effort for periods of up to approximately 90 seconds. The athlete sprinting at the end of a mile run relies heavily on this form of anaerobic energy transfer, which is possible only when glucose breaks down in glycolytic reactions.

Hydrogen Release in Glycolysis

During glycolysis, two pairs of hydrogen atoms are stripped from the substrate and their electrons passed to NAD⁺ to form NADH (Fig. 6.8, reaction 6). Normally, if these electrons were processed directly through the respiratory chain, three molecules of ATP would be generated for each molecule of NADH oxidized (P/O ratio = 3). The mitochondrion, however, is impermeable to the NADH formed in the cytosol during glycolysis. Consequently, the electrons from extramitochondrial NADH are transferred to a carrier and shuttled indirectly into the mitochondrion. Within the cells of the heart, kidney, and liver, this extramitochondrial hydrogen (NADH) produces NADH in the mitochondrion (a mechanism termed the **malate-aspartate shuttle**). This results in the production of three molecules of ATP from the oxidation of each molecule of NADH formed in glycolysis. In skeletal muscle and brain cells, however, the electrons from extramitochondrial NADH are passed to FAD to form

FADH₂ in the mitochondrion (a mechanism termed the **glycerol-phosphate shuttle**). This electron transfer occurs at a point below the first formation of ATP (refer to Fig. 6.5A). *Thus, in skeletal muscle, two, rather than three, ATP molecules are formed when cytosolic NADH is oxidized by the respiratory chain (P/O ratio = 2). Because two molecules of NADH are formed during glycolysis, four molecules of ATP are generated aerobically by subsequent electron transport–oxidative phosphorylation.*

Formation of Lactic Acid

During moderate levels of energy metabolism, the mitochondrial capacity for oxidative metabolism is adequate, and sufficient oxygen is available to the cells. Consequently, the hydrogens (electrons) stripped from glucose and carried by NADH are oxidized within the mitochondria and passed to oxygen to form water. Any lactic acid that is formed is oxidized by other tissues at its rate of formation. In a biochemical sense, a "steady state" (or, more precisely, a **"steady rate"**) exists because hydrogen is oxidized at about the same rate as it becomes available. Biochemists frequently refer to this condition as **aerobic glycolysis,** with pyruvate being the end product.

During strenuous exercise, when energy demands exceed either the oxygen supply or its rate of utilization, the rate of production of hydrogen joined to NADH exceeds the rate at which it can be processed through the respiratory chain. Continued release of anaerobic energy in glycolysis depends on the availability of NAD⁺ for the oxidation of 3-phosphoglyceraldehyde (refer to reaction 6, Fig. 6.8); otherwise, the rapid rate of glycolysis would grind to a halt. Under the conditions of **anaerobic glycolysis,** NAD⁺ is regenerated as pairs of "excess" hydrogens combine with pyruvate in one additional step catalyzed by the enzyme **lactic dehydrogenase (LDH).** This forms lactic acid in the reversible reaction indicated in Figure 6.9.[a]

---

[a] The "onset" of anaerobic energy metabolism is reflected in the accumulation of lactic acid, not simply its production. This is because at rest and during moderate exercise, some lactic acid is continually formed by the energy metabolism of red blood cells that contain no mitochondria, and by limitations imposed by enzyme activity within other tissues such as muscle fibers with high glycolytic capacity. However, any lactic acid formed in this manner is readily oxidized at its rate of formation by neighboring muscle fibers with high oxidative capacity or by more distant tissues such as the heart. In such cases, lactic acid does not accumulate because its removal rate equals its rate of production. This ability for lactate clearance or "turnover" during exercise is well developed in endurance-trained athletes.[12]

The temporary storage of hydrogen with pyruvate is a unique aspect of energy metabolism because it provides a ready "sump" for the excess hydrogen end product of anaerobic glycolysis. Also, once lactic acid forms in the muscle, it diffuses rapidly into the blood, where it is buffered to form lactate, and is then transported from the site of energy metabolism. In this way, glycolysis can proceed to supply additional anaerobic energy for ATP resynthesis. This avenue for extra energy is only temporary because the regeneration of ATP cannot keep pace with its utilization, and the capacity for exercise diminishes. Fatigue is largely mediated by increased acidity (and perhaps the effect of the lactate anion itself), which inactivates various enzymes involved in energy transfer and interferes with the muscle's contractile properties.[2, 9, 13] However, increases in acidity (decreased pH) do not singularly explain the decrement in exercise capacity during heavy physical effort.[10]

Lactic acid should not be viewed as a metabolic "waste product." Rather, it is a valuable source of chemical potential energy that is continually utilized by the body in moderate exercise and accumulates during heavy exercise. The hydrogen atoms attached to the lactic acid that does accumulate are picked up by NAD^+ and are eventually oxidized when sufficient oxygen becomes available, as in recovery or when the pace of exercise is slowed. The remaining pyruvate is then used as an energy source. Figure 6.10 illustrates how the potential energy in the lactate and pyruvate formed in skeletal muscle during exercise can also be conserved by the liver: the carbon skeletons of the lactate and pyruvate molecules are used for the synthesis of glucose in the gluconeogenic processes called the **Cori cycle.** This cycle (which is complemented by the gluconeogenic alanine-glucose cycle described in Chapter 1) provides not only a means for lactate removal but also a means for augmenting blood glucose and muscle glycogen during exercise.[b]

THE KREBS CYCLE

Because the anaerobic reactions of glycolysis release only about 5% of the energy in the glucose molecule, another means is available for extracting the remaining potential energy. This means is provided within the mitochondrion when the pyruvate molecule is **irreversibly** converted to a form of acetic acid called **acetyl-CoA.** This intermediate compound then enters the second stage of carbohydrate breakdown known as the Krebs cycle (named for its discoverer, 1953 Nobel laureate Sir Hans Krebs) or, more descriptively, the citric acid or tricarboxylic acid cycle.[4] As shown schematically in Figure 6.11, a main function of the Krebs cycle is to degrade the acetyl-CoA substrate to carbon dioxide and hydrogen atoms within the mitochondrial matrix. The hydrogen atoms are then oxidized in electron transport–oxidative phosphorylation and ATP subsequently regenerated.

---

[b]During more strenuous endurance exercise when carbohydrate catabolism is high, the glycogen within inactive tissues can become available to meet the needs of active muscle. This active glycogen turnover through the **exchangeable lactate pool** is possible as inactive tissues release lactate into the circulation. This lactate, in turn, is available as a gluconeogenic precursor (via liver and kidneys) to provide added carbohydrate to support blood glucose homeostasis and to provide fuel for exercise.[5, 12]

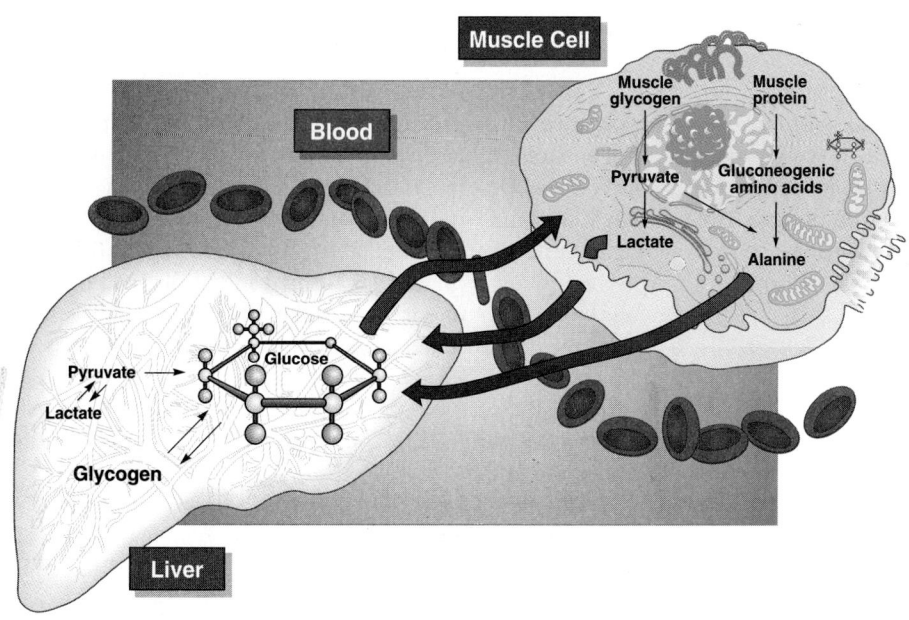

FIGURE 6.10
The Cori cycle is a biochemical process that takes place in the liver in which the lactic acid released from the active muscles is synthesized to glucose. This gluconeogenic process provides the body with an option for maintaining its limited carbohydrate reserves.

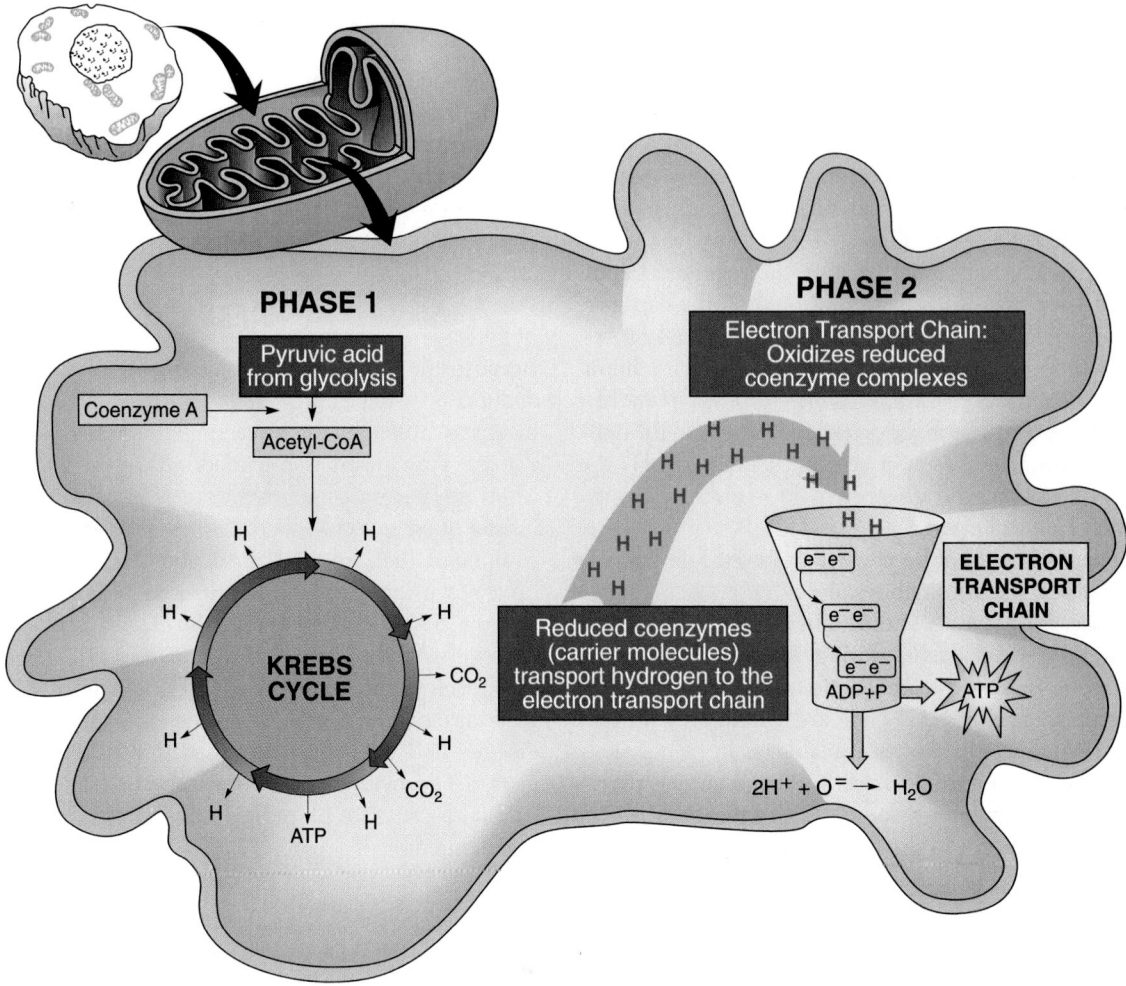

FIGURE 6.11

Phase 1: In the mitochondrion, the Krebs cycle generates hydrogen atoms during the breakdown of acetyl-CoA. *Phase 2:* Significant quantities of ATP are regenerated when these hydrogens are oxidized via the aerobic process of electron transport–oxidative phosphorylation.

As shown in Figure 6.12, pyruvate is prepared for entrance into the Krebs cycle by joining with the vitamin B derivative coenzyme A (A for acetic acid) to form the two-carbon compound **acetyl-CoA.** *This is the point of entry for all metabolic fuels into the Krebs cycle.* In the process, two hydrogen atoms are released and their electrons transferred to NAD^+, and one molecule of carbon dioxide is formed as follows:

$$Pyruvate + NAD^+ + CoA \longrightarrow$$
$$Acetyl\text{-}CoA + CO_2 + NADH + H^+$$

When the acetyl portion of acetyl-CoA condenses with the four-carbon **oxaloacetate,** it forms **citrate** (the same citrate or citric acid found in citrus fruits), a six-carbon compound that then proceeds through the Krebs cycle. The cycle is continued because the original oxaloacetate molecule is retained and joins with a new acetyl fragment.

For each acetyl-CoA molecule oxidized in the Krebs cycle, two carbon dioxide molecules and four pairs of hydrogen atoms are cleaved from the substrate. One molecule of ATP is also regenerated directly by substrate-level phosphorylation in Krebs cycle reactions (refer to reaction 7, Fig. 6.12). As summarized at the bottom of Figure 6.12, for the two pyruvate molecules formed in glycolysis, a total of four hydrogen atoms are released in the formation of acetyl-CoA, and 16 hydrogen atoms are released in the Krebs cycle. *In essence, the most important function of the Krebs cycle is the generation of electrons (hydrogens) for transfer to the respiratory chain by means of NAD^+ and, in one instance, FAD.*

Note that molecular oxygen does not participate directly in the reactions of the Krebs cycle. The major portion of the chemical energy in pyruvate is transferred to ADP through the aerobic process of electron transport–oxidative phosphorylation. As long as the oxygen supply is adequate and enzymes and substrate are available, NAD$^+$ and FAD are regenerated and Krebs cycle aerobic metabolism proceeds unimpeded. The three components of aerobic metabolism are:

- The Krebs cycle,
- Electron transport, and
- Oxidative phosphorylation.

TOTAL ENERGY TRANSFER FROM GLUCOSE CATABOLISM

The pathways for energy transfer during the breakdown of a glucose molecule in skeletal muscle are summarized in Figure 6.13. A net of two ATP molecules are formed from substrate-level phosphorylation in glycolysis, and, similarly, two ATP molecules are generated during acetyl-CoA degra-

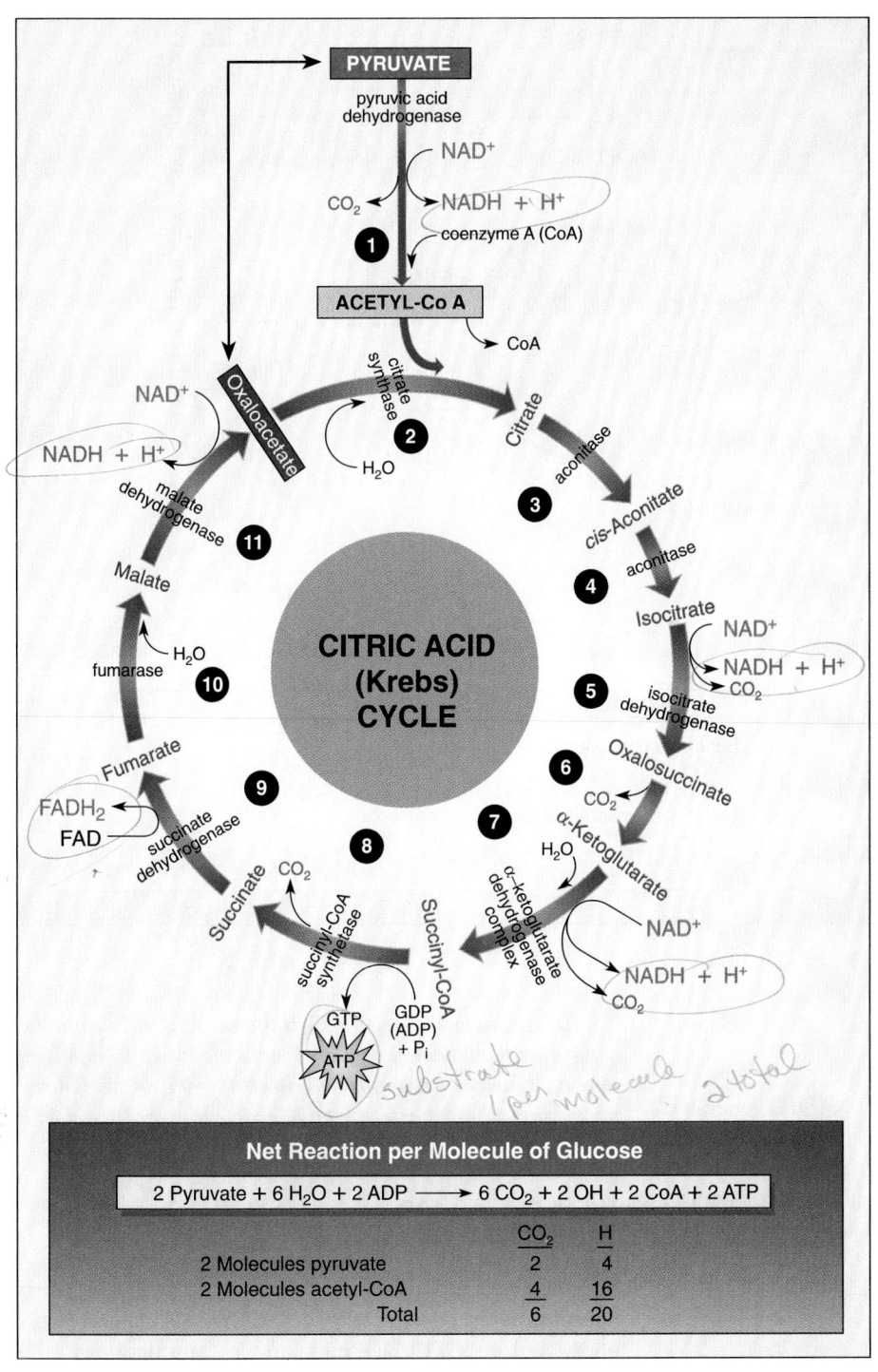

FIGURE 6.12

"Flow sheet" for the release of hydrogen atoms and carbon dioxide in the mitochondrion during the breakdown of one molecule of pyruvate. All values have been doubled when computing the net gain of hydrogen atoms and carbon dioxide because two molecules of pyruvate are formed from one glucose molecule in glycolysis.

Net Reaction per Molecule of Glucose

2 Pyruvate + 6 H_2O + 2 ADP ⟶ 6 CO_2 + 2 OH + 2 CoA + 2 ATP

	CO_2	H
2 Molecules pyruvate	2	4
2 Molecules acetyl-CoA	4	16
Total	6	20

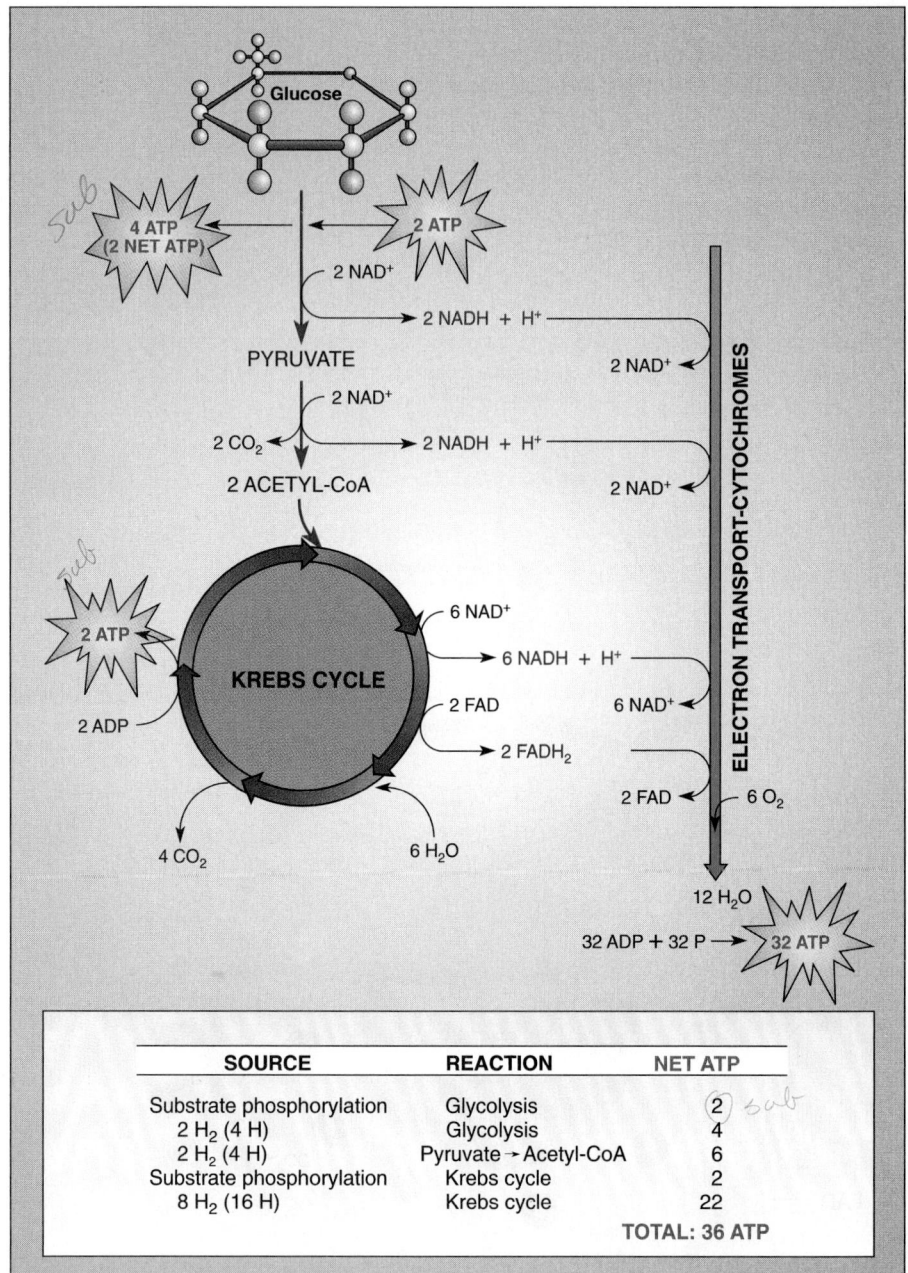

FIGURE 6.13

A net yield of 36 ATP results from energy transfer during the complete oxidation of one glucose molecule in skeletal muscle through glycolysis, the Krebs cycle, and electron transport.

SOURCE	REACTION	NET ATP
Substrate phosphorylation	Glycolysis	2
2 H_2 (4 H)	Glycolysis	4
2 H_2 (4 H)	Pyruvate → Acetyl-CoA	6
Substrate phosphorylation	Krebs cycle	2
8 H_2 (16 H)	Krebs cycle	22
		TOTAL: 36 ATP

dation in the Krebs cycle. The 24 hydrogen atoms released can be accounted for as follows:

- Four extramitochondrial hydrogens (2 NADH) generated in glycolysis yield 4 ATP (6 ATP in heart, kidney, and liver).
- Four hydrogens (2 NADH) released in the mitochondria as pyruvate is changed to acetyl-CoA yield 6 ATP.
- Twelve of the 16 hydrogens (6 NADH) released in the Krebs cycle yield 18 ATP.
- Four hydrogens joined to FAD (2 $FADH_2$) in the Krebs cycle yield 4 ATP.

Thirty-six molecules of ATP is the net ATP yield from the complete breakdown of a glucose molecule in skeletal muscle; four ATP molecules are formed directly from substrate-level phosphorylation (glycolysis and Krebs cycle), whereas 32 ATP molecules are generated during oxidative phosphorylation.

What Regulates Energy Metabolism?

Under normal conditions, the transfer of electrons and subsequent release of energy are tightly coupled to ADP phosphorylation. In general, unless ADP is available and phosphorylated to ATP, electrons do not shuttle down the respiratory chain to oxygen. Enzymatic regulatory control of glycolysis and the Krebs cycle is modulated by compounds that either inhibit or activate enzymes at key control points in the oxidative pathways.[10] Each pathway has at least one enzyme that is considered "rate-limiting." More specifically, ATP and NADH act as enzyme inhibitors, while ADP and NAD$^+$ serve as activators. These roles make considerable sense because such chemical feedback enables the metabolic level to adjust rapidly to the cells' energy needs. Within the resting cell, the concentration of ATP is considerably greater than the concentration of ADP (about 500:1). However, decreased ATP:ADP and intramitochondrial NADH:NAD$^+$ ratios (as would occur at the beginning of exercise) signal a need for increased metabolism of stored nutrients. On the other hand, at relatively low levels of energy demand, high ratios of ATP:ADP and NADH:NAD$^+$ are maintained and the rate of energy metabolism is blunted accordingly.[1]

ENERGY RELEASE FROM LIPID

Stored lipid represents the body's most plentiful source of potential energy. Relative to other nutrients, the quantity of lipid available for energy is almost unlimited. The actual lipid fuel reserves in a typical young adult male amount to about 90,000 to 110,000 kcal (23,800 kJ) of energy. In contrast, the carbohydrate energy reserve is about 2% of this total, or approximately 2000 kcal (8400 kJ).

SOURCES FOR LIPID CATABOLISM

Sources for lipid catabolism include the following:

- Triglycerides stored directly within the muscle cell, particularly the high-oxidative (slow-twitch) fibers.
- Circulating triglycerides in lipoprotein complexes, which are hydrolyzed by lipoprotein lipase on the surface of a tissue's capillary endothelium.
- Circulating free fatty acids mobilized from triglycerides in adipose tissue.

Prior to energy release from lipid, the triglyceride molecule is hydrolyzed in the cell's cytosol into its component glycerol and three fatty acid molecules. These fatty acids contain by far the largest portion of the triglyceride's rich potential energy. This reaction of lipid breakdown, or **lipolysis**, is catalyzed by the enzyme **lipase** as follows:

$$\text{Triglyceride} + 3\text{H}_2\text{O} \xrightarrow{\text{lipase}} \text{Glycerol} + 3 \text{ fatty acids}$$

ADIPOCYTES: THE SITE OF LIPID STORAGE AND MOBILIZATION

The most active supplier of fatty acid molecules is adipose tissue, though some lipid is stored in all cells. Fat cells, or **adipocytes,** are specialized for synthesizing and storing triglycerides, with triglyceride droplets occupying as much as 95% of the cell's volume. Once the fatty acids diffuse from the adipocyte into the bloodstream, they bind to plasma albumin as **free fatty acids,** or **FFAs.** FFAs are then delivered to active tissues and are metabolized for energy. Lipid utilization for energy varies closely with blood flow in the active tissue. As blood flow increases, more FFAs are delivered from adipose tissue to active muscle; hence, greater quantities of this nutrient are used for energy. This is particularly the case for slow-twitch muscle fibers, whose ample blood supply and large, numerous mitochondria make them ideal for the process of lipid catabolism.

Circulating triglycerides carried in lipoprotein complexes also provide a lipid source of energy. The hydrolysis of these triglycerides is catalyzed by the enzyme **lipoprotein lipase,** or **LPL.** This enzyme is synthesized within the cell and then is localized on the surface of the surrounding capillaries. The local activity level of LPL facilitates the cell's uptake of fatty acids for use either as energy in muscle or for the resynthesis (re-esterification) of stored triglycerides in muscle and adipose tissue.[17]

The activation of lipase and subsequent lipolysis and mobilization of FFAs from adipose tissue is augmented by the hormones epinephrine, norepinephrine, glucagon, and growth hormone. Injecting epinephrine into the blood, for example, results in a rapid increase in plasma FFAs. Because plasma concentrations of these lipogenic hormones increase during exercise, the muscles receive a continual supply of this rich energy substrate. Lipase activation (and thus the regulation of lipid breakdown) is catalyzed by an intracellular mediator, **adenosine 3′,5′-cyclic monophosphate,** or **cyclic AMP.** Cyclic AMP is activated by the various lipid-mobilizing hormones, which themselves do not enter the cell.[16] Increases in the activity level of skeletal muscle and adipose tissue lipases, as well as biochemical and vascular adaptations in the muscle itself, help explain the enhanced use of lipids for energy during moderate-intensity exercise following training.[7, 8, 11, 17] A more detailed evaluation of hormone regulation during exercise is presented in Chapter 20.

The dynamics of either lipid breakdown or synthesis are linked to the availability of the "building block" fatty acid molecules. After a meal, when energy metabolism is low, digestive processes increase the delivery of free fatty acids and triglycerides to the cell. This increase, in turn, causes triglyceride synthesis through the process of esterification. During moderate exercise, on the other hand, the increased use of fatty acids for energy reduces their concentrations in the cells, stimulating triglyceride breakdown into its glycerol and fatty acid components. Concurrently, hormonal release triggered by exercise stimulates adipose tissue lipolysis, which further augments the delivery of FFAs to the active muscle.

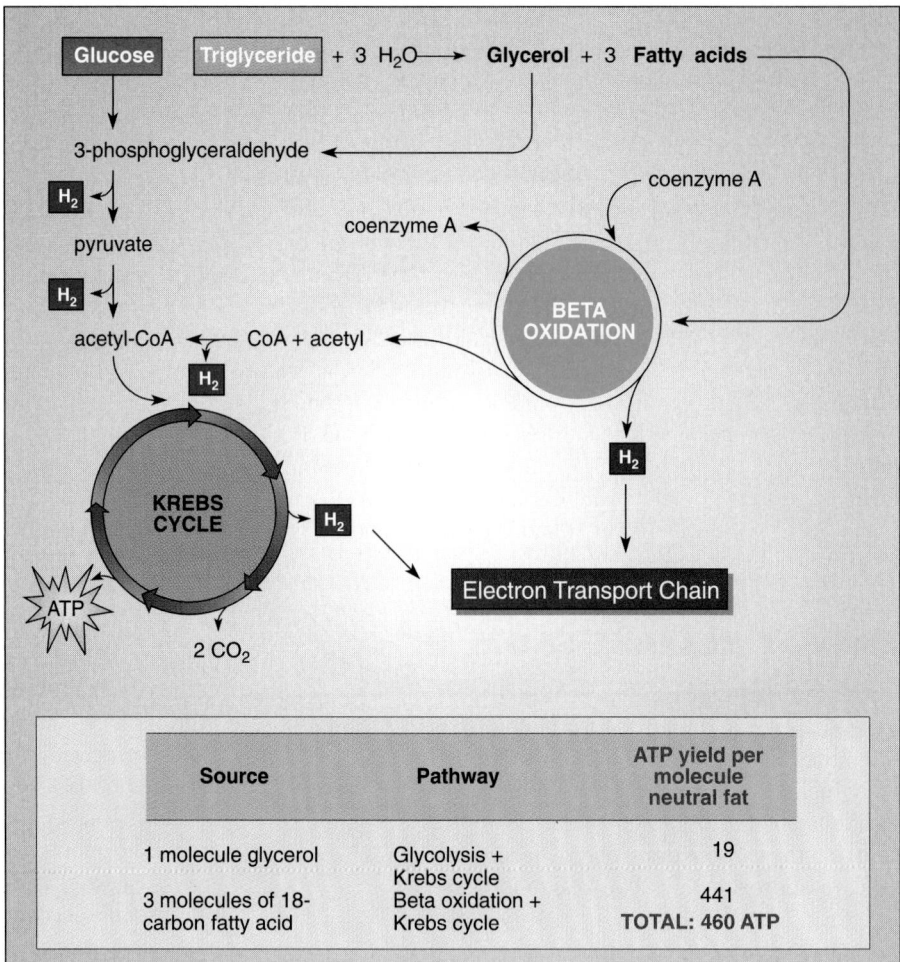

FIGURE 6.14

General scheme for the breakdown of the glycerol and fatty acid fragments of a triglyceride molecule. Glycerol enters the energy pathway during the reactions of glycolysis. The fatty acid fragments are prepared for entrance into the Krebs cycle through the process of β-oxidation. The hydrogen atoms released from glycolysis, β-oxidation, and Krebs cycle metabolism are oxidized via the electron transport chain.

Source	Pathway	ATP yield per molecule neutral fat
1 molecule glycerol	Glycolysis + Krebs cycle	19
3 molecules of 18-carbon fatty acid	Beta oxidation + Krebs cycle	441
		TOTAL: 460 ATP

CATABOLISM OF GLYCEROL AND FATTY ACIDS

Figure 6.14 summarizes the pathways for the degradation of the glycerol and fatty acid fragments of the triglyceride molecule.

Glycerol is accepted into the anaerobic reactions of glycolysis as 3-phosphoglyceraldehyde and is degraded to pyruvate. In this process, ATP is formed via substrate-level phosphorylation and hydrogen atoms are released to NAD^+; pyruvate is then oxidized in the Krebs cycle. In total, 19 ATP molecules are synthesized in the complete breakdown of the glycerol molecule. Glycerol can also serve an important function by providing its carbon skeleton for glucose synthesis. The gluconeogenic role of glycerol is important when carbohydrate is restricted in the diet or during long-term exercise, which can significantly drain glycogen reserves.

Fatty acid breakdown proceeds within the mitochondrion in a process called **β-oxidation.** During the chemical reactions of β-oxidation, the fatty acid molecule is successively cleaved into two-carbon acetyl fragments split from the long chain of the fatty acid. Adenosine triphosphate is used to phosphorylate the reactions, water is added, hydrogens are passed to NAD^+ and FAD, and the acetyl fragment joins with coenzyme A to form acetyl-CoA. This is the same acetyl unit from glucose breakdown that then enters the Krebs cycle for further metabolism. This process is repeated until the entire fatty acid molecule is degraded to acetyl-CoA. The hydrogen atoms released during the β-oxidation of fatty acids are oxidized through the respiratory chain. *It is important to note that the breakdown of fatty acids is directly associated with oxygen uptake.* For β-oxidation to proceed, oxygen must be available to accept hydrogen. Under anaerobic conditions, hydrogen remains with NAD^+ and FAD and lipid catabolism comes to a halt.

TOTAL ENERGY TRANSFER FROM LIPID CATABOLISM

The breakdown of a fatty acid molecule can be outlined as follows:

- β-Oxidation produces NADH and $FADH_2$ from the splitting of the fatty acid molecule into two-carbon acetyl fragments.

- Acetyl-CoA is degraded in the Krebs cycle.
- Hydrogen is oxidized via electron transport–oxidative phosphorylation.

For each 18-carbon fatty acid molecule, a net of 146 ADP molecules are phosphorylated to ATP during β-oxidation and Krebs cycle metabolism. Because each triglyceride molecule contains three fatty acid molecules, 438 ATP molecules (3 × 146 ATP) are formed from the fatty acid component of neutral fat. Also, because 19 molecules of ATP form during glycerol breakdown, a total of 457 molecules of ATP are generated for each triglyceride molecule catabolized for energy. This quantity represents a considerable energy yield considering that only 36 ATP molecules are formed during the catabolism of a glucose molecule in skeletal muscle. With the exception of its carboxyl groups, a fatty acid consists of all hydrocarbons. A glucose molecule, on the other hand, is already in a partly oxidized form because of its relatively large number of oxygen-containing groups. The efficiency of energy conservation for fatty acid oxidation is about 40%, an efficiency value similar to that of glucose.

Depending on a person's nutritional state, level of training, and the intensity and duration of a specific physical activity, between 30 and 80% of the energy for biologic work is usually supplied from intracellular and extracellular lipid molecules.[11, 15] When high-intensity, long-duration physical activity causes significant glycogen depletion, lipid becomes the primary energy fuel during exercise and recovery.[11] Furthermore, prolonged exposure to a high-fat diet brings about enzymatic adaptations that enhance one's capacity for lipid oxidation during exercise.[14]

ENERGY RELEASE FROM PROTEIN

As mentioned in Chapter 1, protein can serve a significant role as an energy substrate during sustained exercise and heavy training. In such a case, the amino acids (primarily the branched-chain amino acids leucine, isoleucine, and valine in addition to glutamine and aspartate) first must be converted to a form that can readily enter the pathways for energy release. This conversion requires the removal of nitrogen from the amino acid molecule. Whereas the main site for this **deamination** is the liver, skeletal muscle also contains the enzymes for removing the nitrogen in an amino acid and passing it to other compounds in a process called **transamination.** For example, the Krebs cycle intermediate α-ketoglutarate can accept a nitrogen-containing amino group (NH_2) to form a new amino acid, glutamate. In this way, the "carbon skeleton" by-products of certain donor amino acids (specifically, the branched-chain amino acids) can be used directly in muscle for energy. In fact, the levels of enzymes for transamination adapt to training; this may further facilitate the use of protein as an energy substrate. Once the amino group is

removed from the amino acid, the remaining carbon skeleton usually is one of the reactive compounds in the Krebs cycle and can contribute to ATP formation. Some amino acids are glucogenic: when deaminated, they yield pyruvate, oxaloacetate, or malate, each of which is an intermediate for glucose synthesis via gluconeogenesis. For example, alanine loses its amino group and gains a double-bond oxygen to form pyruvate. This method for gluconeogenesis is an important adjunct to the Cori cycle for providing glucose during prolonged exercise. It should be noted that although gluconeogenesis provides a metabolic option for synthesizing glucose from noncarbohydrate sources, this process cannot maintain glycogen stores unless dietary carbohydrates are regularly consumed. Other amino acids such as glycine are ketogenic; when deaminated they yield the intermediate acetyl-CoA or acetoacetate. These compounds cannot be used to synthesize glucose but instead can be synthesized to lipids or catabolized for energy in the Krebs cycle.

When protein is used for energy, the nitrogen-containing amino group must be eliminated from the body. In birds, for example, nitrogen is excreted in the form of uric acid. This compound is insoluble in water and thus does not demand the excretion of "obligatory" water. Consequently, birds need relatively little water. In humans, on the other hand, the waste products of protein breakdown must leave the body dissolved in fluid (urine). For this reason, excessive protein catabolism augments the body's fluid needs.

THE METABOLIC MILL— INTERRELATIONSHIPS AMONG CARBOHYDRATE, LIPID, AND PROTEIN METABOLISM

The Krebs cycle plays a much more important role than simply the degradation of pyruvate produced during glucose catabolism. The Krebs cycle provides the means by which fragments of other organic compounds formed from the breakdown of lipids and proteins are effectively metabolized for energy. As illustrated in Figure 6.15, the deaminated residues of excess amino acids enter the Krebs cycle at various intermediate stages, whereas the glycerol fragment of lipid catabolism gains entrance via the glycolytic pathway. Fatty acids are oxidized by β-oxidation to acetyl-CoA, which then enters the Krebs cycle directly.

Although the illustration for the "metabolic mill" depicts the Krebs cycle as the vital link between food energy and the chemical energy of ATP, the Krebs cycle is also a metabolic hub for providing intermediates that cross the mitochondrial membrane into the cytosol to synthesize bionutrients required for growth and maintenance. For example, excess carbohydrates provide the glycerol and acetyl-CoA fragments to which carbon atoms are added, usually two at

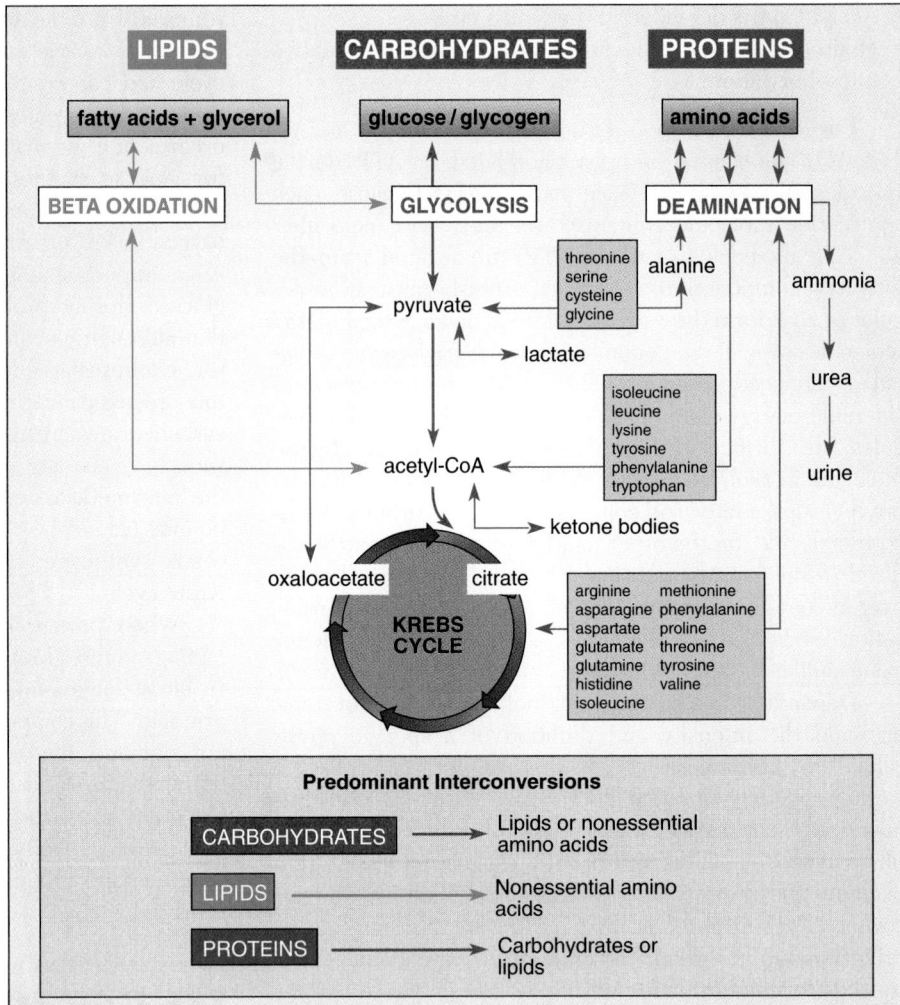

FIGURE 6.15

The "metabolic mill": important inter-conversions between carbohydrates, lipids, and proteins.

a time, for the synthesis of neutral fat. Acetyl-CoA also can function as the starting point for the biosynthesis of cholesterol and other steroid compounds. Because the conversion of pyruvate to acetyl-CoA is not reversible (notice the one-way arrow), fatty acids **cannot** be converted into pyruvate or oxaloacetate to synthesize glucose. However, many of the carbon compounds generated in Krebs cycle reactions provide the organic starting points for synthesizing nonessential amino acids.

LIPIDS BURN IN A CARBOHYDRATE FLAME

An interesting aspect of the metabolic mill is that fatty acid breakdown depends in part on a continual background level of carbohydrate catabolism. Recall that acetyl-CoA enters the Krebs cycle by combining with oxaloacetate to form citrate. This oxaloacetate is generated from pyruvate during carbohydrate breakdown under the control of the enzyme pyruvate carboxylase. The degradation of fatty acids via the Krebs cycle continues only if sufficient oxaloacetate is available to combine with the acetyl-CoA formed during

β-oxidation. Pyruvate formation during glucose metabolism plays an important role in maintaining a proper level of this oxaloacetate intermediate (Fig. 6.15); when the carbohydrate level decreases, the oxaloacetate level may become inadequate. In this sense, "lipids burn in a carbohydrate flame." There is also likely to be a rate limit to fatty acid use by the active muscle. Although aerobic training can greatly enhance this limit, the power generated solely by lipid breakdown is only about half that achieved when carbohydrate provides the chief energy source. Thus, the maximum power output of muscle must decline when muscle glycogen is depleted (for example, because of poor diet or heavy exercise). Just as the hypoglycemic condition is associated with a "central" or neural fatigue, so also is the depletion of muscle glycogen the probable cause of a "peripheral" or local muscle fatigue during exercise. During extreme carbohydrate restriction or depletion, the acetyl-CoA produced in β-oxidation and the FFAs delivered from adipose tissue build up in the extracellular fluids because they cannot enter the Krebs cycle. These compounds are readily converted by the liver to a form of acetone called **ketone bodies,** some of which are excreted in the urine. If this condition, called ketosis, persists, the acid quality of the body fluids can increase to potentially toxic levels.

■SUMMARY■

1. Food nutrients provide the major sources of potential energy for rejoining ADP and phosphate ion to form ATP.

2. The complete breakdown of 1 mole of glucose liberates 689 kcal of energy. Of this, about 263 kcal, or 38%, is conserved in the bonds of ATP, with the remainder dissipated as heat.

3. During glycolytic reactions in the cell's cytosol, a net of 2 ATP molecules are formed in the anaerobic process of substrate-level phosphorylation.

4. During the second stage of carbohydrate breakdown, which occurs within the mitochondrion, pyruvate is converted to acetyl-CoA, which is then processed through the Krebs cycle. The hydrogen atoms released during glucose breakdown are oxidized via the respiratory chain, and the energy generated in this process is coupled to the phosphorylation of ADP.

5. The complete oxidation of glucose in skeletal muscle yields a total of 36 ATP molecules.

6. A biochemical "steady state" or "steady rate" is said to exist when hydrogen atoms are oxidized at the rate they are formed. During heavy exercise, when hydrogen oxidation does not keep pace with its rate of production, pyruvate temporarily combines with hydrogen to form lactic acid. This allows anaerobic glycolysis to proceed for an additional period.

7. The complete breakdown of a lipid molecule yields about 457 molecules of ATP. Fatty acid catabolism is directly associated with oxygen uptake, and such reactions are termed aerobic.

8. Protein also serves as an important energy substrate. After nitrogen is removed from the amino acid molecule during the process of deamination, the remaining carbon skeletons enter various metabolic pathways for the aerobic production of ATP.

9. Numerous interconversions are possible among the food nutrients. Noteworthy exceptions are fatty acids that cannot be used for glucose synthesis.

10. A certain level of carbohydrate breakdown is required for lipids to be continually metabolized for energy in the metabolic mill. To this extent, "lipids burn in a carbohydrate flame."

■REFERENCES■

1. Balban, R.S.: Regulation of oxidative phosphorylation in the mammalian cell. *Am. J. Physiol.,* 258:C377, 1990.

2. Bertocci, L.A., and Gollnick, P.D.: pH effect on mitochondria and individual enzyme function. *Med. Sci. Sports Exerc.,* 17:244, 1985.

3. Bodner, G.M.: Metabolism: Part I. Glycolysis, or the Embden-Myerhoff pathway. *J. Chem. Ed.,* 63:566, 1986.

4. Bodner, G.M.: The tricarboxyclic acid (TCA), citric acid, Krebs cycle. *J. Chem. Ed.,* 63:673, 1986.

5. Brooks, G.A.: Physical activity and carbohydrate metabolism. In *Physical Activity, Fitness, and Health.* C. Bouchard, et al., Eds., Champaign, IL, Human Kinetics, 1994.

6. Chasiotis, D.: Role of cyclic AMP and inorganic phosphate in the regulation of muscle glycogenolysis during exercise. *Med. Sci. Sports Exerc.,* 20:545, 1988.

7. Coggan, A.R., et al.: Plasma glucose kinetics during exercise in subjects with high and low lactate thresholds. *J. Appl. Physiol.,* 73:1873, 1992.

8. Coggan, A.R., et al.: Isotopic estimation of CO_2 production during exercise before and after endurance training. *J. Appl. Physiol.,* 75:70, 1993.

9. Hogan, M.C., et al.: Increased [lactate] in working dog muscle reduces tension development independent of pH. *Med. Sci. Sports Exerc.,* 27:371, 1995.

10. Jacobs, I., et al.: Effects of prior exercise or ammonium chloride ingestion on muscular strength and endurnace. *Med. Sci. Sports Exerc.,* 25:809, 1993.

11. Kiens, B., et al.: Skeletal muscle substrate utilization during submaximal exercise in man: Effect of endurance training. *J. Physiol.,* 469:459, 1993.

12. MacRae, H.S-H., et al.: Effects of training on lactate production and removal during progressive exercise. *J. Appl. Physiol.,* 72:1649, 1992.

13. Mainwood, G.W., and Renaud, J.M.: The effect of acid-base on fatigue of skeletal muscle. *Can. J. Physiol. Pharmacol.,* 63:403, 1985.

14. Mudio, D.M., et al.: Effects of dietary fat on metabolic adjustments to maximal VO_2 and endurance in runners. *Med. Sci. Sports Exerc.,* 26:81, 1994.

15. Romijn, J.A., et al.: Regulations of endogenous fat and carbohydrate metabolism in relation to exercise intensity and duration. *Am. J. Physiol.,* 265:E380, 1993.

16. Shepherd, R.E., and Bah, M.D.: Cyclic AMP regulation of fuel metabolism during exercise: regulation of adipose tissue lipolysis during exercise. *Med. Sci. Sports Exerc.,* 20:531, 1988.

17. Stefanick, M.L., and Wood, P.D.: Physical activity, lipid and lipoprotein metabolism, and lipid transport. In *Physical Activity, Fitness, and Health.* C. Bouchard, et al., Eds., Champaign, IL, Human Kinetics, 1994.

■SUGGESTED READINGS■

Bjorntorp, P.: Importance of fat as a support nutrient for energy: Metabolism of athletes. In *Foods, Nutrition and Sports Performance.* C. Williams and J.T. Devlin (Eds.), London, E. & F.N. Spon, 1992.

Brooks, G.A., et al.: *Exercise Physiology: Human Bioenergetics and its Applications,* 2nd ed. Mountain View, CA, Mayfield, 1996.

Cerretelli, P.: Energy sources for muscular exercise. *Int. J. Sports Med.,* 13 (Suppl. 1):S106, 1992.

Horton, E.S., and Terjung, R.L. (Eds.): *Exercise, Nutrition, and Energy Metabolism,* 2nd ed. New York, Macmillan, 1994.

Lehninger, A.L.: *Bioenergetics: The Molecular Basis of Biological Energy Transformations.* Menlo Park, CA, W.A. Benjamin, 1971.

Lehnigner, A.L., et al.: *Principles of Biochemistry,* 2nd ed. New York, Worth Publishers, 1993.

Marieb, E.N.: *Human Anatomy and Physiology,* 2nd ed. Redwood City, CA, Benjamin Cummings, 1992.

Mott-Smith, M.: *The Concept of Energy Simply Explained.* New York, Dover Press, 1964.

Shils, M.E., et al.: *Modern Nutrition in Health and Disease,* 8th ed. Philadelphia, Lea & Febiger, 1993.

Stryer, L.: *Biochemistry,* 2nd ed. San Francisco, W.H. Freeman, 1988.

Vander, A.J., et al.: *Human Physiology. The Mechanisms of Body Function,* 6th ed. New York, McGraw-Hill, 1993.

Brooks, G.A., et al.: Glycogen synthesis and metabolism of lactic acid after exercise. *Am. J. Physiol.* **224:1162, 1973.**

From the early work of Hill and associates, the elevated recovery oxygen uptake ($\dot{V}_{O_2}$, the so-called "oxygen debt") was believed to represent the oxidation of about one-fifth of the lactic acid produced during exercise to provide the necessary energy to reconvert the remaining lactate to glycogen. The

Female rats served as subjects during two experiments to test the lactic acid-oxygen debt theory. In experiment 1, animals served in either a sedentary group or an exercise group that ran to exhaustion using different combinations of treadmill speed and grade to induce a significant lactic acid production and a large postexercise $\dot{V}_{O_2}$. Following exercise, the animals were killed and measurements were taken of the quantities of glycogen, glucose, and lactic acid in muscle, liver, and blood during a 24-hour recovery. The upper figure displays liver and muscle glycogen concentrations related to time after exhaustive exercise. Compared to sedentary controls *(purple squares)*, little glycogen remained in the muscles and liver at the end of exhaustive exercise. No significant glycogen synthesis occurred in the postexercise period. Moreover, liver glycogen concentration after 24 hours of recovery from exhaustive exercise did not exceed the immediate postexercise values. The pattern for liver glycogen concentration remained essentially the same as that of muscle. Thus, the hypothesis set forth by Hill and colleagues to explain the elevated postexercise $\dot{V}_{O_2}$ could not be confirmed based on the level of glycogen synthesis immediately after exercise.

In a parallel experiment (experiment 2), ^{14}C-labeled lactate was infused into exercise-exhausted and pair-fasted sedentary control rats. Measurements also included the amount of labeled CO_2 during recovery from exhaustive exercise to determine the fate of the injected ^{14}C lactate. The lower figure shows the pattern of labeled CO_2 exhalation in recovery after infusion of labeled lactate. If lactic acid during recovery reconverted to glycogen, little of the injected isotope should have appeared as expired CO_2. In contrast, if the primary pathway included oxidation of lactic acid during recovery from exhaustive exercise, then most of the labeled carbon in the infused lactate would indeed have appeared as $^{14}CO_2$ in expired air. The results were unequivocal: 70 to 90% of the isotope appeared as CO_2. Because no glycogen replenishment occurred immediately after exercise, glycogen synthesis could not be a predominant process during the immediate postexercise recovery period.

Considered in total, lactate production and subsequent glycogen resynthesis in recovery could not be explained by the excess postexercise oxygen consumption (EPOC) originally proposed by Hill and associates in the 1920s to account for the level of anaerobic metabolism (reflected by lactic acid accumulation) during exercise. The work of Brooks directly tested Hill's hypothesis about the fate of lactic acid produced during heavy exercise. Subsequent research has redefined and expanded the explanations for the functions of the EPOC.

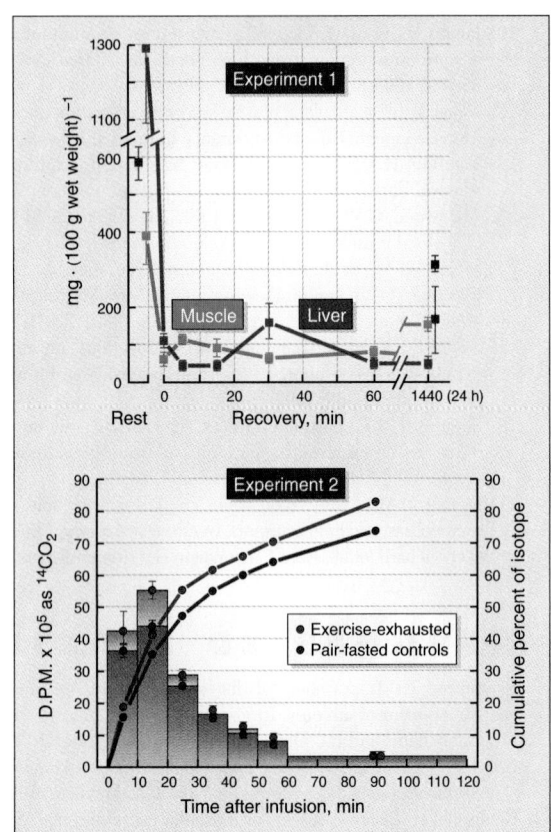

Experiment 1. Liver and muscle glycogen concentrations as a function of time after exhaustive exercise in rats fasted for 10 to 12 hours. *Experiment 2.* Production of labeled CO_2 over time after infusion of ^{14}C-labeled lactate in exercise-exhausted and pair-fasted rats (bar graph, left ordinate). Expiration of labeled CO_2 is also expressed as a cumulative percentage of activity of infused ^{14}C-labeled lactate (line graph, right ordinate).

subsequent research of Margaria and colleagues retained this "lactic acid interpretation" of the elevated $\dot{V}_{O_2}$ in recovery (refer to page 132). Until the publication of this paper by Brooks and coworkers, few investigators had directly challenged the idea that significant glycogen synthesis occurred during the postexercise repayment of the "O_2 debt."

Energy Transfer in Exercise

Compared to all of the complex metabolic functions in the body, increases in physical activity demand by far the greatest amount of energy. During sprinting and swimming, for example, the energy output from the active muscles can be more than 100 times greater than at rest. During less intense but sustained exercise such as marathon running, the energy requirement increases to some 20 to 30 times more than at rest. The relative contributions of the various means of energy transfer differ markedly depending on the intensity and duration of the exercise and the fitness of the participant.

IMMEDIATE ENERGY: THE ATP-CP SYSTEM

Performances of short duration and high intensity such as a 100-yard dash, a 25-yard swim, or heavy weightlifting require an immediate and rapid supply of energy. This energy is provided almost exclusively from the high-energy phosphates or phosphagens ATP and CP stored within the specific muscles activated during the exercise.

Approximately 5 millimoles (mmol) of ATP and 15 mmol of CP are stored within each kilogram of muscle.[35] For a 70-kg person with a muscle mass of 30 kg, the combined total is between 570 and 690 mmol of high-energy phosphates. If we assume that 20 kg of muscle can be activated during "major muscle" exercise, then sufficient stored phosphate energy is available in the recruited muscle mass to walk briskly for 1 minute, run a cross-country race for 20 to 30 seconds, or perform all-out exercises such as sprinting and swimming for about 5 to 6 seconds. (This rate of energy transfer from the high-energy phosphates [and to some degree the anaerobic reactions of glycolysis] is probably between 4 and 8 times the maximal rate of energy transfer from aerobic metabolic reactions.) During the 100-yard dash, for example, maximum speed cannot be maintained for longer than this 5- to 6-second period (because of the slower rate of energy transfer via glycolysis); thus, the winner is often the person who slows down the least during the last portion of the race. In such a situation, the quantity of intramuscular high-energy phosphates may significantly influence one's performance.

All sports require utilization of the high-energy phosphates, but many activities rely almost exclusively on this means for energy transfer. For example, success in football, weightlifting, field events, baseball, or volleyball requires a brief but maximal effort during the performance. It is difficult to imagine an athlete breaking away for the goal in ice hockey or soccer, driving for a layup in basketball, thrusting upward in a pole vault, or performing an end run in football without the capacity to generate energy rapidly from stored high-energy phosphates. This capability of energy transfer is augmented by physical training that stresses brief bursts of power output by the musculature required in the activity. For sustained exercise and for recovery from a prior brief all-out effort, additional energy must be generated for ATP replenishment. To this end, the stored carbohydrate, lipid, and protein nutrients within the cellular fluids and tissue depots stand ready to continually recharge the available pool of high-energy phosphates.

Nuclear Magnetic Resonance Spectroscopy to Study Exercise Muscle Metabolism

Nuclear magnetic resonance (NMR) spectroscopy is a relatively new and exciting noninvasive method for studying intracellular metabolism. The use of radiofrequency energy makes it possible to probe and identify the content of chemical elements and compounds within living tissue. NMR techniques are particularly well suited to continuously measuring the relative concentrations and turnover rates in muscle of the phosphorylated high-energy compounds, as well as other metabolic events that occur during exercise.[8, 46, 48] These measurements can be taken at regular intervals during exercise without the disruptive consequences of the muscle biopsy technique. Figure 7.1A illustrates the NMR method during wrist flexion exercise.[47] The muscles used in the exercise are placed over a superconducting magnet, and the subject exercises under conditions that control for power output, contraction speed, and exercise duration. The concentrations of various biochemically active compounds are determined by applying specific radiofrequency pulses within the strong magnetic field. Figure 7.1B shows the results for ATP, CP (PCr), and inorganic phosphate during rest and low- and moderate-intensity exercise. In NMR spectroscopy, the areas under the peaks correspond to the relative concentrations of the free phosphorous compounds, including the three phosphorus atoms of ATP. Such elegant studies of the ratio of inorganic phosphate (phosphate ion) to creatine phosphate provide insight on the rate of mitochondrial respiration. This technique currently is used to study muscle injury, glycolytic

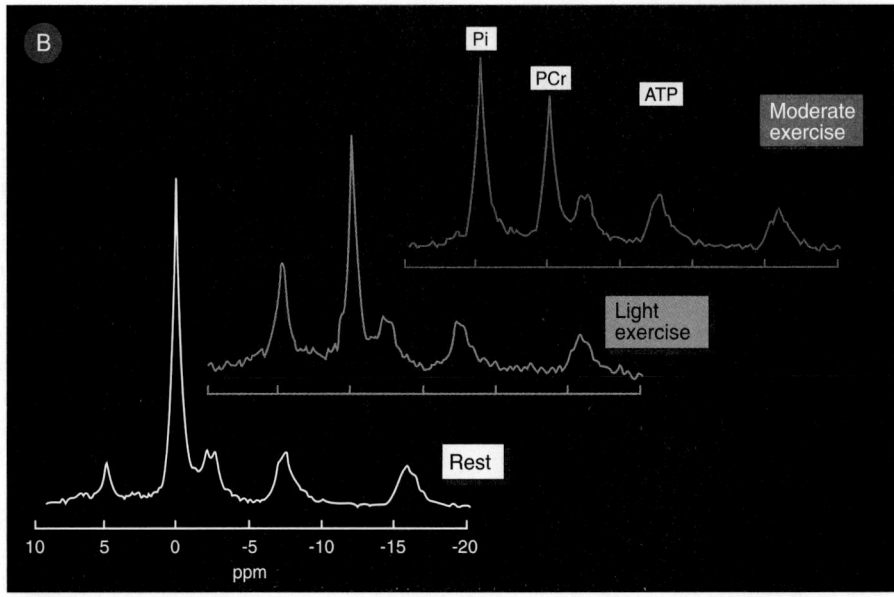

FIGURE 7.1

NMR spectroscopy. **A,** The wrist flexor muscles are placed on a surface coil in a superconducting magnet. The subject grasps a handle attached to an isokinetic dynamometer (constant-velocity, variable-force output). The subject watches a recorder that provides feedback on the level of force produced. **B,** Example of NMR spectroscopy spectra for ATP, PCr, and inorganic phosphate during rest and two levels of exercise. (Modified from original drawing provided by Dr. Kevin K. McCully, Medical College of Pennsylvania, Department of Geriatric Medicine, Philadelphia, PA.)

metabolism, and the effects of training on the intricacies of muscle metabolic function, as well as the relationship between local muscle metabolism and cardiovascular functional capacity and exercise performance.[43]

SHORT-TERM ENERGY: THE LACTIC ACID SYSTEM

The high-energy phosphates must continually be resynthesized at a rapid rate for strenuous exercise to continue beyond a brief period. During such intense exercise, the energy to phosphorylate ADP comes mainly from stored muscle glycogen through anaerobic glycolysis (maximal power output that is about 45% that of the high-energy phosphates), which results in the formation of lactic acid. In a way, this mechanism of lactic acid formation "buys time." It allows for the rapid formation of ATP by substrate-level phosphorylation, even though the oxygen supply is inadequate and/or the energy demands outstrip the muscle's capacity to resynthesize ATP aerobically. This anaerobic energy for ATP resynthesis can be thought of as reserve fuel brought into use when an athlete tries to sprint the last few hundred yards of a mile run. Anaerobic glycolysis also performs the critical role of rapidly supplying energy beyond that available from the stored high-energy phosphates during a 440-yard run or 100-yard swim. *The most rapidly ac-*

cumulated and highest lactate levels are reached during all-out exercise (when the muscles are taxed maximally) that can be sustained for 60 to 180 seconds. As the intensity of such arduous exercise decreases (thereby extending the work period), so do both the rate of accumulation and final level of blood lactate.[39]

Blood Lactate Accumulation

Blood lactate does not accumulate at all levels of exercise. Figure 7.2 illustrates, for endurance athletes and untrained subjects, the general relationship between oxygen uptake, expressed as a percentage of maximum, and blood lactate during light, moderate, and heavy exercise. During light exercise, the energy demands of both groups are adequately met by reactions that consume oxygen. In biochemical terms, the ATP for muscle action is provided predominantly through energy generated by the oxidation of hydrogen. Any lactic acid formed in exercise is rapidly oxidized by the heart and neighboring muscle fibers with high oxidative capacities. As such, the blood lactate level remains fairly stable despite an increase in oxygen uptake.

Blood lactate accumulates and rises in exponential fashion at about 55% of the healthy, untrained person's maximal capacity for aerobic metabolism.[17, 19] The usual explanation for a lactate increase is based on an assumed relative tissue hypoxia during heavy exercise. With a predominance of glycolytic energy metabolism, NADH production exceeds the cell's capacity for shuttling hydrogen atoms (and electrons) down the respiratory chain, regardless of the availability of oxygen. This imbalance in hydrogen release and subsequent oxidation causes pyruvate to accept the excess hydrogens, and lactic acid accumulates.[42]

An alternate explanation for lactic acid buildup is based on research that uses radioactive tracers to label the carbon in the glucose molecule.[9, 21] These studies show that lactic acid is formed continuously at rest and in moderate exercise. Under aerobic conditions, however, lactic acid formation is matched by its rate of removal by other tissues, so blood lactate concentration remains stable. It is only when removal does not match production that blood lactate accumulates. With aerobic training, cellular adaptations provide for a high rate of lactate turnover, so accumulation occurs only at higher exercise levels.[56] Another explanation for lactate ac-

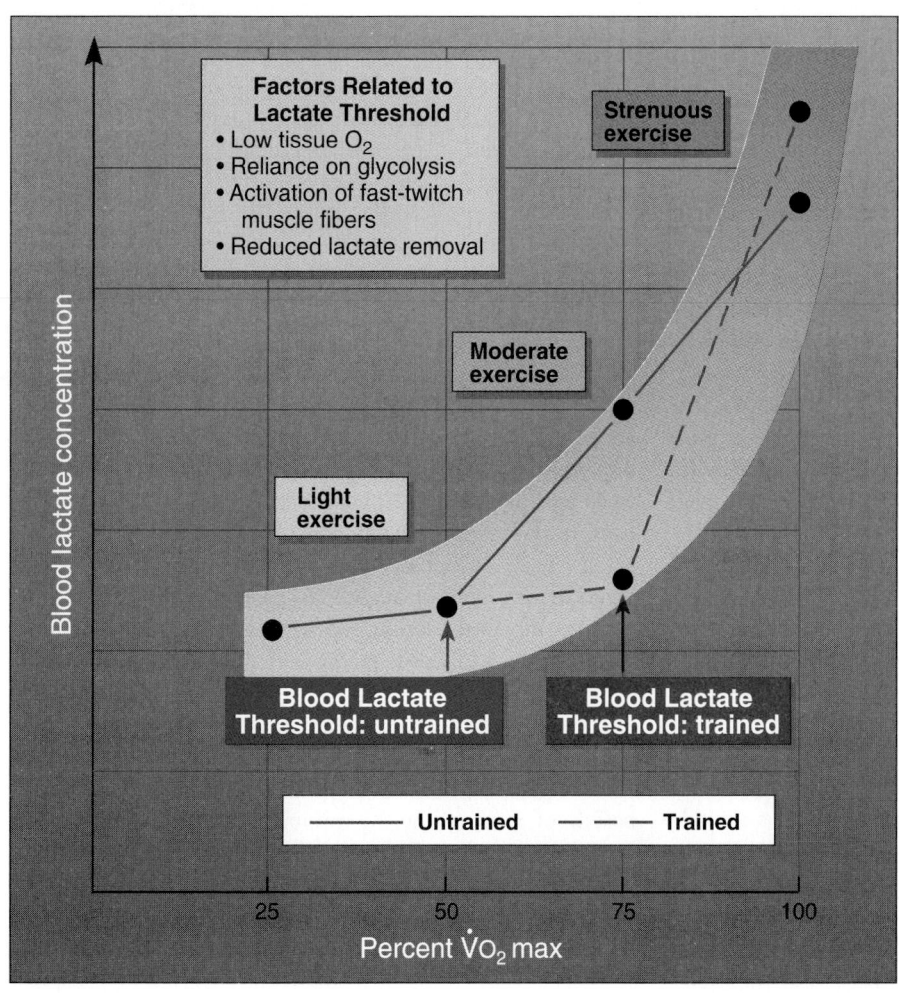

FIGURE 7.2
Blood lactate concentration at different levels of exercise expressed as a percentage of maximal oxygen uptake for trained and untrained subjects.

cumulation is the tendency of the enzyme lactate dehydrogenase (LDH) in fast-twitch muscle fibers to favor the conversion of pyruvic acid to lactic acid. On the other hand, the LDH level in slow-twitch fibers favors the conversion of lactic acid to pyruvic acid. Therefore, recruitment of the fast-twitch fibers (as occurs in more intense exercise) would favor lactate formation independent of tissue oxygenation.

Lactate production accelerates as exercise becomes more intense and the muscle cells can neither oxidize lactate at its rate of production nor meet the additional energy demands aerobically. This pattern is essentially similar for trained subjects except that the threshold for lactate buildup, termed the **blood lactate threshold,** occurs at a higher percentage of the athlete's aerobic capacity.[18, 24, 53, 59] This favorable aerobic response could be a result of the endurance athlete's specific genetic endowment (muscle fiber type), specific local adaptations with training that favor the production of less lactic acid,[15, 34, 58] or a more rapid rate of its removal (lactate clearance or turnover) at any particular level of exercise intensity.[10, 44] For example, it is well documented that capillary density—as well as the size and number of mitochondria—increases with endurance training, as do the concentrations of various enzymes and transfer agents during aerobic metabolism;[26, 34] we should note that this training response may be unimpaired by the aging process.[16] Researchers have also shown that lactate formed in one part of a working muscle can be oxidized by other fibers in the same muscle or by less active neighboring muscle tissue.[38, 40] Such adjustments and training adaptations certainly enhance the cell's capacity to generate ATP aerobically, principally through the breakdown of fatty acids. These aerobic adaptations also conserve glycogen by keeping lactate levels low and may extend the percentage of one's aerobic capacity that can be sustained before reaching the blood lactate threshold.[14, 15, 36] Trained endurance athletes, for example, exercise at intensities that are between 80 and 90% of their maximum capacity for aerobic metabolism.[17, 57] The concept of the blood lactate threshold and its measurement and relation to endurance performance is discussed more fully in Chapter 14.

Lactate-Producing Capacity

Because tissues continually utilize lactate during exercise, the total blood lactate accumulation may significantly underestimate blood lactate production during exercise. However, the ability to generate a high blood lactate level during all-out exercise increases with specific "anaerobic" training and subsequently decreases when training is discontinued. When sprint-power athletes perform maximal short-term exercise, their blood lactate levels are 20 to 30% higher than in untrained subjects who perform similar exercise. The mechanism for this response is unknown, but it is likely a result of differences in motivation accompanying the trained state, as well as an approximate 20% increase in enzymes that regulate glycolysis, specifically phosphofructokinase, which accompanies anaerobic training. Because lactic acid is continuously removed during and after exercise at a rate that varies among individuals, blood lactate measured at a particular time during recovery will not likely give the full picture of an individual's capacity for anaerobic metabolism.[24] The increased intramuscular glycogen stores that accompany the trained state also probably allow for a greater contribution of energy via anaerobic glycolysis. Although enzymes of the anaerobic pathway increase during sprint-power training, the magnitude of such increases are not as impressive as the much greater changes in aerobic enzymes during endurance training.[34, 38]

LONG-TERM ENERGY: THE AEROBIC SYSTEM

Although energy release in glycolysis is rapid and requires no oxygen, relatively little ATP is resynthesized in this manner. Consequently, aerobic reactions provide the important final stage for energy transfer, particularly if vigorous exercise proceeds beyond several minutes' duration.

OXYGEN UPTAKE DURING EXERCISE

The curve in Figure 7.3 illustrates the oxygen uptake (also referred to as the **pulmonary oxygen uptake** because $\dot{V}O_2$ is measured at the level of the lung and not directly at the active muscles) during each minute of a relatively slow jog continued at a steady pace for 10 minutes. Oxygen uptake rises in an exponential fashion (fast component of exercise oxygen uptake shown in the figure) during the first minutes of exercise.[7] A plateau is reached between the third and fourth minute, and thereafter the oxygen uptake remains relatively stable for the duration of the exercise. The flat portion or plateau of the oxygen uptake curve is generally considered the **steady rate** or **steady state.** This steady rate reflects a balance between the energy required by the working muscles and ATP production via aerobic metabolism. In this region, oxygen-consuming reactions supply the energy for exercise; any lactic acid produced is either oxidized or reconverted to glucose, predominantly in the liver and possibly in the kidneys. *Blood lactate does not accumulate to any appreciable extent under steady-rate metabolic conditions.*

Theoretically, once a steady rate has been attained, exercise could continue indefinitely if the individual had the willpower to continue. This hypothetical situation is based, of course, on the premise that a steady rate of aerobic metabolism is the only factor determining one's capacity for sustained submaximal exercise. Other factors, however, also must be considered. Fluid loss and electrolyte depletion often become significant limiting factors, princi-

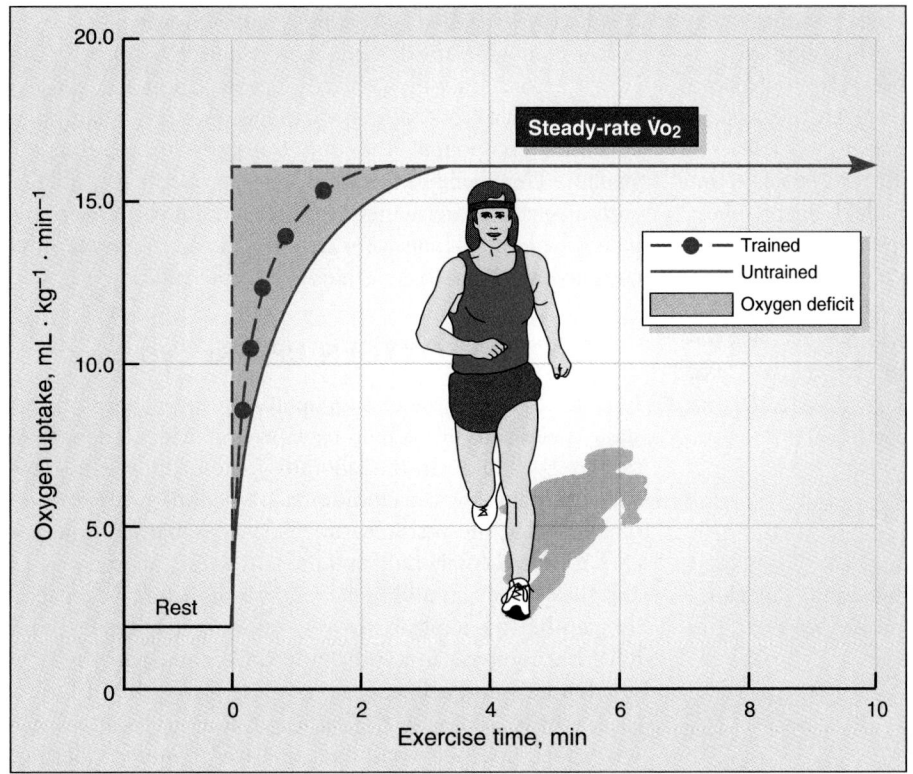

FIGURE 7.3
Time course of oxygen uptake during a continuous jog at a relatively slow pace for endurance-trained and untrained individuals who exercise at the same steady-rate $\dot{V}O_2$. The shaded area indicates the oxygen deficit or the quantity of oxygen that would have been consumed had the oxygen uptake reached a steady rate immediately.

pally during exercise in the heat. Of considerable importance during prolonged exercise is maintaining adequate fuel reserves, particularly liver glycogen and blood glucose for function of the central nervous system, and muscle glycogen to power exercise. Work capacity is dramatically reduced once a muscle's glycogen reserves are depleted.

There are many steady-rate levels. For some, the spectrum of steady rate might range from sitting and watching TV to pushing a power lawn mower. At the upper limit, on the other hand, the elite endurance runner can maintain a steady rate of aerobic metabolism throughout a 26.2-mile run averaging less than 5 minutes per mile or cover a 658-mile ultramarathon averaging 118 miles a day for 5.5 days! These magnificent accomplishments depend largely on how well central circulation can **deliver** oxygen to the working muscles and how well active tissues can **utilize** this oxygen.

Oxygen Deficit

Once exercise begins, the oxygen uptake curve shown in Figure 7.3 does not increase instantaneously to a steady rate. During the beginning or transitional stage of exercise, the oxygen uptake is considerably below the steady-rate level even though the energy requirement presumably remains unchanged throughout the exercise period. This lag in oxygen uptake is not surprising, however, because the en-

ergy for muscular work is always provided directly by the immediate nonaerobic breakdown of ATP. Stated differently, the increase in oxygen uptake resulting from exercise will always lag with energy expenditure because of an initial delay in the production of oxidizable substrate (hydrogen) with which oxygen can combine. Oxygen becomes important only in subsequent energy-transfer reactions when it serves as an electron acceptor and combines with the hydrogens generated in glycolysis, β-oxidation of fatty acids, or the reactions of the Krebs cycle. Within several minutes of submaximal exercise, however, hydrogen production becomes proportional to exercise intensity and oxygen uptake, and a steady rate is achieved in aerobic metabolism.

The oxygen deficit can be viewed quantitatively as the difference between the total oxygen actually consumed during exercise and the total that would have been consumed had a steady rate of aerobic metabolism been reached at the start. The energy provided during this transitional or deficit phase of exercise represents nonaerobic energy (that is, immediate energy from the stored high-energy phosphates plus anaerobic energy from glycolysis) used until a steady rate is reached between oxygen uptake in the active tissues and the energy demands of exercise.

Figure 7.4 depicts the relationship between the size of the oxygen deficit and the contribution of energy from both the ATP-CP and lactic acid energy systems. As shown, the high-energy phosphates are substantially depleted during exercise that generates approximately a 3- to 4-liter oxygen deficit. Consequently, this exercise can continue only on a "pay-as-you-go" basis, with ATP being continually replenished through either the aerobic breakdown of the food nutrients or anaerobic glycolysis. Interestingly, lactic acid begins to increase in exercising muscle well before the high-energy phosphates reach their lowest levels, indicating that glycolysis contributes anaerobic energy during the early stages of vigorous exercise, even before the full utilization of the intramuscular high-energy phosphates. *Energy for exercise is not merely the result of a series of energy systems that "switch on" and "switch off" but, rather, the smooth blending with considerable overlap from one mode of energy transfer to another.*

Oxygen Deficit in the Trained and Untrained

Once the steady rate is attained, oxygen uptake during light and moderate exercise is similar in trained and untrained persons. For the endurance-trained person, however, the steady rate is reached more rapidly and with a smaller oxygen deficit compared to someone who is untrained (see Figure 7.3).[29,31] Consequently, the total oxygen consumed during exercise is greater for the trained person, and, presumably, the anaerobic component of energy transfer is proportionately smaller. This facilitated rate of aerobic metabolism in the early stages of exercise may result from training-induced cellular adaptations, many of which are known to increase the capacity of muscle to generate ATP aerobically.

MAXIMAL OXYGEN UPTAKE ($\dot{V}O_2$max)

Figure 7.5 depicts the oxygen uptake during a series of constant-speed runs up six hills, each progressively steeper than the previous one. (In the laboratory, these "hills" are simulated by increasing the elevation of a treadmill or step bench or increasing the resistance to pedaling a bicycle ergometer.) Each successive hill requires a greater energy output and thus places an additional load on the runner's capacity for aerobic metabolism. During runs up the first several hills, the increase in oxygen uptake is rapid and the new steady-rate value is linear and in direct proportion to exercise severity. Although the runner is able to maintain running speed up the two last hills, the oxygen uptake does not increase as rapidly or to the same extent observed for the previous hills.[51] No increase is noted for the run up the last hill. *The region where oxygen uptake plateaus and shows no further increase or increases only slightly with an additional workload is called the maximal oxygen uptake, maximal oxygen consumption, maximal aerobic power, or simply $\dot{V}O_2$max.* Additional physical work is accomplished only by the energy-transfer reactions of glycolysis with the resulting formation of lactic acid. Under these conditions, the runner soon becomes exhausted and unable to continue.

The $\dot{V}O_2$max value quantitatively expresses a person's **capacity** for aerobic resynthesis of ATP. As such, it is an important factor in determining one's ability to sustain high-intensity exercise for longer than 4 or 5 minutes. The attainment of a high $\dot{V}O_2$max has an important physiologic meaning in addition to its role in supporting sustained energy metabolism because a high aerobic capacity requires the integrated and high-level response of diverse physiologic "support" systems, as illustrated in Figure 7.6. In subsequent chapters, we will discuss various aspects of aerobic power, including its physiologic significance, measurement, and role in exercise performance.

FAST- AND SLOW-TWITCH MUSCLE FIBERS

Using surgical biopsy, which extracts about 20 to 40 mg of tissue (the size of a grain of rice), exercise biochemists have studied the functional and structural characteristics of human skeletal muscle. Two distinct types of muscle fiber have been

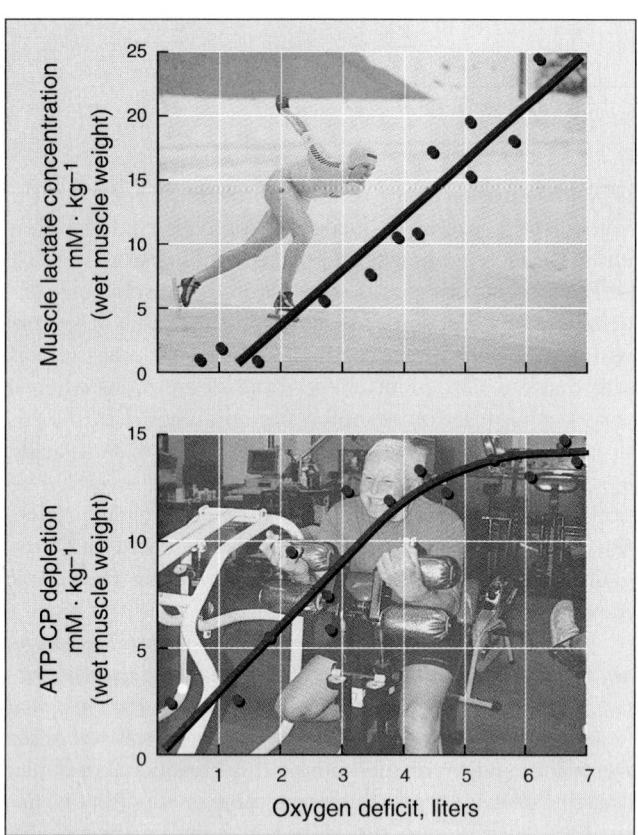

FIGURE 7.4

Muscle ATP and CP depletion and muscle lactate concentration in relation to oxygen deficit. (Adapted from Pernow, B., and Karlsson, J.: Muscle ATP, CP and lactate in submaximal and maximal exercise. In *Muscle Metabolism During Exercise.* B. Pernow and B. Saltin, Eds., New York, Plenum Press, 1971.)

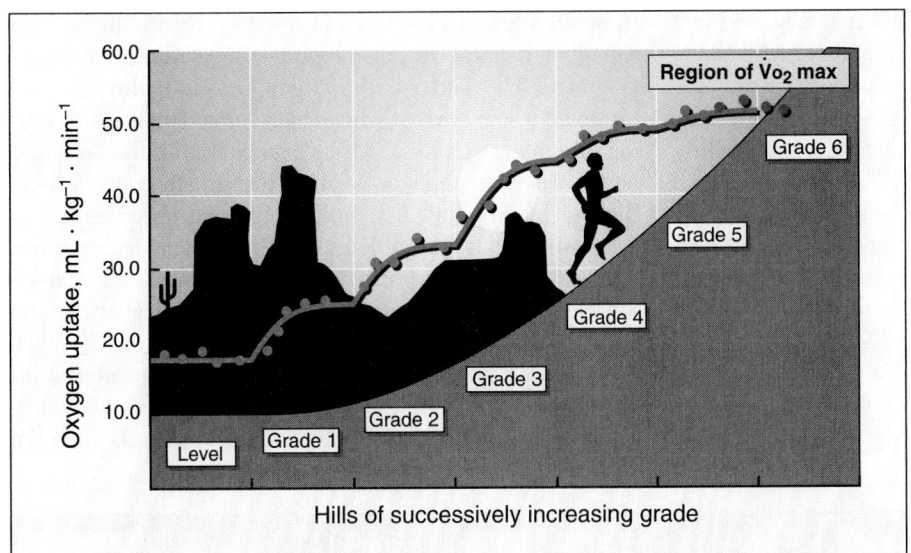

FIGURE 7.5
Maximal oxygen uptake ($\dot{V}O_2$max) is reached while running up hills of increasing grade. This occurs in the region at which a further increase in exercise intensity is not accompanied by an additional increase in oxygen uptake. The dots represent measured values of oxygen uptake during runs up each of the hills.

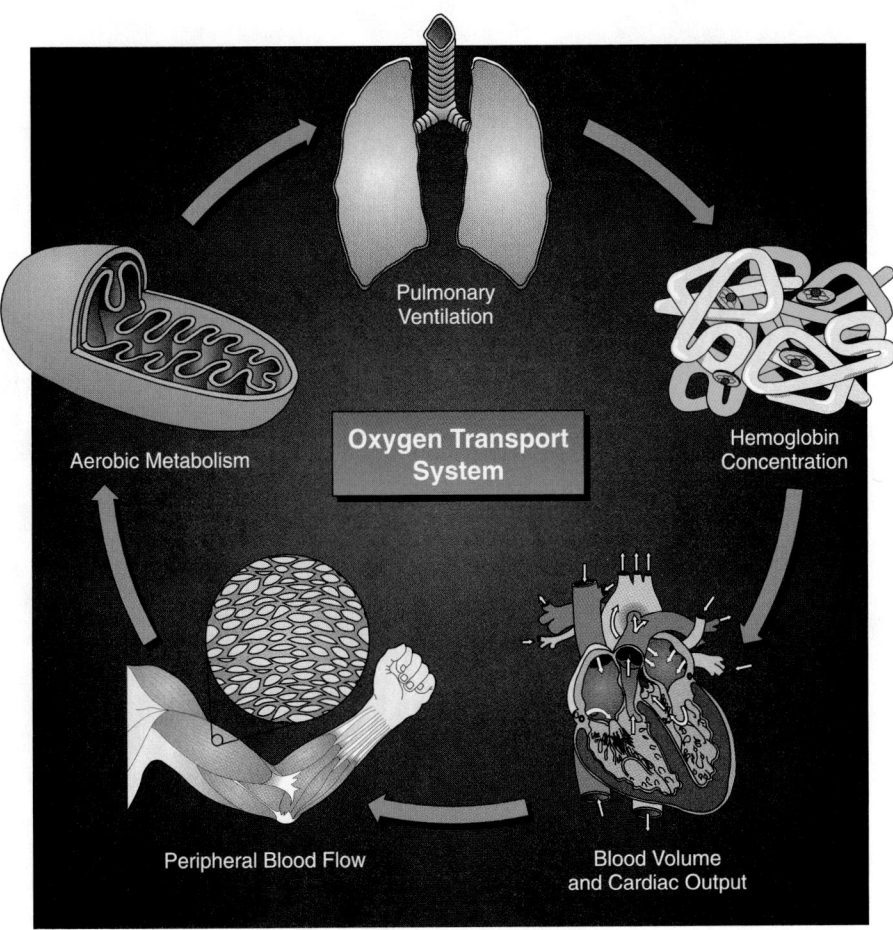

FIGURE 7.6
The aerobic system. The physiological significance of the $\dot{V}O_2$max is related to its dependence upon the functional capacity and integration of the systems required for oxygen supply, transport, delivery, and utilization.

identified in human skeletal muscle. One type is **fast-twitch** (FT), or **type II,** fiber. This fast-contracting fiber has two basic subdivisions and a high capacity for anaerobically producing ATP in glycolysis. Fast-twitch fibers are activated during change-of-pace and stop-and-go activities such as basketball, soccer, and ice hockey, as well as during all-out exercise requiring rapid, powerful movements that depend almost exclusively on the energy generated from anaerobic metabolism.

The second major classification is **slow-twitch** (ST), or **type I,** muscle fiber. This fiber type is predominantly aerobic in its metabolic capacity and has a relatively slow speed of contraction compared to its fast-twitch counterpart. The capacity of slow-twitch fibers to generate ATP aerobically relates intimately to their numerous and large mitochondria and high levels of enzymes required to sustain aerobic metabolism, as in the catabolism of fatty acids. A primary role of slow-twitch muscle fibers is to sustain continuous activities requiring a steady rate of aerobic energy transfer. Data have shown that glycogen depletion occurs primarily in the leg's slow-twitch fibers during fatigue associated with distance running.[27] This pattern of glycogen depletion also has been observed in the arms of wheelchair-dependent athletes during prolonged exercise.[55] More than likely, it is the predominance of slow-twitch muscle fibers that greatly contributes to the high blood lactate thresholds commonly observed among successful endurance athletes.[40, 54] From a practical perspective, however, most sports require relatively slow, sustained muscle actions and bursts of short-term powerful effort, and both types of muscle fibers are recruited. Figure 7.7 illustrates the fiber-type composition of two athletes representing sports that rely on different energy systems and, consequently, different muscle fiber characteristics. For the

FIGURE 7.7

Differences in fiber-type composition between a sprint swimmer and endurance racing cyclist. The type I and type II muscle fibers were sampled from the vastus lateralis muscle and stained for myofibrilar ATPase after incubation at pH 4.3. The type I fibers stain dark, while the type II fibers remain unstained. (Photos and photomicrographs courtesy of Dr. R. Billeter, Department of Anatomy, University of Bern, Switzerland.)

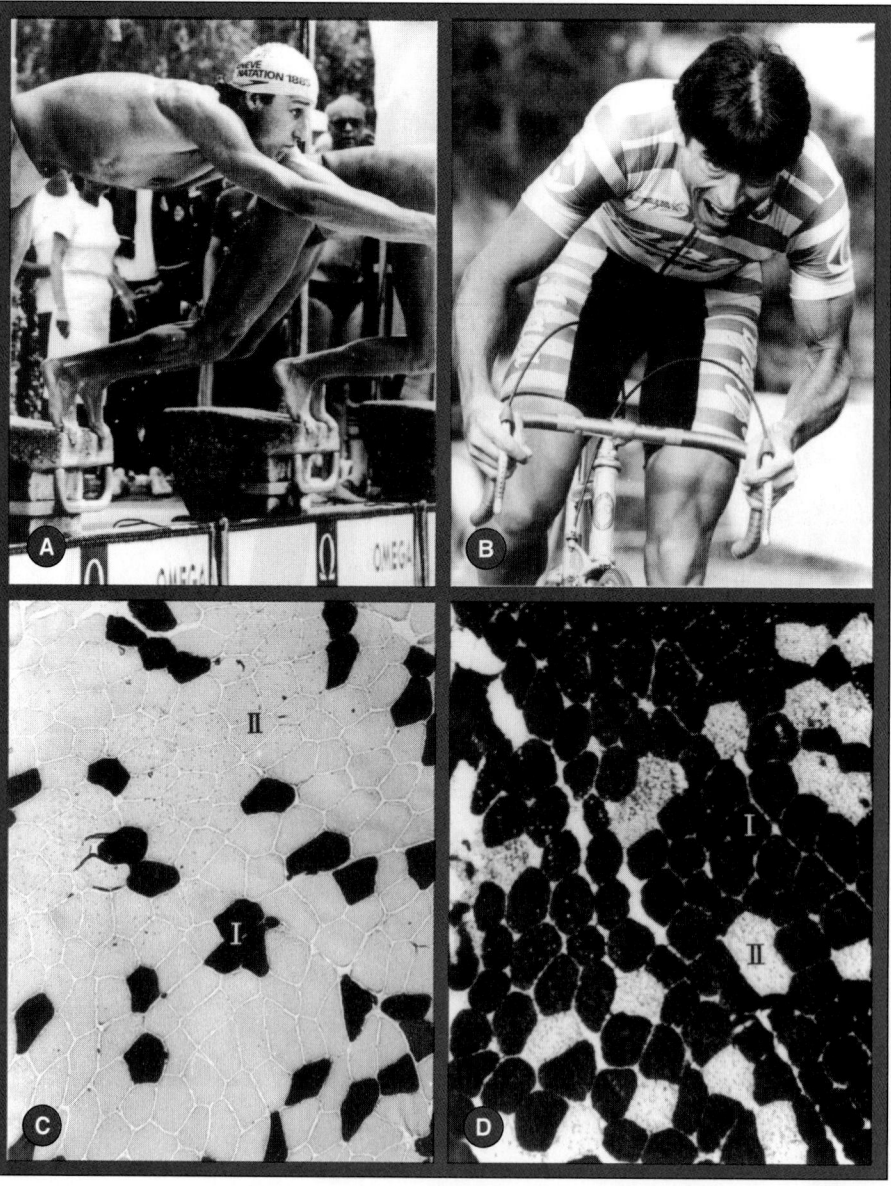

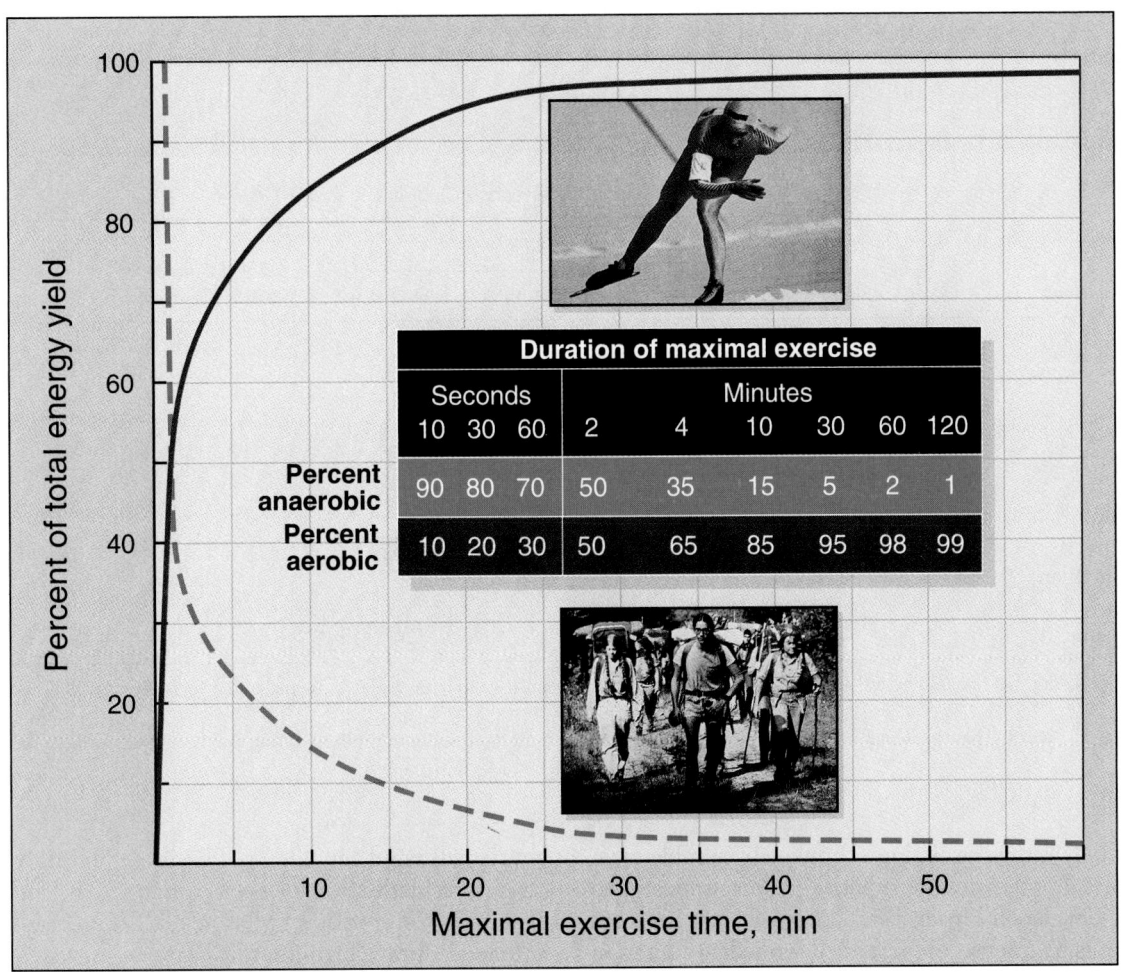

FIGURE 7.8

Relative contributions of aerobic and anaerobic energy metabolism during maximal physical effort of varying durations. Note that two minutes of maximal effort requires about 50% of the energy from both aerobic and anaerobic processes. At a world-class, 4-minute-mile pace, approximately 65% of the energy is derived from aerobic metabolism with the remainder generated from anaerobic processes. A marathon, on the other hand, is powered almost totally by energy derived from aerobic processes. (Adapted from Åstrand, P.O., and Rodahl, K.: *Textbook of Work Physiology.* New York, McGraw-Hill Book Company, 1977.)

50-meter sprint swim champion, type II fibers represent about 80% of the total muscle fibers, whereas the endurance cyclist possesses 80% of the type I variety.

From the preceding discussion, it would seem that a muscle's predominant fiber type is crucial in determining success in certain sports or physical activities. This idea is discussed more fully in Chapter 18, along with other considerations concerning each type of muscle fiber, the various subdivisions and proposed means of classification, and the effects of exercise training.

THE ENERGY SPECTRUM OF EXERCISE

Figure 7.8 illustrates the relative contribution of anaerobic and aerobic energy sources during various durations of maximal exercise. In addition, Table 7.1 lists the approximate

percentage energy yields from these systems of energy transfer, as well as the relative contributions of the major energy fuels during various competitions involving running. Although these data were estimated from laboratory experiments that involved running and bicycling, they easily can be related to other activities by drawing the appropriate time relationships. For example, a 100-meter sprint run is equivalent to any all-out activity lasting about 10 seconds, while an 800-meter run lasts about 2 minutes. All-out exercise for approximately 1 minute includes the 400-meter dash in track, the 100-meter swim, and, possibly, repeated full-court presses at the end of a basketball game.

It is useful to consider energy transfer as a continuum. At one extreme, the total energy for exercise is supplied almost entirely by intramuscular high-energy phosphates. About one-half of the energy needed for intense exercise lasting 2 minutes is supplied by the ATP-CP and lactic acid

Know this chart

TABLE 7.1
AN ESTIMATE OF THE PERCENTAGE CONTRIBUTION OF DIFFERENT FUELS TO ATP GENERATION IN VARIOUS RUNNING EVENTS

		Percentage Contribution to ATP Generation			
		Glycogen			
Event	*Creatine Phosphate*	*Anaerobic*	*Aerobic*	*Blood Glucose (Liver Glycogen)*	*Triglyceride (Fatty Acids)*
100 m	50	50	—	—	—
200 m	25	65	10	—	—
400 m	12.5	62.5	25	—	—
800 m	6	50	44	—	—
1,500 m	a	25	75	—	—
5000 m	a	12.5	87.5	—	—
10,000 m	a	3	97	—	—
Marathon	—	—	75	5	20
Ultra-marathon (80 km)	—	—	35	5	60
24-h race	—	—	10	2	88
Soccer game	10	70	20	—	—

From Newsholme, E.A., et al.: Physical and mental fatigue: metabolic mechanisms and importance of plasma amino acids. *Br. Med. Bull.*, 48:477, 1992.

*a*In such events creatine phosphate will be used for the first few seconds and, if it has been resynthesized during the race, in the sprint to the finish.

systems, whereas the remainder is supplied by aerobic reactions. To excel under these conditions, a person must possess a well-developed capacity for both aerobic and anaerobic metabolism. Intense exercise of intermediate duration performed for 5 to 10 minutes, such as middle-distance running and swimming or basketball, results in a greater demand for aerobic energy transfer. Performances of long duration such as marathon running, distance swimming, cycling, recreational jogging, and hiking require a fairly constant supply of energy derived aerobically and rely little on lactic acid formation.

An understanding of the energy demands of various activities explains in part why a world record holder in the 1-mile run is not necessarily a noted distance runner. Conversely, premier marathon runners are generally unable to run 1 mile in less than 4 minutes, yet can complete 26 miles at a 5-minute per mile pace. The appropriate approach to exercise training includes an analysis of the activity in terms of its specific energy components and training of those systems to ensure optimal adaptations in physiologic and metabolic functions. *An improved capacity for energy transfer usually translates into improved exercise performance.*

OXYGEN UPTAKE DURING RECOVERY: THE SO-CALLED "OXYGEN DEBT"

After exercise, bodily processes do not immediately return to resting levels. After relatively light, short-duration exercise,

recovery is rapid and often proceeds unnoticed. If the activity is particularly stressful, such as running a half-mile race or swimming 200 yards as fast as possible, or if the duration is extended during high-intensity aerobic exercise, considerable time may be required for metabolism to return to the resting level. The variation in recovery from light, moderate, and strenuous exercise is determined by specific metabolic and physiologic processes resulting from each level of effort.[2]

Oxygen uptakes during and while recovering from different intensities of exercise are shown in Figure 7.9. During light exercise (Figure 7.9A), when the oxygen deficit is small and the steady-rate oxygen uptake is reached rapidly, the recovery oxygen uptake also is small as recovery proceeds quickly. In this situation, the magnitude of the recovery oxygen uptake is roughly equal to the size of the oxygen deficit at the beginning of exercise. The rate of recovery follows a logarithmic curve, decreasing by about 50% over each subsequent 30-second period until the oxygen uptake returns to the pre-exercise level. (Note: Oxygen uptake during both steady-rate and non-steady-rate [heavy] exercise, as well as during recovery, can be plotted as a logarithmic function related to time.[7,61] The function either increases [as in exercise] or decreases [as in recovery] by some constant fraction for each unit of time as the oxygen uptake curve approaches a level, or asymptote, value. Consider the example of recovery from 10 minutes of light, steady-rate exercise. If the exercise oxygen uptake of 2000 mL · min^{-1} decreased during recovery by one-half for a 30-second time period, then oxygen uptake would be 1000 mL · min^{-1} at 30 seconds recovery and

500 mL · min⁻¹ at 60 seconds, with a resting value of 250 mL O_2 · min⁻¹ achieved in about 90 seconds.)

With moderate to heavy aerobic exercise (Figure 7.9B), a person takes longer to reach a steady rate; thus, the oxygen deficit is considerably large compared to light exercise. Consequently, more time will be needed for the oxygen uptake to return to the resting level during recovery. Immediately following this more strenuous exercise, there is an initial rapid decline in oxygen uptake (as in recovery from light exercise) followed by a more gradual decline to baseline. In both Figures 7.9A and 7.9B, the oxygen deficit and recovery oxygen uptake are computed using the steady-rate oxygen uptake to represent the oxygen (energy) requirements of the exercises. During the exhausting exercise illustrated in Figure 7.9C, a steady rate of aerobic metabolism cannot be attained. In this situation, anaerobic energy transfer is large, blood lactate accumulates, and considerably more time is needed for complete recovery. During this level of exercise, no steady-rate is achieved because the energy demand exceeds the maximal or peak oxygen uptake, and the true oxygen deficit is difficult to determine.

From each of the illustrations in Figure 7.9, we can see that, regardless of the intensity of the exercise, oxygen uptake during recovery always exceeds the resting value. This excess has commonly been termed the **oxygen debt**. (As discussed later, a more correct term is **recovery oxygen uptake**.) The oxygen debt, indicated by the purple-shaded area under the recovery curve, is calculated as the total oxygen consumed in recovery minus the total oxygen that theoretically would have been consumed at rest during the recovery period if the prior exercise had not been performed. For example, if a total of 5.5 L of oxygen were consumed in recovery until reaching the resting value of 0.310 L per minute, and the recovery required 10 minutes, the oxygen debt would be 5.5 L − [0.310 L × 10 minutes], or 2.4 L. This result means that the preceding exercise caused physiologic alterations during both exercise and recovery to facilitate the uptake of an additional 2.4 L of oxygen before attaining the pre-exercise oxygen uptake. An important assumption that underlies the calculation of the oxygen debt is that resting oxygen uptake has remained essentially unchanged during exercise and recovery. As we shall point out, this assumption is not entirely correct, particularly concerning recovery from strenuous exercise.

The recovery curves in Figure 7.9 illustrate two important characteristics of oxygen uptake during recovery:

- If the prior exercise was primarily aerobic and of relatively short duration (with little disruption in body temperature and the hormonal milieu), about one-half of the total recovery oxygen uptake is repaid within 30 seconds; within several minutes, the recovery is complete as the rate of decline follows a single component exponential decline. This part of the curve is called the **fast component** of recovery oxygen uptake.[5, 50]

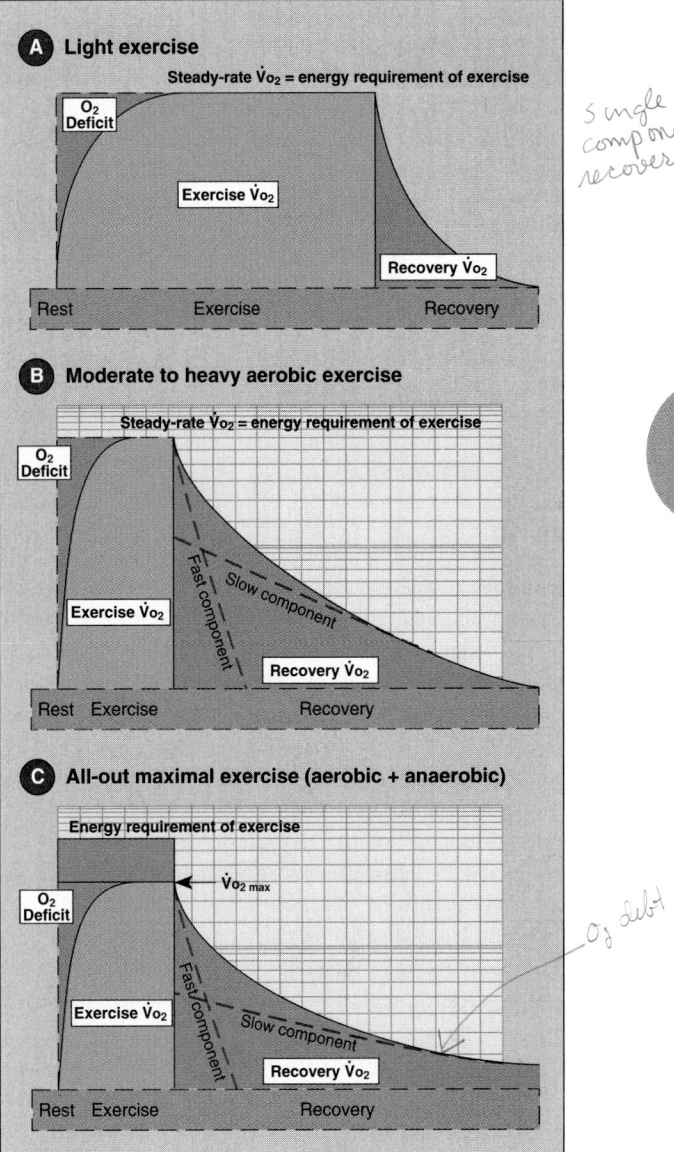

FIGURE 7.9

Oxygen uptake during exercise and in recovery from (**A**) light steady-rate exercise, (**B**) moderate to heavy steady-rate exercise, and (**C**) exhaustive exercise where a steady rate of aerobic metabolism cannot be attained. The first phase of recovery occurs rapidly; the second phase is much slower and may take considerable time to return to the pre-exercise level. Note that during exhaustive exercise, the oxygen requirement of the exercise is greater than the actual exercise oxygen uptake.

- Recovery from strenuous exercise presents a different picture because of a potentially considerable increase in body temperature, blood lactate, and thermogenic hormone levels. In addition to the fast-component phase of the recovery curve, a second, slower phase of recovery exists and is termed the **slow component.** Depending on the intensity and duration of exercise, this phase of recovery may take up to several hours (or even a day) before reestablishing the pre-exercise oxygen uptake level.[4, 28, 50, 52] Even with shorter intermittent bouts of "supermaximal" exercise (for example, three 2-minute bouts at 108% $\dot{V}o_2$max interspersed with 3-minute rests), the recovery oxygen uptake can remain elevated for 1 hour or longer.[1]

METABOLIC DYNAMICS OF RECOVERY OXYGEN UPTAKE

A precise biochemical explanation of recovery oxygen uptake, particularly the role of lactic acid, is not possible because there still is no clear explanation of the specific chemical dynamics of "oxygen debt."[23, 60]

Traditional Concepts

The term oxygen debt was first coined in 1922 by the Nobel Prize scientist Archibald Vivian Hill. A.V. Hill, as well as others, discussed energy metabolism during exercise and recovery in financial-accounting terms.[32] Within this framework, the body's carbohydrate stores were likened to energy "credits." If these stored credits were expended during exercise, then a "debt" was incurred: the greater the energy "deficit" (or use of available stored energy credits), the larger the energy debt incurred. The recovery oxygen uptake was thought to represent the metabolic cost of repaying this debt, hence, the term oxygen debt.

In more concrete terms, the accumulation of lactate during the anaerobic component of exercise represented the utilization of glycogen (the stored energy credit). The ensuing oxygen debt was believed to serve two purposes: (a) to reestablish the original glycogen stores (credits) by resynthesizing approximately 80% of the lactic acid back to glycogen in the liver via the Cori cycle, and (a) to catabolize the remaining lactate through the pyruvic acid–Krebs cycle pathway. The ATP generated in this process presumably was used to power the resynthesis of lactate to glycogen. This early explanation of the dynamics of recovery oxygen uptake often has been termed the "lactic acid theory of oxygen debt."

In 1933, subsequent to the work of Hill, researchers at the Harvard Fatigue Laboratory explained their observations that the initial portion of the recovery oxygen uptake was consumed before blood lactate began to decrease.[45] It was possible to incur an oxygen debt of almost 3 L without an appreciable lactate accumulation. To resolve these findings, two phases of oxygen debt were proposed: (a) **alactic** or **alactacid** oxygen debt (without lactate buildup), and (a) **lactic acid** or **lactacid** oxygen debt associated with elevated blood lactate levels. It is noteworthy that these two explanations were based on speculation because these researchers were unable to measure ATP and CP replenishment, or the relationship between blood lactate and glucose and glycogen levels. For nearly 65 years, the following model has served to explain the energetics of oxygen debt:

- **Alactacid debt**—The alactacid portion of the oxygen debt for recovery from light, steady-rate exercise (Figure 7.9A) or for the rapid phase of recovery from more strenuous exercise (Figure 7.9B and C) was attributed to the restoration of the high-energy phosphates ATP and CP depleted during exercise. It was reasoned that the energy for this restoration came from the aerobic breakdown of food nutrients during recovery. A small portion of the recovery oxygen uptake also was used to reload muscle myoglobin, as well as the hemoglobin in the blood returning from previously active tissues.
- **Lactacid debt**—In keeping with the explanation by A.V. Hill, the major portion of the lactacid oxygen debt was thought to represent the reconversion of lactic acid to glycogen in the liver.

Controversy with Traditional Explanation of Oxygen Debt

Several relationships must be established to show that an aerobic energy deficit in exercise is temporarily compensated for by energy from anaerobic sources that are then resynthesized in recovery (refer to Focus on Research). For example, a moderate relationship exists between the anaerobiosis in exercise (oxygen deficit) and the excess oxygen uptake in recovery (oxygen debt.) To accept the traditional explanation for the lactacid phase of the oxygen debt, it also must be established that the major portion of lactate accumulated in exercise is actually resynthesized to glycogen in recovery as Hill and others had speculated. This has never been shown. In experiments with humans, no substantial replenishment of glycogen was observed 10 minutes after strenuous exercise, even though blood lactate levels were significantly reduced. *Apparently, a major portion of lactic acid is oxidized for energy.*[2, 6] This seems likely because the heart, liver, kidney, and skeletal muscle tissues readily use lactate as an energy substrate during exercise and recovery.[56]

Contemporary Concepts

There is no doubt that the elevated aerobic metabolism in recovery is necessary to restore the body to its pre-exercise condition and is largely the result of the preceding metabolic and physiologic events during exercise. During short-duration light to moderate exercise, recovery oxygen uptake generally serves to replenish the high-energy phosphates depleted by exercise.[2] This process is rapid: it is usually completed within several minutes.[5] During longer-duration (less than 60 minutes), high-intensity aerobic exercise, the recovery oxygen uptake can remain elevated for a considerably longer period.[3, 52] This effect of exercise duration on the magnitude of recovery oxygen uptake during high-intensity aerobic exercise is illustrated in Figure 7.10. Eight women exercised at 70% of $\dot{V}o_2$max for either 20, 40, or 60 minutes. **Excess postexercise oxygen con-**

sumption (EPOC) totaled 8.6 L for the 20-minute exercise and 9.8 L for the 40-minute session, whereas the cost of recovery for the 60-minute workout nearly doubled to 15.2 L. Although lactate accumulation is not associated with this prolonged recovery, other "disequilibriums" in physiologic function are probably operating to keep recovery metabolism elevated (see below).

During exhaustive exercise with a significant anaerobic component and lactate accumulation, some of the recovery oxygen uptake is used to resynthesize a portion of lactate back to glycogen. (This mechanism for gluconeogenesis also takes place during exercise and is noteworthy among trained groups.[21, 44]) The main source for replenishing glycogen, however, is dietary carbohydrate, not resynthesized lactic acid.

A significant portion of the recovery oxygen uptake can be attributed to physiologic processes that actually take place **during** recovery. The considerably larger oxygen debt in relation to oxygen deficit during prolonged aerobic exercise (and exhaustive anaerobic exercise) probably is the result of such factors. Body temperature, for example, rises about 3°C (5.4°F) during a long bout of vigorous aerobic exercise and can remain elevated for several hours during recovery. This has a direct stimulating effect on metabolism, causing an increase in recovery oxygen uptake.[2, 3, 11]

Other factors also affect recovery oxygen uptake. As much as 10% of the recovery oxygen is used to reload the blood as it returns from the exercised muscles. An additional 2 to 5% restores the oxygen dissolved in body fluids and the oxygen bound to myoglobin in the muscle itself. During intense exercise, the volume of air breathed increases to 8 to 10 times above rest and remains elevated for some time in recovery. Thus, the respiratory muscles require more oxygen during recovery than they normally require at rest and can account for about 10% of the total recovery oxygen uptake.[41] The heart also works harder and requires a greater oxygen supply during recovery. Tissue repair and redistribution of the ions calcium, potassium, and sodium within muscle and other body compartments require energy, while the residual effects of the thermogenic hormones epinephrine, norepinephrine, thyroxine, and the glucocorticoids released in exercise can elevate metabolism for a considerable time during recovery.[25] In essence, all of the physiologic systems activated with exercise also need increased oxygen during recovery. *The oxygen debt, or, more accurately, the recovery oxygen uptake or excess postexercise oxygen consumption (EPOC), reflects both the anaerobic metabolism of previous exercise and the respiratory, circulatory, hormonal, ionic, and thermal adjustments that occur during recovery.*

Causes of Excess Postexercise Oxygen Consumption (EPOC) Resulting from Heavy Exercise

- Resynthesize ATP and CP.
- Resynthesize lactate to glycogen (Cori cycle).
- Oxidize lactate in energy metabolism.
- Restore oxygen to blood.
- Thermogenic effects of elevated core temperature.
- Thermogenic effects of hormones, particularly the catecholamines epinephrine and norephinephrine.
- Effects of elevated heart rate, ventilation, and other elevated levels of physiologic function.

IMPLICATIONS OF EPOC FOR EXERCISE AND RECOVERY

An understanding of the dynamics of EPOC provides a basis for structuring intervals of exercise and optimizing recovery. No appreciable lactate accumulates with either steady-rate aerobic exercise or brief 5- to 10-second bouts of all-out effort. Consequently, recovery is rapid (fast component) and exercise can begin again without the hindering effects of fatigue. In contrast, longer periods of anaerobic exercise are performed at the expense of a lactate buildup in the blood and active muscles as well as a significant disruption in physiologic processes. In this situation, recovery oxygen uptake consists of both fast and slow components, and considerably more time is required to achieve complete recovery. This can pose a problem in sports such as basketball, hockey, soccer, tennis, and badminton because a performer pushed to a high level of anaerobic metabolism may not fully recover during brief rest periods, such as time outs, or other rest periods throughout the competition.

Procedures for speeding recovery from exercise generally can be categorized as either **active** or **passive.** For active recovery (often called "cooling-down" or "tapering-off"), submaximal aerobic exercise is performed under the assumption that continued movement in some way prevents

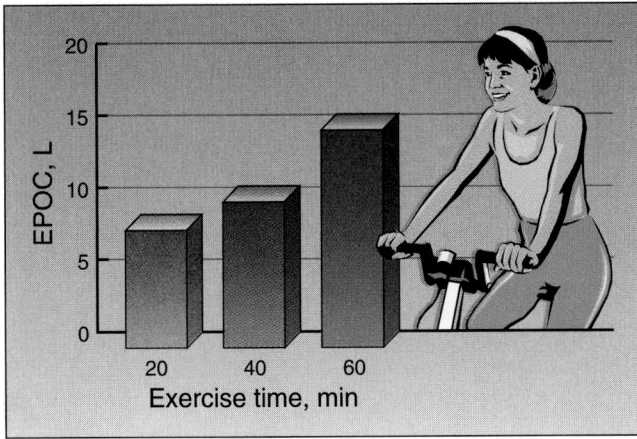

FIGURE 7.10

Total excess postexercise oxygen consumption (EPOC) during a 3-hour recovery from exercise at 70% $\dot{V}O_2$max for 20-, 40-, and 60-minute durations. EPOC for the 60-minute exercise was significantly larger than for the 20- or 40-minute workouts. (From Quinn, T.J., et al.: Postexercise oxygen consumption in trained females: effect of exercise duration. *Med. Sci. Sports Exerc.,* 26:908, 1994.)

muscle cramps and stiffness and facilitates the recovery process. In passive recovery, the person usually lies down under the assumption that complete inactivity reduces resting energy requirements and thus "frees" oxygen for the recovery process. Modifications of active and passive recovery have included the use of massage, cold showers, specific body positions, and the ingestion of cold liquids.

Optimal Recovery from Steady-Rate Exercise

For most people, exercise performed at an oxygen uptake below 50% of $\dot{V}O_2$max generally can be continued at a steady rate with little lactate buildup. Recovery from this exercise entails the resynthesis of high-energy phosphates; replenishment of oxygen in the blood, body fluids, and muscle myoglobin; and a small energy cost to sustain elevated circulation and ventilation. In a situation such as this, recovery is more rapid using passive procedures because exercise would only elevate total metabolism and delay recovery to the resting level.

Optimal Recovery from Non-Steady-Rate Exercise

When exercise intensity exceeds 60 to 75% of $\dot{V}O_2$max, a steady rate of aerobic metabolism no longer is maintained, lactic acid formation in muscle exceeds its rate of removal,

and blood lactate accumulates. As exercise intensity increases, the level of lactate rises sharply and the exerciser soon becomes exhausted. Although the precise mechanisms for fatigue during anaerobic exercise are unclear, the blood lactate level does provide an objective indication of the relative strenuousness of exercise and may also reflect the adequacy of the recovery process.[37] Because the lactate anion causes fatigue in skeletal muscle independent of associated reductions in pH,[33] any procedure that accelerates lactate removal could probably augment subsequent exercise performance.

Blood lactate removal is accelerated by performing active aerobic exercise in recovery.[12, 22, 24] Apparently, the optimal level of recovery exercise is between 29 and 45% of the $\dot{V}O_2$max for bicycle exercise, and 55 to 60% of $\dot{V}O_2$max when the recovery involves treadmill running.[49] Such variation probably is a result of the more localized muscle involvement in bicycling and reflects a lower threshold for lactate accumulation during this form of exercise.[30]

Figure 7.11 illustrates blood lactate recovery patterns for trained males who performed 6 minutes of supermaximal work on a bicycle ergometer. Active recovery involved 40 minutes of continuous exercise at either 35 or 65% of $\dot{V}O_2$max. A combination of 65% (7 minutes) followed by 35% (33 minutes) of $\dot{V}O_2$max also was used to evaluate whether a higher-intensity exercise interval early in recovery would

FIGURE 7.11
Blood lactate concentration following maximal exercise during passive and active exercise recoveries at 35, 65, and a combination of 35 and 65% of $\dot{V}O_2$max. The horizontal gray line indicates the level of blood lactate produced by exercise at 65% of $\dot{V}O_2$max without previous exercise. (Adapted from Dodd, S., et al.: Blood lactate disappearance at various intensities of recovery exercise. *J. Appl. Physiol.: Respirat. Environ. Exerc. Physiol.*, 57:1462, 1984.)

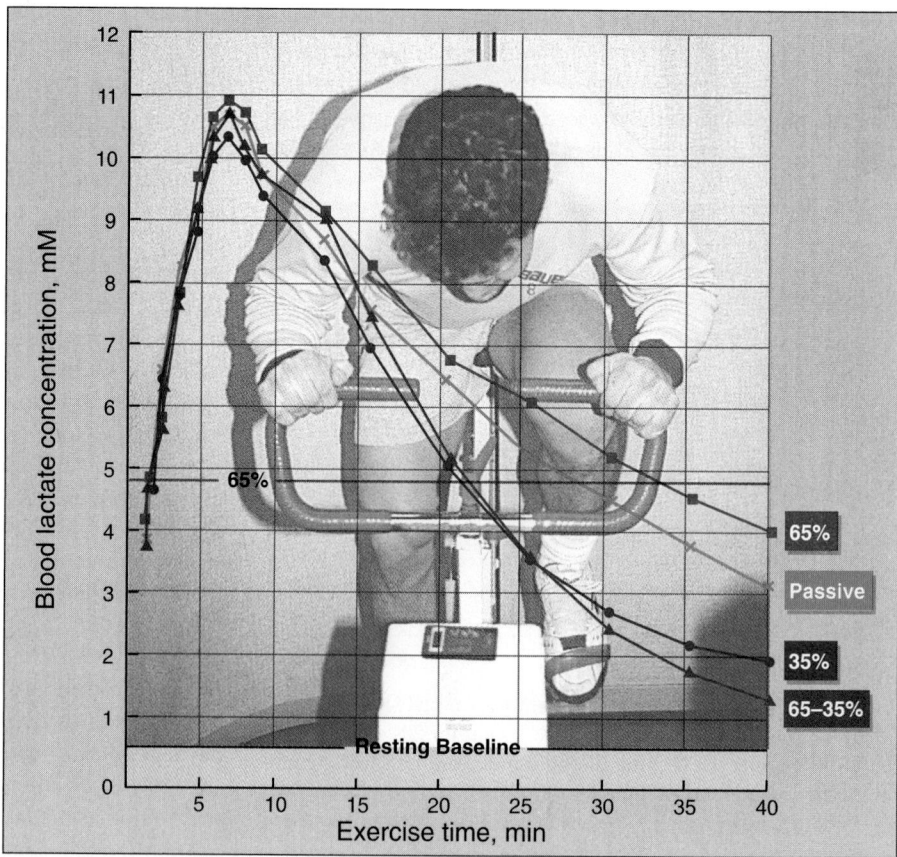

expedite lactate removal from the tissues to the blood.[20] These data clearly show that moderate aerobic exercise during recovery facilitates lactate removal more effectively than passive recovery. The combination of higher-intensity followed by lower-intensity exercise was of no more benefit than a single level of exercise at moderate intensity. Importantly, if recovery exercise is too intense and performed above the lactate threshold, it is of no added benefit and may even prolong recovery by initiating lactate formation. In a practical sense, if left to their own choices, people select their optimal intensities for recovery exercise.

The reasons are not clear for the benefits of active compared to passive recovery. The facilitated removal of lactate with recovery exercise likely is the result of an increased perfusion of blood through "lactate-using" organs such as the liver and heart. In addition, increased blood flow through the muscles during active recovery certainly would enhance lactate removal because this tissue can oxidize lactate via Krebs cycle metabolism.[24]

INTERMITTENT EXERCISE

It is possible to perform a significant amount of typically exhaustive exercise without excessively relying on anaerobic energy transfer through glycolysis and subsequent lactate buildup. One means of achieving this exercise output is by training the aerobic systems to increase one's capacity to sustain heavy exercise aerobically. Dramatic examples of this capability are the performances of elite marathon runners, distance swimmers, and cross-country skiers, many of whom compete in steady rate at oxygen uptakes averaging 4.0 L per minute (and performed at between 85 and 90% of aerobic capacity). Another approach to performing at exercise intensities that would normally cause exhaustion within 3 to 5 minutes if performed continuously is to exercise **intermittently** using pre-established work and rest intervals.[13] This technique is popular in conditioning programs and is known as **interval training.** Here, various work-to-rest intervals incorporating supermaximal exercise are used to overload the various systems of energy transfer. For example, during all-out exercise for up to 8 seconds, the intramuscular high-energy phosphates provide the major portion of energy, and reliance on the glycolytic pathway is minimal. Therefore, recovery is rapid (alactic, fast component), and another bout of heavy exercise can begin after only a brief recovery.

The results of a series of laboratory experiments using various combinations of work and rest intervals during intermittent exercise are summarized in Table 7.2. On one day, the subject ran at a speed that would normally be exhausting within 5 minutes. About 0.8 mile was covered during this continuous run, and the runner attained a maximal oxygen uptake of 5.6 L per minute. A relative state of exhaustion resulting from a high level of anaerobic metabolism was verified by the high blood lactate level shown in the last column of the table. On another day, the same fast

TABLE 7.2
RESULTS OF AN EXPERIMENT DEALING WITH INTERMITTENT EXERCISE

Exercise Rest Periods	Total Distance Run (yards)	Average Oxygen Uptake (L · min⁻¹)	Blood Lactate Level (mg · 100 mL blood⁻¹)
4 min continuous	1422	5.6	150
10 s exercise 5 s rest	7294	5.1	44
10 s exercise 10 s rest	5468	4.4	20
15 s exercise 30 s rest	3642	3.6	16

From data of Christenson, E.H., et al: Intermittent and continuous running. *Acta Physiol. Scand.,* 50:269, 1960, as reported in Åstrand, P.O., and Rodahl, K.: *Textbook of Work Physiology.* New York, McGraw-Hill Book Company, 1970, p. 384.

speed was maintained, but the exercise was performed intermittently using periods of 10 seconds of exercise and 5 seconds of recovery. With a 30-minute protocol of this intermittent exercise, the actual duration of running amounted to 20 minutes and the distance covered was 4 miles compared to less than 5 minutes and 0.8 miles when the run was performed continuously! This capability for exercise is even more impressive if one considers that the blood lactate level remained low even though the oxygen uptake was quite high, averaging 5.1 L per minute, or 91% of V̇o₂max, throughout the 30-minute period. A relative balance had been achieved between the energy requirements of exercise and the level of aerobic energy transfer within the muscle during the work and rest intervals.

Clearly, a specific energy-transfer system can be emphasized and overloaded by manipulating the duration of work and rest intervals. When the rest interval was extended from 5 to 10 seconds, the oxygen uptake averaged 4.4 L per minute; with 15-second work and 30-second recovery intervals, only a 3.6-L oxygen uptake was noted. For each 30 minutes of intermittent exercise, the runner achieved a longer-distance run and a much lower lactate level compared to the same exercise intensity performed continuously. Chapter 21 focuses on the specific application of the principles of intermittent exercise to both aerobic and anaerobic training and sports performance.

■ SUMMARY ■

1. The major pathway for ATP production differs depending on the intensity and duration of exercise. During intense exercise of short duration (100-yard dash, lifting heavy weights), the energy required for exercise already

is present in the intramuscular stores of ATP and CP (immediate energy system). For somewhat less intense exercise of longer duration (1 to 2 minutes), energy is generated mainly from the anaerobic reactions of glycolysis (short-term energy system). As exercise progresses beyond several minutes, the aerobic system predominates and oxygen uptake becomes an important factor (long-term energy system).

2. Humans possess different types of muscle fiber, each with unique metabolic and contractile properties. The two major fiber types are (a) low glycolytic–high oxidative, slow-twitch fibers, and (b) low oxidative–high glycolytic, fast-twitch fibers. Intermediate fibers with overlapping metabolic characteristics of the fast-twitch type are also present.

3. By understanding the energy spectrum of exercise, it is possible to train for specific improvement in the appropriate energy system.

4. A steady rate of oxygen uptake represents a balance between the energy requirements of the active muscles and the aerobic resynthesis of ATP. The term oxygen deficit refers to the difference between the oxygen requirement of exercise and the oxygen actually consumed during exercise.

5. The maximum capacity for the aerobic resynthesis of ATP is quantitatively measured as the maximum oxygen uptake, or $\dot{V}O_2$max. This is one of the most important indicators of a person's ability to sustain high-intensity exercise.

6. When exercise ceases, the oxygen uptake remains elevated above the resting level. This recovery oxygen uptake reflects the metabolic demands of the preceding exercise as well as the physiologic alterations caused by that exercise.

7. Moderate physical activity performed following anaerobic exercise (active recovery) facilitates recovery compared to passive procedures. In most cases, an active recovery is reflected by a faster removal of blood lactate.

■ REFERENCES ■

1. Bahr, R.: Effects of supramaximal exercise on excess postexercise oxygen consumption. *Med. Sci. Sports Exerc.*, 24:66, 1992.
2. Bahr, R.: Excess postexercise oxygen consumption—magnitude, mechanisms and practical implications. *Acta Physiol. Scand. (Suppl),* 605:1, 1992.
3. Bahr, R., and Sejersted, O.M.: Effect of intensity of exercise on excess postexercise oxygen consumption. *Metabolism,* 40:836, 1991.
4. Bahr, R., et al.: Triglyceride/fatty acid cycling is increased after exercise. *Metabolism,* 39:993, 1990.
5. Bangsbo, J., et al.: Anaerobic energy production and O_2 deficit-debt relationship during exhaustive exercise in humans. *J. Physiol.,* 422:539, 1990.
6. Bangsbo, J.P., et al.: Substrates for muscle glycogen synthesis in recovery from intense exercise in man. *J. Physiol.,* 434:423, 1991.
7. Barstow, T.J.: Characterization of $\dot{V}O_2$ kinetics during heavy exercise. *Med. Sci. Sports Exerc.,* 26.:1327, 1994.
8. Bernús, G., et al.: ^{31}P-MRS of quadriceps reveals quantitative differences between sprinters and long-distance runners, *Med, Sci. Sports Exerc.,* 25:479, 1993.
9. Brooks, G.A.: Anaerobic threshold: review of the concept and directions for future research. *Med. Sci. Sports Exerc.,* 17:22, 1985.
10. Brooks, G.A.: Physical activity and carbohydrate metabolism. In *Physical Activity, Fitness, and Health.* C. Bouchard, et al., Eds., Champaign, Ill., Human Kinetics, 1994.
11. Brooks, G.A., et al.: Temperature, skeletal muscle mitochondrial functions and oxygen debt. *Am. J. Physiol.,* 220:1053, 1971.
12. Choi, D., et al.: Effect of passive and active recovery on the resynthesis of muscle glycogen. *Med. Sci. Sports Exerc.,* 26:992, 1994.
13. Christenson, E.H., et al.: Intermittent and continuous running. *Acta Physiol. Scand.,* 50:269, 1960.
14. Coggan, A.R., et al.: Endurance training decreases plasma glucose turnover and oxidation during moderate-intensity exercise in men. *J. Appl. Physiol.,* 68:990, 1990.
15. Coggan, A.R., et al.: Plasma glucose kinetics during exercise in 136subjects with high and low lactate thresholds. *J. Appl. Physiol.,* 73:1873, 1992.
16. Coggan, A.R., et al.: Skeletal muscle adaptations to endurance training in 60- to 70 yr-old men and women. *J. Appl. Physiol.,* 72:1780, 1992.
17. Costill, D.L., et al.: Fractional utilization of the aerobic capacity during distance running. *Med. Sci. Sports,* 5:248, 1973.
18. Coyle, E.F.: Blood lactate threshold in some well trained ischemic heart disease patients. *J. Appl. Physiol.,* 54:18, 1983.
19. Davis, J.A., et al.: Anaerobic threshold alterations caused by endurance training in middle-aged men. *J. Appl. Physiol.,* 46:1039, 1979.
20. Dodd, S., et al.: Blood lactate disappearance at various intensities of recovery exercise. *J. Appl. Physiol.,* 57:1462, 1984.
21. Donovan, C.M., and Brooks, G.A.: Endurance training affects lactate clearance, not lactate production. *Am. J. Physiol.,* 244 (Endocrinol. Metab. 7): E83, 1983.
22. Falk, B., et al.: Blood lactate concentration following exercise: effects of heat exposure and of active recovery in heat-acclimatized subjects. *Int. J. Sports Med.,* 16:7, 1995.
23. Gaesser, G.A., and Brooks, G.A.: Metabolic basis of excess post-exercise oxygen consumption: a review. *Med. Sci. Sports Exerc.,* 16:29, 1984.
24. Gladden, L.B.: Lactate uptake by skeletal muscle. In *Exercise and Sport Sciences Reviews.* Vol. 17, K.B. Pandolf, Ed., New York, Macmillan, 1989.
25. Gladden, L.B., et al.: Norepinephrine increases and canine skeletal muscle $\dot{V}O_2$ during recovery. *Med. Sci. Sports Exerc.,* 14:371, 1982.
26. Gollnick, P.D., and Saltin, B.: Significance of skeletal muscle oxidative enzyme enhancement with endurance training. *Clin. Physiol.,* 2:1, 1983.
27. Gollnick, P.D., et al.: Glycogen depletion patterns in human skeletal muscle fibers after varying types and intensities of exercise. In *Metabolic Adaptation to Prolonged Exercise.* H. Howard and J. Poortmans, Eds., Basel, Birkhausen Verlag, 1975.
28. Gore, C.J., and Withers, R.I.: Effects of exercise intensity and duration on postexercise metabolism. *J. Appl. Physiol.,* 68:2362, 1990.
29. Hagberg, J.M., et al.: Faster adjustment to and recovery from submaximal exercise in the trained state. *J. Appl. Physiol.,* 48:218, 1980.
30. Hermansen, L., and Stensvold, I.: Production and removal of lactate during exercise in man. *Acta Physiol. Scand.,* 86:191, 1972.
31. Hickson, R.C., et al.: Faster adjustment of O_2 uptake to the energy requirement of exercise in the trained state. *J. Appl. Physiol.,* 44:877, 1978.
32. Hill, A.V., et al.: Muscular exercise, lactic acid and the supply and utilization of oxygen. *Proc. R. Soc. Lond. (Biol.),* 96:438, 1924.
33. Hogan, M.C., et al.: Increased [lactate] in working dog muscle reduces tension development independent of pH. *Med. Sci. Sports Exerc.,* 27:371, 1995.

34. Holloszy, J.O., and Coyle, E.F.: Adaptations of skeletal muscle to endurance training and their metabolic consequences. *J. Appl. Physiol.*, 56:831, 1984.

35. Hultman, E.: Studies on muscle metabolism of glycogen and active phosphate in man with special reference to exercise and diet. *Scand. J. Clin. Lab. Invest.*, Suppl. 94, 1967.

36. Ivy, J.L., et al.: Muscle respiratory capacity and fiber type as determinants of lactate threshold. *J. Appl. Physiol.*, 48:523, 1980.

37. Jacobs, I.: Blood lactate: implications for training and sports performance. *Sports Med.*, 3:10, 1986.

38. Jacobs, I., et al.: Sprint training effects on muscle myoglobin, enzymes, fiber types, and blood lactate. *Med. Sci. Sports Exerc.*, 19:368, 1987.

39. Karlsson, J.: Lactate and phosphagen concentrations in working muscle of man. *Acta Physiol. Scand.*, Suppl. 358, 1971.

40. Karlsson, J., and Jacobs, I.: Onset of blood lactate accumulation during muscular exercise as a threshold concept. I. Theoretical considerations. *Int. J. Sports Med.*, 3:190, 1982.

41. Katch, F.I., et al.: The influence of the estimated oxygen cost of ventilation on oxygen deficit and recovery oxygen intake for moderately heavy bicycle ergometer exercise. *Med. Sci. Sports*, 4:71, 1972.

42. Katz, A., and Sahlin, K.: Role of oxygen in regulation of glycolysis and lactate production in human skeletal muscle. In *Exercise and Sport Sciences Reviews*. Vol. 18, K.B. Pandolf, Ed., Baltimore, Williams & Wilkins, 1990.

43. Kent-Braun, J.A., et al.: Human skeletal muscle metabolism in health and disease: utility of magnetic resonance spectroscopy. *Exerc. Sport Sci. Revs.*, 23:305, 1995.

44. MacRae, H.S-H., et al.: Effect of training on lactate production and removal during progressive exercise. *J. Appl. Physiol.*, 72:1649, 1992.

45. Margaria, R., et al.: The possible mechanism of contracting and paying the oxygen debt and the role of lactic acid in muscular contraction. *Am. J. Physiol.*, 106:687, 1933.

46. McCann, D.J., et al.: Phosphocreatine kinetics in humans during exercise and recovery. *Med. Sci. Sports Exerc.*, 27:378, 1995.

47. McCully, K.K., et al.: Application of ^{31}P magnetic resonance spectroscopy to the study of athletic performance. *Sports Med.*, 5:312, 1988.

48. McCully, K.K., et al.: Simultaneous in vivo measurements of HbO_2 saturation and PCr kinetics after exercise in normal humans. *J. Appl. Physiol.*, 77:5, 1994.

49. McLellan, T.M., and Skinner, J.S.: Blood lactate removal during active recovery related to aerobic threshold. *Int. J. Sports Med.*, 3:224, 1982.

50. Poehlman, E.A., et al.: The impact of exercise and diet restriction on daily energy expenditure. *Sports Med.*, 11:78, 1991.

51. Poole, D.C.: $\dot{V}O_2$ slow component: physiological and functional significance. *Med. Sci. Sports Exerc.*, 26:1354, 1994.

52. Quinn, T.J., et al.: Postexercise oxygen consumption in trained females: effect of exercise duration. *Med. Sci. Sports Exerc.*, 26:908, 1994.

53. Seip, R.L., et al.: Perceptual responses and blood lactate concentration: effect of training state. *Med. Sci. Sports Exerc.*, 23:80, 1991.

54. Sjödin, B., and Jacobs, I.: Onset of blood lactate accumulation and marathon running performance. *Int. J. Sports Med.*, 2:23, 1981.

55. Skirnar, G.S., et al.: Glycogen utilization in wheelchair-dependent athletes. *Int. J. Sports Med.*, 3:215, 1982.

56. Stainsby, W.N., and Brooks, G.A.: Control of lactic acid metabolism in contracting muscles and during exercise. In *Exercise and Sport Sciences Reviews*. Vol. 18, K.B. Pandolf, Ed., Baltimore, Williams & Wilkins, 1990.

57. Wasserman, K., et al.: Respiratory physiology of exercise: metabolism, gas exchange and ventilatory control. *Int. Rev. Resp. Physiol.*, 111:149, 1981.

58. Weltman, A.: The lactate threshold and endurance performance. *Adv. Sports Med. Fitness*, 2:91, 1989.

59. Weltman, A., et al.: Reliability and validity of a continuous incremental treadmill protocol for the determination of lactate threshold, fixed blood lactate concentrations and $\dot{V}O_2$ max. *Int. J. Sports Med.*, 11:26, 1990.

60. Weltman, A.: The Blood Lactate Response to Exercise. Current Issues in Exercise Science. Monograph Number 4. Champaign, IL., Human Kinetics, 1995.

61. Whipp, B.J.: The slow component of O_2 uptake kinetics during heavy exercise. *Med. Sci. Sports Exerc.*, 26:1319, 1994.

Krogh, A., and Lindhard, J.: The relative value of fat and carbohydrate as sources of muscular energy. *Biochem. J.* 14:290, 1920.

In this 73-page research report, the Nobel laureate A. Krogh and coauthor J. Lindhard made 220 determinations of respiratory gas exchange from six subjects (including themselves) who consumed varied diets to determine nutrient combustion during rest and exercise. For two days prior to testing, subjects maintained a high-carbohydrate, low-protein diet or a high-lipid, low-protein diet. It was Krogh's idea that different respiratory gas exchange ratios (RERs) for the same exercise performed us-

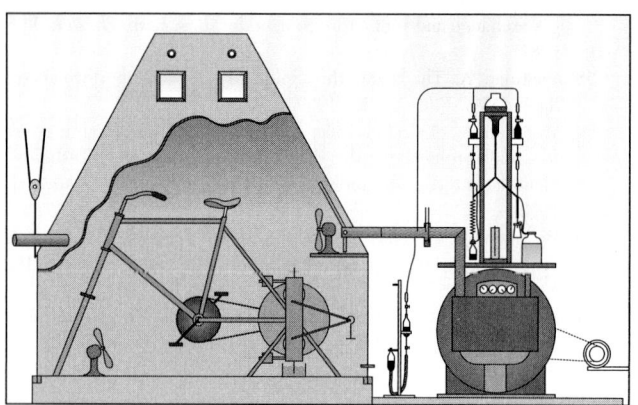

Unique enclosed chamber consisting of a cycle ergometer and two fans. The gas collection apparatus was situated outside and was connected via small-bore tubing. The chamber sat in a water bath to ensure an airtight seal. With this system Krogh collected respiratory gases with an error of less than 1.0%.

ing different diets would indicate the preferential use of a particular fuel substrate.

Krogh made careful measurements of energy expenditure at rest and during 2 hours of cycling exercise using a closed-circuit, air current-flow-through apparatus in common use during that time. A water bath surrounded the chamber to ensure an airtight seal. Subjects rode the stationary bicycle within the chamber with appropriate tubing placed between the subject and a gas collection apparatus outside the chamber (see figure). Typical of Krogh's research, extreme care in data collection ensured high accuracy and reliability of individual

data. The measurements of respiratory gas exchange provided accuracy to within ±1.0%, a remarkable figure considering the hand-made equipment used.

The major findings of the research showed that the energy expended to perform a constant amount of muscular work varied inversely with the RER. This meant that different energy values existed for lipid and carbohydrate; specifically, the energy value per liter of oxygen consumed is less for lipid than for carbohydrate. Although the subjects consumed exclusively either lipid or carbohydrate (with protein held constant), the RER values did not represent combustion of lipid only or carbohydrate only. This permitted determination of the quantitative relationship between the RER and the relative amounts of lipid and carbohydrate catabolized. The researchers showed that the relative amount of energy derived from lipid approximated a straight-line function of the RER.

In a second series of experiments performed on two trained athletes at rest and during exercise, the proportion of carbohydrate to lipid catabolized varied as a function of the relative availabilities of the two substrates. Krogh and Lindhard hypothesized that neither lipid nor carbohydrate exclusively supplied the body's energy requirements during exercise, and that a blend of macronutrients probably served simultaneously as fuel sources during exercise.

Overall, this important experiment showed the following:

1. The efficiency of constant-load exercise increased when using carbohydrate compared to lipid.
2. During severe exercise, subjects performed poorly when lipid (not carbohydrate) served as the preferential nutrient.
3. The preceding diet influences a person's metabolism during rest and in the postabsorptive state.
4. The RER became altered in the transition from rest to moderate exercise, and increased when exercise intensity increased. This indicated greater reliance on carbohydrate as a fuel.
5. Lipid metabolism predominated during the latter portions of 1 hour of constant-load exercise.

Measurement of Human Energy Expenditure

METHODS OF MEASURING THE BODY'S HEAT PRODUCTION

The quantity of energy generated by the body during rest and physical activity can be accurately determined using several different methods. These methods are broadly classified as **direct** and **indirect** calorimetry.

DIRECT CALORIMETRY

All of the metabolic processes that occur in the body result ultimately in the production of heat. Consequently, heat production and metabolism can be viewed in a similar context. Human heat production can be measured directly in a calorimeter similar to the bomb calorimeter, described in Chapter 4, used to determine the energy content of food.

From a historical perspective, the first human calorimeter of major scientific importance was built and perfected by Wesleyan University professors Atwater (a chemist) and Rosa (a physicist) in the 1890s.[1, 17] Their elegant human calorimetric experiments relating energy input to energy expenditure successfully verified the law of the conservation of energy and established the validity of the relationship between direct and indirect calorimetry. The calorimeter, diagramed schematically in Figure 8.1, was a small chamber in which a subject could live, eat, sleep, and exercise on a bicycle ergometer. The experiments lasted from several hours to 13 days, and during some experiments, cycling exercise was performed continuously for up to 16 hours with total energy expenditure exceeding 10,000 kcal! The Atwater-Rosa calorimeter was staffed by 16 people who worked in teams of 8 for 12-hour shifts. The calorimeter consisted of an airtight, thermally-insulated chamber. The heat produced and radiated by the person inside was removed by a stream of cold water that flowed at a constant rate through multiple, large copper "heat absorbers" suspended below the chamber's ceiling. The difference between the temperature of the water entering and leaving the chamber (as measured in 0.01°C with the aid of a microscope mounted along a thermometer) reflected directly the subject's heat production. Humidified air was continually supplied and circulated, and in later experiments, expired carbon dioxide was removed by chemical absorbents. To maintain the normal oxygen supply, oxygen was added to the air before it reentered the calorimeter.

In the 90 years since the seminal papers were published on the Atwater-Rosa human calorimeter, other calorimetric methods have been developed to infer energy expenditure indirectly from metabolic gas exchanges (see next section) in respiration chambers for extended time periods.[5, 8, 12, 13] Methods have also been used to measure metabolic and thermal balance using water flow and air flow calorimeters.[11, 16] The modern space suit worn by astronauts is really a suit calorimeter designed to maintain respiratory gas exchange and thermal balance while the astronaut works for extended periods outside an orbiting space vehicle, on the lunar surface, and, after the turn of the century, constructing space stations or perhaps traveling to other planets.[17]

Direct calorimetry is highly accurate and of great theoretical importance, yet its use is limited. The human calorimeter is relatively expensive to build and maintain and is not applicable to assessing energy expenditures in most sport, recreational, and occupational activities. Its use is highly impractical for large-scale studies in under-developed and poor countries, where there is a great need for total nutritional assessments such as measurements of energy expenditure under a variety of deprivation conditions, particularly undernutrition and starvation.[4]

INDIRECT CALORIMETRY

All energy-releasing reactions in the body ultimately depend on the utilization of oxygen. By measuring a person's oxygen uptake at rest and under conditions of steady-rate exercise, it is possible to obtain an indirect estimate of energy metabolism because the anaerobic energy yield is quite small under such conditions.[2]

Studies using the bomb calorimeter have shown that approximately 4.82 kcal is liberated when a blend of carbohydrate, lipid, and protein is burned in one liter of oxygen. This calorific value for oxygen varies only slightly, even with large variations in the metabolic mixture. Assuming the combustion of a mixed diet, a rounded value of 5.0 kcal per liter of oxygen consumed can be used as an appropriate conversion factor for estimating the body's energy expenditure under steady-rate conditions. This energy-oxygen

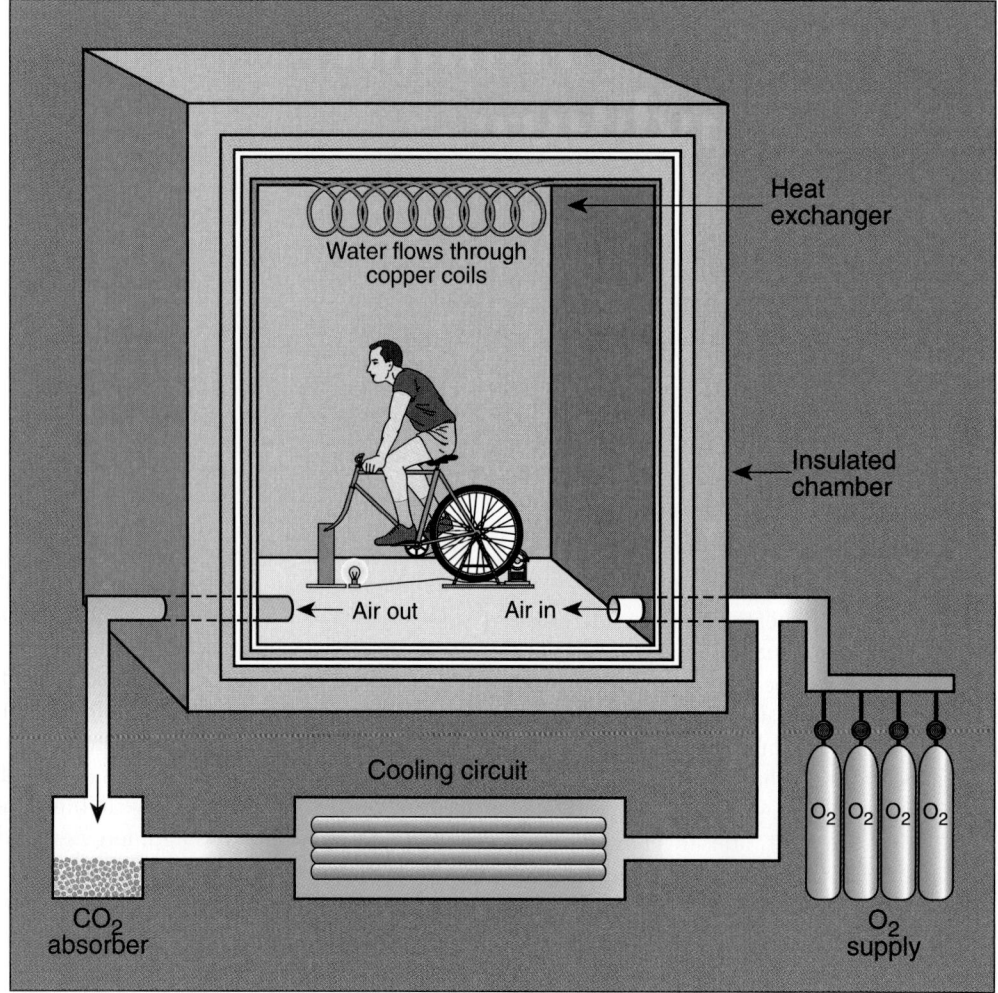

FIGURE 8.1

The body's rate of energy metabolism (heat production) can be measured directly in a human calorimeter. In the Atwater-Rosa calorimeter depicted, a thin sheet of copper lines the interior wall to which heat exchangers are attached overhead and through which cold water is passed. Water cooled to 2°C was passed at a high flow rate (rapidly absorbing the heat radiated from the subject) while the subject exercised. While the subject rested, warmer water was used at a slower flow rate. In the original bicycle ergometer shown in the schematic, the rear wheel was in contact with the shaft of a generator that powered a light bulb. In a later version of the ergometer, the rear wheel was partially constructed of copper. As it rotated through the field of an electromagnet, it produced an electric current from which the power output could be accurately determined. Over the years, various heat-measuring devices have been developed, each based on a different principle of operation. In an **air-flow calorimeter,** the change in air temperature that flows through an insulated space is multiplied by the air's mass and specific heat (including calculations for evaporative heat loss) to provide the rate of heat production. A **water-flow calorimeter** operates in a similar way, except that the change in temperature occurs in water flowing through coils that can be part of a self-contained body suit, such as the space suits worn by astronauts. In **gradient layer calorimetry,** heat produced from a subject flows through a sheet of insulating material (with appropriate piping and cooler water flowing on the outside of the gradient), and the change in temperature that develops across the insulating layer is measured. In **storage calorimetry,** the subject sits in an insulated tank surrounded by a known mass of water at a constant temperature. The heat given off by the subject changes the surrounding water temperature, reflecting heat production.

equivalent of 5.0 kcal per liter is a convenient yardstick for transposing any aerobic physical activity to a caloric frame of reference. In fact, indirect calorimetry through oxygen-uptake measurement is a means to evaluate the caloric stress of most physical activities.

Although the techniques for indirect calorimetry are relatively simple and inexpensive compared to direct measurement of heat production in a human calorimeter, both types of measurement yield comparable results.[15]

Closed-circuit and **open-circuit spirometry** are the two applications of indirect calorimetry.

Closed-Circuit Spirometry

Closed-circuit spirometry, illustrated in Figure 8.2, is used routinely in hospitals and other laboratory settings to estimate resting energy expenditure. The subject breathes from a prefilled container, or spirometer, of 100% oxygen. This equipment constitutes a "closed system" because the person rebreathes only the gas in the spirometer. Carbon dioxide in the exhaled air is absorbed by a canister of soda lime (potassium hydroxide) placed in the breathing circuit. A drum attached to the spirometer revolves at a known speed and records changes in the volume of the system as oxygen is consumed.

During exercise, it is exceedingly difficult to measure oxygen uptake using closed-circuit spirometry. The spirometer is bulky, the subject must remain close to the equipment, the circuit's resistance to the large breathing volumes during exercise is considerable, and the speed of carbon dioxide removal may be inadequate during moderate to heavy exercise. For these reasons, open-circuit spirometry is the most widely used procedure to measure exercise oxygen uptake.

Open-Circuit Spirometry

The open-circuit method provides a relatively simple means for measuring oxygen uptake and indirectly determining energy expenditure. With this method, the subject does not rebreathe from a container of oxygen, as in the closed-circuit method, but instead inhales ambient air with a constant composition of 20.93% oxygen, 0.03% carbon dioxide, and 79.04% nitrogen. The nitrogen fraction also includes a small quantity of inert gases. Because oxygen is used during energy-yielding reactions and carbon dioxide is produced, the exhaled air contains less oxygen and more carbon dioxide than the inhaled air. The difference in composition of the inspired and expired gas volumes reflects the body's constant release of energy through aerobic metabolic reactions.

Three common indirect calorimetry procedures are used to measure oxygen uptake during physical activity:

- Portable spirometry,
- Bag technique, and
- Computerized instrumentation.

Portable Spirometry. The box-shaped portable spirometer shown in Figure 8.3 was originally used to estimate the energy requirements of people working at different industrial jobs and to provide an equitable basis for food rationing in Germany during World War II. The unit weighs about 3 kg and is usually worn on the back. Through a two-way breathing valve, ambient air is inspired, and expired air passes through a gas meter that measures the total expired air volume and collects a small gas sample in a 100-mL butyl rubber bag. This sample is later analyzed for oxygen and carbon dioxide content, and oxygen uptake and energy expenditure are computed for the measurement period.

The attractive aspect of the portable spirometer is that the subject has considerable freedom of movement for a variety of diverse activities such as mountain climbing, downhill skiing, sailing, golf, and gardening. The equipment is

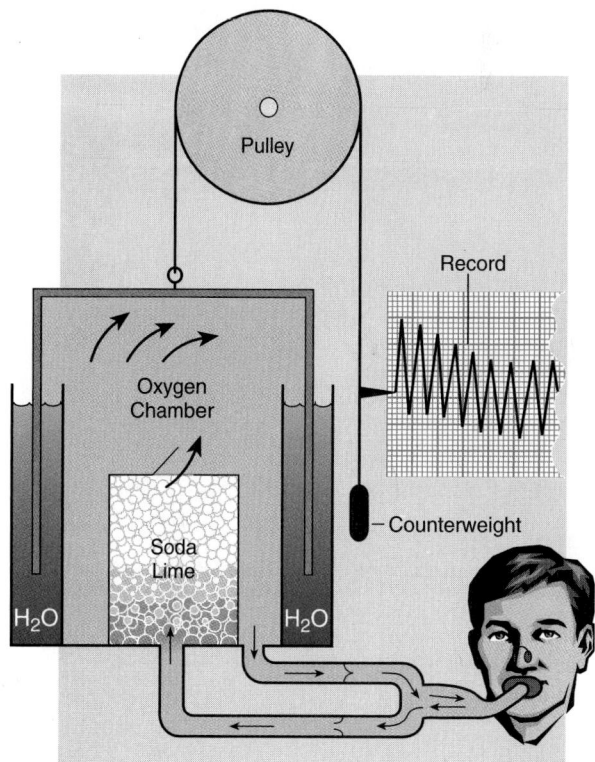

FIGURE 8.2
The closed-circuit method employs a spirometer prefilled with 100% oxygen. The subject breathes from the spirometer, and the expired air's carbon dioxide content is removed as the air is passed through soda lime. Oxygen uptake is computed from the difference between the initial and final volumes of oxygen in the calibrated spirometer during the measurement interval. This method works well for resting conditions or light-intensity exercise. It is inadequate for more intense exercise because of the resistance in the circuit to moving large breathing volumes, and because the production of carbon dioxide exceeds its timely removal by the soda lime absorbent.

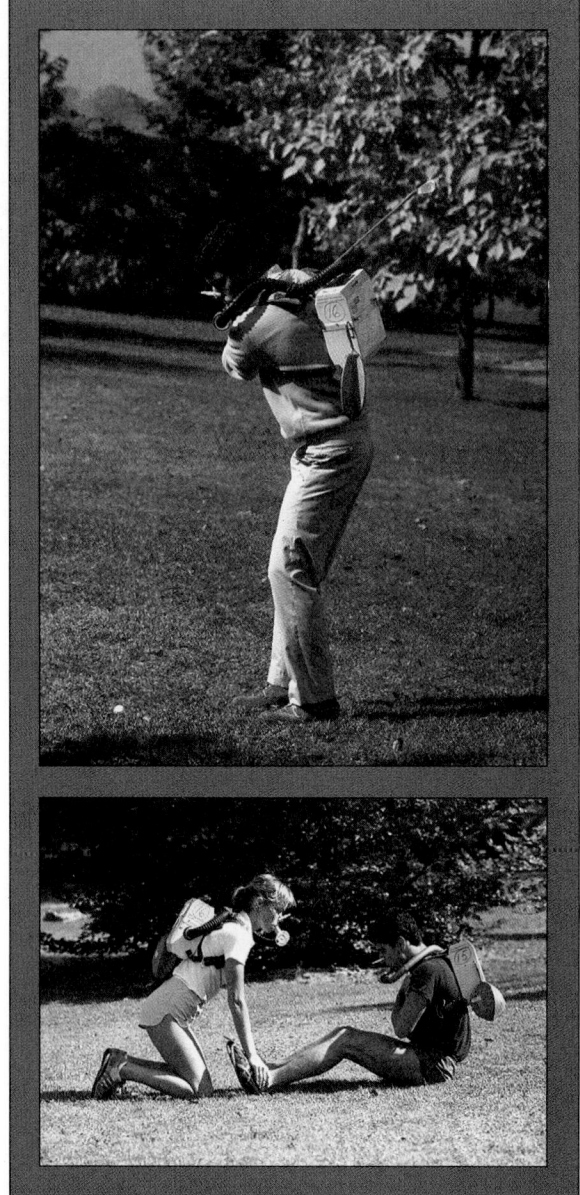

FIGURE 8.3
Portable spirometer used to measure oxygen uptake via the open-circuit method during golf and calisthenics.

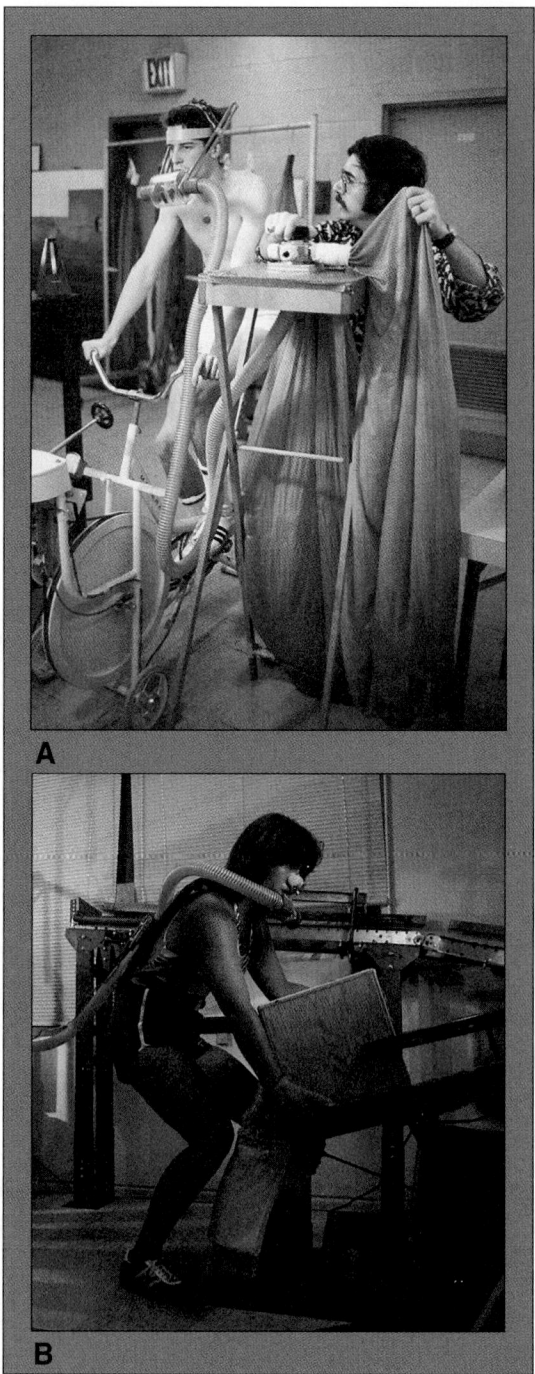

FIGURE 8.4
Measurement of oxygen uptake using open-circuit spirometry (bag technique) during **(A)** stationary cycle ergometer exercise and **(B)** box loading and unloading.

cumbersome during vigorous activity, however, and some questions exist as to the accuracy of air-flow measurements through the meter during heavy exercise and subsequent rapid breathing.

Bag Technique. The bag technique is depicted in Figure 8.4A and B. The subject wears special headgear with a two-way, high-velocity, low-resistance breathing valve. Ambient air is breathed in through one side of the valve while expired air is expelled out the other side. The air then passes into either large canvas or plastic Douglas bags (named for the respiratory physiologist who popularized their use) or rubber meteorological balloons, or directly

through a gas meter, which continually measures the volume of expired air. A small sample of expired air is collected and analyzed for its oxygen and carbon dioxide composition. As with all indirect calorimetric techniques, energy expenditure is computed from oxygen uptake using the appropriate calorific transformation for oxygen.

Computerized Instrumentation. Advances in computer and microprocessor technology enable exercise scientists to efficiently measure metabolic and physiologic responses to exercise. A computer is interfaced with at least three instruments: a system to continually sample the subject's expired air, a flow meter or turbine device to record the volume of air breathed, and oxygen and carbon dioxide analyzers to measure the fractional composition of the expired gas mixture. The computer is programmed to perform the metabolic calculations based on the electronic signals it receives from the instruments. A printed or graphic display of the data is provided throughout the measurement period. More advanced systems include automated blood pressure, heart rate, and temperature monitors as well as computerized programs to regulate the speed, duration, and workload of a treadmill, bicycle ergometer, stepper, rower, or other piece of exercise equipment. The automated-computerized approach yields reproducible and accurate

measurements compared to the more time-consuming Douglas bag or balloon methods previously described.[9,18] Figure 8.5 depicts an example of the automated and computerized measurement of metabolic and physiologic responses during exercise.

The system illustrated in Figure 8.6 provides the wireless telemetric transmission of data for metabolic measurement—pulmonary ventilation and oxygen and carbon dioxide analysis—during a broad range of exercise, sport, and occupational activities. The components are light-weight (less than 2 lb) and miniaturized to fit into a small pack-vest worn around the chest. The system contains a voice-sensitive chip that provides feedback on pacing, duration of exercise, energy expenditure, heart rate, and ventilation. The microprocessor in the unit can store up to several hours of exercise data for later downloading to a computer. Using telemetry, data collection is viewed on line and in real time on a host computer. With proper and frequent calibra-

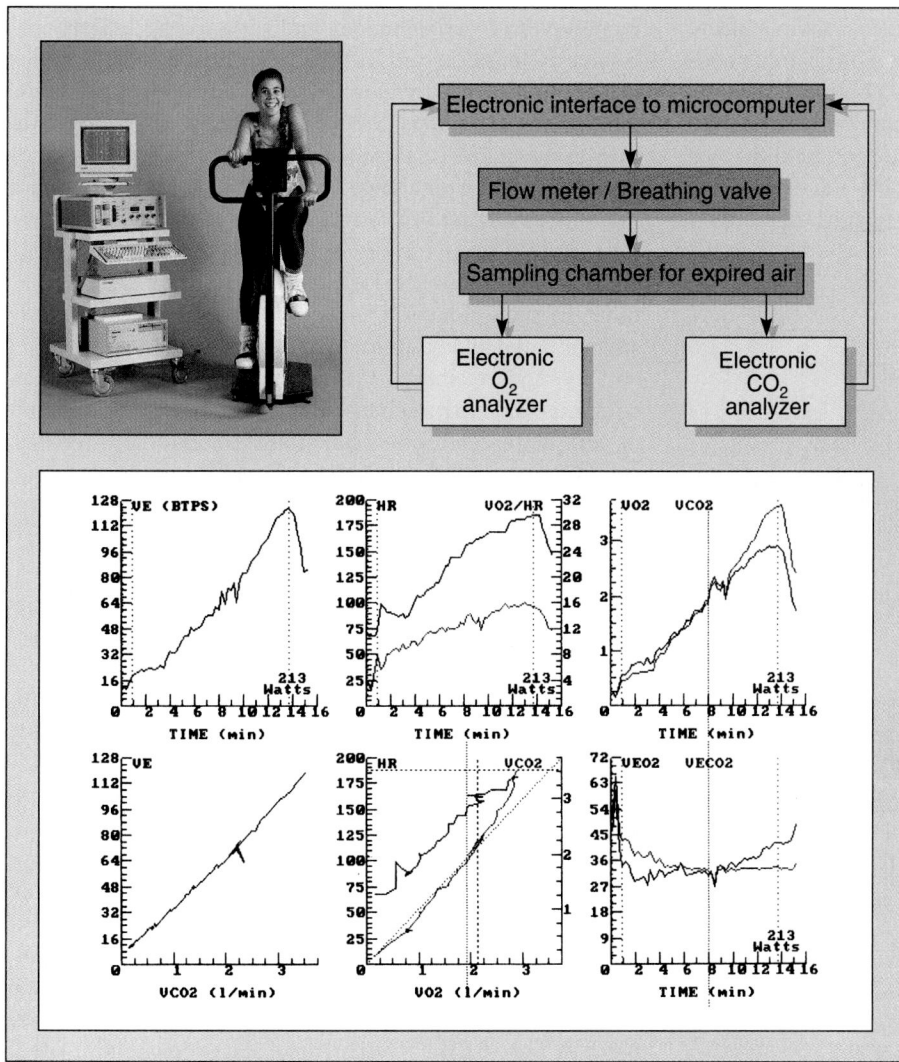

FIGURE 8.5

Computer systems approach to the collection, analysis, and output of physiologic and metabolic data. (Photo courtesy of Fitco, a division of Physio-Dyne Instrument Corporation, Farmingdale, NY.)

tions, such commercially available miniaturized equipment provides reasonable accuracy for quantifying the energy cost "in vivo" of diverse physical activities.[3]

Although there are tremendous advantages to computerized systems in terms of operational ease and rapid data analysis, there are also distinct disadvantages including the relatively high cost of equipment and delays resulting from system breakdowns. And, of course, good results require good data. *Regardless of the apparent sophistication of a particular automated system, the output data are only as good as the accuracy of the measuring device. In large part, this accuracy depends on careful and frequent calibration of the electronic equipment using established reference standards.*

Methods of Calibration

Figure 8.7 illustrates two common chemical procedures for analyzing various gas mixtures of oxygen, carbon dioxide, and nitrogen and for calibrating electronic analyzers. Using the micro-Scholander technique, oxygen and carbon dioxide concentrations in expired air can be measured to an accuracy of 0.015 volume percent.[14] A 0.5-mL "micro" sample of the gas to be analyzed is introduced into a reaction chamber connected to a mercury-containing micrometer burette. The gas sample is then drawn into the reaction chamber by tilting the apparatus without altering the total liquid content of the system. As the sample comes into contact with the oxygen and carbon dioxide absorbents, a measurable quantity of mercury

is released to the system from the burette to maintain the original balance of the gas against the compensating chamber. The vapor tension within the system is maintained by raising and lowering the fluid and absorbents, and changes in gas volume (as absorption takes place) are read directly from the micrometer. The fractional concentrations of oxygen, carbon dioxide, and nitrogen are then computed using standard volumetric computations.

Another technique for gas analysis is the Haldane method.[6] With this analyzer, the gas sample is moved by means of a column of mercury from the initial measuring burette to gas absorption tubes and then back to the burette for remeasurement. The volume decreases when the gas sample comes into contact with the reagent potassium hydroxide, converting it to potassium carbonate as the carbon dioxide is removed from the original gas sample. The gas sample (minus its carbon dioxide) is then brought into contact with pyrogallate, an alkaline solution that captures the oxygen in the sample; this again decreases the volume of the original gas, which is then accurately measured. The volume of gas remaining in the burette is nitrogen.

Before the widespread use of computerized instrumentation to measure oxygen and carbon dioxide fractional concentrations in expired air, all determinations of the body's oxygen uptake used primarily the Scholander or Haldane method of gas analysis. Studies of exercise energy expenditure using indirect calorimetry might involve hundreds of separate analyses for a single experiment, requiring frequent multiple calibrations to verify results. For this and other reasons, studies from early exercise physiology literature only used one or two subjects for energy metabolism studies. Fortunately, such pioneering efforts were conducted carefully and with meticulous attention to instrumentation calibration and method reliability. Unfortunately, undue reliance on computerized instrumentation and "certified" gas calibration in current research often substitutes for the more tedious, yet often more valid, "classic" methods.

DIRECT VERSUS INDIRECT CALORIMETRY

Energy metabolism studies using both direct and indirect calorimetry provide convincing evidence for the validity of the indirect method to estimate energy metabolism. At the turn of the century, the two calorimetric methods were compared in experiments conducted for 40 days on three men living in calorimeters similar to the one shown in Figure 8.1. Their daily caloric outputs averaged 2723 kcal when measured directly by heat production and 2717 kcal when computed indirectly using closed-circuit measures of oxygen uptake. Other experiments with animals and humans based on moderate exercise also demonstrated a close agreement between direct and indirect methods, and in most instances, the difference was less than 1%. It is noteworthy that in the Atwater and Rosa calorimetry experiments, the method error was only 0.2%, a remarkable achievement given that

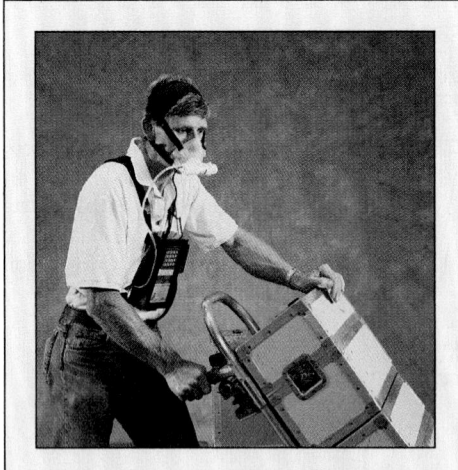

FIGURE 8.6

Miniature metabolic system. The 3 × 6-inch system is worn in a chest-vest containing the electronic instrumentation, battery, oxygen and carbon dioxide sensors, and telemetry connections to a microcomputer that permits infrared transmissions of up to 3 miles to a source computer. The metabolic system weighs approximately 1.13 kg (2.5 lb) and is easily transported during physical activity. (Photo courtesy of AeroSport, Inc., Ann Arbor, MI.)

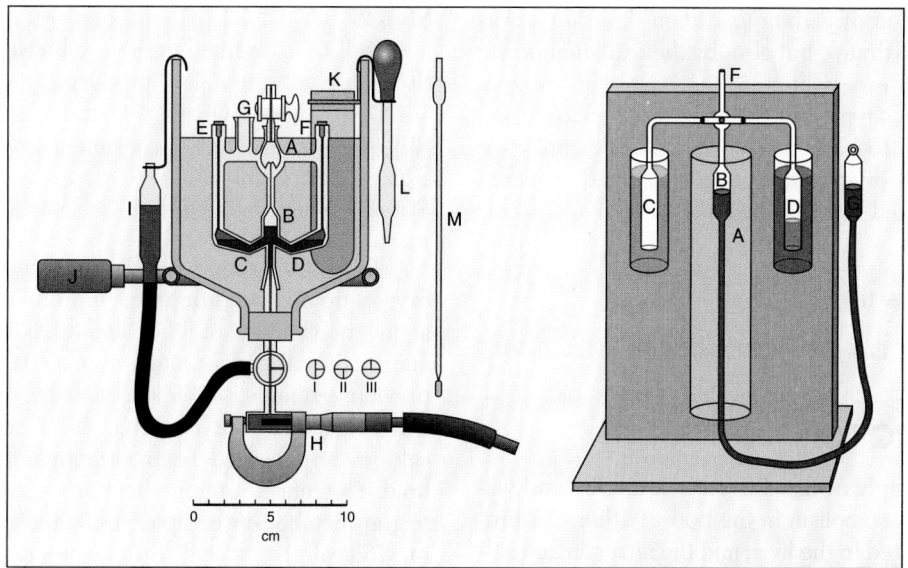

FIGURE 8.7

Two common analytical procedures for gas calibration. *Left.* Micro-Scholander gas analyzer: **(A)** compensating chamber, **(B)** reaction chamber, **(C)** side-arm for CO_2 absorber, **(D)** side-arm for O_2 absorber, **(E and F)** solid vaccine bottle stoppers, **(G)** receptacle for stopcock, **(H)** micrometer burette, **(I)** leveling bulb containing mercury, **(J)** handle for titling apparatus, **(K)** tube for storing the acid rinsing solution, **(L)** pipette for the rinsing acid, and **(M)** transfer pipette. *Right.* Haldane gas analyzer: **(A)** water jacket surrounding the measuring burette, **(B)** calibrated measuring burette containing a thermo-barometer to compensate for changes in temperature and barometric pressure, **(C)** vessel containing CO_2 absorber (potassium hydroxide), **(D)** vessel containing O_2 absorber (pyrogallate), **(E)** glass valve, **(F)** entry for gas sample, and **(G)** mercury leveling bulb. The gas introduced into the burette is lowered into the appropriate CO_2 and O_2 absorbers by alternately lowering and raising the mercury leveling bulb. The CO_2 and O_2 gas volumes are determined by subtracting the initial volume of the gas from the final volume and correcting for the water vapor at a given temperature and atmospheric pressure.

these experiments were conducted using mostly hand-made instruments. They were conducted with a dedication to precise calibration methods long before the availability of electronic instrumentation.

THE RESPIRATORY QUOTIENT (RQ)

Because of inherent differences in the chemical compositions of carbohydrates, lipids, and proteins, different amounts of oxygen are required to oxidize completely the molecule's carbon and hydrogen atoms to the carbon dioxide and water end products. Thus, the quantity of carbon dioxide produced in relation to oxygen consumed varies somewhat depending on the substrate metabolized. This ratio of metabolic gas exchange in the combustion of food is termed the respiratory quotient, or RQ, and is defined as follows:

$$RQ = CO_2 \text{ produced} \div O_2 \text{ consumed}$$

The RQ is useful for evaluating rest and aerobic exercise because it serves as a convenient, though perhaps general, guide to the macronutrient mixture catabolized for energy.[7, 10] Also, because the caloric equivalent for oxygen differs somewhat depending on the nutrient oxidized, one

must know both the RQ and the oxygen uptake to estimate precisely the body's heat production.

RQ FOR CARBOHYDRATE

Because the ratio of hydrogen to oxygen atoms in carbohydrates is always the same as in water, that is, 2:1, all of the oxygen consumed by cells is used to oxidize the carbon in the carbohydrate molecule to carbon dioxide. Consequently, during the complete oxidation of a glucose molecule, six molecules of oxygen are consumed and six molecules of carbon dioxide are produced. The overall equation for this reaction is:

$$C_6H_{12}O_6 + 6\,O_2 \rightarrow 6\,CO_2 + 6\,H_2O$$

Because the gas exchange in this reaction is equal, the RQ for carbohydrate is unity, or 1.00:

$$RQ = 6\,CO_2 \div 6\,O_2 = 1.00$$

RQ FOR LIPID

The chemical composition of lipids differs from carbohydrates because lipids contain considerably fewer oxygen atoms in proportion to atoms of hydrogen. Consequently, when a lipid is catabolized for energy, oxygen is required not only for the oxidation of carbon to carbon dioxide (as was the case for carbohydrate), but also for the oxidation of the hydrogen atoms in excess of their 2:1 ratio with oxygen. When palmitic acid, a typical fatty acid, is oxidized to carbon dioxide and water, 16 carbon dioxide molecules are produced for every 23 oxygen molecules consumed. This exchange is summarized by the equation:

$$C_{16}H_{32}O_2 + 23\ O_2 \rightarrow 16\ CO_2 + 16\ H_2O$$
$$RQ = 16\ CO_2 \div 23\ O_2 = 0.696$$

Generally, the RQ value for lipid is considered to be 0.70.

RQ FOR PROTEIN

Proteins are not simply oxidized to carbon dioxide and water during energy metabolism in the body. Rather, the protein is first deaminated in the liver, and the nitrogen and sulfur fragments are excreted in the urine and feces. The resulting "keto acid" fragments are then oxidized to carbon dioxide and water to provide energy to sustain metabolism. As was the case with lipid breakdown, these short-chain keto acids require, for complete combustion, more oxygen in relation to carbon dioxide produced. The protein albumin oxidizes as follows:

$$C_{72}H_{112}N_2O_{22}S + 77\ O_2 \rightarrow$$
Albumin

$$63\ CO_2 + 38\ H_2O + SO_3 + 9\ CO(NH_2)_2$$
Urea

$$RQ = 63\ CO_2 \div 77\ O_2 = 0.818$$

The general value for the RQ of protein is 0.82.

NONPROTEIN RQ

The RQ computed from the compositional analysis of expired air usually reflects the catabolism of a blend of carbohydrates, lipids, and proteins. The precise contribution of each of these nutrients to the metabolic mixture can be determined. For example, approximately 1 g of urinary nitrogen is excreted for every 6.25 g of protein metabolized for energy. Each gram of excreted nitrogen represents a carbon dioxide production of approximately 4.8 L and an oxygen uptake of approximately 6.0 L. Within this framework, the following example illustrates the stepwise procedure for calculating the **nonprotein** elements in the RQ, that is, that portion of the respiratory exchange not attributed to the combustion of protein but **only** to the combustion of carbohydrate and lipid.

This example is based on data from a subject who consumes 4.0 L of oxygen and produces 3.4 L of carbon dioxide during a 15-minute rest period. During this time, 0.13 g of nitrogen are excreted in the urine.

Step 1. 4.8 L $CO_2 \cdot g^{-1}$ protein catabolized $\times$ 0.13 g = 0.62 L CO_2 produced in the catabolism of protein.

Step 2. 6.0 L $O_2 \cdot g^{-1}$ protein catabolized $\times$ 0.13 g = 0.78 L O_2 consumed in the catabolism of protein.
Step 3. Nonprotein CO_2 produced = 3.4 L CO_2 − 0.62 L CO_2 = 2.78 L CO_2.
Step 4. Nonprotein O_2 consumed = 4.0 L O_2 − 0.78 L O_2 = 3.22 L O_2.
Step 5. Nonprotein RQ = 2.78 ÷ 3.22 = 0.86.

Table 8.1 presents the thermal (energy) equivalents for oxygen uptake for different nonprotein RQ values and the actual percentage of lipid and carbohydrate utilized for energy. For the nonprotein RQ of 0.86 computed in the previous example, 4.875 kcal are liberated per liter of oxygen consumed. For this RQ, 54.1% of the "nonprotein" calories are derived from carbohydrate and 45.9% from lipid. The total 15-minute heat production at rest attributed to the metabolism of lipid and carbohydrate is 15.70 kcal (4.875 kcal $\cdot$ L^{-1} × 3.22 L O_2); the energy from the breakdown of protein is equal to 3.51 kcal (4.5 kcal $\cdot$ L^{-1} × 0.78 L O_2). Consequently, the total energy from both the protein and nonprotein macronutrients during the 15-minute period is 19.21 kcal (15.70 kcal nonprotein + 3.51 kcal protein).

Interestingly, had the thermal equivalent for a mixed diet with an RQ of 0.82 been used in the caloric transformation, or had the RQ had been obtained simply from the total respiratory gas exchange and applied to Table 8.1 without considering the protein component, the estimated energy expenditure during this period would have been about 19.3 kcal (4.825 kcal $\cdot$ L^{-1} × 4.0 L O_2, assuming a mixed diet)—a difference of only 0.5% from the value obtained using the more elaborate and time-consuming method requiring urinary nitrogen analysis.

Although the use of Table 8.1 assumes a nonprotein RQ, in most cases, the gross metabolic RQ calculated without measures of urinary and other nitrogen introduces only minimal error because the contribution of protein to energy metabolism is relatively small.

HOW MUCH FOOD WAS METABOLIZED FOR ENERGY?

The last two columns of Table 8.1 present the conversions for nonprotein RQ to grams of carbohydrate and lipid metabolized per liter of oxygen consumed. For the subject with an RQ of 0.86, this represents approximately 0.62 g of carbohydrate and 0.25 g of lipid. For the 3.22 L of oxygen consumed during the 15-minute period of rest, 2.00 g of carbohydrate (3.22 L O_2 × 0.62) and 0.80 g of lipid (3.22 L O_2 × 0.25) were metabolized for energy.

RQ FOR A MIXED DIET

During activities that range from complete bed rest to mild, aerobic exercise such as walking or slow jogging, the RQ seldom reflects the oxidation of pure carbohydrate or pure lipid. Instead, a mixture of these nutrients is usually used, and the intermediate RQ value is between 0.70 and 1.00. *For most purposes, an RQ of 0.82 from the metabolism of a mixture of 40% carbohydrate and 60% lipid can be assumed, and the caloric equivalent of 4.825 kcal per liter of oxygen can be applied in energy transformations.* Using this midpoint value, the maximum error possible in estimating energy metabolism from oxygen uptake would be only about 4%. Of course, if greater precision is required, the actual RQ can be calculated and Table 8.1 consulted to obtain the exact caloric transformation as well as the percent-

age contribution of carbohydrate and lipid to the metabolic mixture.

RESPIRATORY EXCHANGE RATIO (R)

The application of the RQ is based on the assumption that the exchange of oxygen and carbon dioxide measured at the lungs reflects the actual gas exchange from nutrient catabolism in the cell. This assumption is reasonably valid under steady-rate exercise conditions.[7] However, factors can spuriously alter the exchange of oxygen and carbon dioxide in the

---

TABLE 8.1
THERMAL EQUIVALENTS OF OXYGEN FOR THE NONPROTEIN RESPIRATORY QUOTIENT (RQ), INCLUDING PERCENT KILOCALORIES AND GRAMS DERIVED FROM CARBOHYDRATE AND LIPID

Nonprotein RQ	kcal per $L\,O_2$	Percentage kcal Derived from		Grams per $L\,O_2$	
		Carbohydrate	Lipid	Carbohydrate	Lipid
0.707	4.686	0.0	100.0	0.000	.496
.71	4.690	1.1	98.9	.012	.491
.72	4.702	4.8	95.2	.051	.476
.73	4.714	8.4	91.6	.090	.460
.74	4.727	12.0	88.0	.130	.444
.75	4.739	15.6	84.4	.170	.428
.76	4.750	19.2	80.8	.211	.412
.77	4.764	22.8	77.2	.250	.396
.78	4.776	26.3	73.7	.290	.380
.79	4.788	29.9	70.1	.330	.363
.80	4.801	33.4	66.6	.371	.347
.81	4.813	36.9	63.1	.413	.330
.82	4.825	40.3	59.7	.454	.313
.83	4.838	43.8	56.2	.496	.297
.84	4.850	47.2	52.8	.537	.280
.85	4.862	50.7	49.3	.579	.263
.86	4.875	54.1	45.9	.621	.247
.87	4.887	57.5	42.5	.663	.230
.88	4.899	60.8	39.2	.705	.213
.89	4.911	64.2	35.8	.749	.195
.90	4.924	67.5	32.5	.791	.178
.91	4.936	70.8	29.2	.834	.160
.92	4.948	74.1	25.9	.877	.143
.93	4.961	77.4	22.6	.921	.125
.94	4.973	80.7	19.3	.964	.108
.95	4.985	84.0	16.0	1.008	.090
.96	4.998	87.2	12.8	1.052	.072
.97	5.010	90.4	9.6	1.097	.054
.98	5.022	93.6	6.4	1.142	.036
.99	5.035	96.8	3.2	1.186	.018
1.00	5.047	100.0	0	1.231	.000

From Zuntz, H.: *Pflugers Arch. Physiol.*, 83:557, 1901.

lungs so that the ratio of this gas exchange no longer reflects only the substrate mixture in energy metabolism. Respiratory physiologists have termed the ratio of carbon dioxide produced to oxygen consumed under such conditions—the exchange of oxygen and carbon dioxide at the lungs no longer reflects the oxidation of specific foods in the cells—the respiratory exchange ratio, or R. This ratio is calculated in exactly the same manner as the RQ.

For example, carbon dioxide elimination increases during hyperventilation (refer to Chapter 14) when the breathing response is disproportionate to the metabolic demands of a particular situation. As a result of this overbreathing, the normal level of carbon dioxide in the blood is reduced because the gas is "blown off" in the expired air. This additional carbon dioxide elimination is not accompanied by a corresponding increase in oxygen uptake; thus, there is a rise in the respiratory exchange ratio that cannot be attributed to the oxidation of foodstuff. In such cases, the R usually increases to above 1.00.

Exhaustive exercise presents another situation where the R can rise significantly above 1.00. The lactic acid generated during anaerobic metabolism is buffered, or "neutralized," by sodium bicarbonate in the blood to maintain the proper acid-base balance in the reaction:

$$HLa + NaHCO_3 \rightleftharpoons NaLa + H_2CO_3 \rightleftharpoons$$
$$H_2O + CO_2 \rightleftharpoons Lungs$$

This process produces carbonic acid, a weaker acid (refer to Chapter 14). In the pulmonary capillaries, carbonic acid breaks down to its components, carbon dioxide and water, and the carbon dioxide exits through the lungs. This buffering process adds "extra" carbon dioxide to the expired air above that quantity normally released during energy metabolism, and the R moves toward and above 1.00. In rare instances, the exchange ratio exceeds 1.00 when a person gains body fat through excess intake of dietary carbohydrate. In this lipogenic situation, oxygen is liberated when carbohydrate is converted to lipid as the excess calories are stored in adipose tissue. This "extra" oxygen is then used in energy metabolism; consequently, less atmospheric oxygen is consumed even though the normal metabolic complement of carbon dioxide is released during energy metabolism.

It is also possible to obtain relatively low R values. For example, following exhaustive exercise, carbon dioxide is retained in the cells and body fluids to replenish the bicarbonate that was used to buffer the accumulating lactic acid. This action reduces the expired carbon dioxide without affecting oxygen uptake and may cause the respiratory exchange ratio to dip below 0.70.

METABOLIC CALCULATIONS

Much of the study of exercise physiology involves the measurement of energy metabolism. Measurements of the oxygen and carbon dioxide contents of expired air, together with either the inspired or expired breathing volume, provide the basic data for determining respiratory gas exchange and oxygen uptake and inferring the body's rate of energy expenditure. Appendix C presents the step-by-step method and rationale for metabolic calculations based on experimental data using open-circuit spirometry.

■ SUMMARY ■

1. Direct and indirect calorimetry are the two methods for determining the body's rate of energy expenditure. Using direct calorimetry, the actual heat production is measured in an appropriately insulated calorimeter. Indirect calorimetry infers energy expenditure from measurements of oxygen uptake and carbon dioxide production using the methods of closed-circuit or open-circuit spirometry.

2. Because of its chemical composition, each nutrient requires a different quantity of oxygen uptake in relation to carbon dioxide production during its complete oxidation. The ratio of carbon dioxide produced to oxygen consumed is called the respiratory quotient (RQ) and provides an important clue to the nutrient mixture catabolized for energy. The RQ for carbohydrate is 1.00, for lipid, 0.70, and for protein, 0.82.

3. For each RQ value, there is a corresponding caloric value for each liter of oxygen consumed. This value enables a high degree of accuracy in determining energy expenditure during exercise.

4. Because of the nonmetabolic production of carbon dioxide, as occurs during the buffering of lactic acid, the RQ is not representative of specific substrate utilization during strenuous exercise.

5. The respiratory exchange ratio, or R, reflects the pulmonary exchange of carbon dioxide and oxygen under various physiologic and metabolic conditions that do not fully reflect the macronutrient mixture being catabolized.

■ REFERENCES ■

1. Atwater, W.O., and Rosa, E.B.: Description of a new respiration calorimeter and experiments on the conservation of energy in the human body. Bulletin No. 63, Washington, D.C., U.S. Department of Agriculture, Office of Experiment Stations, Government Printing Office, 1899.

2. Brooks, G.A., et al.: Estimation of anaerobic energy production and efficiency in rats during exercise. *J. Appl. Physiol.*, 56:520, 1984.

3. Crandall, C.G., et al.: Evaluation of the Cosmed K2 portable telemetric oxygen uptake analyzer. *Med. Sci. Sports Exerc.*, 26:108, 1994.

4. Dulloo, A.G., et al.: A low-budget and easy-to-operate room respirometer for measuring daily energy expenditure in man. *Am J. Clin. Nutr.* 48:1367, 1988.

5. Ferraro, R., et al.: Energy cost of physical activity on a metabolic ward in relationship to obesity. *Am J. Clin. Nutr.* 53:1368, 1991.

6. Haldane, J.S., and Priestley, J.G.: *Respiration.* New York, Oxford University Press, 1935.

7. Jansson, E.: On the significance of the respiratory exchange ratio after different diets during exercise in man. *Acta Physiol. Scand.,* 114:103, 1982.

8. Jéquier, E, and Schutz, Y.: Long-term measurements of energy expenditure in humans using a respiration chamber. *Am J. Clin. Nutr.,* 38:989, 1983.

9. Kannagi, T., et al.: An evaluation of the Beckman Metabolic Cart for measuring ventilation and aerobic requirements during exercise. *J. Cardiac Rehab.,* 3:38, 1983.

10. Livesey, G., and Elia, M.: Estimation of energy expenditure, net carbohydrate utilization and net fat oxidization and synthesis by indirect calorimetry: evaluation of errors with special reference to detailed composition of fuels. *Am. J. Clin. Nutr.,* 47:608, 1988.

11. Murgatroyd, R.R., and James, W.P.T.: Energy measurement in man by direct calorimetry. In *Recent Advances in Obesity Research.* Bjorntorp et al. (Eds.), London, John-Libby, 1982.

12. Ravussin, E., et al.: Determinants of 24-hour energy expenditure in man: methods and results using a respiratory chamber. *J. Clin. Invest.,* 78:1568, 1986.

13. Rumpler, W., et al.: Repeatability of 24-hour energy expenditure measurements in humans by indirect calorimetry. *Am J. Clin. Nutr.,* 51:147, 1990.

14. Scholander, P.F.: Analyzer for accurate estimation of respiratory gases in one-half cubic centimeter samples. *J. Biol. Chem.,* 167:235, 1947.

15. Snellen, J.W.: Studies in human calorimetry. In *Assessment of Energy in Health and Disease.* Columbus, Ohio, Ross Laboratories, 1980.

16. Snellen, J.W., et al.: Technical description and performance characteristics of a human whole-body calorimeter. *Med. Biol. Eng. Comput.,* 21:9, 1983.

17. Webb, P.: *Human Calorimeters.* Endocrinology and Metabolism Series, Vol. 7. New York, Praeger Scientific, 1985.

18. Wilmore, J.H., et al.: An automated system for assessing metabolic and respiratory function during exercise. *J. Appl. Physiol.,* 40:619, 1976.

Margaria, R., et al.: The possible mechanisms of contracting and paying the oxygen debt and the role of lactic acid in muscular contraction. *Am. J. Physiol.* **106:689, 1933.**

Hill and colleagues had theorized that the cause for the increased oxygen uptake during recovery (the so-called oxygen debt) occurred from the delayed oxidation of a fraction of the lactic acid

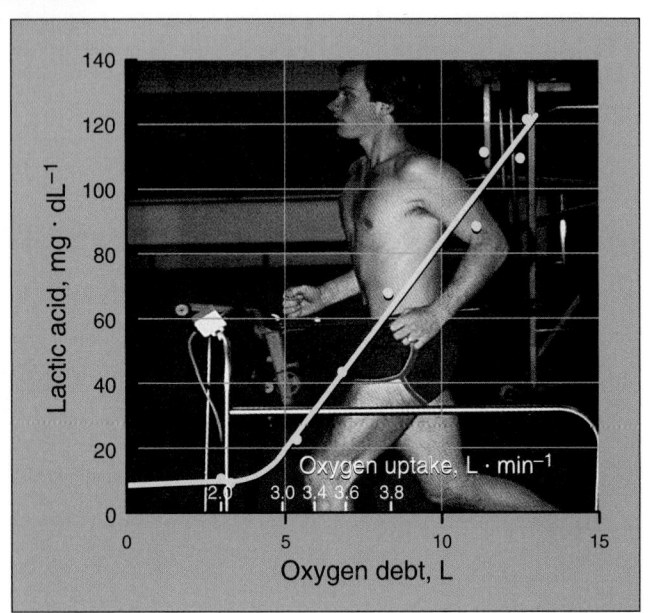

Relation between lactic acid concentration in the blood and oxygen debt (calculated after A.V. Hill), and oxygen uptake at various levels of exercise. Duration of exercise was 10 minutes in each case.

(LA) produced during anaerobic processes in muscular activity. These researchers, however, did not provide direct evidence for quantifying the relationship between the oxygen debt and LA production to confirm their hypothesis.

Margaria and his group of researchers working at the prestigious Harvard Fatigue Laboratory provided the first quantitative evaluation of Hill's theory. The researchers described the time-course characteristics of LA removal, and related this to the oxygen uptake during recovery. The curve for LA removal, described as an exponential function of time, showed a rate of disappearance proportionate to LA content at any time in recovery. The

exact form of the oxygen uptake recovery curve, subdivided into two distinct parts, related to different metabolic events in exercise. The terms "alactic" and "lactacid" oxygen debt described the different portions of the recovery oxygen uptake curve.

Experimental evidence came from one subject observed during 10-minute runs on different occasions. LA, measured at different times during each exercise period from the femoral vein and an arm artery and vein, diffused rapidly and uniformly throughout the body. Blood LA concentration varied proportionally to the body's total LA content. The figure illustrates the relationship between LA concentration in blood during exercise and recovery oxygen uptake. Note that the curve did not begin to deviate from baseline LA levels until the oxygen debt reached 3 to 4 liters. For this subject, this coincided with an exercise $\dot{V}O_2$ of about 3.0 $L \cdot min^{-1}$. The concentration of blood LA (and corresponding oxygen debt) then increased as a linear function of exercise $\dot{V}O_2$. The researchers reasoned that when oxygen debt was less than about 3 L, the LA mechanism remained inactive during exercise. They called this type of exercise "alactic" to signify that the work was performed with minimal LA accumulation. In this case, the $\dot{V}O_2$ would return to resting levels rapidly during recovery. LA accumulated in the blood with exercise of about two-thirds of the maximum aerobic metabolic rate ($\dot{V}O_2max$), thereafter increasing rapidly. LA removal, a slow process, had a velocity constant of 0.02 (one-half removed each 15 minutes).

The researchers concluded that the LA mechanism would play an important role only during strenuous exercise. They also postulated that the total recovery $\dot{V}O_2$ consisted of the sum effect of two distinct mechanisms: a "lactacid" oxygen debt attributable to oxidation of lactic acid, and an amount ("alactic" oxygen debt) occurring at the beginning of recovery unrelated to LA oxidation. This important systematic experiment provided insight into why the recovery $\dot{V}O_2$ remained elevated above baseline values. Subsequent research in the late 1970s further clarified the exact mechanisms underlying the presence of the oxygen debt so eloquently described in this classic 1933 paper.

Human Energy Expenditure During Rest and Physical Activity

Metabolism involves all the chemical reactions of biological molecules within the body, including both synthesis (anabolism) and breakdown (catabolism). Figure 9.1 illustrates that the total daily energy expenditure (TDEE) is influenced by three general factors:

- Resting metabolic rate (includes basal and sleeping conditions plus the added metabolic cost of arousal)
- Thermogenic effect of food consumed
- Energy expended during physical activity and recovery

PART 1
ENERGY EXPENDITURE AT REST

BASAL METABOLIC RATE

A minimum level of energy is required to sustain the body's vital functions in the waking state. This energy requirement is called the **basal metabolic rate,** or **BMR.** The BMR reflects the body's heat production and is determined indirectly by measuring oxygen uptake under fairly stringent conditions. Measurements are made in the postabsorptive state: Food is not eaten for at least 12 hours before testing to avoid an increase in metabolism resulting from the digestion, absorption, and assimilation of the ingested nutrients. To reduce other calorigenic influences, physical activity is also restricted prior to the BMR test. The subject rests supine in a comfortable thermoneutral environment for about 30 minutes, after which time oxygen uptake is measured for a 10-minute period. Values for oxygen uptake during the BMR test usually range between 160 and 290 mL per minute (0.8 and 1.43 kcal · min^{-1}), depending on a variety of factors, especially overall body size and in particular the fat-free body mass (FFM).[13]

The BMR can be used to establish the important energy baseline for constructing a sound program of weight control based on diet, exercise, or the effective combination of both. In most instances, so-called basal values measured under controlled laboratory conditions are only slightly lower than values for resting metabolic rate (RMR) measured under less strict conditions, 3 to 4 hours after a light meal and without prior physical activity. For our purposes, RMR refers to the sum of the metabolic processes of the active cell mass related to the maintenance of normal body functions and regulatory balance during rest. For the typical person, the RMR accounts for about 60 to 75% of the TDEE, while the thermic effects of feeding account for approximately 10%, and physical activity for the remaining 15 to 30%.

METABOLISM AT REST

Scientists in the late 1800s observed that energy metabolism at rest is proportional to the surface area of the body. Consequently, a "surface area law" was proposed to account for individual differences in energy metabolism. In a series of experiments during which the metabolisms of a dog and man were determined over a 24-hour period, the total heat generated by the larger man was about 200% greater than that generated by the dog. When heat production was expressed in relation to surface area, however, the metabolic difference between man and dog was reduced to only about 10%. This finding led to the common practice of expressing resting metabolic rate (energy expenditure) relative to body surface area.

Later studies in the 1920s provided evidence that the surface area formulation did not apply universally to diverse species of temperature-regulating animals. One classic monograph proposed the concept of *metabolic size,* which related basal metabolism to the 0.75 power of body mass.[23] This value of body mass to the 0.75 power holds true not only for humans, but for a wide variety of other mammals and birds differing considerably in body sizes and shapes. Figure 9.2 is a logarithmic plot of body mass (ranging from 0.01 kg to 10,000 kg) and metabolic rate (ranging from 0.1 to 1000 W). This best-fitting straight line describing the relationship between metabolism (expressed as an animal's energy production or oxygen uptake) and body mass truly is a remarkable fit and one of the more striking biological observations related to animal size and physiological function.

Many subsequent studies have demonstrated that indexing the RMR to lean body mass (representing the nonadipose tissue) and fat-free body mass (representing

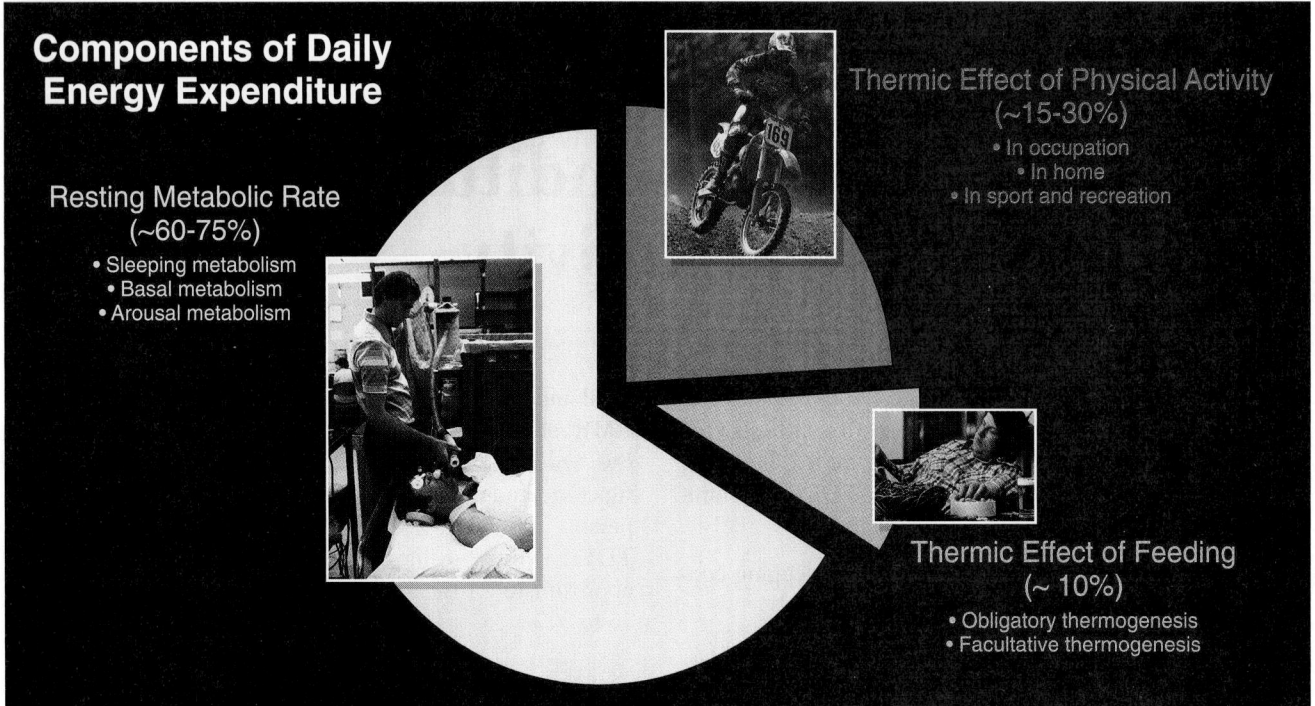

FIGURE 9.1
Components of the total daily energy expenditure.

the nonlipid mass) provides the overall best method for explaining intergender differences in RMR and TDEE. It should be noted, however, that body surface area offers as good an index of RMR as does lean body mass for an individual or group of individuals of the same sex. This is true because of the strong relationships between body surface area and lean body mass within a particular sex. One of the pitfalls to comparing males versus females concerning RMR/surface area is that females have a smaller lean body mass, reflecting a smaller muscle mass component and not necessarily implying a lower proportion of active protoplasmic tissues. Such an interpretation has clinical ramifications, including the promulgation of the so-called "myth of feminine metabolism."[13]

The results of numerous experiments have provided data on average BMR values for men and women of different ages and over a wide range of body weights. These data are presented in Figure 9.3 and expressed as hourly values of heat production per square meter of body surface ($kcal \cdot m^{-2} \cdot h^{-1}$). Whereas these data represent averages established from measurements of large numbers of men and women, an individual's RMR estimated from these curves is generally within 10% of the actual value if obtained from laboratory measurements.

Figure 9.3 reveals that the BMR is about 5 to 10% lower in women than in men. This disparity does not reflect a true sex difference in the metabolic rate of specific tissues; rather, it exists largely because women generally possess more body fat than men of similar size, and fat tissue is metabolically less active than muscle. Changes in body composition, either the decrease in fat-free mass and/or increase in body fat during adulthood,[19] largely explain the 2 to 3% per decade decrease in BMR usually observed through adulthood for both men and women.[5, 22, 44, 55] In comparisons between young and middle-aged endurance-trained men having the same fat-free body masses, measures of BMR were similar for both groups.[34] In addition, there was an accompanying 8% increase in resting metabolism in 50- to 65-year old men who significantly increased their fat-free mass through a program of heavy resistance training.[46] *Such data indicate that regular endurance and resistance exercise can offset the decrease in resting metabolism usually noted with aging.* Furthermore, an 8-week aerobic training program for older individuals resulted in a 10% increase in resting metabolism even though fat-free body mass did not change.[42] This suggests that regular exercise affects factors other than body composition that have a stimulating effect on resting metabolism.

Although variations in body composition largely explain sex differences in BMR, the curves in Figure 9.3 can be used to estimate adequately a person's resting metabolic rate. For example, between the ages of 20 and 40, the BMR of men averages about 38 $kcal \cdot m^{-2} \cdot h^{-1}$, whereas for women the corresponding value is 35 $kcal \cdot m^{-2} \cdot h^{-1}$. For greater precision, the value for a specific age can be read directly from the appropriate curve. The estimated total metabolic rate per

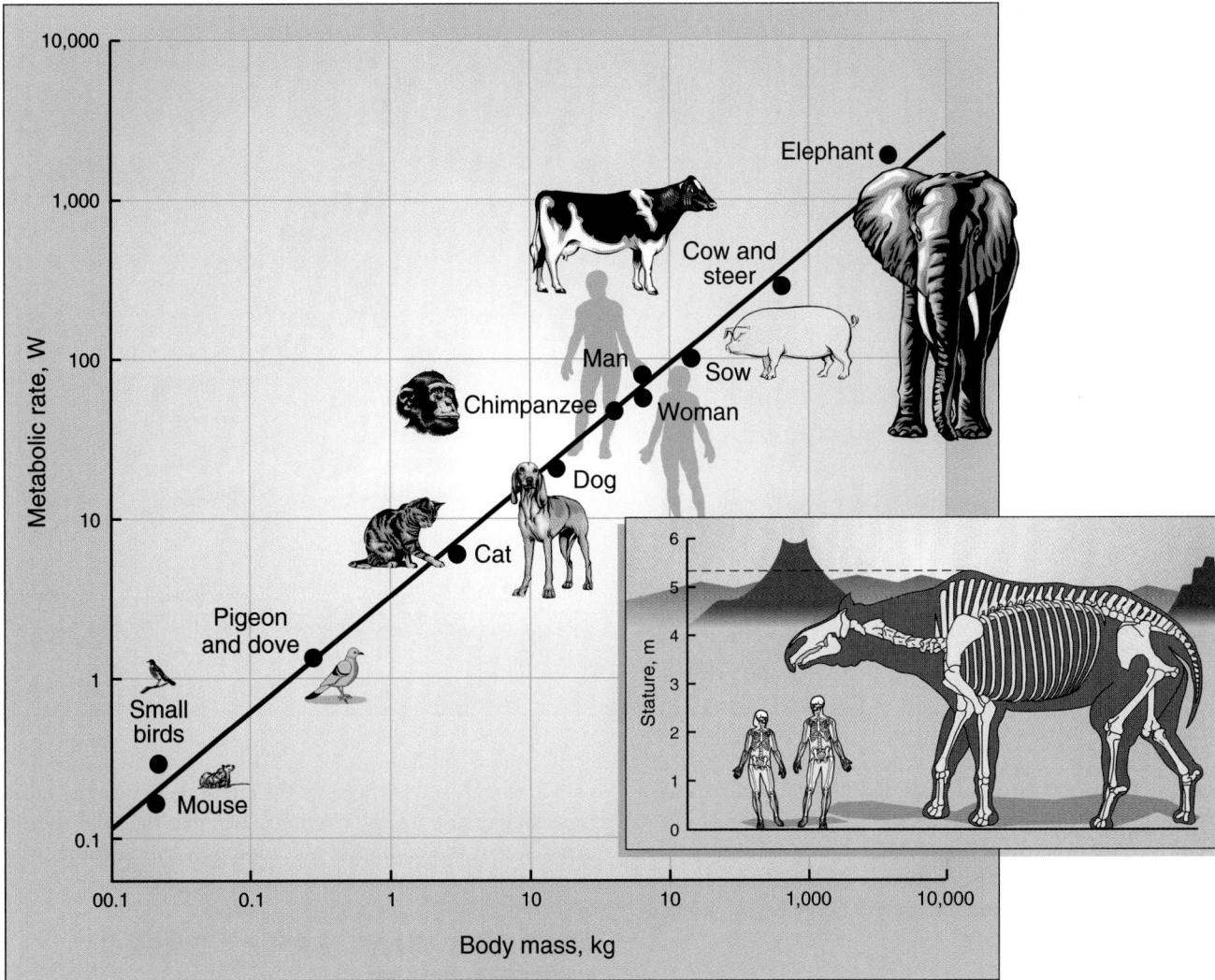

FIGURE 9.2

Metabolic rate from mouse to elephant. Logarithmic plot of body mass and metabolic rate for a variety of birds and mammals differing considerably in body size and shape. Numerous experiments have confirmed the "mouse-to-elephant curve" using body mass$^{0.75}$, whereas metabolic rate is related to body mass$^{0.67}$ as a function of surface area. The schematic insert figure compares the body size of the world's tallest male (2.89 m [9 ft 5¾ in.]) and female (2.48 m [8 ft 1¾ in.]) with the world's largest land mammal (the predecessor of the rhinoceros, *Baluchitherium*), whose body mass was approximately 30 tons at a stature of 5.26 m (17 ft 3 in.). Comparisons between a microorganism (ameoba; mass = 0.1 mg) and a 100-ton blue whale (or the smallest shrew, which is one-tenth the size of a mouse or one-millionth the size of an average-size elephant) illustrate the importance of appropriate scaling procedures when relating physiological variables such as oxygen uptake, heart size, and blood volume to body mass.[47, 50]

hour is obtained by multiplying the BMR value by the person's surface area. This calculation provides important information for determining one's daily energy expenditure as well as the baseline requirement for caloric intake.

Figure 9.4 illustrates a simple method for determining body surface area from stature and body mass. Surface area is determined from the nomogram by locating the appropriate stature on *Scale I* and mass on *Scale II*. These two points are then connected with a straight edge, and the intersection at *Scale III* represents the surface area expressed in square meters. For example, if stature is 185 cm and mass is

75 kg, surface area according to *Scale III* of the nomogram would be 1.98 m².

ESTIMATING DAILY RESTING ENERGY EXPENDITURE

Surface Area

An estimate based on surface area can be made of an individual's daily resting energy expenditure by multiplying the appropriate BMR value in Figure 9.3 by the surface area

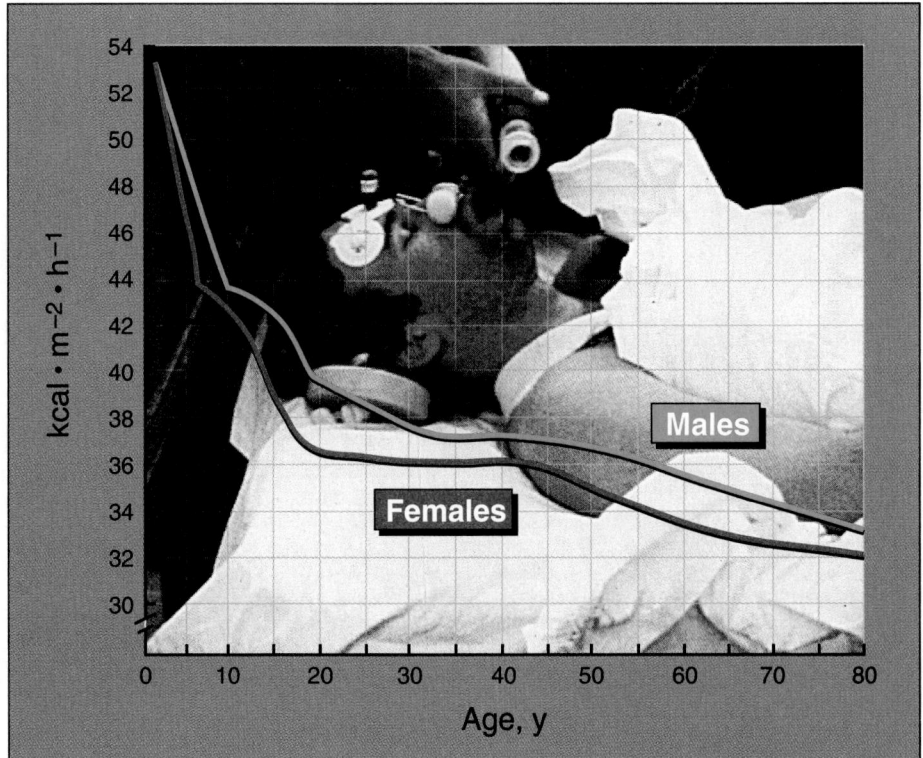

FIGURE 9.3
Basal metabolic rate (BMR) as a function of age and sex. (Data from Altman, P.L., and Dittmer, D.: *Metabolism*. Bethesda, MD, Federation of American Societies for Experimental Biology, 1968.)

computed from stature and mass. For a 55-year-old woman, for example, the estimated BMR is 32 kcal · m^{-2} · h^{-1}. If her surface area were 1.40 m^2, the hourly energy expenditure would be 44.8 kcal per hour (32 kcal × 1.40 m^2). On a daily basis, this amounts to an energy expenditure of 1075 kcal (44.8 kcal × 24).

Fat-Free Body Mass FFM

A relatively easy and more accurate estimate of resting daily energy expenditure (RDEE) can be obtained from Table 9.1 by using FFM to estimate the resting metabolism. The FFM can be estimated using several indirect procedures described in Chapter 27. The generalized equation for RDEE, applicable to males and females over a wide range of body weights, is as follows:

$$RDEE = 370 + 21.6 \, (FFM, kg)$$

For example, a male weighing 90.9 kg (200 lb) with 21% body fat has an estimated FFM of 71.7 kg (158 lb). This translates to an RDEE (using 72 kg) of 1925 kcal, or 8047 kJ (8.05 MJ).

Table 9.2 lists estimates of the absolute and relative energy needs of various body tissues under resting conditions, expressed in terms of oxygen uptake. Note that the brain and skeletal muscles consume about the same total quantity of oxygen during rest, even though the brain weighs only 1.6 kg, while muscle constitutes almost 50% of the body mass. This similarity in metabolism, however, is not the case

with maximal exercise because the energy generated by muscles can increase nearly 120 times, whereas the total energy expended by the brain probably increases only slightly.

FACTORS THAT AFFECT ENERGY EXPENDITURE

Important factors that affect a person's TDEE include physical activity, dietary-induced thermogenesis, climate, and pregnancy and lactation.

PHYSICAL ACTIVITY

As discussed and illustrated throughout this text, *physical activity has by far the most profound effect on human energy expenditure.* World-class athletes, for example, nearly double their daily caloric outputs as a result of 3 or 4 hours of hard training. It is noteworthy that most people can sustain metabolic rates that are 10 times the resting values during "big muscle" exercises such as fast walking, running, and swimming. Under normal circumstances, physical activity accounts for between 15 and 30% of a person's total daily energy expenditure.

DIETARY-INDUCED THERMOGENESIS

For most people, the ingestion of food stimulates energy metabolism. This **dietary-induced thermogenesis** con-

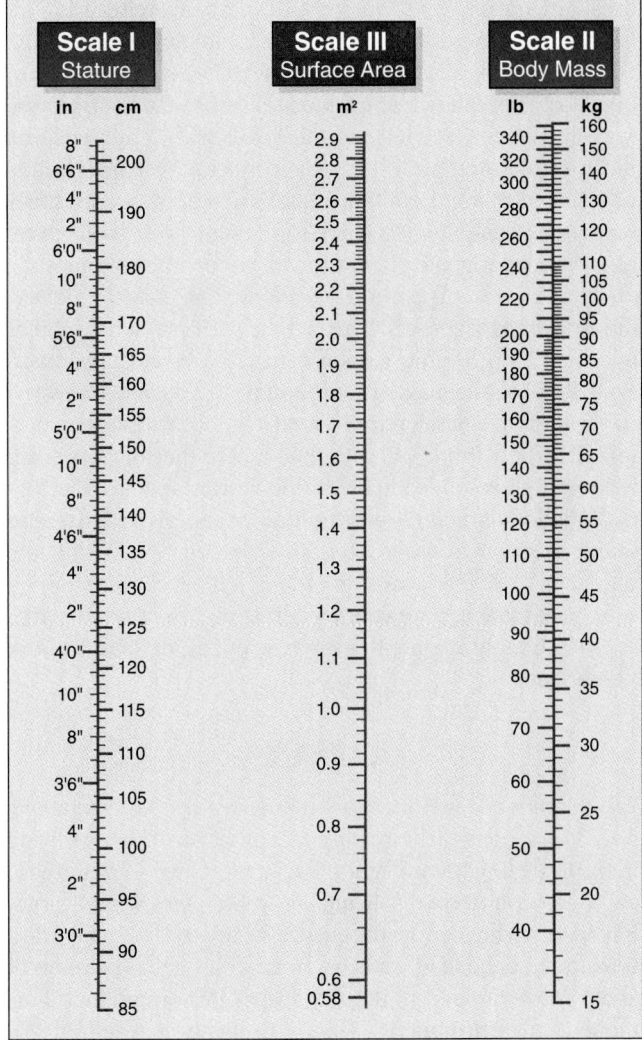

FIGURE 9.4

Nomogram to estimate body surface area from stature and mass. (Reproduced from "Clinical Spirometry" as prepared by Boothby and Sandiford of the Mayo Clinic, through the courtesy of Warren E. Collins, Inc., Braintree, MA.)

TABLE 9.1

ESTIMATION OF RESTING METABOLIC RATE (RMR) BASED ON FAT-FREE BODY MASS[a]

FFM (kg)	RMR (kcal)[b]	FFM (kg)	RMR (kcal)[b]	FFM (kg)	RMR (kcal)[b]
30	1018	58	1623	86	2228
31	1040	59	1644	87	2249
32	1061	60	1666	88	2271
33	1083	61	1688	89	2292
34	1104	62	1709	90	2314
35	1126	63	1731	91	2336
36	1148	64	1752	92	2357
37	1169	65	1774	93	2379
38	1191	66	1796	94	2400
39	1212	67	1817	95	2422
40	1234	68	1839	96	2444
41	1256	69	1860	97	2465
42	1277	70	1882	98	2487
43	1299	71	1904	99	2508
44	1320	72	1925	100	2530
45	1342	73	1947	101	2552
46	1364	74	1968	102	2573
47	1385	75	1990	103	2595
48	1407	76	2012	104	2616
49	1428	77	2033	105	2638
50	1450	78	2055	106	2660
51	1472	79	2076	107	2681
52	1493	80	2098	108	2703
53	1515	81	2120	109	2724
54	1536	82	2141	110	2746
55	1558	83	2163	111	2768
56	1580	84	2184	112	2789
57	1601	85	2206	113	2811

[a]The prediction equation for RMR was derived as the weighted mean of regression constants from studies of large samples of males and females;[13] the method for estimating FFM is presented in Chapter 27.

[b]To convert kcal to kJ, multiply by 4.18; to convert kcal to MJ, multiply by 0.0042.

sists of two components. One component, called **obligatory thermogenesis** (formerly called specific dynamic action, or SDA), is a result of the energy-requiring processes of digesting, absorbing, and assimilating food nutrients. The second component is called **facultative thermogenesis.** This increase in metabolism with food ingestion is related to the activation of the sympathetic nervous system and its stimulating effect on metabolism.

In general, the thermic effect of food reaches a maximum within 1 hour after a meal. While considerable variability exists between individuals, the magnitude of dietary-induced thermogenesis can vary between 10 and 35% of the ingested food energy in normal individuals depending on both the quantity and type of food eaten.[4, 23, 59] A meal of pure protein, for example, elicits a thermic effect that is

nearly 25% of the meal's total calories.[18] This large thermic effect is due mainly to digestive processes as well as the extra energy required by the liver to assimilate and synthesize protein or deaminate certain amino acids and convert them to glucose.

The calorigenic effect of protein ingestion has been used by some people to advocate a high-protein diet for weight reduction. They maintain that because of protein's relatively high thermic effect, fewer calories are ultimately available to the body compared to a meal of similar caloric value but consisting mainly of lipid or carbohydrate. Although this point has some validity, many other factors

TABLE 9.2
OXYGEN UPTAKE OF VARIOUS TISSUES AT REST FOR A 65-KG MAN

Organ	Oxygen Uptake ($mL \cdot min^{-1}$)	Percent of Resting Metabolism
Liver	67	27
Brain	47	19
Heart	17	7
Kidneys	26	10
Skeletal muscle	45	18
Remainder	48	19
	250	100

From data of Passmore, R., and Draper, M.H.: The chemical anatomy of the human body. In *Biochemical Disorders in Human Disease,* 2nd ed. R.H.S. Thompson and E.J. King (Eds.), London, Churchill, 1964.

must be considered in formulating a sound program for weight loss, not least of these the potentially harmful strain on kidney and liver functions that could result from excessive protein intake. Well-balanced nutrition requires a blend of carbohydrate, lipid, and protein as well as appropriate quantities of vitamins and minerals. In addition, if physical activity is added to dietary modification for weight loss, it is important to maintain an adequate carbohydrate intake to power the diverse forms of physical activity.

Research indicates that individuals who have poor control of body mass often have a blunted thermic response to eating, which can contribute to the accumulation of excess body fat.[48, 51, 52, 53] Interestingly, the magnitude of dietary-induced thermogenesis may also be lower in exercise-trained individuals compared to their untrained counterparts.[26, 43, 58] Whereas such a "training effect" probably reflects a calorie-sparing adaptation to conserve energy and glycogen during periods of increased physical activity, it may seem counterproductive to the potential of increased physical activity for weight control. The important point is that for a physically active person, dietary-induced thermogenesis represents only a small portion of the total daily energy expenditure compared to the energy expended through regular physical activity.

CALORIGENIC EFFECT OF FOOD ON EXERCISE METABOLISM

Dietary-induced thermogenesis has been compared in exercising and resting subjects after they had consumed meals of similar size and composition. In one study, six men engaged in moderate exercise on a bicycle ergometer before

breakfast on one day. On separate days, exercise was performed 30 minutes after a breakfast containing either 350, 1000, or 3000 kcal.[7] The following results were obtained: (*a*) breakfast increased resting metabolism by 10%, (*b*) variations in the caloric value of the meal had no influence on the thermic effect, and (*c*) when exercise was performed following a meal of 1000 or 3000 kcal, energy expenditure was larger compared to exercise without prior food ingestion. This calorigenic effect of food was nearly two times the effect at rest. Apparently, exercise augments dietary-induced thermogenesis. This agrees with previous findings in which the thermic response to a 1000-kcal meal averaged 28% of the basal requirement at rest and increased to 56% of the basal requirement when exercise was performed after eating.[35] As with the blunted thermic responses for some obese individuals during rest, it appears that the potentiation of dietary-induced thermogenesis with exercise is not as great in these men and women.[52, 62] Within the framework of the available, though limited, research, it seems reasonable to encourage moderate exercise after eating to possibly augment caloric expenditure and control weight gain.

CLIMATE

Environmental factors can influence resting metabolic rate. For example, the resting metabolisms of people living in tropical climates are generally 5 to 20% higher than those of their counterparts living in more temperate areas. Exercise performed in the heat also imposes a small additional metabolic load, causing an oxygen uptake increase of about 5% compared to the same work performed in a thermoneutral environment. This is probably a result of the thermogenic effect of an elevated core temperature, per se, as well as the additional energy required for sweat-gland activity and altered circulatory dynamics during work in the heat.

Cold environments can have a significant effect on energy metabolism both at rest and during exercise, the extent of which depends largely on a person's body fat content and the effectiveness of clothing worn. During extreme cold stress at rest, metabolic rate can double or triple as shivering commences and the body generates heat in an attempt to maintain a stable core temperature. The effects of cold stress during exercise are most evident in cold water because it is quite difficult to maintain a stable core temperature in such an environment.[32, 56]

PREGNANCY

Considering the increased number of women involved in physically demanding exercise, sports, and occupations, including those in the military and public safety, it is important to establish prudent guidelines concerning exercise during pregnancy.[2, 54] Researchers are only now beginning to understand the impacts of exercise, training, and environmental stress on both mother and fetus. One area of interest is the degree to which pregnancy affects the metabolic cost and physiologic strain imposed by exercise. In one earlier investigation, 13 women were studied over a period spanning from month 6 of pregnancy to 6 weeks after gestation.[24] Physiologic measures taken every 4 weeks included heart rate and oxygen uptake during bicycle and treadmill exercise. The increased heart rate and oxygen uptake during walking coincided with body weight increases in pregnancy, whereas exercise heart rate and oxygen uptake did not change during weight-supported bicycle exercise over the study period. *These and other findings suggest that maternal cardiovascular dynamics follow normal response patterns and that moderate exercise presents no greater physiologic stress to the mother than that imposed by the additional weight gain and possible encumbrance of fetal tissue.*[3, 20] Furthermore, the absolute value for aerobic capacity ($L \cdot min^{-1}$) does not appear to be compromised by pregnancy.[29, 49] As pregnancy progresses, however, the increase in maternal body weight adds significantly to exercise effort during weight-bearing exercises such as walking, jogging, and stair climbing and may adversely affect the economy of effort.[39] Pregnancy, particularly in its later stages, also increases pulmonary ventilation at a given submaximal exercise level.[60] This maternal "hyperventilation" has been attributed to the direct stimulating effects of the hormone progesterone and an increased sensitivity to carbon dioxide.[39, 61] Table 9.3 summarizes important maternal metabolic and cardiorespiratory adaptations during pregnancy.

Effects of Exercise on Fetus

Another area of concern among exercise specialists and physicians is the effect of vigorous maternal exercise on the developing fetus. The proposed hypothetical risks of acute maternal exercise to which repeated exposures could result in altered fetal growth and development include:[61]

- Reduced placental blood flow and accompanying fetal hypoxia,
- Fetal hyperthermia, and
- Reduced fetal glucose supply.

Certainly, any factor that might temporarily compromise fetal blood supply is of concern when counseling pregnant women about exercise. Although human research in this area is obviously sparse, other species of mammals have been studied. In one investigation, treadmill exercise to exhaustion caused a drop in both uterine blood flow and arterial oxygen pressure in near-term pregnant ewes.[9] Despite this potentially negative response, oxygen uptake by the uteroplacental tissues and fetus was maintained by a facilitated unloading of oxygen from the available blood supply. However, a significant reduction was noted in fetal oxygen supply in animals having one umbilical artery tied off to re-

strict placental circulation.[17] The researchers concluded that under normal conditions, vigorous maternal exercise was well tolerated by the fetus, but it could be potentially harmful to a fetus experiencing limited umbilical circulation.

Status of Current Opinion

Thirty to forty minutes of moderate aerobic exercise by a previously active, healthy, low-risk woman during an uncomplicated pregnancy does not compromise fetal oxygen supply or acid-base status or produce other adverse effects to mother or fetus.[27, 40, 53a] Performed on a regular basis, such exercise not only maintains cardiovascular fitness but can actually produce a training effect.[25, 41, 45, 60] Hormonal action of the sympathetic nervous system during strenuous exercise probably diverts some blood away from the uterus and visceral organs for preferential distribution to active muscles. This could pose a hazard to a fetus with restricted placental blood flow. Thus, it is prudent for a pregnant woman to exercise in moderation, especially if the pregnancy is compromised to any degree. In addition, exercise late in pregnancy may magnify the normal maternal hypoglycemic response by increasing glucose uptake by maternal skeletal muscle; in the extreme, this response could adversely affect glucose supply to the fetus.[6, 10, 57]

It also is possible that a decrease in uterine blood flow or an elevation in maternal core temperature with extended exercise, particularly under environmental heat stress, could

---

TABLE 9.3
IMPORTANT METABOLIC AND CARDIORESPIRATORY ADAPTATIONS DURING PREGNANCY

- Blood volume increases 40 to 50%; hemodilution causes reduced hemoglobin concentration
- Increase in blood volume causes dilation of left ventricle
- Slight increase in oxygen uptake at rest and during submaximal, weight-supported exercise such as stationary cycling
- Substantial increase in oxygen uptake during weight-bearing exercise such as walking and running
- Increased heart rate during submaximal exercise
- Essentially no change in $\dot{V}O_2max$ ($L \cdot min^{-1}$)
- Increased ventilatory response at rest and during submaximal exercise
- Possible magnified hypoglycemic response during exercise, especially late in pregnancy
- Possible blunted sympathetic nervous system responses to exercise in late gestation

Modified from Wolfe, L.A., et al.: Maternal exercise, fetal well-being and pregnancy outcome. *Exerc. Sport Sci. Rev.*, 22:145, 1994.

compromise the dissipation of heat from the fetus through the placenta.[21, 33] Because hyperthermia can negatively affect fetal development (for example, increase the risk of neural tube defect), especially during the first trimester of pregnancy,[36] it is recommended that, in warm weather, pregnant women exercise in the cool part of the day and for shorter intervals while maintaining regular fluid intake. Within this framework, aquatic exercise would serve as an ideal form of maternal exercise.

It is currently recommended that for an uncomplicated pregnancy, current fitness level and ability should guide a woman's exercise habits throughout pregnancy and in the postpartum period. Regular aerobic exercise can play an important role in maintaining functional capacity and general well-being during pregnancy. It may also contribute to optimizing overall weight gain during the later stages of pregnancy.[12] It is unclear, however, whether extremes of maternal exercise are of any benefit to either the mother or the developing fetus or whether exercise during pregnancy enhances the course of pregnancy, including labor, delivery, and outcome.[8, 11, 21, 25] Beginning 6 to 8 weeks postpartum, regular exercise has no deleterious effect on the volume or composition of lactation and significantly improves the mother's level of aerobic fitness.[15, 28]

■ SUMMARY ■

1. One's daily energy expenditure is the sum total of the basal and resting metabolisms, thermogenic influences (particularly the thermic effect of food), and energy generated during physical activity.

2. The BMR is the minimum energy required to maintain vital functions in the waking state and is measured under strictly controlled laboratory conditions. The BMR is only slightly lower than the resting metabolic rate (RMR) and is proportionate to the surface area of the body.

3. The RMR also is related to age (it decreases) and generally is larger for men than women. These disparities are largely due to variations in fat-free body mass. In fact, RMR can be predicted quite accurately from fat-free body mass in men and women who vary considerably in body size.

4. Different organs expend different amounts of energy during rest and exercise. At rest, muscles generate about 20% of the total energy expenditure. During all-out exercise, however, the energy expended by skeletal muscle can increase to more than 100 times above its resting value.

5. Four major factors that affect a person's metabolic rate are physical activity, dietary-induced thermogenesis, climate, and pregnancy. The greatest influence comes from physical activity.

6. For the previously active, healthy woman, moderate aerobic exercise does not appear to compromise fetal

oxygen supply. It remains unclear, however, whether extremes of maternal exercise are beneficial to the course of pregnancy or to the child in the early period after birth.

PART 2

ENERGY EXPENDITURE DURING PHYSICAL ACTIVITY

CLASSIFICATION OF PHYSICAL ACTIVITIES BY ENERGY EXPENDITURE

All of us at one time or another have engaged in some type of physical work that we would classify as exceedingly "difficult." This might have included walking up a long flight of stairs, shoveling snow for 90 minutes, running a block to catch a bus, digging a deep trench to fix an underground pipe, skiing through a blizzard, or hiking up a steep mountain. Intensity and duration are two important factors affecting the physical difficulty or strenuousness of a particular task. For example, the same number of calories may be required to complete a 26.2-mile marathon at various speeds. One runner, however, might expend a considerable rate of energy running at maximum pace (about 80% of $\dot{V}O_2$max) and complete the race in a little more than 2.5 hours. Another runner of equal fitness might select a slower, more comfortable pace (about 55% of $\dot{V}O_2$max) and complete the run in 3.5 hours. In this example, the **intensity** of effort is the factor distinguishing the manner for completing the task. In another situation, two people may run at the same speed, but one person may run twice as long as the other. In this situation, exercise **duration** becomes the important consideration in classifying the physical effort.

Several classification systems have been proposed for rating sustained physical activity in terms of its strenuousness. One recommendation is that work tasks be classified by the ratio of energy required for the task to the resting energy requirement.[1] This system uses the **physical activity ratio,** or **PAR,** to classify physical activities. **Light work** for men is defined as that eliciting an oxygen uptake (or energy expenditure) as great as three times the resting requirement; **heavy work** is categorized as that requiring six to eight times the resting metabolism; whereas **maximal work** is any task requiring an increase in metabolism to nine times or more above rest. As a frame of reference, most industrial jobs and household tasks require less than three times the resting energy expenditure.

For women, the work classifications above are slightly lower owing to their generally lower aerobic capacities. It is noteworthy that energy expenditure standards for categorizing the strenuousness of occupational tasks are somewhat lower than would be applied to general exercise. This is so because industrial work is usually prolonged, often requiring the use of small muscle mass, and performed under varying and often stressful environmental conditions and physical constraints.

The MET

The five-level classification system presented in Table 9.4 is based on the energy required by untrained men and women performing different physical activities, including a broad range of occupational tasks.[16] Because 5 kcal is approximately equal to 1 L of oxygen consumed, it is also possible to present this five-stage classification in terms of liters of oxygen consumed per minute ($L \cdot min^{-1}$), milliliters of oxygen per kilogram of body mass per minute ($mL \cdot kg^{-1} \cdot min^{-1}$), or **METs,** *a MET being defined as a multiple of the resting metabolic rate.* Thus, 1 MET is equivalent to a resting oxygen uptake of about 250 mL per minute for an average man and 200 mL per minute for an average woman. Work performed at 2 METs requires twice the resting metabolism, or about 500 mL of oxygen per minute for a man, 3 METs is three times the resting energy expenditure, and so on. For a slightly more accurate classification that accounts for variations in body size, the MET is usually expressed in terms of oxygen uptake per unit of body mass, with 1 MET equal to approximately $3.6 \text{ mL} \cdot \text{kg}^{-1} \cdot \text{min}^{-1}$.

Table 9.5 presents a classification system for characterizing the intensity of leisure physical activity for abso-lute (multiples of resting metabolism) and relative (percentage of $\dot{V}O_2max$) intensity. The categorization for exercise intensity in absolute terms (METs) is adjusted lower with age to account for the general "aging effect" on aerobic capacity.

DAILY RATES OF AVERAGE ENERGY EXPENDITURE

Table 9.6 displays daily energy expenditure averages for men and women living in the United States. The "average" man between the ages of 23 and 50 expends between 2700 and 3000 kcal per day, whereas his female counterpart expends between 2000 and 2100 kcal. As seen in the bottom portion of this table, nearly 75% of the average person's day, regardless of sex, is spent in activities requiring only a light energy expenditure. For most men and women, energy expenditure rarely climbs significantly above the resting level, with walking being the most prevalent form of physical activity. Indeed, U.S. citizens have all too appropriately been termed *Homo sedentarius*.

EFFECT OF BODY MASS

Body mass is an important factor that affects the energy expended in many forms of exercise. The energy cost of a particular exercise is generally higher for heavier people, especially for **weight-bearing exercises** such as walking and running, during which the person must transport his or her body mass. The effect of body mass is illustrated in

---

TABLE 9.4
FIVE-LEVEL CLASSIFICATION OF PHYSICAL ACTIVITY BASED ON EXERCISE INTENSITY[a]

Level	Energy Expenditure			
	Men			
	$kcal \cdot min^{-1}$	$L \cdot min^{-1}$	$mL \cdot kg^{-1} \cdot min^{-1}$	METs
Light	2.0–4.9	0.40–0.99	6.1–15.2	1.6–3.9
Moderate	5.0–7.4	1.00–1.49	15.3–22.9	4.0–5.9
Heavy	7.5–9.9	1.50–1.99	23.0–30.6	6.0–7.9
Very heavy	10.0–12.4	2.00–2.49	30.7–38.3	8.9–9.9
Unduly heavy	12.5–	2.50–	38.4–	10.0–
	Women			
	$kcal \cdot min^{-1}$	$L \cdot min^{-1}$	$mL \cdot kg^{-1} \cdot min^{-1}$	METs
Light	1.5–3.4	0.30–0.69	5.4–12.5	1.2–2.7
Moderate	3.5–5.4	0.70–1.09	12.6–19.8	2.8–4.3
Heavy	5.5–7.4	1.10–1.49	19.9–27.1	4.4–5.9
Very heavy	7.5–9.4	1.50–1.89	27.2–34.4	6.0–7.5
Unduly heavy	9.5–	1.90–	34.5–	7.6–

[a]$L \cdot min^{-1}$ based on 5 kcal per liter of oxygen; $mL \cdot kg^{-1}$ based on 65-kg man and 55-kg woman; one **MET** is equivalent to the average resting oxygen uptake.

TABLE 9.5
CHARACTERIZATION OF THE INTENSITY OF LEISURE ACTIVITY IN RELATION TO AGE

Categorization	Relative intensity (% $\dot{V}O_2$ max)	Absolute intensity (METs)			
		Young	Middle-aged	Old	Very old
Rest	<10	1.0	1.0	1.0	1.0
Light	<35	<4.5	<3.5	<2.5	<1.5
Fairly light	<50	<6.5	<5.0	<3.5	<2.0
Moderate	<70	<9.0	<7.0	<5.0	<2.8
Heavy	>70	>9.0	>7.0	>5.0	>2.8
Maximal	100	13.0	10.0	7.0	4.0

From Bouchard, C., et al.: *Exercise, Fitness, and Health: A Consensus of Current Knowledge.* Champaign, IL, Human Kinetics, 1990.

TABLE 9.6
AVERAGE RATES OF ENERGY EXPENDITURE FOR MEN AND WOMEN LIVING IN THE UNITED STATES[a]

	Age (y)	Body Mass		Stature		Energy Expenditure (kcal)
		(kg)	(lb)	(cm)	(in)	
Males	15–18	66	145	176	69	3000
	19–24	72	160	177	70	2900
	25–50	79	174	176	70	2900
	51+	77	170	173	68	2300
Females	15–18	55	120	163	64	2200
	19–24	58	128	164	65	2200
	25–50	63	138	163	64	2200
	50+	65	143	160	63	1900

Average Time Spent During the Day

Activity	Time (h)
Sleeping and lying down	8
Sitting	6
Standing	6
Walking	2
Recreational Activity	2

Data from Food and Nutrition Board, National Research Council: *Recommended Dietary Allowances,* revised. Washington, DC, National Academy of Sciences, 1989.
[a]The information in this table was designed for the maintenance of practically all healthy people in the United States.

Figure 9.5, which demonstrates that the energy cost of walking increases directly with body mass. For people of the same body mass, the variation in oxygen uptake is so small that the energy expended while walking can be predicted from body mass with high accuracy.

Body mass will influence energy metabolism during weight-bearing exercise regardless of whether a person gains weight "naturally," in the form of body fat, or through an acute added load, such as sports equipment or a weighted vest on the torso.[14, 37] During **weight-supported exercise** such as stationary cycling, the influence of body mass on energy cost is much less extreme (about 5% higher in cycling because of the extra energy required to lift the heavier lower limbs). Certainly, for overweight people who want to use

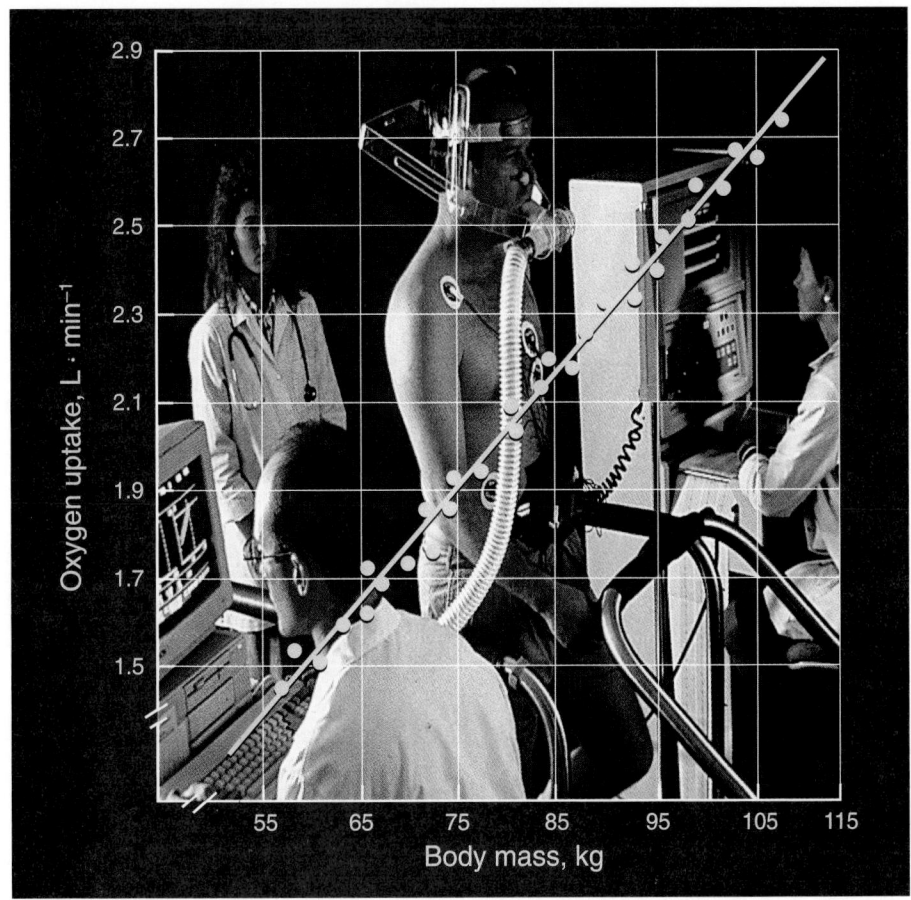

FIGURE 9.5

Relationship between body mass and oxygen uptake measured during sub-maximal, brisk treadmill walking. (From Applied Physiology Laboratory, Queens College, NY. Photo courtesy of Dr. Jay Graves, Exercise Science Department, Syracuse University, Syracuse, NY.)

exercise to lose weight, weight-bearing forms of exercise can provide a considerable caloric expenditure.

The energy cost for cross-country running ranges from 8.2 kcal per minute for a 50-kg person to almost twice as much, 16.0 kcal, for a person weighing 98 kg. If, however, the energy requirement is expressed in relation to body mass as $kcal \cdot kg^{-1} \cdot min^{-1}$, this variation is essentially eliminated, and the energy cost averages about 0.164 $kcal \cdot kg^{-1} \cdot min^{-1}$. By expressing energy cost in this manner (that is, per unit of body mass), we greatly reduce the differences between individuals regardless of age, race, sex, or body mass. The **total** number of calories expended by the heavier person, however, is still considerably larger than that expended by a lighter counter-part, simply because the body mass must be transported during the activity, requiring proportionately more total energy.

USE OF HEART RATE TO ESTIMATE ENERGY EXPENDITURE

For each person, heart rate and oxygen uptake tend to be linearly related throughout a wide range of aerobic exercises. If this precise relationship is known, the exercise heart rate can be used to estimate oxygen uptake (and then to compute energy expenditure) during similar forms of physical activity. This approach has been used when the oxygen uptake could not be measured during the actual activity.

The data for two members of a nationally ranked women's basketball team during a laboratory treadmill running test are presented in Figure 9.6. For each woman, the heart rate increased linearly, with an increase in oxygen uptake being accompanied by a proportionate increase in heart rate. However, even though both heart rate–oxygen uptake lines are linear, the same heart rate does not correspond to the same level of oxygen uptake for both women because the slope or rate of change of the line differs considerably among people. For a given increase in oxygen uptake, the heart rate of subject B increases to a much smaller extent than that of subject A. The significance of this difference and its relation to cardiovascular fitness are discussed in Chapters 11, 17, and 21. The important point is that if heart rate is known, oxygen uptake often can be estimated with reasonable accuracy. For player A, an exercise heart rate of 140 beats per minute corresponds to an oxygen uptake of 1.08 L per minute, whereas the same heart rate for player B is associated with a 1.60-L oxygen uptake. Heart rates obtained using radiotelemetry during actual basketball competition then were applied to each

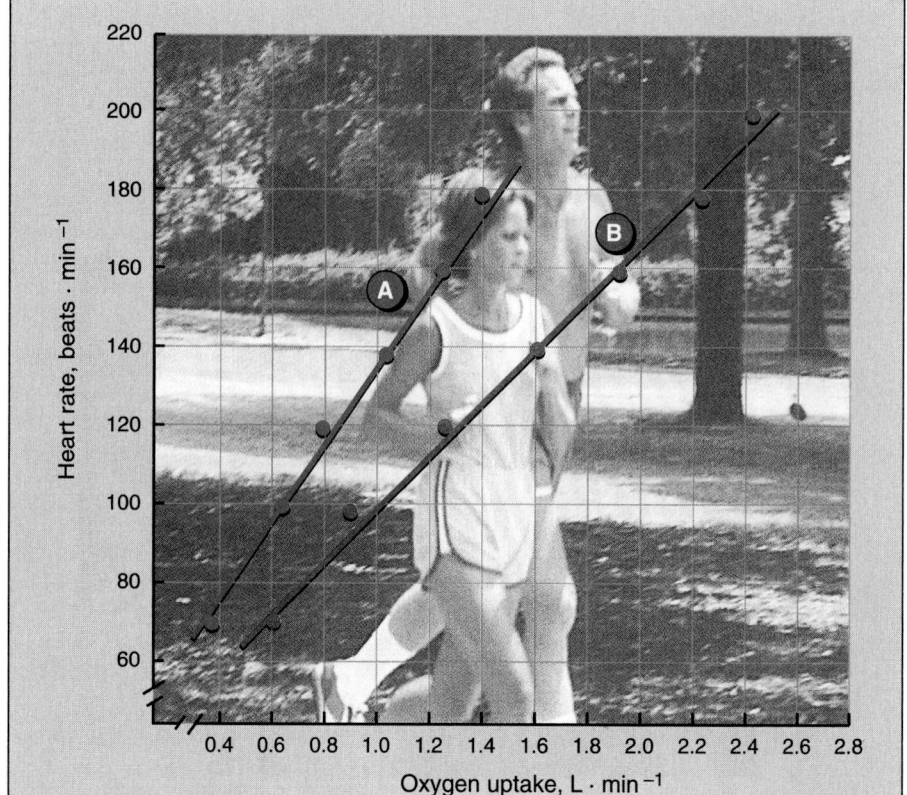

FIGURE 9.6

Linear relationship between heart rate and oxygen uptake measured during a graded exercise test on a motor-driven treadmill in two collegiate basketball players of different aerobic fitness levels. (Data from Laboratory of Applied Physiology, Queens College, NY.)

player's "HR-$\dot{V}O_2$ line" to provide a general estimate of energy expenditure under game conditions.[31]

Although the technique for using heart rate to estimate energy expenditure is practical, it is of limited use for research purposes because its validity has yet to be adequately established for more than a few general activities. One of the major problems is determining the degree of similarity between the laboratory test used to establish the heart rate–oxygen uptake line and the specific activity to which it is applied. For one thing, factors other than oxygen uptake can influence the heart rate response to exercise. These factors include environmental temperature, emotions, previous food intake, body position, muscle groups exercised, continuity of the exercise, or whether the muscles are acting statically or in a more dynamic manner. During an activity such as aerobic dance, for example, heart rates while dancing at a particular oxygen uptake are significantly higher than heart rates at the same oxygen uptake while using a treadmill.[38] During arm exercise or when muscles are acting statically in a straining-type exercise, heart rates are **consistently higher** compared to dynamic leg exercise at any particular submaximal oxygen uptake. Consequently, when heart rate during upper body or static exercise is applied to a heart rate–oxygen uptake line developed during running or cycling, the result is an **overprediction** of the actual oxygen uptake.[30]

■ SUMMARY ■

1. Different classification systems exist for rating the strenuousness of physical activities. These include ratings based on (*a*) the ratio of the energy cost of the task to the resting energy requirement, (*b*) the oxygen requirement in $mL \cdot kg^{-1} \cdot min^{-1}$, or (*c*) multiples of the resting metabolic rate, or METs.

2. The average daily energy expenditure is estimated to be 2700 to 2900 kcal for men and 2000 to 2100 for women between the ages of 15 and 50 years. There is considerable variability among people in daily energy expenditure largely related to their physical activity levels.

3. It is possible to classify different occupations and athletic groups by daily energy expenditure. Within any classification, there is great variability because of energy expended during a person's leisure-time recreational pursuits. In addition, heavy individuals expend more total energy during a given physical activity than their lighter counterparts.

4. While heart rate provides a good indication of the relative strenuousness of physical activity, its usefulness is limited in predicting oxygen uptakes and caloric expenditures for diverse forms of exercise.

■ REFERENCES ■

1. Ainsworth, B.E., et al.: Compendium of physical activities: classification of energy costs of human physical activities. *Med. Sci. Sports Exerc.*, 25:71, 1993.

2. American College of Obstetricians and Gynecologists: *Technical Bulletin. Exercise During Pregnancy and the Postnatal Period.* Washington, DC, ACOG, 1985.

3. Artal, R., et al.: Exercise in pregnancy: maternal cardiovascular and metabolic responses in normal pregnancy. *Am. J. Obstet. Gynecol.*, 140:123, 1981.

4. Belko, A., et al.: Effect of energy and protein intake and exercise intensity on the thermic effect of food. *Am. J. Clin. Nutr.*, 43:863, 1986.

5. Bemben, M.G., et al.: Age-related patterns in body composition for men aged 20-79 yr. *Med. Sci. Sports Exerc.*, 27:264, 1995.

6. Bonnen, A., et al.: Substrate and endocrine responses during exercise at selected stages of pregnancy. *J. Appl. Physiol.*, 73:134, 1992.

7. Bray, G.: The acute effects of food intake on energy expenditure during cycle ergometry. *Am. J. Clin. Nutr.*, 27:254, 1974.

8. Carpenter, M.W.: Physical activity, fitness, and health of the pregnant mother and fetus. In *Physical Activity, Fitness, and Health.* C. Bouchard, et al. (Eds.), Champaign, IL, Human Kinetics, 1994.

9. Clapp, J.F., III.: Acute exercise stress in the pregnant ewe. *Am. J. Obstet. Gynecol.*, 136:489, 1980.

10. Clapp, J.F. III: Thermoregulatory and metabolic responses to jogging prior to and during pregnancy. *Med. Sci. Sports Exerc.*, 19:124, 1987.

11. Clapp, J.F., III, and Dickstein, S.: Endurance exercise and pregnancy outcome. *Med. Sci. Sports Exerc.*, 16:556, 1984.

12. Clapp, J.F., and Little, K.D.: Effect of recreational exercise on pregnancy weight gain and subcutaneous fat deposition. *Med. Sci. Sports Exerc.*, 27:170, 1995.

13. Cunningham, J.J.: Body composition and resting metabolic rate: the myth of feminine metabolism. *Am. J. Clin. Nutr.*, 36:721, 1982.

14. Cureton, K.J., and Sparling, P.B.: Distance running performance and metabolic responses to running in men and women with excess weight experimentally equated. *Med. Sci. Sports*, 12:288, 1980.

15. Dewey, K.G., et al.: A randomized study of the effects of aerobic exercise by lactating women on breast-milk volume and composition. *N. Engl. J. Med.*, 330:449, 1994.

16. Durnin, J.V.G.A., and Passmore, R.: *Energy, Work and Leisure.* London, Heinmann, 1967.

17. Emmanouilides, G.C., et al.: Fetal responses to maternal exercise in sheep. *Am. J. Obstet. Gynecol.*, 112:130, 1982.

18. Flatt, J.B.: Energetics of intermediary metabolism. In *Assessment of Energy Metabolism in Health and Disease.* Columbus, OH, Ross Laboratories, 1980.

19. Going, S., et al.: Aging and body composition: biological changes and methodological issues. *Exerc. Sport Sci. Revs.*, 23:459, 1995.

20. Hutchinson, P.L., et al.: Metabolic and circulatory responses to running during pregnancy. *Phys. Sportsmed.*, 9:55, 1981.

21. Jarrett, J.C., and Spellacy, W.N.: Jogging during pregnancy: an improved outcome? *Obstet. Gynecol.*, 61:705, 1983.

22. Keys, A., et al.: Basal metabolism and age of adult men. *Metabolism*, 22:579, 1973.

23. Kleiber, M.: *The Fire of Life: An Introduction to Animal Energetics.* Huntington, NY, Krieger, 1975.

24. Knuttgen, H.G., and Emerson, K., Jr.: Physiological response to pregnancy at rest and during exercise. *J. Appl. Physiol.*, 36:549, 1974.

25. Kulpa, P.J., et al.: Aerobic exercise in pregnancy. *Am. J. Obstet. Gynecol.*, 156:1395, 1987.

26. LeBlanc, J., et al.: Hormonal factors in reduced post prandial heat production of exercise trained subjects. *J. Appl. Physiol.*, 56:772, 1984.

27. Lokey, E.A., et al.: Effects of physical exercise on pregnancy outcomes: a meta-analytic review. *Med. Sci. Sports Exerc.*, 23:1234, 1991.

28. Lovelady, C.A., et al.: Effects of exercise on plasma lipids and metabolism of lactating women. *Med. Sci. Sports Exerc.*, 27:22, 1995.

29. Lotgering, F.K., et al.: Maximal aerobic exercise in pregnant women: heart rate, O_2 consumption, CO_2 production, and ventiltion. *J. Appl. Physiol.*, 70:1016, 1991.

30. Maas, S., et al.: The validity of the use of heart rate in estimating oxygen consumption in static and in combined static/dynamic exercise. *Ergonomics*, 32:141, 1989.

31. McArdle, W.D., et al.: Aerobic capacity, heart rate, and estimated energy cost during women's competitive basketball. *Res. Q.*, 42:178, 1971.

32. McArdle, W.D., et al.: Metabolic and cardiovascular adjustment to work in air and water at 18, 25 and 33°C. *J. Appl. Physiol.*, 40:85, 1976.

33. McMurray, R.G., and Katz, V.L.: Thermoregulation in pregnancy. *Sports Med.*, 10:146, 1990.

34. Meredith, C.N., et al.: Body composition and aerobic capacity in young and middle-aged endurance-trained men. *Med. Sci. Sports Exerc.*, 19:557, 1987.

35. Miller, D.S., et al.: Gluttony 2: Thermogenesis in overeating man. *Am. J. Clin. Nutr.*, 20:1223, 1967.

36. Milunsky, A., et al.: Maternal heat exposure and neural tube defects. *JAMA*, 268:882, 1992.

37. Montgomery, D.L., et al.: The effect of added weight on ice hockey performance. *Phys. Sportsmed.*, 10:91, 1982.

38. Parker, S.B., et al.: Failure of target heart rate to accurately monitor intensity during aerobic dance. *Med. Sci. Sports Exerc.*, 21:230, 1989.

39. Pivarnik, J.M., et al.: Physiological and perceptual responses to cycle and treadmill exercise during pregnancy. *Med. Sci. Sports Exerc.*, 23:470, 1991.

40. Pivarnik, J.M., et al.: Maternal respiration and blood gases during aerobic exercise performed at moderate altitude. *Med. Sci. Sports Exerc.*, 24:868, 1992.

41. Pivarnik, J.M., et al.: Effects of maternal aerobic fitness on cardiorespiratory responses to exercise. *Med. Sci. Sports Exerc.*, 25:993, 1993.

42. Poehlman, E.T., and Danforth, E., Jr.: Endurance training increases metabolic rate and norepinephrine appearance rate in older individuals. *Am. J. Physiol.*, 261:E233, 1991.

43. Poehlman, E.T., et al.: Resting metabolic rate and post prandial thermogenesis in highly trained and untrained males. *Am. J. Clin. Nutr.*, 47:793, 1988.

44. Poehlman, E.T., et al.: Endurance exercise in aging humans: effects on energy metabolism. *Exerc. Sport Sci. Rev.*, 22:751, 1994.

45. Potteiger, J.A., et al.: From parturition to a marathon: a 16-week study of an elite runner. *Med. Sci. Sports Exerc.*, 25:673, 1993.

46. Pratley, R., et al.: Strength training increases resting metabolic rate and norepinephrine levels in healthy 50- to 65-yr-old men. *J. Appl. Physiol.*, 73:133, 1994.

47. Reiss, M.J.: *The Allometry of Growth and Reproduction.* Cambridge, Cambridge University Press, 1989.

48. Rothwell, N.J., and Stock, M.J.: Luxuskonsumption, diet-induced thermogenesis and brown fat: the case in favor. *Clin. Sci.*, 64:64, 1983.

49. Sady, M.A., et al.: Cardiovascular response to maximal cycle exercise during pregnancy and at two and seven months postpartum. *Am. J. Obstet. Gynecol.*, 162:1181, 1990.

50. Schmidt-Nielsen, K.: *Scaling. Why is Animal Size so Important?* Cambridge, Cambridge University Press, 1984.

51. Schutz, Y., et al.: Diet induced thermogenesis measured over a whole day in obese and non-obese women. *Am. J. Clin. Nutr.*, 40:542, 1984.

52. Segal, K.R., et al.: Thermic effects of food and exercise on lean and obese men of similar lean body mass. *Am. J. Physiol.*, 252:E110, 1987.

53. Shetty, P.S., et al.: Post prandial thermogenesis in obesity. *Clin. Sci.*, 60:519, 1981.

53a. Sternfeld, B., et al.: Exercise during pregnancy and pregnancy outcome. *Med. Sci. Sports Exerc.*, 27:634, 1995.

54. Simpson, J.L.: Are physical activity and employment related to preterm birth and low birth weight? *Am. J. Obstet. Gynecol.*, 168:1231, 1993.

55. Steen, B.: Body composition and aging. *Nutr. Rev.*, 46:45, 1988.

56. Toner, M.M., and McArdle, W.D.: Human thermoregulatory responses to acute cold stress with special reference to water immersion. In *Handbook of Physiology, Envir. Physiol.* In press, 1996.

57. Treadway, J.L., and Young, J.C.: Decreased glucose uptake in fetus after maternal exercise. *Med. Sci. Sports Exerc.*, 21:140, 1989.

58. Trembly, A., et al.: Diminished dietary thermogenesis in exercise-trained human subjects. *Eur. J. Appl. Physiol.*, 52:1, 1983.

59. Tuckerman, M.M., and Turco, S.J.: *Human Nutrition.* Philadelphia, Lea & Febiger, 1983.

60. Wolfe, L.A., et al.: Effects of pregnancy and chronic exercise on respiratory responses to graded exercise. *J. Appl. Physiol.*, 76:1928, 1994.

61. Wolfe, L.A., et al.: Maternal exercise, fetal well-being and pregnancy outcome. *Exerc. Sport Sci. Rev.*, 22:145, 1994.

62. Zahorska-Markiewicz, B.: Thermic effect of food and exercise in obesity. *Eur. J. Appl. Physiol.*, 44:231, 1980.

Mahadeva, K., et al.: Individual variations in the metabolic cost of standardized exercises: The effects of food, age, sex and race. *J. Physiol.* 121:225, 1953.

In early studies of exercise metabolism, few experiments dealt with human energy requirements during different forms of exercise, especially the influence of body size, age, sex, and skill. We now know that such contributing factors are important for exercise prescription and for estimating energy expenditure to maintain energy balance for weight control.

The research of Mahadeva and colleagues, one of the first large-scale "energy cost" studies, focused attention on energy expenditure in two common forms of exercise: (a) stepping, in which measurable external work occurs in raising the body mass, and (b) level, constant-rate walking. Multiple observations were made on 50 subjects, aged 13 to 79 years old and having body mass ranging from 48 to 110 kg. There were 35 males, 15 females, 41 "Europeans," and 9 "Asians." Measurements included basal and resting metabolic rates using indirect calorimetry with the Douglas bag method of open-circuit spirometry. Exercise studies were made using the portable Kofranyi-Michaelis gas meter (see p. 141). Subjects stepped to a metronome cadence of 15 up-and-down cycles per minute for 10 minutes on a 10-inch (25.4-cm) stool. Subjects also walked on an indoor track for 10 minutes at a speed of 3 mph (4.8 km $\cdot$ hr^{-1}).

The two graphs show the relationship and corresponding regression line between energy expenditure and body mass for each activity (C, energy expenditure in kilocalories per 10 minutes; W, body mass in kilograms). For walking and stepping, energy expenditure was directly proportional to body mass. Separate analyses by age, sex, race, and previous diet showed that these variables contributed little to the precision in predicting the metabolic cost of the activities. This important work in exercise energy expenditure indicated that in any physical activity that involves moving the body mass (that is, weight-bearing exercise), the metabolic energy cost is directly proportional to the body mass (refer to pp. 159–161).

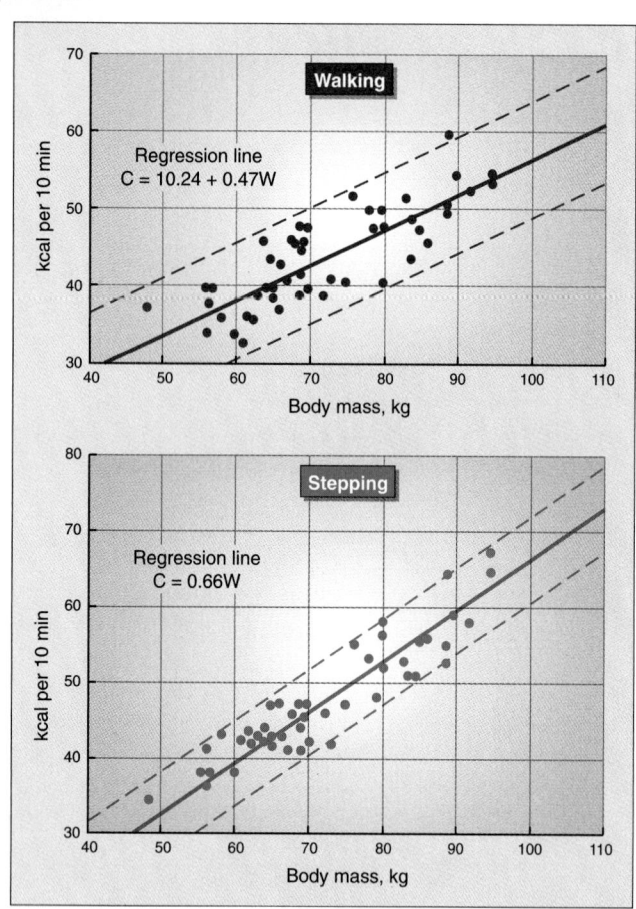

Top, Energy expenditure in kilocalories per 10 minutes as a function of body mass during walking at 3 mph. The *dashed lines* show twice the standard error of estimate. *Bottom,* Energy expenditure in kilocalories per 10 minutes as a function of body mass during stepping. The *dashed lines* show twice the standard error of estimate.

Energy Expenditure During Walking, Jogging, Running, and Swimming

The total energy expended each day depends largely on the type and duration of one's physical activity. The following sections detail the energy expenditure for the popular activities walking, running, and swimming. Aside from being competitive in nature, these exercises take on special significance for their roles in weight control, physical conditioning, and health maintenance and rehabilitation.

GROSS AND NET ENERGY EXPENDITURE

The following example illustrates the use of oxygen uptake to estimate the energy requirement of swimming. A 25-year-old man swimming for 40 minutes at a moderate, steady pace requiring an oxygen uptake of 2.0 L per minute consumes a total of 80 L of oxygen. The oxygen uptake can be transposed to an energy value by using the approximate calorific transformation of 5.0 kcal per liter of oxygen consumed. Thus, the swimmer expends about 400 kcal (80 L O_2 × 5 kcal) during the swim. This, however, is not the cost of the swim per se because this total, or **gross energy expenditure,** also includes energy expended had the person only rested and not swum. To obtain a clearer picture of the true cost of the exercise, or the **net energy expenditure,** one estimates the resting metabolism and subtracts this from the gross energy cost of the exercise as follows:

Net energy expenditure = Gross energy expenditure − Resting energy expenditure (for equivalent time period)

Knowing the swimmer's size (mass, 65 kg; stature, 174 cm), we can compute from the nomogram in Figure 9.4 a surface area of 1.78 m². Multiplying this value by the average BMR for young men of 38 kcal · m^{-2} · h^{-1} (Fig. 9.3) results in an estimated resting energy expenditure of 67.6 kcal per hour (1.78 m² × 38 kcal), or about 45 kcal for the 40-minute swim. The energy expended solely for the swim is then computed as gross energy expenditure (400 kcal) minus the 40-minute resting value (45 kcal). This results in a net energy expenditure for swimming of 355 kcal.

During constant-load exercise at light to moderate intensity, oxygen uptake rises rapidly in the first several minutes and then levels off and remains fairly constant thereafter. When exercise stops, oxygen uptake decreases rapidly, with the recovery value being approximately equal to the oxygen deficit incurred over the first few minutes of exercise. Total energy expenditure can therefore be estimated from only one or two measures of oxygen uptake during the steady-rate phase of aerobic exercise. During activities with considerable variation in pace, such as tennis, soccer, or basketball, more frequent measures of oxygen uptake must be made to obtain an accurate estimate of the total energy expenditure. During vigorous exercise, when the energy requirements exceed the capacity for aerobic energy transfer, considerable energy is generated anaerobically and blood lactate accumulates. In this situation, estimates of energy cost require measurements of oxygen uptake during exercise and recovery. The precision of these estimates is limited, however, because heavy anaerobic exercise produces physiologic alterations that keep the oxygen uptake elevated for a prolonged period during recovery (refer to Chapter 7). The elevated oxygen uptake does not reflect the true energy cost of the exercise per se and can inflate the actual estimate as much as 10% compared to the same exercise performed aerobically.

MOVEMENT ECONOMY AND MECHANICAL EFFICIENCY DURING EXERCISE

The concept of efficiency considers the relationship between input and resulting output. In a figurative comparison to economics, efficiency of operation parallels the cost required to produce goods in relation to the money generated from the sale of such goods. We might also liken human efficiency of operation to the auto industry, which always strives to optimize the aerodynamic designs of its vehicles to improve efficiency of operation and the important miles-per-gallon rating. Efficiency of human movement is a relation of the amount of energy required to perform a particular task to the actual work accomplished. In a sense, this evaluation occurs when assessing the ease of movement of elite athletes. One does not need a trained eye to qualitatively discriminate the ease, efficiency, or economy of effort when comparing elite swimmers, skiers, cyclists, and dancers to less skilled counterparts who seemingly expend considerable "wasted energy" performing the same task.

ECONOMY OF MOVEMENT

A common method for assessing differences between individuals in their **economy of movement** requires evaluating the oxygen consumed while the subject performs a particular exercise at a set power output or speed.[71] This approach applies to steady-rate exercise, during which the oxygen uptake closely mirrors the energy expended. For example, at a given submaximal speed of running, cycling, or swimming, an individual with greater economy of movement consumes less oxygen. Economy takes on considerable importance during longer-duration exercise, where success largely depends on the aerobic capability of the individual and the oxygen requirements of the task. All else being equal, any adjustment in training that improves the economy of effort translates directly into improved performance.[34] Figure 10.1 relates running economy to endurance performance in elite athletes of comparable aerobic fitness. Clearly, athletes with greater running economies achieve better performance: the relationship is strong. In a statistical sense, approximately 64% of the total variation in 10-km running performance among athletes can be explained by the variations in running economy.[49]

There is no single biomechanical factor that accounts for individual differences in running economy.[12, 41] Significant variation in economy observed at a particular running speed occurs even among trained runners.[15, 50, 54] In general, improvements in running economy can result from long-term

programs of run training.[16, 20] Short-term training that emphasizes only the "proper techniques" of running (that is, arm movements and body alignment) probably does not improve running economy.[35] Recent research indicates, however, that distance runners lacking an economical stride-length pattern benefit from a short-term program of audio-visual feedback that focuses on optimizing stride length.[53]

Indirect evidence from studies of cycling indicates that muscle fiber-type distribution may affect the economy of effort. During submaximal cycling, the exercise economies of well-trained cyclists varied as much as 15%.[17] An important component of this variation was differences in muscle fiber types in the working muscles. Those cyclists exhibiting the greater economy also possessed the greater percentage of slow-twitch, type I muscle fiber in their legs. This suggests that the type I fiber acts with greater mechanical efficiency than the type II fiber.[18]

MECHANICAL EFFICIENCY

Another way to evaluate the relationship between energy input and resulting power output in exercise is to compute the actual **mechanical efficiency** of the movements. Mechanical efficiency is the percentage of total chemical energy expended that contributes to external work, the remainder being lost as heat. Within this context:

$$\text{Mechanical efficiency (\%)} = \text{Actual mechanical work accomplished} \div \text{Input of energy} \times 100$$

The actual external work accomplished or energy output is expressed as force acting through a vertical distance (F × D) and usually recorded as foot pounds or kilogram meters (kg · m). This is fairly easy to determine during cycle ergometry or exercises that require lifting the body mass, such as stair climbing or bench stepping. During horizontal walking or running, the computation of external work output is not possible because external work is not accomplished: The reciprocal movements of the legs and arms negate each other and the body achieves no net gain in terms of vertical distance. If a person walks or runs up a grade, the work component can be estimated from body mass and the vertical distance, or lift, achieved during the exercise period. The energy input portion of the efficiency equation is commonly inferred from the steady-rate oxygen uptake during the exercise. To obtain common units for expressing work, the oxygen uptake is converted to energy units (roughly 1.0 L O_2 = 5.0 kcal; see Table 8.1 for precise calorific transformations based on RQ), which are then converted to units of work (1 kcal = 3087 ft · lb or 426.4 kg · m in a perfect machine with no loss in efficiency).

For example, suppose 13,300 kg · m of work is generated during a 15-minute ride on a stationary bicycle, and the net oxygen consumed to achieve this work totals 25 L (RQ = 0.88). To create common units of measurement, the oxygen consumed is converted to a corresponding work output. From

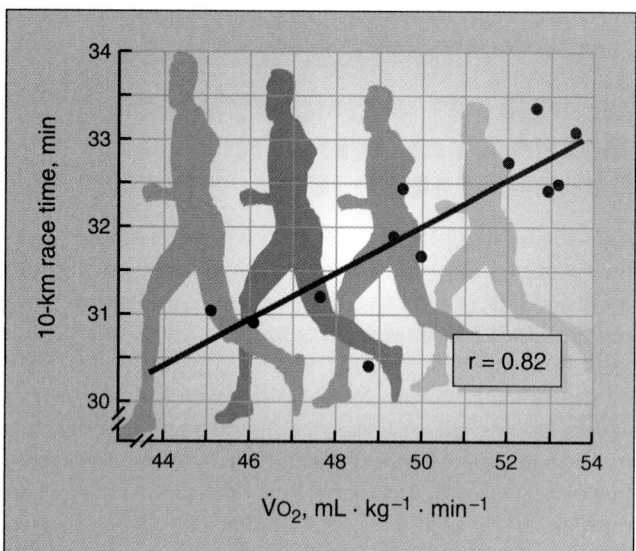

FIGURE 10.1

Relationship between submaximal oxygen uptake at 268 m · min⁻¹ and 10-km race time in elite male runners of comparable aerobic capacity. (From Morgan, D.W., and Craib, M.: Physiological aspects of running economy. *Med. Sci. Sports Exerc.*, 24:456, 1992.)

Table 8.1, note that for an RQ of 0.88, each liter of oxygen uptake generates an energy equivalent of 4.9 kcal. Therefore, 25 L of oxygen uptake generates 122.5 kcal of energy (25 × 4.9 kcal) during the 15-minute ride. The work equivalent of 1 kcal is 426.4 kg · m in a perfectly efficient machine, so the work input is computed as 52,234 kg · m (122.5 × 426.4 kg · m). Mechanical efficiency is computed as follows:

$$\text{Mechanical efficiency} = (13,300 \text{ kg} \cdot \text{m} \div 52,234 \text{ kg} \cdot \text{m}) \times 100 = 25.5\%$$

As with all machines, the efficiency of the human body for producing mechanical work is considerably less than 100%. The biggest factor that affects efficiency is the energy required to overcome internal and external friction. This is essentially wasted energy because it does not accomplish work; consequently, work output is always less than work input. In general, the efficiency of human locomotion in walking, running, and cycling ranges between 20 and 30%.

ENERGY EXPENDITURE DURING WALKING

Walking is the most common form of exercise. For most people, it represents the major physical activity outside the realm of sedentary living. Figure 10.2 displays the research from five countries on the energy expenditure of men who walked at speeds ranging from 1.0 to 10 km per hour (0.62 to 6.2 mph). The relationship between walking speed and oxygen uptake is approximately linear between speeds of 3.0 and 5.0 km per hour (1.86 and 3.10 mph); at faster speeds, walking economy decreases and the relationship curves upward, indicating a disproportionate increase in energy expenditure with increasing speed. This explains why, per unit distance traveled, the total calories expended are greater at these faster, less efficient walking speeds.[8, 24]

INFLUENCE OF BODY MASS

At horizontal walking speeds ranging between 3.2 and 6.4 km per hour (2.0 and 4.0 mph), energy expenditure of people who differ in body mass can be predicted accurately using an equation based on the combined data in Figure 10.2 and other studies.[1, 23, 58] The energy expenditure values are listed in Table 10.1; they are generally accurate to within 15% of the actual energy expenditure for both men and women. On a daily basis, therefore, estimates of the energy expended in walking could be in error by only about

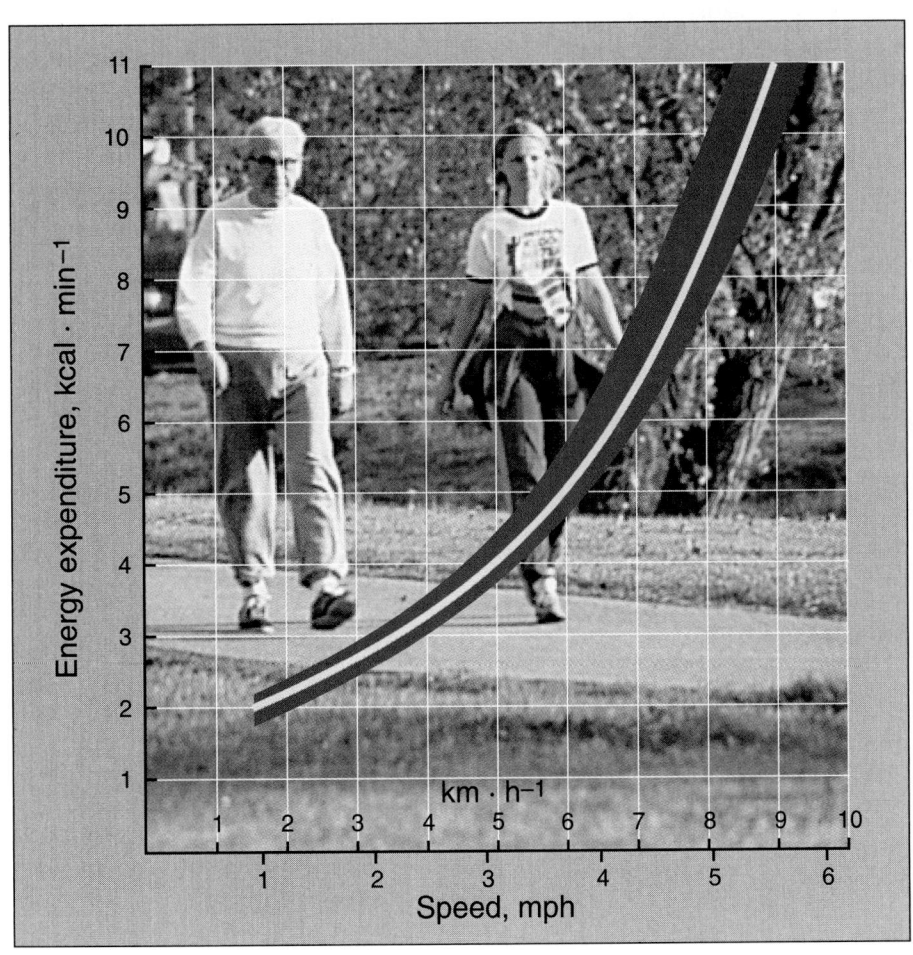

FIGURE 10.2
Energy expenditures while walking on a level surface at different speeds. The line is a compilation of representative average values from various studies reported in the literature.

50 to 100 kcal, assuming that the person walks 2 hours each day. The table is easy to use, formulated on sound research, and relatively accurate for assessing the caloric cost of walking at speeds indicated and for body masses up to 91 kg (200 lb). For heavier individuals, extrapolations can be made but with some loss in accuracy.

EFFECTS OF TERRAIN AND WALKING SURFACE

The influence of terrain and surface on the energy cost of walking is summarized in Table 10.2. Economy is similar for level walking on a grass track or a paved surface. Walking in the sand, however, is almost twice as costly as walking on a hard surface, while walking in soft snow elevates the metabolic cost threefold compared to similar walking on a treadmill.[65] Certainly, a brisk walk along a beach or in freshly fallen snow would provide an excellent exercise stress in programs designed to "burn" calories or improve physiologic fitness.

In another series of experiments, the energy cost of treadmill walking at 2.93 km per hour (1.8 mph) and 5.86 km per hour (3.6 mph) was no different from normal walking on a hard surface at the same speeds.[61] This indicates that people can generate essentially the same exercise stress either by walking on a level surface or walking at the same speed and distance on an exercise treadmill. Such results also lend support to the use of laboratory data to quantify human energy expenditure in "real-life" situations.

Downhill Walking

For most of us, walking the downhill portion of a mountain hike or golf course is a welcome relief in terms of exertion compared to the uphill portion of the exercise. Downhill walking (or running) is a form of **negative work,** during which the body's center of mass is displaced in a downward vertical direction with each step cycle; this leads to a decrease in the total potential energy of the system. Consequently, at the same speed and magnitude (that is, percent grade), it is less costly to perform exercise that utilizes the eccentric muscle actions of negative work compared to the concentric actions of positive work.

Figure 10.3 illustrates the net oxygen cost of both level and negative grade walking at constant speeds of either 90 or 105 $m \cdot s^{-1}$.[70] Compared with walking on level ground, progressive negative grade walking results in a decreasing oxygen cost down to -9% for speeds of 90 $m \cdot min^{-1}$

TABLE 10.2
EFFECT OF DIFFERENT TERRAIN ON THE ENERGY EXPENDITURE OF WALKING BETWEEN 5.2 AND 5.6 KM · H^{-1}

Terrain	Correction Factor[a]
Paved road (similar to grass track)	0.0
Plowed field	1.5
Hard snow	1.6
Sand dune	1.8

First entry from Passmore, R., and Durnin, J.V.G.A.: Human energy expenditure. *Physiol. Rev.*, 35:801, 1955. Last three entries from Givoni, B., and Goldman, R.F.: Predicting metabolic energy cost. *J. Appl. Physiol.*, 30:429, 1971.
[a]The correction factor is a multiple of the energy expenditure for walking on a paved road or grass track. For example, the energy cost of walking in a plowed field is 1.5 times that of walking on a paved road.

TABLE 10.1
PREDICTION OF ENERGY EXPENDITURE (KCAL · MIN^{-1}) FROM SPEED OF LEVEL WALKING AND BODY MASS^a

Speed		Body Mass						
mph	km · h^{-1}	kg 36 / lb 80	45 / 100	54 / 120	64 / 140	73 / 160	82 / 180	91 / 200
2.0	3.22	1.9	2.2	2.6	2.9	3.2	3.5	3.8
2.5	4.02	2.3	2.7	3.1	3.5	3.8	4.2	4.5
3.0	4.83	2.7	3.1	3.6	4.0	4.4	4.8	5.3
3.5	5.63	3.1	3.6	4.2	4.6	5.0	5.4	6.1
4.0	6.44	3.5	4.1	4.7	5.2	5.8	6.4	7.0

Data from Passmore, R., and Durnin, J.V.G.A.: Human energy expenditure. *Physiol. Rev.*, 35:801, 1955.
^{a}How to use the table: A 120-lb (54-kg) person who walks at 3.0 mph (4.83 km · h^{-1}) expends 3.6 kcal · min^{-1}. A total of 216 kcal would be expended if the person walked for 60 minutes.

and −12% for speeds of 105 m · min⁻¹. At the more severe negative grades, however, the energy cost begins to increase. This added oxygen cost for walking down the more steep grades is attributed to the additional energy required to resist or "brake" the body from the pull of gravity while attempting to maintain a proper and safe walking rhythm.

EFFECTS OF FOOTWEAR

It is considerably more costly to carry weights on the feet or ankles than to carry a similar weight attached to the torso. For example, with a weight equal to 1.4% of body mass placed on the ankles, the energy cost of walking increases an average of 8%, or nearly 6 times more than if the same weight were carried on the torso.[33] In a practical sense, the energy cost of walking and running is significantly increased by wearing boots compared to running shoes. Simply adding an additional 100 g to each shoe causes a 1% increase in oxygen uptake during moderate running. The implications of these findings in the design of running shoes, hiking and climbing boots, and work boots traditionally required in professions such as mining, forestry, fire fighting, and the military is clear—small changes in shoe weight produce meaningful changes in the economy of locomotion. The cushioning properties of shoes also affect movement economy.[57] A softer-soled running shoe has reduced the

oxygen cost of running at a moderate speed by about 2.4% compared to a similar shoe with a firmer cushioning system, even though the pair of softer-soled shoes was 31 g heavier.[26]

Figure 10.4 displays the heart rate and oxygen uptake of eight women during a 15-minute treadmill run at 90% of aerobic capacity (average speed of 3.3 m · s⁻¹) while wearing training shoes (midsole constructed of ethyl vinyl acetate [EVA] and polyurethane [PU]; average mass, 538 g) and racing flats (midsole constructed of only EVA; average mass, 311 g).[29] At the start of the run, both heart rate and oxygen uptake were significantly higher while wearing the training shoes; thereafter, the heart rate and oxygen uptake

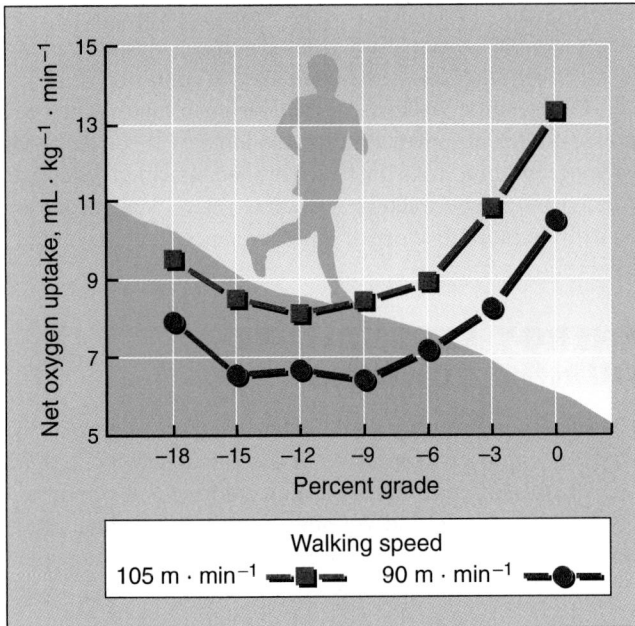

FIGURE 10.3

Net oxygen costs of level and downhill walking at grades between −3 and −18% and speeds between 90 and 105 m · min⁻¹. *Percent grade* reflects the vertical distance moved downward per unit horizontal distance traversed. (From Wanta, D.M., et al.: Metabolic response to graded downhill walking. *Med. Sci. Sports Exerc.*, 25:159, 1993.)

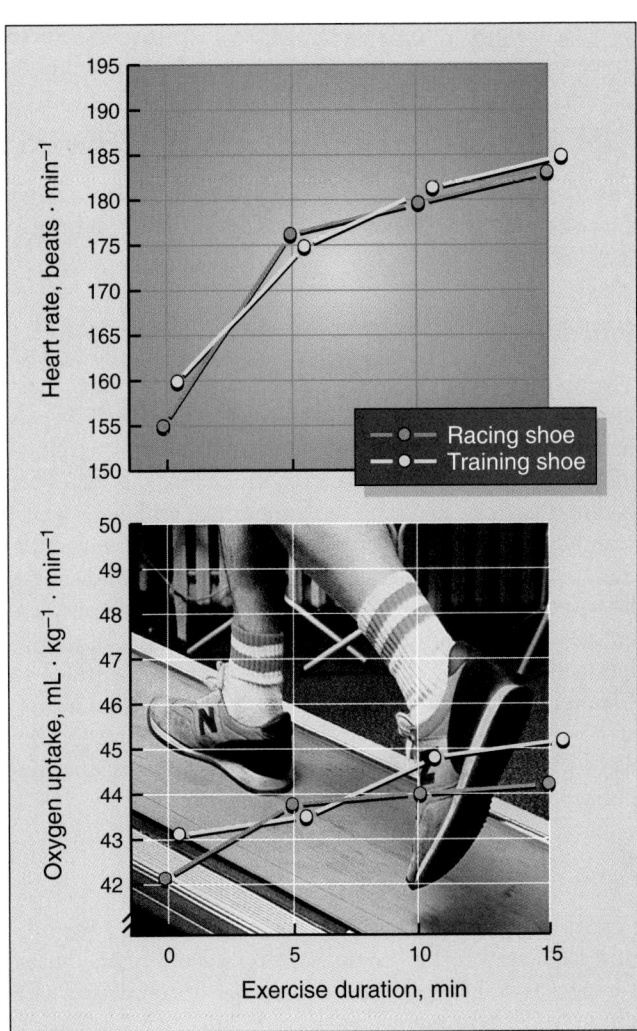

FIGURE 10.4

Heart rate (*Top*) and oxygen uptake (*Bottom*) during a 15-minute training run with subjects wearing training shoes or running flats. The measurements, taken at 90% of V̇O₂max, represent 8 females running on a level treadmill at an average speed of 3.3 m · s⁻¹. (From Hamill, J., et al.: Effects of shoe type on cardiorespiratory responses and rear foot motion during treadmill running. *Med. Sci. Sports Exerc.*, 20:515, 1988.)

continued to increase, but with no significant difference in these variables between the two shoe conditions. The runners were unable to discern differences in perceived effort during runs with the two pairs of shoes, even though the cumulative increase in oxygen uptake of 1.3% while wearing the training shoes would theoretically translate to a $2.4 \text{ mL} \cdot \text{kg}^{-1} \cdot \text{min}^{-1}$ higher total energy expenditure during a 10-km run performed in 40 minutes. What is unknown is whether the differences in shoe construction (added mediolateral stability with the heavier shoe compared to the lighter but less stable racing shoe) actually would translate to improved track performance. A major concern with the lighter but less stable shoe is the increased possibility of lower extremity injury. The answer to this concern lies in further research with different combinations of midsole materials and designs, coupled with physiological and performance indices in men and women of different training status and ability.

USE OF HAND-HELD AND ANKLE WEIGHTS

The impact force on the leg while running is equal to about 3 times body mass, whereas the level of leg shock walking is only 30% of this value.

Walking

The use of ankle weights can increase the energy cost of walking to values usually observed for running.[48] This is beneficial for those who desire to use only walking as a low-impact training modality yet require intensities of effort higher than can be achieved at normal walking speeds. Hand-held weights and upper-body exercise also increase the energy cost of walking.[9, 22, 27] There is some indication, however, that this procedure disproportionately elevates exercise systolic blood pressure, perhaps as a result of the effects of upper body exercise on blood pressure (refer to Chapter 15) and the elevated intramuscular tension associated with gripping the weight. This factor would restrict the use of hand-held weights for individuals with existing hypertension or coronary heart disease.

Running

Considering the relatively small increase in energy expenditure facilitated by the use of hand or ankle weights during running, it would seem more desirable to simply increase the unweighted running speed or distance. This would reduce the injury potential from increased impact force caused by weights and eliminate the added discomfort of carrying the weights.[14]

COMPETITION WALKERS

The energy expenditures of five Olympic-caliber walkers were studied at various speeds while the subjects walked and ran on a treadmill.[47] In actual competition, the walking speed of these athletes averaged $13.0 \text{ km} \cdot \text{h}^{-1}$ (11.5 to 14.8 $\text{km} \cdot \text{h}^{-1}$ [7.1 to 9.2 mph]) over distances ranging from 1.6 to 50 km. This was a relatively fast speed, because the winner of the 20-km walk at the 1988 Korea Olympics averaged a record $14.4 \text{ km} \cdot \text{h}^{-1}$ (8.9 mph) during a 12.4-mile walk (the world-record walk, set in 1994 by Bernardo Segura of Mexico, averaged 6 minutes 24 seconds per mile!). As illustrated in Figure 10.5, the break point in the economy of locomotion between walking and running for these race-walkers is between 8.0 and 9.0 $\text{km} \cdot \text{h}^{-1}$. These data, plus biomechanical evidence, indicate that the crossover speed—when running becomes more economical than walking—is about the same for both conventional and competitive styles of walking (Figure 10.6).[11] In addition, the oxygen uptakes for race-walkers during treadmill walking at competition speeds were only slightly lower than the highest oxygen uptakes achieved during treadmill running. Although the relationship between oxygen uptake and walking at speeds greater than 8 km per hour (4.97 mph) was approximately linear, the slope of the line was twice as steep compared to running at the same speeds. These athletes were able to walk at velocities up to 16 km · h^{-1} (9.94 mph) and attain oxygen uptakes as high as those achieved while running; *the economy of walking faster than 8 km per hour was one-half of that for running at the same speeds.* The attainment of similar values for $\dot{V}O_2$max during both race-walking and running in the elite competitors further supports the model for aerobic **training specificity** because aerobic capacity in untrained subjects during walking is generally 5 to 15% lower compared to running.[28, 44]

Competition walkers can achieve such high yet uneconomical rates of movement, unattainable with conventional walking, by using a distinctive modified walking technique. Among elite race-walkers, variations in walking economy contribute more to successful performance than in competitive running.[28]

ENERGY EXPENDITURE DURING RUNNING

Energy expenditure for running has been quantified in two ways: (*a*) during performance of the actual activity, and (*b*) on a treadmill, where speed and grade can be precisely controlled. Jogging and running are essentially qualitative terms related to the speed at which the movement is performed. At identical speeds, a distance runner is running at a much lower percentage of aerobic capacity than an untrained runner even though their oxygen uptakes while running may be similar. Thus, the demarcation between what is considered jogging and running depends on the fitness level of the participant: a jog for one person could be a run for another.

Independent of fitness, however, it is more economical from an energy standpoint to discontinue walking and begin

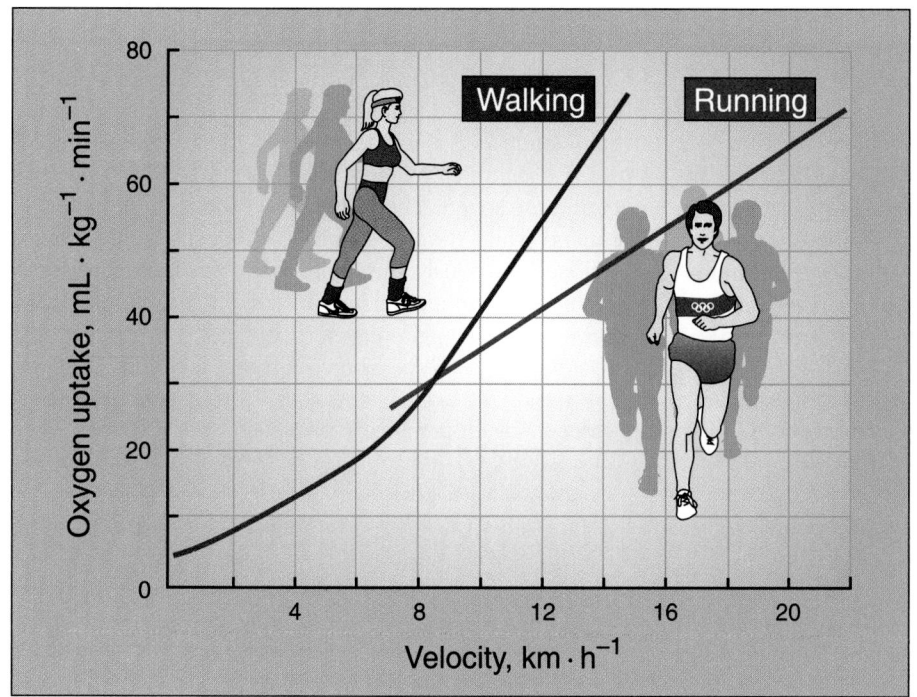

FIGURE 10.5

Relationship between oxygen uptake and horizontal velocity for walking and running in competition walkers. (Adapted from Menier, D.R., and Pugh, L.G.C.E.: The relation of oxygen intake and velocity of walking and running in competition walkers. *J. Physiol.*, 197: 717, 1968.)

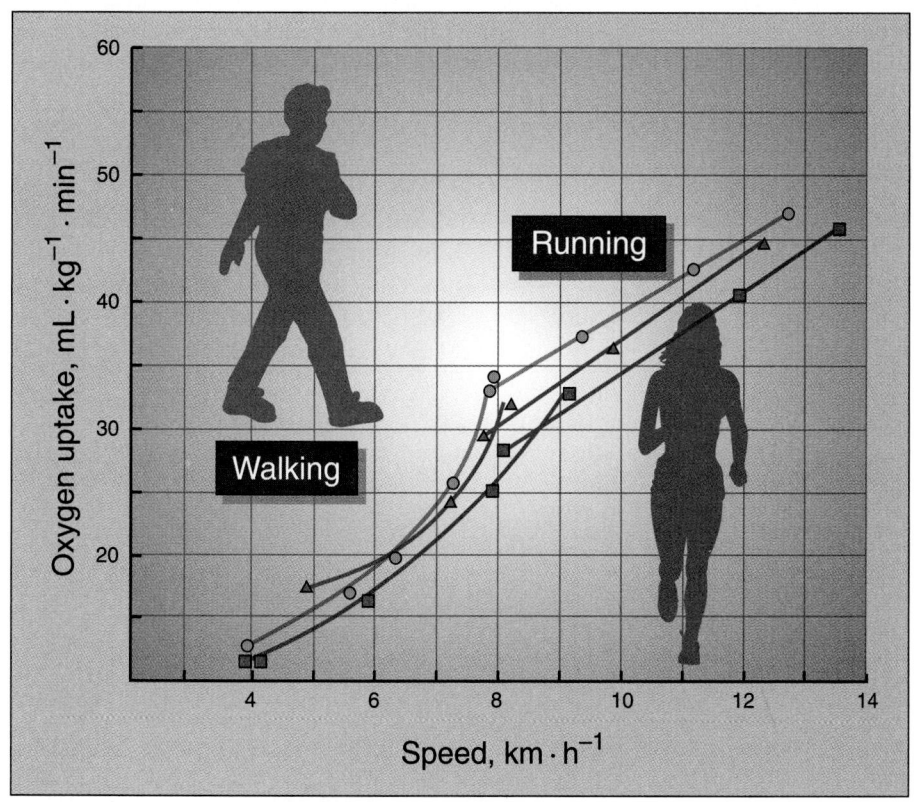

FIGURE 10.6

Relationship between oxygen uptake and speed of horizontal walking and running in men and women. Different symbols represent values from various research studies. (From Falls, H.B., and Humphrey, L.D.: Energy cost of running and walking in young women. *Med. Sci. Sports.*, 8:9, 1976.)

running at speeds greater than about 8 km · h⁻¹ (5 mph). This is illustrated in Figure 10.6, which illustrates the relationship between oxygen uptake and horizontal walking and running for men and women at speeds between 4 and 14 km · h⁻¹ (2.5 and 8.7 mph). In the data depicted by the triangles,[39] the lines relating oxygen uptake and speed intersect at a running speed of 8.0 km · h⁻¹ (5.0 mph), whereas for competition walkers, shown by the squares,[47] the "break point" in locomotion economy occurs at about 8.7 km · h⁻¹ (5.4 mph).

THE ECONOMY OF RUNNING FAST OR SLOW

The data for running given in Figure 10.6 illustrate an important principle concerning running speed and energy expenditure. *Because the relationship between oxygen uptake and running speed is linear, the total caloric cost of running a given distance at a steady-rate oxygen uptake is about the same regardless of whether the pace is fast or slow.* Simply stated, running a mile at 10 mph requires about twice the energy per minute as running a mile at 5 mph; however, at the faster speed running the mile takes 6 minutes, while running at the slower speed takes twice as long, or 12 minutes. Consequently, the energy cost of the mile is about the same. This is true not only for horizontal running but also for running at grades that range from −45 to +15%.[21, 39] *During horizontal running, the net energy cost (that is, excluding the resting requirement) per kilogram of body mass per kilometer traveled is approximately 1 kcal, or 1 kcal · kg^{-1} · km^{-1}.* Thus, for a person weighing 78 kg, the net energy cost of running 1 km would be about 78 kcal, regardless of running speed. Expressed in terms of oxygen uptake, this amounts to 15.6 L of oxygen consumed per kilometer (1 L O_2 = 5 kcal). In comparing the net energy costs of locomotion per unit distance traveled, it is well documented that it is more costly to run than to walk a given distance.[5]

ENERGY COST VALUES

Table 10.3 presents values for the net energy expended during running for 1 hour at various speeds. Speed is expressed in kilometers per hour and miles per hour as well as the number of minutes required to complete 1 mile at a particular running speed. The values in bold are the net calories expended while running 1 mile for a given body mass; as mentioned previously, this energy requirement is fairly constant and independent of running speed. *Thus, for a person who weighs 62 kg, running a 26.2-mile marathon requires approximately 2600 kcal regardless of whether the run is completed in just over 2 hours, 3 hours, or 4 hours!*

For a heavier person, the energy cost per mile increases proportionally. This fact certainly supports the role of exercise as a caloric stress for the relatively unfit, overfat person who wants to increase energy expenditure for weight control. For example, if a 102-kg person jogs 5 miles each day at a comfortable pace, 163 kcal is expended for each mile completed, or a total of 815 kcal for the 5-mile run. Increasing or decreasing the speed (within the broad range of steady-rate paces) simply alters the duration of the exercise period; it has little effect on the total energy expended.

Table 10.4 summarizes the data from various studies on the energy expenditure for horizontal and grade walking and running on a solid surface. The energy requirement is ex-

TABLE 10.3
NET ENERGY EXPENDITURE PER HOUR OF HORIZONTAL RUNNING RELATED TO VELOCITY AND BODY MASS[a]

Body Mass		$km \cdot h^{-1b}$	8	9	10	11	12	13	14	15	16
		mph	4.97	5.60	6.20	6.84	7.46	8.08	8.70	9.32	9.94
		min per mile	12:00	10:43	9:41	8:46	8:02	7:26	6:54	6:26	6:02
(kg)	(lb)	kcal per mile									
50	110	**80**	400	450	500	550	600	650	700	750	800
54	119	**86**	432	486	540	594	648	702	756	810	864
58	128	**93**	464	522	580	638	696	754	812	870	928
62	137	**99**	496	558	620	682	744	806	868	930	992
66	146	**106**	528	594	660	726	792	858	924	990	1056
70	154	**112**	560	630	700	770	840	910	980	1050	1120
74	163	**118**	592	666	740	814	888	962	1036	1110	1184
78	172	**125**	624	702	780	858	936	1014	1092	1170	1248
82	181	**131**	656	738	820	902	984	1066	1148	1230	1312
86	190	**138**	688	774	860	946	1032	1118	1204	1290	1376
90	199	**144**	720	810	900	990	1080	1170	1260	1350	1440
94	207	**150**	752	846	940	1034	1128	1222	1316	1410	1504
98	216	**157**	784	882	980	1078	1176	1274	1372	1470	1568
102	225	**163**	816	918	1020	1122	1224	1326	1428	1530	1632
106	234	**170**	848	954	1060	1166	1272	1378	1484	1590	1696

[a]The table is interpreted as follows: For a 50-kg person, the *net* energy expenditure for running for 1 hour at 8 km · h^{-1} or 4.97 mph is 400 kcal; this speed represents a 12-minute per mile pace. Thus, 5 miles would be run in 1 hour and 400 kcal would be expended. If the pace was increased to 12 km · h^{-1}, 600 kcal would be expended during the hour of running.
[b]Running speeds are expressed as kilometers per hour (km · h^{-1}), miles per hour (mph), and minutes required to complete each mile (min per mile). The values in **boldface type** are the *net* calories expended to run 1 mile for a given body mass, independent of running speed.

TABLE 10.4
ENERGY REQUIREMENTS (METs) FOR HORIZONTAL AND GRADE WALKING AND RUNNING ON A SOLID SURFACE

Horizontal and Grade Walking

% Grade	mph	1.7	2.0	2.5	3.0	3.4	3.75
	$m \cdot min^{-1}$	45.6	53.7	67.0	80.5	91.2	100.5
0		2.3	2.5	2.9	3.3	3.6	3.9
2.5		2.9	3.2	3.8	4.3	4.8	5.2
5.0		3.5	3.9	4.6	5.4	5.9	6.5
7.5		4.1	4.6	5.5	6.4	7.1	7.8
10.0		4.6	5.3	6.3	7.4	8.3	9.1
12.5		5.2	6.0	7.2	8.5	9.5	10.4
15.0		5.8	6.6	8.1	9.5	10.6	11.7
17.5		6.4	7.3	8.9	10.5	11.8	12.9
20.0		7.0	8.0	9.8	11.6	13.0	14.2
22.5		7.6	8.7	10.6	12.6	14.2	15.5
25.0		8.2	9.4	11.5	13.6	15.3	16.8

Horizontal and Grade Jogging/Running
Outdoors on solid surface

% Grade	mph	5	6	7	7.5	8	9	10
	$m \cdot min^{-1}$	134	161	188	201	215	241	268
0		8.6	10.2	11.7	12.5	13.3	14.8	16.3
2.5		10.3	12.3	14.1	15.1	16.1	17.9	19.7
5.0		12.0	14.3	16.5	17.7	18.8		
7.5		13.9	16.4	18.9				
10.0		15.5	18.5					

Modified from American College of Sports Medicine: *Guidelines for Exercise Testing and Prescription*, 3rd ed. Philadelphia, Lea & Febiger, 1986.

pressed in **MET** units, which represent multiples of the resting metabolic rate. Each MET represents the equivalent of about 3.6 mL $O_2 \cdot kg^{-1} \cdot min^{-1}$.

STRIDE LENGTH, STRIDE FREQUENCY, AND SPEED

Running   *BioMech*

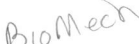

Running speed can be increased in one of three ways: (*a*) by increasing the number of steps each minute (**stride frequency**), (*b*) by increasing the distance between steps (**stride length**), or (*c*) by increasing **both** the length and frequency of strides. Although the third option may seem the obvious way to increase running speed, several experiments have provided objective data concerning this question.

In 1944, the stride pattern was evaluated for the Danish champion in the 5- and 10-km running events.[8] At a running speed of 9.3 km per hour (5.8 mph), this athlete's stride frequency was 160 per minute with a corresponding stride length of 97 cm (38.2 in.). When running speed was

increased 91% to 17.8 km $\cdot$ h^{-1} (11.1 mph), stride frequency increased only 10% to 176 per minute, whereas an 83% increase to 168 cm was observed in stride length. Figure 10.7A displays the interaction between stride frequency and stride length as running speed increases. Doubling the speed from 10 to 20 km $\cdot$ h^{-1} increases stride length by 85%, whereas stride frequency only increases about 9%. Increasing speed above 23 km $\cdot$ h^{-1} (14.3 mph), however, is achieved mainly by augmenting stride frequency. *As a general rule, running speed is increased mainly by lengthening the stride. Only at faster speeds does stride frequency become important.*

COMPETITION WALKING

The competitive walker does not increase speed in the same way as a runner. Figure 10.7B illustrates the stride length–stride frequency relationship for an Olympic 10-km medal winner walking at speeds from 10 to 14.4 km $\cdot$ h^{-1}. When walking speed increased from 10 to 14.4 km $\cdot$ h^{-1}, the stride frequency increased by 27% and the stride length in-

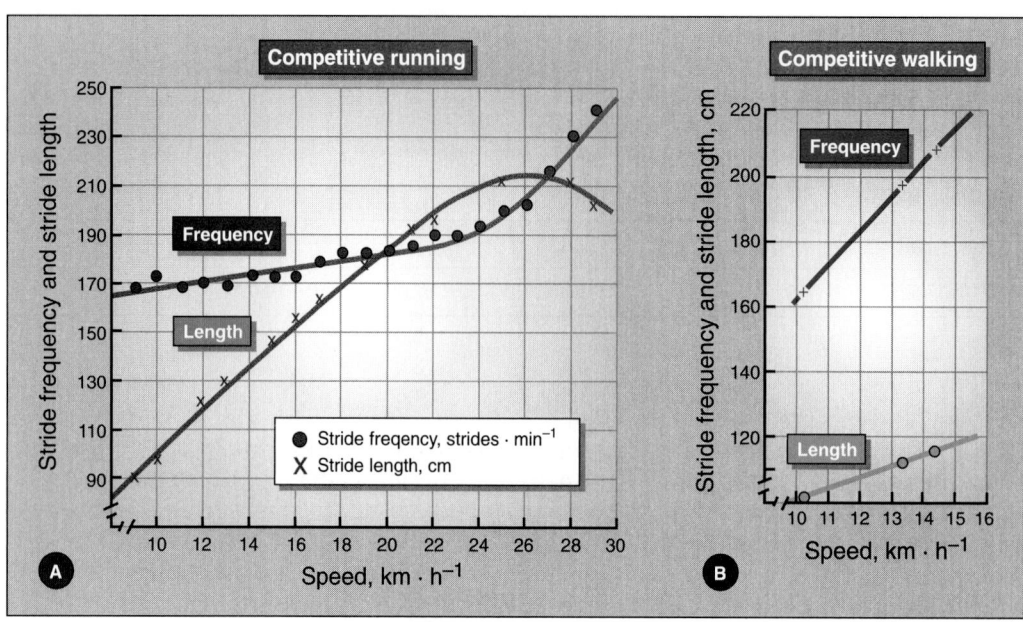

FIGURE 10.7

A, Stride frequency and stride length plotted as a function of running speed. **B,** Data for an Olympic walker during race-walking. (From Hogberg, P.: Length of stride, stride frequency, flight period and maximum distance between the feet during running with different speeds. *Int. Z. Angew. Physiol.*, 14:431, 1952.)

creased by 13%. At faster speeds, there was an even greater increase in stride frequency, because—unlike running, during which the body glides through the air—competitive walking requires that the back foot remain on the ground until the front foot makes contact. Thus, lengthening the stride becomes a difficult and ineffective means to increase speed. Owing to this standardization of style in competitive walking, additional energy must be expended to move the leg rapidly forward; this requires a corresponding involvement of the trunk and arm musculature and explains why it is more economical from an energy standpoint to run than to walk at speeds greater than 8 or 9 km per hour (Figure 10.6).

OPTIMUM STRIDE LENGTH

Running at a constant speed can be performed at an optimum combination of stride length and frequency. This optimum depends largely on the person's mechanics, or "style" of running, and cannot be determined from body measurements.[13] Nevertheless, it is generally more costly to overstride than to understride. Figure 10.8 relates oxygen uptake to different stride lengths altered by a subject while running at a relatively fast speed of 14 km · h⁻¹ (8.7 mph).

For this runner, a stride length of 135 cm was associated with the lowest oxygen uptake, 3.35 L per minute. Oxygen uptake increased 8% when stride length was shortened to 118 cm; a 12% increase in oxygen uptake was noted when the distance between steps was lengthened to 153 cm. The curve in the inset graph shows a similar pattern for oxygen uptake when running speed increased to 16 km per hour

and stride lengths varied between 135 and 169 cm. Decreasing this runner's stride length from an optimum of 149 cm to 135 cm increased oxygen uptake by 4.1%, while lengthening the stride to 169 cm increased the aerobic requirement nearly 13%. As might be expected, the most economical stride length for a particular running speed was usually the one selected by the subject (marked in the figure by an *X*). Lengthening the stride above the optimum caused a larger increase in oxygen uptake than using a shorter-than-optimum length. Thus, urging a runner who shows signs of fatigue to "Lengthen your stride!" to maintain speed is actually counterproductive in terms of oxygen cost.

It is probably best to let well-trained runners run at the stride length they have selected through years of running.[30] In keeping with the concept that the body attempts to achieve a level of "minimum effort," this generally produces the most economical running performance, reflecting an individual's unique body size, inertia of limb segments, and anatomic development.[12, 48a, 48b] *Consequently, there is no "best" style characteristic of elite runners.* Biomechanical analysis may help the athlete correct minor irregularities in movement patterns while running.[56] To the competitive runner, even minor improvement in movement economy may eventually translate into improved performance.

RUNNING ECONOMY: CHILDREN AND ADULTS, TRAINED AND UNTRAINED

In general, boys and girls are less economical runners than adults because they require 20 to 30% more oxygen per unit of body mass to run at a particular speed.[20, 35] Such differences have been attributed to greater stride frequencies and shorter stride lengths among children, as well as differences in body mechanics that could reduce movement economy.[25, 36, 63] As demonstrated in Figure 10.9*B*, running economy improves steadily during years 10 to 18. This partly explains the relatively poor performance of young children in distance running and their progressive improvement in endurance performance through adolescence, although their aerobic capacity in relation to body mass (mL $O_2 \cdot kg^{-1} \cdot min^{-1}$; Figure 10.9*A*) remains relatively constant during this time.[19, 20]

When running at a particular speed, elite adolescent and adult endurance runners generally have lower oxygen uptakes than less trained or less successful counterparts of the same age.[34, 42, 54] In fact, distance athletes as a group run 5 to 10% more economically than well-trained middle-distance runners.[15] For trained runners, economy values and biomechanical characteristics during running remain fairly stable from day to day, even during high-intensity exercise.[51, 52]

AIR RESISTANCE

Anyone who has run into a headwind intuitively knows that more energy is expended trying to maintain a given pace under such conditions than when running in calm air or with the wind at one's back. The magnitude of the effect of air resistance on the energy cost of running varies with three factors: (*a*) air density, (*b*) the runner's projected surface area, and (*c*) the square of the runner's velocity. Depending on speed, overcoming air resistance can require 3 to 9% of the total energy cost of running in calm air.[31, 59] Running into a

headwind creates an additional energy expense. As shown in Figure 10.10, the average oxygen uptake while running at 15.9 $km \cdot h^{-1}$ in calm conditions was 2.92 L per minute. This number increased 5.5%, to 3.09 L per minute, against a 16-$km \cdot h^{-1}$ (9.9-mph) "headwind" and increased to 4.1 L per minute against the strongest wind (41 mph)—an additional 41% expenditure of energy to maintain running velocity!

Drafting: Often a Wise Position

The negative effect of air resistance and headwind on the energy cost of running confirms the wisdom of athletes who choose to run in a more aerodynamically desirable position directly behind a competitor, a technique called **drafting.** For example, running 1 m behind another runner at a speed of 6 $m \cdot s^{-1}$ decreases the total energy expenditure by about 7%.[59] Drafting at this speed could save about 1 second for each 400 m covered during a race. The beneficial effect of drafting on the economy of effort also has been observed for cross-country skiing and bicycling.[6, 45] Bicycling at 40 $km \cdot h^{-1}$ on a calm day requires that about 90% of the power generated be used to overcome air resistance. At this speed, reductions in energy expenditure of 26 to 38% are possible when a competitor closely follows another cyclist.[37]

Some may argue that the negative effects of running into a headwind are counterbalanced by one's return with the tail wind. This is not the case, however, as the energy cost of cutting through a headwind is significantly greater than the corresponding reduction in oxygen uptake resulting from an equivalent wind velocity at one's back. Wind tunnel tests have shown that clothing modifications or even trimming one's hair can improve aerodynamics and reduce

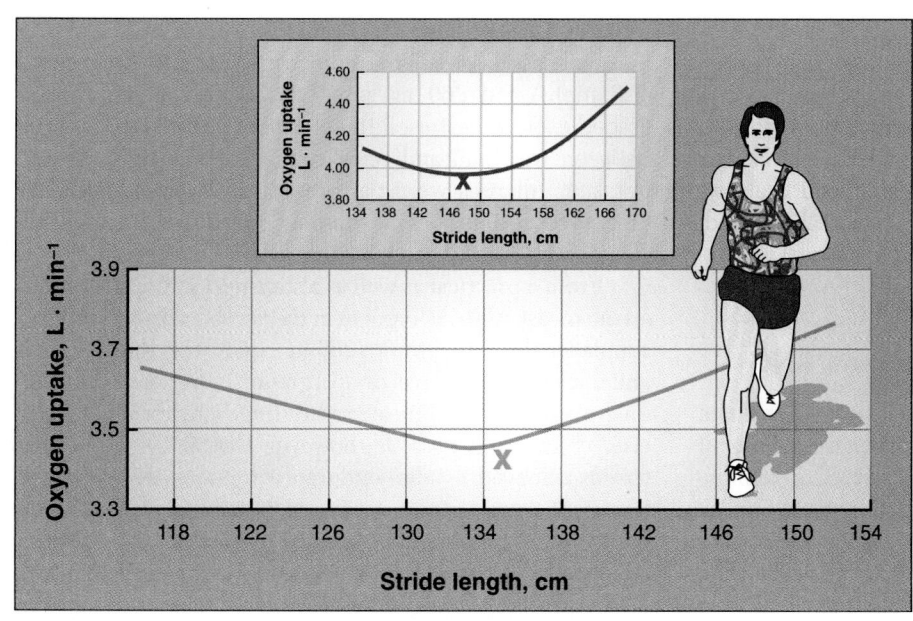

FIGURE 10.8

Oxygen uptake while running at 14 $km \cdot h^{-1}$ as affected by different stride lengths. The inset graph is a plot of oxygen uptake at a faster speed of 16 $km \cdot h^{-1}$. (From Hogberg, P.: Length of stride, stride frequency, flight period and maximum distance between the feet during running with different speeds. *Int. Z. Angew. Physiol.*, 14:431, 1952.)

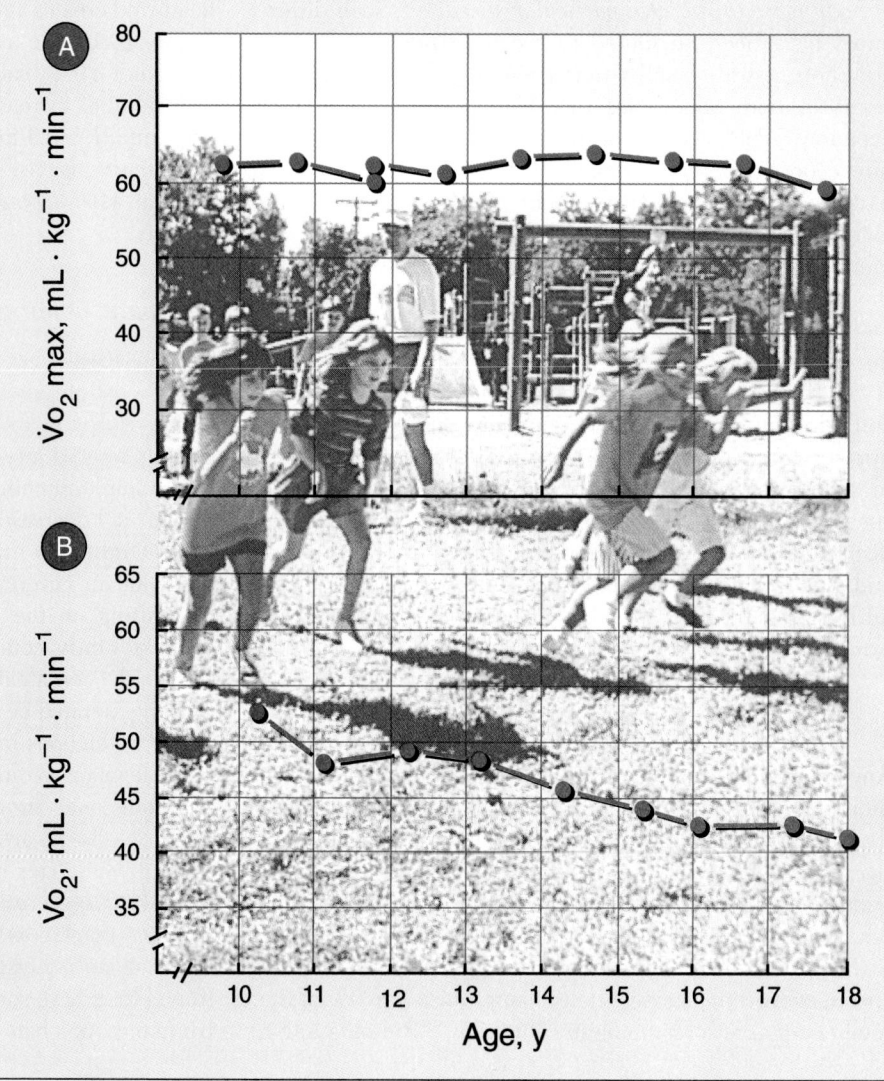

FIGURE 10.9

Effects of growth on (**A**) aerobic capacity and (**B**) submaximal oxygen uptake during running at 202 m · min⁻¹. (Adapted from Daniels, J., et al.: Differences and changes in V̇o₂ among runners 10 to 18 years of age. *Med. Sci. Sports,* 10:200, 1978.)

the effects of air resistance as much as 6%. This could translate into a significant improvement in running performance.[3] At higher altitudes, wind velocity has less effect on energy expenditure than at sea level because of the reduced air density at higher elevations. For example, the oxygen cost of competitive skating at a particular speed is always lower at high altitudes than at sea level.[2] In all likelihood, this altitude effect also applies to other sports such as running, cross-country skiing, and cycling.

TREADMILL VERSUS TRACK RUNNING

Although the treadmill is used almost exclusively to evaluate the physiology of running, one could question the validity of this procedure for determining the energetics of running and relating this to competitive track performance. For example, is the energy required to run at a given speed on a treadmill the same as that required to run on a track in calm weather? To answer this question, eight distance runners

were studied on both a treadmill and track at three submaximal speeds of 180 m · min⁻¹ (6.7 mph), 210 m · min⁻¹ (7.8 mph), and 260 m · min⁻¹ (9.7 mph), and during a graded exercise test used to determine possible differences between treadmill and track running on maximal oxygen uptake.[46] All runs were performed under calm air conditions. The results for one running speed and for maximal exercise are summarized in Table 10.5.

From a practical as well as a statistical standpoint, there are no measurable differences in the aerobic requirements of submaximal running (up to 286 m · min⁻¹) on the treadmill and track (either on level or up a grade), or between the maximal oxygen uptakes measured during both forms of exercise.[3, 46] It is still possible, however, that at faster running speeds achieved by elite endurance runners, the impact of air resistance on a calm day is considerable and the oxygen cost of track running may be greater compared to "stationary" running on a treadmill at the same fast speed. This is certainly the case in activities requiring the athlete to move at

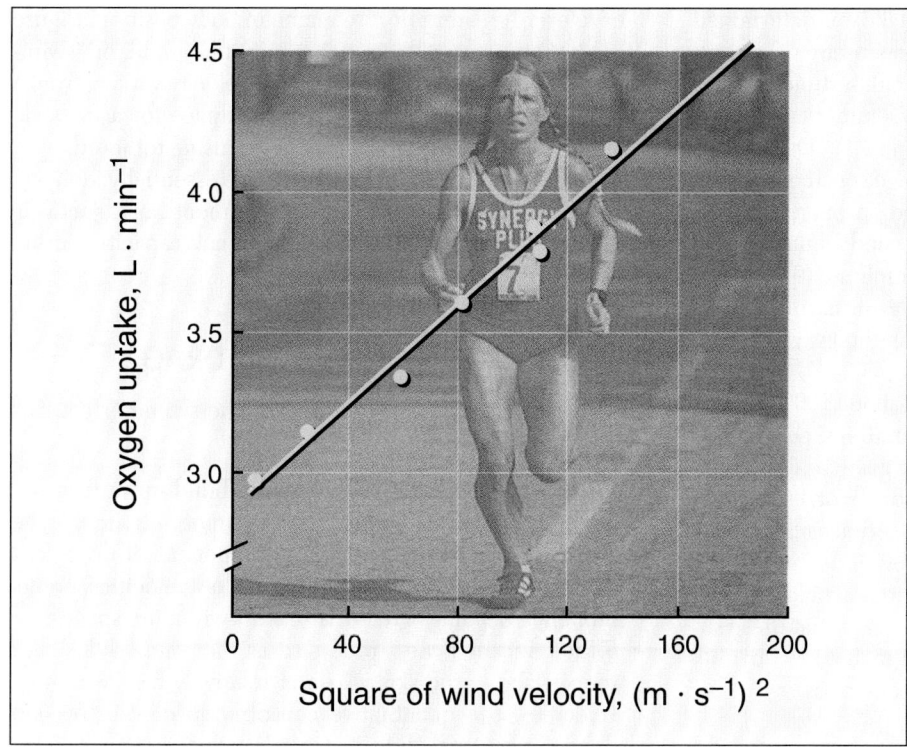

FIGURE 10.10
Oxygen uptake as a function of the square of the wind velocity while running at 15.9 km · h⁻¹ against various headwinds. (From Pugh, L.G.C.E.: Oxygen intake and treadmill running with observations on the effect of air resistance. *J. Physiol.*, 207:823, 1970.)

TABLE 10.5
COMPARISON OF AVERAGE METABOLIC RESPONSES DURING TREADMILL AND TRACK RUNNING

Measurement	Treadmill	Track	Difference
Submaximal Exercise			
Oxygen uptake,			
mL · kg⁻¹ · min⁻¹	42.2	42.7	0.5
Respiratory exchange ratio	0.89	0.87	−0.02
Running speed, m · min⁻¹	213.7	216.8	3.1
Maximal Exercise			
Oxygen uptake, L · min⁻¹	4.40	4.44	0.04
mL · kg⁻¹ · min⁻¹	66.9	66.3	−0.6
Ventilation, L · min⁻¹, BTPS	142.5	146.5	4.0
Respiratory exchange ratio	1.15	1.11	−0.04

Adapted from McMiken, D.F., and Daniels, J.T.: Aerobic requirements and maximum aerobic power in treadmill and track running. *Med. Sci. Sports*, 8:14, 1976.

high velocities such as in cycling and speed skating, in which the retarding effects of air resistance become considerable. This forces the athlete to focus on factors that improve aerodynamics such as clothing, equipment, and body position.

MARATHON RUNNING

In 1988, the Ethiopian Belayneh Densimo set the world record in the marathon with a time of 2 h:06 min:50 s. The average speed of just under 4 min:53 s per mile over the 26.2-mile course truly is an outstanding achievement in human performance capacity. Not only does this blistering pace require a steady-rate oxygen uptake that exceeds the aerobic capacity of most male college students, it also represents an average of approximately 75 to 90% of the marathoner's aerobic power being sustained for just over 2 hours!

Two distance runners were measured during a marathon to determine the energy expenditure per minute and the total caloric cost of the run.[40] Oxygen uptake was determined every 3 miles using the bag technique of open-circuit spirometry illustrated in Figure 8.4. Their marathon times were 2 h:36 min:34 s ($\dot{V}O_2$max = 70.5 mL · kg^{-1} · min^{-1}) and 2 h:39 min:28 s ($\dot{V}O_2$max = 73.9 mL · kg^{-1} · min^{-1}). During the run, the first runner maintained an average speed of 270.5 m per minute (10.0 mph), which required an oxygen uptake equal to 80% of his $\dot{V}O_2$max. For the second runner, whose average speed was slower at 266.1 m per minute (9.92 mph), the aerobic requirement averaged 78.3% of maximum. For both men, the energy cost to run the marathon was between 2300 and 2400 kcal.

For distance runners who train at about 100 miles, or slightly less than the distance of four marathons, per week at close to competitive speeds, the weekly exercise caloric expenditure is approximately 10,000 kcal, or about 4 to 5 times more than a sedentary adult. For the serious marathoner who trains year-round, the total energy expended in training for 4 years prior to an Olympic competition would be close to 2 million calories! Thus, it is not surprising that these superior, endurance-trained athletes have such a low quantity of body fat (averaging less than 4% of body mass).

SWIMMING

Swimming differs in several important aspects from walking or running. One obvious difference is that energy must be expended to maintain buoyancy and, at the same time, generate horizontal movement through the use of the arms and legs, either in combination or separately. Other differences include the requirements for overcoming the **drag forces** that impede the forward movement of a swimmer through a fluid. The amount of drag depends on the fluid medium and the size, shape, and velocity of the swimmer. All of these factors contribute to a total mechanical efficiency in front-crawl swimming that ranges between only 5 and 9.5%.[69] *Within this framework, the energy cost of swimming a given distance is about four times greater than the cost of running the same distance.*

METHODS OF MEASUREMENT

For short swims such as 25 yards swum at different velocities, subjects need not breathe during the swim, and energy expenditure is estimated from the oxygen uptake during 20 to 40 minutes of recovery. For longer swims, including 12- to 14-hour endurance events, we can compute energy expenditure from oxygen uptake, which is measured using open-circuit spirometry, during portions of the actual swim. In studies conducted in the pool, the researcher walks alongside the swimmer and carries the portable gas-collection equipment (Figure 10.11E).[43] For another form of swimming exercise study, illustrated in Figure 10.11A, the subject remains stationary and attached, or "tethered," to a cable and pulley system by a belt worn around the waist.[38] Periodic increases in the amount of weight attached to the cable force the swimmer to exert greater effort to maintain body position. Figure 10.11B–D shows a subject swimming in a flume, or "swimming treadmill." Water circulates at a velocity varying from a slow swimming speed to a near-record pace for a freestyle sprint. Aerobic capacity measurements using tethered, free, or flume swimming techniques produce essentially identical values.[7] Any of these modes of measurement can objectively evaluate the aerobic system's functional capacity during swimming.

ENERGY COST AND DRAG

The total drag force encountered by the swimmer consists of three components:

- **Wave drag**—caused by waves that build up in front of, and form hollows behind, the swimmer as he or she moves through the water. This component of drag does not significantly affect swimming at slow velocities, but its influence becomes greater at faster swimming speeds.
- **Skin friction drag**—produced as the water slides over the surface of the skin. Even at relatively fast swimming velocities, the quantitative contribution of skin friction drag to the total drag is probably small. However, research supports the common practice of swimmers "shaving down" to reduce skin friction drag, thus decreasing energy cost.[64]
- **Viscous pressure drag**—caused by the pressure differential created in front of and behind the swimmer, which contributes substantially to counter-propulsive efforts at slow velocities. Viscous pressure drag, caused by the separation of the thin sheet of water, or boundary layer, forms adjacent to the swimmer. Its effect is probably reduced in highly skilled swimmers who have learned to "streamline" their stroke mechanics, reducing the separation region by moving it closer to the trailing edge of the water. This is similar to an oar slicing through the water with the blade parallel rather than perpendicular to the water flow.

Ways to Reduce Effect of Drag Force

Figure 10.12 depicts a curvilinear relationship between body drag and swimming velocity as the swimmer is towed through the water. As velocity increases above 0.8 m · s^{-1}, drag is reduced if the legs and arms are supported by flotation devices that place the body in a more "hydrodynamically" desirable horizontal position. Generally, the drag force is about 2 to 2.5 times higher in swimming than in passive towing.[67]

Wet suits worn by triathletes during the swim portion of a triathlon result in a 14% reduction in body drag.[68] Improved swimming economy largely explains the significantly faster swim times of athletes using wet suits. As in running, cross-country skiing, and cycling, the technique of drafting in swimming (following closely behind

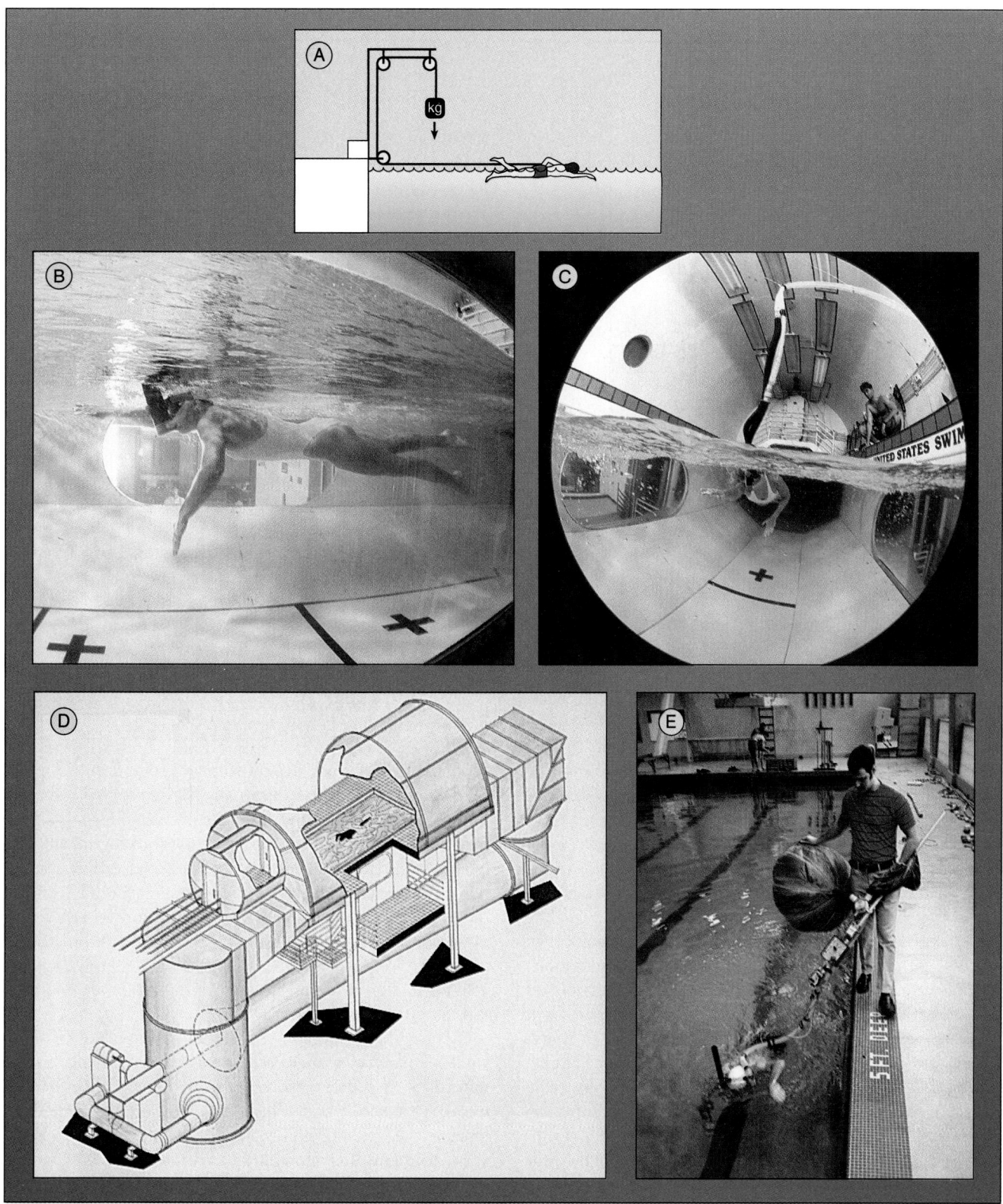

FIGURE 10.11

A, Measurement of energy expenditure during tethered swimming. **B–D,** Swimming treadmill. An environmental chamber surrounding the swimming treadmill controls atmospheric pressure (and other environmental conditions) during swimming. Using the swimming treadmill, researchers conduct physiological and biomechanical experiments during swimming that simulate actual performance conditions. The underwater viewing area provides a convenient means for directly observing swimming performance related to stroke mechanics. **E,** Open-circuit spirometry used to measure oxygen uptake during front-crawl swimming. (Schematic and photos courtesy of the United States Swimming International Center for Aquatic Research, Colorado Springs, CO.)

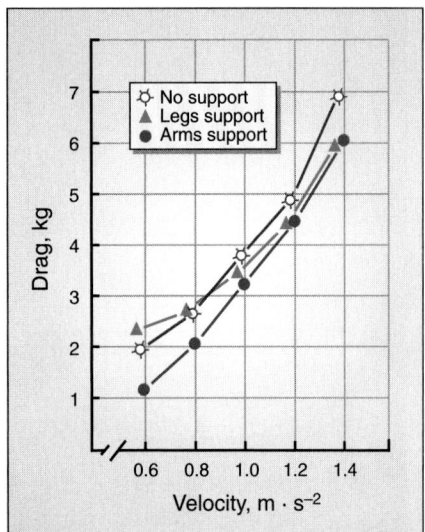

FIGURE 10.12
Drag force in three different prone positions related to towing velocity. (From Holmér, I.: Energy cost of arm stroke, leg kick, and the whole stroke in competitive swimming styles. *Eur. J. Appl. Physiol.*, 33:105, 1974.)

the wake of a lead swimmer) reduces the physiologic demands of the swim.[4] This enables an endurance swimmer such as a triathlete or ocean racer to conserve energy and possibly improve performance toward the end of the competition.

ENERGY COST, SWIMMING VELOCITY, AND SKILL

Elite swimmers can swim a particular stroke at a given velocity with lower oxygen uptakes than relatively untrained or recreational swimmers. Highly skilled swimmers use more of the energy generated per stroke to overcome drag forces; thus, they cover a greater distance per stroke than less skilled swimmers who waste considerable energy just moving water.[66] Figure 10.13A compares the oxygen uptakes and velocities for the breaststroke, back crawl, and front crawl at three levels of ability. One subject was a recreational swimmer who did not participate in swim training; the trained subject swam on a daily basis and was a top Swedish swimmer; the elite swimmer was a European champion. Except during the breaststroke, the elite swimmer, at a given speed, had a lower oxygen uptake than his trained and untrained counterparts. Figure 10.13B demonstrates that, for the two trained athletes swimming at any speed, the breaststroke was the most costly, followed by the backstroke, with the front crawl being the least "expensive" of the three strokes. As a result of marked accelerations and decelerations within the stroke cycle, the energy expended for the butterfly and breaststroke nearly doubles that

needed for the front and back crawl at similar swimming velocities.[66]

EFFECTS OF WATER TEMPERATURE

Relatively cold water places the swimmer under thermal stress and brings about metabolic and cardiovascular adjustments different from those observed in warmer water.[32] These adaptive responses primarily serve to maintain a stable core temperature by compensating for considerable heat flow from the body, particularly at water temperatures below 25°C (77°F). Body heat loss occurs most frequently in lean swimmers, who benefit less from the insulatory effects of greater subcutaneous fat accumulation.[55]

Figure 10.14 illustrates oxygen uptake during breaststroke swimming at water temperatures of 18°, 26°, and 33°C. Regardless of swimming speed, the highest oxygen uptakes occurred in cold water. The "extra" oxygen cost of swimming in cold water results primarily from the energy expended in shivering as the body attempts to regulate core temperature. It appears that, for individuals of average body composition, the optimal water temperature for competitive swimming varies from 28° to 30°C (82° to 86°F). Within this temperature range, the metabolic heat generated during exercise transfers easily to the water, yet the gradient for heat flow is not so extreme to cause increases in energy cost or reductions in core temperature from cold stress.

EFFECTS OF BUOYANCY: MEN VERSUS WOMEN

Women of all ages possess, on average, a significantly higher percentage of body fat than men. Because fat floats and muscle and bone sink in water, the average woman gains a hydrodynamic lift and expends less energy to stay afloat than her male counterpart. More than likely, sex differences in percent body fat and, thus, body buoyancy partially explain the greater swimming economy observed for women.[62] For example, women swim a given distance at about 30% lower total energy cost than men. Expressed another way, women achieve higher swimming velocities than men at the same level of energy expenditure.

The greater peripheral distribution of body fat in women compared to men causes their legs to float high in the water, making them more horizontal, or "streamlined," whereas the leaner legs of men tend to swing down and float lower in the water.[10] This lowering of the legs to a deeper position increases body drag and reduces swimming economy (refer to Figure 10.12). Such differences in flotation, including the significantly smaller body size of women, which also reduces drag, contribute to the "sex difference" in swimming economy.[66] The potential hydrodynamic benefits that women possess become noteworthy with longer distances because swimming economy and body insulation contribute significantly to success. The world record for swimming the

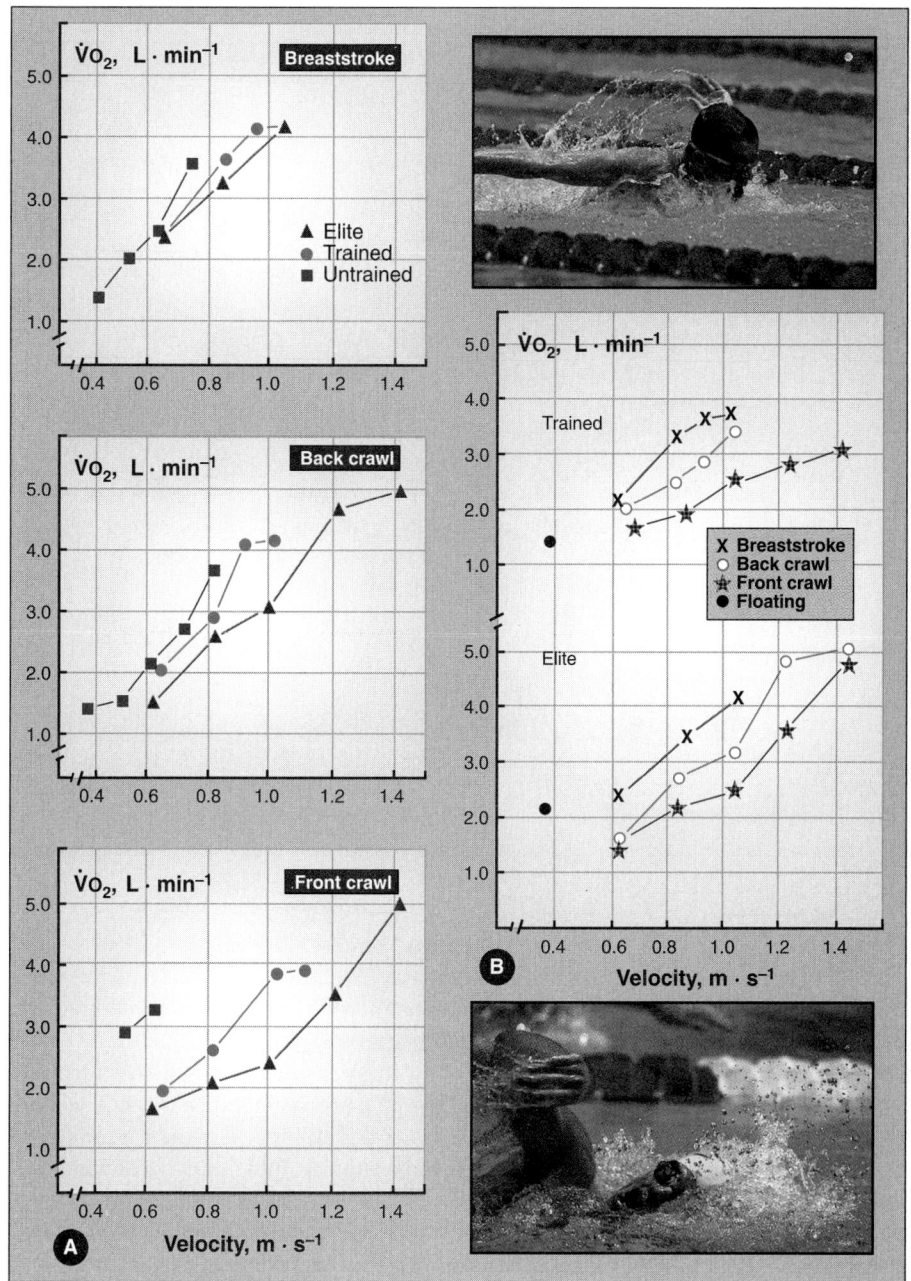

FIGURE 10.13

A, Oxygen uptake related to speed for the breaststroke, front crawl, and back crawl in subjects at three levels of skill ability. **B,** Oxygen uptake for two trained swimmers during three competitive strokes. (From Holmér, I.: Oxygen uptake during swimming in man. *J. Appl. Physiol.*, 33:502, 1972. Photos courtesy of John Urbanchek, varsity men's swim coach, University of Michigan, Ann Arbor.)

English Channel established in 1978 by female champion Penny Dean (7 h:40 min) remained intact until 1994, when it was lowered 23 minutes by male swimmer Chad Hundeby.

ENDURANCE SWIMMERS

Distance swimming in ocean water can pose a severe metabolic and physiologic challenge. In one study of nine distance swimmers, data included measurements taken under race conditions in a salt-water pool at swimming speeds ranging from 2.6 to 4.9 km · h^{-1}.[60] During the race, competitors main-tained a constant stroke rate and pace until the last few hours, when fatigue set in. From detailed observations of one male subject, the average speed of 2.85 km per hour during a 12-hour swim required an average oxygen uptake of 1.7 L O$_2$ · min^{-1}, or an equivalent energy expenditure of 8.5 kcal · min^{-1}. Consequently, the gross caloric requirement for the 12-hour swim was about 6120 kcal (8.5 kcal × 60 min × 12 h). The net caloric cost of swimming the English Channel, assuming a resting energy expenditure of 1.2 kcal · min^{-1} (0.260 L O$_2$ · min^{-1}), exceeded 5200 kcal, or about twice the number of calories consumed while running a marathon.

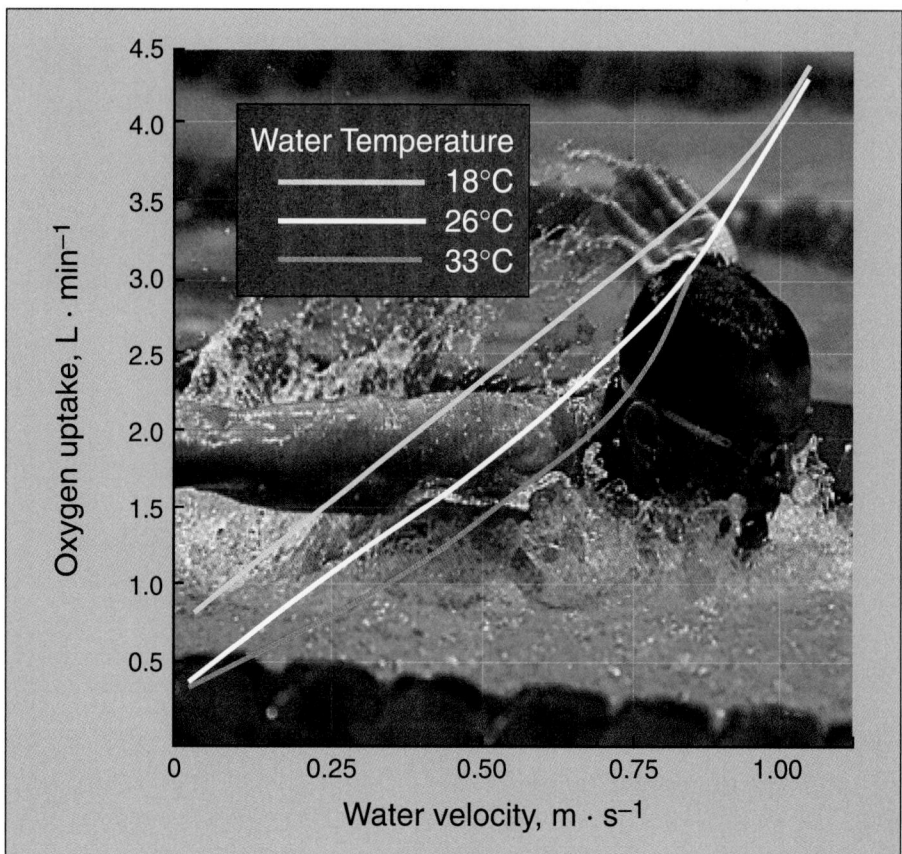

FIGURE 10.14

Energy expenditure for the breaststroke at three water temperatures related to swimming velocity. (From Nadel, E.R., et al.: Energy exchanges of swimming man. *J. Appl. Physiol.*, 36:465, 1974. Photo courtesy of John Urbanchek, University of Michigan, Ann Arbor.)

■ SUMMARY ■

1. Energy expenditure can be expressed in gross as well as net terms. Total or gross values include the resting energy requirement, whereas net energy expenditure is the energy cost of the activity per se, excluding the resting value.

2. The relationship between walking speed and oxygen uptake is essentially linear. Walking surface also has an effect because walking on sand requires about twice the energy expenditure of walking on firm surfaces. A larger energy cost exists for heavier people during such weight-bearing exercises.

3. At speeds exceeding 8 km · h^{-1}, running is more economical than walking from an energy standpoint.

4. For many people, hand-held and ankle weights increase the energy cost of walking to values usually observed for running. This factor benefits those wanting to use walking alone as a low-impact form of exercise training.

5. The total caloric cost of running a given distance at a steady-rate oxygen uptake remains essentially the same regardless of whether the pace is fast or slow. During horizontal running, the net energy expenditure approximates 1 kcal · kg^{-1} · km^{-1}.

6. Generally, less energy is required to shorten the running stride and increase stride frequency to maintain a constant running speed than to lengthen the stride and reduce its frequency. An individual subconsciously "selects" the combination of stride length and frequency that favors optimal economy.

7. Energy expended to overcome air resistance accounts for 3 to 9% of the cost of running in calm air. This percentage increases considerably if a runner attempts to maintain pace while running into a brisk headwind.

8. Children generally require significantly more oxygen while running to transport their body mass than adults. This relatively lower running economy accounts for the poor endurance performance of children compared to adults of similar aerobic capacity.

9. The energy required to run a given distance or speed on a treadmill is about the same as that required to run on a track under identical environmental conditions.

10. The energy expended while swimming a given distance is about four times greater than that expended while running the same distance because the swimmer expends considerable energy maintaining buoyancy and overcoming drag forces that impede forward movement.

11. There are significant differences between men and women in body drag, mechanical efficiency, and net oxygen uptake during swimming. Women swim a given distance at about a 30% lower energy cost than men.

12. Elite swimmers expend fewer calories to swim a given stroke at any velocity. The optimal water temperature for most competitive swimming averages 28° to 30°C (82° to 86°F).

■ REFERENCES ■

1. American College of Sports Medicine: *Guidelines for Exercise Testing and Prescription.* 4th ed., Philadelphia, Lea & Febiger, 1991.
2. Åstrand, P.O., and Rodahl, K.: *Textbook of Work Physiology.* 3rd ed., New York, McGraw-Hill, 1986.
3. Bassett, D.R., et al.: Aerobic requirements of overground versus treadmill running. *Med. Sci. Sports Exerc.,* 17:477, 1985.
4. Bassett, D.R., Jr., et al.: Metabolic responses to drafting during front crawl swimming. *Med. Sci. Sports Exerc.,* 23:744, 1991.
5. Bhambhani, Y., and Singh, M.: Metabolic and cinematographic analysis of walking and running in men and women. *Med. Sci. Sports Exerc.,* 17:131, 1985.
6. Bilodeau, B., et al.: Effect of drafting on heart rate in cross-country skiing. *Med. Sci. Sports Exerc.,* 26:637, 1994.
7. Bonen, A., et al.: Maximal oxygen uptake during free, tethered, and flume swimming. *J. Appl. Physiol.,* 48:232, 1980.
8. Bøje, O.: Energy production, pulmonary ventilation, and length of steps in well-trained runners working on a treadmill. *Acta Physiol. Scand.,* 7:362, 1944.
9. Butts, N.K., et al.: Energy costs of walking on a dual-action treadmill in men and women. *Med. Sci. Sports Exerc.,* 27:121, 1995.
10. Campaigne, B.N.: Body fat distribution in females: metabolic consequences and implications for weight loss. *Med. Sci. Sports Exerc.,* 22:291, 1990.
11. Cavagna, G.A., and Franzetti, P.: Mechanics of competition walking. *J. Physiol. (London),* 315:243, 1981.
12. Cavanagh, P.R., and Kram, R.: Mechanical and muscular factors affecting the efficiency of human movement. *Med. Sci. Sports Exerc.,* 17:326, 1985.
13. Cavanagh, P.R., and Kram, R.: Stride length in distance running: velocity, body dimensions, and added mass effects. *Med. Sci. Sports Exerc.,* 21:467, 1989.
14. Claremont, A.P., and Hall, S.J.: Effects of extremity loading on energy expenditure and running mechanics. *Med. Sci. Sports Exerc.,* 20:161, 1988.
15. Conley, D.L., and Krahenbuhl, G.S.: Running economy and distance running performance of highly trained athletes. *Med. Sci. Sports Exerc.,* 12:357, 1980.
16. Conley, D.L., et al.: Training for aerobic capacity and running economy. *Phys. Sportsmed.,* 9:107, 1981.
17. Coyle, E.F., et al.: Physiological and biomechanical factors associated with elite endurance cycling performance. *Med. Sci. Sports Exerc.,* 23:93, 1991.
18. Coyle, E.F., et al.: Cycling efficiency is related to the percentage of Type I muscle fibers. *Med. Sci. Sports Exerc.,* 24:782, 1992.
19. Cunningham, D.A.: Development of cardiorespiratory function in circumpubertal boys: a longitudinal study. *J. Appl. Physiol.,* 56:302, 1984.
20. Daniels, J., et al.: Differences and changes in $\dot{V}O_2$ among runners 10 to 18 years of age. *Med. Sci. Sports,* 10:200, 1978.
21. Davies, C.T.M., et al.: The physiological responses to running downhill. *Eur. J. Appl. Physiol.,* 32:187, 1974.
22. Evans, B.W., et al.: Metabolic and hemodynamic responses to walking with hand weights in older individuals. *Med. Sci. Sports Exerc.,* 26:1047, 1994.
23. Falls, H.B., and Humphrey, L.D.: Energy cost of running and walking in young women. *Med. Sci. Sports,* 8:9, 1976.
24. Fellingham, G.W., et al.: Calorie cost of walking and running. *Med. Sci. Sports,* 10:132, 1978.

25. Fortney, V.L.: The kinematics of the running pattern of two, four, and six year old children. *Res. Q. Exerc. Sport,* 54:126, 1983.
26. Frederick, E.C., et al.: Lower oxygen demands of running in soft-soled shoes. *Res. Q. Exerc. Sport,* 57:174, 1986.
27. Graves, J.E., et al.: The effect of hand-held weights on the physiological responses to walking exercise. *Med. Sci. Sports Exerc.,* 19:260, 1987.
28. Hagberg, J.M., and Coyle, E.F.: Physiological determinants of endurance performance as studied in competitive race walkers. *Med. Sci. Sports Exerc.,* 15:287, 1983.
29. Hamill, J., et al.: Effects of shoe type on cardiorespiratory responses and rear foot motion during treadmill running. *Med. Sci. Sports Exerc.,* 20:515, 1988.
30. Heinert, L.D., et al.: Effect of stride length variation on oxygen uptake during level and positive grade treadmill running. *Res. Q. Exerc. Sport,* 59:127, 1988.
31. Hill, A.V.: The air resistance to a runner. *Proc. R. Soc. Lond. (Biol.),* 102:380, 1927.
32. Holmér, I.: Physiology of swimming man. In *Exercise and Sport Sciences Reviews,* Vol. 7. R.S. Hutton and D.I. Miller (Eds.), Philadelphia, Franklin Institute Press, 1980.
33. Jones, B.H., et al.: Energy cost of walking and running in boots and shoes. *Ergonomics,* 27:895, 1984.
34. Joyner, M.J.: Physiological limiting factors and distance running: influence of gender and age on record performance. *Exerc. Sport Sci. Rev.,* 21:103, 1993.
35. Krahenbuhl, G.S., and Pangrasi, R.: Characteristics associated with running performance in young boys. *Med. Sci. Sports Exerc.,* 5:488, 1983.
36. Krahenbuhl, G.S., and Williams, T.J. Running economy: Changes with age during childhood and adolescence. *Med. Sci. Sports Exerc.,* 24:462, 1992.
37. Kyle, C.R.: Ergogenics of bicycling. In *Perspectives in Exercise Science and Sports Medicine.* Vol. 4: Ergogenics: Enhancement of Performance in Exercise and Sport. D.R. Lamb and M.H. Williams (Eds.), Madison, WI, Brown and Benchmark, 1991.
38. Magel, J.R., et al.: The specificity of swim training on maximum oxygen uptake. *J. Appl. Physiol.,* 36:753, 1974.
39. Margaria, R., et al.: Energy cost of running. *J. Appl. Physiol.,* 18:367, 1963.
40. Maron, M., et al.: Oxygen uptake measurements during competitive marathon running. *J. Appl. Physiol.,* 40:836, 1976.
41. Martin, P.E., and Morgan, D.W.: Biomechanical considerations for economical walking and running. *Med. Sci. Sports Exerc.,* 24:467, 1992.
42. Mayers, N., and Gutin, B.: Physiological characteristics of elite prepubertal cross-country runners. *Med. Sci. Sports,* 11:172, 1979.
43. McArdle, W.D., et al.: Metabolic and cardiorespiratory response during free swimming and treadmill walking. *J. Appl. Physiol.,* 30:733, 1971.
44. McArdle, W.D., et al.: Comparison of continuous and discontinuous treadmill and bicycle tests for $\dot{V}O_2$max. *Med. Sci. Sports,* 5:156, 1973.
45. McCole, S.D., et al.: Energy expenditure during bicycling. *J. Appl. Physiol.,* 68:748, 1990.
46. McMiken, D.F., and Daniels, J.T.: Aerobic requirements and maximum aerobic power in treadmill and track running. *Med. Sci. Sports,* 8:14, 1976.
47. Menier, D.R., and Pugh, L.G.C.E.: The relation of oxygen intake and velocity of walking and running in competition walkers. *J. Physiol. (London),* 197:717, 1968.
48. Miller, J.E., and Stamford, B.A.: Intensity and energy cost of weighted walking vs. running for men and women. *J. Appl. Physiol.,* 62:1947, 1987.
48a. Minetti, A.E., et al.: Mechanical determinants of the minimum energy cost of gradient running in humans. *J. Exp. Biol.,* 195:211, 1994.

48b. Minetti, A.E., et al.: Effects of stride frequency on mechanical power and energy expenditure of walking. *Med. Sci. Sports Exerc.*, 27:1195, 1995.

49. Morgan, D.W., and Craib, M.: Physiological aspects of running economy. *Med. Sci. Sports Exerc.*, 24:456, 1992.

50. Morgan, D.W., et al.: Ten kilometer performance and predicted velocity at $\dot{V}O_2$max among well-trained male runners. *Med. Sci. Sports Exerc.*, 21:78, 1989.

51. Morgan, D.W., et al.: Variability in running economy and mechanics among trained runners. *Med. Sci Sports Exerc.*, 23:378, 1991.

52. Morgan, D.W., et al: Daily variability in running economy among well-trained male and female distance runners. *Res. Q. Exerc. Sport.*, 65:72, 1994.

53. Morgan, D.W., et al.: Effect of step length optimization on the aerobic demand of running. *J. Appl. Physiol.*, 77:245, 1994.

54. Morgan, D.W., et al.: Variation in the aerobic demand of running among trained and untrained subjects. *Med. Sci. Sports Exerc.*, 27:404, 1995.

55. Nadel, E., et al.: Energy exchanges of swimming man. *J. Appl. Physiol.*, 36:465, 1974.

56. Nelson, R.C., and Gregor, R.J.: Biomechanics of distance running: a longitudinal study. *Res. Q.*, 47:471, 1976.

57. Nigg, B.M., and Anton, A.: Energy aspects for elastic and viscous shoe soles and playing surfaces. *Med. Sci. Sports Exerc.*, 27:92, 1995.

58. Pandolf, K.B., et al.: Predicting energy expenditure with loads while standing or walking very slowly. *J. Appl. Physiol.*, 43:577, 1977.

59. Pugh, L.G.C.E.: Oxygen uptake in track and treadmill running with observations on the effect of air resistance. *J. Physiol. (London)*, 207:823, 1970.

60. Pugh, L.G.C.E., and Edholm, O.G.: The physiology of channel swimmers. *Lancet*, 2:761, 1955.

61. Ralston, H.J.: Comparison of energy expenditure during treadmill walking and floor walking. *J. Appl. Physiol.*, 15:1156, 1960.

62. Rennie, D.W., et al.: Energetics of swimming in man. In *Swimming II*. L. Lewille and J. Clarys (Eds.), Baltimore, University Park Press, 1975.

63. Rowland, T.W., et al.: Physiologic responses to treadmill running in adult and prepubertal males. *Int. J. Sports Med.*, 8:292, 1987.

64. Sharp, R.L., and Costill, D.L.: Influence of body hair removal on physiological responses during breaststroke swimming. *Med. Sci. Sports Exerc.*, 21:576, 1989.

65. Smolander, J., et al.: Cardiorespiratory strain during walking in snow with boots of differing weights. *Ergonomics*, 32:319, 1989.

66. Toussaint, H.M., and Hollander, A.P.: Energetics of competitive swimming: implications for training programs. *Sports Med.*, 18:384, 1994.

67. Toussaint, H.M., et al.: Active drag related to velocity in male and female swimmers. *J. Biomechanics*, 21:435, 1988.

68. Toussaint, H.M., et al.: Effect of triathlon wet suit on drag during swimming. *Med. Sci. Sports Exerc.*, 21:325, 1989.

69. Toussaint, H.M., et al.: The mechanical efficiency of front crawl swimming. *Med. Sci. Sports Exerc.*, 22:402, 1990.

70. Wanta, D.M., et al.: Metabolic response to graded downhill walking. *Med. Sci. Sports Exerc.*, 25:159, 1993.

71. Williams, K.R., and Cavanagh, P.R.: Relationship between distance running mechanics, running economy, and performance. *J. Appl. Physiol.*, 63:1236, 1987.

Mitchell, J.H. et al.: The physiological meaning of the maximal oxygen intake test. *J. Clin. Invest.* **37:538, 1958.**

In the 1920s, A.V. Hill and colleagues—and in latter years other scientists—considered the maximal oxygen uptake ($\dot{V}O_2$max) the single best measure of cardiorespiratory capacity. Hill asserted that $\dot{V}O_2$max "was physiologically restricted owing to thelimitation of the circulatory and respiratory

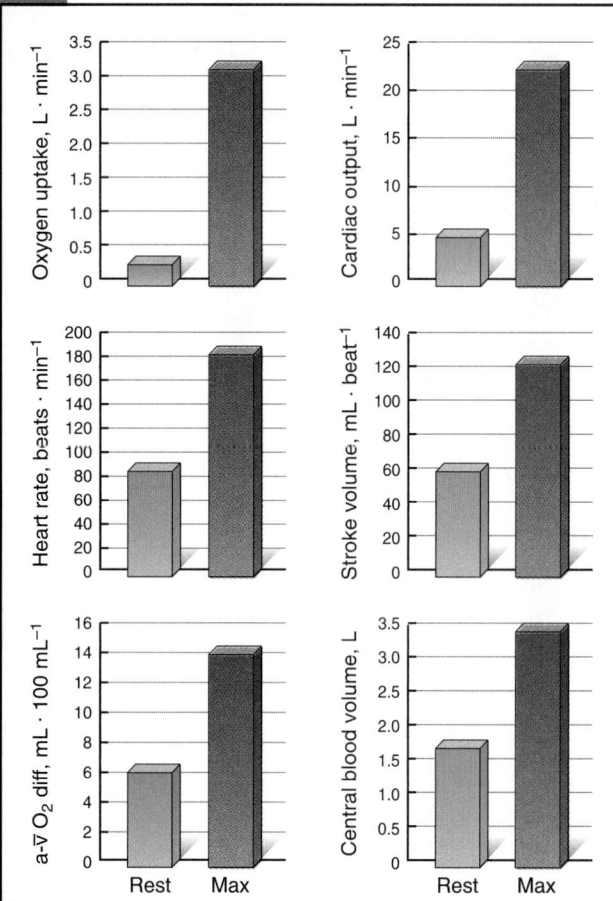

Magnitude of changes in cardiovascular dynamics (arteriovenous oxygen difference, heart rate, oxygen uptake, stroke volume, and blood volume) in 15 normal subjects between rest and exercise at the maximal oxygen uptake.

systems." This assertion, however, had not been tested experimentally because the interplay among circulation, ventilation, and blood-gas parameters had not yet been established. Mitchell and colleagues directly examined the relationships among $\dot{V}O_2$max and various cardiovascular-pulmonary parameters to more fully describe and understand the physiological significance of the $\dot{V}O_2$max.

Sixty-five men performed graded, discontinu-ous treadmill exercise to the point of $\dot{V}O_2$max. Subgroups of subjects participated in several different protocols up to volitional exhaustion. Measurements included cardiac output and a-$\bar{v}$ O_2 difference by the dye dilution technique; blood gases; and central blood volume. Two of the findings were methodological but nevertheless important. First, the $\dot{V}O_2$max served as a reproducible measure *"if rigid criteria for determining the point at which the maximal value has been attained are applied."* For 15 subjects, the reliability coefficient (r) for $\dot{V}O_2$max scores equaled 0.92 with a standard error of measurement of ±7% for predicting an individual's maximal value. Second, a "peaking over" or "plateauing" criterion established for attainment of $\dot{V}O_2$max serves as an important conceptual standard applied to $\dot{V}O_2$max testing in diverse forms of exercise. This standard is presented below:

"Plots of oxygen intake against workload for the entire material showed that, until a maximal value was attained, oxygen intake rose 142 ±44 mL with each increase in workload. If the rise was less than 142 minus 88 (twice the standard deviation), or 54 mL, the final value was accepted as the maximal intake, the assumption being that the subject had attained his true maximal value or had reached the beginning of a plateau and could not increase his intake very much more."

The findings endorsed the view that the $\dot{V}O_2$max depended almost exclusively on the functional capacity of the cardiovascular system (cardiac output and a-$\bar{v}$ O_2 difference) and not on the accommodation of left ventricular output by the vascular bed. No significant change occurred in arterial oxygen tension from rest to heavy work; the slight arterial desaturation often observed in heavy exercise occurred by a decrease of blood pH and the resulting Bohr effect on hemoglobin saturation. The maintenance of arterial oxygen tension during heavy exercise argued against the possibility that pulmonary factors were a "weak link" in determining $\dot{V}O_2$max. In essence, the researchers maintained that an adequate arterial oxygen tension gradient always exits from the alveoli to the blood and from the blood to the active tissues.

This study confirmed the importance of the $\dot{V}O_2$max test as an indicator of central circulatory function (cardiac capacity) and to a lesser degree the capacity of peripheral or local factors reflected by the a-$\bar{v}$ O_2 difference. Based on this research, the measure of $\dot{V}O_2$max became the "benchmark" to quantify cardiovascular functional capacity and aerobic "fitness."

Individual Differences and Measurement of Energy Capacities

Although we all possess the capability for anaerobic and aerobic energy metabolism, the capacity for each form of energy transfer varies considerably among individuals. This between-person variability underlies the concept of **individual differences** in metabolic capacity for exercise. Furthermore, each person's capacity for energy transfer (and for many physiologic functions) is not simply a general factor; instead, it depends highly on the mode of exercise during which it is trained and evaluated.[62, 63, 71, 80] A high maximal oxygen uptake in running, for example, does not necessarily ensure a similar level of metabolic power when different muscle groups are exercised, as in swimming and rowing. This is an example of **specificity** of metabolic capacity. However, some individuals with high aerobic power in one activity also possess above average aerobic power in other activities. This is an illustration of the **generality** of metabolic function. Often, there is considerable specificity when comparisons are made among the body's three distinct means of energy transfer, as illustrated in Figure 11.1. The non-overlapped areas represent specificity of metabolic function while overlapped areas represent generality. For each of the energy systems, specificity exceeds generality; for example, it would be rare to find a person who possesses high energy-generating capacity for such diverse performances as running or swimming sprint, middle-distance, and long-distance events.

Because of exercise specificity, training to achieve a high aerobic power would contribute little to one's capacity to generate energy anaerobically, and vice versa. The effects of exercise training also are highly specific for neuromuscular patterning and demands. *Terms such as "speed," "power," and "endurance" must therefore be viewed carefully within the context of the specific movement patterns and the specific metabolic and physiologic requirements of the activity.*

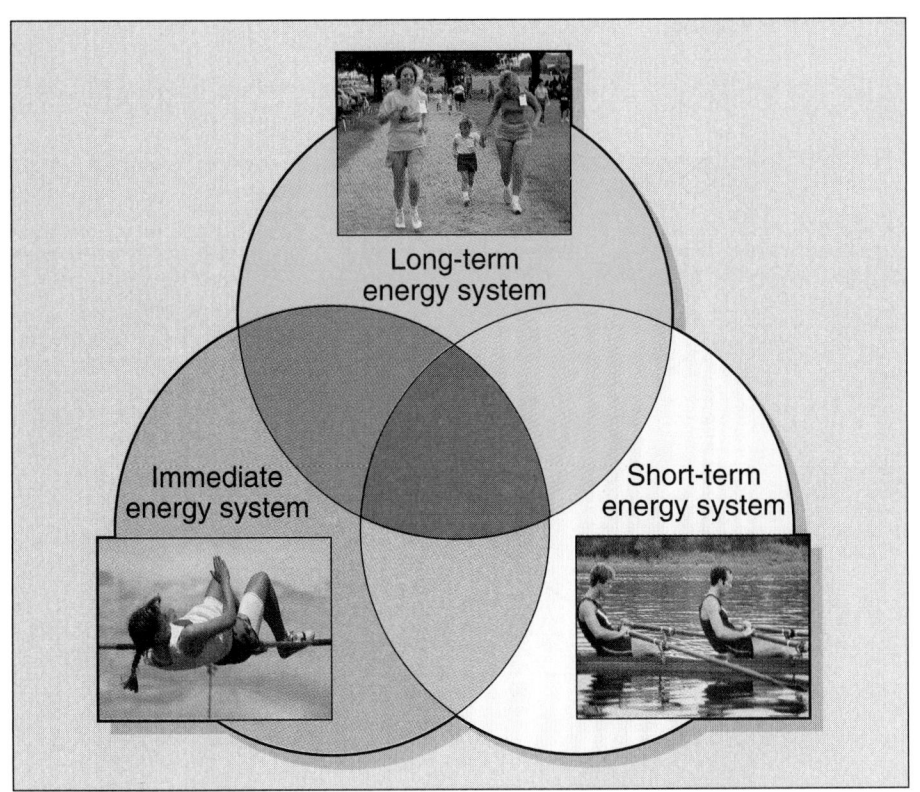

FIGURE 11.1
Illustration to represent the specificity-generality concept of the three energy systems. If only two systems are considered, their overlap represents generality, and the remainder is specificity.

In this chapter, the capacity of the three energy-transfer systems discussed in Chapters 6 and 7 are evaluated, with special reference to individual differences, specificity, and measurement.

OVERVIEW OF ENERGY-TRANSFER CAPACITY DURING EXERCISE

All-out exercise for up to 2 minutes is powered mainly by the **immediate** and **short-term energy systems.** Both of these systems operate anaerobically because their transfer of chemical energy does not require molecular oxygen. Generally, a greater reliance is placed on anaerobic energy for fast movement or when there is increased resistance to movement at a given speed. This is demonstrated in Figure 11.2, which illustrates the relative involvement of the anaerobic and aerobic energy-transfer systems for different durations of all-out exercise. When movement begins at either fast or slow speed, ATP and CP, the intramuscular high-energy phosphates, provide immediate and anaerobic energy for muscle action. After the first few seconds of movement, an increasingly greater proportion of energy for ATP resynthesis is generated by the glycolytic pathways. For exercise to continue, a progressively greater demand is placed on aerobic metabolism. All physical activities and sports can be classified on the anaerobic-to-aerobic continuum. Some activities rely predominantly on a single system of energy transfer, whereas most physical activity requires the capacity of more than one energy system, depending on intensity and duration. Of course, the higher the intensity and shorter the duration, the greater the demand will be on anaerobic energy transfer.

ANAEROBIC ENERGY TRANSFER: THE IMMEDIATE AND SHORT-TERM ENERGY SYSTEMS

EVALUATION OF THE IMMEDIATE ENERGY SYSTEM

Sports such as football, weightlifting, and other brief, all-out activities requiring an almost instantaneous energy release rely almost exclusively on energy derived from the muscle's pool of high-energy phosphates.[44, 45, 88] Performance tests that cause maximal activation of the ATP-CP energy system have been developed to provide practical "field tests" for evaluating the capacity of this immediate means of energy transfer. Two assumptions underlying tests to estimate the power-generating capacity of high-energy phosphates are: (*a*) at maximal power output all ATP is regenerated by the ATP-CP system and, accordingly, the magnitude of power generated during this time depends on the energy-transfer capacity of this system; and (*b*) there is enough ATP and CP to support maximal performance for about 6 seconds. These tests are generally referred to as **power tests.** Power in this context is defined as the time-rate of doing work and is computed as:

$$P = (F \times D) \div T$$

where F is the force generated, D is the distance through that the force is moved, and T is the duration of the exercise. Power can be expressed in **watts**—one watt equals 0.73756 ft · lb · sec^{-1}, 0.01433 kcal · min^{-1}, 1.341 × 10^{-3} hp (or 0.0013 hp), or 6.12 kg · m · min^{-1}.

FIGURE 11.2

The three systems of energy transfer and their percentage contribution to total energy output during all-out exercise of different durations.

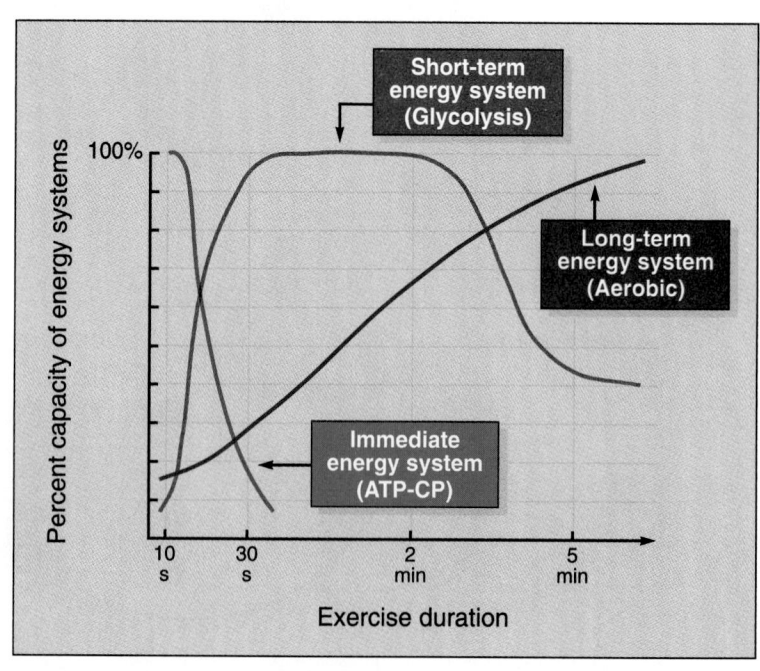

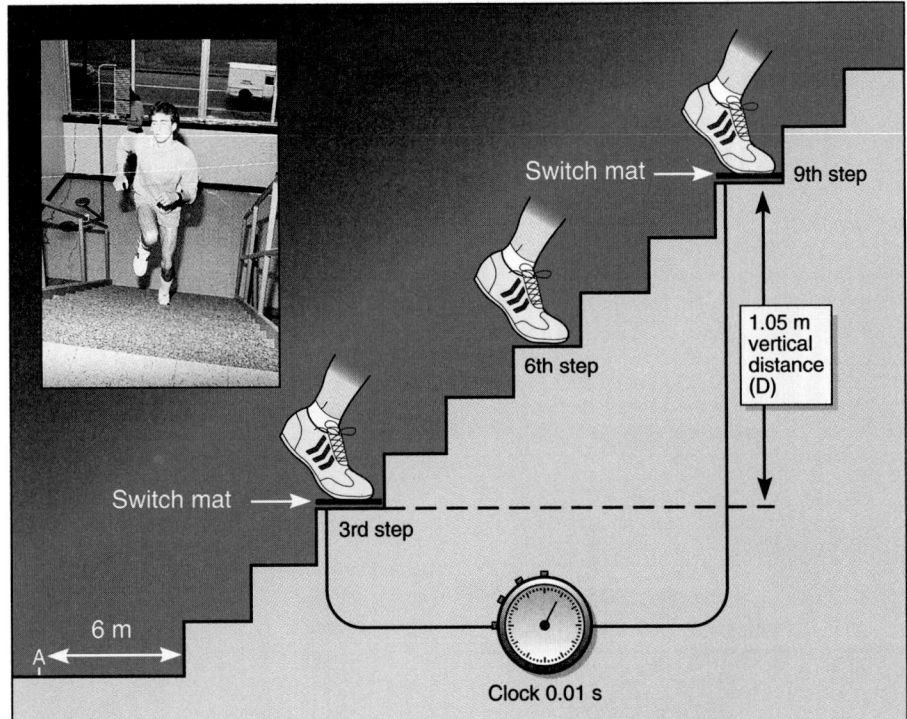

FIGURE 11.3
Stair-sprinting power test. The subject begins at point A and runs as rapidly as possible up a flight of stairs, taking three steps at a time. The time needed to cover the distance between stairs 3 and 9 is recorded to the nearest 0.01 second using electric switch mats placed on the steps. Power output is the product of the subject's mass (F) and vertical distance covered (D), divided by the time (T).

Stair-Sprinting Power Tests

Researchers have proposed that muscular power can be measured by having the subject sprint up a flight of stairs as illustrated in Figure 11.3.[43,66] The subject runs up a staircase as fast as possible, taking three steps at a time. The external work accomplished in this test is the total vertical distance the body mass is lifted up the stairs; this distance for six stairs is usually about 1.05 m. The power output of a 65-kg woman who traverses six steps in 0.52 second would be computed as follows:

$$F = 65 \text{ kg}$$

$$D = 1.05 \text{ m}$$

$$T = 0.52 \text{ s}$$

$$\text{Power} = (65 \text{ kg} \times 1.05 \text{ m}) \div 0.52 \text{ s}$$

$$\text{Power} = 131.3 \text{ kg} \cdot \text{m} \cdot \text{s}^{-1} \ (1287 \text{ watts})$$

Because the power score in the stair-sprinting test is influenced significantly by the person's body mass, a heavier person who has achieved the same speed as several other individuals will necessarily have a higher power score. This implies that the heavier person has the more highly developed immediate energy system. However, because there is no direct evidence to support this contention, caution is urged in interpreting differences in stair-sprinting power scores and inferring individual differences in ATP-CP energy-transfer capacity. *The test may be better suited to evaluating individuals of similar body mass or evaluating* *the same individuals before and after specific training designed to develop leg power output from the immediate energy system (assuming no change in body mass).*

Jumping-Power Tests

Jump tests such as the popular **Sargent jump-and-reach test** or a **standing broad jump** have been common elements in many physical fitness test batteries. The Sargent jump is scored as the difference between a person's standing reach and the maximum jump-and-touch height.[89] For the broad jump, the score is the horizontal distance covered in a leap from a semicrouched position. Although both tests purport to measure leg power, they probably fail to achieve this goal. For one thing, in the jump tests, power is generated to propel the body from the crouched position only while the feet are in contact with the surface. *It is doubtful whether this extremely brief period is sufficient to evaluate a person's ATP and CP energy transfer capacity.* Also, no relationship has been established between jump-test scores and actual ATP-CP levels or depletion patterns in those muscles activated during the test.

If jump tests are used as measures of immediate anaerobic power, then particular attention should be given to the methodology for obtaining such information. The data displayed in Figure 11.4 are for repeated trials of the vertical jump and standing long jump. For the vertical jump trials, ten consecutive jumps were made from a force platform with the hands on the hips during the crouch and jump to

FIGURE 11.4

Ten consecutive vertical jump trials (no arm swing) of male collegiate baseball players and long-jump performances (with and without arm swing) of female collegiate soccer players. Prior to testing, subjects stretched for 3 minutes and performed light calisthenics. Subjects were exhorted to make a maximal effort during all jumps. There was a 7.5% improvement in vertical jump between trials 1 and 10; for the standing broad jump, the improvement was 7.0% from trial 1 to trial 10 with arm swing and 15.5% without arm swing. (Vertical jump data courtesy of Jeff Smith, and long jump data courtesy of Jesse Sutella. Human Performance Laboratory, Exercise Science Department, University of Massachusetts, Amherst, 1996.)

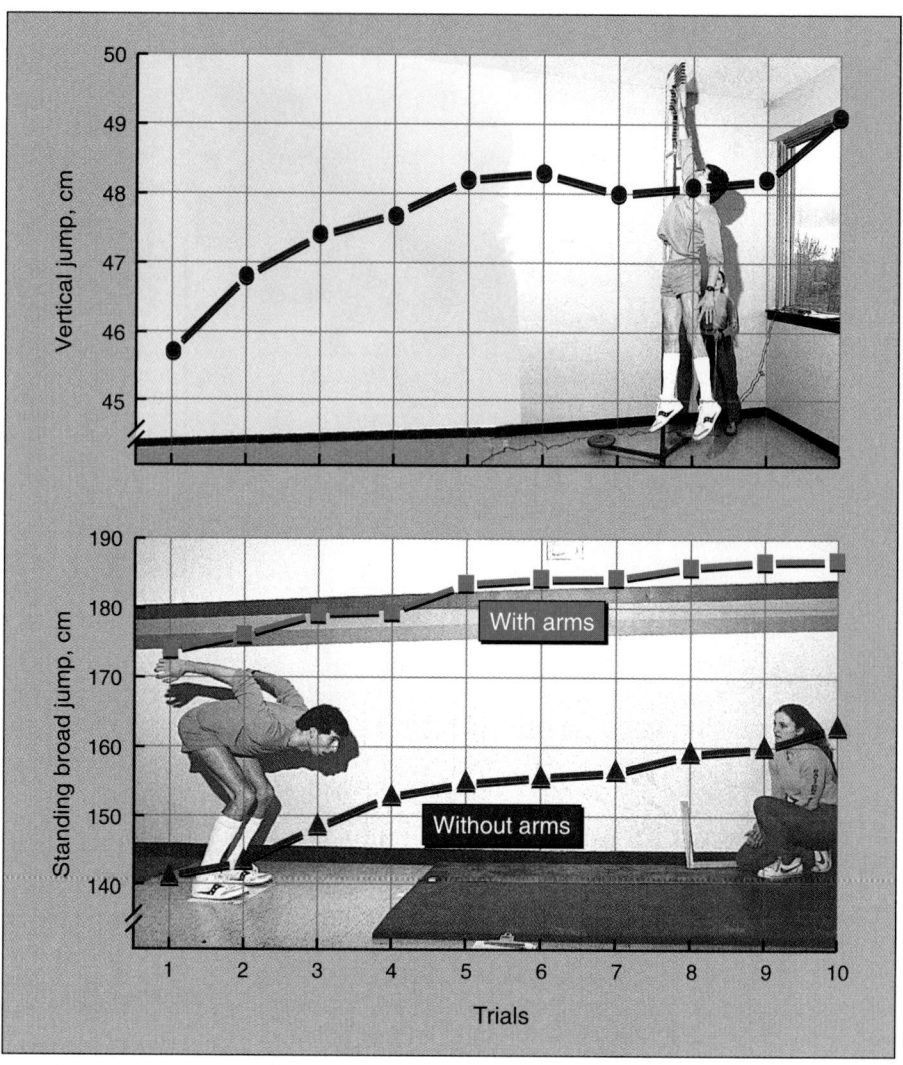

eliminate arm movement that would significantly augment vertical displacement. A 1-minute rest was allotted between the successive trials. A significant underestimation of peak power occurs if only 2 or 3 jumps are administered. Whether the progressive increase in power with repeated jumps results from a "warming-up" effect or from improved neuromuscular activation has not been established. The important point from a testing perspective is to allow for enough trials to establish a person's true power score.

Other Power Tests

As indicated in Figure 11.2, any performance involving all-out exercise of 6 to 8 seconds duration can probably be considered indicative of the person's capacity for immediate power from the high-energy phosphates in the specific muscles activated. In addition to stair-sprinting and jump tests, other examples of such tests are sprint running or cycling, shuttle runs, or even certain more localized movements such as arm cranking.

Interrelationships among Power Tests. If the various power tests measure the same "general" metabolic capacity, then individuals ranking high on one test should rank correspondingly high on a second or third different test. Although information on this topic is incomplete, the available data indicate that those who do well on one power performance test tend to do well on another, but the relationship generally is not strong. Table 11.1 shows the interrelationship (expressed statistically as a correlation coefficient) between several tests intended to measure immediate power output. The relationship ranges from poor to good, indicating some commonality between tests and suggesting that each may be measuring a general metabolic capability. Of practical significance is the fairly strong relationship between scores on the stair-sprinting power test and the 40-yard dash. *This indicates that almost the same information can be obtained through a test involving sprint running on a track as through the more elaborate set-up in the stair sprint.*

Several factors may explain why the interrelationship among the other test scores is not high. *For one* thing, *human performance is highly task-specific.* From a metabolic and performance standpoint, this means that the best sprint runner is not necessarily the best sprint swimmer, sprint cyclist, "stair sprinter," or "arm cranker." Even though the energy to power each performance is generated by the same metabolic reactions, these reactions are isolated within the specific muscles activated by the exercise. The requirement of a different neuromuscular and skill component for each specific test also causes the scores to be more variable.

Besides evaluating changes in an athlete's performance that result from specific training, power tests are excellent for self-testing and motivation and often provide the actual exercise for training the immediate energy system. In football, for example, the 40-yard dash is often used in training and as a criterion to evaluate a player's speed. Although many types of "speed" are required in football, 40-yard dash test scores will likely provide relevant information for evaluating a player, even though it has not yet been established to what degree 40-yard speed in a straight line is related to overall football ability for players at similar positions! A run test of shorter distance (up to 20 yards) or with frequent changes in direction may be a more suitable performance measure of speed in football.

Physiologic Evaluation of the ATP-CP Energy System

Several physiologic and biochemical measures have been used in addition to performance estimates of the energy-generating capacity of the immediate energy system. These include estimating (a) the size of the intramuscular ATP-CP pool, (b) depletion rates of ATP and CP in response to all-out exercise of short duration, (c) the oxygen deficit calculated from the oxygen uptake curve, and (d) the alactic (fast component) portion of recovery oxygen uptake.[51, 113] Of these measures, the depletion rate of ATP and CP appears to be the most direct estimate and correlates highly with performance estimates of the immediate energy system. In reality, however, it is difficult to obtain precise biochemical data during all-out exercise of brief duration. Consequently, we must rely on the face validity of the various specific performance measures as true markers of one's capacity for ATP-CP energy transfer.

EVALUATION OF THE SHORT-TERM ENERGY SYSTEM

As depicted in Figure 11.2, when all-out exercise continues for longer than a few seconds, increasingly more energy for ATP resynthesis is generated from the short-term energy system through the anaerobic reactions of glycolysis. This is not to say that aerobic metabolism is unimportant at this stage of exercise or that the oxygen-consuming reactions have not "switched on." To the contrary, Figure 11.2 illustrates an increase in the contribution of aerobic energy transfer early in the exercise. It is during short-term, all-out exercise that the energy requirement significantly exceeds the energy generated by the oxidation of hydrogen in the respiratory chain. Consequently, anaerobic glycolysis predominates, and large quantities of lactic acid accumulate in the active muscle and, ultimately, in the blood. *The level of blood lactate is the most common indicator of the activation of the short-term energy system.*

Unlike tests for maximal oxygen uptake, no specific criteria exist to indicate that a person has attained a maximal anaerobic effort. It is likely that one's score on such a test is highly influenced by self-motivation and the testing environment.[107] Despite the difficulty in objectifying a person's true anaerobic power capacity, performance test scores are reproducible from day to day, particularly if the test is given under controlled, standardized conditions.[25]

Performance Tests for Anaerobic Power

Performances requiring substantial activation of the short-term energy system demand maximal exercise for up to 3 minutes.[6, 45] All-out runs and cycling have usually been used to assess anaerobic capacity, as have weightlifting (repetitive lifting of a certain percentage of maximum) and shuttle-runs. Because test performance is influenced by factors such as age, sex, skill, motivation, and body size, it is difficult to select a suitable criterion test and develop appropriate norms for evaluating anaerobic power capacity. It does not appear, however, that intramuscular glycogen lev-

TABLE 11.1
CORRELATIONS AMONG TESTS PURPORTING TO MEASURE IMMEDIATE NONAEROBIC POWER OUTPUT FROM THE INTRAMUSCULAR HIGH-ENERGY PHOSPHATES

Variables	40-yd Dash	Sargent Jump and Reach	Bicycle Power Test
Stair-sprinting power test	−0.88[a]	0.56	0.69
40-yd dash	—	−0.48[a]	−0.62[a]
Sargent jump and reach	—	—	0.31

From the Applied Physiology Laboratory, University of Michigan, Ann Arbor (N = 31 males).

[a]A negative correlation coefficient means that for the group of individuals, a high score earned on one test is associated with a low score on the other test. For the correlations with the 40-yd dash, a negative correlation means a good performance on one test is associated with a low 40-yd run time, and a low score in running (time) is a good performance.

els above the normal affect test performance or the final level of lactate accumulation.[97a] Also, because of exercise specificity, short-term anaerobic capacity for an upper body activity like rowing or swimming should not be assessed with a test that makes maximum use of the leg muscles. *The performance test must be similar to the activity for which the energy capacity is being evaluated.* In many cases, the actual activity can serve as the test.

An all-out cycling test of short duration used to estimate the power and capacity of the anaerobic energy systems was first described in 1973 as the **Katch test**.[51] This work was subsequently extended and resulted in a test in which the frictional resistance against the flywheel was preset at a high load (6 kg for men and 5 kg for women); subjects attempted to turn as many revolutions as possible in 40 seconds.[52] Revolution rate was recorded continuously, with the peak cycling power representing the subject's **anaerobic power** and the total work accomplished representing **anaerobic capacity**. A later modification of this procedure, the **Wingate test**, involves 30 seconds of all-out supermaximal exercise performed on either an arm-crank or leg-cycle ergometer.[6, 41] The resistance to pedaling is based on body mass (0.075 kg resistance per kilogram body mass) and is applied within 3 seconds after the initial inertia and unloaded frictional resistance of the ergometer are overcome. **Peak power** is the highest mechanical power generated during any 3- to 5-second period of the test; **average power** output is the arithmetic average of the total power generated during the 30-second test period. **Rate of fatigue** can also be computed as the rate of decline in power relative to the peak value. As in the Katch test, the assumption underlying this test is that the value for peak power output represents the energy-generating capacity of the high-energy phosphates, while the average power value reflects glycolytic capacity.[40] Normative standards for average and peak power outputs in young-adult, physically active men and women during cycling exercise in the Wingate test are presented in Table 11.2.[67] These performance scores are reproducible, and validity is moderate when compared to a variety of other measures of anaerobic capacity.[78] Some of the highest reported all-out cycle ergometer power scores have been achieved by elite volleyball and ice hockey players.

Figure 11.5 presents the relative contribution of each energy system during three all-out cycle ergometer tests of anaerobic power, each having a different duration. The lower portion gives the results estimated in kilojoules of total energy, and the upper portion presents the data as the percent contribution of each system to the total work accomplished. Note the progressive change in the percentage contribution of each energy system as the duration of effort changes.

Lower in Children. The explanation is yet unknown for the relatively poor performance of children on this test compared to adolescents and young adults. It is possible that

TABLE 11.2
PERCENTILE NORMS FOR AVERAGE POWER AND PEAK POWER FOR PHYSICALLY ACTIVE YOUNG ADULT MEN AND WOMEN

% Rank	Average Power Watts (W)		Peak Power Watts (W)	
	Male	Female	Male	Female
90	662	470	822	560
80	618	419	777	527
70	600	410	757	505
60	577	391	721	480
50	565	381	689	449
40	548	367	671	432
30	530	353	656	399
20	496	336	618	376
10	471	306	570	353

	$W \cdot kg\ BW^{-1}$		$W \cdot kg\ BW^{-1}$	
	Male	Female	Male	Female
90	8.24	7.31	10.89	9.02
80	8.01	6.95	10.39	8.83
70	7.91	6.77	10.20	8.53
60	7.59	6.59	9.80	8.14
50	7.44	6.39	9.22	7.65
40	7.14	6.15	8.92	6.96
30	7.00	6.03	8.53	6.86
20	6.59	5.71	8.24	6.57
10	5.98	5.25	7.06	5.98

From Maud, P.J., and Schultz, B.B.: Norms for the Wingate anaerobic text with comparisons in another similar test. *Res. Q. Exerc. Sport*, 60:144, 1989.

both lower intramuscular glycogen concentrations and a slower rate of glycogen utilization in children during exercise provide part of the answer.[26, 40]

Sex Differences. As with most measures of physiologic capacity and exercise performance, large sex differences exist between men and women in anaerobic power capacity during exercise when they are compared on an absolute basis.[27, 86] On the surface, these observations seem to be readily explained by the clear differences between the sexes in factors that affect power-output capacity, such as body mass, muscle mass, and fat-free body mass. Consequently, the sex difference in anaerobic capacity should be greatly reduced or even eliminated if the exercise performance is expressed in relation to some component of body mass or body composition. Such data should offer insight into whether there is a true sex effect on a muscle's capacity to generate energy anaerobically during exercise.

Available data indicate that the significant difference in anaerobic power between women and men **cannot** be fully explained by sex differences in body composition, physique, muscular strength, or neuromuscular factors.[68, 79] For example, for a given fat-free leg volume, the peak oxygen deficit (a valid measure of anaerobic capacity[5, 73]) during supermaximal cycling exercise has been shown to be significantly higher in men than in women.[105] These differences averaged about 20% even though the estimated differences between the sexes in active muscle mass had been considered. Similar observations have been made for anaerobic exercise capacity in children and adolescents.[86, 98] This "sex effect" is particularly apparent for the lower body musculature[79] and is not eliminated when performance scores are corrected for differences in body composition.

Such findings suggest the possibility of a real biologic difference in anaerobic exercise capacity between the sexes. If this is true, physical testing that focuses on this fitness component would enlarge the typically expected performance differences between men and women. This effect would **not** be eliminated by adjusting performance to body size or composition. Of relevance to the occupational setting

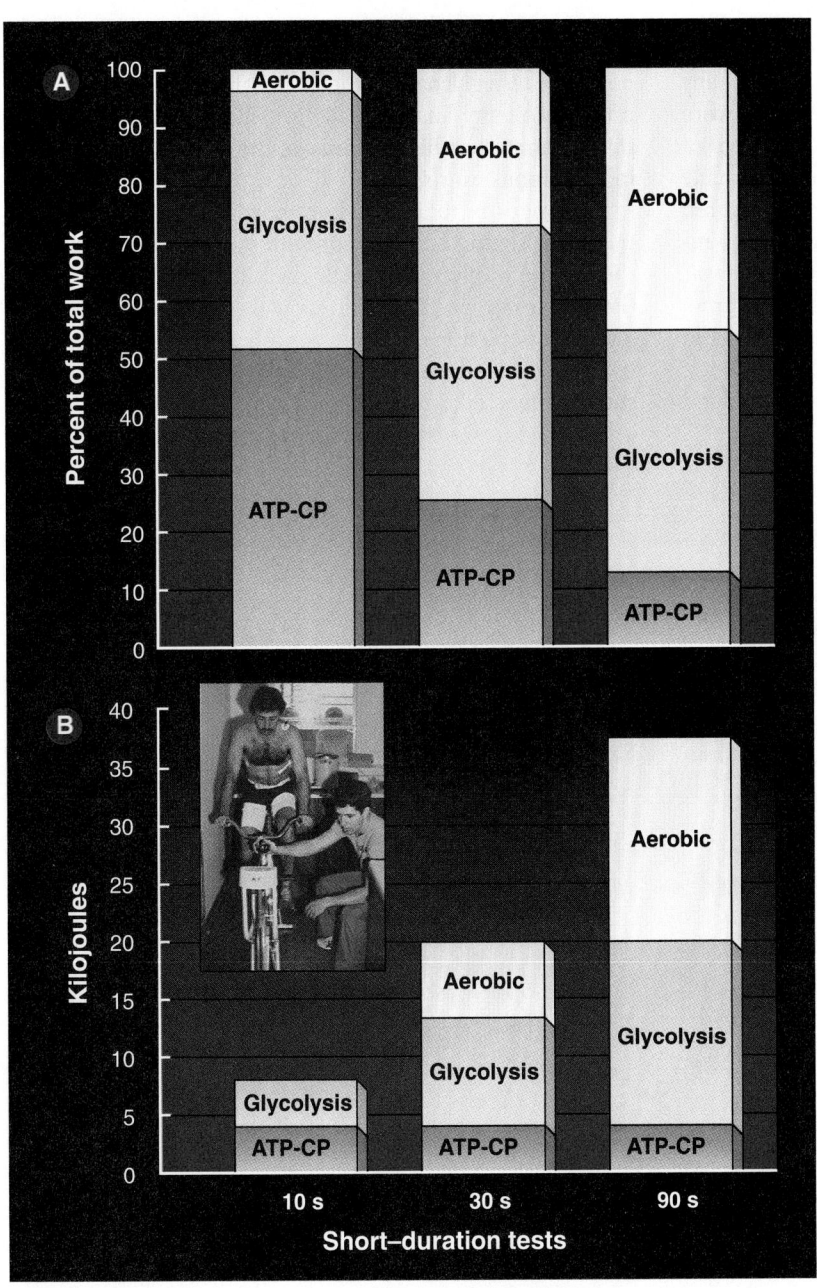

FIGURE 11.5
Relative contribution of each of the energy systems to the total work accomplished in three tests of short duration. **A,** Percent of total work output. **B,** Total kilojoules of energy. Test results based on Katch test protocol (see p. 194). (Data from the Applied Physiology Laboratory, University of Michigan, Ann Arbor.)

is the justifiable concern that physical testing involving significant all-out anaerobic exercise would exacerbate sex differences in performance scores and magnify the adverse impact on females.

Blood Lactate Levels

As demonstrated previously in Figure 7.2, the blood lactate level remains low and stable during steady-rate exercise requiring up to about 55% of the maximum oxygen uptake. As the $\dot{V}O_2$max is approached, there is a precipitous rise in the level of blood lactate.

The data in Figure 11.6 were obtained from 10 college males who, participating in the Katch test, performed nine all-out bicycle ergometer rides of different durations and on different days. The subjects were highly motivated: many were involved in conditioning programs and some were varsity athletes. They were unaware of the duration of each test but were instructed and urged to turn as many revolutions as possible. Venous blood-lactate was measured before and immediately after the test and throughout recovery. The plotted points are the average blood lactate values for each test. Blood lactate levels increased in direct proportion to the duration (and total work output) of the all-out exercise. At the end of the 3-minute cycling bout, blood lactate averaged 140 mg for each 100 mL of blood (16 to 17 mmol).

Glycogen Depletion

Because the short-term energy system is powered mainly by glycogen stored in the specific muscles activated by an exercise, glycogen depletion patterns in these muscles also provide an indication of the glycolytic contribution to exercise. Figure 11.7 illustrates that the rate of glycogen depletion in the quadriceps femoris muscle during bicycle exercise is closely related to exercise intensity. Following steady-rate exercise at about 30% of $\dot{V}O_2$max, a considerable muscle glycogen reserve remains, even after 180 minutes of exercise. This is because relatively large quantities of fatty acid are used as energy and the drain is only moderate on stored glycogen. The most rapid and pronounced glycogen depletion is observed at the two heaviest supermaximal workloads. This outcome makes sense from a metabolic standpoint because glycogen is the only stored macronutrient that provides energy anaerobically for ATP resynthesis; clearly, this substrate has high priority in the "metabolic mill" during strenuous exercise.

Changes in total muscle glycogen, such as those illustrated in Figure 11.7, may not offer a precise indication of the degree of glycogen breakdown in specific fibers within the active muscle. Depending on the intensity of exercise, glycogen depletion occurs selectively in either fast- or slow-twitch muscle fibers.[83] For example, during all-out exercise such as repeated 1-minute sprints on a bicycle ergometer at a heavy load, fast-twitch fibers that are activated provide

FIGURE 11.6

Pedaling a stationary bicycle ergometer at one's highest possible power output causes blood lactate to increase in direct proportion to the duration of exercise for up to 3 minutes. Each value represents the average of 10 subjects. (Data from the Applied Physiology Laboratory, University of Michigan, Ann Arbor.)

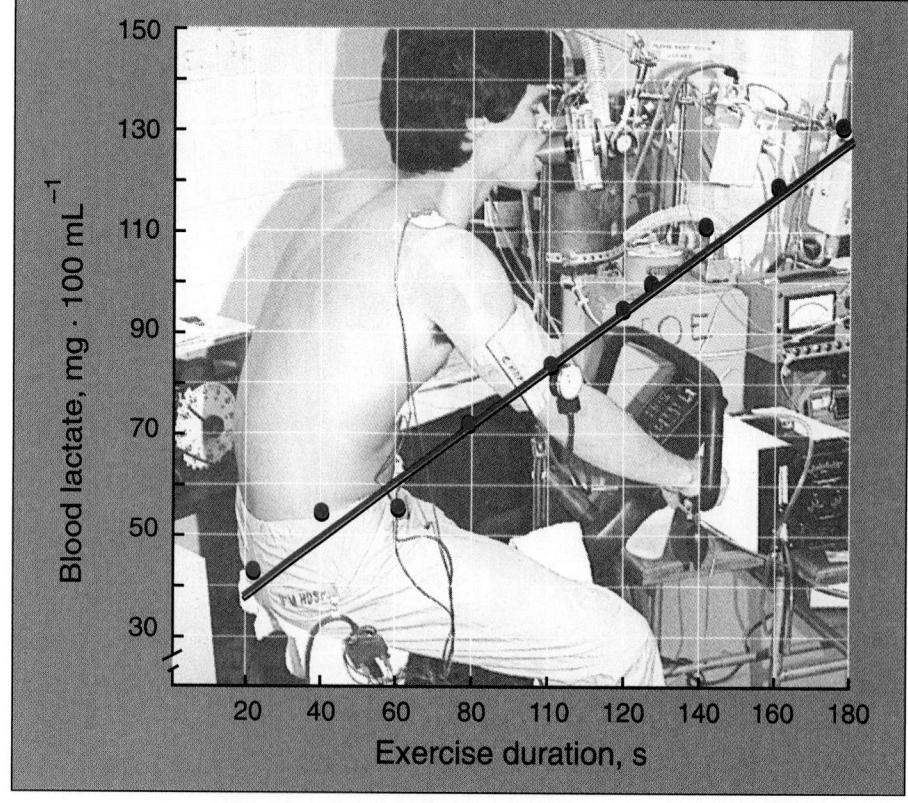

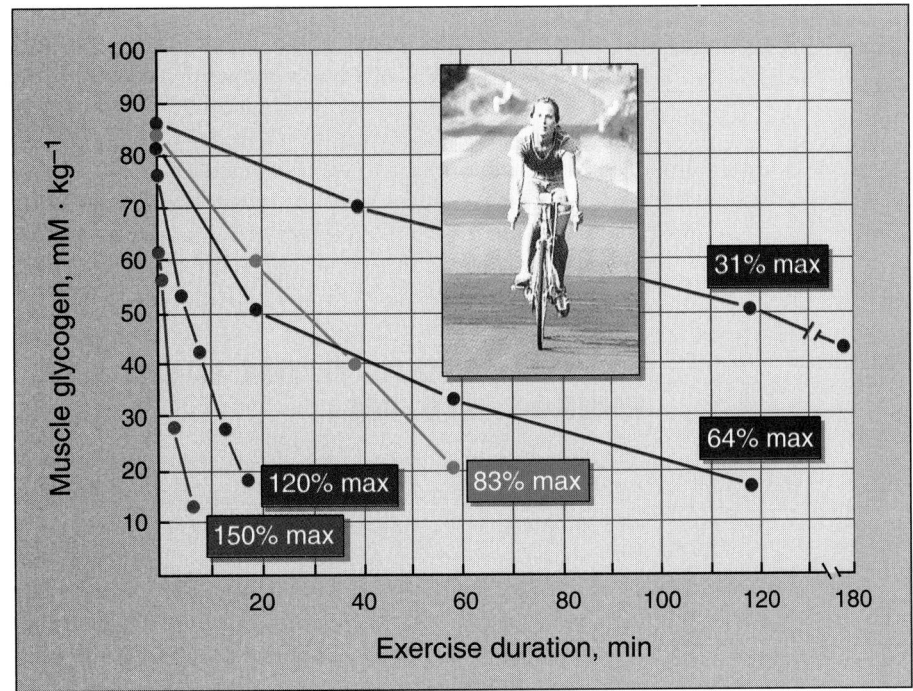

FIGURE 11.7
Glycogen depletion from the vastus lateralis portion of the quadriceps femoris muscle during bicycle exercise of different intensities and durations. Exercise at 31% of $\dot{V}o_2$max (the lightest workload) caused some depletion of muscle glycogen, but the most rapid and largest depletion occurred during exercise that ranged between 83% and 150% of $\dot{V}o_2$max. (Adapted from Gollnick, P.D.: Selective glycogen depletion pattern in human muscle fibers after exercise of varying intensity and at varying pedaling rates. *J. Physiol.*, 241:45, 1974.)

most of the power for the exercise. Because of the anaerobic nature of this effort, the glycogen content in these fibers becomes almost totally depleted. In contrast, during moderately heavy prolonged aerobic exercise such as distance running, the slow-twitch fibers are always the first to become glycogen-depleted.[35] This specificity in glycogen utilization (and depletion) makes it difficult to evaluate the glycolytic involvement of specific fibers from the changes in a muscle's total glycogen content before and after exercise.

INDIVIDUAL DIFFERENCES IN ANAEROBIC ENERGY-TRANSFER CAPACITY

Several factors contribute to differences among individuals in the capacity to generate short-term anaerobic energy. These factors include previous training, motivation, and the capacity to buffer acid metabolites.

Effects of Training

A comparison of biochemical factors related to anaerobic metabolism for trained and untrained subjects is presented in Figure 11.8. After short-term maximal exercise on the bicycle ergometer, the trained subjects always exhibited higher levels of muscle lactic acid and blood lactate as well as greater depletion of muscle glycogen. These results support the belief that training for short-term, all-out exercise enhances one's capacity to generate energy from the glycolytic system.[21, 31] This finding is important because, in sprint- and middle-distance activities, individual differences in anaerobic capacity (as reflected by a high level of blood

lactate accumulation) can account for considerable variation in exercise performance.

Buffering of Acid Metabolites

When anaerobic energy-transfer predominates, lactic acid accumulates and the acidity of muscle and blood increases. This has a dramatic negative effect on the intracellular environment and the contractile capability of active muscles.[34] This factor has led to speculation that anaerobic training may enhance short-term energy capacity by increasing the body's alkaline reserve. Such a training adaptation would theoretically enable greater lactic acid production because it could be buffered more effectively. Although this reasoning seems appealing, only a small increase in alkaline reserve has been noted in athletes compared to sedentary counterparts. Furthermore, there is no appreciable change in alkaline reserve following hard physical training. *The consensus is that trained people have a buffering capability that is within the range expected for healthy untrained individuals.*

It is interesting that high-intensity anaerobic exercise performance can be enhanced by temporarily altering the acid-base balance in the direction of alkalosis.[106] This enhanced performance was achieved through ingestion of a buffering solution of sodium bicarbonate prior to an 800-meter race. The significantly faster run times were accompanied by higher levels of blood lactate and extracellular H^+ concentration, suggesting an increased anaerobic energy contribution to this exercise. More is said in Chapter 23 concerning the possible ergogenic effects of this procedure.

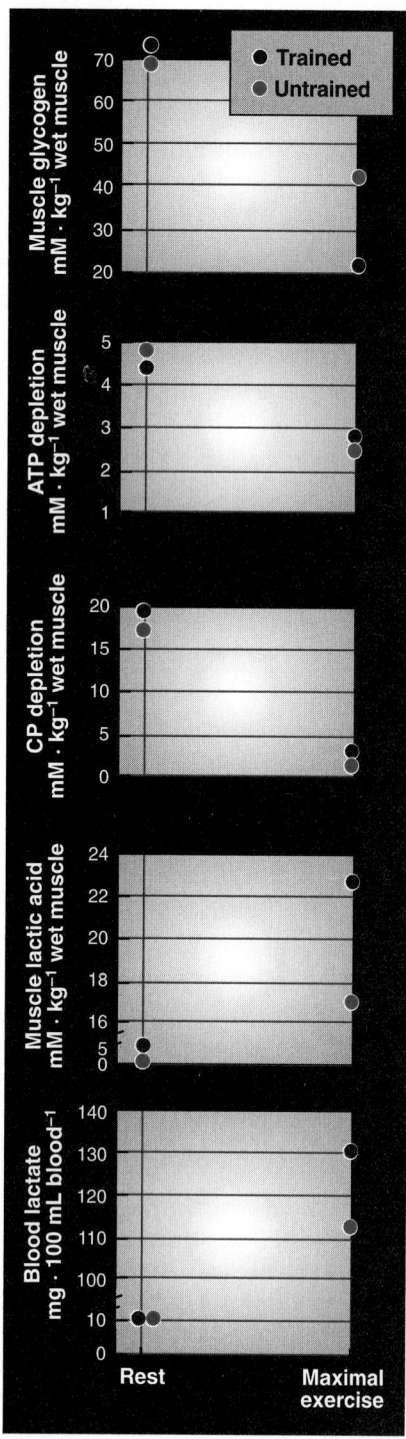

FIGURE 11.8

Depletion of anaerobic substrates (ATP, CP, and glycogen) and increases in muscle and blood lactate during short-term maximal exercise in trained and untrained subjects. The trained subjects exhibited a greater increase in anaerobic metabolism (higher lactate levels) and a more pronounced depletion in muscle glycogen, while the reductions in the high-energy phosphates ATP and CP were essentially the same as for the nontrained. (From Karlsson, J., et al.: Muscle metabolites during submaximal and maximal exercise in man. *Scand. J. Clin. Invest.*, 26:382, 1971.)

Motivation

Individuals with a higher "pain tolerance," "toughness," or ability to "push" beyond the discomforts of fatiguing exercise definitely accomplish more anaerobic work. These people usually achieve greater levels of blood lactate generation and glycogen depletion. They also score higher on tests of short-term energy capacity. Motivational factors, which are difficult to categorize or quantify, undoubtedly play a key role in superior performance at all levels of competition.

AEROBIC ENERGY: THE LONG-TERM ENERGY SYSTEM

As illustrated in Figure 11.9, athletes who excel in endurance sports generally have a large capacity for aerobic energy transfer. The maximal oxygen uptakes recorded for competitors in distance running, swimming, bicycling, and cross-country skiing are almost double those of sedentary men and women.[3, 42] This is not to say that the $\dot{V}O_2$max is the only determinant of endurance performance. Other factors, principally those at the local tissue level such as capillary density, enzymes, mitochondrial size and number, and muscle fiber type, exert a strong influence on a muscle's capacity to sustain a high level of aerobic exercise.[39] The $\dot{V}O_2$max does, however, provide important information on the capacity of the long-term energy system. In addition, this measure has significant physiologic meaning in that attaining a high $\dot{V}O_2$max requires the integration of a high level of ventilatory, cardiovascular, and neuromuscular functions (see Figure 7.6). *This makes $\dot{V}O_2$max a fundamental measure in exercise physiology.*

MEASUREMENT OF MAXIMAL OXYGEN UPTAKE

Maximal oxygen uptake can be determined using a variety of exercises that activate large muscle groups as long as the intensity and duration of the effort are sufficient to engage maximal aerobic energy transfer. The usual exercise modes include treadmill running or walking, bench stepping, and stationary cycling. Aerobic capacity also has been measured during free, tethered, and flume swimming,[10, 61] swim-bench ergometry,[32] in-line skating,[101] simulated arm-leg climbing,[16] rowing,[18] ice skating,[29] and arm-crank and wheelchair exercise.[90, 97, 99] Considerable research effort has been directed toward developing and standardizing tests for maximal aerobic power and establishing $\dot{V}O_2$max norms in relation to age, sex, state of training, and body size.

Criteria for $\dot{V}O_2$max

To be reasonably sure that a person has reached the maximum capacity for aerobic metabolism during exercise (that is, achieved a "true" $\dot{V}O_2$max), a leveling-off or peaking-over

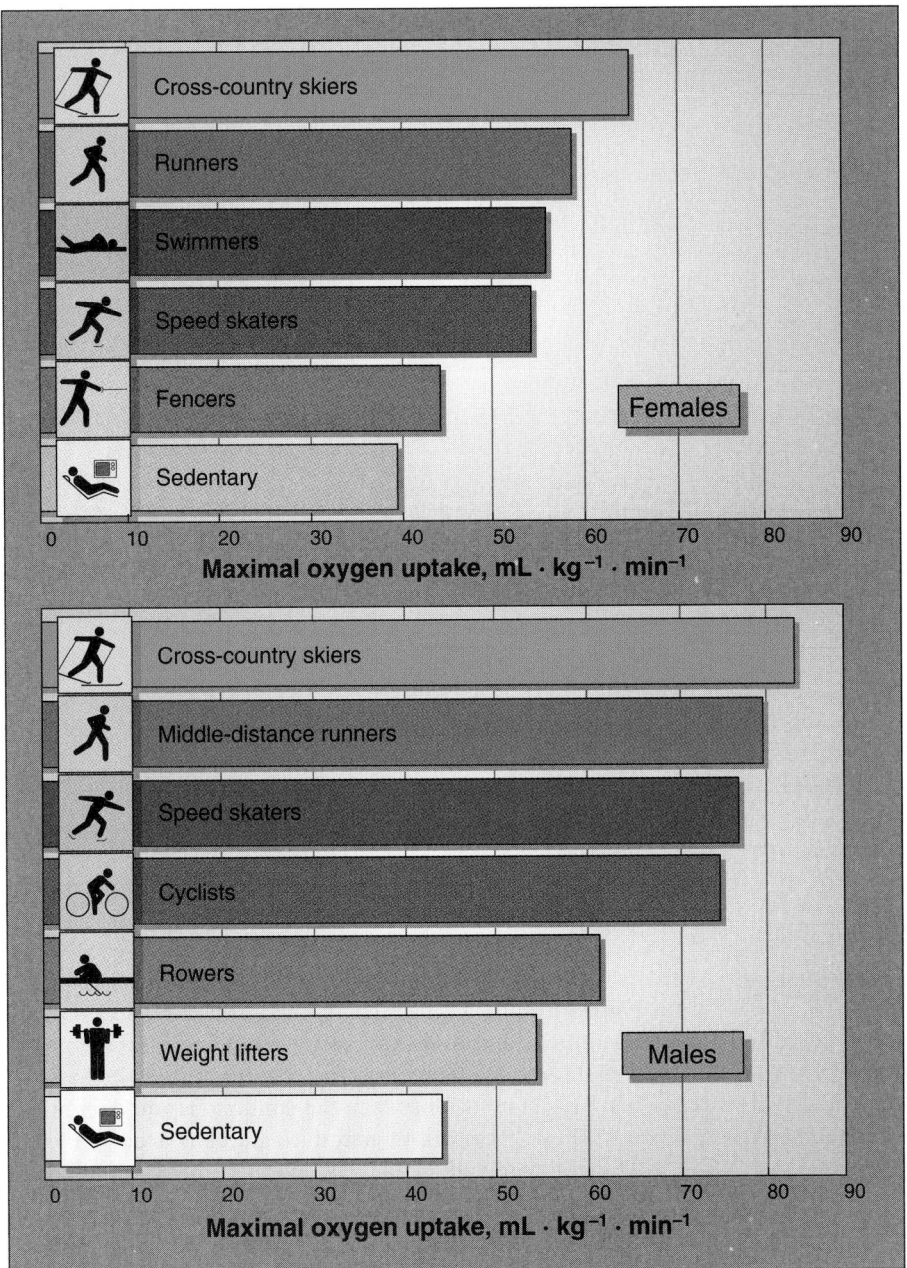

FIGURE 11.9

Maximal oxygen uptake of male and female Olympic-caliber athletes in different sports categories compared to healthy sedentary subjects. (Adapted from Saltin, B., and Åstrand, P.O.: Maximal oxygen uptake in athletes. *J. Appl. Physiol.*, 23:353, 1967.)

in oxygen uptake should be demonstrated (Figure 11.10), although agreement on a precise standard for this criterion remains elusive.[39a] When leveling off is not seen, or the test performance appears to be limited by local muscular factors rather than central circulatory dynamics, the term **peak oxygen uptake, or peak $\dot{V}O_2$,** is used. *Peak $\dot{V}O_2$ refers to the highest value of oxygen uptake measured during the test.*

The $\dot{V}O_2$max test shown in Figure 11.10 involved a progressive increase in treadmill exercise intensity. The test was terminated when the subject would not complete the full duration of a particular work block. For the average oxygen uptake values of 18 subjects plotted in this figure, the highest oxygen uptake was reached before the subjects attained their maximum exercise level. This peaking-over criterion verifies that the $\dot{V}O_2$max has been reached.

In many instances, however, a peaking-over in oxygen uptake is not readily observed at the higher exercise levels in adults, and it is quite uncommon in children.[85] Often, the highest oxygen uptake is recorded in the last minute of exercise. Consequently, less stringent $\dot{V}O_2$max criteria have been suggested, regardless of age, based on changes in oxygen uptake with increasing exercise intensity. In such a case, $\dot{V}O_2$max is considered to have been reached when oxygen uptake fails to increase by some value that is usually expected based on previous observations using the particular

FIGURE 11.10

Peaking over in oxygen uptake with increasing intensity during treadmill exercise. Each point represents the average oxygen uptake of 18 sedentary males. The region at which oxygen uptake fails to increase the expected amount, or even decreases slightly with increasing exercise intensity, represents the $\dot{V}O_2$max. (Data from the Applied Physiology Laboratory, University of Michigan, Ann Arbor. Photo courtesy of J. Graves, Exercise Science Laboratory, Syracuse University.)

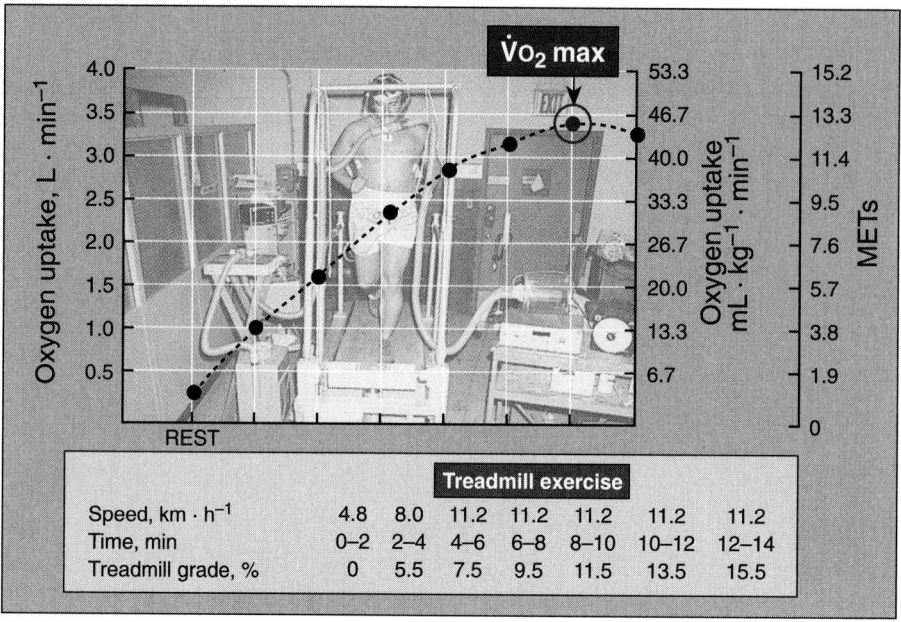

			Treadmill exercise				
Speed, km · h⁻¹	4.8	8.0	11.2	11.2	11.2	11.2	11.2
Time, min	0–2	2–4	4–6	6–8	8–10	10–12	12–14
Treadmill grade, %	0	5.5	7.5	9.5	11.5	13.5	15.5

test.[1, 39a, 76, 95] It is also argued that to accept an oxygen uptake value as maximum, blood lactate levels should reach 70 or 80 mg per 100 mL of blood (about 8 to 10 mmol) or higher. Less precise but more easily measured secondary criteria are attainment of the age-predicted maximum heart rate (refer to Figure 21.6) or a respiratory exchange ratio (R) in excess of 1.00.

TESTS OF MAXIMAL OXYGEN UPTAKE

Numerous tests have been devised and standardized for measuring $\dot{V}O_2$max. Performance on these tests is generally independent of strength, speed, body size, and skill, with the exception of specialized tests such as swimming, rowing, and ice skating.

The $\dot{V}O_2$max test may require a single continuous 3- to 5-minute supermaximal effort, but it usually consists of progressive increments in effort (**graded exercise**) to the point at which the subject will no longer continue to exercise. Some researchers have termed this end point "exhaustion." However, it is the person exercising who terminates the test. This decision is often influenced by a variety of psychological or motivational factors that may not necessarily reflect true physiologic strain. Considerable urging and prodding are often required to get subjects to the point at which acceptable criteria for either $\dot{V}O_2$max or peak $\dot{V}O_2$ attainment can be demonstrated. Practical experience has shown that high levels of motivation and anaerobic output generally are required to demonstrate a plateau in oxygen uptake during a graded exercise test to volitional termination. This poses a special difficulty for untrained people in particular who do not normally perform strenuous exercise and experience its associated discomforts.

Comparison of Tests

Maximal oxygen uptake tests are usually performed:

- Continuously—with no rest between exercise increments, or
- Discontinuously—with the subject resting several minutes between exercise periods.

The data in Table 11.3 reflect the results of a systematic comparison of $\dot{V}O_2$max scores measured using six common continuous and discontinuous treadmill and bicycle protocols.[71] Although there was only an 8-mL difference in maximal oxygen uptake between the continuous and discontinuous bicycle tests, the $\dot{V}O_2$max during cycling averaged 6.4 to 11.2% below values demonstrated on the treadmill. The largest difference between any of the three treadmill running tests was only 1.2%. The walking test, on the other hand, elicited $\dot{V}O_2$max scores about 7% higher than values on the bicycle but 5% lower than the average for the three running tests.

A common complaint of subjects participating in both the continuous and discontinuous bicycle tests was a feeling of intense local discomfort in the thigh muscles during heavy exercise. Many subjects stated that this was the major factor limiting their ability to continue exercising. During the walking test, subjects experienced local discomfort in the lower back and calf muscles, especially when walking at the more severe treadmill grades. Local muscular discomfort was not common in the running tests, and subjects complained more of a general fatigue usually categorized as feeling "winded." For ease of administration, the continuous treadmill run appears to be the preferred test of aerobic capacity for large numbers of healthy subjects. The total time to administer the test averaged a little over 12 minutes, whereas the discontinuous running test averaged about 65 minutes. Subjects seemed to tolerate the continuous test well and preferred the shorter time period. Research indicates that $\dot{V}O_2$max can be reached using a continuous protocol when exercise intensity is increased progressively in 15-second intervals.[28] With this approach, the total test time for either bicycle or treadmill exercise averages only about 5 minutes.

Commonly Used Treadmill Protocols. Six treadmill protocols commonly used to assess aerobic capacity in both normal individuals and cardiac patients are summarized in Figure 11.11. A feature common to these tests is the manipulation of exercise duration and treadmill speed and grade. The Harbor treadmill protocol (example *F*), referred to as a **ramp test,** is a unique application. In this procedure, the grade is increased each minute for up to 10 minutes by a constant amount between 1 and 4% depending on the exerciser's fitness. This relatively quick procedure elicits a linear increase in oxygen uptake to the maximum level and is well tolerated by both healthy subjects and cardiac patients.[17, 23, 103]

Can a Test Protocol Be Manipulated to Increase $\dot{V}O_2$max?

When a person has completed a maximal oxygen uptake test, we assume that the tester has made every attempt to "push" the subject to the near-limits of performance. This effort can take the form of verbal and peer encouragement as well as a monetary incentive. Following the test, if the usual physiological criteria are met, it is assumed that the test score will represent the "true" $\dot{V}O_2$max. Figure 11.12 illustrates the results of an experiment during which 44 either sedentary or trained men and women performed a continuous treadmill $\dot{V}O_2$max test (*Max 1*) to the point at which they would no longer continue exercising ("exhaustion"). The subjects recovered for two minutes and then performed

a second test for $\dot{V}O_2$max (*Max 2*). During the recovery from *Max 1*, the treadmill grade was lowered at least 2.5% below the final grade of the previous test, and the running speeds were reduced from 183 m · min^{-1} to 150 m · min^{-1} for the trained subjects and from 150 m · min^{-1} to 100 m · min^{-1} for sedentary subjects.

After two minutes of active recovery, treadmill speed was increased to the *Max 1* test speed for 30 seconds, and percent grade was then increased to the final grade of *Max 1*. Every 2 minutes thereafter, the treadmill grade was increased until the subject once again terminated the test. During both tests, strong verbal encouragement was provided, particularly over the last minutes of the tests when it was apparent that the end point was imminent. The average $\dot{V}O_2$max score was 1.4% higher (statistically significant) on the second test. This difference of 48 mL (0.7 mL · kg^{-1} · min^{-1} for a typical subject), while small, was almost twice as large as that normally obtained between the two final oxygen uptake values of either a continuous or discontinuous test. Thus, a "booster" test following a normally administered test of aerobic capacity can increase slightly the final oxygen uptake. Considerable attention should be given to how tests are administered.

FACTORS THAT AFFECT MAXIMAL OXYGEN UPTAKE

Many factors influence the maximal oxygen uptake score. The most important of these are mode of exercise, heredity, state of training, body size and composition, sex, and age.

Mode of Exercise

It is generally accepted that variations in $\dot{V}O_2$max during different forms of exercise reflect the quantity of muscle mass activated.[9, 59] For experiments in which $\dot{V}O_2$max is determined on the same subjects during different exercise modes, the highest values are generally obtained during

---

TABLE 11.3
AVERAGE MAXIMAL OXYGEN UPTAKES FOR 15 MALE COLLEGE STUDENTS DURING CONTINUOUS AND DISCONTINUOUS TESTS ON THE TREADMILL AND BICYCLE ERGOMETER[a]

Variable	Bike, discontinuous	Bike, continuous	Treadmill, discontinuous walk-run	Treadmill, continuous walk	Treadmill, discontinuous run	Treadmill, continuous run
$\dot{V}O_2$max, mL · min^{-1}	3691 ± 453	3683 ± 448	4145 ± 401	3944 ± 395	4157 ± 445	4109 ± 424
$\dot{V}O_2$max, mL · kg^{-1} · min^{-1}	50.0 ± 6.9	49.9 ± 7.0	56.6 ± 7.3	566 ± 7.6	55.5 ± 7.6	55.5 ± 6.8

Adapted from McArdle, W.D., et al.: Comparison of continuous and discontinuous treadmill and bicycle tests for max $\dot{V}O_2$. *Med. Sci Sports.,* 5:156, 1973.

[a]Values are means ± standard deviations.

FIGURE 11.11

Six treadmill protocols commonly used to measure maximal oxygen uptake. **A,** *Naughton protocol.* Three-minute exercise periods of increasing intensity alternate with 3 minutes of rest. The exercise periods vary in grade and speed. **B,** *Åstrand protocol.* The speed is constant at 5 mph. After 3 minutes at 0% grade, the grade is increased 2½% every 2 minutes. **C,** *Bruce protocol.* Grade and/or speed are changed every 3 minutes. The 0% and 5% grades are omitted in healthier subjects. **D,** *Balke protocol.* After 1 minute at 0% grade and 1 minute at 2% grade, the grade is increased 1% per minute, all at a speed of 3.3 mph. **E,** *Ellestad protocol.* The initial grade is 10% and the later grade is 15% while the speed is increased every 2 or 3 minutes. **F,** *Harbor protocol.* After 3 minutes of walking at a comfortable speed, the grade is increased at a constant preselected amount each minute: 1%, 2%, 3%, or 4%, so that the subject reaches $\dot{V}O_2max$ in approximately 10 minutes. (From Wasserman, K., et al.: *Principles of Exercise Testing and Interpretation.* 2nd ed., Philadelphia, Lea & Febiger, 1994.)

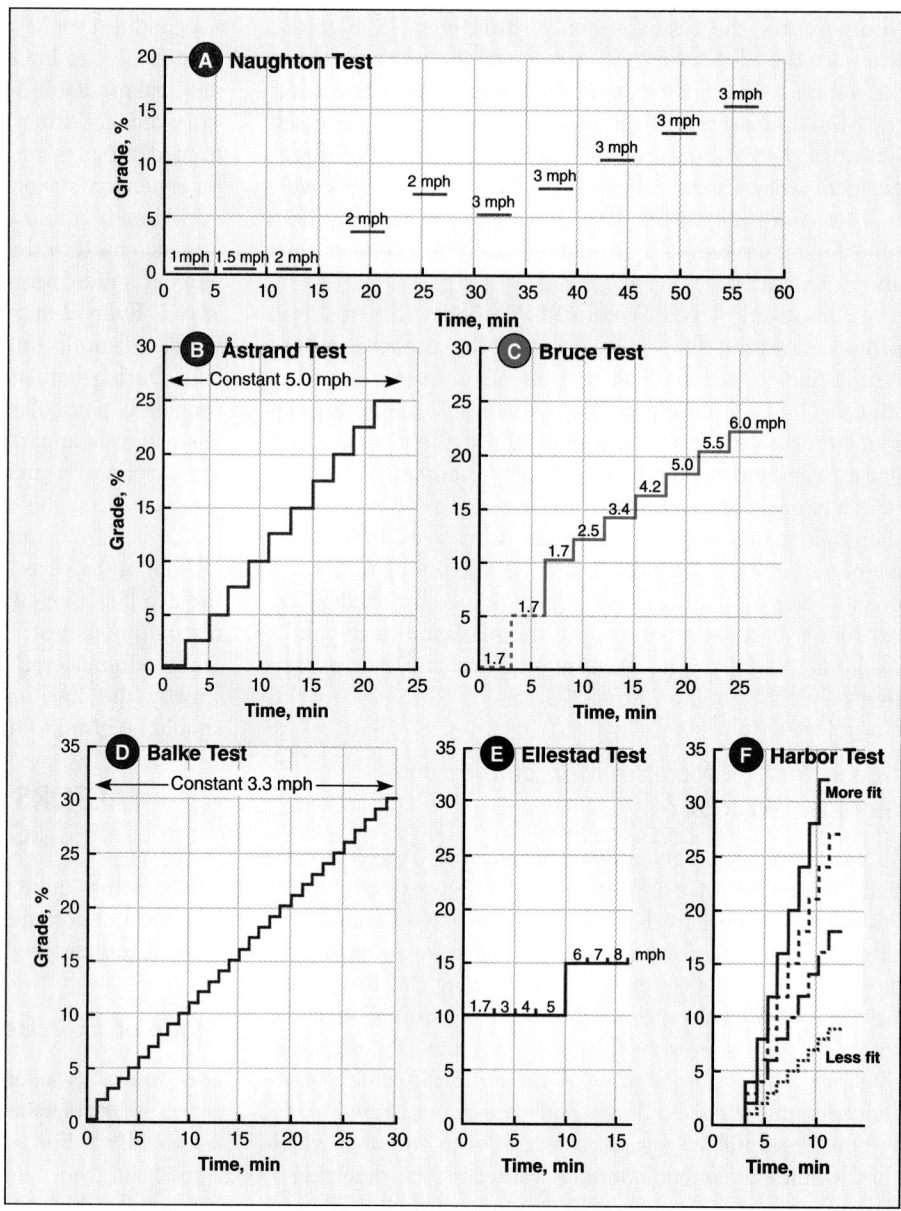

treadmill exercise. Bench-stepping, however, has produced $\dot{V}O_2max$ scores identical to treadmill values and significantly higher than those obtained on the bicycle ergometer.[46] During arm-crank exercise, the aerobic capacity value reaches only about 70% of one's capacity on the treadmill.[97] For skilled but untrained swimmers, the maximal oxygen uptake during swimming is usually about 20% below treadmill values.[61, 72] A definite **test specificity** is evident for this form of exercise because trained collegiate swimmers achieve $\dot{V}O_2max$ values while swimming that are only 11% below their treadmill values,[69] and some elite competitive swimmers can equal or even exceed their treadmill $\dot{V}O_2max$ scores during swimming tests.[61] Similarly, a distinct exercise specificity is noted for competitive

race-walkers who achieve oxygen uptakes while walking that are similar to their $\dot{V}O_2max$ values during treadmill running.[74] Furthermore, if competitive cyclists are permitted to cycle at the fast pedaling frequencies of competition, they too achieve $\dot{V}O_2max$ values equivalent to their treadmill scores.[36, 94]

In the laboratory, the treadmill is the apparatus of choice for determining $\dot{V}O_2max$ in healthy subjects. Exercise intensity is easily determined and regulated. Compared to other forms of exercise, the treadmill allows subjects to more easily meet one or more of the criteria needed to establish that $\dot{V}O_2max$ has actually been attained. In field experiments, bench-stepping and cycle ergometry are suitable alternatives.

Heredity

A knowledge of the interaction of inherited factors (DNA sequence variation) and exercise is crucial to understanding the individual variations in training responsiveness as well as the anticipated health-related benefits to be derived from regular physical activity.[12] Questions concerning the relative contribution of natural endowment **(genotype)** to physiologic function and exercise performance **(phenotype)** have been frequently raised.[2] For example, to what extent did heredity determine the extremely high aerobic capacities of the endurance athletes in Figure 11.9? Are these exceptionally high levels of functional capacity simply the results of intensive training? Although the answers are far from complete, researchers have indeed focused on the contribution of genetics to individual differences in physiologic and metabolic capacity.

In earlier investigations, studies were made of 15 pairs of identical twins (who presumably have the same heredity because they come from the same fertilized egg) and 15 pairs of fraternal twins (who, like ordinary siblings, result from the separate fertilization of two eggs) raised in the same city and having parents of similar socioeconomic backgrounds. Researchers concluded that heredity alone accounted for up to 93% of the observed differences in aerobic capacity as measured by the $\dot{V}O_2$max! In addition, the capacity of the short-term energy system of glycolysis was shown to be approximately 81% genetically determined, and the maximum heart rate was shown to be approximately 86% genetically determined.[56, 57] Subsequent investigations of larger groups of brothers, fraternal twins, and identical twins have indicated a significant but smaller effect of inherited factors on aerobic capacity and endurance performance.[15]

Genetic effect is currently estimated at about 10 to 30% for $\dot{V}O_2$max, 50% for maximum heart rate, and 70% for physical working capacity.[14, 82] Identical twins have similar muscle fiber composition, whereas fiber type varies widely between fraternal twins and brothers.[60] With muscular strength, about 40% of the variation among people is believed to be a result of genetic factors.[81] Table 11.4 summarizes the current estimation of genetic contribution to some important health-related fitness components. Though future research may determine an upper limit of genetic de-

TABLE 11.4
ESTIMATED GENETIC CONTRIBUTION TO INDIVIDUAL DIFFERENCES IN IMPORTANT COMPONENTS OF HEALTH-RELATED PHYSICAL FITNESS

Fitness Component	Genetic Contribution
• $\dot{V}O_2$max	20–30%
• Submaximal Exercise Response	20–30%
• Muscular Fitness	20–30%
• Blood Lipid Profile	30–50%
• Resting Blood Pressure	30%
• Total Body Fat	25%
• Regional Fat Distribution	30%
• Habitual Activity Level	30%

Modified from Bouchard, C., and Perusse, L.: Heredity, activity level, fitness, and health. in *Physical Activity, Fitness, and Health.* Champaign, IL, Human Kinetics, 1994.

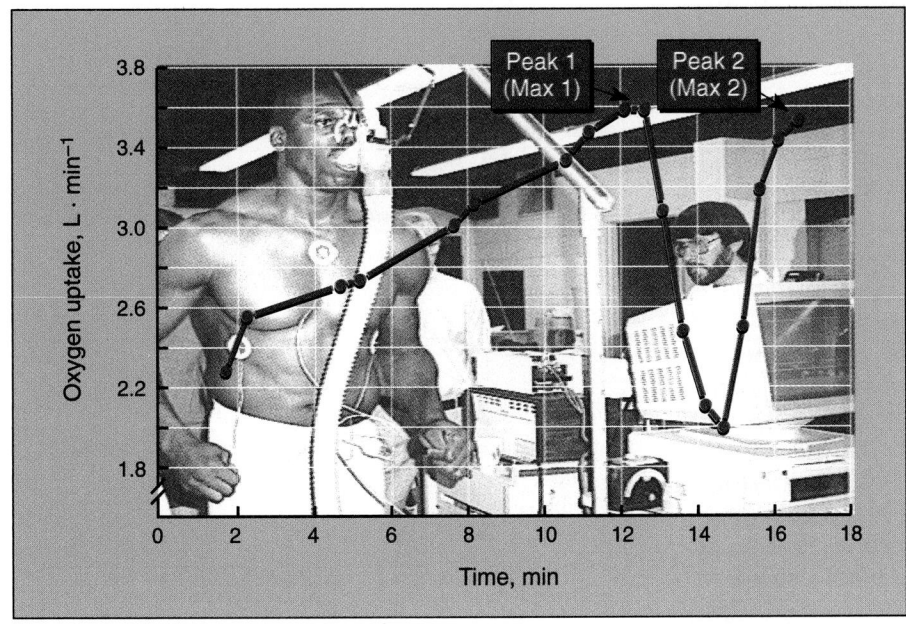

FIGURE 11.12
Oxygen uptake plotted as a function of time during repeat treadmill $\dot{V}O_2$max tests in 44 men and women. *Peak 1* refers to the highest oxygen uptake during the first test *(Max 1)* and *Peak 2* is the highest oxygen uptake during the repeat test *(Max 2)*. (Data from: Keller, B.A.: The influence of body size variables on gender differences in strength and maximum aerobic capacity. Unpublished doctoral dissertation, University of Massachusetts, Amherst, 1989. Data presented at 1991 ACSM meeting and published as an abstract. Keller, B., and Katch, F.I.: It is not valid to adjust gender differences in aerobic capacity and strength for body mass or lean body mass. *Med. Sci. Sports Exerc.,* 23:S167, 1991.)

termination, we can assume at this time that inherited factors significantly contribute to physiologic function and exercise performance and to the components of health-related physical fitness.[11, 12]

Trainability and Genes. Of two individuals in the same exercise program, one person might show 10 times the improvement of the other. It is now apparent that much of our sensitivity to maximal aerobic and anaerobic power training, as well as the adaptations of most of our muscle enzymes, is genotype dependent.[13, 15, 37, 84, 92] In other words, both members of a pair of twins generally show the same training response. While a vigorous program of physical training will enhance a person's level of fitness regardless of genetic background, it is clear that the limits for developing fitness capacity are linked to natural endowment. Genetic makeup plays such a predominant role in determining the training response that it is almost impossible to predict a particular individual's response to a given training stimulus.

State of Training

The $\dot{V}O_2$max score must be evaluated relative to the subject's state of training at the time of measurement. Normally, maximal oxygen uptake will vary between 5 and 20% depending on whether a person is "in shape" or "out of shape" at the time of measurement. The influence of training on aerobic capacity is discussed in Chapter 21.

Sex

The $\dot{V}O_2$max for women is typically 15 to 30% below that of men.[100] Even among trained endurance athletes, the sex difference ranges between 15 and 20%.[7] These differences, however, are considerably larger if the $\dot{V}O_2$max is expressed as an absolute value (L · min^{-1}) rather than relative to body mass (mL · kg^{-1} · min^{-1}).[104] Among world-class male and female cross-country skiers, for example, a 43% lower $\dot{V}O_2$max value for women (6.54 versus 3.75 L · min^{-1}) becomes 15% lower (83.8 versus 71.2 mL · kg^{-1} · min^{-1}) when the body masses of the athletes are used in the ratio expression.

The apparent sex difference in $\dot{V}O_2$max has generally been ascribed to differences in body composition (discussed in next section) and hemoglobin concentration. Untrained young adult women, for example, generally possess about 26% body fat whereas the corresponding value for men averages 15%.[48] Although trained athletes have lower percentages of fat, trained women still possess significantly more body fat than their male counterparts. Thus, the average male can generate more total aerobic energy simply because he possesses more muscle mass and less fat than the average female. Probably because of their higher level of testosterone, men also have a 10 to 14% greater concentration of hemoglobin than women. This difference in the oxygen-carrying capacity of the blood potentially enables men to circulate more oxygen during exercise, increasing their aerobic capacities compared to women.[109]

Although lower body fat and higher hemoglobin evidently provide the male with greater aerobic power, other factors must be considered to explain fully the differences between the sexes. One possible explanation is the difference in the normal physical activity level of the "average" male compared to that of the "average" female. It can be convincingly argued that, because of social constraints, the opportunities for women to participate in extracurricular athletic activities, as well as many recreational pursuits, have been considerably less than those for men. Among prepubertal children, boys are significantly more active in daily life than girls of the same age.[33] Despite these factors, the aerobic capacities of active females are generally higher than those of sedentary males. Female cross-country skiers have $\dot{V}O_2$max scores that are 40% higher than those of untrained males.[7] Even among the so-called "normal" population, there is considerable variability within sexes, and the $\dot{V}O_2$max scores for many women exceed the values for men.

Body Size and Composition

An estimated 69% of the differences in $\dot{V}O_2$max scores among individuals can be explained simply by variations in body mass.[111] Thus, it is usually not meaningful to compare exercise performance or absolute values of oxygen uptake among individuals who differ in body size or composition. This factor has led to the common practice of expressing oxygen uptake in terms of its relation to surface area, body mass, fat-free body mass, or limb volume. As illustrated in Table 11.5, for an untrained man and woman differing considerably in body mass, the difference in $\dot{V}O_2$ is 43% when it is expressed in liters per minute. When expressed in relation

**TABLE 11.5
DIFFERENT WAYS OF EXPRESSING
OXYGEN UPTAKE**

Variable	Female	Male	Female vs. Male % difference
$\dot{V}O_2$max, L · min^{-1}	2.00	3.50	−43
$\dot{V}O_2$max, mL · kg^{-1} · min^{-1}	40.0	50.0	−20
$\dot{V}O_2$max, mL · kgFFM^{-1} · min^{-1}	53.3	58.8	−9
Body mass, kg	50	70	−29
Percent body fat	25	15	+67
Fat-free body mass, kg	37.5	59.5	−37

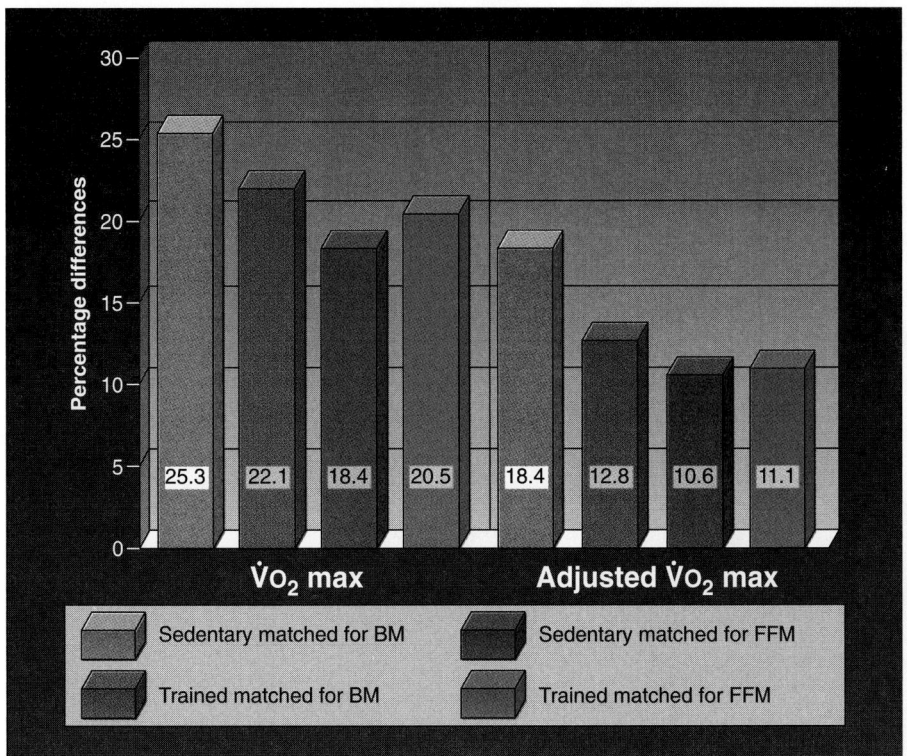

FIGURE 11.13
Percentage differences in $\dot{V}O_2$max, including the adjustment for hemoglobin (*Adjusted $\dot{V}O_2$max*), in sedentary and trained males and females matched for body mass (BM) and fat-free body mass (FFM). (From Keller, B.A.: The influence of body size variables on gender differences in strength and maximum aerobic capacity. Unpublished doctoral dissertation, University of Massachusetts, Amherst, 1989.)

to body mass ($mL \cdot kg^{-1} \cdot min^{-1}$), the $\dot{V}O_2$ value for the woman is still about 20% lower than that for the man. If aerobic capacity is expressed in relation to fat-free body mass, however, the difference between the two subjects is reduced still more. When oxygen uptake values during maximal arm-cranking exercise were corrected for variations in arm and shoulder size, no difference in peak $\dot{V}O_2$ was observed between the sexes.[102] *These findings suggest that the difference in aerobic capacity between men and women is largely a function of the size of the contracting muscle mass.* On the other hand, one must not be misled into believing that simply expressing the aerobic or endurance performance capacity in terms of some measure of body composition will automatically "adjust" such criterion measures to a "sex-neutral" state. The crucial test is to ascertain whether the sex differences are real (that is, biological in origin) or a result factors other than true inherited characteristics.

An Argument for Biological Differences between Sexes. The traditional ways of expressing oxygen uptake presented in Table 11.5 do not necessarily answer the question of whether sex differences in oxygen uptake are biologically inherent or fully attributable to differences in muscle mass and body composition.[108] This uncertainty exists because statistical adjustments may not truly "eliminate" sex differences: they simply express the criterion trait, such as aerobic capacity or muscular strength, relative to whatever divisor is used (for example, body mass, fat-free body mass, or muscle cross-sectional area).

An experimental approach to evaluating this important topic would be to compare the physiologic responses and capacities of men and women who do not differ in body size, body composition, or training history. Such a comparison would eliminate the need to express oxygen uptake as a ratio score relative to body size or composition. Consequently, if such traits were matched and body size were no longer a factor, it follows that there should be no sex differences in aerobic capacity. To evaluate this hypothesis, 10 pairs of sedentary and endurance-trained men and women were compared for aerobic capacity after being matched in age, stature, body mass, fat-free body mass, and prior training history.[53] In addition, the aerobic capacity was adjusted for the observed sex difference in hemoglobin concentration. Figure 11.13 illustrates the effect of sex matching for either body mass or fat-free body mass on the percentage difference in aerobic capacity measured during an incremental treadmill running test. The differences in aerobic capacity between men and women matched for body mass were 25.3% (sedentary) and 22.1% (trained). After adjustment for differences in hemoglobin concentration (*Adjusted $\dot{V}O_2$max*), sex differences persisted: they were reduced slightly to 18.4% for the sedentary group and 12.8% for the trained group. When the groups were matched for fat-free body mass, the sex differences were still substantial, averaging 18.4% for the sedentary group and 20.5% for the trained group. When these differences in aerobic capacity were adjusted for hemoglobin concentration, the sex differences

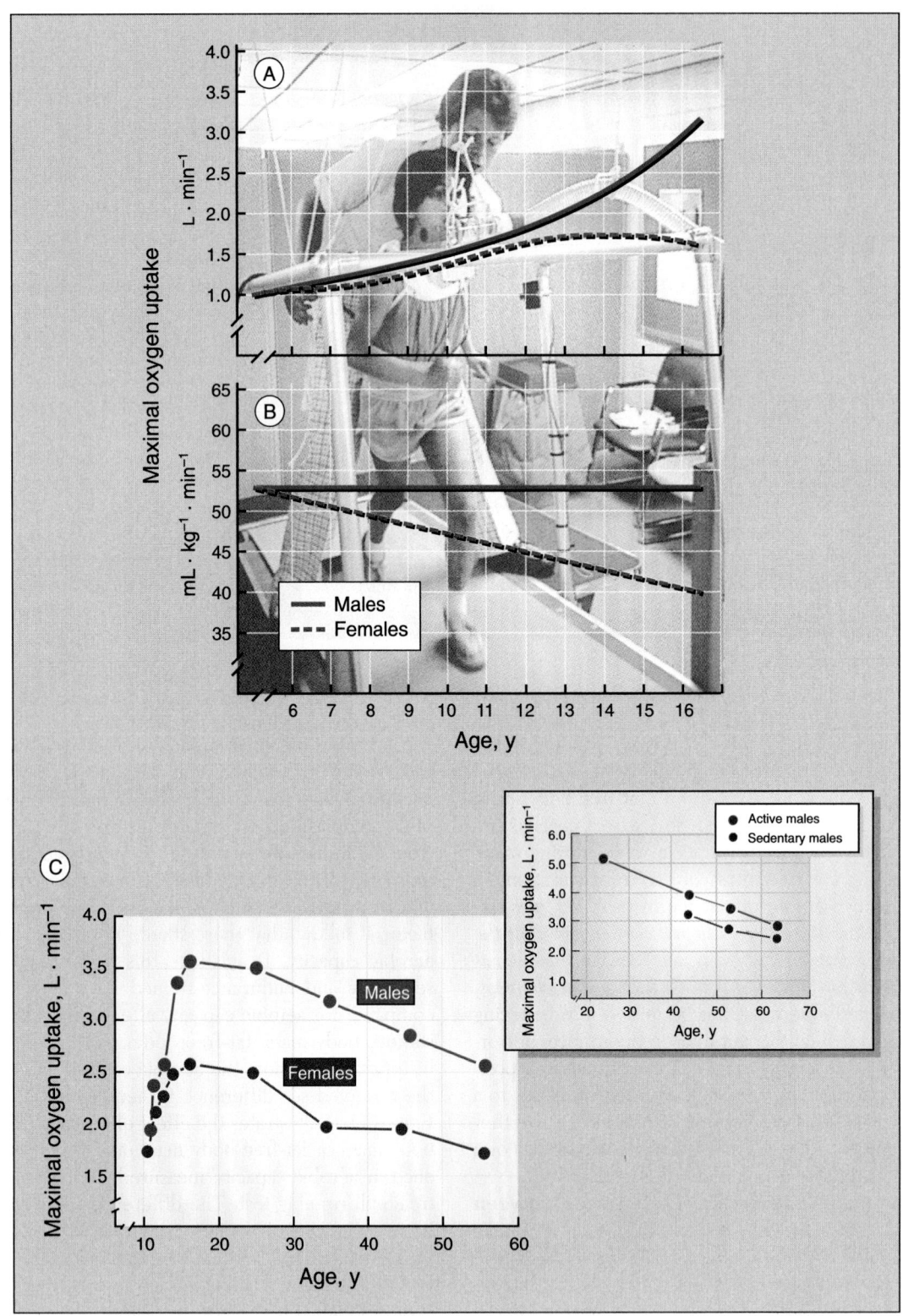

FIGURE 11.14

Maximal oxygen uptake in relation to age in boys and girls and men and women. (**A** and **B** from Krahenbuhl, G.S., et al.: Developmental aspects of maximal aerobic power in children. In *Exercise and Sport Sciences Reviews.* Vol. 13, Terjung, R.L. [Ed.], New York, Macmillan, 1985. **C** modified from Hermansen, L.: Individual differences. In *Fitness, Health, and Work Capacity. International Standards for Assessment.* Larson, L.A. [Ed.], New York, Macmillan, 1974. The inset graph in **C** was redrawn from tabled data of Åstrand, P.O., and Rodahl, K.R.: *Textbook of Work Physiology.* New York, McGraw-Hill, 1970.)

were reduced somewhat but still averaged about 11% for both groups.[54]

These findings suggest that a portion of the sex difference in aerobic capacity may be biologically inherent and unalterable. This is not to say that aerobic capacity cannot be significantly affected by training—of course, it can. Rather, these results suggest that it may be inappropriate to expect "sex-free" differences in aerobic capacity. In Chapter 22, data are presented on sex differences in muscular strength based on experiments with males and females having the same body size and composition.

Age

Maximal oxygen uptake is not spared the effects of aging.[47, 91, 93] Although inferences from cross-sectional studies of people of different ages are somewhat limited, the available data provide insight into the possible effects of aging on physiologic function. Figure 11.14 illustrates data from various studies on age trends in aerobic capacity of children and adults.

Children. Figures 11.14A and B illustrate age trends in the absolute and relative aerobic capacities of boys and girls aged 6 to 16.

- Absolute values—The $\dot{V}O_2$max values in $L \cdot min^{-1}$ (Figure 11.14A) for boys and girls are similar until about age 12; at age 14, the $\dot{V}O_2$max value for boys averages about 25% larger than that for girls, and by age 16, the difference exceeds 50%. This difference is generally attributed to the development of a greater muscle mass in boys as well as a sex difference in daily physical activity.
- Relative values—For boys, average aerobic capacity in $mL \cdot kg^{-1} \cdot min^{-1}$ (Figure 11.14B) remains level at about 52 $mL \cdot kg^{-1} \cdot min^{-1}$ from age 6 to 16; for females, the line slopes downward with age, reaching about 40 $mL \cdot kg^{-1} \cdot min^{-1}$ at age 16, a value that is 32% below that of their male counterparts. This difference is probably a result of the greater accumulation of body fat in females; this extra fat must be transported but does not contribute to an enhanced capacity for aerobic metabolism.[8, 58]

Adults. *After age 25, $\dot{V}O_2$max declines steadily at a rate of about 1% per year so that, by age 55, it is about 27% below values reported for 20-year-olds* (Figure 11.14C). The data in the insert graph indicate that while active adults retain a relatively high $\dot{V}O_2$max at all ages, there is still a progressive decline in aerobic power with advancing years. In one study of 8 women averaging about 80 years of age, $\dot{V}O_2$max averaged 13.4 $mL \cdot kg^{-1} \cdot min^{-1}$, or about 3.7 METs.[30] There is strong evidence to indicate, however, that one's habitual level of physical activity has far more influence on aerobic capacity than chronological age per se.[75] The age-related effects on physiologic function are discussed more fully in Chapter 30.

TESTS TO PREDICT AEROBIC CAPACITY

The direct measurement of $\dot{V}O_2$max requires an extensive laboratory and specialized equipment as well as considerable subject motivation. Consequently, these tests are not suitable for measuring large groups of untrained subjects outside of the laboratory. In addition, such strenuous exercise could pose a hazard to adults who are not medically cleared or who are asked to exercise without appropriate safeguards or supervision. In view of these considerations, tests have been devised to **predict** $\dot{V}O_2$max from performance measures such as walking and running endurance or from heart rate measured during or immediately after exercise.[19, 38, 110, 112] The tests are easy to administer, can be used with large groups of men or women, and usually require only submaximal exercise.

WALKING TESTS

With interest in "fitness walking" reaching a peak in the 1980s, walking tests were developed to predict $\dot{V}O_2$max. The following equation can be used to predict $\dot{V}O_2$max from walking speed and other variables in men and women:[55]

$$\dot{V}O_2max = 6.9652 + (0.0091 \times Wt) - (0.0257 \times Age) + (0.5955 \times Sex) - (0.224 \times T1) - (0.0115 \times HR1\text{-}4)$$

For this equation, $\dot{V}O_2$max is in liters per minute; Wt is body weight in pounds; Age is in years; Sex: 0 = female, 1 = male; T1 is time for the 1-mile track walk expressed as minutes and hundredths of a minute; and HR1-4 is the heart rate in beats per minute taken immediately at the end of the last quarter-mile.

The equation for $\dot{V}O_2$max, expressed in milliliters per kilogram per minute, is:

$$\dot{V}O_2max = 132.853 - (0.0769 \times Wt) - (0.3877 \times Age) + (6.315 \times Sex) - (3.2649 \times T1) - (0.1565 \times HR1\text{-}4)$$

For these equations, the multiple correlation for predicting $\dot{V}O_2$max from 1-mile walking performance is R = 0.92, with a standard error of prediction of ± 0.335 $L \cdot min^{-1}$ (4.4 $mL \cdot kg^{-1} \cdot min^{-1}$). This means that about 68% of the people tested will have an actual $\dot{V}O_2$max within either 0.335 $L \cdot min^{-1}$ or 4.4 $mL \cdot kg^{-1} \cdot min^{-1}$ of the predicted value. Because the group studied ranged in age from 30 to 69 years, this prediction method is probably applicable to a large segment of the adult population.

The following data for a 30-year-old female illustrate the test's use:

$$Body\ weight = 155.5\ lb$$
$$T1 = 13.56\ min$$
$$HR1\text{-}4 = 145\ beats \cdot min^{-1}$$

Substituting in the equation to predict $\dot{V}O_2$max in $mL \cdot kg^{-1} \cdot min^{-1}$:

$$\dot{V}O_2max = 132.853 - (0.0769 \times 155.5) - (0.3877 \times 30.0) + (6.315 \times 0) - (3.2649 \times 13.56) - (0.1565 \times 145)$$

$$\dot{V}O_2max = 132.853 - (11.96) - (11.63) + (0) - (44.27) - (22.69)$$

$$\dot{V}O_2max = 42.3 \ mL \cdot kg^{-1} \cdot min^{-1}$$

ENDURANCE RUNS

Like walking tests, runs of various durations or distances are used to evaluate aerobic fitness.[4, 19, 49, 50] Such tests are based on the reasonable notion that the distance one can run in a specified time (in excess of 5 or 6 minutes) is determined by that person's ability to maintain a high, steady-rate level of oxygen uptake. This ability, in turn, is largely influenced on one's maximum capacity to generate energy aerobically. Based on this rationale, a field performance test was devised in 1959 to evaluate aerobic fitness of military personnel.[4] For this test, the subjects were required to run as far as possible in 15 minutes. In a 1968 study by Cooper, the run time was shortened to 12 minutes.[19]

In his original validation of the 12-minute test, Cooper observed a strong correlation between the $\dot{V}O_2max$ values of Air Force personnel and the distances they could run-walk in 12 minutes. A correlation coefficient of r = 0.90 was reported between the 12-minute run-walk distance and the $\dot{V}O_2max$ values ($mL \cdot kg^{-1} \cdot min^{-1}$) in 47 men varying considerably in age (17 to 54 years), body mass (52 to 123 kg), and $\dot{V}O_2max$ (31 to 59 $mL \cdot kg^{-1} \cdot min^{-1}$). This same correlation also was observed in 9 ninth-grade boys.[24] Other investigators, however, have been unable to demonstrate such a strong relationship between "Cooper test" scores and aerobic capacity. One study, for example, measured 11- to 14-year-old boys and reported a correlation of r = 0.65.[64] For a group of 26 female athletes, the correlation between the run-walk scores and $\dot{V}O_2max$ values was r = 0.70,[65] and for 36 untrained college women, a similar correlation of r = 0.67 was observed.[49]

It is noteworthy that a simple correlation of run-walk scores to $\dot{V}O_2max$ does not take into account the interaction of factors such as age and body mass. These variables are themselves related to both run-walk times and $\dot{V}O_2max$ scores. When the original data of Cooper were restricted to the same age range as those in the preceding study of 36 women, the computed correlation coefficient was reduced dramatically—from r = 0.90 to r = 0.59!

Predictions of aerobic capacity should be approached with caution when they are based on running performance. The need to establish a consistent level of motivation and effective pacing is critical with inexperienced subjects. Some individuals may achieve an optimal pace such that they do not run too fast in the early part of a run and, therefore, do not slow down or even stop as a result of lactic-acid buildup as the test progresses. Other individuals, however, may begin too slowly and continue that way, causing their final performance scores to reflect inappropriate pacing or motiva-

tion rather than physiologic capacity. In addition, $\dot{V}O_2max$ is not the only variable that determines endurance running performance. Factors such as body mass and body fatness, running economy, and the all-important percentage of aerobic capacity that can be sustained without blood lactate buildup contribute significantly to successful running.[20, 22, 49]

PREDICTIONS BASED ON HEART RATE

Common tests to predict $\dot{V}O_2max$ use exercise or postexercise heart rate during a standardized regimen of submaximal exercise performed either on a bicycle ergometer, treadmill, or step test. These tests make use of the essentially linear relationship between heart rate and oxygen uptake during various intensities of light to moderately heavy aerobic exercise. The slope of the line used in this relationship (that is, rate of heart rate increase) reflects the individual's efficiency in cardiovascular response and level of aerobic fitness. The $\dot{V}O_2max$ can then be estimated by drawing a straight line through several submaximal points that relate heart rate and oxygen uptake (or exercise intensity), then extending this HR-$\dot{V}O_2$ line to some assumed maximum heart rate for the particular age group.

Figure 11.15 illustrates the application of this **extrapolation procedure** to trained and untrained subjects. The HR-$\dot{V}O_2$ line was drawn from four submaximal measures during graded bicycle ergometer exercise. Although each person's HR-$\dot{V}O_2$ line tends to be linear, the **slope** of the individual lines can differ considerably. Consequently, a person of relatively high aerobic fitness can perform more intense exercise (achieve higher oxygen uptake) before reaching a heart rate of 140 or 160 beats per minute than a less "fit" person. Also, because heart rate increases linearly with exercise intensity, the person with the smallest heart rate increase tends to have the highest exercise capacity and, hence, the highest $\dot{V}O_2max$. For the two subjects illustrated in Figure 11.15, $\dot{V}O_2max$ was predicted by extrapolating the HR-$\dot{V}O_2$ line to a heart rate of 195 beats per minute— the assumed maximum heart rate for subjects of college age.

The accuracy of predicting $\dot{V}O_2max$ from submaximal exercise heart rate is limited by the following assumptions:

• *Linearity of heart rate–oxygen uptake (exercise intensity) relationship.* This assumption is met to a large degree, particularly for various intensities of light to moderate exercise. In some subjects, however, the heart rate–oxygen uptake line curves, or asymptotes, at the heavier workloads in a direction that indicates a larger than expected increase in oxygen uptake per unit increase in heart rate. The oxygen uptake actually increases more than would be predicted through linear extrapolation of the HR-$\dot{V}O_2$ line. Thus, the predicted $\dot{V}O_2max$ of these subjects would be underestimated.

• *Similar maximum heart rates for all subjects.* The standard deviation from average maximum heart rate for in-

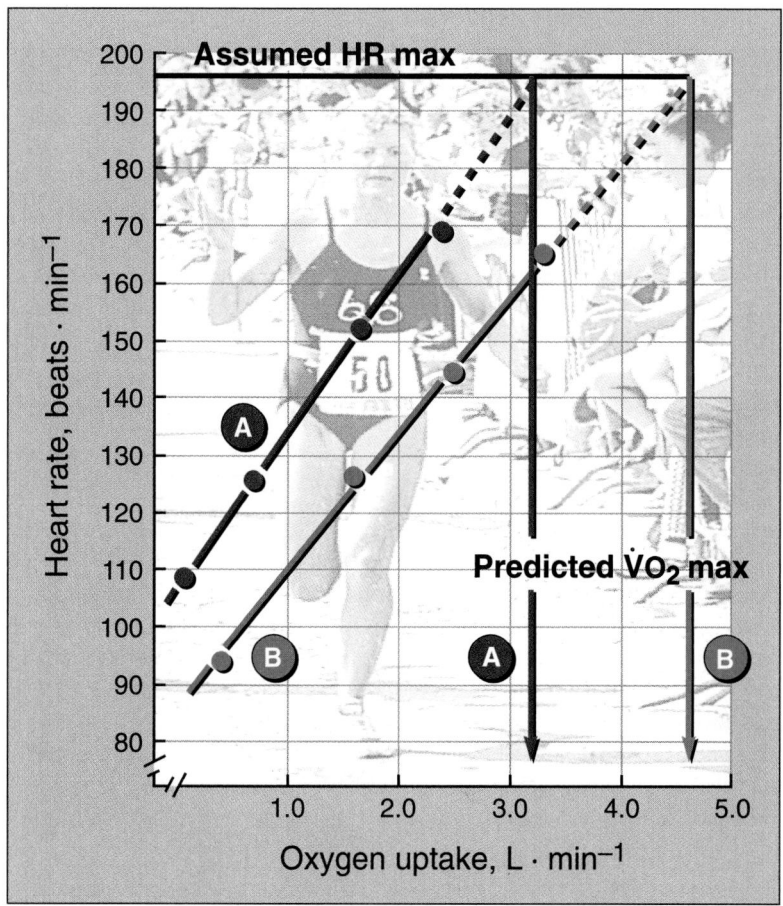

FIGURE 11.15
Extrapolating the linear relationship between submaximal heart rate and oxygen uptake to $\dot{V}O_2$max during graded exercise in an untrained and endurance trained subject.

dividuals of the same age is approximately ±10 beats per minute. Therefore, the $\dot{V}O_2$max of a person with an actual maximum heart rate of 185 beats per minute would be overestimated if the HR-$\dot{V}O_2$ line were extrapolated to 195 or 200 beats per minute. The opposite would occur for a subject with an actual maximum heart rate of 210 beats per minute. Maximum heart rate also decreases with age. Unless this age effect is considered, older subjects will consistently be overestimated if we assume a maximum heart rate of 195 beats per minute, which is only appropriate for 25-year-olds. More is said in Chapter 30 concerning the effect of age on maximum heart rate.

• *Assumed constant economy or mechanical efficiency during exercise.* In cases where submaximal oxygen uptake is not measured but instead estimated from the external workload, the predicted $\dot{V}O_2$max may be in error by the magnitude of variability in the exercise economy. A subject with poor exercise economy (oxygen uptake in submaximal exercise higher than assumed) will be underestimated in terms of $\dot{V}O_2$max because heart rate will be elevated due to the added oxygen cost of the uneconomical exercise. The variations in economy among individuals during walking or cycling does not usually exceed ±6%; for bench stepping, the variation can be about 10%, and this is not related to age, leg length, fitness, or degree of body fatness.[96]

In addition, seemingly small modifications in test procedures can have profound effects on the metabolic cost of the exercise. Simply allowing individuals to support themselves with the treadmill handrails, for example, can reduce the oxygen cost of exercise by as much as 30%.[114]

• *Small day-to-day variations in heart rate.* Even under highly standardized conditions, the day-to-day variation in heart rate is about ±5 beats per minute at a particular submaximal exercise level.

Within the framework of these limitations, the $\dot{V}O_2$max predicted from submaximal heart rate is generally within 10 to 20% of the person's actual value. While this is not acceptable accuracy for research purposes, these tests are well suited to purposes of screening and classifying subjects in terms of aerobic fitness. This technique also has been successfully applied in estimating aerobic capacity during pregnancy.[87]

THE STEP TEST

Heart rate during recovery from a standardized stepping exercise provides a practical means of classifying people for aerobic fitness. With the use of "prediction equations" applied to step-test results, $\dot{V}O_2$max can also be estimated with a reasonable degree of accuracy.

We have used a simple 3-minute step test (The Queens College step test) to evaluate the heart rate responses of thousands of college men and women.[70] The test was developed using gymnasium bleachers (16¼ inches high) so that large numbers of students could be tested at the same time. Each stepping cycle was performed to a four-step cadence, "up-up-down-down." The women performed 22 complete step-ups per minute, regulated by a metronome set at 88 beats per minute. Because the average man tended to be more fit for step-up exercise, the cadence was set at 24 step-ups per minute, or 96 beats per minute on the metronome. The step test was begun after a brief demonstration and practice period. At the completion of stepping, the students remained standing, and pulse rates were measured for a 15-second period, 5 to 20 seconds into recovery. Recovery heart rate was converted to beats per minute (15-second HR × 4) and compared to the established percentile rankings presented in Table 11.6.

Based on the essentially linear relationship between heart rate and oxygen uptake during exercise, one would expect a person with a low heart rate on the step test to be further away from $\dot{V}O_2$max than someone with a relatively high heart rate response. In other words, the lower the heart rate response to a standard exercise task, the higher the $\dot{V}O_2$max should be. To evaluate the validity of the step test as a measure of a person's aerobic capacity, we measured the $\dot{V}O_2$max

of a group of young adult men and women who had also performed the step test. For the women, the relationship between each subject's $\dot{V}O_2$max and step-test score is shown in Figure 11.16. The results clearly indicated that knowledge of a person's $\dot{V}O_2$max could be obtained from the step test score. Subjects with a high recovery heart rate tended to have a lower maximal oxygen uptake, whereas a faster recovery (lower heart rate) tended to be associated with a relatively high $\dot{V}O_2$max. To enable us to predict the $\dot{V}O_2$max ($mL \cdot kg^{-1} \cdot min^{-1}$) from step-test results for similar groups of men and women, the following equations were derived:

Men:
$$\dot{V}O_2max = 111.33 - (0.42 \times \text{step-test pulse rate, beats} \cdot min^{-1})$$

Women:
$$\dot{V}O_2max = 65.81 - (0.1847 \times \text{step-test pulse rate, beats} \cdot min^{-1})$$

To simplify these conversions, the "Predicted $\dot{V}O_2$max" columns of Table 11.6 present the maximal oxygen uptake values for men and women as predicted from recovery heart rate scores. For predictive accuracy, we can be 95% confident that the predicted $\dot{V}O_2$max will be within about ±16% of the person's true $\dot{V}O_2$max.

When a high degree of accuracy is required, the maximal oxygen uptake should be measured directly in the laboratory using an appropriate, graded exercise test. When this

TABLE 11.6
PERCENTILE RANKINGS FOR STEP TEST RECOVERY HEART RATE (HR) AND PREDICTED MAXIMAL OXYGEN UPTAKE FOR MALE AND FEMALE COLLEGE STUDENTS

Percentile Ranking	Recovery HR, Female	Predicted $\dot{V}O_2max$ ($mL \cdot kg^{-1} \cdot min^{-1}$)	Recovery HR, Male	Predicted $\dot{V}O_2max$ ($mL \cdot kg^{-1} \cdot min^{-1}$)
100	128	42.2	120	60.9
95	140	40.0	124	59.3
90	148	38.5	128	57.6
85	152	37.7	136	54.2
80	156	37.0	140	52.5
75	158	36.6	144	50.9
70	160	36.3	148	49.2
65	162	35.9	149	48.8
60	163	35.7	152	47.5
55	164	35.5	154	46.7
50	166	35.1	156	45.8
45	168	34.8	160	44.1
40	170	34.4	162	43.3
35	171	34.2	164	42.5
30	172	34.0	166	41.6
25	176	33.3	168	40.8
20	180	32.6	172	39.1
15	182	32.2	176	37.4
10	184	31.8	178	36.6
5	196	29.6	184	34.1

From McArdle, W.D., et al.: Percentile norms for a valid step test in college women. *Res. Q.*, 44:498, 1973

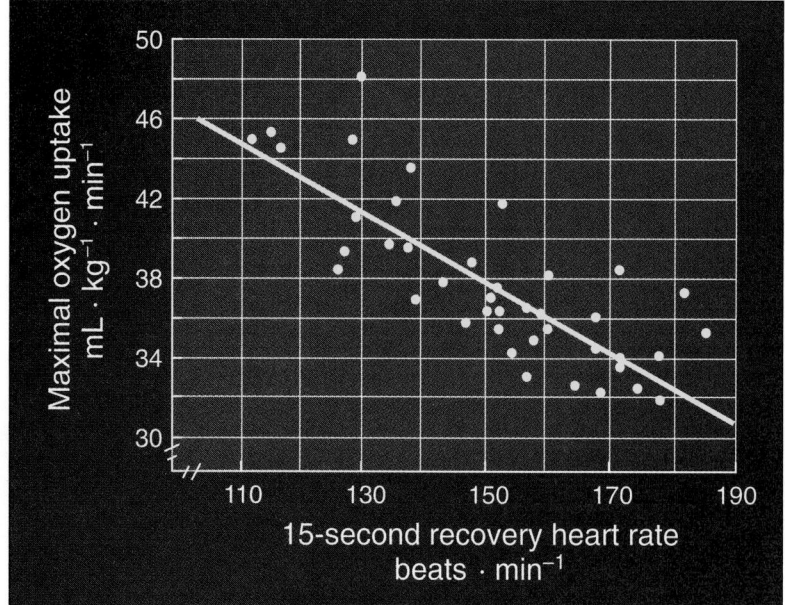

FIGURE 11.16

Scattergram and line of "best fit" relating step-test heart rate scores and maximal oxygen uptakes in college women. (From McArdle, W.D., et al.: Reliability and interrelationships between maximal oxygen uptake, physical work capacity, and step test scores in college women. *Med. Sci. Sports,* 4:182, 1972.)

is impractical, or when accuracy can be compromised somewhat, prediction tests are useful for classification purposes.

■ SUMMARY ■

1. The concepts of individual differences and specificity are important to understanding capacities for anaerobic and aerobic power. Individual differences refers to the real differences among individuals in contrast to the instability of a measure for any one person. Specificity refers to metabolic and physiologic functions that are not general in nature but, rather, dependent on a host of factors.

2. The contributions of anaerobic and aerobic energy transfer depend largely on the intensity and duration of exercise. During strength and power-sprint activities, energy transfer primarily involves the immediate and short-term anaerobic energy systems. The long-term aerobic energy system becomes progressively more important during activities that last longer than 2 minutes.

3. The capacity of each energy system can be estimated using appropriate physiologic measurements and performance tests. These tests can be used to evaluate the capacity at a particular time or show changes consequent to specific training programs.

4. The stair-sprinting test is commonly used to measure the power capacity of the intramuscular high-energy phosphates. Peak power and average power output capacity from the glycolytic pathway can be evaluated using the 30-second, all-out Wingate test. Interpretations of test results must take into consideration the exercise specificity principle.

5. Training status, motivation, and acid-base regulation are factors that contribute to individual differences in the capacities of the immediate and short-term energy systems.

6. The maximal oxygen uptake provides reproducible and important information on the power of the long-term aerobic energy system as well as the functional capacity of various physiologic support systems. Consideration of the type and amount of exercise performed and related physiologic functioning is required to ensure that a "true" $\dot{V}O_2$max score has been attained.

7. The maximal aerobic power is influenced by heredity, state and type of training, age, sex, and body composition. Each factor contributes uniquely to an individual's $\dot{V}O_2$max.

8. The result of expressing aerobic capacity in terms of some ratio of body size or composition (for example, $mL \cdot kg^{-1} \cdot min^{-1}$, or $mL \cdot kg\,FFM^{-1} \cdot min^{-1}$) does not answer the question as to whether true sex differences exist in maximal oxygen uptake. It is possible that a portion of the sex difference in aerobic capacity is a sex-linked, inherited trait.

9. Tests to predict $\dot{V}O_2$max from submaximal physiological and performance data are generally useful for classification purposes. However, they are only as good as the validity of the assumptions underlying their use for prediction. These assumptions include linearity of the HR-$\dot{V}O_2$ relationship, a constant exercise economy, and a relatively small day-to-day variation in exercise heart rate.

10. Field methods for predicting $\dot{V}O_2$max should be viewed with an understanding of the limitations of the assumptions underlying their use. When used and interpreted properly, however, field methods provide useful information in the absence of more valid laboratory methods.

■ REFERENCES ■

1. Armstrong, N., and Welsman, J.R.: Assessment and interpretation of aerobic fitness in children and adolescents. *Exerc. Sport Sci. Rev.*, 22:435, 1994.

2. Åstrand, P.O., and Rodhal, K.: *Textbook of Work Physiology.* New York, McGraw-Hill, 1986.

3. Åstrand, P.O., and Saltin, B.: Maximal oxygen uptake and heart rate in various types of muscular activity. *J. Appl. Physiol.*, 16:977, 1961.

4. Balke, B., and Ware, R.W.: An experimental study of fitness of Air Force personnel. *U.S. Armed Forces Med. J.*, 10:675, 1959.

5. Bangsbo, J., et al.: Anaerobic energy production and O_2 deficit-debt relationship during exhaustive exercise in humans. *J. Physiol. (Lond)*, 422:539, 1990.

6. Bar-Or, O.: The Wingate anaerobic test: An update on methodology, reliability, and validity. *Sports Med.*, 4:381, 1987.

7. Bergh, V.: The influence of body mass in cross-country skiing. *Med. Sci. Sports Exerc.*, 19:324, 1987.

8. Beunen, G., and Malina, R.: Growth and physical performance relative to timing of the adolescent spurt. In *Exercise and Sport Sciences Reviews.* Vol 16, K.B. Pandolf (Ed.), New York, Macmillan, 1988.

9. Blomquist, C.G., et al.: Similarity of the hemodynamic responses to static, and dynamic exercise of small muscle groups. *Circ. Res.*, 48(Suppl. I):87, 1982.

10. Bonen, A., et al.: Maximal oxygen uptake during free, tethered, and flume swimming. *J. Appl. Physiol.*, 48:232, 1980.

11. Bouchard, C., and Lortie, J.: Heredity and human performance. *Sports Med.*, 1:38, 1984.

12. Bouchard, C., and Pérusse, L.: Heredity, activity level, fitness, and health. In *Physical Activity, Fitness, and Health.* C. Bouchard, et al. (Eds.), Champaign, IL, Human Kinetics, 1994.

13. Bouchard, C., et al.: Aerobic performance in brothers, dizygotic and monozygotic twins. *Med. Sci. Sports Exerc.*, 18:639, 1986.

14. Bouchard, C., et al.: Genetic effects in human skeletal muscle fiber type distribution and enzyme activities. *Can. J. Physiol. Pharmacol.*, 64:125, 1986.

15. Bouchard, C., et al.: Genetics of aerobic and anaerobic performance. *Exerc. Sport Sci. Rev.*, 20:27, 1992

16. Brahler, C.J., and Blank, S.E.: VersaClimbing elicits higher $\dot{V}O_2$max than does treadmill running or rowing ergometry. *Med. Sci. Sports Exerc.*, 27:249, 1995.

17. Buchfuhrer, M.J., et al.: Optimizing the exercise protocol for cardiopulmonary assessment. *J. Appl. Physiol.*, 55:1558, 1983.

18. Carey, P., et al.: Comparison of oxygen uptake during maximal work on the rowing ergometer. *Med. Sci. Sports*, 6:101, 1974.

19. Cooper, K.: Correlation between field and treadmill testing as a means for assessing maximal oxygen intake. *JAMA*, 203:201, 1968.

20. Costill, D.L.: Physiology of marathon running. *JAMA*, 221:1024, 1972.

21. Cunningham, D., and Faulkner, J.A.: The effect of training on aerobic and anaerobic metabolism during a short exhaustive run. *Med. Sci. Sports*, 1:65, 1969.

22. Cureton, K.J., et al.: Effect of experimental alterations in excess weight on aerobic capacity and distance running performance. *Med. Sci. Sports*, 10:194, 1978.

23. Davis, J.A., et al.: Effect of ramp slope on measurement of aerobic parameters from the ramp exercise test. *Med. Sci. Sports Exerc.*, 14:339, 1982.

24. Doolittle, T.L., and Bigbee, R.: The twelve-minute run-walk: a test of cardiorespiratory fitness of adolescent boys. *Res. Q.*, 39:41, 1968.

25. Dotan, R., and Bar-Or, O.: Climatic heat stress and performance in the Wingate anaerobic test. *Eur. J. Appl. Physiol.*, 44:237, 1980.

26. Eriksson, B.O.: Muscle metabolism in children: a review. *Acta Paediatr. Scand.* (Suppl.), 283:20, 1980.

27. Esbjornsson, B., et al.: Fast-twitch fibers may predict anaerobic performance in both females and males. *Int. J. Sports Med.*, 14:257, 1993.

28. Fairshter, R.D., et al.: A comparison of incremental exercise tests during cycle and treadmill ergometry. *Med. Sci. Sports Exerc.*, 15:549, 1983.

29. Ferguson, R.J., et al.: A maximal oxygen uptake test during ice skating. *Med. Sci. Sports*, 1:207, 1969.

30. Foster, V.L., et al.: The reproducibility of VO_2max, ventilatory, and lactate threshold in elderly women. *Med. Sci. Sports Exerc.*, 18:425, 1986.

31. Fournier, M.: Skeletal muscle adaptation in adolescent boys: endurance training and detraining. *Med. Sci. Sports Exerc.*, 14:453, 1982.

32. Gergley, T., et al.: Specificity of arm training on aerobic power during swimming and running. *Med. Sci. Sports Exerc.*, 16:349, 1984.

33. Gilliam, T.B., et al.: Physical activity patterns as determined by heart rate monitoring in 6–7 year-old children. *Med. Sci. Sports Exerc.*, 13:65, 1981.

34. Gollnick, P.D., and Saltin, B.: Significance of skeletal muscle oxidative enzyme enhancement with endurance training. *Clin. Physiol.*, 2:1, 1982.

35. Gollnick, P.D., et al.: Glycogen depletion pattern in human skeletal muscle fiber after heavy exercise. *J. Appl. Physiol.*, 34:615, 1973.

36. Hagberg, J.M., et al.: Comparison of three procedures for measuring VO_2max in competitive cyclists. *Eur. J. Appl. Physiol.*, 39:47, 1978.

37. Hammel, P., et al.: Heredity and muscle adaptation to endurance training. *Med. Sci. Sports Exerc.*, 18:690, 1986.

38. Hermiston, R., and Faulkner, J.A.: Prediction of maximal oxygen uptake by stepwise regression technique. *J. Appl. Physiol.*, 30:833, 1971.

39. Holloszy, J.O., and Coyle, E.F.: Adaptations of skeletal muscle to endurance exercise and their metabolic consequences. *J. Appl. Physiol.*, 56:831, 1984.

39a. Howley, E.T., et al.: Criteria for maximal oxygen uptake: review and commentary. *Med. Sci. Sports Exerc.*, 27:1292, 1995.

40. Inbar, O., and Bar-Or, O.: Anaerobic characteristics in male children and adolescents. *Med. Sci. Sports Exerc.*, 18:264, 1986.

41. Jacobs, I., et al.: Lactate in human skeletal muscle after 10 and 30s of supramaximal exercise. *J. Appl. Physiol.*, 55:365, 1983.

42. Joyner, M.J.: Physiological limiting factors and distance running: influence of gender and age on record performances. *Exerc. Sport Sci. Rev.*, 21:103, 1993.

43. Kalamen, J.L.: Measurement of maximum muscular power in man. Unpublished doctoral dissertation, Ohio State University, Columbus, 1968.

44. Karlsson, J., and Saltin, B.: Lactate, ATP, and CP in working muscles during exhaustive exercise in man. *J. Appl. Physiol.*, 29:598, 1970.

45. Karlsson, J., et al.: Muscle metabolites during submaximal and maximal exercise in man. *Scand. J. Clin. Lab. Invest.*, 26:385, 1971.

46. Kasch, F.W., et al.: A comparison of maximal oxygen uptake by treadmill and step test procedures. *J. Appl. Physiol.*, 21:1387, 1966.

47. Kasch, F.W., et al.: A longitudinal study of cardiovascular stability in active men aged 45 to 65 years. *Phys. Sportsmed.*, 16:117, 1988.

48. Katch, F.I., and McArdle, W.D.: *Introduction to Nutrition, Exercise, and Health.* 4th ed., Philadelphia, Lea & Febiger, 1993.

49. Katch, F.I., et al.: Maximal oxygen intake, endurance running performance, and body composition in college women. *Res. Q.*, 44:301, 1973.

50. Katch, F.I., et al.: Relationship between individual differences in steady pace endurance running performance and maximal oxygen intake. *Res. Q.*, 44:206, 1973.

51. Katch, V.L.: Kinetics of oxygen uptake and recovery for supramaximal work of short duration. *Int. Z. Angew. Physiol.*, 31:197, 1973.

52. Katch, V.L., et al.: Optimal test characteristics for maximal anaerobic work on the bicycle ergometer. *Res. Q.*, 48:319, 1977.

53. Keller, B.A.: The influence of body size variables on gender differences in strength and maximum aerobic capacity. Unpublished doctoral dissertation, University of Massachusetts, Amherst, 1989.

54. Keller, B., and Katch, F.I.: It is not valid to adjust gender differences in aerobic capacity and strength for body mass or lean body mass. *Med. Sci. Sports Exerc.*, 23:S167, 1991.

55. Kline, G., et al.: Estimation of $VO_{2\,max}$ from a one-mile track walk, gender, age, and body weight. *Med. Sci. Sports Exerc.*, 19:253, 1987.

56. Klissouras, V.: Heritability of adaptive variation. *J. Appl. Physiol.*, 31:338, 1971.

57. Klissouras, V., et al.: Adaptation to maximal effort: genetics and age. *J. Appl. Physiol.*, 35:288, 1973.

58. Krahenbuhl, G.S., et al.: Developmental aspects of maximal aerobic power in children. In *Exercise and Sport Sciences Reviews.* R.L. Terjung (Ed.), New York, Macmillan, 1985.

59. Lewis, S.F., et al.: Cardiovascular responses to exercise as functions of absolute and relative work load. *J. Appl. Physiol.,* 54:1314, 1983.

60. Lortie, G., et al.: Muscle fiber type composition and enzyme activities in brothers and monozygotic twins. In *Proceedings of the 1984 Olympic Scientific Congress.* Vol. 4, R.M. Malina and C. Bouchard (Eds.), *Sport and Human Genetics,* Champaign, IL, Human Kinetics Publishers, 1986.

61. Magel, J.R., and Faulkner, J.A.: Maximum oxygen uptake of college swimmers. *J. Appl. Physiol.,* 22:929, 1967.

62. Magel, J.R., et al.: Specificity of swim training on maximum oxygen uptake. *J. Appl. Physiol.,* 38:151, 1975.

63. Magel, J.R., et al.: Metabolic and cardiovascular adjustment to arm training. *J. Appl. Physiol.,* 45:75, 1978.

64. Maksud, M.G., and Coutts, K.D.: Application of the Cooper twelve-minute run-walk to young males. *Res. Q.,* 42:54, 1971.

65. Maksud, M.G., et al.: Energy expenditure and Vo_2max of female athletes during treadmill exercise. *Res. Q.,* 47:692, 1976.

66. Margaria, R., et al.: Measurement of muscular power (anaerobic) in man. *J. Appl. Physiol.,* 21:1662, 1966.

67. Maud, P.J., and Schultz, B.B.: Norms for the Wingate anaerobic test with comparisons in another similar test. *Res. Q. Exerc. Sport,* 60:144, 1989.

68. Mayhew, J.L., and Salm, P.C.: Gender differences in anaerobic power tests. *Eur. J. Appl. Physiol.,* 60:133, 1990.

69. McArdle, W.D., et al.: Metabolic and cardiorespiratory response during free swimming and treadmill walking. *J. Appl. Physiol.,* 30:733, 1971.

70. McArdle, W.D., et al.: Reliability and inter-relationships between maximal oxygen intake, physical work capacity, and step-test scores in college women. *Med. Sci. Sports,* 4:182, 1972.

71. McArdle, W.D., et al.: Comparison of continuous and discontinuous treadmill and bicycle tests for max Vo_2. *Med. Sci. Sports,* 5:156, 1973.

72. McArdle, W.D., et al.: Specificity of run training on Vo_2max and heart rate changes during running and swimming. *Med. Sci. Sports,* 10:16, 1978.

73. Medbo, J.L., et al.: Anaerobic capacity determined by maximal accumulated oxygen deficit. *J. Appl. Physiol.,* 64:50, 1988.

74. Menier, D.R., and Pugh, L.G.C.E.: The relation of oxygen intake and velocity of walking in competition walkers. *J. Physiol. (London),* 197:717, 1968.

75. Meredith, C.N., et al.: Body composition and aerobic capacity in young and middle-aged endurance-trained men. *Med. Sci. Sports Exerc.,* 19:557, 1987.

76. Mitchell, J., et al.: The physiological meaning of the maximal oxygen intake test. *J. Clin. Invest.,* 37:538, 1958.

77. Naughton, J., et al.: Treadmill exercise in assessment of patients with cardiac disease. *Am. J. Cardiol.,* 30:757, 1972.

78. Nebelsick-Gullett, L.J., et al.: A comparison between methods of measuring anaerobic work capacity. *Ergonomics,* 31:1413, 1988.

79. Nindl, B.C., et al.: Lower and upper body anaerobic performance in male and female adolescent athletes. *Med. Sci. Sports Exerc.,* 27:235, 1995.

80. Pechar, G.S., et al.: Specificity of cardiorespiratory adaptation to bicycle and treadmill training. *J. Appl. Physiol.,* 36:753, 1974.

81. Pérusse, L., et al.: Inter-generation transmission of physical fitness in the Canadian population. *Can. J. Sport Sci.,* 13:8, 1988.

82. Pérusse, L., et al.: Genetic and environmental influences on level of habitual physical activity and exercise participation. *Am. J. Epidemiol.,* 129:1012, 1989.

83. Piehl, K.: Glycogen storage and depletion in human skeletal muscle fibers. *Acta Physiol. Scand.* (Suppl.), 402:1, 1974.

84. Prud'homme, D., et al.: Sensitivity of maximal aerobic power to training is genotype-dependent. *Med. Sci. Sports Exerc.,* 16:489, 1984.

85. Rowland, T.W.: Does peak Vo_2 reflect Vo_2max in children? *Med. Sci. Sports Exerc.,* 25:689, 1993.

86. Saavedra, C., et al.: Maximal anaerobic performance of the knee extensor muscles during growth. *Med. Sci. Sports Exerc.,* 23:1083, 1991.

87. Sady, S.P., et al.: Prediction of Vo_2max during cycle exercise in pregnant women. *J. Appl. Physiol.,* 65:657, 1988.

88. Saltin, B.: Metabolic fundamentals in exercise. *Med. Sci. Sports,* 5:137, 1973.

89. Sargent, D.A.: Physical test of man. *Am. Phys. Ed. Rev.,* 26:188, 1921.

90. Sawka, M.N.: Physiology of upper body exercise. *Exerc. Sport. Sci. Rev.,* 14:175, 1986.

91. Schulman, S.P., and Gerstenblith, G.: Cardiovascular changes with aging: The response to exercise. *J. Cardiopulmonary Rehabil.,* 19:12, 1989.

92. Simoneau, J.A., et al.: Inheritance of human skeletal muscle and anaerobic capacity adaptation to high-intensity intermittent training. *Int. J. Sports Med.,* 7:167, 1986.

93. Stamford, B.A.: Exercise in the elderly. In *Exercise and Sport Sciences Reviews.* Vol. 16, New York, Macmillan, 1988.

94. Strømme, S.B., et al.: Assessment of maximal aerobic power in specially trained athletes. *J. Appl. Physiol.,* 42:833, 1977.

95. Taylor, H.L., et al.: Maximal oxygen intake as an objective measure of cardiorespiratory performance. *J. Appl. Physiol.,* 8:73, 1955.

96. Thomas, S.G., et al.: Sources of variation in oxygen consumption during a stepping task. *Med. Sci. Sports Exerc.,* 25:139, 1993.

97. Toner, M.N., et al.: Cardiorespiratory responses to exercise distributed between the upper and lower body. *J. Appl. Physiol.,* 54:1403, 1983.

97a. Vandenberghe, K., et al.: No effect of glycogen level on glycogen metabolism during high intensity exercise. *Med. Sci. Sports Exerc.,* 27:1278, 1995.

98. Van Praagh, E., et al.: Gender difference in relationships of anaerobic power output to body composition in children. *Pediatr. Exerc. Sci.,* 2:336, 1990.

99. Veeger, H.E.J., et al.: Peak oxygen uptake and maximal power output of Olympic wheelchair-dependent athletes. *Med. Sci. Sports Exerc.,* 23:1201, 1991.

100. Vogel, J.A., et al.: An analysis of aerobic capacity in a large United States population. *J. Appl. Physiol.,* 60:494, 1986.

101. Wallick, M.E., et al.: Physiological responses to in-line skating compared to treadmill running. *Med. Sci. Sports Exerc.,* 27:242, 1995.

102. Washburn, R.A., and Seals, D.R.: Peak oxygen uptake during arm cranking in men and women. *J. Appl. Physiol.,* 56:954, 1984.

103. Wasserman, K., et al.: *Principles of Exercise Testing and Interpretation.* Philadelphia, Lea & Febiger, 1987.

104. Wells, C.L., and Plowman, S.A.: Sexual differences in athletic performance: biological or behavioral? *Phys. Sportsmed.,* 11:52, 1983.

105. Weyand, P.G., et al.: Peak oxygen deficit during one- and two-legged cycling in men and women. *Med. Sci. Sports Exerc.,* 25:584, 1993.

106. Wilkes, D., et al.: Effect of acute induced metabolic alkalosis on 800-m racing time. *Med. Sci. Sports Exerc.,* 4:277, 1983.

107. Wilmore, J.H.: Influence of motivation on physical work capacity and performance. *J. Appl. Physiol.,* 24:459, 1968.

108. Winter, E.M., et al.: Maximal exercise performance and lean leg volume in men and women. *J. Sports Sci.,* 9:3, 1991.

109. Woodson, R.D.: Hemoglobin concentration and exercise capacity. *Am. Rev. Resp. Dis.* (Suppl.), 129:72, 1984.

110. Wyndham, C.H.: Submaximal tests for estimating maximum oxygen uptake. *Can. Med. Assoc. J.,* 96:736, 1967.

111. Wyndham, C.H., and Hegns, A.J.A.: Determinants of oxygen consumption and maximum oxygen intake of Caucasians and Bantu males. *Int. Z. Angew. Physiol.,* 27:51, 1969.

112. Wyndham, C.H., et al.: Studies of the maximum capacity of men for physical effort. Part I. A comparison of methods of assessing the maximum oxygen intake. *Int. Z. Angew. Physiol.,* 22:285, 1966.

113. Yamamoto, S.H., et al.: Quantitative estimation of anaerobic and oxidative energy metabolism and contraction characteristics in intact human skeletal muscle in response to electrical stimulation. *Clin. Physiol.,* 3:227, 1983.

114. Zeimetz, G.A., et al.: Quantifiable changes in oxygen uptake, heart rate, and time to target heart rate when hand support is allowed during treadmill exercise. *J. Cardiac Rehab.,* 11:525, 1985.

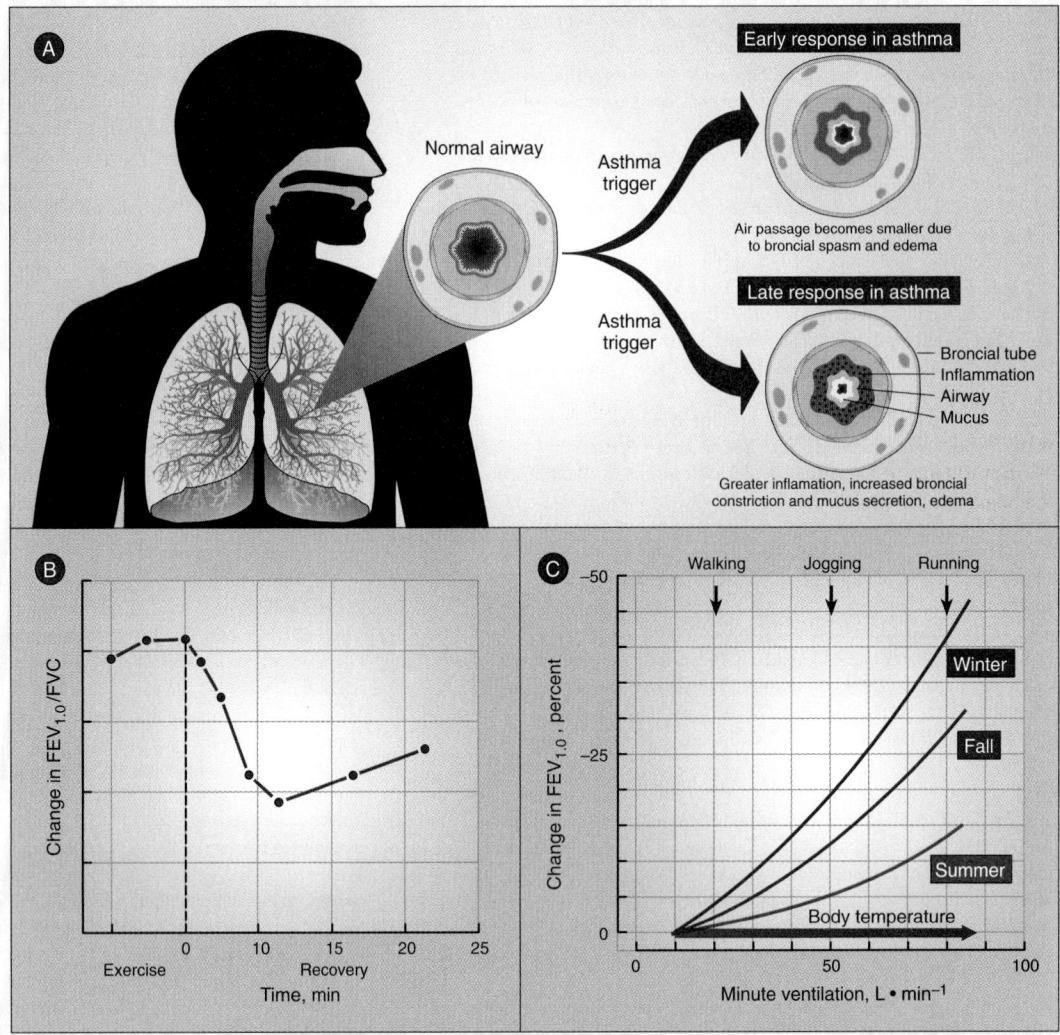

"THE VENTILATORY AND CARDIOVASCULAR

SYSTEMS PROVIDE THE ACTIVE

MUSCLES WITH A CONTINUOUS

STREAM OF NUTRIENTS AND OXYGEN

TO SUSTAIN A HIGH ENERGY OUTPUT

Systems of Energy Delivery and Utilization

Many sport, recreational, and occupational activities require a moderately intense yet sustained energy release. This energy for the phosphorylation of adenosine diphosphate (ADP) to adenosine triphosphate (ATP) is provided by the aerobic breakdown of carbohydrates, lipids, and proteins. Unless a steady rate is achieved between oxidative phosphorylation and the energy requirements of the activity, an anaerobic-aerobic energy imbalance develops, lactic acid accumulates, tissue acidity increases, and fatigue quickly ensues. The ability to sustain a high level of physical activity without undue fatigue depends on two factors:

- The capacity and integration of the physiologic systems for oxygen delivery.
- The capacity of the specific muscle cells to generate ATP aerobically.

Understanding the role of the ventilatory, circulatory, muscular, and endocrine systems during exercise described in this section enables one to appreciate individual differences in aerobic exercise capacity. Knowledge of the energy requirements and corresponding physiologic adjustments to exercise also provides a sound basis for formulating a proper training program and evaluating the effectiveness of such training.

Dejours, P.: The regulation of breathing during muscular exercise in man. A neurohumoral theory. In *The Regulation of Human Respiration*. Cunningham, D.J.C., and Lloyd, B.B. (eds.). Oxford, England: Blackwell, 1963.

Early theories concerning the mechanisms for increases in pulmonary ventilation during exercise centered on either P_{CO_2}, arterial blood pH, or reflex

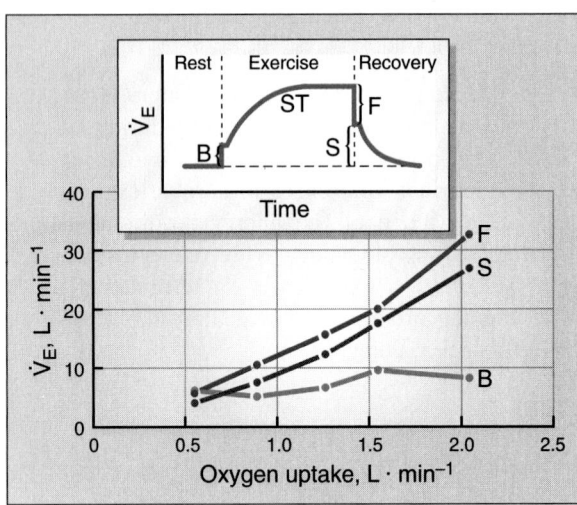

The inset graph plots ventilation during exercise and recovery in mild exercise. Portion *B* is the immediate, rapid increase at the onset of exercise, *ST* is the more gradual rise to a steady state, *F* is the quick fall when exercise stops, and *S* represents the slower return of ventilation to pre-exercise levels. The main graph shows the magnitude of the contribution of each of these ventilatory response components in relation to the exercise oxygen uptake. Both the *F* (neurogenic) and *S* (humoral) components in exercise recovery increase with the intensity of the preceding exercise; the fast component at the start of exercise *(B)* increases with exercise intensity much less than either *F* or *S* in recovery. These data show an increase in the neurogenic and humoral controls; their relative contributions change with exercise intensity.

stimulation originating from muscle receptors. Dejours suggested that no factor by itself regulated breathing during exercise, but instead believed in a multiplicity of contributing factors. He hypothesized that exercise hyperpnea depended on humoral (or circulatory) and neurogenic stimuli that varied during the phase of exercise and recovery.

Dejours' observations (see figure) of the time course of minute ventilation ($\dot{V}_E$) during the transitions from rest to exercise to recovery revealed a consistent pattern. When a subject initiates exercise, $\dot{V}_E$ increases abruptly. The increase begins

within the same ventilatory cycle coinciding with the start of exercise. Some 10 to 20 seconds later, a slow increase occurs to an eventual steady state. When exercise stops, $\dot{V}_E$ declines abruptly, then remains fairly constant for 20 to 30 seconds, and finally decreases progressively to the resting value.

Dejours concluded that respiratory dynamics in exercise consist of a combination of rapid (fast component) and slow (slow component) responses that occur at different stages of exercise. He proposed that different physiologic factors control the two ventilatory components. The fast component consists of two factors: a cerebral factor involving a series of impulses from the psychomotor area of the brain to the respiratory center in the medulla, and an extrathoracic mechanoreceptive stimulus arising from "muscle proprioceptors" in the exercising body parts. Two mechanisms control the slower-responding component of ventilation during exercise and recovery. The first, reflexive in nature, originates from muscle chemoreceptors sensitive to progressive physiochemical changes that muscle undergoes during exercise. The second controlling factor includes a humoral mechanism. The humoral factor was based on experiments of leg blood flow occlusion in which $\dot{V}_E$ fell below resting levels, without hypocapnea and hyperoxia, thus demonstrating the dependence of $\dot{V}_E$ on blood-borne factors (humoral control).

Dejours stressed the interrelationship between the fast and slow components of exercise ventilation. Reflex and presumably cortical factors control the fast change of ventilation at the start of exercise. In contrast, humoral factors, and possibly an increase of neurogenic control, control the slower increase in ventilation during the first minute of exercise. The latter steady-state response is probably related to increases in reflex, mechanoreceptive drive through local physical and chemical changes in the medium bathing the peripheral mechanoreceptors, or positive interactions between neurogenic and humoral drives. At the end of exercise, neurogenic control diminishes and ventilation slows. After this abrupt decrease, control of ventilation occurs exclusively by humoral factors.

Dejours' basic conclusions led to fundamental explanations of pulmonary ventilation during exercise and recovery. More recent research (refer to Fig. 14.4) points to several different factors to explain exercise hyperpnea and provides a more comprehensive model for ventilatory control with exercise and recovery.

Pulmonary Structure and Function

Chapters 12, 13, and 14 detail the process of pulmonary ventilation and gas transport and elaborate on the mechanisms by which oxygen is supplied and extracted from the external environment and exchanged for almost equal quantities of carbon dioxide. This capability for pulmonary ventilation contributes significantly to the regulation of the internal environment at rest and during physical activity.

SURFACE AREA AND GAS EXCHANGE

If the oxygen supply of humans depended only on diffusion through the skin, it would be impossible to sustain the basal energy requirement, let alone the 3- to 4-L gas exchange necessary each minute to run at a pace of 5 minutes per mile in a 26.2-mile marathon. Within the relatively compact human body, the requirements for gas exchange are met by the remarkably effective **ventilatory system**. This system, depicted in Figure 12.1, regulates the gaseous state of the body's "external" environment to provide effective aeration of body fluids.

ANATOMY OF VENTILATION

Ambient air is brought into and exchanged with the air in the lungs through the process of **pulmonary ventilation.** Air entering the nose and mouth flows into the conductive portion of the ventilatory system, where it is adjusted to body temperature, filtered, and almost completely humidified as it passes through the **trachea.** This air-conditioning process continues as the inspired air passes into two **bronchi,** the large tubes that serve as primary conduits into each of the lungs. The bronchi further divide into numerous **bronchioles,** which conduct the inspired air through a tortuous and narrow route until it eventually mixes with the existing air in the **alveolar ducts.** These ducts are completely surrounded by microscopic **alveoli,** which are the terminal branches of the respiratory tract.

THE LUNGS

The lungs provide the separating surface between the blood and the surrounding alveolar gaseous external environment. Their major function is **gas exchange;** the lungs transfer oxygen from the air into the venous blood and move carbon dioxide from this blood into the alveolar chambers, where it

is subsequently expelled into ambient air. Although an adult's lung volume varies between an average of 4 and 6 L (approximately the amount of air contained in a basketball), its surface area is considerable. The lungs of an average-sized person weigh approximately 1 kg; however, if spread out as shown in Figure 12.2, this tissue would cover a surface of between 50 and 100 square meters. The lung tissue is approximately 20 to 50 times larger than the body's external surface and would cover about one-half of a tennis court or an entire badminton court.

The highly vascularized, moist surface of the lungs fits within the relatively small confines of the chest cavity by means of numerous infoldings; the lung membranes actually fold over onto themselves. The interface for the aeration of blood is considerable; at rest, a single red blood cell is contained in the pulmonary capillaries for only about 0.5 to 1.0 second and traverses about two to three individual alveoli. During any one second of maximal exercise, probably no more than 1 pint of blood is contained in the fine network of blood vessels within the lung tissue.

THE ALVEOLI

The lungs contain more than 300 million alveoli. These elastic, thin-walled, membranous sacs (approximately 0.3 mm in diameter) provide the vital surface for gas exchange between the lung tissue and the blood. Alveolar tissue has the largest blood supply of any organ in the body. Millions of short, thin-walled capillaries and alveoli lie side by side; air moves along one side and blood along the other. Gaseous diffusion occurs through the extremely thin barrier of these alveolar and capillary cells (approximately 0.3 μm in some areas), and this diffusion distance is essentially maintained throughout varying levels of exercise. Also, small pores (called pores of Kohn) within each alveolus enable the interchange of gas between adjacent alveoli. This provides the indirect ventilation of some alveoli that are damaged or blocked as a result of chronic obstructive lung diseases such as emphysema.

During each minute at rest, approximately 250 mL of oxygen leaves the alveoli and enters the blood and approximately 200 mL of carbon dioxide diffuses in the opposite direction. During heavy exercise in endurance athletes, nearly 25 times this quantity of oxygen is transferred across the alveolar membrane. *The primary function of pulmonary ventilation during rest and exercise is to maintain a fairly constant and favorable concentration of oxygen and carbon*

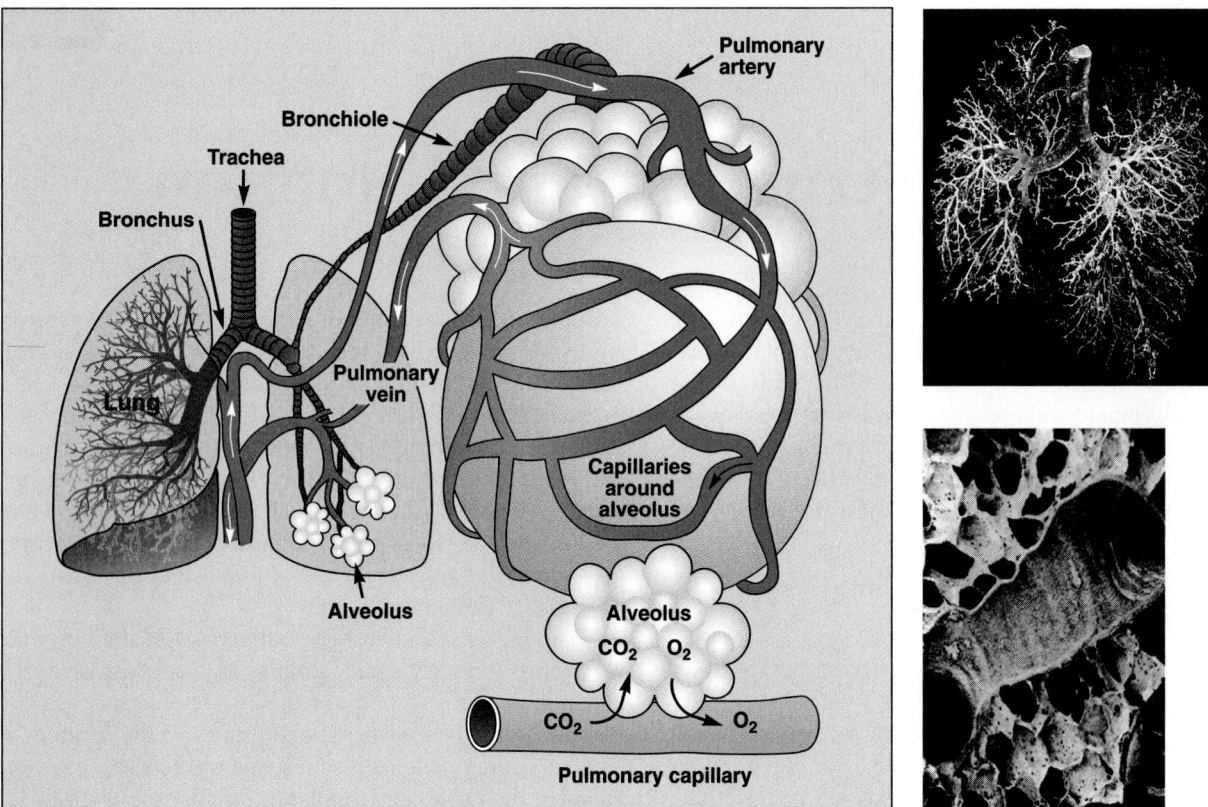

FIGURE 12.1

Left, A general view of the ventilatory system showing the respiratory passages, alveoli, and gas exchange function in an alveolus. *Top right,* A cast of the human lungs from the trachea to the terminal bronchioles; the alveoli are not shown. *Bottom right,* A section of lung tissue showing individual alveoli; the holes in the alveolar wall are the pores of Kohn. The pulmonary capillaries run in the walls of the alveoli. (Bottom images from West, J.B.: *Respiratory Physiology—The Essentials,* 5th ed. Baltimore, Williams & Wilkins, 1995.)

dioxide in the alveolar chambers. This ensures effective gaseous exchange before the blood leaves the lungs to be transported throughout the body.

MECHANICS OF VENTILATION

The physical principle that underlies the dynamics of breathing is illustrated in Figure 12.3. Two lung-shaped balloons are suspended in a jar in which the glass bottom has been replaced by a thin rubber membrane. The volume of the jar increases when the membrane is pulled down. This causes the air pressure within the jar to become less than the ambient air outside the jar; as a result, air rushes in, causing the balloons to inflate. Conversely, as the elastic membrane recoils, pressure in the jar temporarily increases and air rushes out. A considerable volume of air can be exchanged within the balloons in a given time period if there is an increase in the depth and rate of the descent and ascent of the rubber membrane. This is essentially how ambient air and alveolar air are exchanged in the lungs.

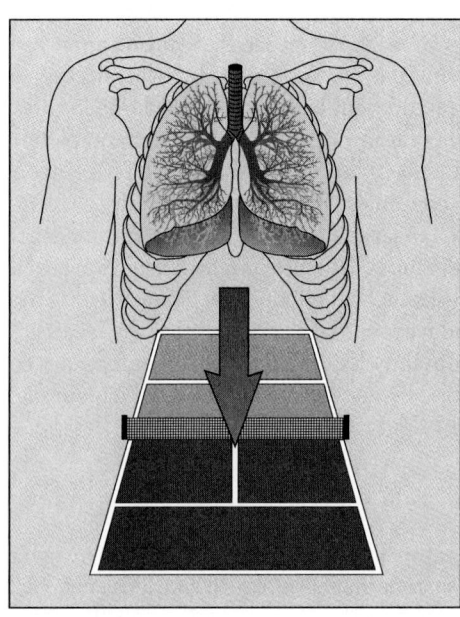

FIGURE 12.2

The lungs provide a large surface for gas exchange.

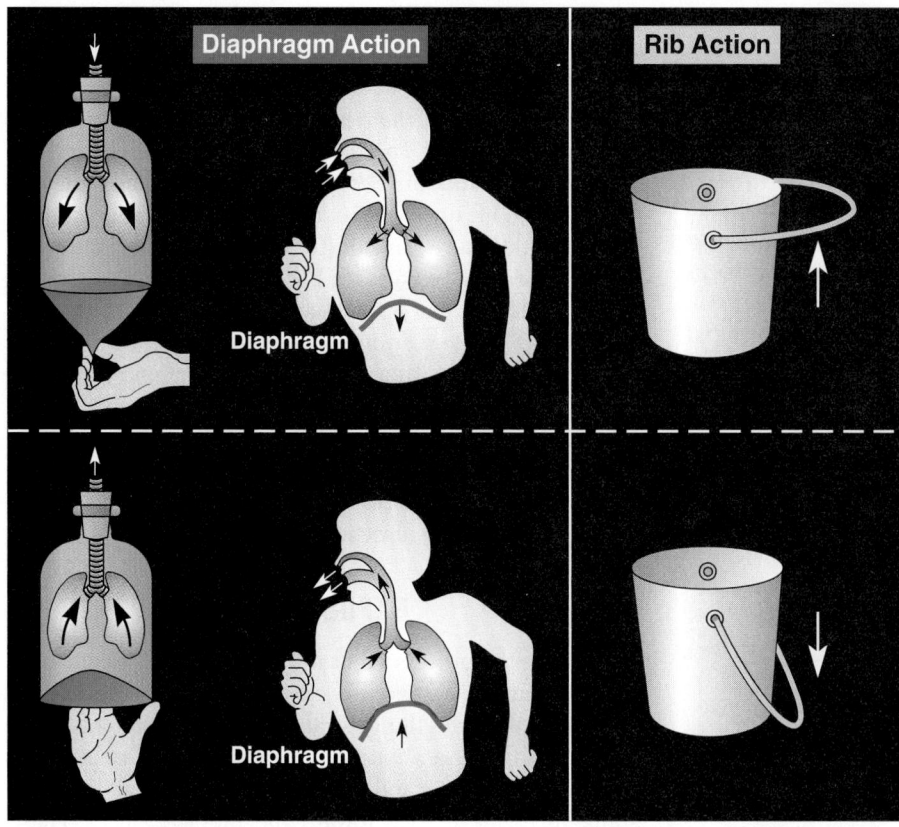

FIGURE 12.3
Mechanics of breathing. During *inspiration,* the chest cavity increases in size because of the raising of the ribs and lowering of the diaphragm and air moves into the lungs. In this process, there are increases in the anterior-posterior (A-P) and vertical diameters of the rib cage. Approximately 70% of lung expansion is due to A-P enlargement, and 30% is due to diaphragmatic movement. From a muscular standpoint, the external intercostal muscles become active and the internal intercostal muscles relax. During *exhalation,* the ribs swing down and the diaphragm returns to a relaxed position. This reduces the volume of the thoracic cavity and air rushes out. The movement of the jar's rubber bottom causes air to enter and exit the two balloons, simulating the action of the diaphragm. The movement of the bucket handle simulates the action of the ribs. Muscles that elevate the thorax are called muscles of inspiration (diaphragm, external intercostal muscles, sternocleidomastoids, scapular elevators and anterior serrati scleni, and spinal erector muscles); muscles that depress the thorax are known as muscles of expiration (abdominal muscles, internal intercostal muscles, posterior inferior serrati).

The ventilatory system can be subdivided into two parts (Fig. 12.4): a conducting zone, which includes the trachea and the terminal bronchioles; and a transitional and respiratory zone, which includes the respiratory bronchioles, the alveolar ducts, and the alveoli. Because there are no alveoli in the structures of the conducting zone, this space is known as the **anatomic dead space** (see page 228). The respiratory zone occupies about 2.5 to 3.0 L and comprises the largest portion of the total lung volume. When air is brought into the lungs, it literally flows down the trachea to the terminal bronchi, much like water flowing in bulk through a hose. However, when the air reaches the smaller air passages in the transitional zone, the tremendous increase in the surface of this area significantly decreases the forward velocity of the airflow down into the alveoli. This concept in the relationship between airway generation (forward velocity) and total cross-sectional area of various portions of the lung tissue is illustrated in Figure 12.5. When air reaches the terminal bronchioles, there is a large increase in the tissue cross section. At this stage, diffusion is the chief way in which the gases are distributed across the alveolar membranes, and there is a rapid equilibration of gases on each side of the alveolar-capillary membrane. Gas diffusion is governed by **Fick's law,** which states that the rate of gas transfer through a sheet of tissue is proportional to the tissue area, a diffusion constant, and the difference between the pressure of the gas on each side of the membrane and is inversely proportional to the thickness of the tissue. The diffusion constant (D) is proportional to the gas solubility (S) and inversely proportional to the square root of the molecular weight (MW) of the gas ($D \propto S \div \sqrt{MW}$). On a per-molecule basis, carbon dioxide (MW = 44) diffuses about 20 times as fast through thin membranous tissues as oxygen (MW = 32) because carbon dioxide has a higher solubility, even though the MW of carbon dioxide is relatively close to the MW of oxygen.

The lungs are not merely suspended in the chest cavity as in the example with the balloons (Fig. 12.3). Instead, the pressure differential between the air in the lungs and the lung-chest wall interface causes the lungs to adhere to the chest wall and literally follow its every movement. Therefore, any change in the volume of the thoracic cavity causes a corresponding change in lung volume. The lungs depend on accessory means for altering their volume because they contain no muscles. The volume of the lungs is altered during **inspiration** and **expiration** by the action of voluntary muscles.

INSPIRATION

A large, dome-shaped sheet of musculofibrous tissue called the **diaphragm** serves the same purpose as the rubber membrane of the jar in Figure 12.3. This muscle makes an airtight separation between the abdominal and thoracic cavities but provides a series of openings through which the esophagus, blood vessels, and nerves pass. During inspiration, the diaphragm muscle contracts, flattens, and moves downward toward the abdominal cavity as much as 10 cm. This movement causes the chest cavity to become elongated and enlarged. Consequently, the air in the lungs expands and its pressure, referred to as **intrapulmonic pressure,** reduces to slightly below atmospheric pressure. The lungs inflate as air is literally sucked in through the nose and mouth; the degree of filling depends on the magnitude of inspiratory movements. In healthy men, the maximum pressure generated by the inspiratory muscles ranges between 80 and 140 mm Hg.[36] Inspiration is complete when thoracic cavity expansion ceases and the intrapulmonic pressure increases to equal ambient atmospheric pressure.

During exercise, the ribs and sternum also assist in the action of inspiration. The contraction of the **scaleni** and **external intercostal** muscles between the ribs causes the ribs to rotate and lift up and away from the body.[20] This action is similar to the movement of the handle lifted up and away from the side of a bucket (see Fig. 12.3 [*right*]). The descent of the diaphragm, the upward swing of the ribs, and the outward thrust of the sternum cause the volume of the chest cavity to increase with a subsequent inhalation of ambient air. Athletes often bend forward from the waist to facilitate breathing following an exhausting exercise. This probably serves two purposes: (*a*) it facilitates the flow of blood to the heart, and (*b*) it minimizes the antagonistic effects of gravity on the usual upward direction of inspiratory movements.

EXPIRATION

Expiration, the process of air movement out of the lungs, is predominantly a passive process during rest and light exercise. It results from the natural recoil of the stretched lung tissue and the relaxation of the inspiratory muscles. This causes the sternum and ribs to swing down and the diaphragm to move back toward the thoracic cavity. These movements decrease the size of the chest cavity and compress alveolar gas so that air moves out through the respiratory tract and into the atmosphere. Expiration is complete when the compressive forces of the expiratory musculature are no longer acting and intrapulmonic pressure decreases to atmospheric pressure. During ventilation in heavy exercise, the **internal intercostal** and **abdominal** muscles act powerfully on the ribs and abdominal cavity to facilitate the reduction of thoracic dimensions. Thus, exhalation occurs more rapidly and to a more pronounced extent.

No major differences are observed in ventilatory mechanics between men and women or among people of different ages. At rest in the supine position, most people are "abdominal" or diaphragmatic breathers, whereas in the upright position, the action of the ribs and sternum becomes more apparent.[61] The rapid alterations in thoracic volume required during heavy exercise are accomplished mainly through the movement of the rib cage. This suggests that the muscles of the ribs are capable of more rapid action than the diaphragm and the abdominal muscles. The position of the head and back naturally adapted by long-distance runners (forward lean from the waist, neck flexed, and head extended forward with mandible parallel to the ground) favors pulmonary ventilation during heavy exercise.[28]

Valsalva Maneuver. Aside from their normal role in pulmonary ventilation, the expiratory muscles also are important in the ventilatory maneuvers of coughing and sneezing, as well as in stabilizing the abdominal and chest cavities during lifting of heavy objects. In quiet breathing, the intra-

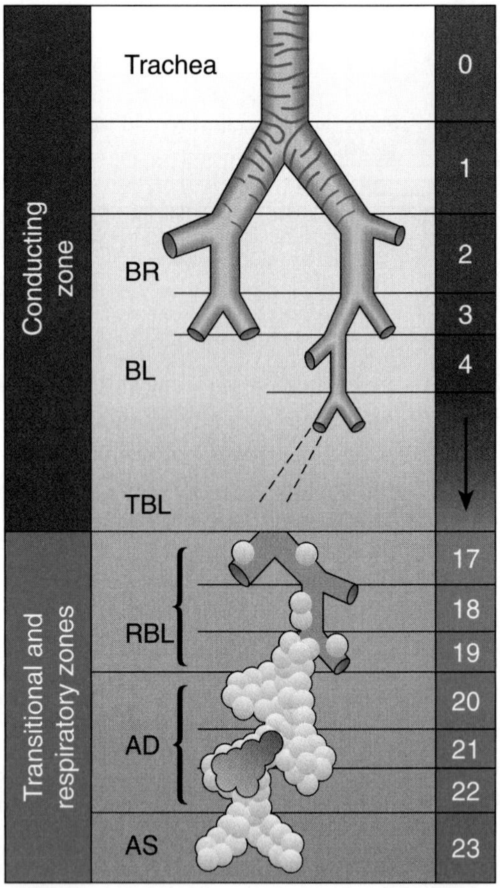

FIGURE 12.4

Separation of human lung tissue into a series of discrete zones designated as conduction zones (zones 1 through 16) and transitional and respiratory zones (zones 17 through 23). *BR,* bronchus; *BL,* bronchiole; *TBL,* terminal bronchiole; *RBL,* respiratory bronchiole; *AD,* alveolar duct; *AS,* alveolar sac. (Modified from West, J.B.: *Respiratory Physiology—The Essentials,* 5th ed. Baltimore, Williams & Wilkins, 1995.)

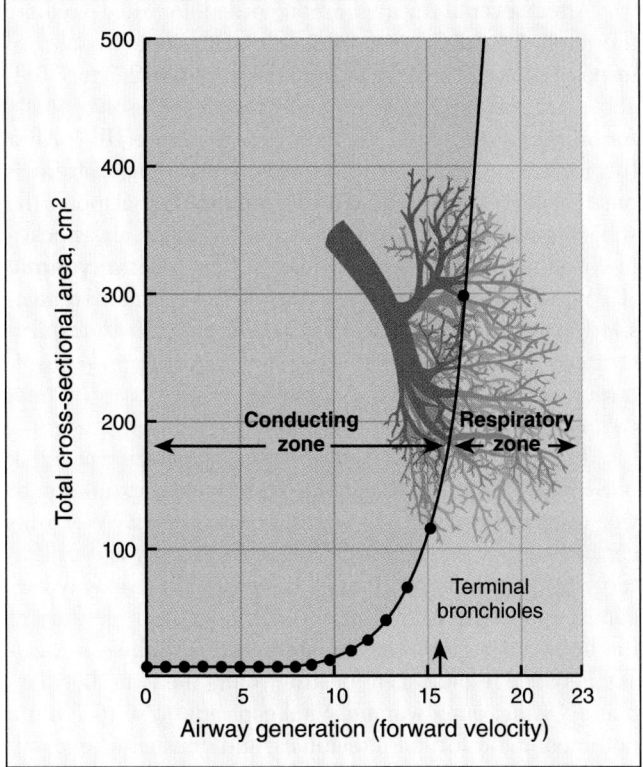

FIGURE 12.5

Airflow in the lungs plotted as a function of total cross-sectional tissue area. The forward velocity of airflow during an inspiration decreases markedly because of the tremendous increase in tissue cross-sectional area beginning in the region of the terminal bronchioles. (Modified from West, J.B.: *Respiratory Physiology—The Essentials,* 5th ed. Baltimore, Williams & Wilkins, 1995.)

pulmonic pressure may fall only about 3 mm Hg during the inspiratory cycle and rise a similar amount above atmospheric pressure during exhalation. If, however, the **glottis** (the narrowest part of the larynx through which air passes into and out of the trachea) is closed after a full inspiration and the expiratory muscles are maximally activated, the compressive force of exhalation can increase the **intrathoracic pressure** by more than 150 mm Hg above atmospheric pressure, with a somewhat higher pressure within the abdominal cavity.[27] This forced exhalation against a closed glottis, termed the **Valsalva maneuver,** commonly occurs in weight lifting and other activities that require a rapid and maximum application of force for a short duration. The fixation of the abdominal and chest cavities with this maneuver enhances the action of the muscles attached to the chest.

Physiologic Consequences of the Valsalva Maneuver.
As illustrated in Figure 12.6, the increased intrathoracic pressure during a Valsalva maneuver is transmitted through the thin walls of the veins that pass through the thoracic region. Because venous blood is under relatively low pressure, these veins are compressed and there is a significant reduc-

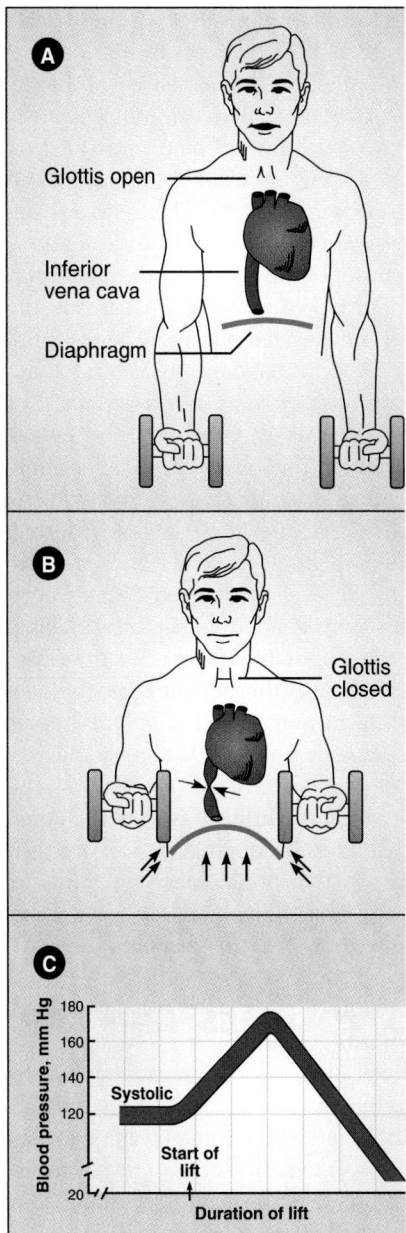

FIGURE 12.6

The Valsalva maneuver significantly reduces the return of blood to the heart. This occurs because the increase in intrathoracic pressure collapses the vein (inferior vena cava) that passes through the chest cavity. **A,** Normal breathing. **B,** Straining exercise with accompanying Valsalva maneuver. **C,** Blood pressure response before and during straining exercise.

tion in the return of blood to the heart. With exercise involving straining, venous return is reduced and arterial blood pressure subsequently decreases, which can diminish blood supply to the brain. This can produce dizziness, "spots before the eyes," and even fainting. When the glottis is opened and intrathoracic pressure is released, normal blood flow is reestablished (with perhaps even an "overshoot" in flow).[62, 65]

With the onset of a Valsalva maneuver at the start of the lift (Fig. 12.6C), blood pressure rises abruptly (within the first heart cycle after the maneuver) as the elevated intrathoracic pressure forces blood from the heart into the arterial system; stroke volume and blood pressure then fall sharply to below the resting level due to the reduced return of blood from the thoracic veins.[16, 35] This temporary increase in blood pressure within the heart and arteries of the chest at the immediate onset of the Valsalva maneuver is compensated for by a proportionate pressure increase on the outside walls caused by the elevated intrathoracic pressure.

The Valsalva maneuver usually accompanies straining muscular efforts, such as in isometric and heavy resistance exercise. However, it probably is not the cause of the dramatic hemodynamic response to such exercise. This is most likely because straining exercise greatly increases resistance to blood flow in the active muscles during the sustained muscle action.[22] Intramuscular fluid pressure increases linearly with all levels of isometric force up to the muscle's maximum force-generating capacity.[60] This produces a significant **rise** both in arterial blood pressure and in the heart's workload throughout exercise, independent of the Valsalva maneuver.[39] It is for this reason (and not the Valsalva maneuver per se) that individuals with cardiovascular disease should refrain from straining exercises such as isometrics or heavy lifting. Performing more rhythmic muscular activity results in a steady blood flow with only moderate increases in arterial blood pressure and subsequent strain on the heart. The blood pressure response in exercise is discussed more fully in Chapter 15.

LUNG VOLUMES AND CAPACITIES

The various lung volume measurements that reflect one's ability to increase the depth of breathing are illustrated in Figure 12.7, including average values for lung volumes for men and women. To obtain these measurements, the subject rebreathes through a recording spirometer similar to that described in Chapter 8 (Fig. 8.2) for measuring oxygen uptake by the closed-circuit method. As with many anatomic and physiologic measurements, lung volumes vary with age, sex, and body size, but especially with stature. *Therefore, lung volumes should only be evaluated in relation to established standards that account for these factors.*

STATIC LUNG VOLUMES

The bell of the spirometer shown in Figure 12.7 falls and subsequently rises as air is inhaled and exhaled to provide a record of the ventilatory volume and breathing rate. The volume of air moved during either the inspiratory or expiratory phase of each breath is termed **tidal volume** (TV) and is indicated by the rise or fall of the spirometer during the first portion of the record. Under resting conditions, tidal volumes usually range between 0.4 and 1.0 L air per breath.

After several tracings are recorded for tidal volume, the subject inspires as deeply as possible after a normal inspiration. This additional volume of about 2.5 to 3.5 L above the inspired tidal air represents the reserve ability for inhalation or **inspiratory reserve volume** (IRV). After the measurement of IRV, the normal breathing pattern is once again established. After a normal exhalation, the subject continues to exhale and forces as much air as possible from the lungs. This is the **expiratory reserve volume** (ERV), which ranges between 1.0 and 1.5 L for an average-sized man. *During exercise, encroachment on both inspiratory and expiratory reserve volumes, particularly the inspiratory volume, provides a considerable increase in tidal volume.*

The total volume of air that can be voluntarily moved in one breath, from full inspiration to maximum expiration or vice versa, is termed the **forced vital capacity** (FVC). This consists of the tidal volume plus the inspiratory and expiratory reserve volumes. Although values for vital capacity vary considerably with body size, as well as with the position of the body during the measurement, average values are usually between 4 and 5 L in healthy young men and between 3 and 4 L in young women. Vital capacities of 6 to 7 L are not uncommon for tall individuals, and unusually large values have been reported for a professional football player (7.6 L) and an Olympic gold medalist in cross-country skiing (8.1 L).[3, 69] The large lung volumes of such athletes generally reflect genetic influences and body size characteristics, because static lung volumes cannot be changed with exercise training to any great degree.

Residual Lung Volume. Even upon exhaling as deeply as possible, a volume of air remains in the lungs. This volume that cannot be exhaled is the **residual lung volume** (RLV). It averages between 0.8 and 1.2 L for women and between 0.9 and 1.4 L for men, although values between 0.96 and 2.46 L have been reported for apparently healthy professional football players.[69] Residual lung volume tends to increase with age, whereas the inspiratory and expiratory reserve volumes become proportionally smaller. The loss in breathing reserve and the concomitant increase in residual volume are generally attributed to a decrease in the elastic components of the lung tissue with aging. This, however, is not entirely an aging phenomenon per se, as evidence indicates that regular aerobic training may blunt the decline in static and dynamic lung functions associated with aging.[26]

The residual lung volume serves an important physiologic function because it prevents the lungs from being fully "emptied." This allows an uninterrupted exchange of gas between the blood and alveoli, thus preventing fluctuations in blood gases during phases of the breathing cycle, including deep breathing. The residual lung volume plus the vital capacity constitute the **total lung capacity** (TLC).

The residual lung volume cannot be measured directly from spirographic tracings but can be determined by several

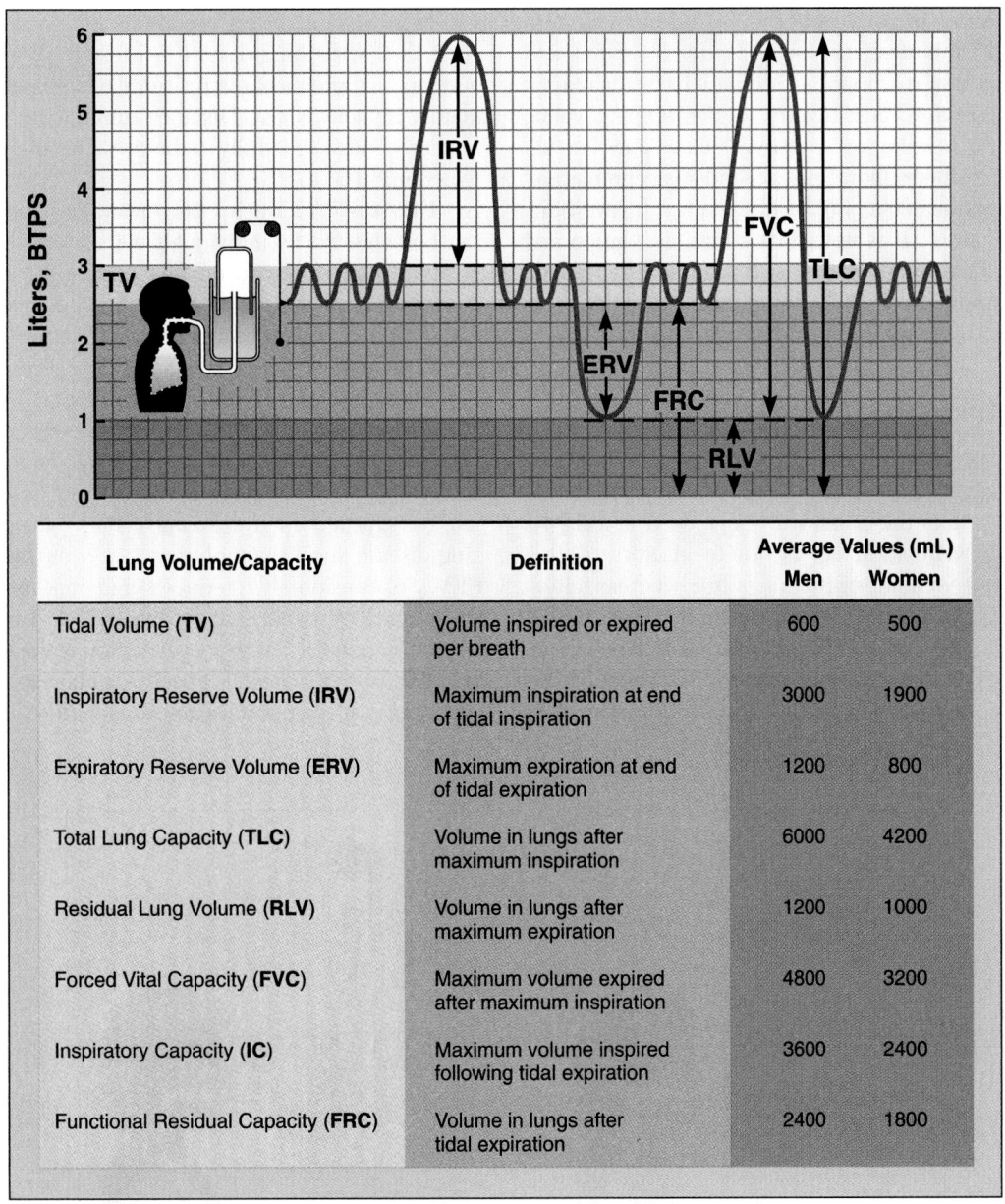

Lung Volume/Capacity	Definition	Average Values (mL)	
		Men	Women
Tidal Volume (**TV**)	Volume inspired or expired per breath	600	500
Inspiratory Reserve Volume (**IRV**)	Maximum inspiration at end of tidal inspiration	3000	1900
Expiratory Reserve Volume (**ERV**)	Maximum expiration at end of tidal expiration	1200	800
Total Lung Capacity (**TLC**)	Volume in lungs after maximum inspiration	6000	4200
Residual Lung Volume (**RLV**)	Volume in lungs after maximum expiration	1200	1000
Forced Vital Capacity (**FVC**)	Maximum volume expired after maximum inspiration	4800	3200
Inspiratory Capacity (**IC**)	Maximum volume inspired following tidal expiration	3600	2400
Functional Residual Capacity (**FRC**)	Volume in lungs after tidal expiration	2400	1800

FIGURE 12.7

Static measurements of lung volumes.

indirect techniques that involve rebreathing a known volume of gas containing either helium or pure oxygen. With the **helium dilution method,** the subject expires normally; the air remaining in the lungs at this end-normal expiration position is called the **functional residual capacity** (FRC) and includes the known expiratory reserve volume and the unknown residual volume. The subject then rebreathes a known helium mixture for approximately 5 minutes. Expired carbon dioxide is absorbed, and the exact amount of oxygen consumed is replaced continuously to maintain a constant rebreathing volume. The functional residual lung volume can be computed easily from the dilution of the original helium mixture. This volume minus the expiratory

reserve volume is equal to the residual lung volume. The **oxygen dilution method** is more rapid than the helium method, although it is similar in principle.[68] In this technique, the residual volume is determined from the dilution of the lung's original nitrogen concentration. Dilution is achieved by the rapid rebreathing of a volume of approximately 5 L of 100% oxygen. The dilution principle for the measurement of residual lung volume is illustrated in Figure 12.8.

Effects of Previous Exercise. The residual lung volume is temporarily increased during and in recovery from an acute bout of both short- and long-term exercise.[21, 44] In one study, residual lung volume increased during recovery following a maximal treadmill test by 21% after 5 minutes, by 17% after 15 minutes, and by 12% after 30 minutes.[10] Although the precise reason for an increase in residual lung volume with exercise (that reverts to the original value within 24 hours) is unknown, possible factors may be the closure of the small peripheral airways and an accumulation of pulmonary extravascular fluid with exercise (preventing complete exhalation). It is noteworthy that any temporary increase in residual lung volume could significantly impact subsequent computations of body volume via hydrostatic weighing for body composition studies (see Chapter 27).

DYNAMIC LUNG VOLUMES

In appraising the adequacy of pulmonary ventilation, the important consideration is the ability to sustain high levels of airflow rather than the quantity of air moved in a single breath. Dynamic ventilation depends on two factors: (a) the maximum "stroke volume" of the lungs (the vital capacity), and (b) the speed that this volume can be moved (the breathing rate). The velocity of airflow, in turn, depends on the resistance of the respiratory passages to the smooth flow of air and the resistance of both the chest and lung tissue to a change in shape during breathing. Pulmonary reserve is so great that when lung disease is present, patients rarely experience symptoms of distress until a large part of their ventilatory capacity is lost. Distance running can be engaged in regularly and successfully in the presence of mild airway obstruction.[41]

FEV-to-FVC Ratio. Normal values for vital capacity can be achieved by individuals with severe lung disease if no time limit is placed on this ventilatory maneuver. For this reason, physicians usually obtain a more "dynamic" measurement of lung function, such as the percentage of the forced vital capacity that can be expired in 1.0 second. This measurement of **forced expiratory volume** (FEV) provides an indication of expiratory power and overall resistance to air movement in the lungs and is symbolized as $\mathbf{FEV_{1.0}/FVC}$. *Normally, about 85% of the vital capacity can be expelled in 1.0 second.* With severe obstructive lung disease such as emphysema or bronchial asthma, the $FEV_{1.0}$ is considerably reduced and may often represent less than 40% of the vital capacity.[43, 63] Usually, the demarcation point for airway obstruction is the point at which less than 70% of the vital capacity can be expired in 1.0 second.[59] Examples of pulmonary function tests for $FEV_{1.0}$ and

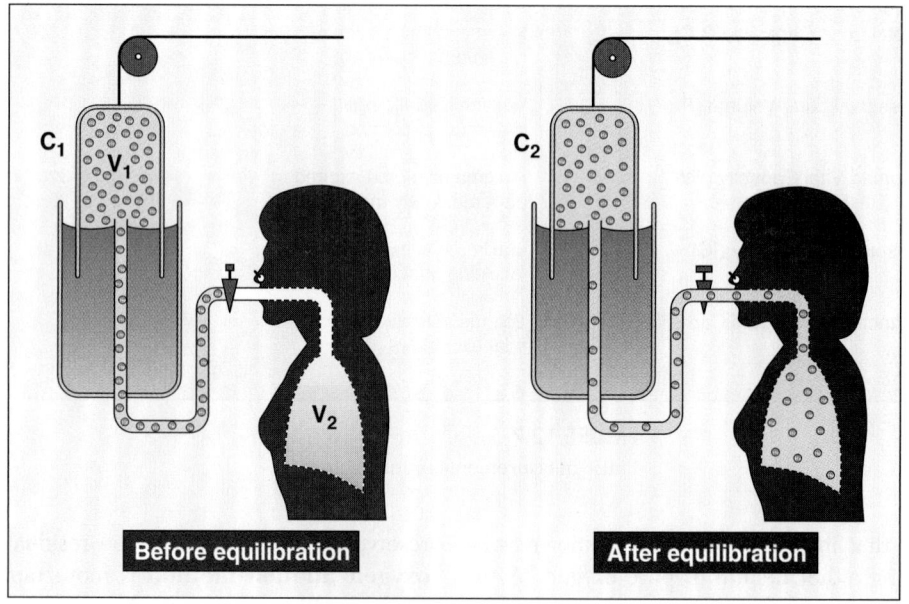

FIGURE 12.8

Application of the dilution principle to assess residual lung volume. In this procedure, the subject exhales to the unknown residual lung volume and then breathes from a known initial volume and concentration of a gas such as oxygen or helium (e.g., 5.0 L of a known concentration of the criterion gas). In this example, the known gas is helium. After a short period of deep, rapid breathing, the unknown, helium-free volume in the subject's lungs has been mixed with the known concentration of helium in the known volume that is rebreathed. An equilibrium is reached between the gases in the spirometer and the gases in the subject's residual volume. During the rebreathing process, oxygen is continually added to the spirometer to replace that consumed by the body during rebreathing (and carbon dioxide is absorbed from the spirometer). The residual lung volume is computed from the concentration-volume relationship, in which the initial helium volume (V_1) × initial helium concentration (C_1) is equal to the final gas volume (V_2) × final helium concentration (C_2). The previously unknown residual lung volume (V_2) is determined from the relationship $V_1 (C_1 - C_2)/C_2$. The final gas volume is corrected to body temperature and pressure saturated (BTPS) using the constants from Appendix C.

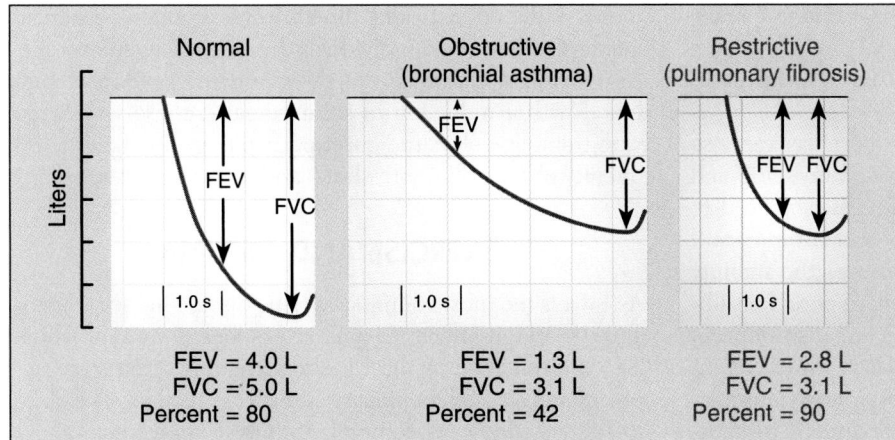

FIGURE 12.9

Examples of spirometric tracings during standard pulmonary function tests for $FEV_{1.0}$ and FVC in individuals with normal dynamic lung function and in patients with either obstructive or restrictive lung disease. (Modified from West, J.B.: *Respiratory Physiology—The Essentials*, 5th ed. Baltimore, Williams & Wilkins, 1995.)

FVC in individuals with normal lung function and with obstructive and restrictive lung disease are shown in Figure 12.9.

Maximum Voluntary Ventilation. Another dynamic test of ventilatory capacity requires rapid and deep breathing for 15 seconds. This 15-second volume is then extrapolated to the volume that would have been breathed if the subject had continued for 1 minute and represents the **maximum voluntary ventilation** (MVV). The MVV is usually approximately 25% higher than the ventilation volume observed during maximal exercise because the ventilatory system is not stressed maximally in exercise. The MVV of healthy, college-aged men is usually between 140 and 180 L · min^{-1}, and values for women are between 80 and 120 L · min^{-1}. MVV in male members of the United States Nordic Ski Team averaged 192 L · min^{-1}; the individual high MVV was 239 L · min^{-1}.[25] Patients with obstructive lung disease, on the other hand, can achieve only about 40% of the MVV considered normal for their age and size.[37] Specific exercise training of the ventilatory musculature improves the strength and endurance of these muscles and increases the MVV in both normal persons and pulmonary patients.[1, 57, 63] In patients with chronic pulmonary disease, this training adaptation allows enhanced capacity for exercise with less physiologic strain.[17, 53] An important benefit of either general exercise training or specific ventilatory muscle training for patients with chronic obstructive lung disease is the progressive desensitization to the feeling of breathlessness and a greater self-control of respiratory symptoms.[51]

LUNG FUNCTION, TRAINING, AND EXERCISE PERFORMANCE

Although some measurements of lung function are sensitive indices of the severity of obstructive and restrictive lung disease and do increase somewhat in patients and normal persons with training, they are of little use in predicting fitness or exercise performance if the values fall within the normal range. For example, no difference was noted between the average vital capacities of prepubescent and Olympic wrestlers, middle-distance athletes, and untrained, healthy subjects.[52, 55, 58] Furthermore, players from a professional football team averaged only 94% of their predicted vital capacity; the defensive backs achieved only 83% of values predicted "normal" for their body size.[69] Somewhat surprisingly, values for both static and dynamic lung function of accomplished marathon runners and other endurance-trained athletes were **no different** than values for untrained controls of comparable body size.[26, 42]

Swimming and diving may be more conducive to the development of larger-than-normal static lung volumes. In these sports, the inspiratory muscles are strengthened as they work against the additional resistance of the weight of the water compressing the thorax. This may explain the relatively large vital capacities reported for skin divers and competitive swimmers.[9, 13, 18]

The inability to predict the exercise performance of healthy individuals from measurements of lung function was demonstrated for a large group of teenage boys and girls after summer camp.[19] When lung volumes and capacities were adjusted for body size, they showed no relationship to various track performances, including distance running. Similarly, for marathon runners, essentially no difference existed between the athletes' lung function measurements and the values of sedentary subjects of similar body size (see Table 12.1).[34, 42] When variations in body size are considered, there is no relationship between maximal oxygen uptake and either vital capacity or maximum ventilation volume for healthy, untrained subjects.[24]

Although fatigue in strenuous exercise is frequently related to feeling "out of breath" or "winded," it appears that the normal capacity for pulmonary ventilation does not limit exercise performance. The larger-than-normal lung volumes and breathing capacities of some athletes can probably be attributed to genetic endowment, although some variation may reflect strengthened respiratory muscles due to specific exercise training.

Training May Benefit Ventilatory Endurance. *Inspiratory muscle fatigue does occur as a result of high-intensity, prolonged exercise.*[4, 14, 15, 29, 33] Whereas exercise training may have little effect on the maximum static and dynamic measurements of lung function, it is beneficial to improving one's ability to sustain high levels of **submaximal** ventilation.[7, 45, 57] Endurance training improves the stability of the body's internal milieu during a standard period of submaximal exercise. Consequently, there is less disruption in whole-body hormonal and acid-base balance, which might negatively impact the function of the inspiratory musculature.[32] Also, the ventilatory muscles benefit directly from exercise training. For example, 20 weeks of regular run training improved the ventilatory muscle endurance (less lactic acid produced during ventilation exercise) by approximately 16% in healthy adult men and women. This enhanced function may be due partly to the documented increase in aerobic enzyme levels and oxidative capacity of the ventilatory muscles with training.[50, 54] Research also has shown an increased capacity of the inspiratory muscles to generate force and sustain a given level of inspiratory pressure following exercise training.[15] These adaptations would reduce the level of lactic acid generated by the ventilatory muscles of untrained subjects who ventilate to levels observed in heavy exercise.[46] This would also reduce the feelings of local pulmonary discomfort and breathlessness often observed among the untrained individuals during prolonged exercise. An enhanced endurance of the ventilatory muscles, combined with a reduction in submaximal exercise ventilation with training, delays the onset of diaphragmatic fatigue frequently observed in both short- and long-term exercise.[12, 38]

EXERCISE AND ASTHMA

Asthma is the most common chronic disease in the industrialized world; it affects 12 million Americans, most of whom are children. The medical costs of treating asthma are approximately 6.5 billion dollars annually. A high level of physical fitness does not confer immunity from asthma; about 11% of the U.S. athletes who competed in the 1984 Olympic Games suffered from this ailment.[67] This obstructive pulmonary disease is characterized by hyperirritability of the pulmonary airways followed by bronchial spasm, edema, and mucus secretion, which are accompanied by symptoms of chest tightness, coughing, wheezing, and/or shortness of breath (Fig. 12.10).

Unfortunately, for approximately 80 to 90% of persons with asthma and 30 to 50% of those suffering from allergic rhinitis and hay fever, exercise is a potent stimulus for bronchoconstriction (or **exercise-induced bronchospasm**).[40, 48] With exercise, catecholamines from the sympathetic nervous system are released to produce a relaxation effect on the smooth muscle of the pulmonary airways. As shown in Figure 12.10A, the initial bronchodilation with exercise occurs in both the normal person and the individual with asthma. In the individual with asthma, however, bronchodilation is then followed by bronchospasm, excessive mucus secretion, and subsequent bronchoconstriction. An acute episode of airway obstruction is often apparent within 5 to 15 minutes after exercise (Fig. 12.10B); recovery usually occurs spontaneously between 30 and 90 minutes. One technique for detecting an exercise-induced asthmatic response is simply to provide progressive increments of exercise. A spirometric evaluation of FVC and $FEV_{1.0}$ is made after each period of exercise, and during 10 to 20 minutes of recovery. Generally, a 10 to 15% reduction in pre-exercise values for $FEV_{1.0}/FVC$ confirms the diagnosis of exercise-induced bronchospasm.[30, 48]

Sensitivity to Thermal Gradients. Many mechanisms are postulated for the bronchospastic response to exercise.[66] One of the more attractive theories relates to the rate and magnitude of alterations in heat and water exchange in the tracheobronchial tree brought on by increased exercise ventilation. As the incoming breath of air moves down the respiratory tract, heat and water are transferred from the respiratory tract as the air is warmed and humidified. The net effect of the thermal flux generated by this air-conditioning process is a cooling of the respiratory mucosa. There also may be a change in the osmolality of its cells, causing mast-cell degranulation and the release of chemical

---

TABLE 12.1
ANTHROPOMETRIC DATA, PULMONARY FUNCTION, AND RESTING MINUTE VENTILATION IN 20 MARATHON RUNNERS AND CONTROL SUBJECTS

Measure	Runners	Controls	Difference[a]
Anthropometric			
Age, y	27.8	27.4	0.4
Stature, cm	175.8	176.7	0.9
Surface area, m²	1.82	1.89	0.07
Pulmonary Function			
FVC, L	5.13	5.34	0.21
TLC, L	6.91	7.13	0.22
$FEV_{1.0}$, L	4.32	4.47	0.15
$FEV_{1.0}/FVC$, %	84.3	83.8	0.5
MVV, $L \cdot min^{-1}$	179.8	176.0	3.8
Resting Ventilation			
$\dot{V}_E$ $L \cdot min^{-1}$	11.9	11.9	0.9
Breathing rate, breaths $\cdot min^{-1}$	10.9	11.1	0.2
Tidal volume, L	1.16	1.06	0.10

From Mahler, D.A., et al.: Ventilatory responses at rest and during exercise in marathon runners. *J. Appl. Physiol.*, 52:388, 1982.
[a]Differences not statistically significant.

mediators that trigger bronchoconstriction. It is also postulated that hyperemia of the airway wall's microcirculation causes edema, which constricts the airway, independent of any constriction by bronchial smooth muscle.[48] Regardless of the mechanism, however, large volumes of incompletely conditioned inspired air in heavy exercise place a tremendous burden on the smaller airways of the tracheobronchial tree, to the extent that a significant decrease in mucosal temperature occurs. A quantitative association exists between heat loss from the airways during exercise and the subsequent constriction of the bronchioles in the susceptible asthmatic.[11] After exercise, airway cooling is fol-

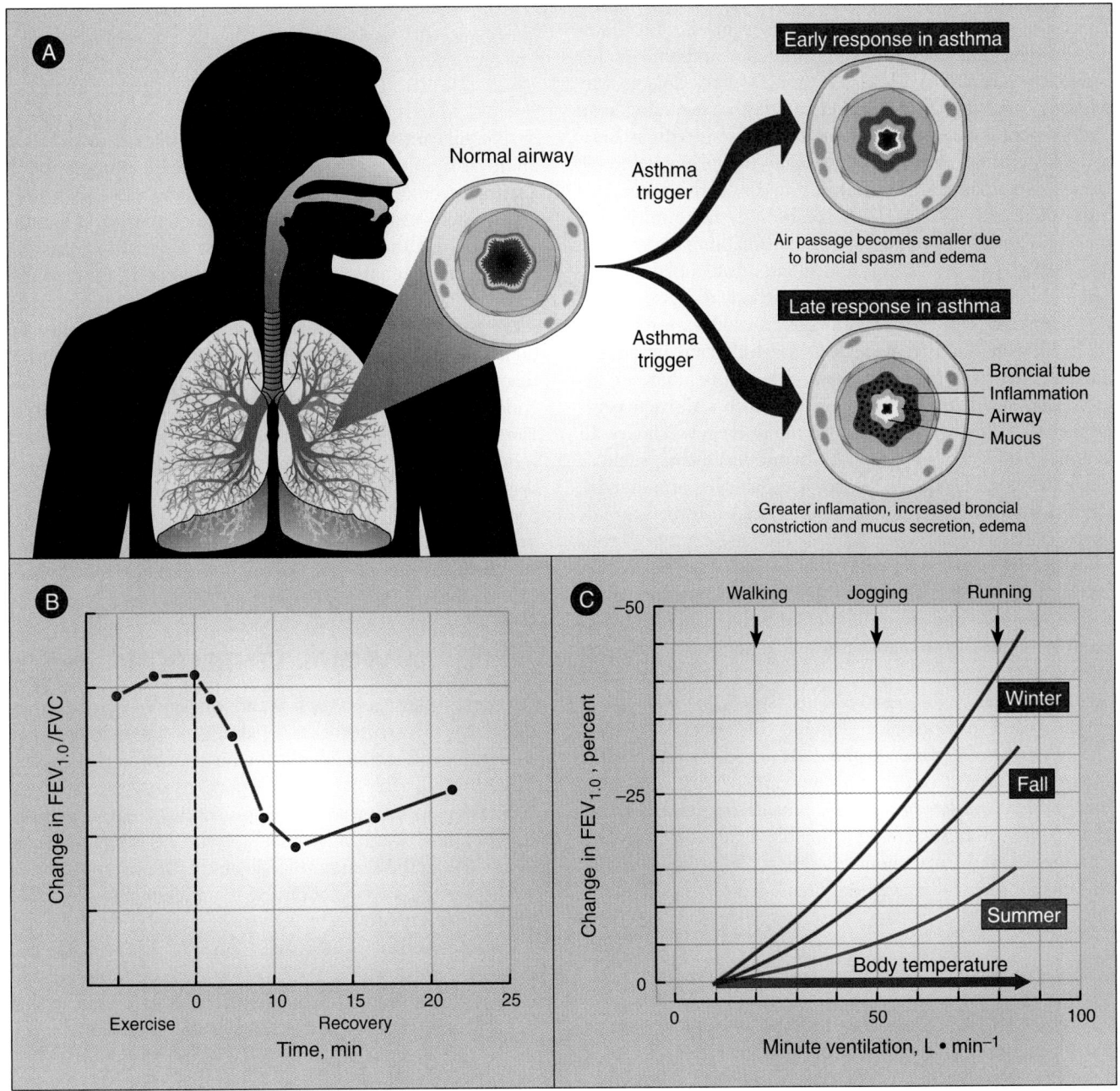

FIGURE 12.10

A, The typical response to an asthma attack. **B,** The pattern of dynamic lung function ($FEV_{1.0}/FEV$) during an episode of exercise-induced bronchospasm. **C,** The interaction between exercise intensity (walking, jogging, running) and the characteristics of the environment. Note that in **C,** the maximal obstruction occurs when dry air at low temperature (e.g., in winter) is inhaled and the minimal obstruction occurs when hot, humid air (e.g., in summer) is inspired. (**C** modified from McFadden, E.R., Jr., and Gilbert, I.A.: Current concepts in exercise-induced asthma. *N. Engl. J. Med.,* 330:1362, 1994.)

lowed by abrupt rewarming as pulmonary ventilation rapidly declines. It is likely that the thermal gradient provided by this combination of airway cooling and subsequent rewarming stimulates the bronchospastic process in susceptible individuals.[8, 47]

The Environment Makes a Difference. As illustrated in Figure 12.10C, exercise-induced bronchospasm is blunted when exercise is performed in a humid rather than a dry environment. This occurs regardless of air temperature.[6, 31, 48] The bronchospastic response in one study was totally abolished when the patients inhaled ambient air that was fully saturated with water vapor.[64] This explains why walking or jogging on a warm, humid day or swimming in an indoor pool is often well tolerated by persons with asthma, whereas outdoor winter sports usually trigger an asthmatic attack. The benefit of swimming to the asthma-sensitive individual may not simply be the humid environment but may be the interrupted nature of the breathing pattern and the lower total ventilation and greater catecholamine response with this predominantly upper body exercise.[31]

Light to moderate continuous warmup exercise for 15 to 30 minutes is beneficial to the asthmatic because it initiates a "refractory period" in which subsequent intense exercise does not trigger as severe a bronchoconstrictive response.[48, 56] This benefit may continue as long as 2 hours. In addition, effective medications (**bronchodilators** such as theophylline or β_2 agonists, as well as inhaled heparin therapy, or **anti-inflammatory agents** such as inhaled corticosteroids or cromolyn sodium) are available to limit the degree of bronchoconstriction in those who wish to exercise on a regular basis; these medications do not affect exercise performance.[30]

A clearer understanding of the factors related to exercise-induced bronchospasm will ultimately enable the physician to "prescribe" the optimum environment and exercise intensity for persons with asthma to obtain both physical and psychological benefits of regular exercise. *Although exercise training cannot eliminate or cure an asthmatic condition, it can increase pulmonary airflow reserve and reduce ventilatory work by potentiating bronchodilation during exercise.* This may enable asthmatics to maintain high airflow throughout exercise for more efficient endurance in physical activity despite an impaired pulmonary function.

POSTEXERCISE COUGHING

Exercise is frequently associated with a dryness in the throat and coughing during the recovery period. This is common following exercise in cold weather, during which considerable water loss from the respiratory tract can occur. The phenomenon of postexercise coughing is directly related to the overall respiratory water loss (rather than respiratory heat loss) associated with the large ventilatory volumes during exercise.[5]

PULMONARY VENTILATION
MINUTE VENTILATION

During quiet breathing at rest, the normal breathing rate is approximately 12 breaths per minute and the average tidal volume is approximately 0.5 L air per breath. Consequently, the volume of air breathed each minute, or **minute ventilation** ($\dot{V}E$), is 6 L.

$$\text{Minute ventilation } (\dot{V}E) = \text{Breathing rate} \times \text{Tidal volume}$$
$$= 12 \cdot \text{min}^{-1} \times 0.5 \text{ L}$$
$$= 6 \text{ L} \cdot \text{min}^{-1}$$

Significant increases in minute ventilation result from an increase in either the rate or depth of breathing or both. During strenuous exercise, the breathing rate of healthy young adults usually increases to between 35 and 45 breaths per minute, although rates as high as 60 to 70 breaths per minute have been measured in elite athletes during maximal exercise. Tidal volumes of 2.0 L and higher are common during exercise. With such increases in breathing rate and tidal volume, the exercise minute ventilation easily can reach 100 L (or about 17 times the resting value). In male endurance athletes, minute ventilation may increase to 160 L $\cdot$ min^{-1} in response to maximal exercise. Ventilation volumes of 200 L have been reported in several research studies, and a high volume of 208 L was observed in a professional football player during maximal bicycle exercise.[69] *Even with these large minute ventilations, tidal volumes for both trained and untrained individuals rarely exceed 60% of vital capacity.*

ALVEOLAR VENTILATION

A portion of the air in each breath does not enter the alveoli and, therefore, is not involved in gaseous exchange with the blood. This air, which fills the nose, mouth, trachea, and other nondiffusable conducting portions of the respiratory tract, is contained within the **anatomic dead space**. In healthy individuals, this volume averages 150 to 200 mL (or about 30% of the resting tidal volume). The composition of dead-space air is almost identical to ambient air, except that it is fully saturated with water vapor.

Because of the dead-space volume, only about 350 mL of the 500 mL inspired tidal volume at rest enters into and mixes with the existing alveolar air. This does not mean that only 350 mL of air enters and leaves the alveoli with each breath. On the contrary, if the tidal volume is 500 mL, then 500 mL of air enters the alveoli but only 350 mL of this is fresh air. This represents about one-seventh of the total air in the alveoli. Such a relatively small and seemingly inefficient **alveolar ventilation** prevents drastic changes in alveolar air composition and ensures a consistency in arterial blood gases throughout the entire breathing cycle.

TABLE 12.2
RELATIONSHIP BETWEEN TIDAL VOLUME, BREATHING RATE, AND BOTH TOTAL AND ALVEOLAR MINUTE VENTILATION

Condition	Tidal Volume (mL)	×	Breathing Rate (breaths · min⁻¹)	=	Minute Ventilation (mL · min⁻¹)	−	Dead Space Minute Ventilation (mL · min⁻¹)	=	Alveolar Minute Ventilation (mL · min⁻¹)
Shallow breathing	150		40		6000		(150 mL × 40)		0
Normal breathing	500		12		6000		(150 mL × 12)		4200
Deep breathing	1000		6		6000		(150 mL × 6)		5100

Minute ventilation does not always reflect alveolar ventilation (see Table 12.2). In the first example of shallow breathing, the tidal volume is reduced to 150 mL, but it still is possible to achieve a 6-L minute ventilation if the breathing rate is increased to 40 breaths per minute. The same 6-L minute volume can be achieved by decreasing the breathing rate to 12 breaths per minute and increasing the tidal volume to 500 mL. On the other hand, by doubling tidal volume and halving the ventilatory rate, as in the example of deep breathing, a 6-L minute ventilation is again achieved. Each of these ventilatory adjustments, however, drastically affects alveolar ventilation. In the example of shallow breathing, all that has been moved or ventilated is the dead-space air, without any alveolar ventilation. In the other examples, breathing is deeper and a larger portion of each breath enters into and mixes with alveolar air. It is the alveolar ventilation that determines the gaseous concentrations at the alveolar-capillary membrane.

Dead Space versus Tidal Volume. The preceding examples of alveolar ventilation were oversimplified because a constant dead space was assumed despite changes in tidal volume. Actually, the anatomic dead space increases as tidal volume becomes larger; it can double during deep breathing due to some stretching of the respiratory passages with a fuller inspiration.[2] However, this increase in dead space is still proportionately less than the increase in tidal volume. *Consequently, deeper breathing provides more effective alveolar ventilation than a similar minute ventilation achieved only through an increase in breathing rate.*

Physiologic Dead Space. Adequate gas exchange between the alveoli and the blood requires an alveolar ventilation that is well matched to the quantity of blood perfusing the pulmonary capillaries. At rest, approximately 4.2 L of air normally ventilates the alveoli each minute, whereas an average of 5.0 L of blood flows through the pulmonary capillaries. In this instance, the ratio of alveolar ventilation to pulmonary blood flow, termed the **ventilation-perfusion ratio,** is approximately 0.8 (4.2 ÷ 5.0). This ratio means that each liter of pulmonary blood flow is matched by an alveolar ventilation of 0.8 L. In light exercise, the ventilation-perfusion ratio is maintained at approximately 0.8, whereas in heavy exercise, there is a disproportionate increase in alveolar ventilation. In healthy individuals, the ventilation-perfusion ratio may increase to more than 5.0 with a fairly uniform distribution of pulmonary blood flow to ensure adequate aeration of the blood returning in the venous circulation.

In certain instances, a portion of the alveoli may not function adequately in gas exchange due to either (*a*) an underperfusion of blood or (*b*) an inadequate ventilation relative to the alveolar surface. This portion of the alveolar volume with a poor ventilation-perfusion ratio is termed the **physiologic dead space.** As illustrated in Figure 12.11, the physiologic dead space in the healthy lung is small and can be considered negligible. Physiologic dead space, however, can increase to as much as 50% of the tidal volume. This occurs with either **inadequate perfusion** during hemorrhage or blockage of the pulmonary circulation by an embolism or with **inadequate ventilation** that occurs in emphysema, asthma, and pulmonary fibrosis. When a relatively large physiologic dead space results from a decreased functional alveolar surface, as occurs in emphysema, excessive ventilation is noted, even at low exercise levels. Many of these patients are unable to achieve their maximal circulatory capacity because of ventilatory muscle fatigue from excessive ventilation. Adequate gas exchange becomes impossible when the total dead space of the lung exceeds 60% of lung volume.

Rate versus Depth. Alveolar ventilation in exercise results from an increase in both the rate and depth of breathing. In moderate exercise, well-trained athletes maintain alveolar ventilation by increasing tidal volume with only a small increase in breathing rate.[23] With deeper breathing, alveolar ventilation increases from 70% of the total minute ventilation at rest to over 85% of the exercise ventilation. As shown in Figure 12.12, the increase in exercise tidal volume

FIGURE 12.11
Distribution of tidal volume in a healthy subject at rest. Tidal volume includes about 350 mL of ambient air that mixes with alveolar air, 150 mL of air in the larger air passages (anatomic dead space), and a small portion of air distributed to either poorly ventilated or poorly perfused alveoli (physiologic dead space).

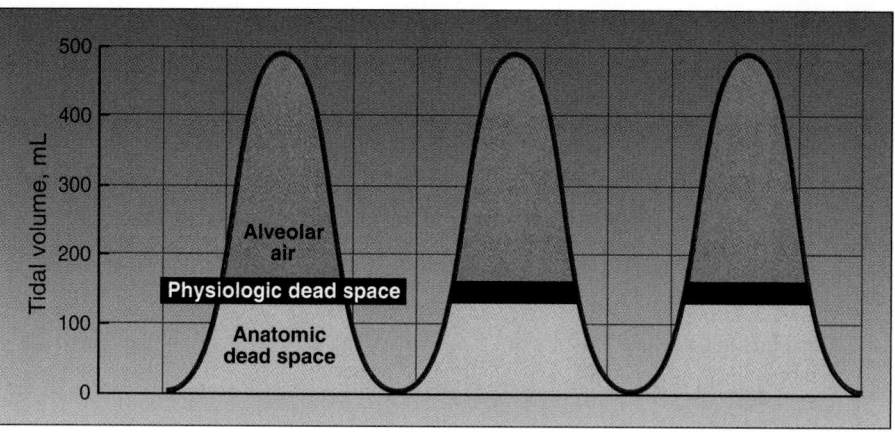

FIGURE 12.12
Tidal volume and subdivisions of pulmonary air at rest and during exercise.

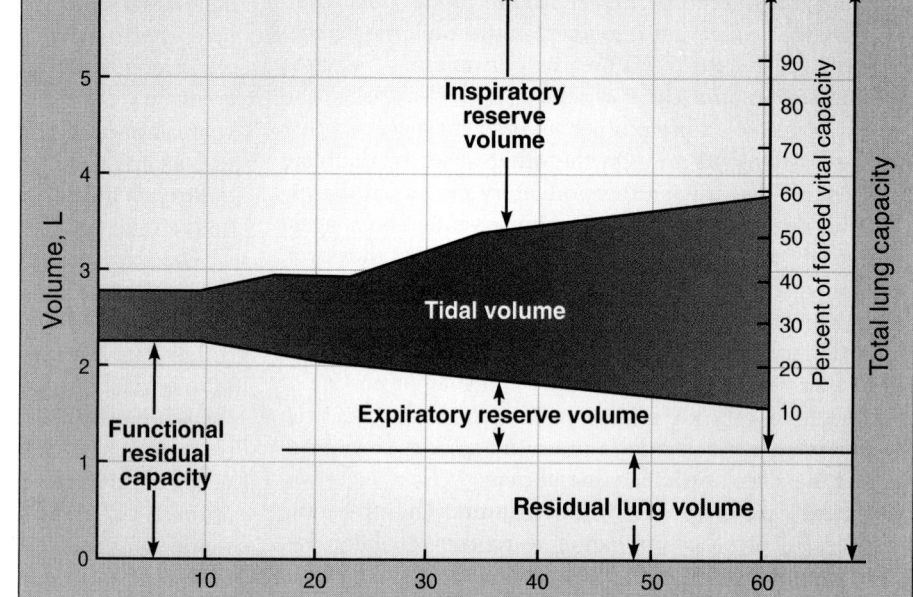

is largely due to encroachment on the inspiratory reserve volume with an accompanying but smaller decrease in the end-expiratory level. With more intense exercise, the increase in tidal volume begins to plateau at approximately 60% of the vital capacity; minute ventilation increases further through increases in breathing frequency. These adjustments occur unconsciously. Each person develops a "style" of breathing in which the breathing frequency and tidal volume are blended to provide effective alveolar ventilation. Any conscious attempt to modify breathing during general physical activities such as running is of no benefit in terms of performance. Conscious manipulation of breathing is usually detrimental

to the exquisitely regulated physiologic adjustments to exercise. *At rest and during exercise, a healthy person should breathe in the manner that seems most natural.*

■ SUMMARY ■

1. The lungs provide a large surface between the body's internal fluid environment and the gaseous external environment. During any 1 second of exercise, probably no more than 1 pint of blood is contained in the pulmonary capillaries.

2. Pulmonary ventilation is regulated to maintain a favorable concentration of alveolar oxygen and carbon dioxide to ensure adequate aeration of the blood flowing through the lungs.

3. Pulmonary airflow depends on small pressure differences between ambient air and air within the lungs. These differences are brought about by the muscles that act to alter the dimensions of the chest cavity.

4. A forced exhalation against a closed glottis is called a Valsalva maneuver. This causes a large pressure increase within the chest and abdominal cavities, which compresses the thoracic veins, thereby reducing venous return to the heart. The straining muscular effort that usually accompanies the Valsalva maneuver temporarily elevates blood pressure and places an added workload on the heart. Therefore, individuals with heart and vascular disease should refrain from straining exercises such as heavy weight lifting and isometric muscle actions.

5. Lung volumes vary with age, sex, and body size (especially stature) and should only be evaluated in relation to established norms based on these factors.

6. Tidal volume increases during exercise by encroachment on both the inspiratory and expiratory reserve volumes. Air still remains in the lungs during maximal exhalation, even when a person breathes to vital capacity. This residual lung volume allows an uninterrupted exchange of gas during all phases of the breathing cycle.

7. Forced expiratory volume and maximum voluntary ventilation provide a dynamic picture of the ability to sustain a high level of airflow and serve as excellent screening tests to detect possible lung disease.

8. Tests of static and dynamic lung function are of little use in predicting fitness and exercise performance if the values fall within a normal range.

9. Exercise-induced bronchospasm is an obstructive lung disorder that is associated with the rate and magnitude of airway cooling and subsequent rewarming. This response is greatly reduced when humidified air is breathed during exercise. Exercise training cannot "cure" the asthmatic condition, but it can increase airflow reserve and reduce the work of breathing during physical activity.

10. Minute ventilation is a function of breathing rate and tidal volume. It averages 6 to 10 L $\cdot$ min^{-1} at rest and may increase to as high as 200 L $\cdot$ min^{-1} during maximal exercise.

11. Alveolar ventilation is the portion of the minute ventilation that enters the alveoli and is involved in gaseous exchange with the blood.

12. The ventilation-perfusion ratio is the ratio of alveolar minute ventilation to pulmonary blood flow. This indicates that each liter of pulmonary blood is matched by an alveolar ventilation of 0.8 L. During heavy exercise, alveolar ventilation in healthy individuals increases dis-proportionately and the ventilation-perfusion ratio may reach 5.0.

13. At rest and during exercise, a healthy person should breathe in a manner that seems most natural.

■ REFERENCES ■

1. Akabas, S.R., et al: Metabolic and functional adaptation of the diaphragm to training with resistive loads. *J. Appl. Physiol.,* 66:529, 1989.
2. Asmussen, E., and Nielsen, M.: Physiological dead-space and alveolar gas pressures at rest and during muscular exercise. *Acta Physiol. Scand.,* 38:1, 1956.
3. Åstrand, P.O., and Rodahl, K.: *Textbook of Work Physiology.* New York, McGraw-Hill, 1986.
4. Babcock, M.A., et al.: Hypoxic effects on exercise-induced diaphragmatic fatigue in normal healthy humans. *J. Appl. Physiol.,* 78:82, 1995.
5. Banner, A.S., et al.: Relation of respiratory water loss to coughing after exercise. *N. Engl. J. Med.,* 311:883, 1984.
6. Bar-Or, O., and Inbar, O.: Swimming and asthma–benefits and deleterious effects. *Sports Med.,* 14:397, 1992.
7. Bender, P.R., and Martin, B.J.: Maximal ventilation for exhausting exercise. *Med. Sci. Sports Exerc.,* 17:164, 1985.
8. Berk, J.L., et al.: Cold-induced bronchoconstriction: role of cutaneous reflexes vs. direct airway effects. *J. Appl. Physiol.,* 63:659, 1987.
9. Bjurström, R.L., and Schoene, R.B.: Control of ventilation in elite synchronized swimmers. *J. Appl. Physiol.,* 63:1019, 1987.
10. Buno, M.J., et al.: The effect of an acute bout of exercise on selected pulmonary function measurements. *Med. Sci. Sports Exerc.,* 13:290, 1981.
11. Busse, W.: Exercise induced asthma. *Am. J. Med.,* 68:471, 1980.
12. Bye, R.T.P., et al.: Ventilatory muscles during exercise in air and oxygen in normal men. *J. Appl. Physiol.,* 56:464, 1984.
13. Carey, C.R., et al.: Effects of skin diving on lung volumes. *J. Appl. Physiol.,* 8:19, 1955.
14. Chevrolet, J.C., et al.: Alterations in inspiratory and leg muscle force and recovery pattern after a marathon. *Med. Sci. Sports Exerc.,* 25:501, 1993.
15. Clanton, T.L., et al.: Effects of swim training on lung volumes and inspiratory muscle conditioning. *J. Appl. Physiol.,* 62:39, 1987.
16. Clifford, P.S., et al.: Arterial blood pressure response to rowing. *Med. Sci. Sports Exerc.,* 26:715, 1994.
17. Cooper, C.B.: Determining the role of exercise in patients with chronic pulmonary disease. *Med. Sci. Sports Exerc.,* 27:147, 1995.
18. Cordain, L., et al.: Lung volumes and maximal respiratory pressures in collegiate swimmers and runners. *Res. Q. Exerc. Sport,* 61:70, 1990.
19. Cummings, G.R.: Correlation of athletic performance with pulmonary function in 13 to 17 year old boys and girls. *Med. Sci. Sports Exerc.,* 1:140, 1969.
20. Farkas, G.A., et al.: Contractile properties of intercostal muscles and their functional significance. *J. Appl. Physiol.,* 59:528, 1985.
21. Farrell, P.A., et al.: The course of lung volume changes during prolonged treadmill exercise. *Med. Sci. Sports Exerc.,* 15:319, 1983.
22. Gaffney, F.A., et al.: Cardiovascular and metabolic responses to static contraction in man. *Acta Physiol. Scand.,* 138:249, 1990.
23. Grimby, G.: Respiration in exercise. *Med. Sci. Sports Exerc.,* 1:9, 1969.
24. Grimby, G., and Soderholm, B.: Spirometric studies in normal subjects. *Acta Med. Scand.,* 173:199, 1963.
25. Hanson, J.S.: Maximal exercise performance in members of the U.S. Nordic Ski Team. *J. Appl. Physiol.,* 33:592, 1973.
26. Hagberg, J.M., et al.: Pulmonary function in young and older athletes and untrained men. *J. Appl. Physiol.,* 65:101, 1988.
27. Harman, E.A., et al.: Intra-abdominal and intra-thoracic pressures during lifting and jumping. *Med. Sci. Sports Exerc.,* 20:195, 1988.

28. Hass, F., et al.: Effect of upper body posture on forced inspiration and expiration. *J. Appl. Physiol.*, 52:879, 1982.

29. Hill, N. et al.: Effect of an endurance triathlon on pulmonary function. *Med. Sci. Sports Exerc.*, 11:1260, 1991.

30. Hough, D.O., and Dec, K.L.: Exercise-induced asthma and anaphylaxis. *Sports Med.*, 18:162, 1994.

31. Inbar, O., et al.: The effect of prone immersion on bronchial responsiveness in children with asthma. *Med. Sci. Sports Exerc.*, 25:1098, 1993.

32. Johnson, B.D., et al.: Mechanical constraints on exercise hyperpnea in endurance athletes. *J. Appl. Physiol.*, 73:874, 1992.

33. Johnson, B.D., et al.: Exercise induced diaphragmatic fatigue in healthy humans. *J. Physiol. (Lond.)*, 460:385, 1993.

34. Kaufmann, D.A., et al.: Pulmonary function of marathon runners. *Med. Sci. Sports Exerc.*, 6:114, 1974.

35. Lassen, A., et al.: Cardiovascular responses to static contractions in man with topical nerve blockade. *J. Physiol. (Lond.)*, 409:333, 1989.

36. Leech, J.A., et al.: Respiratory pressures and function in young adults. *Am. Rev. Respir. Dis.*, 128:17, 1983.

37. Levison, H., and Cherniack, R.: Ventilatory cost of exercise in chronic obstructive pulmonary disease. *J. Appl. Physiol.*, 25:21, 1968.

38. Loke, J., et al.: Respiratory muscle fatigue after marathon running. *J. Appl. Physiol.*, 52:821, 1982.

39. MacDougall, J.D., et al.: Arterial blood pressure response to resistance exercise. *J. Appl. Physiol.*, 58:785, 1985.

40. Mahler, D.: Exercise-induced asthma. *Med. Sci. Sports Exerc.*, 25:554, 1993.

41. Mahler, D.A., et al.: Exercise performance in marathon runners with airway obstruction. *Med. Sci. Sports Exerc.*, 13:284, 1981.

42. Mahler, D.A., et al.: Ventilatory responses at rest and during exercise in marathon runners. *J. Appl. Physiol.*, 52:388, 1982.

43. Mahler, D.A., and Harper, A.: Prediction of peak oxygen consumption in obstructive airway disease. *Med. Sci. Sports Exerc.*, 20:574, 1988.

44. Maron, M.B., et al.: Alterations in pulmonary function consequent to competitive marathon running. *Med. Sci. Sports Exerc.*, 11:244, 1979.

45. Martin, B.J., and Stager, J.M.: Ventilation endurance in athletes and non-athletes. *Med. Sci. Sports Exerc.*, 13:21, 1981.

46. Martin, B.J., et al.: Anaerobic metabolism in the respiratory muscles during exercise. *Med. Sci. Sports Exerc.*, 16:82, 1984.

47. McFadden, E.R.: Exercise-induced asthma; recent approaches. *Chest*, 93:1282, 1988.

48. McFadden, E.R., Jr., and Gilbert, I.A.: Current concepts in exercise-induced asthma. *N. Engl. J. Med.*, 330:1362, 1994.

49. Mckenzie, D.C., et al.: The protective effects of continuous and interval exercise in athletes with exercise-induced asthma. *Med. Sci. Sports Exerc.*, 26:951, 1994.

50. Moore, R.L., and Gollnick, P.D.: Response of ventilatory muscles of the rat to endurance training. *Pflugers Arch.*, 92:268, 1982.

51. Moser, K., et al.: Results of a comprehensive rehabilitation program; physiological and functional effects on patients with chronic obstructive pulmonary disease. *Arch. Intern. Med.*, 140:1596, 1980.

52. Newman, F., et al.: A comparison between body size and lung function of swimmers and normal school children. *J. Physiol. (Lond.)*, 156:9, 1961.

53. Pardy, R.L., et al.: Respiratory muscle training compared with physiotherapy in chronic airflow limitation. *Am. Rev. Respir. Dis.*, 123:421, 1981.

54. Powers, S., et al.: Diaphragmatic fiber type specific adaptation to endurance exercise. *Respir. Physiol.*, 89:195, 1992.

55. Rasch, P.J., and Brandt, J.W.A.: Measurement of pulmonary function in United States Olympic free style wrestlers. *Res. Q.*, 28:279, 1957.

56. Reiff, D.B., et al.: The effect of prolonged submaximal warm-up exercise on exercise-induced asthma. *Am. Rev. Respir. Dis.*, 139:479, 1989.

57. Robinson, E.P., and Kjeldgaard, J.M.: Improvement in ventilatory muscle function with running. *J. Appl. Physiol.*, 52:1400, 1982.

58. Sady, S., et al.: Physiological characteristics of high-ability prepubescent wrestlers. *Med. Sci. Sports Exerc.*, 6:72, 1984.

59. Schapira, R.M., et al.: The value of expiratory time in the physical diagnosis of obstructive airway disease. *JAMA*, 270:731, 1993.

60. Sejersted, O.N., et al.: Intramuscular fluid pressure during isometric contraction of human skeletal muscle. *J. Appl. Physiol.*, 56:287, 1984.

61. Sharp, J.T., et al.: Relative contributions of rib cage and abdomen to breathing in normal subjects. *J. Appl. Physiol.*, 39:609, 1975.

62. Smith, M.A.: Assessment of beat to beat changes in cardiac output during the Valsalva maneuver using bioimpedence cardiology. *Clin. Sci.*, 72:423, 1987.

63. Sonne, L.J., and Davis, J.A.: Increased exercise performance in patients with severe COPD following inspiratory resistive training. *Chest*, 81:436, 1982.

64. Strauss, R.H., et al.: Influence of heat and humidity on the airway obstruction induced by exercise in asthma. *J. Clin. Invest.*, 61:433, 1978.

65. Ten Harkel, A.D.J., et al.: Assessment of cardiovascular reflexes: influence of posture and period of preceding rest. *J. Appl. Physiol.*, 68:147, 1990.

66. Virant, F.S.: Exercise-induced bronchospasm: epidemiology, pathophysiology, and therapy. *Med. Sci. Sports Exerc.*, 24:851, 1992.

67. Voy, R.O.: The U.S. Olympic committee experience with exercise-induced bronchospasm, 1984. *Med. Sci. Sports Exerc.*, 18:328, 1986.

68. Wilmore, J.H.: A simplified method for the determination of residual lung volume. *J. Appl. Physiol.*, 27:96, 1969.

69. Wilmore, J.H., and Haskell, W.L.: Body composition and endurance capacity of professional football players. *J. Appl. Physiol.*, 33:564, 1972.

Whipp, B.J., and Wasserman, K.: Effect of body temperature on the ventilatory response to exercise. *Respir. Phyisiol.* **87:354, 1970.**

Neurogenic reflexes originating in the exercising limbs and cerebral cortex, combined with humoral mechanism acting via the known peripheral or central chemoreceptors, serve as important mechanisms for increasing and regulating pulmonary ventilation during exercise. Additional

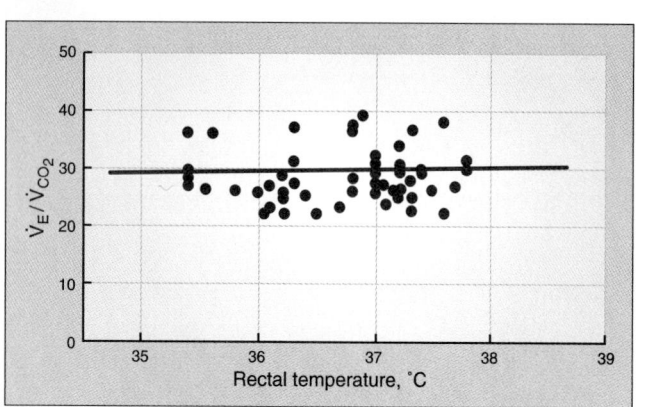

Ventilatory equivalent for CO_2 ($\dot{V}E/\dot{V}CO_2$) during graded exercise at various rectal temperatures. Core temperature, as reflected by rectal temperature, has little independent effect on the ventilatory response to exercise.

mechanisms include temperature changes in exercise that act directly on hypothalamic regulatory neurons or indirectly by increasing the sensitivity to stimuli of the peripheral and/or central chemoreceptors. Because hyperthermia (core temperature increases of more than 1°C) induces hyperventilation and a concomitant hypocapnia (reduced arterial PCO_2), these researchers studied the rela-

tionship between body temperature and the ventilatory response to graded exercise.

Eight fit men (aged 20 to 44 years) completed two identical graded exercise protocols (6-minute work periods in increments of 343 kg · m · min⁻¹) on a cycle ergometer under both normal and hypothermic conditions. To induce hypothermia, subjects took cold showers for 60 to 90 minutes (water temperature 16° ± 1°C) prior to exercising. The cold shower reduced rectal temperature by approximately 3°C. For subjects who were visibly shivering, a 1-minute warm shower given at the end of the cold shower eliminated the shivering response. This brief warming did not appreciably affect hypothermia, because rectal temperature remained unchanged.

Measurements included oxygen uptake ($\dot{V}O_2$), carbon dioxide production ($\dot{V}CO_2$), and ventilation volume ($\dot{V}E$) each minute during exercise. The figure presents the ventilatory equivalent for CO_2 ($\dot{V}E/\dot{V}CO_2$) plotted against rectal temperature under both conditions. Because ventilation during exercise is more closely related to $\dot{V}CO_2$ than $\dot{V}O_2$, the $\dot{V}E/\dot{V}CO_2$ permitted comparisons of ventilation normalized to a subject's CO_2 production. The $\dot{V}E/\dot{V}CO_2$ during exercise remained unaffected by body temperature—shown by the nearly horizontal plot of the data. Also, the $\dot{V}O_2$, $\dot{V}CO_2$, and $\dot{V}E$ did not differ significantly during normothermic and hypothermic conditions. The authors reasoned that if body temperature had a specific ventilatory stimulus during exercise (independent of some function of $\dot{V}CO_2$), then elevation in $\dot{V}E/\dot{V}CO_2$ would occur at higher body temperatures. The results ruled out changes in core temperature as an important independent stimulus to minute ventilation during exercise.

Gas Exchange and Transport

The body's supply of oxygen depends on the **concentration** and **pressure** of this gas in ambient air. Ambient air remains relatively constant in composition, comprising approximately 20.93% oxygen, 79.04% nitrogen (including small quantities of other inert gases that behave physiologically as nitrogen), 0.03% carbon dioxide, and usually small quantities of water vapor. The gas molecules move at relatively high speeds and exert a pressure against any surface with which they come in contact. At sea level, the pressure of these air molecules is sufficient to raise a column of mercury to a height of 760 mm or 29.9 inches.[a] The barometric reading varies somewhat with changing weather conditions and is considerably lower at higher altitudes (see Chapter 24).

PART 1
GASEOUS EXCHANGE IN THE LUNGS AND TISSUES

CONCENTRATIONS AND PARTIAL PRESSURES OF RESPIRED GASES

The molecules of each specific gas in a mixture of gases exerts their own **partial pressure**. The total pressure of the mixture is the sum of the partial pressures of the individual gases. Partial pressure is computed as:

$$\text{Partial pressure} = \frac{\text{Percent}}{\text{concentration}} \times \frac{\text{Total pressure}}{\text{of gas mixture}}$$

AMBIENT AIR

Table 13.1 lists the volumes, percentages, and partial pressures of the gases in dry ambient air at sea level. The partial pressure of oxygen is 20.93% of the total pressure of 760 mm Hg exerted by air, or 159 mm Hg (20.93/100 × 760 mm Hg); the random movement of the minute quantity of carbon dioxide exerts a pressure of only 0.23 mm Hg (0.03/100 × 760 mm Hg), while the molecules of nitrogen exert a pressure that raises the mercury in a manometer to about 600 mm (79.04/100 × 760 mm Hg). Partial pressure is usually denoted by a P in front of the gas symbol. The partial pressures at sea level for the principal components of ambient air are as follows: oxygen (P_{O_2}), 159 mm Hg; carbon dioxide (P_{CO_2}), 0.2 mm Hg; and nitrogen (P_{N_2}), 601 mm Hg.

TRACHEAL AIR

Air becomes completely saturated with water vapor when it enters the nasal cavities and mouth and passes down the respiratory tract. This vapor dilutes the inspired air mixture somewhat. At a body temperature of 37°C, for example, the pressure of water molecules in humidified air is 47 mm Hg; this leaves 713 mm Hg (760 − 47 mm) as the total pressure exerted by the inspired dry air molecules. Consequently, the effective P_{O_2} in **tracheal air** is reduced by about 10 mm Hg from its ambient value of 159 mm Hg to 149 mm Hg [0.2093 (760 − 47 mm Hg)]. The humidification process exerts little effect on the inspired P_{CO_2} because of the negligible contribution of carbon dioxide to inspired air.

ALVEOLAR AIR

The composition of alveolar air differs considerably from the incoming breath of moist ambient air because carbon dioxide is continually entering the alveoli from the blood, whereas oxygen is leaving the lungs to be carried throughout the body. As shown in Table 13.2, alveolar air contains approximately 14.5% oxygen, 5.5% carbon dioxide, and about 80.0% nitrogen. After subtracting the vapor pressure of moist alveolar gas, the average alveolar P_{O_2} becomes 103 mm Hg [0.145 (760 − 47 mm Hg)] and 39 mm Hg [0.055 (760 − 47 mm Hg)] for P_{CO_2}. *These values represent the average pressures exerted by oxygen and carbon dioxide molecules against the alveolar side of the alveolar-capillary membrane.* They are not physiologic constants but vary somewhat with the phase of the ventilatory cycle and the adequacy of ventilation in various portions of the lung. Recall that a relatively

---

[a] The **torr**—named after the Italian physicist and mathematician Evangelista Torricelli (1608–1647), who invented the barometer—is not an SI unit, but is commonly used to express gas pressure. One torr is the pressure sufficient to support a 1-mm column of mercury 1 mm high at 0°C against the standard acceleration of gravity at 45° north latitude (980.6 cm · s^{-2}). One standard atmosphere equals 760 torr.

large volume of air remains in the lungs after each normal exhalation. This functional residual capacity serves as a damper, so each incoming breath of air has only a small effect on the composition of alveolar air. This explains why the partial pressures of alveolar gases remain relatively stable.

TABLE 13.1
PARTIAL PRESSURE AND VOLUME OF THE GASES IN DRY AMBIENT AIR AT SEA LEVEL

Gas	Percentage	Partial Pressure[a] (mm Hg)	Volume of Gas (mL · L⁻¹)
Oxygen	20.93	159	209.3
Carbon dioxide	0.03	0.2	0.4
Nitrogen	79.04[b]	600	790.3

[a]At 760 mm Hg ambient air pressure.
[b]Includes 0.93% argon and other trace rare gases.

TABLE 13.2
PARTIAL PRESSURE AND VOLUME OF DRY ALVEOLAR GASES AT SEA LEVEL (37°C)

Gas	Percentage	Partial Pressure[a] (mm Hg)	Volume of Gas (mL · L⁻¹)
Oxygen	14.5	103	145
Carbon dioxide	5.5	39	55
Nitrogen[b]	80.0	571	800
Water vapor		47	

[a]At 760 − 47 mm Hg alveolar gas pressure.
[b]Nitrogen occupies a slightly greater percentage of alveolar air than ambient air because, under most metabolic conditions, less carbon dioxide is produced in relation to oxygen consumed (i.e., the respiratory quotient [$RQ = \dot{V}CO_2 \div \dot{V}O_2$] is less than 1.00). Because of this exchange imbalance, the nitrogen percentage increases.

MOVEMENT OF GAS IN AIR AND FLUIDS

In accordance with **Henry's law** (named after William Henry, an English chemist, 1775–1836), two factors determine the amount of gas that dissolves in a fluid:

- The **pressure differential** between the gas above the fluid and that dissolved in the fluid, and
- The **solubility** of the gas in the fluid

PRESSURE

Oxygen molecules continually strike the surface of the water in the three chambers illustrated in Figure 13.1. Because the pure water in chamber A contains no oxygen (P = 0 mm Hg), a large number of oxygen molecules enter the water and become dissolved in it. Because dissolved gas molecules also move randomly, some oxygen molecules leave the water. In chamber B, the net movement of oxygen is still into the fluid from the gaseous state. Eventually, however, the number of molecules entering and leaving the fluid becomes equal, as occurs in chamber C. When this happens, the gas pressures equilibrate, with no net diffusion of oxygen either into or out of the water. Conversely, if the pressure of dissolved oxygen molecules exceeds the pressure of the free gas in the air, oxygen leaves the fluid until a new pressure equilibrium is reached.

SOLUBILITY

For two different gases at identical pressures, the number of molecules moving into or out of a fluid is determined by the solubility of each gas. For each unit of pressure favoring diffusion, approximately 25 times more carbon dioxide than oxygen moves into (or from) a fluid. Viewed in another way, equal quantities of oxygen and carbon dioxide enter or leave a fluid under significantly different pressure gradients for each gas. This is precisely what takes place in the body.

FIGURE 13.1
Solution of oxygen in water. **A,** When oxygen first comes in contact with pure water. **B,** After the dissolved oxygen is halfway to equilibrium with gaseous oxygen. **C,** Equilibrium is established between the oxygen in air and in water.

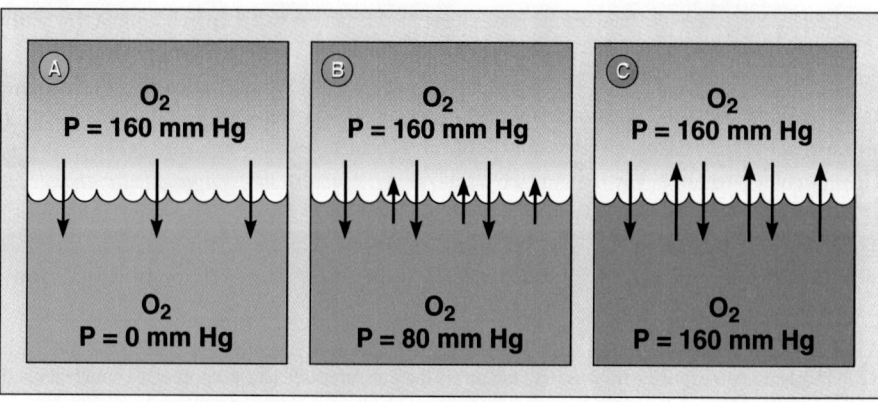

GAS EXCHANGE IN THE LUNGS AND TISSUES

The exchange of gases between the lungs and the blood, as well as their movement at the tissue level, is due entirely to the passive process of diffusion. Figure 13.2 illustrates the pressure gradients favoring gas transfer in the body at rest.

GAS EXCHANGE IN THE LUNGS

At rest, the pressure of oxygen molecules of 100 mm Hg in the alveoli is about 60 mm Hg greater than in the venous blood (40 mm Hg) entering the pulmonary capillaries. Consequently, oxygen dissolves and diffuses through the alveolar membrane into the blood. Carbon dioxide, on the other hand, exists under a slightly greater pressure in returning venous blood than it does in the alveoli. Thus, there is a net diffusion of carbon dioxide from the blood into the lungs. Although the pressure gradient of 6 mm Hg for carbon dioxide diffusion is small compared to the pressure gradient for oxygen, adequate transfer of carbon dioxide occurs rapidly due to its high solubility in plasma. Nitrogen, which is neither utilized nor produced in metabolic reactions, remains essentially unchanged in alveolar-capillary gas.

The process of gas exchange is so rapid in the healthy lung that to reach an equilibrium between blood and alveolar gas takes only about 0.25 second, or at about one-third of the blood's transit time through the lungs. For most people, even in intense exercise, the time it takes for red blood cells to pass through the pulmonary capillaries is maintained within half the time at rest. One important reason for this relatively slow velocity of pulmonary blood flow is that, with increasing exercise intensity, the pulmonary capillaries can increase the volume of blood contained within them by about 3 times the resting value.[2] With complete aeration, the blood leaving the lungs for delivery throughout the body contains oxygen at a pressure of approximately 100 mm Hg and carbon dioxide at 40 mm Hg, and these values vary little during vigorous exercise.[b]

In pulmonary disease, the gas transfer capacity of the blood-gas membrane is impaired due to a buildup of a pollutant layer or thickening of the alveolar membrane or a reduction of alveolar surface. This extends the time before alveolar capillary gas attains equilibration. When the added demand for gas exchange occurs with exercise, adequate aeration cannot be achieved and exercise performance is severely compromised.

GAS TRANSFER IN THE TISSUES

In the tissues, where oxygen is consumed in energy metabolism and an almost equal amount of carbon dioxide is produced, gas pressures can differ considerably from those in arterial blood. At rest, the average P_{O_2} in the fluid immediately outside a muscle cell is about 40 mm Hg, and the cellular P_{CO_2} averages 46 mm Hg. In heavy exercise, however, the pressure of oxygen molecules in the muscle tissue may fall toward 0 mm Hg,[18] whereas the pressure of carbon dioxide approaches 90 mm Hg. *The pressure differences between gases in the plasma and those in the tissues establish the gradients for diffusion.* Oxygen leaves the blood and diffuses toward the metabolizing cell, while carbon dioxide flows from the cell into the blood. This blood then passes into the venous circuit (venules and veins) and is returned to the heart to be pumped to the lungs. Diffusion rapidly begins once again as the blood enters the dense capillary network of the lungs. The body does not attempt to rid itself completely of carbon dioxide. To the contrary, as the blood leaves the lungs with a P_{CO_2} of 40 mm Hg, it still contains about 50 mL of carbon dioxide in each 100 mL of blood. As discussed in the next chapter, this small amount of "background-level" carbon dioxide is vital because it provides the chemical basis to control breathing through its stimulating effect on the neurons of the pons and medullary centers of the brainstem. This collection of neural tissue in the brain is known as the **respiratory center.**

If it were not for our capacity to breathe, some average pressure would be reached between alveolar and blood gases and diffusion would cease. By bringing in another breath of air, the oxygen content of the alveoli increases, whereas the carbon dioxide becomes diluted. *Because alveolar ventilation is adjusted to metabolic demands, the composition of alveolar gas remains remarkably constant, even during strenuous exercise that increases oxygen uptake and carbon dioxide output up to 25 times.*

■ S U M M A R Y ■

1. Gas molecules diffuse in the lungs and tissues down their concentration gradients from an area of higher concentration (higher pressure) to one of lower concentration (lower pressure).
2. The partial pressure of a specific gas in a mixture of gases is proportional to the concentration of the gas and the total pressure exerted by the mixture.

---

[b]The P_{O_2} of arterial blood is usually slightly lower than the alveolar P_{O_2}, because some blood in the alveolar capillaries may pass through poorly ventilated alveoli. Also, the blood leaving the lungs is joined by venous blood from the bronchial and cardiac circulations. This small amount of poorly oxygenated blood is termed **venous admixture.** Although its effect is small in healthy individuals, it does reduce the arterial P_{O_2} slightly below that in pulmonary end-capillary blood.

FIGURE 13.2

Pressure gradients for gas transfer in the body at rest. In **A**, the Po_2 and Pco_2 of ambient, tracheal, and alveolar air are shown along with these gas pressures in venous and arterial blood and muscle tissue. Movement of gas at the alveolar-capillary and tissue-capillary membranes is always from an area of higher partial pressure to one of lower partial pressure. The time required for gas exchange is shown in **B**. At rest, blood remains in the pulmonary and tissue capillaries for about 0.75 s. In pulmonary disease (*dashed line*), the rate of gas transfer across the alveolar-capillary membrane is impaired, thus prolonging the time for equilibration of gases. During maximal exercise, the transit time is reduced to about 0.4 s, but this is usually still adequate in the healthy lung for complete aeration of the blood. The details of gas exchange (diffusion) between the capillaries and the tissues are illustrated in **C**.

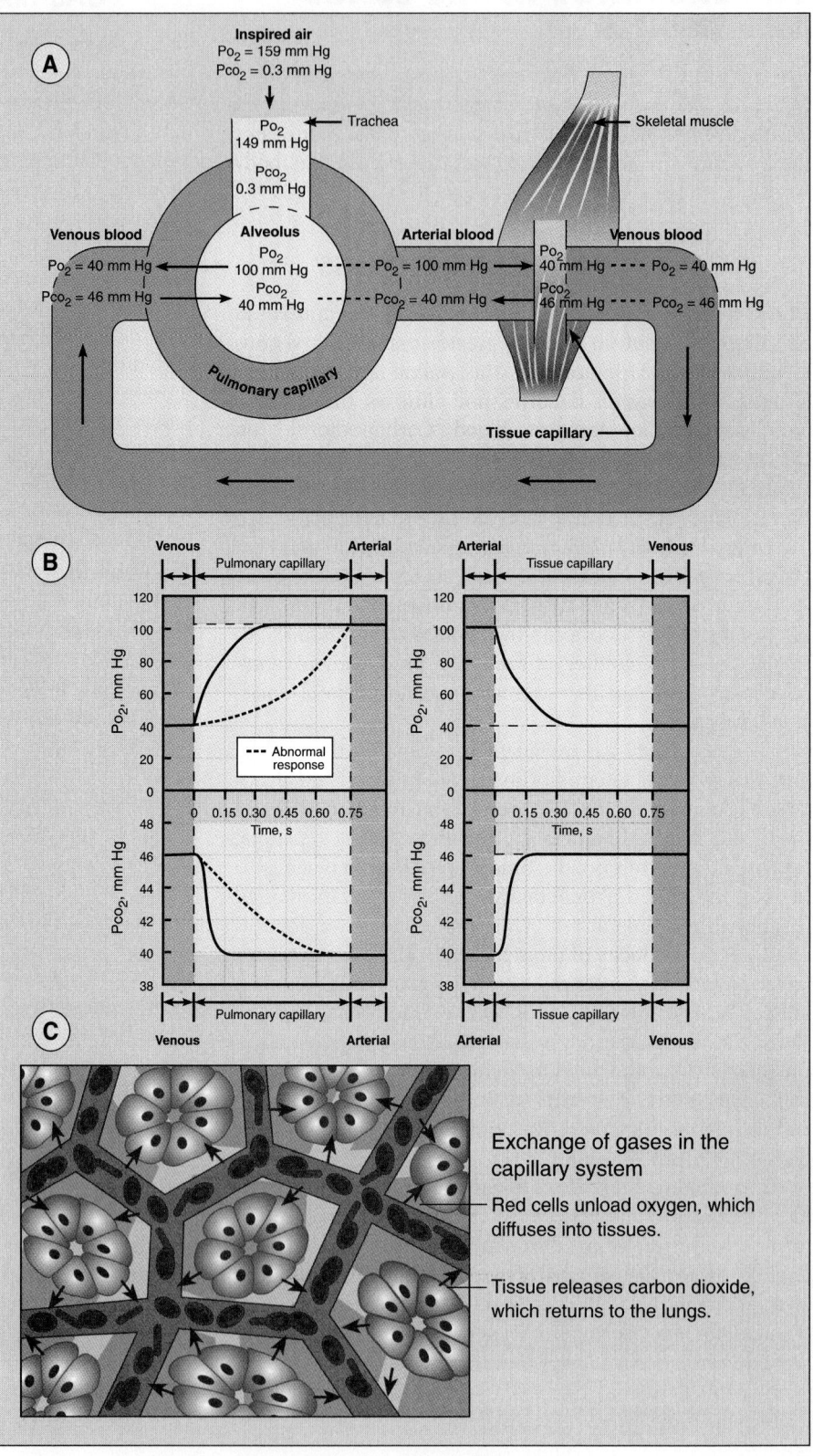

Exchange of gases in the capillary system

Red cells unload oxygen, which diffuses into tissues.

Tissue releases carbon dioxide, which returns to the lungs.

3. Henry's law states that the quantity of gas that dissolves in a fluid is determined by its pressure gradient and solubility. Because the solubility of carbon dioxide in plasma is about 25 times greater than that of oxygen, large amounts of carbon dioxide move into and out of body fluids down a relatively small diffusion (pressure) gradient.

4. At rest and during exercise, adjustments in alveolar ventilation occur so the composition of alveolar gas remains remarkably constant. Oxygen pressure is maintained at about 100 mm Hg and carbon dioxide pressure at 40 mm Hg. Because venous blood contains oxygen at lower pressure and carbon dioxide at higher pressure than alveolar gas, oxygen diffuses into the blood and carbon dioxide diffuses into the lungs.

5. Gas exchange is so rapid in the healthy lung that equilibrium occurs at about the midpoint of the blood's transit through the pulmonary capillaries. Even with vigorous exercise, the velocity of blood flow through the lungs generally does not restrict the full loading of oxygen and unloading of carbon dioxide.

6. In the tissues, the diffusion gradient favors the movement of oxygen from the capillaries to the tissues and carbon dioxide from the cells to the blood. During exercise, these gradients expand, and oxygen and carbon dioxide diffuse rapidly.

PART 2
TRANSPORT OF OXYGEN

TRANSPORT OF OXYGEN IN THE BLOOD

Oxygen is carried in the blood in one of two ways:

• In physical solution dissolved in the fluid portion of the blood, or

• In loose combination with hemoglobin, the iron-protein compound in the red blood cell

OXYGEN IN SOLUTION

Because oxygen is not particularly soluble in fluids, its concentration in the body fluids is low. At an alveolar P_{O_2} of 100 mm Hg, only about 0.3 mL of gaseous oxygen dissolves in each 100 mL of blood (0.003 mL for each additional 1 mm Hg increase in P_{O_2}); this is equivalent to 3 mL of oxygen per liter of blood. Because the blood volume of an averaged-sized person is about 5 L, 15 mL of oxygen is carried dissolved in the fluid portion of the blood (3 mL per liter × 5). Unfortunately, this is only enough oxygen to sustain life for about 4 seconds! Viewed from a somewhat different perspective, if oxygen alone in physical solution was

available to the body, about 80 L of blood would have to be circulated each minute to supply the resting oxygen requirements. This rate is about 2 times higher than the maximum blood flow ever recorded for an exercising human!

As occurs for carbon dioxide, the small quantity of oxygen transported in physical solution serves several important physiologic functions. The random movement of dissolved oxygen molecules establishes the P_{O_2} of the blood and tissue fluids. This pressure plays a role in the regulation of breathing; it also determines the loading of hemoglobin in the lungs and the subsequent release of oxygen in the tissues.

OXYGEN COMBINED WITH HEMOGLOBIN

Metallic compounds are present in the blood of many species of animals and serve to augment the blood's oxygen-carrying capacity. In humans, this compound is **hemoglobin,** the iron-containing globular protein pigment illustrated in Figure 13.3. About 280 million hemoglobin molecules are crowded into each of the body's more than 25 trillion red blood cells; this concentration of hemoglobin permits the blood to carry 65 to 70 times more oxygen than is normally dissolved in plasma. Thus, in each liter of blood, about 197 mL of oxygen is temporarily "captured" by hemoglobin. Each of the four iron atoms in the hemoglobin molecule can loosely bind one molecule of oxygen in the following reversible reaction:

$$Hb_4 + 4O_2 \rightleftarrows Hb_4O_8$$

This reaction requires no enzymes; it occurs without a change in the valence of Fe^{2+}, as would occur in the more permanent process of oxidation. *The oxygenation of hemoglobin to oxyhemoglobin depends entirely on the partial pressure of oxygen in solution.*

Oxygen-Carrying Capacity of Hemoglobin

In men, there is approximately 15 to 16 g of hemoglobin in each 100 mL of blood. The value is about 5 to 10% less for women and averages about 14 g per 100 mL of blood. This sex difference accounts to some degree for the lower aerobic capacity of women relative to men, even after considering differences in body mass and body fat. The reason for the difference may be the stimulating effects on red blood cell production of the "male" hormone testosterone.

Each gram of hemoglobin can combine loosely with 1.34 mL of oxygen. Thus, if the hemoglobin content of the blood is known, its oxygen-carrying capacity can easily be calculated as follows:

$$\begin{array}{ccc} \text{Blood's oxygen} & & \\ \text{capacity} & = & \text{Hemoglobin} \\ \text{(mL} \cdot \text{100 mL blood)}^{-1} & & \text{(g} \cdot \text{100 mL blood)}^{-1} \end{array} \times \begin{array}{c} \text{Oxygen capacity} \\ \text{of hemoglobin} \end{array}$$

$$20 \text{ mL O}_2 \quad = \quad 15 \quad \times 1.34 \text{ mL O}_2 \cdot \text{g}^{-1}$$

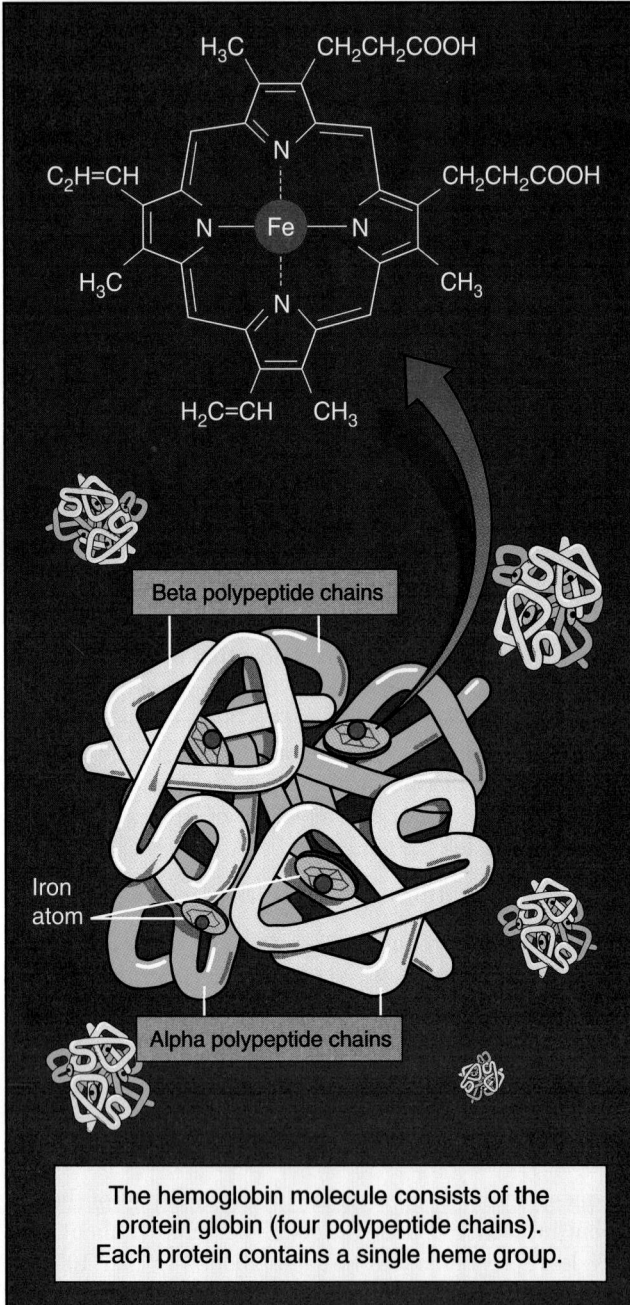

The hemoglobin molecule consists of the protein globin (four polypeptide chains). Each protein contains a single heme group.

FIGURE 13.3

The hemoglobin molecule consists of the protein globin, which is composed of four subunit polypeptide chains. Each of these polypeptides contains a single heme group with its single iron atom that acts as a "magnet" for oxygen.

TABLE 13.3
HEMOGLOBIN (Hb) LEVELS AND EXERCISE HEART RATE RESPONSES OF NORMAL SUBJECTS AND ANEMIC SUBJECTS PRIOR TO AND FOLLOWING SUPPLEMENTAL IRON TREATMENT

Subjects	Hb (g per 100 mL blood) (Average)	Peak Exercise Heart Rate (Average)
Normal		
Men	14.3	119
Women	13.9	142
Iron-Deficient Men		
Pretreatment	7.1	155
Post-treatment	14.0	113
Iron-Deficient Women		
Pretreatment	7.7	152
Post-treatment	12.4	123
Iron-Deficient Men		
Preplacebo	7.7	146
Post-placebo	7.4	137
Iron-Deficient Women		
Preplacebo	8.1	154
Post-placebo	8.4	144

From Gardner, G.W., et al.: Cardiorespiratory, hematological, and physical performance responses of anemic subjects to iron treatment. *Am. J. Clin. Nutr.*, 28:982, 1975.

On average, approximately 20 mL of oxygen would be carried with the hemoglobin in each 100 mL of whole blood when its hemoglobin is fully saturated with oxygen; that is, when all of the hemoglobin is converted to HbO_2.[c]

Anemia affects oxygen transport. The blood's oxygen transport capacity changes only slightly with normal variations in hemoglobin content. On the other hand, a significant decrease in the iron content of the red blood cell, as occurs in **iron-deficiency anemia,** reduces the blood's oxygen-carrying capacity and correspondingly reduces a person's capacity for sustaining even mild aerobic exercise.[5] The data in Table 13.3 were obtained from 29 iron-deficient anemic men and women with low hemoglobin levels. They were placed in one of two groups; one group received intramuscular injections of iron over an 80-day period, while the placebo group received similar

---

[c]Physiologists often use the term volume percent (vol%) to describe the content of oxygen in blood. In this regard, volume percent refers to the amount in milliliters of a gas that can be extracted (in a vacuum) from a 100-mL sample of either whole blood (with plasma) or packed red blood cells. While the oxygen capacity of a sample of packed human red blood cells is 45.7 vol%, it is significantly higher for species of mammals that reside at high altitudes. The capacity of packed red blood cells to hold oxygen is about 58 vol% for the llama and vicuña, two members of the camel family that work at altitudes between 15,000 and 17,000 feet. This is particularly advantageous at high altitudes, where the arterial Po_2 may fall to only 40 mm Hg. In this environment, human whole blood will hold oxygen at 14 vol%, while the capacity of vicuña blood is 29% higher at 18 vol%!

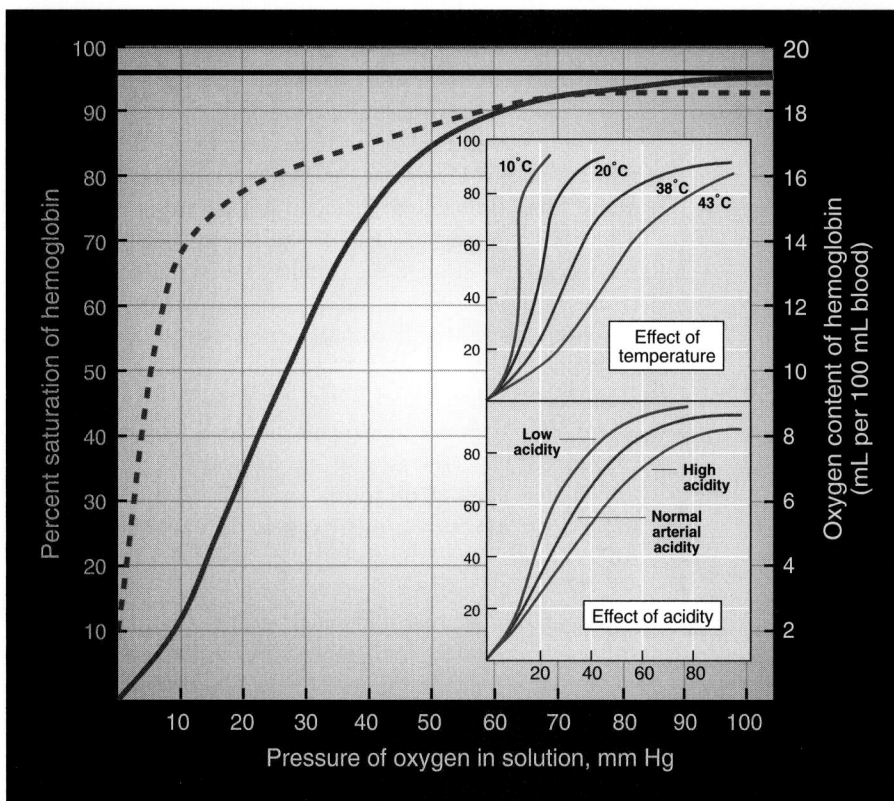

FIGURE 13.4

The oxyhemoglobin dissociation curve. Indicated are the percent saturation of hemoglobin (*solid line*) and myoglobin (*dashed line*) in relation to oxygen pressure. The right ordinate shows the quantity of oxygen carried in each 100 mL of blood under normal conditions. The inset curves illustrate the effects of temperature and acidity in altering hemoglobin's affinity for oxygen (Bohr effect). The bold horizontal line at the top indicates percent saturation of hemoglobin at the average sea-level alveolar P_{O_2}.

intramuscular injections of a colored saline solution. A third group with normal hemoglobin levels served as controls. All groups were tested during exercise prior to the experiment and after 80 days of either iron therapy or placebo treatment. The results show clearly that the anemic group given the iron supplement improved significantly in exercise response compared to their non-supplemented counterparts. Peak heart rate measured during a 5-minute stepping performance decreased from 155 to 113 beats per minute for men and from 152 to 123 beats per minute for women. This translated into an average of 15% more oxygen delivered per heart beat.

P_{O_2} and Hemoglobin Saturation

The binding of oxygen to hemoglobin is known as cooperative binding because when an oxygen molecule binds to the iron atom in one of the four globin chains (Fig. 13.3), it becomes progressively easier for the next molecules to bind. This aspect of cooperative binding is explained by the sigmoid shape of the oxygen saturation curve for hemoglobin.

Figure 13.4 shows the **oxyhemoglobin dissociation curve,** which illustrates the saturation of hemoglobin with oxygen at various P_{O_2} values, including that of normal alveolar-capillary gas (P_{O_2} = 100 mm Hg). Shown on the

right ordinate of this dissociation curve is the quantity of oxygen carried in each 100 mL of normal blood at a particular plasma P_{O_2} value. Dissociation curves are usually established by exposing about 280 to 320 mL of blood in a sealed glass vessel (tonometer) to various pressures of oxygen. Once the blood-gas mixture at a particular pH has equilibrated in a water bath of known temperature, the oxygen content and percent saturation of the blood are determined. Percent saturation is calculated as:

$$\text{Percent saturation} = \frac{\text{O}_2 \text{ combined with hemoglobin}}{\text{O}_2 \text{ capacity of hemoglobin}} \times 100$$

P_{O_2} IN THE LUNG

So far, it has been assumed that hemoglobin becomes fully saturated with oxygen when exposed to alveolar gas. *This is not exactly the case, however, because hemoglobin is about 98% saturated with oxygen at the average sea level alveolar P_{O_2} of 100 mm Hg.* By applying this partial pressure value of 100 mm Hg to the right ordinate of Figure 13.4, it is seen that for each 100 mL of blood leaving the lungs, hemoglobin carries about 19.7 mL of oxygen. Clearly, any additional increase in alveolar P_{O_2} contributes little to the quantity of oxygen already com-

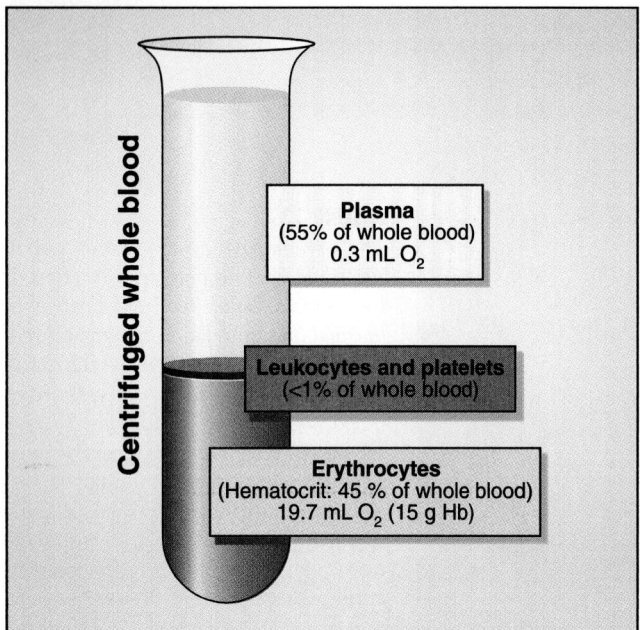

FIGURE 13.5
Major components of whole blood, including the quantity of oxygen carried in each 100 mL of blood (Hb, hemoglobin).

bined with hemoglobin. In addition to the oxygen bound to hemoglobin, the plasma of each 100 mL of arterial blood contains about 0.3 mL of oxygen in solution. Thus, for healthy individuals who breathe ambient air at sea level, approximately 20.0 mL of oxygen is carried in each 100 mL of blood leaving the lungs; 19.7 mL is bound to hemoglobin and 0.3 mL is dissolved in plasma. Figure 13.5 displays the percentage composition of centrifuged whole blood for plasma and red blood cells (called the **hematocrit**), including representative values for the quantity of oxygen carried in each component.

It is common in some athletic competitions to see an athlete breathing a gas mixture of concentrated oxygen following strenuous exercise. Based on the oxyhemoglobin dissociation curve, there really is little chance that the additional pressure of supplemental oxygen inhaled at either sea level or low altitude could markedly augment the delivery of oxygen to the tissues. This topic is discussed in more detail in Chapter 23 on ergogenic aids.

Figure 13.4 also shows that the saturation of hemoglobin changes little until the pressure of oxygen declines to about 60 mm Hg. This flat, upper portion of the oxyhemoglobin dissociation curve provides a margin of safety to ensure that the arterial blood is adequately loaded with oxygen. Even if the alveolar PO_2 decreases to 75 mm Hg, as could occur with certain lung diseases or when one travels to a higher altitude, the saturation of hemoglobin is only lowered by about 6%. At an alveolar PO_2 of 60 mm Hg, hemoglobin is still 90% saturated with oxygen! Below this pressure, however, there is a sharp decrease in the quantity of oxygen that combines with hemoglobin.

PO_2 IN THE TISSUES

At rest, the PO_2 in the cell fluids is approximately 40 mm Hg. Dissolved oxygen from the plasma diffuses across the capillary membrane through the tissue fluids into the cells. This reduces plasma PO_2 below the PO_2 in the red blood cell, and hemoglobin is unable to maintain its high oxygen saturation. The released oxygen ($HbO_2 \rightarrow Hb + O_2$) moves out of the blood cells through the capillary membrane and into the tissues.

At the tissue-capillary PO_2 at rest (PO_2 = 40 mm Hg), hemoglobin holds about 70% of its original total oxygen (Fig. 13.4). When blood leaves the tissues, it carries about 15 mL of oxygen in each 100 mL of blood, as about 5 mL of oxygen has been released to the tissues. This difference in the oxygen content of arterial and mixed venous blood is termed the **arteriovenous oxygen difference**, or **a-v̄ O_2 difference**.

The a-v̄ O_2 difference at rest normally averages 4 to 5 mL of oxygen per 100 mL of blood. The large quantity of oxygen still remaining with hemoglobin provides an "automatic" reserve so the cells can immediately obtain oxygen should the metabolic demands suddenly increase. As the cell's need for oxygen increases in exercise, the tissue PO_2 becomes reduced and a larger quantity of oxygen is rapidly released. During vigorous exercise, when the extracellular PO_2 decreases to about 15 mm Hg, only about 5 mL of oxygen remains bound to hemoglobin. As a result, the a-v̄ O_2 difference increases to 15 mL of oxygen per 100 mL of blood. When the tissue PO_2 falls to about 3 mm Hg during exhaustive exercise, virtually all of the oxygen is released from the blood that perfuses the active tissues. This occurs even without any increase in local blood flow, and the amount of oxygen released to the muscles increases almost three times above that normally supplied at rest—just by a more complete unloading of hemoglobin.

The Bohr Effect

The solid line in Figure 13.4 represents the oxyhemoglobin dissociation curve under resting physiologic conditions at an arterial pH of 7.4 and tissue temperature of 37°C. The inset curves depict other important characteristics of hemoglobin. For example, any increase in acidity, temperature, or concentration of carbon dioxide causes the dissociation curve to shift significantly downward and to the right. This phenomenon is called the **Bohr effect** after its discoverer, Christian Bohr, the father of Nobel physicist Niels Bohr. The Bohr effect reflects an alteration in the molecular structure of hemoglobin. It describes the reduced effectiveness of hemoglobin to hold oxygen, particularly in the PO_2 range of 20 to 50 mm Hg. The Bohr effect is particularly important in vigorous exercise because even more oxygen is released to the tissues due to the accompanying increases in metabolic heat, carbon dioxide, and blood lactate. At the

PO_2 in the alveoli, however, the Bohr effect becomes negligible on pulmonary capillary blood, allowing hemoglobin to load completely with oxygen as blood passes through the lungs, even during maximal exercise.

Red Blood Cell 2,3-DPG

The compound **2,3-diphosphoglycerate,** or 2,3-DPG, is produced within the red blood cell during the anaerobic reactions of glycolysis. (Because the red blood cell contains no mitochondria, its energy is supplied solely by the anaerobic reactions of glycolysis; this contributes to the level of plasma lactate at rest.) 2,3-DPG binds loosely with subunits of the hemoglobin molecule, thus reducing its affinity for oxygen. This causes more oxygen to be released to the tissues for a given decrease in PO_2.[3]

Individuals with cardiopulmonary disorders, and those who live at high altitudes, have an increased level of red blood cell 2,3-DPG.[11] This apparently provides a compensatory adjustment to facilitate oxygen release to the cells. The presence of 2,3-DPG would also aid in oxygen transfer to the muscles during strenuous exercise.[9] Conflicting results have been reported in comparing the 2,3-DPG level of trained and untrained subjects.[4, 12, 16] Significantly higher resting levels of this metabolic intermediate were observed in two groups of athletes than in untrained subjects.[19] The level of 2,3-DPG increased by 15% for the middle-distance runners following maximal exercise of short duration. Prolonged steady-rate exercise, on the other hand, produced a small decrease in 2,3-DPG in endurance athletes. These data support the idea that increases in 2,3-DPG with intense exercise (and perhaps training) reflect an adaptive response to augment oxygen delivery to active tissues. More than likely, the effect of different types of exercise on the level of this compound reflects the specific metabolic demands of exercise. Furthermore, females have significantly higher levels of red blood cell 2,3-DPG compared to male counterparts of similar fitness status and activity level. This possible sex difference might compensate for the lower hemoglobin levels routinely noted among females.[14]

MYOGLOBIN, THE MUSCLE'S OXYGEN STORE

Myoglobin, a globular protein, is an iron-containing compound found in skeletal and cardiac muscle, and functions as a storage site for oxygen. Myoglobin was the first protein whose structural details were uncovered by the process of x-ray crystallography. The molecule contains a peptide backbone and, embedded within it, the heme group with its metallic Fe_2^+. Reddish muscle fibers have a high concentration of this respiratory pigment, whereas fibers deficient in myoglobin appear pale or white.[13] Myoglobin is similar to hemoglobin because it also combines reversibly with oxygen; however, each myoglobin molecule contains only one iron atom, in contrast to hemoglobin, which contains four atoms. Myoglobin adds additional oxygen to the muscle in the reaction:

$$Mb + O_2 \rightarrow MbO_2$$

Oxygen Released at Low Pressures

Aside from its function as an "extra" source of oxygen in muscle, myoglobin probably facilitates the transfer of oxygen to the mitochondria, especially in the beginning of exercise and during intense exercise when there is a considerable drop in cellular PO_2.[21] From the dissociation curve for myoglobin shown in Figure 13.4 (dashed line), the line is not s-shaped as is the case with hemoglobin, but instead forms a rectangular hyperbola. What this means is that there is a steep rise in the amount of saturation in relation to PO_2 until an asymptote is approached. The curve then levels off, with very little change in saturation over a broad range of PO_2 values. In comparing the oxygen saturation curves for myoglobin and hemoglobin, it is seen that myoglobin binds and retains oxygen at low pressures much more readily than hemoglobin. During rest and moderate levels of exercise, myoglobin retains a high saturation with oxygen. For example, at a PO_2 of 40 mm Hg, myoglobin retains 95% of its oxygen. The greatest quantity of oxygen is released from MbO_2 when the tissue PO_2 drops below 5 mm Hg. Unlike hemoglobin, acidity, carbon dioxide, and temperature do not affect the oxygen-binding affinity of myoglobin, so it does not demonstrate a "Bohr effect."

Effects of Training

As might be expected, slow-twitch muscle fibers that have a high capacity to generate ATP aerobically contain relatively large quantities of myoglobin. In animals, the myoglobin level of muscle is also related to the animal's level of physical activity.[6, 10, 15] The leg muscles of active hunting dogs, for example, contain more myoglobin than the muscles of sedentary house pets;[20] this is also the case for grazing cattle compared to cattle that are penned.[17] What remains unclear is whether myoglobin levels can be enhanced in humans as part of the adaptive response to training.[1, 7, 8]

■ SUMMARY ■

1. Hemoglobin, the iron-protein pigment in the red blood cell, permits whole blood to carry about 65 times more oxygen than is carried in physical solution dissolved in the plasma.
2. The small amount of oxygen dissolved in plasma exerts molecular movement and establishes the partial pressure of oxygen in the blood. This determines the loading of hemoglobin at the lungs (oxygenation) and its unloading at the tissues (deoxygenation).

3. The blood's oxygen transport capacity varies only slightly with normal variations in hemoglobin content. Iron-deficiency anemia, however, significantly decreases the blood's oxygen-carrying capacity and consequently reduces aerobic exercise performance.

4. The "s" shape of the oxyhemoglobin dissociation curve shows that hemoglobin saturation changes very little until the PO_2 falls below 60 mm Hg. Because this low pressure occurs in the tissues, the quantity of oxygen bound to hemoglobin falls sharply. Thus, oxygen is released rapidly from capillary blood and flows into the tissues in response to the cells' increased metabolic demands.

5. At rest, only about 25% of the blood's total oxygen is released to the tissues; the remaining 75% returns "unused" to the heart in the venous blood. This difference, called the arteriovenous oxygen difference, indicates that an "automatic" reserve of oxygen exists so cells can rapidly obtain oxygen should there be a sudden increase in metabolic demands.

6. Increases in acidity, temperature, carbon dioxide concentration, and red blood cell 2,3-DPG cause alterations in the molecular structure of hemoglobin, thereby reducing its effectiveness to hold onto its oxygen. Because exercise accentuates these factors, the release of oxygen to the tissues is further facilitated.

7. In skeletal and cardiac muscle, the iron-protein pigment myoglobin acts as an "extra" oxygen store that releases its oxygen at low PO_2. During strenuous exercise, when cellular PO_2 is considerably decreased, myoglobin probably facilitates oxygen transfer to the mitochondria.

PART 3
TRANSPORT OF CARBON DIOXIDE

TRANSPORT OF CARBON DIOXIDE IN THE BLOOD

Once carbon dioxide is formed in the cell, its only means for "escape" is through the process of diffusion and subsequent transport in the venous blood on its way to the lungs. There are three ways that carbon dioxide is carried in the blood. As with oxygen, a small amount of carbon dioxide is carried in physical solution in the blood plasma. Carbon dioxide also combines with hemoglobin during transport, and a large fraction joins with water for delivery to the lung as **bicarbonate.** Figure 13.6 illustrates the various means of transporting carbon dioxide from the tissues to the lungs.

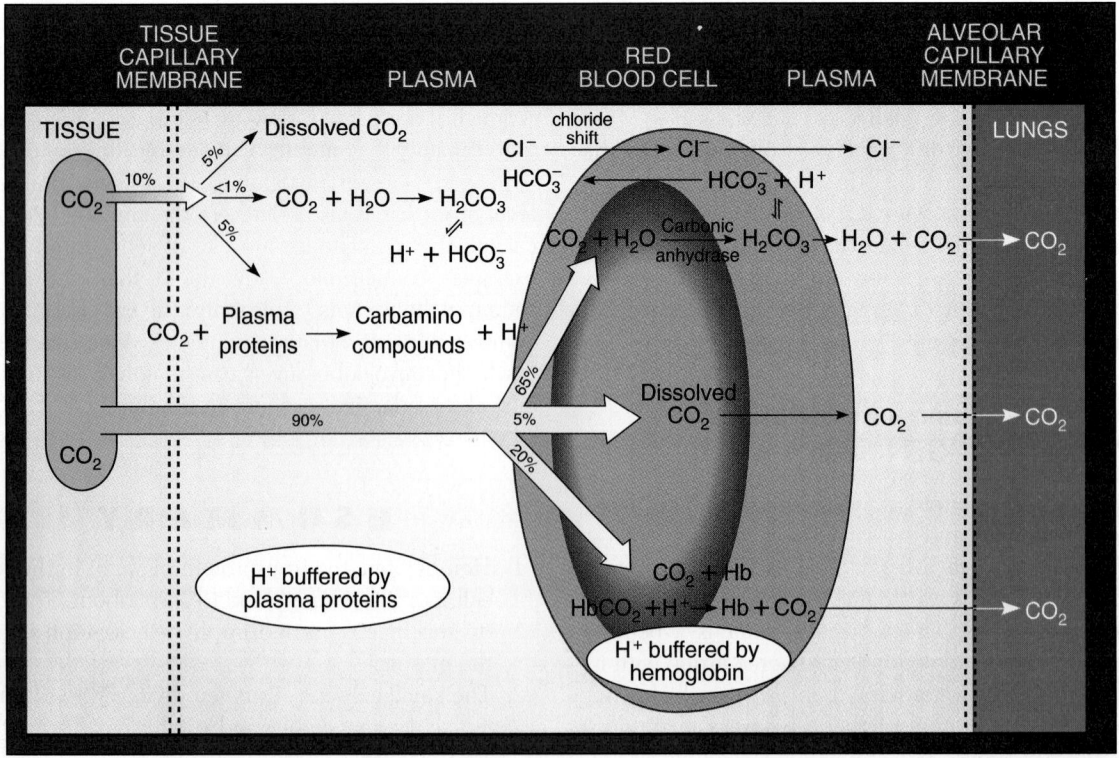

FIGURE 13.6

Transport of carbon dioxide in the plasma and red blood cells as dissolved CO_2, bicarbonate, and carbamino compounds. By far, the greatest amount of carbon dioxide combines with water to form carbonic acid.

CARBON DIOXIDE TRANSPORT IN SOLUTION

Approximately 5% of the carbon dioxide formed during energy metabolism moves in solution as free carbon dioxide in the plasma. *Although this quantity is relatively small, it is the random movement of the dissolved carbon dioxide molecules that establishes the P_{CO_2} in the blood.*

CARBON DIOXIDE TRANSPORT AS BICARBONATE

Carbon dioxide in solution combines with water to form carbonic acid in the following reversible reaction:

$$CO_2 + H_2O \rightleftharpoons H_2CO_3$$

This reaction is slow, and little carbon dioxide would be carried in this form without the action of **carbonic anhydrase,** a zinc-containing enzyme in the red blood cell. This catalyst accelerates the union of a mole of carbon dioxide and water per mole of enzyme to a rate of about 800,000 times a second or about 5,000 times faster than would normally occur without this enzyme. The reaction reaches equilibrium while the blood cell is still moving through the tissue's capillary.

Once carbonic acid is formed in the tissues, most of it ionizes into hydrogen ions (H^+) and bicarbonate ions (HCO_3^-) as follows:

In Tissues

$$CO_2 + H_2O \xrightarrow{\text{carbonic anhydrase}} H_2CO_3 \rightarrow H^+ + HCO_3^-$$

The H^+, buffered by the protein portion of hemoglobin, maintains the pH of the blood within relatively narrow limits (see "Acid-Base Regulation," Chapter 14). Because HCO_3^- remains quite soluble in blood, it diffuses from the red blood cell into the plasma in exchange for the chloride ion (Cl^-) that moves into the blood cell to maintain ionic equilibrium. This is known as the "chloride shift"; it causes the Cl^- content of the erythrocytes in venous blood to be higher than in the red blood cells of arterial blood, particularly during exercise.

Sixty to eighty percent of the total carbon dioxide exists as plasma bicarbonate. The bicarbonate is formed in accordance with the law of mass action; as tissue P_{CO_2} increases, carbonic acid is formed rapidly. Conversely, in the lungs, carbon dioxide leaves the blood, lowering the plasma P_{CO_2}. This disturbs the equilibrium between carbonic acid and the formation of bicarbonate ions. As a result, H^+ and HCO_3^- recombine to form carbonic acid. In turn, carbon dioxide and water reform and carbon dioxide exits through the lungs as follows:

In Lungs

$$H^+ + HCO_3^- \rightarrow H_2CO_3 \xrightarrow{\text{carbonic anhydrase}} CO_2 + H_2O$$

Because the plasma HCO_3^- is lowered in the pulmonary capillaries, the Cl^- moves from the red blood cell back into the plasma.

CARBON DIOXIDE TRANSPORT AS CARBAMINO COMPOUNDS

At the tissue level, carbon dioxide reacts directly with the amino acid molecules of blood proteins to form carbamino compounds. This is particularly true for the globin portion of hemoglobin, which carries about 20% of the body's carbon dioxide as follows:

$$CO_2 + \underset{\text{(Hemoglobin)}}{HbNH} \rightarrow \underset{\text{(Carbaminohemoglobin)}}{HbNHCOOH}$$

The formation of carbamino compounds is reversed as the plasma P_{CO_2} is lowered in the lungs. This causes carbon dioxide to move into solution and enter the alveoli. Concurrently, the oxygenation of hemoglobin reduces its binding ability for carbon dioxide. The interaction between oxygen loading and carbon dioxide release is termed the **Haldane effect.** This phenomenon facilitates the removal of carbon dioxide in the lung.

■ SUMMARY ■

1. A small amount of carbon dioxide is carried as free carbon dioxide in solution in the plasma. This dissolved carbon dioxide establishes the P_{CO_2} of the blood, which affects important physiologic functions.
2. The major quantity of carbon dioxide is transported in chemical combination with water and forms bicarbonate as follows:

$$CO_2 + H_2O \rightarrow H_2CO_3 \rightarrow H^+ + HCO_3^-$$

In the lungs, this reaction is reversed and carbon dioxide leaves the blood and enters the alveoli.
3. About 20% of the body's carbon dioxide combines with blood proteins, including hemoglobin, to form carbamino compounds.

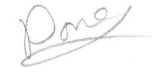

■ REFERENCES ■

1. Coyle, E.F., et al.: Time course of loss of adaptations after stopping prolonged intense endurance training. *J. Appl. Physiol.,* 57:1857, 1984.
2. Dempsey, J.A.: Is the lung built for exercise? *Med. Sci. Sports Exerc.,* 18:143, 1986.
3. Dempsey, J.A., et al.: Muscular exercise, 2,3-DPG and oxy-hemoglobin affinity. *Int. J. Physiol.,* 30:34, 1971.
4. Fornaini, G., et al.: Glucose utilization in human erythrocytes during physical exercise. *Med. Sci. Sports Exerc.,* 13:323, 1981.
5. Gardner, G.W., et al.: Cardiorespiratory, hematological and physical performance responses of anemic subjects to iron treatment. *Am. J. Clin. Nutr.,* 28:982, 1975.
6. Hickson, R.C.: Skeletal muscle cytochrome c and myoglobin, endurance, and frequency of training. *J. Appl. Physiol.,* 51:746, 1981.
7. Jacobs, I.: Sprint training effects on muscle myoglobin, enzymes, fiber types, and blood lactate. *Med. Sci. Sports Exerc.,* 19:368, 1987.
8. Jansson, E., et al.: Myoglobin in the quadriceps femoris muscle of competitive cyclists and untrained men. *Acta Physiol. Scand.,* 114:627, 1982.

9. Klein, J.P., et al.: Hemoglobin affinity for oxygen during short-term exhaustive exercise. *J. Appl. Physiol.,* 48:236, 1980.

10. Lawrie, R.A.: Effect of enforced exercise on myoglobin in muscle. *Nature,* 171:1069, 1953.

11. Lenfant, C., et al.: Effect of altitude on oxygen binding by hemoglobin and on organic phosphate levels. *J. Clin. Invest.,* 47:2652, 1968.

12. Lijnen, P., et al.: Erythrocyte 2,3-diphosphoglycerate and serum enzyme concentrations in trained and sedentary men. *Med. Sci. Sports Exerc.,* 18:174, 1986.

13. Nemeth, P.M., and Lowry, O.H.: Myoglobin in individual human skeletal muscle fibers of different types. *J. Histochem. Cytochem.,* 32:1211, 1984.

14. Pate, R.R., et al.: A physiological comparison of performance-matched female and male distance runners. *Res. Q. Exerc. Sport,* 56:245, 1985.

15. Pattengale, P.K., and Holloszy, J.O.: Augmentation of skeletal muscle myoglobin by a program of treadmill running. *Am. J. Physiol.,* 213:783, 1967.

16. Rand, P.W., et al.: Influence of athletic training on hemoglobin-oxygen affinity. *Am. J. Physiol.,* 224:1334, 1973.

17. Shenk, J.H., et al.: Spectrophotometric characteristics of hemoglobins. *J. Biol. Chem.,* 105;741, 1934.

18. Stainsby, W.N., and Otis, A.B.: Blood flow, blood oxygen tension, oxygen uptake and oxygen transport in skeletal muscle. *Am. J. Physiol.,* 206:858, 1964.

19. Taunton, J.E., et al.: Alterations in 2,3-dpg and P_{50} with maximal and submaximal exercise. *Med. Sci. Sports,* 6:238, 1974.

20. Whipple, G.H.: The hemoglobin of striated muscle. 1. Variations due to age and exercise. *Am. J. Physiol.,* 76:693, 1926.

21. Wittenberg, B.A., et al.: Role of myoglobin in the oxygen supply to red skeletal muscle. *J. Biol. Chem.,* 250:9038, 1975.

Wasserman, K., and McIlroy, M.B.: Detecting the threshold of anaerobic metabolism in cardiac patients during exercise. *Am. J. Cardiol.* 14:844, 1964.

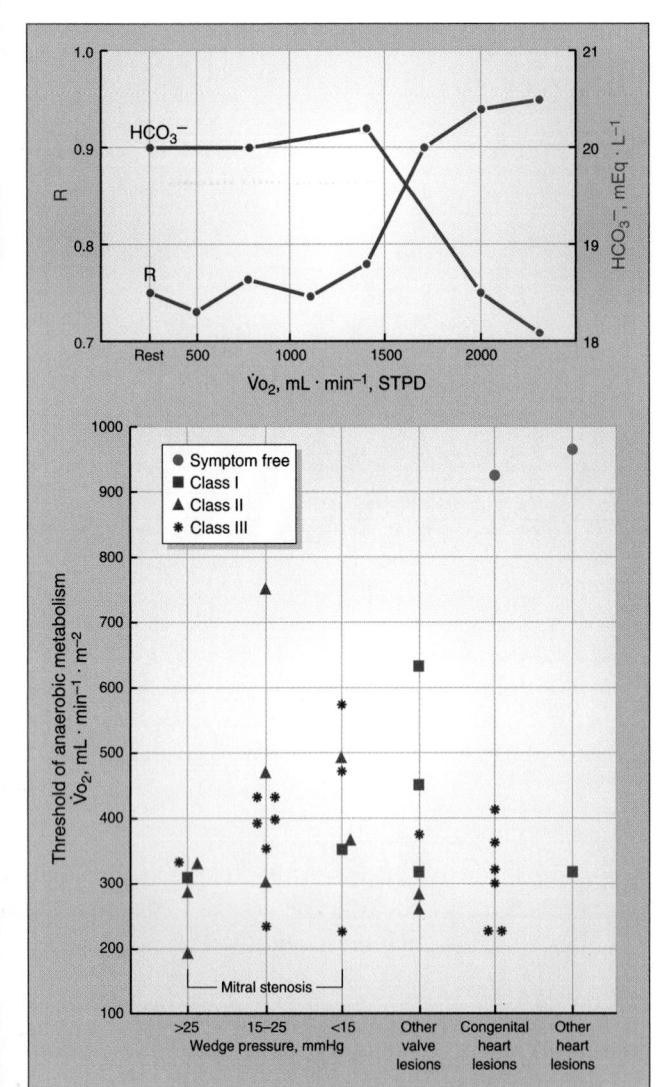

Top, Change in respiratory exchange ratio (R) and plasma bicarbonate (HCO_3^-) from rest and during continuous graded exercise in one subject. *Bottom,* Threshold of anaerobic metabolism in 37 patients with heart disease.

ity for sustained aerobic exercise. The pioneering work of Wasserman and colleagues presented the rationale and methodology using simple respiratory gas exchange data for detecting the onset of anaerobic metabolism; they named this point the "anaerobic threshold." These researchers argued that the threshold of anaerobic metabolism during exercise could be detected in one of three ways: (*a*) as an increase in the blood lactate concentration, (*b*) as a decrease in arterial blood bicarbonate and pH, and (*c*) as an increase in the respiratory gas exchange ratio (R). A method that uses R has the advantage of avoiding blood sampling procedures while at the same time using equipment common to exercise physiology laboratories.

Subjects performed a standardized graded exercise test by pedaling a cycle ergometer or walking on a treadmill for 4-minute exercise intervals. Measurements included heart rate, minute ventilation, $\dot{V}o_2$, and end-tidal CO_2 and N_2 concentrations. R was calculated from end-tidal gas concentrations. In the upper figure, a sigmoid curve was obtained by plotting R from the last 30 seconds of each exercise level against $\dot{V}o_2$. The inflection point at the beginning of the steepest part of this curve, called the *threshold* of anaerobic metabolism, indicates the $\dot{V}o_2$ level where anaerobic metabolism became significant. The anaerobic threshold corresponds to the level where bicarbonate concentration in arterial blood decreased and blood lactate concentration increased.

The lower figure shows the anaerobic threshold data for 37 patients with heart disease. Subjects with the lowest fitness attained anaerobic threshold at a lower $\dot{V}o_2$ (i.e., at a lower exercise intensity). From a clinical perspective, the researchers postulated that the ventilatory gas exchange ratio during exercise would be a useful measure of cardiovascular function, answering the question of how much exercise a patient could perform before cardiovascular function failed to meet the tissues' oxygen requirements. Instead of administering a maximal test or using techniques that require blood sampling and analysis, a researcher or clinician could use a relatively simple noninvasive procedure to determine the threshold of anaerobic metabolism during graded exercise.

Detecting when anaerobiosis occurs during exercise is valuable for evaluating a person's capabil-

Dynamics of Pulmonary Ventilation

PART 1

REGULATION OF PULMONARY VENTILATION

CONTROL OF VENTILATION

The rate and depth of breathing are exquisitely adjusted in response to the body's metabolic needs. The mechanisms for this regulation, however, are complex and not fully understood. Intricate neural circuits relay information from higher centers in the brain, from the lungs, and from other sensors throughout the body to contribute to the control of ventilation.[4] In addition, the gaseous and chemical states of the blood that bathes the medulla and chemoreceptors in the aorta and carotid arteries act to mediate alveolar ventilation. As a result, in healthy individuals, relatively constant alveolar (and arterial) gas pressures are maintained throughout a broad range of exercise intensities. Figure 14.1 is a schematic representation of the input for ventilatory control.

NEURAL FACTORS

The normal respiratory cycle results from the inherent activity of inspiratory neurons, the cell bodies of which are located in the medial portion of the **medulla.** These neurons activate the diaphragm and intercostal muscles, causing the lungs to inflate. The inspiratory neurons cease firing because of their own self-limitations and because of the inhibitory influence of expiratory neurons that are also located in the medulla. The normal rhythm of medullary neurons is influenced by both inhibitory and excitatory signals from throughout the body. As the lungs inflate, for example, stretch receptors in lung tissue are also stimulated, particularly in the bronchioles. These receptors act through afferent fibers to inhibit inspiration and stimulate expiration. As the inspiratory muscles relax, exhalation occurs by the passive recoil of the stretched lung tissue and raised ribs. The activation of expiratory neurons and associated muscles that further facilitate expiration is synchronized with this passive phase. As expiration proceeds, the inspiratory center is progressively released from inhibition and once again becomes active.

The inherent activity of the respiratory center alone cannot account for the smooth pattern of breathing in response to metabolic demands. A neural "command center" in the hypothalamus integrates input from descending neurons in the higher locomotor areas of the cerebral hemispheres, the pons, and other regions of the brain to affect the duration and intensity of the inspiratory cycle. At the same time, ascending neural signals initiated by mechanical and/or chemical changes from active muscles provide peripheral feedback control via the cerebellum to the respiratory center to influence the ventilatory adjustment to physical activity.

HUMORAL FACTORS

Pulmonary ventilation at rest is largely regulated by the chemical state of the blood. Variations in arterial P_{O_2}, P_{CO_2}, acidity, and temperature activate sensitive neural units in the medulla and arterial system that adjust ventilation to maintain arterial blood chemistry within narrow limits.

Plasma P_{O_2} and Peripheral Chemoreceptors. Inhalation of a gas mixture containing 80% oxygen greatly increases alveolar P_{O_2} and causes an approximate 20% reduction in minute ventilation. Conversely, ventilation increases if the inspired oxygen concentration is reduced below ambient levels, particularly if the alveolar P_{O_2} falls below 60 mm Hg. As shown in Figure 13.4, at this P_{O_2}, hemoglobin saturation begins to fall considerably.

Sensitivity to reduced oxygen pressure does not reside in the respiratory center. Instead, the primary site for detecting arterial hypoxia and initiating a ventilatory response is the peripheral **chemoreceptors.**[61] As illustrated in Figure 14.2, these specialized neurons, weighing only a few milligrams, are located in the arch of the aorta and at the branching of the carotid arteries in the neck. These **carotid bodies** are strategically positioned to monitor the state of arterial blood just before it perfuses the brain. A decrease in arterial P_{O_2}, as would occur when one ascends to high altitude or in pulmonary disease, activates the aortic and carotid chemoreceptors to increase alveolar ventilation. These receptors alone protect the organism against reduced oxygen pressure in inspired air.

In addition to providing the early warning system against a reduced arterial P_{O_2}, the peripheral chemoreceptors also stimulate ventilation in exercise, even though reductions in arterial P_{O_2} do not normally occur. This is probably the result of the stimulating effects on carotid discharge of increased carbon dioxide, temperature, and acidity, as

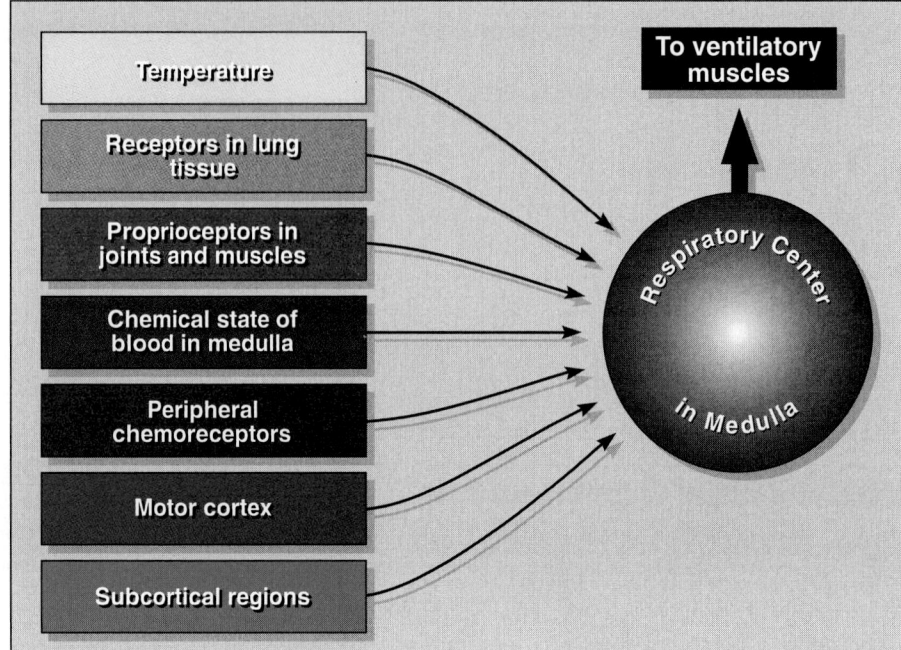

FIGURE 14.1
Schematic representation of various factors that affect the control of pulmonary ventilation by the medulla.

well as the increased potassium concentrations in arterial blood during exercise.[20, 66]

Plasma P_{CO_2} and H^+ Concentration. *At rest, the most important respiratory stimulus is the carbon dioxide pressure in arterial plasma.* Small increases in P_{CO_2} in the inspired air cause large increases in minute ventilation. For example, the resting ventilation is almost doubled by increasing the inspired P_{CO_2} to just 1.7 mm Hg (0.22% CO_2 in inspired air).

The regulation of ventilation by arterial P_{CO_2} is not mediated by the action of molecular carbon dioxide per se. Instead, ventilation seems to be controlled by plasma acidity, which varies directly with the blood's CO_2 content. As discussed previously in this text, carbonic acid, formed from the union of carbon dioxide and water, rapidly dissociates to bicarbonate ions and hydrogen ions. Inspiratory activity is stimulated by the increase in hydrogen ions, particularly in the cerebrospinal fluid that bathes the respiratory areas.

HYPERVENTILATION AND BREATH-HOLDING

If a breath-hold takes place after a normal exhalation, it takes approximately 40 seconds before the urge to breathe becomes so strong that one is forced to inspire. This desire to breathe is mainly due to the stimulating effects of increased arterial P_{CO_2} and H^+ concentration and **not** to the decreased P_{O_2} in the breath-hold condition.[17] The "break

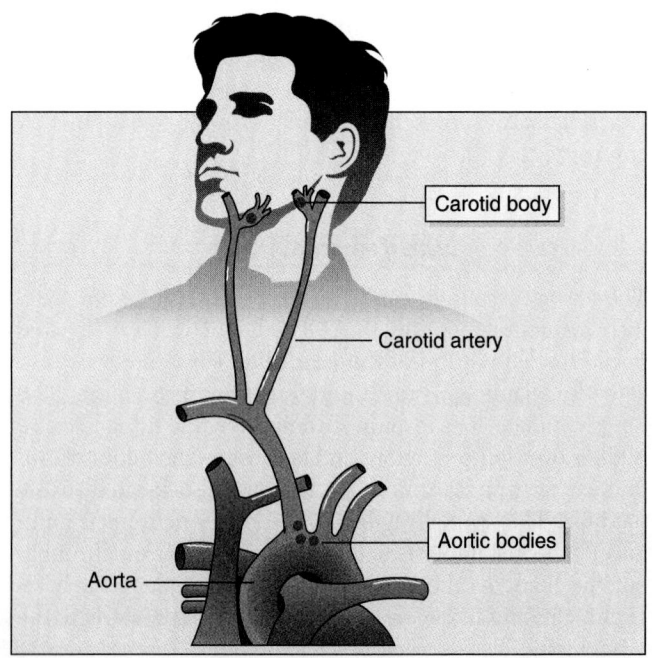

FIGURE 14.2
Aortic and carotid cell bodies that are sensitive to reduced arterial P_{O_2} and increased P_{CO_2} and H^+ and potassium concentrations are located in the aortic arch and bifurcation of the carotid arteries. These peripheral chemoreceptors provide the body's first line of defense against arterial hypoxia, such as would occur in pulmonary disease and ascent to high altitude. They also contribute to the regulation of exercise hyperpnea through the influence of CO_2 and H^+ concentration.

point" for the breath-hold corresponds to an increase in arterial P_{CO_2} to approximately 50 mm Hg.

If, before breath-holding, ventilation is consciously increased above the normal level, the composition of alveolar air changes and becomes more like ambient air. As a result of this overbreathing, or **hyperventilation,** alveolar P_{CO_2} may decrease from its normal value of 40 mm Hg to approximately 15 mm Hg. This creates a considerable diffusion gradient for the runoff of CO_2 into the alveoli from the venous blood that enters the pulmonary capillaries. Consequently, a larger-than-normal quantity of CO_2 leaves the blood and reduces the arterial P_{CO_2}. This extends the duration of breath-hold until the arterial P_{CO_2} and/or H^+ concentration rise to a level that again stimulates ventilation.

Hyperventilation and subsequent breath-hold are used by swimmers and divers to improve performance. In sprint swimming, for example, it is undesirable mechanically to roll the body and turn the head during the breathing phase of the stroke. Consequently, many sprinters hyperventilate on the starting blocks to prolong the breath-hold during the swim. In sport diving, the intention of hyperventilation is the same as in competitive swimming—to extend breath-hold time. In this sport, however, the results can be tragic.[16] As the length and depth of the dive increase, the oxygen content of the blood can be reduced to critically low values before arterial P_{CO_2} rises sufficiently to stimulate breathing and signal ascent to the surface. This can cause the diver to lose consciousness before reaching the surface of the water. Hyperventilation and other factors related to diving are discussed in Chapter 26.

REGULATION OF VENTILATION IN EXERCISE

CHEMICAL CONTROL

Neither chemical stimuli nor any other single mechanism can entirely explain the increased ventilation, or **hy-perpnea,** that occurs in physical activity. It now seems that the classic feedback control of resting ventilation via oxygen-mediated and carbon dioxide–mediated mechanisms is **not** the major factor in exercise hyperpnea.[20] Even when artificial changes are made in inspired P_{O_2} and P_{CO_2} (as well as in plasma acidity), increases in minute ventilation are not nearly as large as those observed during vigorous exercise.

The venous and alveolar P_{CO_2} and alveolar P_{O_2} in relation to oxygen uptake during a graded exercise test are illustrated in Figure 14.3. As exercise intensity increases, alveolar (arterial) P_{O_2} is **not** reduced to an extent that would increase ventilation through a major chemoreceptor stimulation. The large ventilatory volumes during vigorous exercise cause the alveolar P_{O_2} to rise above the average resting value of 100 mm Hg. This increase during heavy exercise may actually hasten the oxygenation of blood in the alveolar capillaries. Pulmonary ventilation during light and moderate exercise is closely coupled with metabolism in a manner that is proportional to oxygen uptake and carbon dioxide production.[63] Under these conditions, the alveolar (and arterial) P_{CO_2} is generally maintained at approximately 40 mm Hg. During strenuous exercise, with its anaerobic component, carbon dioxide and subsequent H^+ concentration increase, which provides an additional ventilatory stimulus. This often **reduces** alveolar P_{CO_2}, sometimes to as low as 25 mm Hg.[33] This causes a decrease in arterial P_{CO_2} that reduces the ventilatory drive from carbon dioxide during exercise.

Based on the alterations in alveolar and arterial gas pressures during exercise, one might question how the peripheral chemoreceptors exert their influence on ventilation during exercise. A possible explanation is the pattern of ventilation that causes the alveolar and capillary P_{CO_2} to be slightly lower at the end of inhalation and higher at the end of exhalation. Even though the **average** levels of arterial oxygen, carbon dioxide, and pH are well regulated during moderate exercise, the cyclic oscillations in these chemical factors during breathing may be detected by the chemore-

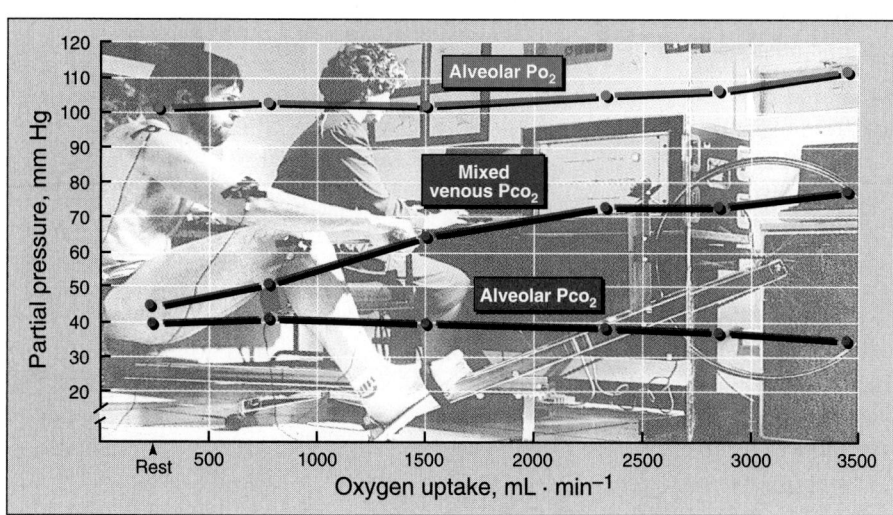

FIGURE 14.3

The values for P_{CO_2} in mixed venous blood that enters the lungs and the alveolar P_{O_2} and P_{CO_2} relate to oxygen uptake during graded exercise. Alveolar P_{O_2} and P_{CO_2} remain near resting levels during a broad range of exercise intensities. (Data from the Laboratory of Applied Physiology, Queens College, Flushing, NY. Photo courtesy of Dr. Peter Cavanaugh, Pennsylvania State University, University Park, PA.)

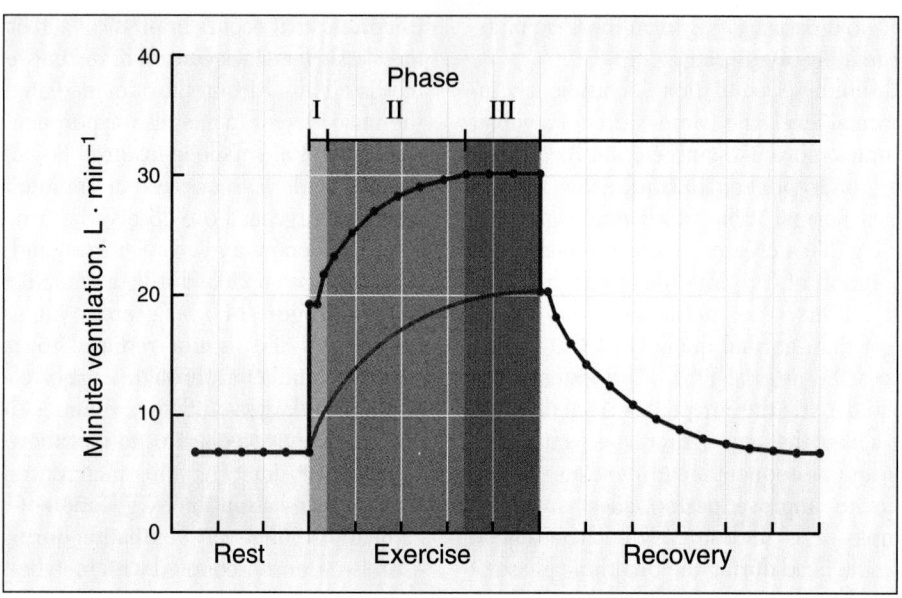

FIGURE 14.4

The three phases of exercise hyperpnea. *Phase I:* rapid increase and brief plateau due to central command drive and input from active muscles. *Phase II:* slower exponential rise begins approximately 20 seconds after onset of exercise. Central command continues, along with feedback from active muscles plus the added effect of short-term potentiation of respiratory neurons. *Phase III:* major regulatory mechanisms have reached stable values; added input from peripheral sources, principally the chemoreceptors and core temperature, provides the "fine tuning" of the ventilatory response. The lower graph depicts the contribution of central neuronal short-term potentiation and rising arterial H^+ concentration to the respiratory response. (Modified from Eldridge, F.L.: Central integration of mechanisms in exercise hyperpnea. *Med. Sci. Sports Exerc.,* 26:319, 1994.)

ceptors to influence exercise ventilation. Chemoreceptor detection may be facilitated by an increased sensitivity of the chemoreceptors in exercise.

NONCHEMICAL CONTROL

The rapidity of the ventilatory response at the onset and cessation of exercise strongly suggests that this portion of exercise hyperpnea is mediated by input other than changes in arterial P_{CO_2} and H^+ concentration.

Neurogenic Factors. Neurogenic factors for ventilatory control include both cortical and peripheral influences.

• **Cortical influence:** The respiratory neurons in the medulla are stimulated by neural outflow from regions of the motor cortex and by cortical activation in anticipation of exercise. This cortical outflow acts in concert with the demands of exercise to contribute to the abrupt increase in ventilation.

• **Peripheral influence:** The ventilatory adjustment to exercise is influenced by sensory input from joints, tendons, or muscles. Although such peripheral receptors have not been identified, experiments involving passive limb movements, electrical stimulation of muscles, and voluntary exercise with the muscle's blood flow occluded support the existence of such mechanoreceptors in producing a reflex hyperpnea.

Influence of Temperature. An increase in body temperature has a direct stimulating effect on the neurons of the respiratory center, which in turn exerts some control over ventilation during prolonged exercise. The rapid rise in ventilation at the start of exercise and the sharp decline at the end of exercise, however, occur too quickly to be accounted for by changes in core temperature.

INTEGRATED REGULATION

During Exercise. *The control of breathing during exercise is not the result of a single factor but is the combined and perhaps simultaneous effect of several chemical and neural stimuli.*[20, 66] The dynamics of minute ventilation at the onset, early phase, and late stages of moderate exercise and during recovery are shown in Figure 14.4. This ventilatory response pattern occurs in three phases. In **Phase I,** the neurogenic stimuli from the cerebral cortex (central command), combined with feedback from the active limbs, stimulate the ventilatory controller (medulla) to cause the abrupt increase in ventilation as exercise begins. This cortical and locomotor peripheral input continues throughout the exercise period. After a short plateau (approximately 20 seconds), minute ventilation then rises exponentially **(Phase II)** to reach a steady level in relation to the demands for metabolic gas exchange. This phase of exercise ventilation is regulated by central command input and factors intrinsic to neurons of the respiratory control system. The activity of these respiratory neurons brings about a short-term potentiation of neurons in the medulla that augments their responsiveness to the same continuing stimulation. This brings the minute ventilation to a new, higher level. It also is likely that some regulation during Phase II is provided by input from the peripheral chemoreceptors in the carotid bodies.[66] The final phase of control (**Phase III**) involves a "fine tuning" of the steady-state ventilation through peripheral sensory feedback mechanisms. The modulation of alveolar gas pressures in this phase is maintained by central and reflex chemical stimuli, especially those provided by temperature, carbon dioxide, and H^+ concentration through their effect on the chemoreceptors. Some regulatory input also is provided by reflexes related to pulmonary blood flow and the movement of the lung and respiratory muscles.

In Recovery. The initial rapid decrease in ventilation when exercise stops represents the abrupt removal of both the central command drive and the input from previously active muscles. More than likely, the slower phase of the recovery reflects the gradual removal of the short-term potentiation of the respiratory center and the re-establishment of the body's normal metabolic, thermal, and chemical milieu.

∎ S U M M A R Y ∎

1. The normal respiratory cycle results from the inherent activity of neurons in the medulla. Superimposed on this neural output are intricate neural circuits that relay information from higher brain centers, from the lungs, and from other sensors throughout the body.

2. At rest, alveolar ventilation is controlled through several chemical factors that act directly on the respiratory center or modify its activity through chemoreceptors. The most important factors are the level of arterial P_{CO_2} and the H^+ concentration. A drop in arterial oxygen pressure, as would occur during ascent to high altitude or in severe pulmonary disease, also provides a stimulus to breathing.

3. Hyperventilation significantly lowers arterial P_{CO_2} and H^+ concentration. This prolongs breath-hold time until normal levels of carbon dioxide and acidity are reached to stimulate breathing. Extended breath-hold by hyperventilation should not be practiced during underwater swimming because the consequences can be deadly.

4. Ventilatory adjustments to exercise are augmented by nonchemical regulatory factors. These factors include (*a*) cortical activation in anticipation of exercise and outflow from the motor cortex when exercise begins, (*b*) peripheral sensory input from mechanoreceptors in joints and muscles, and (*c*) increases in body temperature.

5. The ventilatory response to exercise occurs in three phases. In Phase I, cortical stimulus plus feedback for active limbs cause the abrupt increase in ventilation as exercise begins; ventilation then rises exponentially in Phase II to reach a steady level in relation to exercise demands; Phase III involves a "fine tuning" of the steady-state ventilation through peripheral sensory feedback mechanisms.

PART 2
PULMONARY VENTILATION DURING EXERCISE

VENTILATION AND ENERGY DEMANDS

Physical activity affects oxygen uptake and carbon dioxide production more than any other form of physiologic stress. With exercise, large amounts of oxygen diffuse from the alveoli into the venous blood returning to the lungs while a considerable quantity of carbon dioxide moves from the blood into the alveoli. Concurrently, alveolar ventilation increases to maintain the proper gas concentrations for rapid gas exchange.

VENTILATION IN STEADY-RATE EXERCISE

The relationship between oxygen uptake and minute ventilation during various levels of exercise up to the maximal oxygen uptake is illustrated in Figure 14.5. During light to moderate exercise, ventilation increases **linearly** with oxygen uptake and carbon dioxide production, averaging between 20 and 25 L of air for each liter of oxygen consumed. Under these conditions, ventilation increases mainly through an increase in tidal volume, whereas breathing frequency takes on a more important role at higher exercise levels. With these ventilatory adjustments, there is complete aeration of blood because the alveolar P_{O_2} and P_{CO_2} levels remain near resting values. The transit time for blood in the pulmonary capillaries is still slow enough for the complete equilibration of the lung-blood gases (see Fig. 13.3).

The ratio of minute ventilation to oxygen uptake is termed the **ventilatory equivalent** and is symbolized $\dot{V}_E/\dot{V}_{O_2}$. In healthy young adults, this ratio is usually maintained at approximately 25 to 1 (that is, 25 L of air breathed per liter of oxygen consumed) during submaximal exercise up to approximately 55% of the maximal oxygen uptake.[62] The ventilatory equivalent is higher in children and averages approximately 32 L.[54] The mode of exercise also affects the ventilatory equivalent. During prone swimming, for example, the $\dot{V}_E/\dot{V}_{O_2}$ ratios are significantly lower than for running at all levels of energy expenditure.[43] This is due to the restrictive nature of swimming on breathing and could pose a problem in providing adequate gas exchange at maximal

FIGURE 14.5

Pulmonary ventilation, blood lactate, and oxygen uptake during graded exercise to maximum. The dashed line represents the extrapolation of the linear relationship between $\dot{V}_E$ and $\dot{V}_{O_2}$ during submaximal exercise. The lactate threshold is the highest exercise intensity or level of oxygen uptake that is not associated with an elevation in blood lactate concentration. It is detected by the point at which the relation between $\dot{V}_E$ and $\dot{V}_{O_2}$ deviates from linearity, indicated as the point of ventilatory threshold. (OBLA represents the point of lactate increase above a 4.0 mM baseline.) Respiratory compensation is a further increase in ventilation to counter the falling pH in heavy anaerobic exercise.

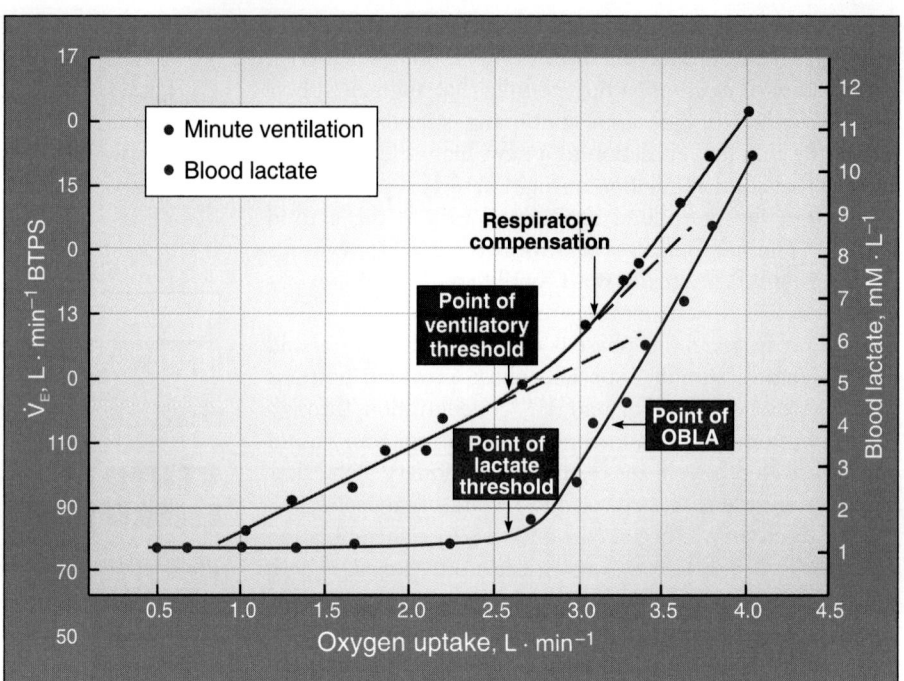

VENTILATION IN NON–STEADY-RATE EXERCISE

During more intense submaximal exercise, the minute ventilation takes a sharp upswing and increases disproportionately in relation to oxygen uptake. As a result, the ventilatory equivalent may reach values as high as 35 or 40 L of air per liter of oxygen consumed.

Onset of Blood Lactate Accumulation. During steady-rate exercise, aerobic metabolism is matched to the energy requirements of the active muscles. Under these conditions, there is little or no accumulation of blood lactate. *The term **lactate threshold** refers to the highest exercise level (intensity) or level of oxygen uptake that is not associated with an elevation in blood lactate concentration above the pre-exercise level (or an increase less than 1.0 mM).*[65] The region in which blood lactate shows a systematic increase equal to or above a level of 4.0 mM is termed the point of **onset of blood lactate accumulation** or simply **OBLA**.[55, 68] Often, the terms lactate threshold and OBLA are used interchangeably (as we do below), although their precise points of demarcation in terms of exercise intensity are operationally different. To some, the 4.0-mM value for OBLA implies a maximum exercise intensity that a person can sustain for a prolonged period. In reality, this maximum stable lactate level is probably quite variable among individuals.[15]

swimming velocities. This may partly explain the generally lower maximal oxygen uptake achieved during swimming compared to running.[40]

Almost all of the lactic acid generated in anaerobic metabolism is buffered to lactate in the blood by sodium bicarbonate in the following reaction:

$$\text{Lactic acid} + NaHCO_3 \longrightarrow Na\ Lactate + H_2CO_3$$
$$\updownarrow$$
$$H_2O + CO_2$$

The excess, nonmetabolic carbon dioxide released in this reaction stimulates pulmonary ventilation, and CO_2 is exhaled into the atmosphere.

Controversy exists regarding the exact cause of the OBLA. It is often assumed that it represents a distinct point for the onset of muscle anaerobiosis. However, blood lactate values do not always reflect the lactic acid concentration in specific muscles.[25] Lactate accumulation may result not only from muscle anaerobiosis but also from a decreased lactate clearance in total or an increased lactic acid production in specific fibers within a muscle. Although caution is urged in interpreting too broadly the specific metabolic significance of the OBLA, it generally is considered to reflect the start of the exponential accumulation of lactic acid in the active muscle.[28]

Because blood lactate accumulation is associated with changes in carbon dioxide production (respiratory exchange ratio) via buffering, blood pH, bicarbonate, and H^+ concentration, these variables have been used to indirectly assess OBLA.[32, 62] Although these measures are indeed related to OBLA, it is doubtful that any one of them should be used independently to precisely denote the onset of anaerobic metabolism in active muscle. Nevertheless, it is common to use "bloodless" techniques such as changes in the R, $\dot{V}E/\dot{V}O_2$, or various fractional concentrations of expired gas during incremental exercise to signal the onset of metabolic acidosis. Even if the association between metabolic events and ventilatory dynamics is not causal in nature, much useful information about exercise performance has resulted with application of these indirect evaluation procedures.

Specificity of the Point of OBLA. As with many measures of physiologic function and exercise performance, OBLA is specific to the exercise task. Differences in OBLA occur when comparing bicycle, treadmill, and arm-crank exercise at all levels of oxygen uptake. More than likely, this results from variations in the muscle mass activated in the specific form of exercise. At a particular exercise level or submaximal oxygen uptake, for example, the metabolic rate per unit of active muscle mass is higher in arm-crank and bicycle exercise than in treadmill walking or running. Therefore, the OBLA would be reached at a lower exercise level during bicycling and arm-crank exercise.[19, 36] *This indicates that different forms of exercise should not be used interchangeably to determine and quantify the point of OBLA.*

Some Independence Between OBLA and $\dot{V}O_2$max. As discussed in Chapter 7, blood lactate in a trained individual begins to accumulate not only at a higher level of submaximal oxygen uptake but also at a higher percentage of aerobic capacity compared to someone who is untrained. For both children and adults, training can improve the point of OBLA **without** a concomitant increase in the $\dot{V}O_2$max.[18, 24, 35, 42] This indicates that the OBLA and $\dot{V}O_2$max are determined by somewhat different factors. The muscle mass activated during exercise and the muscle fiber type, capillary density, mitochondrial size and number, and alterations in a muscle's enzymatic and oxidative capabilities play a major role in establishing the percentage of aerobic capacity that can be sustained in exercise with little lactate accumulation.[10, 27, 64] The absolute quantity of muscle mass activated and the functional capacity of the cardiovascular system are important determining factors in achieving a high aerobic capacity.

A lack of close association between aerobic capacity and OBLA has been shown in a study of trained cardiac patients compared to trained healthy counterparts.[12] Although the patients with impaired cardiac function (i.e., a blunted capacity for maximal blood flow) had a significantly lower $\dot{V}O_2$max than the healthy individuals, the patients were able to run at the same speed (and achieve essentially the same endurance performance) as the healthy individuals without an accumulation of blood lactate. As shown in Figure 14.6, these patients maintained nearly a metabolic steady rate while running at a speed that elicited their $\dot{V}O_2$max. The point of OBLA represented 100% of $\dot{V}O_2$max!

OBLA and Endurance Performance. Two important factors influence endurance performance:

- The maximal capacity to consume oxygen as reflected by the $\dot{V}O_2$max
- The maximal level for steady rate exercise or OBLA

Traditionally, exercise physiologists have used the $\dot{V}O_2$max as the yardstick to gauge one's capacity for endurance exercise. Although this measurement generally relates to exercise performance, it does not fully explain success. This is because longer-duration, high-intensity exercise is not performed at the $\dot{V}O_2$max. *For men and women, the exercise intensity at the point of OBLA is a consistent and powerful predictor of performance in aerobic exercise.*[13, 21, 37, 57] This is clearly illustrated in a study of competitive race walkers.[23] Here, the race-walking velocity at the point of lactate accumulation was highly correlated to 20-km performance. The race-walking velocity at OBLA predicted race performance to within 0.6% of the actual time! The results were similar in a more recent study of elite cyclists in which cycling power output at the lactate threshold was highly correlated (r = 0.93) to the average absolute power output maintained during a 1-hour ride in the laboratory.[14] This laboratory measurement, in turn, was a strong predictor of performance in an actual 40-km road race. In many studies, changes in endurance performance with training are often more closely related to the training-induced changes in the exercise level for OBLA than to the changes in $\dot{V}O_2$max.[2, 58, 64]

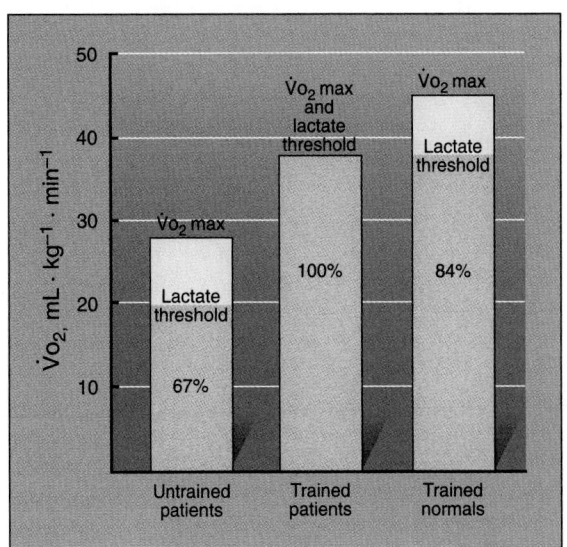

FIGURE 14.6
Lactate threshold in relation to the $\dot{V}O_2$max in trained and untrained patients with coronary artery disease and in healthy, trained subjects. (From Coyle, E.F., et al.: Blood lactate threshold in some well-trained ischemic heart disease patients. *J. Appl. Physiol.,* 54:18, 1983.)

ENERGY COST OF BREATHING

The relationship between pulmonary ventilation and oxygen uptake in healthy people during rest and submaximal exercise and its division into ventilatory and nonventilatory components are shown in Figure 14.7.[39] At rest and during light exercise, the oxygen requirement of breathing is small, averaging 1.9 to 3.1 mL of oxygen per liter of air breathed, or approximately 4% of the total energy expenditure. As the breathing rate and tidal volume increase, the energy cost rises to between 2.1 and 4.5 mL of oxygen per liter of ventilation.[9] The contribution of the oxygen cost of ventilation to the oxygen deficit and recovery oxygen uptake also has been estimated during moderately heavy steady-rate exercise.[34] The energy cost of breathing accounts for approximately 19% of the oxygen deficit and 11% of the recovery oxygen uptake (Fig. 14.8A). These results indicate that the oxygen cost of ventilation has an approximately twofold greater influence on oxygen deficit than on the recovery oxygen uptake. The reason for the smaller contribution of ventilation cost to the total cost of recovery is that the minute ventilation volume declines exponentially at the end of exercise in the same manner as recovery oxygen uptake (Fig. 14.8B). This is not the case in the beginning of exercise, during which ventilation increases at a greater rate than the oxygen uptake.

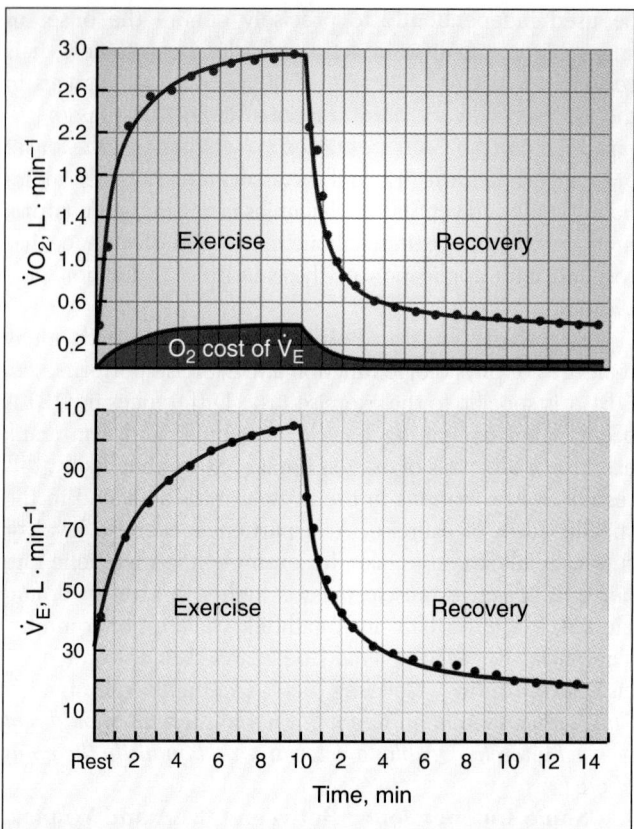

FIGURE 14.8

A, Estimated oxygen cost of ventilation on oxygen deficit and recovery oxygen uptake. For the 33 subjects, the steady-rate oxygen uptake averaged 2.9 L · min^{-1} during the 10 minutes of bicycle ergometer exercise at 1,080 kg · m · min^{-1}. The exercise and recovery oxygen cost values are indicated by the shaded area under the curves. **B,** Two-component exponential curve for exercise and recovery minute ventilation. (Modified from Katch, F.I., et al.: The influence of the estimated oxygen cost of ventilation on oxygen deficit and recovery oxygen intake for moderately heavy bicycle ergometer exercise. *Med. Sci. Sports Exerc.*, 4:71, 1972.)

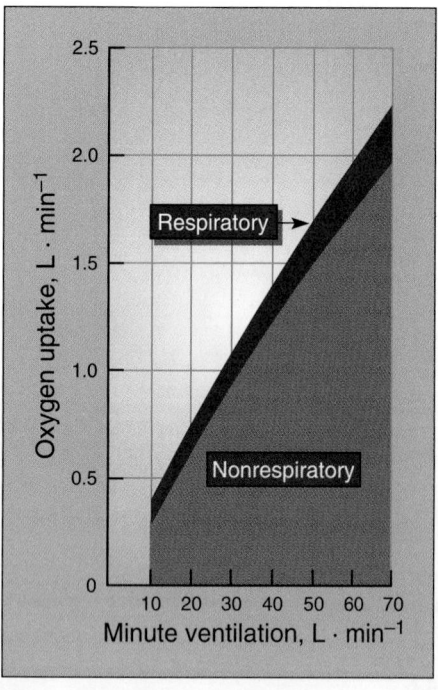

FIGURE 14.7

Relationship between minute ventilation and total oxygen uptake and its respiratory and nonrespiratory components during submaximal exercise in healthy subjects. (From Levison, H., and Cherniak, R.: Ventilatory cost of exercise in chronic obstructive pulmonary disease. *J. Appl. Physiol.*, 25:21, 1968.)

During exercise that elicits $\dot{V}O_2$max, as much as 8 to 11% of the total oxygen uptake is required for respiratory muscle work. At this exercise level, the inspiratory muscles are using approximately 40 to 60% of their maximum capacity to generate pressure (force).[1] It has yet to be demonstrated whether the energy cost of ventilation during the heavy exercise associated with extreme levels of aerobic fitness actually limits endurance capacity.

RESPIRATORY DISEASE

The healthy person rarely senses the effort to breathe, even during moderate exercise. In individuals with respiratory disease, however, the work of breathing can become an exhaustive exercise in itself. In patients with chronic obstructive lung disease (COPD), the increased resistance to exhalation may increase the cost of breathing at rest to three times the normal value; during light exercise, it may increase to as much as 10 mL of oxygen for each liter of air breathed.[39] In severe pulmonary disease, the cost of breathing may easily reach 40% of the total exercise oxygen uptake. This encroaches on the oxygen available to the active, nonrespiratory muscle mass and seriously limits the exercise capacity of individuals with this disease. Although little or no improvement is seen in measures of pulmonary function or disease status in patients with COPD after exercise training, benefits do occur. Increased exercise capacity, reduced dyspnea, and enhanced psychological state are important positive results of regular exercise for these individuals.[6]

CIGARETTE SMOKING

The research relating smoking habits to exercise performance is meager, although most endurance athletes avoid cigarettes for fear of hindering performance due to a "loss of wind." Chronic cigarette smokers tend to be less physically active and have lower levels of fitness than their nonsmoking counterparts.[56] For some unknown reason, cigarette smoking increases one's dependence on carbohydrates for energy at rest and during sustained exercise.[11] Smokers also show a decrease in dynamic lung function, which, in severe instances, is manifest in chronic obstructive lung disorders. Such pathologic processes usually take some time to develop. Therefore, in young smokers, chronic alterations in lung function may be minimal and insignificant in terms of their effect on physical performance. Other more acute effects of cigarette smoking may adversely affect exercise capacity.

Acute Effects. Airway resistance at rest increases as much as threefold in both chronic smokers and nonsmokers

following 15 puffs on a cigarette during a 5-minute period.[44] This added resistance to breathing lasts an average of 35 minutes and probably only has a minor effect during light exercise, in which the cost of breathing is small. During vigorous exercise, however, this residual effect of smoking could be detrimental because the additional cost of breathing might become prohibitive. The increase in peripheral airway resistance with smoking is mainly caused by the vagal reflex (possibly triggered from sensory stimulation of minute particles in cigarette smoke) and partially by the stimulation of parasympathetic ganglia by nicotine.[45]

The oxygen cost of breathing was studied in six habitual smokers immediately after they smoked two cigarettes and 1 day after abstinence from tobacco.[53] The subjects ran on a treadmill at a speed and grade that required approximately 80% of the $\dot{V}O_2$max. Ventilation during the "smoking" and "nonsmoking" runs was then increased in two ways: (a) subjects voluntarily hyperventilated during the run (Voluntary HV) and (b) hyperventilation was induced by increasing alveolar P_{CO_2} by having subjects breathe through a large-diameter tube that increased the anatomic dead space by approximately 1400 mL (Dead Space HV). The oxygen cost of the "extra" breathing was then determined as the difference between the normal oxygen uptake and the oxygen uptake in the hyperventilation experiments.

As shown in Table 14.1, the oxygen cost of breathing decreased between 13 and 79% as a result of abstinence. During exercise at 80% of $\dot{V}O_2$max, the energy requirement of breathing averaged 14% of the exercise oxygen uptake after smoking and only 9% in the nonsmoking trials for the heaviest smokers. Also, heart rates averaged 5 to 7% lower during exercise following 1 day of cigarette abstinence, and all subjects reported that they felt better exercising in the non-

TABLE 14.1
THE OXYGEN COST OF HYPERVENTILATION (HV) IN "SMOKING" AND "NONSMOKING" EXERCISE THAT REPRESENTS APPROXIMATELY 80% OF EACH SUBJECT'S $\dot{V}O_2$ MAX[a]

| | Smoking | | | | Nonsmoking | | | |
| | Voluntary HV | | Dead Space HV | | Voluntary HV | | Dead Space HV | |
Subject	$\dot{V}_E$ (L · min⁻¹)	Cost (mL · L⁻¹)	$\dot{V}_E$ (L · min⁻¹)	Cost (mL · L⁻¹)	$\dot{V}_E$ (L · min⁻¹)	Cost (mL · L⁻¹)	$\dot{V}_E$ (L · min⁻¹)	Cost (mL · L⁻¹)
1	26.4	15.1	18.9	12.7	22.7	11.4	23.0	6.5
2	39.0	10.3	28.1	5.9	42.6	11.3	41.3	4.8
3	22.8	7.9	27.2	7.0	23.8	7.2	22.8	5.7
4	36.3	5.0	28.7	5.6	44.7	3.8	18.6	−1.6[a]
5	52.7	13.5	26.7	12.4	75.2	6.1	22.8	5.7
6	22.4	8.5	27.3	1.1	23.2	3.4	30.1	3.0
Average	32.6	10.1	26.2	7.4	38.7	7.2	26.5	4.0

From Rode, A., and Shephard, R. J.: The influence of cigarette smoking upon the oxygen cost of breathing in near-maximal exercise. *Med. Sci. Sports Exerc.*, 3:51, 1971
[a]The implication of the "negative" cost of $\dot{V}_E$ in this subject is that the added dead space reduced the cost of the normal exercise ventilation.

smoking condition. It appears that a substantial reversibility of the increased cost of breathing with smoking occurs in chronic smokers with only **1 day of abstinence.** Therefore, if an athlete is unable to eliminate smoking completely, it should at least be stopped the day before a competition.

A Blunted Heart Rate Response. A paradox exists between the maximal exercise capacity of cigarette smokers and their submaximal response to exercise. Recent research has shown that maximal test duration during graded exercise (longer time reflects higher aerobic fitness) is significantly less in smokers than nonsmokers.[56] Despite this poorer performance in maximal testing, exercise test duration to a submaximal heart rate of 130 beats per minute was significantly longer for the smokers. This indirect submaximal estimate of exercise capacity indicated a higher fitness level among the smokers, i.e., more exercise accomplished before a predetermined heart rate was reached. This blunted heart rate response of smokers to submaximal exercise may be the result of an altered sensitivity in autonomic neural control due to cigarette smoking.[38] These findings indicate that one's smoking status should be considered when evaluating fitness data based on the submaximal heart rate response to standard exercise such as a step test or heart rate prediction test. If this is is not considered, then a smoker's fitness status would be overestimated because the heart rate would be lower (blunted response) and the prediction of fitness would be higher.

ADAPTATIONS IN BREATHING WITH TRAINING

Aerobic training brings about several changes in pulmonary ventilation during maximal and submaximal exercise.

- **Maximal exercise:** Maximal exercise ventilation increases with improvements in maximal oxygen uptake. This makes sense physiologically, because any increase in aerobic capacity results in a larger oxygen requirement and correspondingly larger production of carbon dioxide that must be eliminated through increased alveolar ventilation.

- **Submaximal exercise:** Following only several weeks of training, a considerable **reduction** in the ventilatory equivalent is observed during submaximal exercise. Consequently, a smaller amount of air is breathed at a particular oxygen uptake, thereby reducing the percentage of the total oxygen cost of exercise attributable to breathing.[7] Theoretically, this is important in endurance exercise for two reasons: (*a*) it reduces the fatiguing effects of exercise on the ventilatory musculature and (*b*) any oxygen freed from use by the respiratory muscles becomes available to the active muscles.[8, 31]

The mechanism for the training adaptations in pulmonary ventilation during submaximal exercise is unclear. These changes, however, have been consistently observed in studies of adolescents and in both young and older individuals.[22, 29, 60] In general, the tidal volume becomes **larger** and breathing frequency is **reduced.** Consequently, air remains in the lungs for a longer period of time between breaths, which results in an increased extraction of oxygen from the inspired air. For example, the exhaled air of trained individuals contains only 14 to 15% oxygen during submaximal exercise, whereas the expired air of untrained persons contains approximately 18% at the same exercise level. This translates to the well-known observation that the untrained person must ventilate proportionately more air to achieve the same submaximal oxygen uptake.

The ventilatory response is **specific** to the type of exercise, and the physiological adaptations are **specific** to the form of exercise used in training. When subjects performed arm and leg exercises, the ventilation equivalent was always greater during arm exercise than leg exercise (Fig. 14.9).[51]

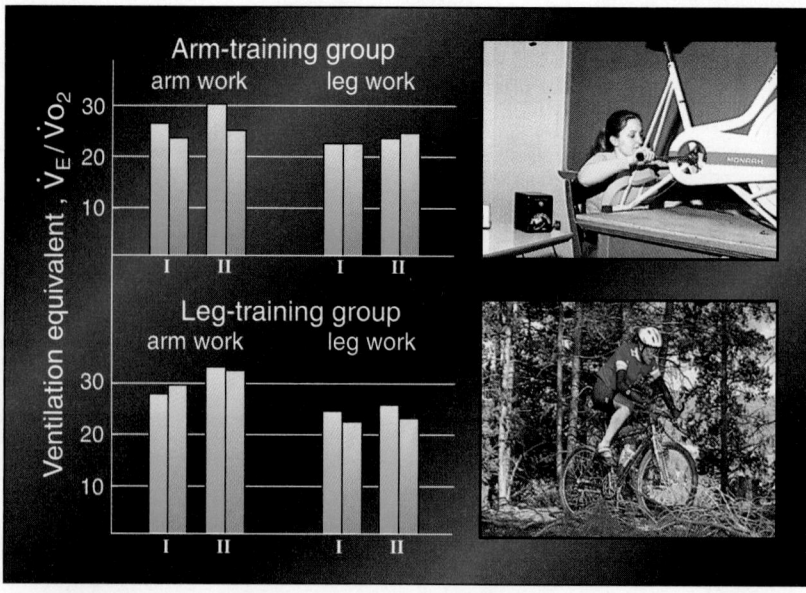

FIGURE 14.9
Ventilation equivalents during light (I) and heavy (II) submaximal arm and leg exercise before and after arm training (*top*) and leg training (*bottom*). Yellow-green bars indicate posttraining values. (From Rasmussen, B., et al.: Pulmonary ventilation, blood gases, and blood pH after training of the arms and the legs. *J. Appl. Physiol.*, 38:250, 1975.)

As expected, the ventilatory equivalent was reduced with exercise training. However, this reduction was noted **only** with exercise that used the specifically trained muscles. For the group trained by arm-crank ergometry, the ventilation equivalent was reduced only during arm exercise and vice versa for the leg-trained group. This training adaptation was closely related to a less pronounced rise in blood lactate and heart rate during the specific training exercise. This suggests that the ventilatory adjustment to training partly results from local adaptations in the specific muscles trained through exercise. A lower lactic acid production with training would remove the drive to ventilation from the carbon dioxide produced in the buffering process.

DOES VENTILATION LIMIT AEROBIC POWER AND ENDURANCE?

The adaptability of the structural and functional components of the pulmonary system to chronic exercise training are considerably less than adaptations observed for the cardiovascular and neuromuscular systems.[3] Currently, considerable interest exists in studying how this lack of pulmonary system "plasticity" affects aerobic exercise performance, particularly at the extreme levels in elite endurance athletes.

If one's ability to breathe during exercise is inadequate, then the relationship between pulmonary ventilation and oxygen uptake would curve in a direction opposite to that indicated in Figure 14.5, and the the $\dot{V}E/\dot{V}O_2$ ratio would decrease. Such a response, which is common in patients with COPD, would indicate a **failure** of ventilation to keep pace with oxygen uptake; in this situation, one truly would "run out of breath." During heavy exercise, healthy individuals actually tend to overbreathe in relation to oxygen uptake. This overbreathing was clearly illustrated in Figure 14.3, which showed that the ventilation increase during strenuous exercise generally results in a **decrease** in alveolar PCO_2, with a concomitant but small **increase** in alveolar PO_2. Even during maximal exercise, a considerable breathing reserve exists because minute ventilation represents only approximately 60 to 85% of a healthy person's maximum capacity for breathing.[5, 41] *Such findings indicate that pulmonary function is probably not a "weak link" in the oxygen transport system of healthy individuals who have an average to moderately high aerobic capacity.*

An Important Exception. In elite endurance athletes (in whom cardiovascular and muscular adaptations to training have reached exceptional levels), the pulmonary system may be taxed maximally or even lag behind the functional capacity of the other "aerobic systems" and pose a resistance to the transport of oxygen.[48-50, 52, 67] For example, when highly trained endurance athletes exercised at near maximal oxygen uptakes (more than 65 mL · kg^{-1} · min^{-1}; Fig. 14.10), the pressure differential between alveolar and arterial oxygen widened in some athletes to more than

30 mm Hg.[30] As a result, arterial oxygen saturation fell below the 90% level, with a corresponding arterial PO_2 below 75 mm Hg. These data indicate that, at extremely high levels of aerobic metabolism, some athletes are unable to achieve complete aeration of the blood in the pulmonary capillaries. Possible causes for arterial desaturation during maximal exercise in elite athletes include: (*a*) an inequality between alveolar ventilation and blood perfusion (known as the **ventilation-perfusion ratio**) within the lung or specific portions of the lung; (*b*) shunting of blood between the venous and arterial circulation, thus bypassing areas for diffusion; and, perhaps the most likely reason, (*c*) failure to achieve an end-capillary equilibrium between alveolar gas pressure and the pressure of gases in blood that perfuses the pulmonary capillaries. This diffusion limitation would be due to the rapid blood flow achieved by endurance athletes through a relatively normal-sized pulmonary capillary volume. The reason for the potentiation of this desaturation effect among older endurance athletes is unknown.[50]

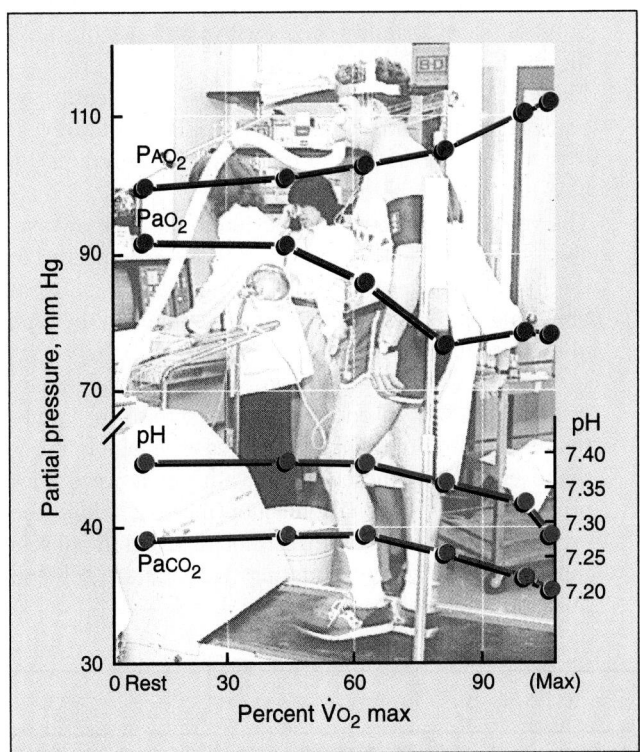

FIGURE 14.10

Average values for blood gas pressures (PaO_2 and $PaCO_2$), acid-base status (pH), and difference between alveolar (PAO_2) and arterial (PaO_2) oxygen pressure in eight male athletes during graded exercise up to $\dot{V}O_2$ max. Note the widening of the (A-a)O_2 gradient and the fall in PaO_2 during maximal exercise. (From Johnson, B.D., et al.: Mechanical constraints on exercise hyperpnea in endurance athletes. *J. Appl. Physiol.*, 73:874, 1992.)

■ SUMMARY ■

1. During light to moderate exercise, pulmonary ventilation increases linearly with oxygen uptake. The ventilatory equivalent ($\dot{V}E/\dot{V}O_2$) is maintained at approximately 20 to 25 L of air breathed per liter of oxygen consumed.

2. In nonsteady-rate exercise, ventilation increases disproportionately with increases in oxygen uptake, and the ventilatory equivalent may reach 35 or 40 L.

3. The eventual sharp upswing in ventilation during incremental exercise provides a "bloodless" means for estimating the onset of blood lactate accumulation. This submaximal measure is believed to reflect the onset of anaerobiosis in the active muscles. Consequently, an important aspect of aerobic fitness can be evaluated without significant metabolic acidosis or severe cardiovascular strain.

4. In healthy individuals, the oxygen cost of breathing is relatively small, even during the most severe exercise. In those with respiratory disease, however, the work of breathing is excessive and alveolar ventilation often becomes inadequate.

5. Airway resistance greatly increases after cigarette smoking. This increases the cost of breathing, which could be detrimental to performance during prolonged exercise. Substantial reversibility occurs with just 1 day of smoking abstinence.

6. Exercise training generally reduces the ventilatory equivalent in submaximal exercise. This "conserves" oxygen because the cost of breathing is lowered during a particular exercise task.

7. The ventilatory response is specific to the type of exercise, and the physiological adaptations are specific to the form of exercise used in training. A more efficient breathing pattern is generally observed only in the type of exercise used in training.

8. In individuals of average aerobic fitness, pulmonary ventilation is not taxed in maximal exercise to a point that would limit optimal alveolar gas exchange in maximal exercise. For the endurance athlete, however, improvements in pulmonary function may lag behind the exceptional adaptations in cardiovascular and muscle function, thereby compromising the aeration of blood during maximal effort.

PART 3
ACID-BASE REGULATION

BUFFERING

Substances that dissociate in solution and release H^+ are called **acids,** whereas compounds that can pick up or accept H^+ to form hydroxide ions (OH^-) are **bases.** The term **buffering** is used to designate reactions that minimize changes in H^+ concentration, and the chemical or physiologic mechanisms that prevent this change are termed **buffers**.

The pH is a quantitative measure of the acidity or alkalinity (basicity) of a liquid solution. Specifically, pH refers to the concentration of protons or H^+. Solutions with relatively more H^+ than OH^- have a pH below 7.0 and are termed acidic, and vice versa for basic solutions whose pH is above 7.0. Chemically pure (distilled) water is considered neutral, with equal amounts of H^+ and OH^-, and thus has a pH of 7.0. The pH scale shown in Figure 14.11 was devised in 1909 by the Danish chemist Sören Sörensen. It ranges from +1.0 to +14.0. There is an inverse relation between pH and the concentration of H^+. Because the pH scale is logarithmic, a one-unit change in pH is associated with a tenfold change in H^+ concentration. For example, lemon juice and gastric juice (pH = 2.0) have 1,000 times greater H^+ concentration than black coffee (pH = 5.0), whereas hydrochloric acid (pH = 1.0) has approximately 1,000,000 times the H^+ concentration of blood (pH = 7.4).

The pH of body fluids ranges from a low of 1.0 for the digestive acid hydrochloric acid to a slightly basic pH of between 7.35 and 7.45 for arterial and venous blood and most other body fluids. An increase in pH above the normal average of 7.4 is the direct result of a decrease in H^+ concentration (increase in pH) and is termed **alkalosis.** Conversely, an increase in H^+ concentration (decrease in pH) is referred to as **acidosis.** In the body, the acid-base quality of fluids must be regulated within narrow limits because metabolism is highly sensitive to the H^+ concentration of the reacting medium. Three mechanisms regulate the pH of the internal environment: (*a*) chemical buffers, (2) pulmonary ventilation, and (3) renal function.

CHEMICAL BUFFERS

The body's chemical buffering system consists of a weak acid and the salt of that acid. The bicarbonate buffer, for example, consists of the weak acid, **carbonic acid,** and the salt of that acid, **sodium bicarbonate.** Carbonic acid is formed when bicarbonate binds H^+. As long as the H^+ concentration remains elevated, the reaction produces the weak acid because the excess H^+ ions are bound in accordance with the general reaction:

$$H^+ + Buffer \rightarrow H\text{-Buffer}$$

If, however, the concentration of H^+ decreases (as occurs during hyperventilation, when plasma carbonic acid decreases because carbon dioxide is eliminated from the blood), the buffering reaction moves in the opposite direction and H^+ ions are released:

$$H^+ + Buffer \leftarrow H\text{-Buffer}$$

Much of the carbon dioxide generated in energy metabolism reacts with water to form the relatively weak car-

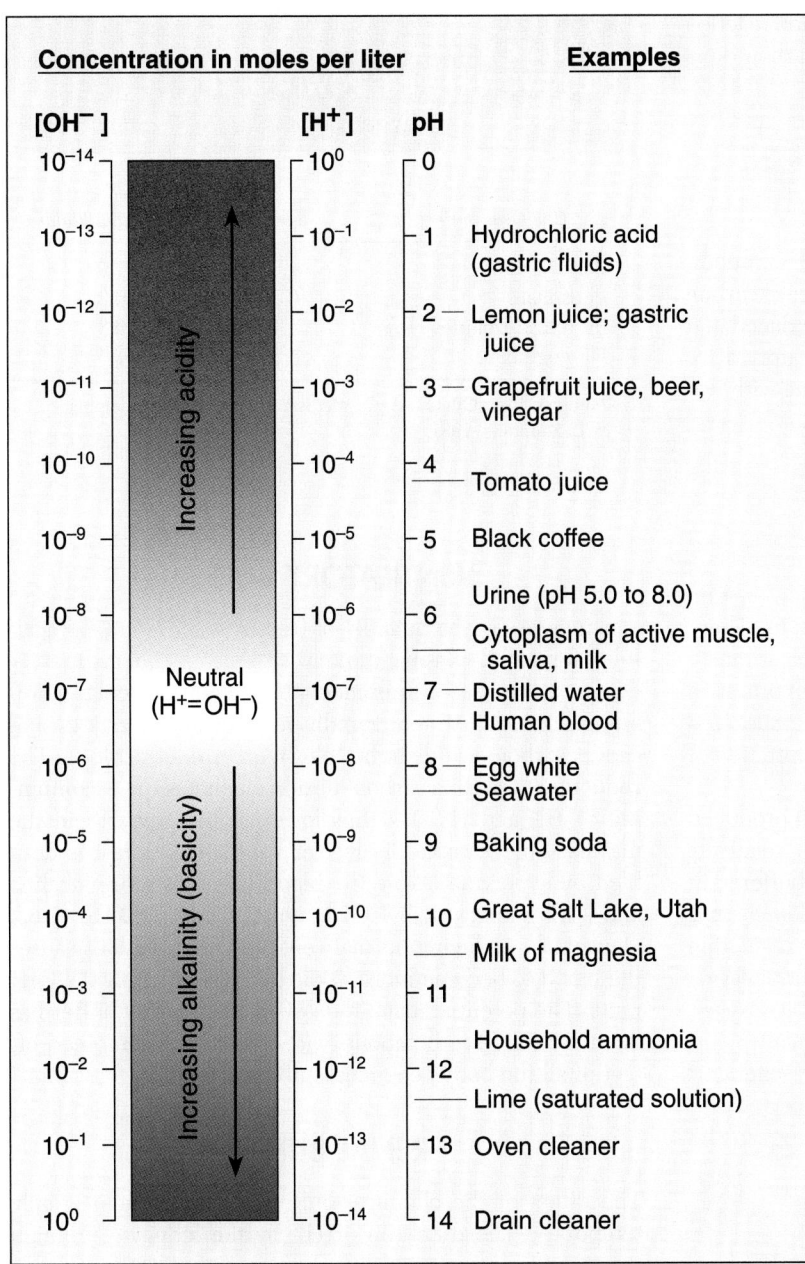

Concentration in moles per liter

| [OH⁻] | [H⁺] | pH | Examples |

$[OH^-]$ $[H^+]$ pH

Increasing acidity

Neutral
($H^+ = OH^-$)

Increasing alkalinity (basicity)

$[OH^-]$	$[H^+]$	pH	Examples
10^{-14}	10^{0}	0	
10^{-13}	10^{-1}	1	Hydrochloric acid (gastric fluids)
10^{-12}	10^{-2}	2	Lemon juice; gastric juice
10^{-11}	10^{-3}	3	Grapefruit juice, beer, vinegar
10^{-10}	10^{-4}	4	Tomato juice
10^{-9}	10^{-5}	5	Black coffee
10^{-8}	10^{-6}	6	Urine (pH 5.0 to 8.0) Cytoplasm of active muscle, saliva, milk
10^{-7}	10^{-7}	7	Distilled water Human blood
10^{-6}	10^{-8}	8	Egg white Seawater
10^{-5}	10^{-9}	9	Baking soda
10^{-4}	10^{-10}	10	Great Salt Lake, Utah Milk of magnesia
10^{-3}	10^{-11}	11	Household ammonia
10^{-2}	10^{-12}	12	Lime (saturated solution)
10^{-1}	10^{-13}	13	Oven cleaner
10^{0}	10^{-14}	14	Drain cleaner

FIGURE 14.11
The pH scale is a quantitative measure of the acidity or alkalinity (basicity) of a liquid solution. Blood pH normally is maintained at the slightly alkaline pH of 7.4. Values for blood pH rarely fall below a pH of 6.9, even during the most vigorous exercise.

bonic acid. This then dissociates to H^+ and HCO^-. Likewise, lactic acid, a stronger acid, reacts with sodium bicarbonate to form sodium lactate and carbonic acid; in turn, carbonic acid dissociates and increases the H^+ concentration of the extracellular fluids. Other organic acids such as fatty acids dissociate and liberate H^+, as do the sulfuric and phosphoric acids produced during protein breakdown.

CHEMICAL BUFFERS

Bicarbonate, phosphate, and protein chemical buffers provide the rapid first line of defense in maintaining consistency in the acid-base quality of the internal environment.

Bicarbonate Buffer. The bicarbonate buffer system consists of carbonic acid and sodium bicarbonate in solution. In the buffering process, for example, hydrochloric acid (a strong acid) is changed into the much weaker carbonic acid by combining with sodium bicarbonate in the reaction:

$$HCl + NaHCO_3 \rightarrow NaCl + H_2CO_3 \longleftrightarrow H^+ + HCO_3^-$$

This buffering process results only in a slight reduction in pH. As mentioned previously, sodium bicarbonate in the plasma exerts a strong buffering action on lactic acid. This causes the formation of sodium lactate and carbonic acid. Any additional increase in H^+ concentration brought about by carbonic acid dissociation causes the dissociation reaction to move in the opposite direction. As a result, carbon dioxide is released into solution as follows:

Acidosis

$$H_2O + CO_2 \leftarrow H_2CO_3 \leftarrow H^+ + HCO_3^-$$

An increase in plasma carbon dioxide or H^+ immediately stimulates ventilation to eliminate the "excess" carbon dioxide. Conversely, if the H^+ concentration is reduced and the body fluids become more alkaline, the ventilatory drive is inhibited, carbon dioxide is retained to combine with water, and the acidity is normalized.

Alkalosis

$$H_2O + CO_2 \rightarrow H_2CO_3 \rightarrow H^+ + HCO_3^-$$

Phosphate Buffer. The phosphate buffering system consists of phosphoric acid and sodium phosphate. These chemicals act in a manner similar to that of the bicarbonate system. The phosphate buffer is particularly important in regulating the acid-base balance in the kidney tubules and intracellular fluids, in which there is a high concentration of phosphates.

Protein Buffer. Although the carbonic acid produced by the union of water and carbon dioxide is a relatively weak acid, the H^+ released when it dissociates is buffered in the venous blood. *By far, hemoglobin is the most important H^+ acceptor for this function.* Its potency for regulating acidity is almost six times greater than the other plasma proteins. In addition, when hemoglobin releases its oxygen to the cells, it becomes a weaker acid. This, in turn, increases its affinity for binding with H^+. The H^+ generated from the formation of carbonic acid in the erythrocyte combines readily with deoxygenated hemoglobin (Hb^-) in the reaction:

$$H^+ + Hb^-(Protein) \rightarrow HHb$$

Intracellular tissue proteins also contribute to the regulation of plasma pH. Some amino acids have free acidic radicals that, when dissociated, form OH^-, which can react with H^+ to form water.

Relative Power of the Chemical Buffers. The relative power of the different chemical buffers in the blood, as well as in blood and interstitial fluids combined, is shown in Table 14.2. As a frame of reference, the buffering power of the bicarbonate system is given the value of 1.00.

PHYSIOLOGIC BUFFERS

The second line of defense in acid-base regulation are the pulmonary and renal systems, which provide a buffering function only when a change in pH has already occurred.

TABLE 14.2
RELATIVE BUFFERING POWER OF THE CHEMICAL BUFFERS

Chemical Buffer	Blood	Blood Plus Interstitial Fluids
Bicarbonate	1.0	1.0
Phosphate	0.3	0.3
Proteins (excludes Hb)	1.4	0.8
Hemoglobin	5.3	1.5

Modified from Guyton, A. C.: *Medical Physiology*. Philadelphia, W.B. Saunders, 1981.

VENTILATORY BUFFER

Any increase in the quantity of free H^+ (acidity) in extracellular fluid and plasma directly stimulates the respiratory center and causes it to immediately increase alveolar ventilation. This adjustment rapidly reduces alveolar P_{CO_2} and causes carbon dioxide to be "blown off" from the blood. The reduction in plasma carbon dioxide facilitates the recombining of H^+ and HCO_3^-, thus lowering the free H^+ in the plasma. For example, if alveolar ventilation at rest is doubled by hyperventilation, the blood becomes more alkaline and pH increases by 0.23 units from 7.40 to 7.63. Conversely, reducing normal ventilation by one-half causes the blood to become more acidic by approximately 0.23 pH units. The potential magnitude of the ventilatory buffer has been estimated to be about twice that of the combined effect of all the body's chemical buffers.

RENAL BUFFER

The effect of the chemical buffers on excess acid is only temporary. The excretion of H^+ by the kidneys, although time consuming, is important in maintaining the body's buffer reserve or **alkaline reserve.** To this end, the kidneys are the body's final defense. Acidity can be controlled in the renal tubules through complex chemical reactions that involve the secretion of ammonia and H^+ into the urine and the reabsorption of alkali, chloride, and bicarbonate.

EFFECTS OF EXERCISE AND TRAINING

The regulation of pH becomes progressively more difficult in strenuous exercise, during which H^+ is increased from both carbon dioxide and lactic acid formation. This is particularly apparent during repeated periods of all-out intermittent exercise of short duration, during which blood lactate values can reach 30 mM (approximately 270 mg of lactate per 100 mL of blood) or more.[26] As illustrated in Figure 14.12, a negative linear relationship exists between blood lactate concentration and blood pH.[47] In these experiments, blood lactate varied between 0.8 mM at rest (pH 7.43) and 32.1 mM during exhaustive exercise (pH 6.80). In active muscle, pH is even lower, falling to a pH of approximately 6.4 or lower at the point of exhaustion.[59]

These data indicate that humans are able **temporarily** to tolerate pronounced disturbances in acid-base balance during maximal exercise, at least to a blood pH as low as 6.80 (one of the lowest values ever reported for a human). Acidosis at a pH below 7.00 is not without consequences; in-

dividuals with acidosis can experience nausea, headache, and dizziness, as well as pain in the muscles involved in exercise.

Does Training Improve Buffering Capacity? It is well known that vigorous anaerobic training enables individuals to tolerate higher blood lactate levels (and lower pH values) than were possible before such training. It is tempting to speculate that anaerobic training has a positive effect on the body's capacity for acid-base regulation, perhaps through the enhancement of chemical buffers or the alkaline reserve. However, it has never been shown that buffering capacity becomes enhanced through exercise training. Improved acid tolerance (in the blood) following heavy training probably is due to motivational factors; the repeated stress of anaerobic exercise training probably "toughens" one's tolerance to the extreme discomfort of the acidic condition.

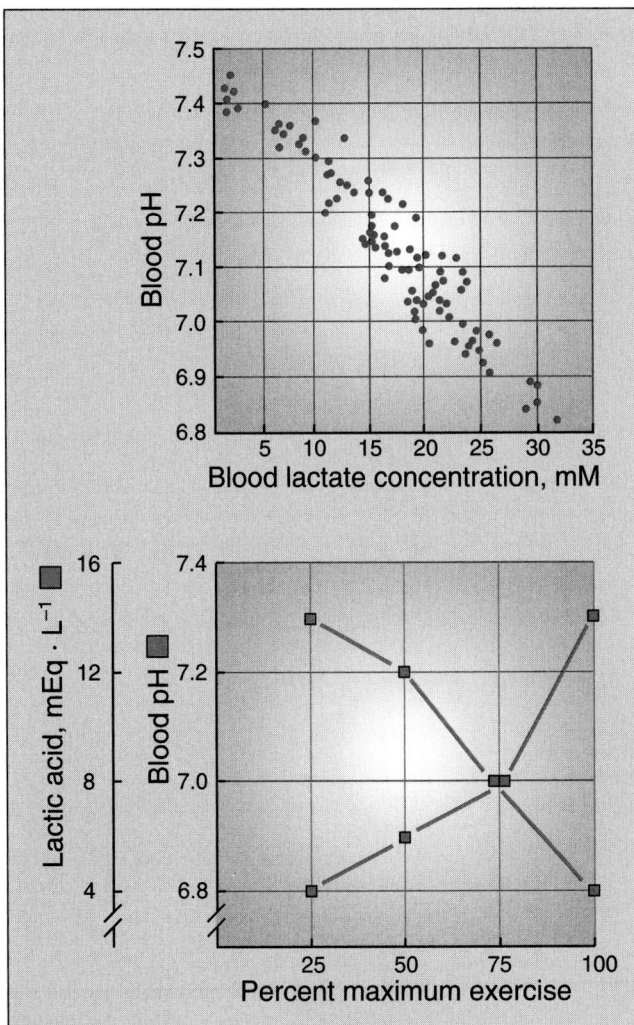

FIGURE 14.12

Top, The relationship between blood pH and blood lactate concentration at rest and during increasing intensities of short-duration exercise up to the maximum. (From Osnes, J.B., and Hermansen, L.: Acid-base balance after maximal exercise of short duration. *J. Appl. Physiol.,* 32:59, 1972.) *Bottom,* Blood pH and blood lactate concentration in relation to exercise intensity expressed as a percent of maximum. As blood lactate increases, there is an accompanying decrease in blood pH.

■ SUMMARY ■

1. The acid-base quality of the body fluids is normally regulated within narrow limits by the chemical and physiologic buffer systems.
2. The bicarbonate, phosphate, and protein chemical buffers provide the rapid first line of defense in acid-base regulation. These buffers consist of a weak acid and the salt of that acid. In an acidic condition, their action converts a strong acid to a weaker acid and a neutral salt.
3. When the chemical buffer system is stressed, the lungs and kidneys are able to regulate pH. Changes in alveolar ventilation rapidly alter the free H^+ in extracellular fluids. In response to increased acidity, the renal tubules act as the body's final defense by secreting H^+ into the urine and reabsorbing bicarbonate.
4. Anaerobic exercise creates an increased demand for buffering, and pH regulation becomes progressively more difficult. From available evidence, it does not seem that exercise training per se enhances the body's overall buffering capacity.

■ REFERENCES ■

1. Aaron, E.A., et al.: Oxygen cost of exercise hyperpnea: implications for performance. *J. Appl. Physiol.,* 75:1818, 1992.
2. Acevedo, E.O., and Goldfarb, A.H.: Increased training intensity effects on plasma lactate, ventilatory threshold, and endurance. *Med. Sci. Sports Exerc.,* 21:563, 1989.
3. Babcock, M.A., and Dempsey, J.A.: Pulmonary system adaptations: limitations to exercise. In *Physical Activity, Fitness, and Health.* Edited by C. Bouchard, et al. Champaign, IL, Human Kinetics, 1994.
4. Bianchi, A.L., et al.: Central control of breathing in mammals: neuronal circuitry, membrane properties, and neurotransmitters. *Physiol. Rev.,* 75:1, 1995.

5. Bye, P.T.P., et al.: Ventilatory muscles during exercise in air and oxygen in normal men. *J. Appl. Physiol.*, 56:464, 1984.

6. Carter, R., et al.: Exercise training in patients with chronic obstructive pulmonary disease. *Med. Sci. Sports Exerc.*, 24:281, 1991.

7. Casaburi, R., et al.: Effect of endurance training on possible determinants of V̇o₂ during heavy exercise. *J. Appl. Physiol.*, 62:199, 1987.

8. Chevrolet, J.C., et al.: Alterations in inspiratory and leg muscle force and recovery pattern after a marathon. *Med. Sci. Sports Exerc.*, 25:501, 1993.

9. Coast, J.R., et al.: Ventilatory work and oxygen consumption during exercise and hyperventilation. *J. Appl. Physiol.*, 74:793, 1993.

10. Coggan, A.R., et al.: Plasma glucose kinetics during exercise in subjects with high and low lactate thresholds. *J. Appl. Physiol.*, 73:1873, 1992.

11. Colberg, S.R., et al.: Increased dependence on blood glucose in smokers during rest and sustained exercise. *J. Appl. Physiol.*, 76:26, 1994.

12. Coyle, E.F., et al.: Blood lactate threshold in some well-trained ischemic heart disease patients. *J. Appl. Physiol.*, 54:18, 1983.

13. Coyle, E.F., et al.: Determinants of endurance in well trained cyclists. *J. Appl. Physiol.*, 64:2622, 1988.

14. Coyle, E.F., et al.: Physiological and biomechanical factors associated with elite endurance cycling performance. *Med. Sci. Sports Exerc.*, 23:93, 1991.

15. Coyle, E.F.: Integration of the physiological factors determining endurance performance in athletes. *Exerc. Sport Sci. Rev.*, 23:25, 1995.

16. Craig, A.B., Jr.: Principles and problems of underwater swimming and diving. *Med. Sci. Sports Exerc.*, 8:171, 1976.

17. Craig, A.B., Jr.: Principles and problems of underwater diving. *Phys. Sportsmed.*, 8(3):72, 1980.

18. Davis, C., et al.: Effect of 40 weeks of endurance training on anaerobic threshold. *Int. J. Sports Med.*, 3:208, 1982.

19. Davis, J.A., et al.: Anaerobic threshold and maximal aerobic power for three modes of exercise. *J. Appl. Physiol.*, 41:544, 1976.

20. Eldridge, F.L.: Central integration of mechanisms in exercise hyperpnea. *Med. Sci. Sports Exerc.*, 26:319, 1994.

21. Farrell, P.A., et al.: Plasma lactate accumulation and distance running performance. *Med. Sci. Sports Exerc.*, 11:338, 1979.

22. Fringer, M.N., and Stull, G.A.: Changes in cardiorespiratory parameters during periods of training and detraining in young adult females. *Med. Sci. Sports Exerc.*, 6:20, 1974.

23. Hagberg, J.M., and Coyle, E.F.: Physiological determinants of endurance performance as studied in competitive racewalkers. *Med. Sci. Sports Exerc.*, 15:287, 1983.

24. Henritze, J., et al.: Effects of training at and above the lactate threshold and maximal oxygen uptake. *Eur. J. Appl. Physiol.*, 54:84, 1985.

25. Hermansen, L.: Lactate production during exercise. In *Muscle Metabolism During Exercise*. Edited by B. Pernow and B. Saltin. New York, Plenum Press, 1971.

26. Hermansen, L.: Effect of metabolic changes on force generation in skeletal muscle during maximal exercise. In *Human Muscle Fatigue: Physiological Mechanisms*. London, Pitman Medical, 1981.

27. Holloszy, J.O, and Coyle, E.F.: Adaptations of skeletal muscle to endurance exercise and their metabolic consequences. *J. Appl. Physiol.*, 56:834, 1984.

28. Ivy, J.L., et al,: Progressive metabolite changes in individual muscle fibers with increasing work rates. *Am. J. Physiol.*, 252:C630, 1987.

29. Jirka, Z., and Adamus, M.: Changes of ventilation equivalents in young people in the course of three years of training. *J. Sports Med.*, 5:1, 1965.

30. Johnson, B.D., et al.: Mechanical constraints on exercise hyperpnea in endurance athletes. *J. Appl. Physiol.*, 73:874, 1992.

31. Johnson, B.D., et al.: Exercise induced diaphragmatic fatigue in healthy humans. *J. Physiol. (Lond.)*, 460:385, 1993.

32. Jones, N.L., and Ehrsam, R.E.: The anaerobic threshold. In *Exercise and Sport Sciences Reviews*. Vol. 10. Edited by R. L. Terjung. Philadelphia, Franklin Institute, 1982.

33. Jones, N.L.: Dyspnea in exercise. *Med. Sci. Sports Exerc.*, 16:14, 1984.

34. Katch, F.I., et al.: The influence of the estimated oxygen cost of ventilation on oxygen deficit and recovery oxygen intake for moderately heavy bicycle ergometer exercise. *Med. Sci. Sports Exerc.*, 4:71, 1972.

35. Kohrt, W.M., et al.: Longitudinal assessment of responses by triathletes to swimming, cycling, and running. *Med. Sci. Sports Exerc.*, 21:569, 1989.

36. Koyal, S.N., et al.: Ventilatory responses to the metabolic acidosis of treadmill and cycle ergometry. *J. Appl. Physiol.*, 40:864, 1976.

37. Kumagi, S., et al.: Relationship of the anaerobic threshold with the 5 km, 10 km, and 10 mile races. *Eur. J. Appl. Physiol.*, 49:13, 1982.

38. Laustiola, K.E., et al.: Cigarette smoking alters sympathoadrenal regulation by decreasing the density of beta₂-adrenoceptors. A study of monitored smoking cessation. *J. Cardiovasc. Pharmacol.*, 17:923, 1991.

39. Levison, H., and Cherniack, R.: Ventilatory cost of exercise in chronic obstructive pulmonary disease. *J. Appl. Physiol.*, 25:21, 1968.

40. Magel, J.R., et al.: Specificity of swim training on maximum oxygen uptake. *J. Appl. Physiol.*, 38:151, 1975.

41. Mahler, D.A., et al.: Ventilatory responses at rest and during exercise in marathon runners. *J. Appl. Physiol.*, 52:388, 1982.

42. Mahon, A.D., and Vaccaro, P.: Ventilatory threshold and V̇o₂max changes in children following endurance training. *Med. Sci. Sports Exerc.*, 21:425, 1989.

43. McArdle, W.D., et al.: Metabolic and cardiorespiratory response during free swimming and treadmill walking. *J. Appl. Physiol.*, 30:733, 1971.

44. Nadel, J.A., and Comroe, J.H.: Acute effects of inhalation of cigarette smoke on airway resistance. *J. Appl. Physiol.*, 16:713, 1961.

45. Nakamura, M., et al.: Acute effects of cigarette smoke inhalation on peripheral airways in dogs. *J. Appl. Physiol.*, 58:27, 1985.

46. Nye, P.C.G.: Identification of peripheral chemoreceptor stimuli. *Med. Sci. Sports Exerc.*, 26:311, 1994.

47. Osnes, J.B., and Hermansen, L.: Acid-base balance after maximal exercise of short duration. *J. Appl. Physiol.*, 32:59, 1972.

48. Powers, S.K., et al.: Incidence of exercise induced hypoxemia in elite endurance athletes at sea level. *Eur. J. Appl. Physiol.*, 58:298, 1988.

49. Powers, S.K., et al.: Effects of incomplete pulmonary gas exchange on V̇o₂max . *J. Appl Physiol.*, 66:2491, 1989.

50. Préfaut, C., et al.: Exercise-induced hypoxemia in older athletes. *J. Appl. Physiol.*, 76:120, 1994.

51. Rasmussen, R., et al.: Pulmonary ventilation, blood gases and blood pH after training of the arms and the legs. *J. Appl. Physiol.*, 38:250, 1975.

52. Rasmussen, J., et al.: Muscle mass effect on arterial desaturation after maximal exercise. *Med. Sci. Sports Exerc.*, 23:1349, 1991.

53. Rode, A., and Shephard, R.J.: The influence of cigarette smoking upon the oxygen cost of breathing in near-maximal exercise. *Med. Sci. Sports Exerc.*, 3:51, 1971.

54. Rowland, T.W., and Green, G.M.: Physiological responses to treadmill exercise in females: adult-child differences. *Med. Sci. Sports Exerc.*, 20:474, 1988.

55. Seip, R.L., et al.: Perceptual responses and blood lactate concentration: effect of training state. *Med. Sci. Sports Exerc.*, 23:80, 1991.

56. Sidney, S., et al.: Cigarette smoking and submaximal exercise test duration in a biracial population of young adults: the CARDIA study. *Med. Sci. Sports Exerc.*, 25:911, 1993.

57. Tanaka, K., et al.: Relationship of anaerobic threshold and onset of blood lactate accumulation with endurance performance. *Eur. J. Appl. Physiol.*, 52:51, 1983.

58. Tanaka, K., et al.: A longitudinal assessment of anaerobic threshold and distance-running performance. *Med. Sci. Sports Exerc.*, 16:278, 1984.

59. Taylor, D.J., et al.: Energetics of human muscle: exercise-induced ATP depletion. *Magn. Reson. Med.*, 3:44, 1986.

60. Tzankoff, S.P., et al.: Physiological adjustments to work in older men as affected by physical training. *J. Appl. Physiol.*, 33:346, 1972.

61. Ward, S.: Assessment of peripheral chemoreflex contributions to exercise hyperpnea in humans. *Med. Sci. Sports Exerc.,* 26:303, 1994.

62. Wasserman, K., et al.: Respiratory physiology of exercise: metabolism, gas exchange and ventilatory control. In *Respiratory Physiology III.* Vol. 23. International Review of Physiology. Edited by J.G. Widdicombe. Baltimore, University Park Press, 1981.

63. Wasserman, K., et al.: *Principles of Exercise Testing and Interpretation.* 2nd Ed. Philadelphia, Lea & Febiger, 1994.

64. Weltman, A.: *The Blood Lactate Response to Exercise.* Champaign, IL, Human Kinetics, 1995.

65. Weltman, A., et al.: Reliability and validity of a continuous incremental treadmill protocol for the determination of lactate threshold, fixed blood lactate concentrations and $\dot{V}O_2$max. *Int. J. Sports Med.,* 11:26, 1990.

66. Whipp, B.J.: Peripheral chemoreceptor control of exercise hyperpnea in humans. *Med. Sci. Sports Exerc.,* 26:337, 1994.

67. Williams, J.H., et al.: Hemoglobin desaturation in highly trained athletes during heavy exercise. *Med. Sci. Sports Exerc.,* 18:168, 1986.

68. Yoshida, T., et al.: Blood lactate parameters related to aerobic capacity and endurance performance. *Eur. J. Appl. Physiol.,* 56:7, 1987.

Karvonen, M.J., et al.: The effects of training on heart rate: a longitudinal study. *Ann. Med. Exp. Biol. Fenn.* 35:307, 1957.

For many years, research focused on endurance exercise to develop and maintain cardiorespiratory fitness. While mode, frequency, duration, type, and intensity of exercise all influence the exercise prescription, exercise intensity serves as the most important consideration. However, experts have hotly debated the most effective method to determine optimal exercise intensity to induce a training response. The study by Karvonen and colleagues provided a simple method using heart rate (HR) to gauge appropriate training intensity.

type (treadmill running), duration of exercise (30 minutes), frequency of training (4 or 5 days per week), and length of training (4 weeks). Three different heart rates served as criterion measures: training heart rate (THR), the heart rate measured during each training session; resting heart rate (RHR), measured every morning in bed, before the subject got up during the training period; and maximal heart rate (MHR), determined before and after the 4 weeks of training.

Because the study aimed to keep training intensity constant, there were periodic increases in running speed so THR would not decrease as cardiovascular fitness improved. The researchers' method for calculating THR, now known as the *"Karvonen method"* or HR reserve method, makes use of the subject's exercise HR increase above RHR in relation to the difference between the MHR and RHR. The basic formula to calculate THR at a given percentage training intensity ($\%T_{INT}$) is as follows:

$$THR = [(MHR - RHR) \times \%T_{INT}] + RHR$$

The formula to calculate $\%T_{INT}$ at a known THR is as follows:

$$\%T_{INT} = (THR - RHR) \div (MHR - RHR) \times 100$$

If one wished to know his THR at $\%T_{INT} = 70\%$, and knows that he has an MHR of 170 beats · min^{-1} and an RHR of 52 beats · min^{-1}, then THR equals 135 beats · min^{-1}: $[(170 - 52) \times 0.70] + 52 = 135$. Conversely, if the THR is known one can calculate the $\%T_{INT}$: $(135 - 52) \div (170 - 52) \times 100 = 70\%$.

The researchers showed that if THR served as an indicator of training intensity, the "borderline" between effective and ineffective training would slightly exceed the 60% T_{INT}. They therefore recommended that to induce a "training effect," THR must be at least 60% T_{INT} and preferably 70% T_{INT}. The figure graphically displays the results from a typical subject. In this example, THR approximated 136 beats · min^{-1} or 71% of his available heart rate range. The top panel displays the change in running speed required to maintain the same THR.

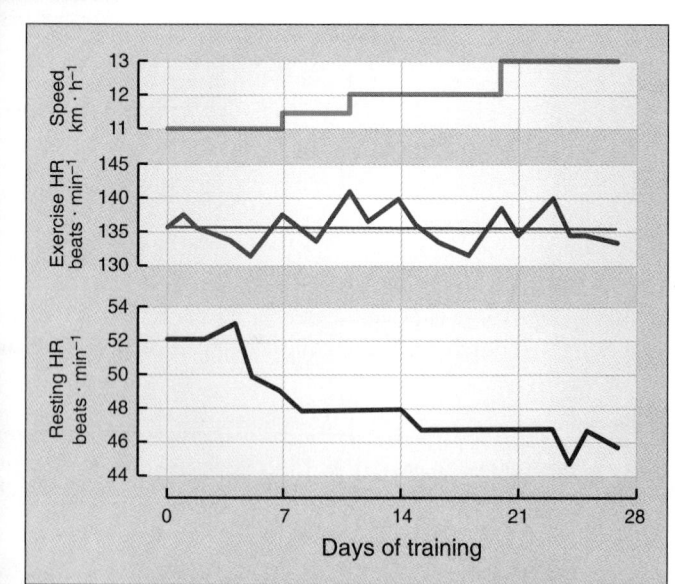

The concept and calculations of effective training intensity using HR developed by Karvonen had a major impact on the field of exercise training.

The researchers used exercise training at different intensities to determine the influence of resting, exercise, and maximal heart rate on the training response of six young adult (20- to 23-year-old) male medical students. The study's unique aspect included constancy of exercise

The Cardiovascular System

The **cardiovascular system** integrates the body as a unit. It provides the active muscles with a continuous stream of nutrients and oxygen to sustain a high energy output. Conversely, by-products of metabolism are rapidly removed by the circulation from the site of energy release.

Chapters 15, 16, and 17 explore the process of circulation, particularly its role in oxygen delivery during exercise, and examine the basic differences in cardiovascular dynamics between trained and untrained men and women. Oxygen transport, coupled with the capacity of active muscles to generate adenosine triphosphate (ATP) aerobically, ultimately sets the maximum level for aerobic energy transfer during exercise.

COMPONENTS OF THE CARDIOVASCULAR SYSTEM

The cardiovascular system is a continuous system consisting of a pump, a high-pressure distribution circuit, exchange vessels, and a low-pressure collection and return circuit. If stretched out in a line, the 100,000 miles of blood vessels of an average-sized adult would circle the earth four times. A schematic view of this system, including the main arteries in an adult, is presented in Figure 15.1. The tabular data show the distribution of blood within the circulatory system, both in absolute and percentage terms. Note that approximately 60% of the total blood volume is contained within the small arteries, veins, and capillaries of the systemic circulation, whereas approximately 7% is contained within the heart muscle.

THE HEART

The heart provides the impetus for blood flow. It is situated in the midcenter of the chest cavity; about two-thirds of its mass lies to the left of the body's midline. Although this four-chambered muscular organ weighs less than a pound, it beats so steadily and powerfully that the force generated during its 40 million beats per year could lift its owner 100 miles above the earth. At rest, the heart's output of blood is approximately 1,400 gallons daily, or 37 million gallons over a 72-year lifetime. Even for a person of average physical fitness, the maximum output of blood from this remarkable organ in 1 minute is greater than the fluid output from a household faucet turned wide open!

The heart muscle, or **myocardium,** is a form of striated muscle similar to skeletal muscle. The individual fibers, however, are multinucleated cells interconnected in a latticework fashion. Consequently, when one cell is stimulated or depolarized, the action potential speeds through the myocardium to all cells, causing the heart to function as a unit.

The structural details of the heart as a pump are shown in Figure 15.2. Functionally, the heart can be viewed as two separate pumps. The hollow chambers that compose the right side of the heart (right heart) perform two important functions:

- Receive blood returning from all parts of the body.
- Pump blood to the lungs for aeration by way of the **pulmonary circulation.**

The left side of the heart (left heart) also performs two important functions:

- Receives oxygenated blood from the lungs.
- Pumps blood into the thick-walled, muscular aorta for distribution throughout the body in the **systemic circulation.**

A thick, solid muscular wall or interventricular septum separates the left and right sides of the heart. The **atrioventricular valves** situated in the heart provide a one-way flow of blood from the right atrium to the right ventricle (**tricuspid valve**) and from the left atrium to the left ventricle (**mitral or bicuspid valve**). The **semilunar valves** located in the arterial wall just outside the heart prevent blood from flowing back into the heart between contractions. The relatively thin-walled, sac-like atrial chambers serve as primer or "booster" pumps to receive and store blood during the period of ventricular contraction. Approximately 70% of the blood returning to the atria flows directly into the ventricles before the atria contract. The simultaneous contraction of both atria then forces the remaining blood into their respective ventricles directly below. Almost immediately after atrial contraction, the ventricles contract and force blood into the arterial system.

As ventricular pressure builds, the atrioventricular valves snap closed. All heart valves remain closed between 0.02 and 0.06 seconds. This brief interval of rising ventricular tension, during which the heart volume and muscle fiber

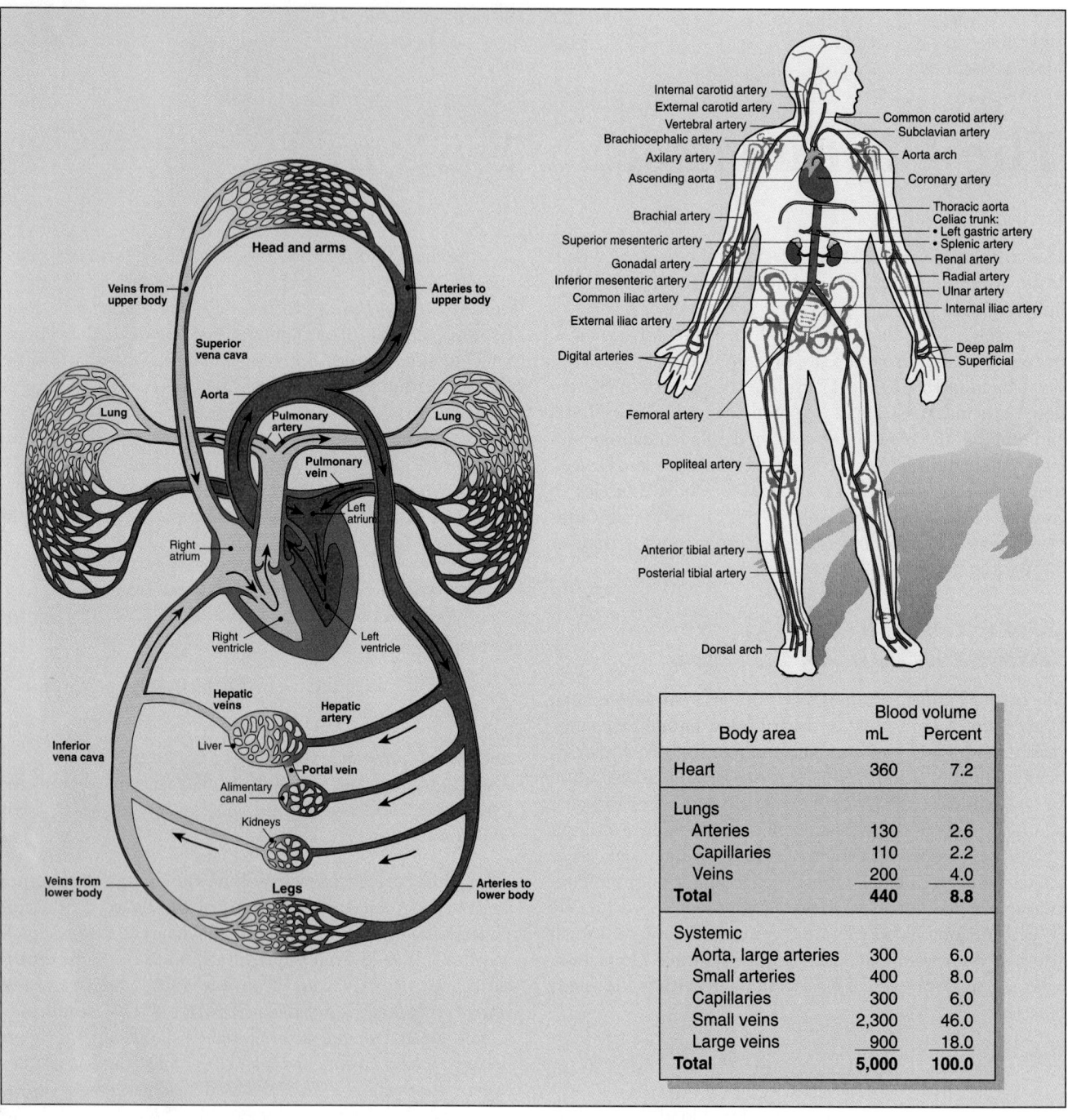

The following table shows the estimated distribution of the total blood volume:

Body area	Blood volume mL	Percent
Heart	360	7.2
Lungs		
Arteries	130	2.6
Capillaries	110	2.2
Veins	200	4.0
Total	**440**	**8.8**
Systemic		
Aorta, large arteries	300	6.0
Small arteries	400	8.0
Capillaries	300	6.0
Small veins	2,300	46.0
Large veins	900	18.0
Total	**5,000**	**100.0**

FIGURE 15.1

Left, Schematic view of the cardiovascular system that consists of the heart and the pulmonary and systemic vascular circuits. The dark shading shows the oxygen-rich arterial blood, whereas the deoxygenated venous blood is somewhat paler. In the pulmonary circuit, the situation is reversed, and oxygenated blood returns to the heart in the right and left pulmonary veins. *Right,* Main arteries in the adult systemic circulation. The table shows the estimated distribution of the total blood volume in the pulmonary and systemic vascular circuits of an adult male of average size at rest.

length remain unchanged, represents the heart's **isovolumetric contraction period.** Blood is ejected from the heart when the ventricular pressure exceeds the arterial pressure. By the nature of the spiral and circular arrangement of bands of cardiac muscle, blood is virtually "wrung out" of the heart with each contraction.

THE ARTERIAL SYSTEM

The Arteries. The arteries are the high-pressure tubing that conducts oxygen-rich blood to the tissues. As depicted in Figure 15.3, the arteries are composed of layers of connective tissue and smooth muscle. The walls of these vessels are so thick that no gaseous exchange takes place between arterial blood and the surrounding tissues. Blood pumped from the left ventricle into the highly muscular yet elastic **aorta** is distributed throughout the body via a network of arteries and smaller arterial branches called **arterioles.** The walls of arterioles are composed of circular layers of smooth muscle that either constrict or relax to regulate blood flow in the periphery. It is the ability of these "resistance vessels" to alter dramatically their internal diameter that provides a rapid and effective means for regulating blood flow through the vascular circuit. This redistribution function is particularly important during exercise because blood can be diverted to active muscles from areas that can temporarily compromise their blood supply. The inset table of Figure 15.3 lists average values for the diameter of the various blood vessels and the corresponding values for the velocity of blood that flows through them.

Blood Pressure. A surge of blood enters the aorta with each contraction of the left ventricle. Because the peripheral vessels do not permit blood to "run off" into the arterial system as rapidly as it is ejected from the heart, a portion of this blood is "stored" in the aorta. This creates pressure within the entire arterial system and causes a pressure wave to travel down the aorta to the remote branches of the arterial tree. This stretch and subsequent recoil of the arterial wall during a cardiac cycle can be felt readily as the characteristic "pulse" in any superficial artery of the body. In healthy individuals, the pulse rate and heart rate are identical. *In essence, arterial blood pressure is a function of the arterial blood flow per minute (i.e., the cardiac output) and the vascular or peripheral resistance to that flow.* This relationship is expressed as follows:

Blood pressure = Cardiac output × Total peripheral resistance

Systolic Blood Pressure. At rest, the highest pressure generated by the heart is approximately 120 mm Hg during the contraction or **systole** of the left ventricle. The point of reference for this measurement is usually the brachial artery at the level of the right atrium. **Systolic blood pressure** provides an estimate of the work of the heart and of the strain against the arterial walls during ventricular contraction. During the heart's relaxation phase, when the aortic valves close, the natural elastic recoil of the arterial system provides for a continuous head of pressure to maintain a steady flow of blood into the periphery until the next surge of blood.

Diastolic Blood Pressure. During **diastole** or the relaxation phase of the cardiac cycle, arterial blood pressure decreases to approximately 70 or 80 mm Hg. **Diastolic**

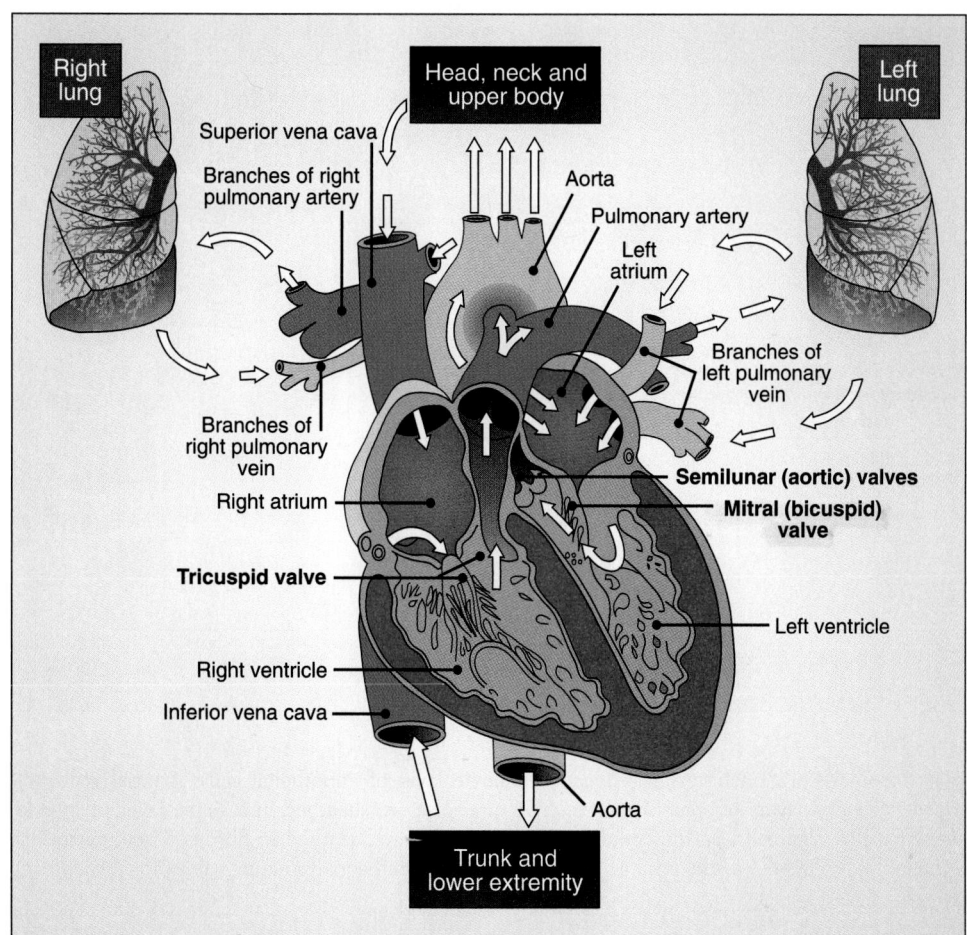

Right lung

Superior vena cava

Branches of right pulmonary artery

Head, neck and upper body

Aorta

Pulmonary artery

Left atrium

Left lung

Branches of left pulmonary vein

Branches of right pulmonary vein

Right atrium

Tricuspid valve

Right ventricle

Inferior vena cava

Semilunar (aortic) valves

Mitral (bicuspid) valve

Left ventricle

Aorta

Trunk and lower extremity

FIGURE 15.2

The heart. The heart's valves provide the one-way flow of blood as indicated by the arrows.

blood pressure provides an indication of **peripheral resistance** or the ease with which blood flows from the arterioles into the capillaries. When peripheral resistance is high, the pressure within the arteries after systole is not rapidly dissipated and thus remains elevated for a large portion of the cardiac cycle. The measurement of systolic and diastolic blood pressure by the common auscultation method is illustrated in Figure 15.4.

Mean Arterial Pressure. In young, healthy adults at rest, the systolic blood pressure averages approximately 120 mm Hg and the diastolic pressure is 80 mm Hg. Because the heart remains in diastole longer than it does in systole, the average or **mean arterial pressure (MAP)** is slightly less than simply the average of the systolic and diastolic pressures and, at rest, averages approximately 93 mm Hg. The MAP represents the average force exerted by the blood against the walls of the arteries during the entire cardiac cycle. The MAP is estimated as follows:

MAP = Diastolic BP + [0.333 (Systolic − Diastolic BP)]

For example, for a person with a diastolic blood pressure of 89 mm Hg and a systolic pressure of 127 mm Hg, the MAP would be 89 + [0.333 (127 − 89)] or 102 mm Hg.

Cardiac Output and Total Peripheral Resistance. The basic hemodynamic equation that relates blood pressure to cardiac output and total peripheral resistance can be rearranged to illustrate the factors that determine either cardiac output or total peripheral resistance as follows:

Cardiac Output = Blood Pressure ÷ Total Peripheral Resistance

Total Peripheral Resistance = Blood Pressure ÷ Cardiac Output

For example, the change in the total resistance to blood flow from rest to exercise can be determined from the MAP (computed from the systolic and diastolic blood pressure) and cardiac output. Suppose the systolic blood pressure at rest is 120 mm Hg, the diastolic pressure is 80 mm Hg (MAP = 93.3 mm Hg), and the cardiac output is 5.0 L · min^{-1}. Substituting these values in the formula for total peripheral resistance gives a value of 18.7 mm Hg per liter of blood flow (93.3 mm Hg ÷ 5.0 L · min^{-1}). During exercise, when systolic pressure increases considerably more than the diastolic pressure and cardiac output can increase six to eight times the value at rest, the resistance to

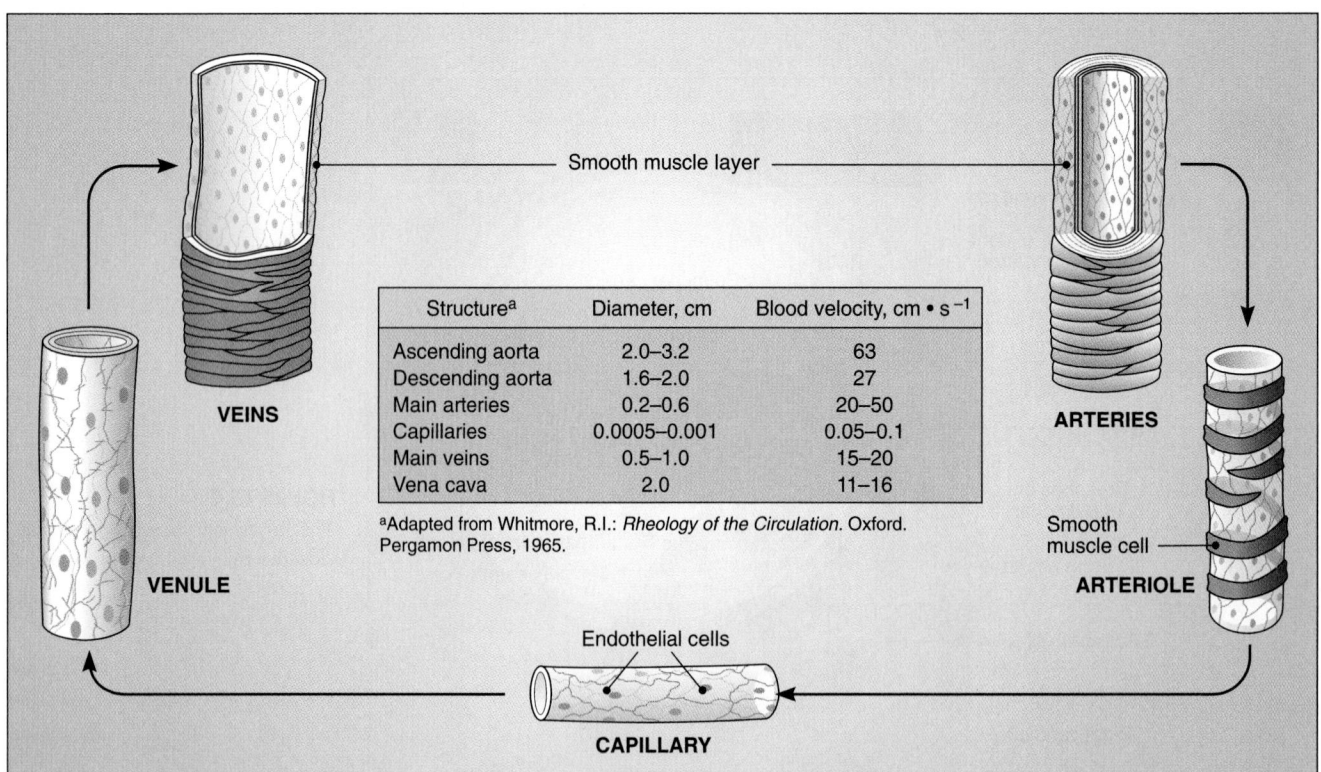

Structure[a]	Diameter, cm	Blood velocity, cm · s^{-1}
Ascending aorta	2.0–3.2	63
Descending aorta	1.6–2.0	27
Main arteries	0.2–0.6	20–50
Capillaries	0.0005–0.001	0.05–0.1
Main veins	0.5–1.0	15–20
Vena cava	2.0	11–16

[a]Adapted from Whitmore, R.I.: *Rheology of the Circulation.* Oxford. Pergamon Press, 1965.

FIGURE 15.3

The structure of the walls of the various blood vessels. Each vessel is lined by a single layer of endothelial cells. Arterial walls are surrounded by fibrous tissue and wrapped in several layers of smooth muscle. The arterioles are sheathed in a single layer of muscle cells; capillaries consist of only one layer of endothelial cells. In the venule, endothelial cells are sheathed in fibrous tissue, and veins also possess a layer of smooth muscle. The table displays the average values for vessel diameter and corresponding values for the velocity of blood flow.

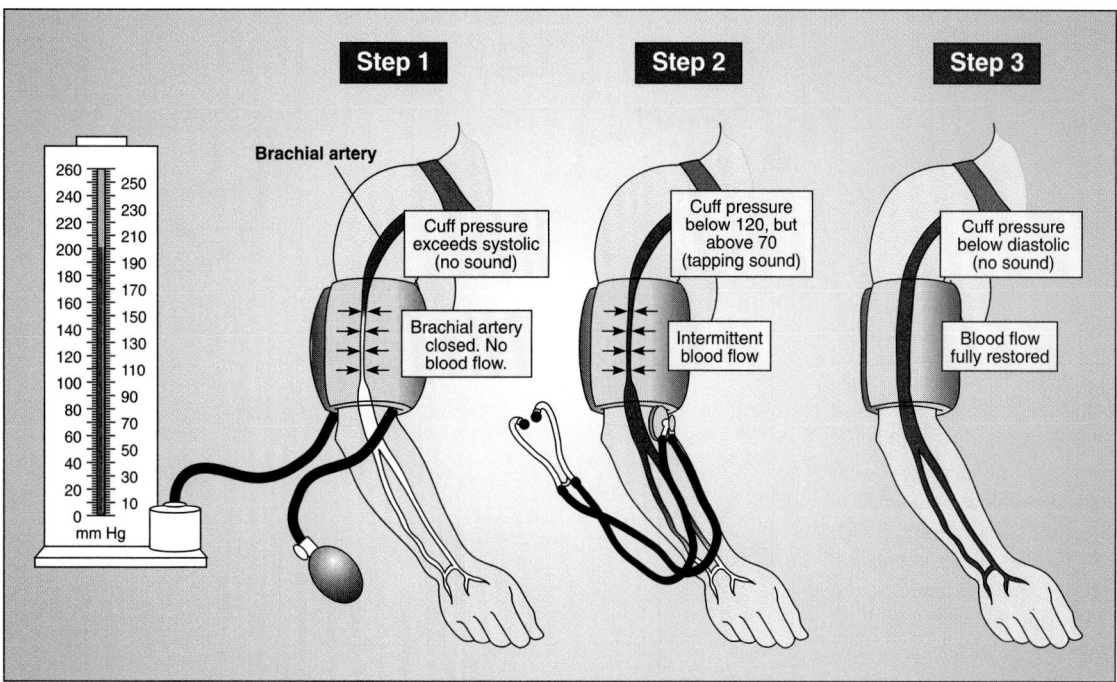

FIGURE 15.4

Measurement of blood pressure at the brachial artery by the auscultatory method. *Step 1,* A pressure cuff or sphygmomanometer is inflated so its pressure exceeds the systolic pressure within the artery. Blood flow is occluded and a brachial pulse (at the elbow fossa) cannot be felt (palpated) or heard (auscultated). Note the restriction to blood flow through the brachial artery. *Step 2,* The pressure within the cuff is reduced by small increments and the examiner listens until a faint sound occurs. This sound represents blood flowing through the brachial artery. The systolic pressure is the pressure exerted on the walls of the artery when the first soft tapping sounds occur. *Step 3,* As the pressure in the cuff is lowered further, distinct sounds continue to be heard as blood flows through the artery for longer portions of the cardiac cycle. Diastolic pressure refers to the pressure in the artery when the sounds are greatly muffled or disappear.

peripheral blood flow can **decrease** dramatically. For example, if the exercise cardiac output is 35.0 L · min⁻¹ and MAP is 130 mm Hg (systolic = 210 mm Hg; diastolic = 90 mm Hg), then resistance to blood flow in the systemic circulation would be 3.71 mm Hg per liter per minute, or 5 times **less** compared to resting conditions.

THE CAPILLARIES

The arterioles continue to branch and form smaller and less muscular vessels called **metarterioles.** These end in a network of microscopic blood vessels (approximately 0.01 mm in diameter) called capillaries. These vessels generally contain approximately 5% of the total blood volume. The average diameter of a capillary is 7 to 10 μm (approximately ¹⁄₁₀₀ of a millimeter). As was shown in Figure 15.3, the capillary wall usually consists of a single layer of endothelial cells. Some capillaries are so narrow that they provide room for only one blood cell to squeeze through at a time. In many instances, the proliferation of capillaries is so extensive that their walls actually abut the membranes of the surrounding cells. The capillary density of human skeletal muscle is estimated to be between 2,000 and 3,000 capillaries

per square millimeter of tissue. This density is even greater in heart muscle, in which no cell lies farther than 0.008 mm from its nearest capillary.

Blood Flow in Capillaries. The diameter of a capillary opening is controlled by a ring of smooth muscle, the **precapillary sphincter,** that encircles the vessel at its origin. The constriction and relaxation action of this sphincter is extremely important in exercise because it provides a localized means for regulating blood flow within a specific tissue to meet its metabolic requirements.

A generalized view of what takes place within the capillaries of muscle during rest and exercise is shown in Figure 15.5. At rest, many more capillary channels are available than are actually used. For this particular example in the gastrocnemius muscle, blood flow each minute averages approximately 5 mL for every 100 g of muscle tissue. Thus, if the muscle weighed 600 g, then approximately 30 mL of blood would flow through it each minute. During exercise, blood flow increases rapidly and dramatically as previously "unused" capillaries are opened. This dilation of precapillary sphincters is brought about by the action of the driving force of increased local blood pressure, as well as by intrinsic neural control and local metabolic factors related to exercise.

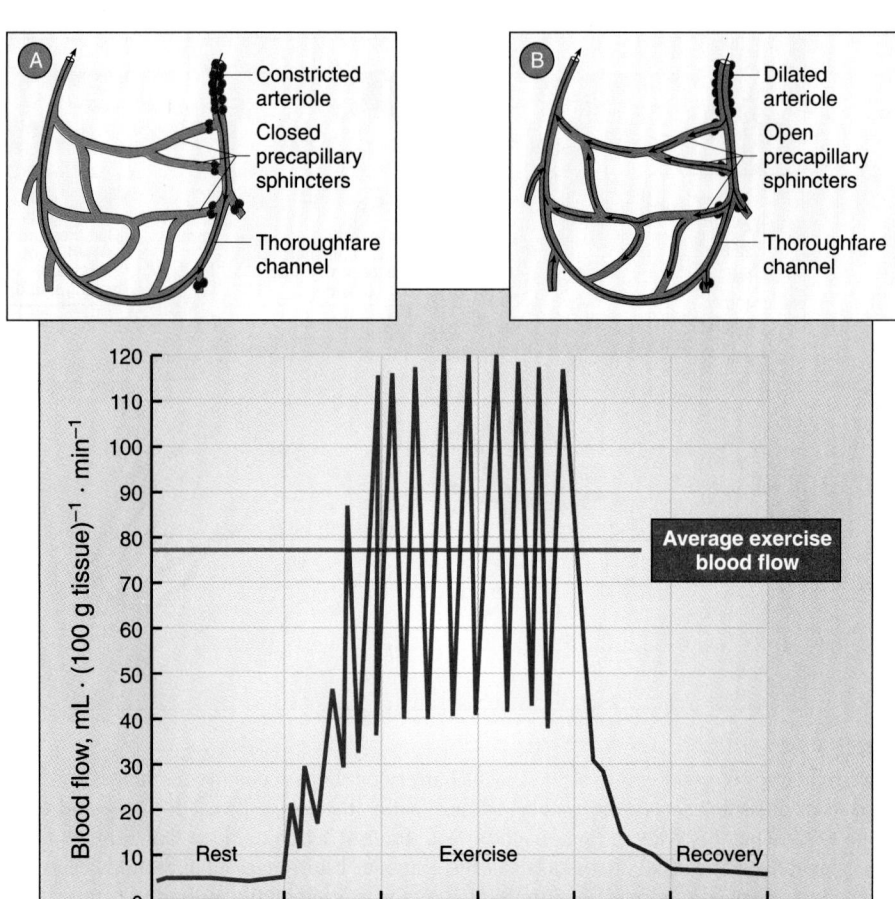

FIGURE 15.5

Blood flow in capillaries at rest (**A**) and during exercise (**B**). The bottom figure shows the pulsatile pattern of blood flow at rest, during exercise, and when exercise ceases. A major factor that augments local blood flow is the dilation of the active muscle's arterioles, which directs blood through the surrounding vascular circuit. Capillary diameter, red blood cell size, and blood viscosity all affect capillary blood flow.

During strenuous exercise, a sustained local blood flow can be increased by 15 to 20 times the resting value or between 450 and 600 mL each minute for the gastrocnemius muscle.

Branching of the capillary microcirculation increases the cross-sectional area of these peripheral vessels to about 800 times that of the 1-inch-diameter aorta. Because the velocity of blood flow is inversely proportional to the vasculature's cross section,[a] there is a progressive decrease in velocity as blood moves toward and into the capillaries. As a result, it takes approximately 1.5 seconds for a blood cell to pass through an average-sized capillary. The total surface area of the capillary walls is more than 100 times greater than the external surface of the average adult. When this tremendous surface area is combined with a slow rate of blood flow (approximately 0.5 to 1.0 mm · sec^{-1} at rest), an extremely effective means exists for exchange between the blood and the tissues.

THE VEINS

The continuity of the vascular system is maintained as the capillaries feed deoxygenated blood at almost a trickle into the **venules** or small veins with which they merge. Blood flow then increases somewhat because the cross-sectional area of the venous system is now less than that of the capillaries. The smaller veins in the lower portion of the body eventually empty into the body's largest vein, the **inferior vena cava,** which returns blood to the right atrium from the abdomen, pelvis, and lower extremities. Venous blood coming from tributary blood vessels in the head, neck, shoulder regions, thorax, and part of the abdominal wall flows into the 7-cm-long **superior vena cava** and joins the inferior vena cava at heart level. This mixture of blood draining from the upper and lower body, called **mixed venous blood,** then enters the upper part of the right atrium and descends into the right ventricle, where it then is pumped through the pulmonary artery to the lungs. Gas exchange takes place in the alveolar-capillary network of the lungs; the blood then returns in the pulmonary veins to the left side of the heart to once again begin its passage through the body.

[a]Velocity, cm · sec^{-1} = Volume of flow, cm^3 · sec^{-1} ÷ Cross-sectional area, cm^2.

As illustrated in Figure 15.6, blood pressure and blood flow vary considerably in the systemic circulation. In the aorta and the large arteries, blood pressure fluctuates between 120 and 80 mm Hg during the cardiac cycle. The pressure then falls in direct proportion to the resistance encountered in the vascular circuit. For example, the blood at the arteriole end of the capillaries exerts an average pressure of only 30 mm Hg. As blood enters the venules, the impetus for blood flow is almost entirely lost. The pressure falls to approximately 0 mm Hg by the time blood reaches the right atrium. Because the venous system operates under relatively low pressure, the walls of the veins are much thinner and less muscular than the thicker-walled and less distensible arteries (see Fig. 15.3).

Venous Return. The low pressure of venous blood poses a special problem that is partly solved by a unique characteristic of veins. As shown in Figure 15.7, the thin, membranous, flaplike **valves** spaced at short intervals within the vein permit a one-way blood flow toward the heart. Due to the low pressure in the venous circuit, veins are easily compressed by the smallest muscular contractions or even by the minor pressure changes within the chest cavity with breathing. The alternate compression and relaxation of the veins, as well as the one-way action of their valves, provide a "milking" action similar to the heart's action. Compression of the veins imparts considerable energy for blood flow, whereas the "diastole" of these vessels enables them to refill as blood flows toward the heart. If valves were not present, blood would tend to pool, as it sometimes does in the veins of the extremities, and people would faint every time they stood up because of a reduction in cerebral blood flow.

An Active Vasculature. The veins are not merely passive conduits. At rest, the venous system normally contains approximately 65% of the total blood volume; therefore, the veins are considered capacitance vessels and serve as **blood reservoirs.** A slight increase in the tension or tone of the smooth muscle layer alters the diameter of the venous tree to produce a rapid redistribution of blood from peripheral veins toward the central blood volume returning to the heart. This gives the venous system an important role as an active blood reservoir to either retard or deliver blood to the systemic circulation.

Varicose Veins. Sometimes the valves within a vein become defective and fail to maintain the one-way flow of blood. This condition is called **varicose veins.** It usually occurs in the surface veins of the lower extremities owing to the force of gravity that retards blood flow in the upright posture.[11] Because these surface vessels have little external support from surrounding tissues, blood gathers, they become excessively distended and painful, and circulation from the affected area is actually impaired. In severe cases, the venous wall becomes inflamed and may degenerate (a condition called phlebitis). The vessel is then removed either surgically or nonsurgically by means of injected solutions that irritate the vessel's surface membranes,

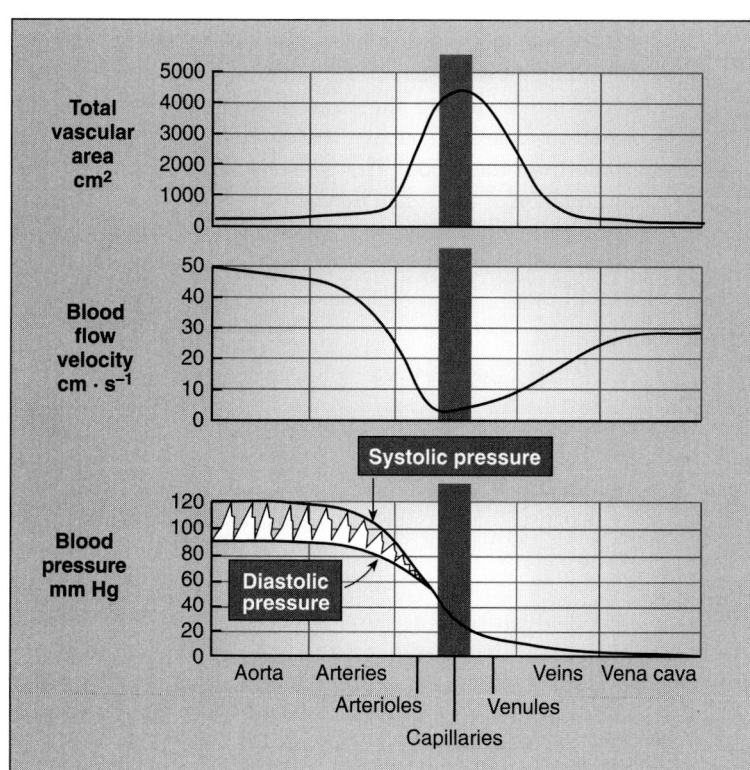

FIGURE 15.6
Blood flow and blood pressure in the systemic circulation. Note that blood pressure within the arterial system is inversely related to the total vascular area (resistance) in that section of the vascular tree.

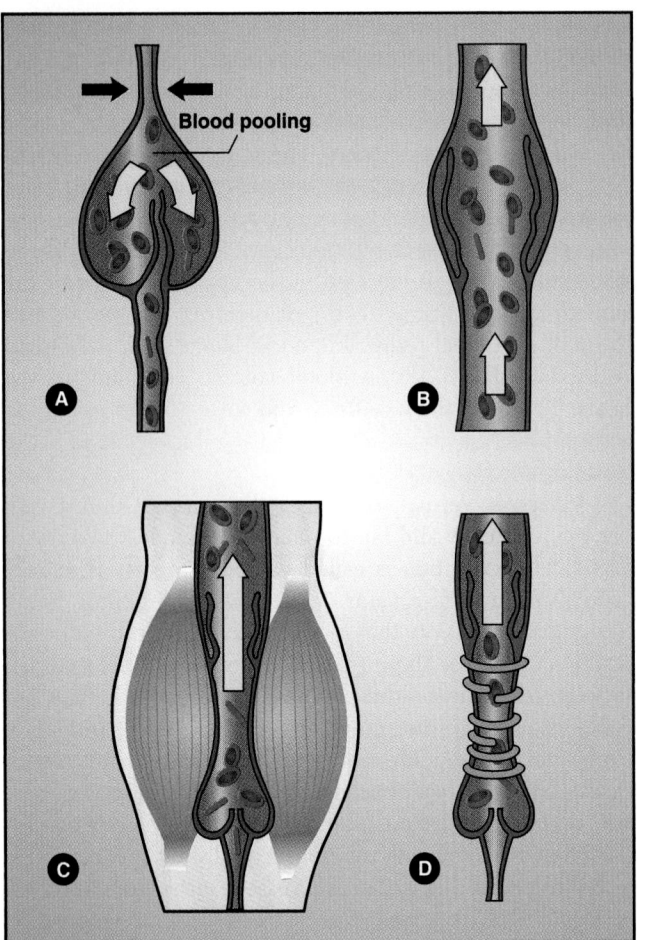

FIGURE 15.7
The valves in veins (**A**) prevent the backflow of blood but (**B**) do not hinder the normal one-way flow of blood. Blood can be propelled through veins by nearby active muscle (**C**) or by the contraction of smooth muscle bands within the veins themselves (**D**).

causing a portion of the vein to collapse, fuse, and eventually shrivel up. The body then reroutes the blood to the deeper veins.

Individuals who have varicose veins should probably avoid excessive straining exercises often used in resistance training. During such sustained, nonrhythmic muscle actions, both the muscle and ventilatory "pumps" are unable to contribute significantly to venous return. The increased abdominal pressure associated with straining also impedes venous return. All of these factors act to cause blood to pool in the veins of the lower body, which can aggravate an existing varicose-vein condition. Although exercise training cannot prevent the occurrence of varicose veins, regular and rhythmic physical activity may minimize complications be-

cause repeated muscle actions keep blood moving toward the heart.[52]

Venous Pooling. The rhythmic action of muscular activity and consequent compression of the vascular tree are so important to venous return that many people faint when forced to maintain an upright posture without movement. The classic "tilt table" experiment demonstrates this point. A subject lays supine and strapped on a table that can pivot to different positions. Heart rate and blood pressure are stable as long as the person remains horizontal. When the table is tilted vertically, an uninterrupted column of blood exists from heart to toes. This creates a hydrostatic force of about 80 to 100 mm Hg, which causes blood to pool in the lower extremities. This results in a backup of fluid in the capillary bed that then seeps into the surrounding tissues to cause swelling or **edema.** As a consequence, venous return is reduced and blood pressure declines; at the same time, the heart rate accelerates and venoconstriction is initiated to counter the effects of venous pooling. If the upright position is maintained, the subject eventually faints due to insufficient cerebral blood supply.[b] Tilting the person either horizontally or head down immediately restores circulation and consciousness is regained rapidly.

The pressurized suits worn by test pilots and special support stockings also aid in reducing the hydrostatic shift of blood to the veins of the lower extremities in the upright position. A similar supportive effect can be achieved in upright exercise in a swimming pool because the external support of the water facilitates venous return to the heart.

The Active Cool Down. The preceding discussion of venous pooling provides a sound rationale for the practice of continuing to walk or jog at a slow pace after strenuous exercise. Such moderate exercise in recovery, popularly known as "cooling down," facilitates blood flow through the vascular circuit (including the heart) during recovery. As discussed in Chapter 7, active recovery also aids in removing lactate from the blood. There also is an indication that the continuation of mild exercise during recovery may blunt any possible deleterious effects following exercise on cardiac function of elevated catecholamines epinephrine and norepinephrine.[10]

HYPERTENSION

Systolic pressure at rest may be as high as 250 or even 300 mm Hg in individuals whose arteries have become "hardened" because fatty materials have deposited within the walls (or because the vessel's connective tissue layer has thickened), or whose arterial system offers excessive resistance to blood flow in the periphery due to nervous strain or kidney malfunction. The diastolic pressure may also be elevated

---

[b]Ancient warriors, although unaware of the physiological mechanism involved, tied captured enemies in the standing position to a stake, where they were left unattended. Without much movement, the person would eventually perish, mainly due to a pooling of blood in the lower extremities, which caused an inadequacy of venous return.

above 90 mm Hg. Such high blood pressure, or **hypertension,** imposes a chronic strain on the cardiovascular system. As much as 95% of hypertension is of unknown cause.

One of every three to four persons will have abnormally high blood pressure at some time during their lives; the disease is prevalent among African Americans.[48] Presently, approximately 50 million Americans have systolic pressures over 140 mm Hg or diastolic pressures over 90 mm Hg (values generally considered **borderline** for hypertension) and/or are currently taking hypertensive medication. Each year, an additional 2 million Americans join this group.[53] Uncorrected hypertension can lead to heart failure, myocardial infarction, or stroke. Just a 2 mm Hg reduction in systolic blood pressure can reduce deaths from stroke by 6% and heart disease by 4%. Blood pressure should be checked at periodic intervals because elevated blood pressure can progress unnoticed for years. It can, however, be effectively treated with lifestyle changes and by medications that reduce extracellular fluid volume or peripheral resistance to blood flow. Beneficial lifestyle changes such as prudent diet, weight control, and moderate exercise performed on a regular basis are more desirable than the pharmacological approach for treating mild hypertension. This is because of possible harmful side effects of drug therapy on other risk factors for coronary artery disease.[29]

EFFECTS OF REGULAR EXERCISE

Systolic and diastolic blood pressure can be lowered by approximately 6 to 10 mm Hg with regular aerobic exercise for many previously sedentary men and women, regardless of age. These results have been observed with normotensive and hypertensive subjects both at rest and during exercise.[2, 23, 30, 55] Regular aerobic exercise as preventive medicine contributes to controlling the tendency for blood pressure to increase over time in individuals at risk for hypertension.[43] This prevention role is important because even when elevated blood pressure is normalized, the disease risk remains higher than it would be if the person had never become hypertensive.

The effects of exercise training on blood pressure are the most impressive in most patients with moderate or "borderline" hypertension.[1, 8, 26, 40] As indicated in Table 15.1, the average resting systolic pressure of seven middle-aged male patients decreased from 139 to 133 mm Hg following 4 to 6 weeks of interval training. At similar submaximal exercise levels, systolic pressure decreased from 173 to 155 mm Hg, while diastolic pressure also was reduced from 92 to 79 mm Hg. Consequently, mean arterial exercise blood pressure was reduced by approximately 14% following training. Similar findings were observed for an apparently healthy yet borderline hypertensive group of 37 middle-aged men following 6 months of exercise.[7] For a group of older men and women with hypertension aged 60 to 70 years, a 9-month program of low-intensity aerobic exercise lowered systolic blood pressure by 20 mm Hg and diastolic pressure by 12 mm Hg.[26]

The precise mechanism for the exercise training effect on lowering blood pressure is not known. Significant contributing factors may include:

- A reduced activity of the sympathetic nervous system with training. This would contribute to a decrease in peripheral resistance to blood flow and a subsequent reduction in blood pressure.[12, 14]
- An altered renal function to facilitate the elimination of sodium by the kidneys to subsequently reduce fluid volume and blood pressure.[34, 55]

TABLE 15.1
MEASURES OF BLOOD PRESSURE AT REST AND DURING SUBMAXIMAL EXERCISE BEFORE AND AFTER 4 TO 6 WEEKS OF TRAINING IN SEVEN MIDDLE-AGED PATIENTS WITH CORONARY HEART DISEASE[a]

| | Rest | | | Submaximal Exercise | | |
| | Average Value | | Difference (%) | Average Value | | Difference (%) |
Measure[a]	Before	After		Before	After	
Systolic blood pressure (mm Hg)	139	133	−4.3	173	155	−10.4
Diastolic blood pressure (mm Hg)	78	73	−6.4	92	79	−14.1
Mean blood pressure (mm Hg)	97	92	−5.2	127	109	−14.3

Modified from Clausen, J. P., et al.: Physical training in the management of coronary artery disease. *Circulation* 40:143, 1969.
[a]Blood pressure was measured directly by a pressure transducer inserted into the brachial artery.

Not all research supports the wisdom of exercise in treating hypertension. For example, studies with various animal models for hypertension have not demonstrated a dramatic or consistent benefit of regular regimens of forced exercise.[19] Even when regular exercise is shown to lower blood pressure in humans, the studies often contain methodological shortcomings and inadequate design.[50] The most glaring weakness is usually the lack of an appropriate control group of individuals who have their blood pressure measured but do not exercise. *Despite these concerns and limitations, a prudent recommendation is to include regular exercise and weight loss as a first line of defense in most therapeutic programs to manage borderline hypertension.*[1, 32] Even if exercise is ineffective in normalizing blood pressure, aerobic training confers health benefits independent of the blood pressure effect. In one study, aerobically fit individuals with hypertension had a 60% lower mortality rate than their unfit normotensive peers.[4] The increased mortality associated with elevated blood pressure was entirely overcome by the higher fitness level. For more severe and resistant elevations in blood pressure, a combination of diet, weight loss, increased exercise, and pharmacological therapies may be required.

BLOOD PRESSURE AND EXERCISE

STATIC AND DYNAMIC RESISTANCE EXERCISE

Straining exercise, especially during the concentric (shortening) phase of the muscle action, mechanically compresses the peripheral arterial system. This causes a sustained reduction in muscle perfusion (dramatic increase in total peripheral resistance) that is in direct proportion to the percentage of the maximum force capacity exerted. Consequently, sympathetic nervous system activity, cardiac output, and mean arterial pressure increase dramatically in an attempt to restore muscle blood flow.[21, 27] The magnitude of this response is directly related to the intensity of effort and the size of the muscle mass involved.[20, 39]

Research has focused on comparing the blood pressure responses during static and dynamic resistance exercise.[17, 36] In a study from one of our laboratories, the blood pressure of normotensive subjects was measured directly with a pressure transducer connected to a catheter inserted into the femoral artery.[18] Three forms of exercise were evaluated: (*a*) isometric bench press performed at 25, 50, 75, and 100% of the maximal voluntary contraction (MVC); (*b*) free-weight bench press performed at 25 and 50% of the isometric MVC; and (*c*) hydraulic resistance bench press exercise performed "all out" for 20 seconds at slow and fast speeds. The results displayed in Table 15.2 illustrate clearly that all three forms of exercise dramatically increase blood pressure and the corresponding workload of the heart (see Rate-Pressure Product, p. 280). Other research also indicates that exercise requiring a large muscle mass and greater relative strain elicits the greatest blood pressure response.[17, 51] As discussed in Chapter 16, this response is due to a greater stimulation of the cardiovascular center by the active areas of the motor cortex and a large peripheral feedback to this center from the contracting muscle mass.

The acute cardiovascular strain with heavy resistance exercise could be harmful to individuals who have heart and vascular disease, particularly for those untrained in this form of exercise. For these people, more rhythmic forms of moderate exercise are desirable and beneficial. Figure 15.8

TABLE 15.2

COMPARISON OF PEAK SYSTOLIC AND DIASTOLIC BLOOD PRESSURE DURING VARIOUS PERCENTAGES OF MAXIMUM VOLUNTARY CONTRACTION (MVC) IN ISOMETRIC AND BENCH PRESS, FREE-WEIGHT, AND HYDRAULIC RESISTANCE EXERCISE

Condition	*Isometric*[a] (% MVC)				*Free Weight Bench Press*[b] (% MVC)		*Hydraulic Bench Press*[c]	
	25	50	75	100	25	50	Slow	Fast
Peak systolic, mm Hg	172	179	200	225	169	232	237	245
Peak diastolic, mm Hg	106	116	135	156	104	154	101	160

Values are averages for seven subjects. Data from reference 18 and unpublished data, Human Performance Laboratory, Department of Exercise Science, University of Massachusetts, Amherst, MA.
[a]Open glottis (no Valsalva maneuver); average of two trials; contraction time 2 to 3 seconds; arm position that of bench-press exercise with hands just slightly above chest.
[b]The weight lifted was either 25 or 50% of previously determined isometric maximum action.
[c]Performed on Hydra-Fitness chest-press apparatus at dial setting 3 (slow) and 5 (fast) for 20 seconds of repeated maximal actions.

presents a generalized comparison between blood pressure at rest and during rhythmic aerobic exercise and heavy resistance exercise using a relatively small and large muscle mass.

CHRONIC EFFECTS OF RESISTANCE TRAINING

Although resistance exercise causes a greater rise in blood pressure than lower-intensity dynamic movement, it does not bring about any long-term increase in the resting blood pressure.[9, 16, 44] Furthermore, a regular program of resistance training blunts the blood pressure response to this form of exercise. Trained body builders, for example, show smaller increases in systolic and diastolic blood pressure with resistance exercise than both novice body builders and untrained individuals.[16] This blunted blood pressure response after training is particularly evident when a person exercises at the same absolute load during the pretraining and posttraining measures.[37] Regarding the effect on hypertension, most research indicates that standard resistance training is less effective in lowering resting blood pressure than programs of regular aerobic exercise,[2, 14, 42] although some positive effects of resistance training have been reported.[25, 57] Heavy resistance exercise is not recommended as the only form of training to lower blood pressure in hypertensive individuals.[1]

STEADY-RATE EXERCISE

During rhythmic muscular activity such as jogging, swimming, and bicycling, dilation of the blood vessels in the active muscles decreases total peripheral resistance, thus enhancing blood flow through large portions of the peripheral vasculature. The alternate contraction and relaxation of the muscles also provide an effective force to propel blood through the vascular circuit and return it to the heart. The increased blood flow during rhythmic steady-rate exercise causes systolic pressure to rise rapidly during the first few minutes of exercise. The blood pressure then levels off at approximately 140 to 160 mm Hg with probably no difference between sexes.[15] As exercise continues, systolic pressure may gradually decline as the arterioles in the muscles continue to dilate and there is a reduction in peripheral resistance to blood flow. The diastolic blood pressure remains relatively unchanged during this exercise.

GRADED EXERCISE

The general pattern for systolic and diastolic blood pressure during continuous, graded treadmill exercise is illustrated in Figure 15.9. After the initial rapid rise from the resting level, systolic blood pressure increases linearly with exercise intensity, whereas diastolic pressure remains stable or increases slightly at the higher levels of exercise. This re-

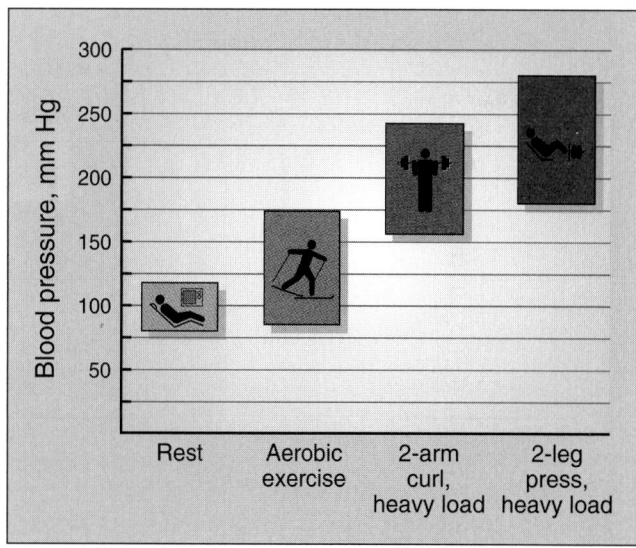

FIGURE 15.8
The blood pressure response is magnified significantly during heavy resistance exercise (higher with legs than arms) compared to rhythmic, continuous aerobic exercise.

sponse is similar for both trained and sedentary subjects. During maximum exercise performed by healthy, fit men and women, the systolic blood pressure may increase to 200 mm Hg or higher, despite significant reductions in total peripheral resistance.[39] This response is most likely due to the large output of blood from the heart during maximal exercise.

BLOOD PRESSURE IN UPPER BODY EXERCISE

As shown in Table 15.3, at a given percentage of the maximal oxygen uptake, systolic and diastolic blood pressures are considerably higher when work is performed with the arms than with the legs.[45, 54] This is because the smaller muscle mass and vasculature of the arms offer greater resistance to blood flow than the larger mass and vasculature of the legs.[5] This form of exercise clearly represents greater cardiovascular strain because the work requirement of the myocardium is increased considerably. For individuals with cardiovascular dysfunction, these observations support the use of exercise requiring large muscle groups, such as walking, bicycling, and running, in contrast to unregulated exercises that engage a rather limited muscle mass such as shoveling, overhead hammering, or even arm-crank exercises.[17a, 38] If a systematic program of arm exercise is used for training patients with coronary heart disease, the workloads must be established based on the person's response to this form of exercise and not from some exercise stress test prescription that uses bicycling or running. The cardiovascular adjustment to arm exercise is discussed further in Chapter 17.

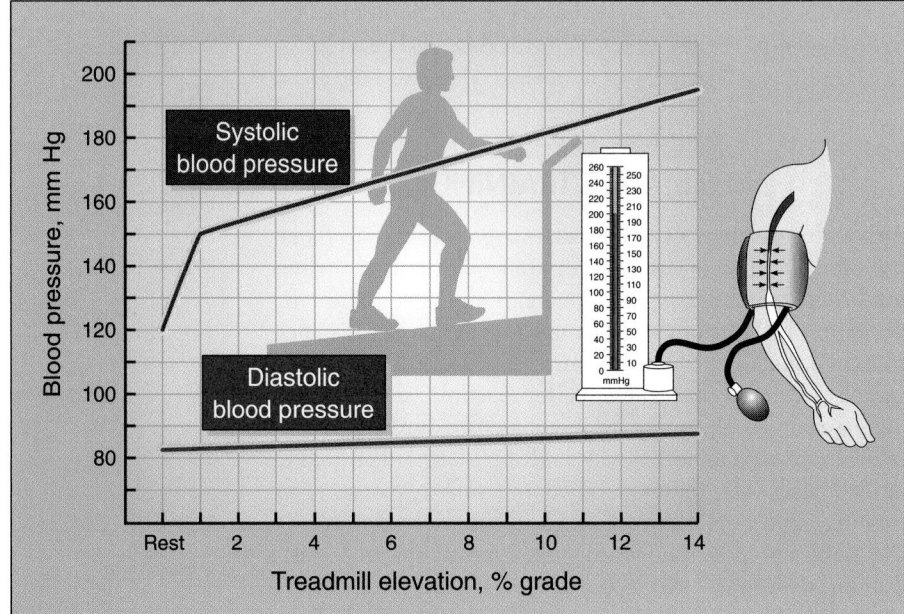

FIGURE 15.9
Generalized response for systolic and diastolic blood pressure during continuous, graded treadmill exercise testing.

TABLE 15.3
COMPARISON OF SYSTOLIC AND DIASTOLIC BLOOD PRESSURE DURING ARM AND LEG EXERCISE AT SIMILAR PERCENTAGES OF THE MAXIMAL OXYGEN UPTAKE

Percent of $\dot{V}o_2max$	Systolic Pressure (mm Hg)		Diastolic Pressure (mm Hg)	
	Arms	Legs	Arms	Legs
25	150	132	90	70
40	165	138	93	71
50	175	144	96	73
75	205	160	103	75

From Åstrand, P. O., et al: Intra-arterial blood pressure during exercise with different muscle groups. *J. Appl. Physiol.*, 20:253, 1965.

IN RECOVERY

After a period of sustained submaximal exercise, systolic blood pressure is temporarily reduced below pre-exercise levels for both normotensive and hypertensive individuals.[31, 47] This **hypotensive response** to previous exercise can last for up to 12 hours into recovery and occurs in response to both low and moderate intensity aerobic exercise.[46] One mechanism proposed for postexercise hypotension is that when aerobic exercise ceases, there is a prolonged period during which a significant quantity of blood remains pooled in the visceral organs and/or lower limbs.[6] This reduces the central blood volume, which causes a lowering of systemic arterial blood pressure. These findings further support the use of exercise as an important nonpharmacologic line of defense in treating hypertension and would justify participating in several periods of moderate physical activity interspersed throughout the day.

BODY INVERSION

Many people use gravity-inversion devices to hang in the upside-down position with the belief that this maneuver can offer relaxation, facilitate a strength-training response, or relieve lower back pain. Although it has never been demonstrated that inverting the body is of any practical or physiologic benefit, it is now apparent that it can cause a significant elevation in both systolic and diastolic blood pressure. In one study of 50 normotensive men and women, body inversion caused systolic blood pressure to rise from an average of 114 mm Hg to nearly 140 mm Hg, whereas diastolic pressure increased from 76 to 91 mm Hg.[35] In addition, these changes continued throughout the 3-minute duration of the inversion maneuver. Such a hypertensive response during inversion at rest in healthy individuals, as well as significant increases in intraocular pressure, raises concern about the possible consequences of inversion for hypertensive people and the prudence of recommending exercise in this position without closely monitoring the blood-pressure response.

THE HEART'S BLOOD SUPPLY

Although more than 2000 gallons of blood flow through the heart's chambers each day, none of its nourishment passes directly into the myocardium. This is because there are no direct circulatory channels within the heart's chambers leading to its tissues. Instead, the heart muscle has an elaborate circulatory network of its own. As shown in Figure 15.10, these vessels form a visible, crownlike network called the **coronary circulation** that arises from the top portion of the heart.

The right and left coronary arteries are derived from the upper part of the ascending portion of the aorta. Their openings are situated in the aorta just above the semilunar valves at a point at which the oxygenated blood leaves the left ventricle. These arteries then curl around the heart's surface; the right coronary artery supplies predominantly the right atrium and ventricle, whereas the greatest volume of blood flows in the left coronary artery to the left atrium and ventricle and a small part of the right ventricle. These vessels divide and eventually form a dense capillary network

within the myocardium. Blood then leaves the tissues of the left ventricle through the **coronary sinus;** blood from the right ventricle exits via the **anterior cardiac veins,** which empty directly into the right atrium.

With each heart beat, the driving force of the heart pushes a portion of blood into the coronary arteries. At rest, normal blood flow to the myocardium is 200 to 250 mL per minute; this represents approximately 5% of the heart's total output.

MYOCARDIAL OXYGEN UTILIZATION

At rest, the oxygen utilization of the myocardium is high in relation to its blood flow, as about 70 to 80% of the oxygen is extracted from the blood that flows in the coronary vessels.

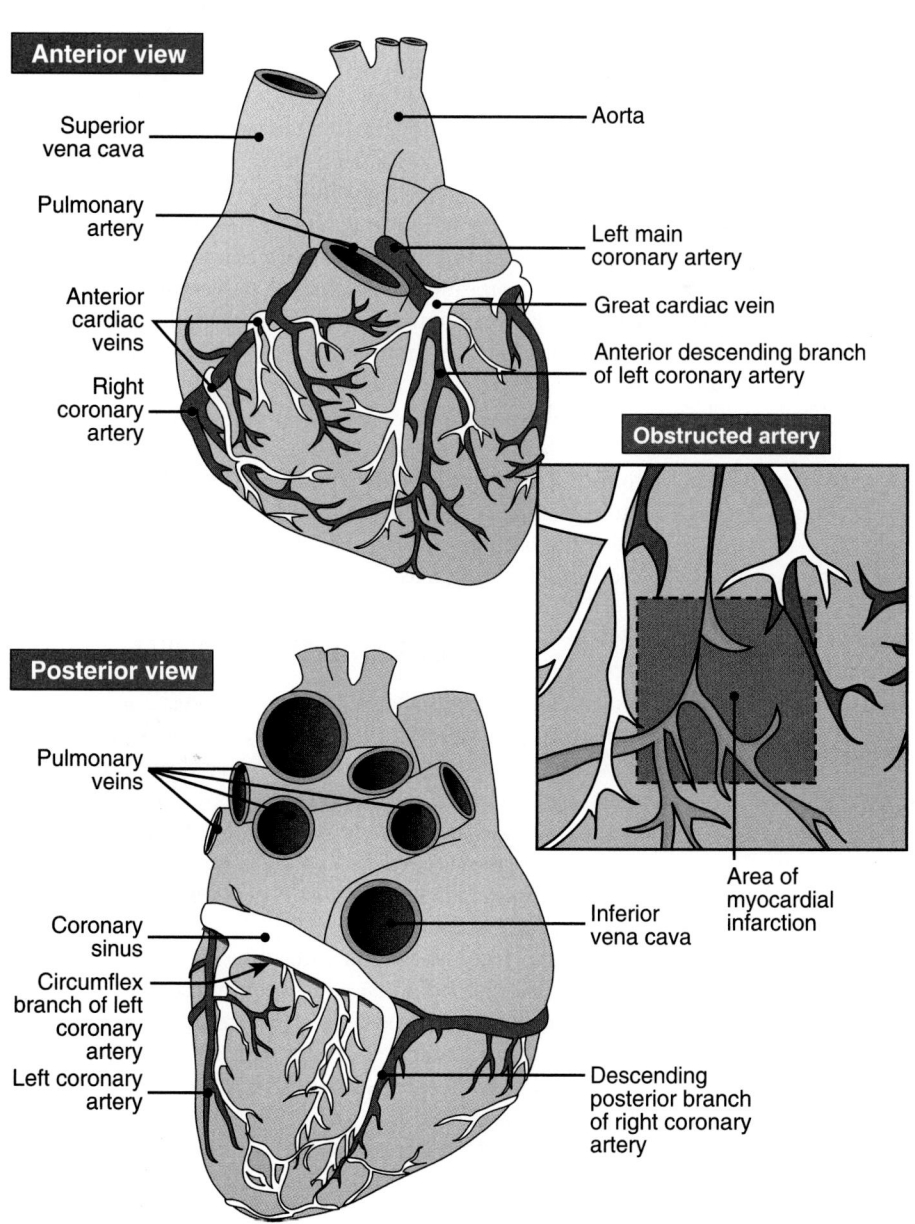

Anterior view

Superior vena cava
Pulmonary artery
Anterior cardiac veins
Right coronary artery

Aorta
Left main coronary artery
Great cardiac vein
Anterior descending branch of left coronary artery

Obstructed artery

Area of myocardial infarction

Posterior view

Pulmonary veins
Coronary sinus
Circumflex branch of left coronary artery
Left coronary artery

Inferior vena cava
Descending posterior branch of right coronary artery

FIGURE 15.10
Anterior and posterior view of the coronary circulation. Arteries are shaded dark and veins are unshaded. The insert figure illustrates a myocardial infarction resulting from the blockage of a coronary vessel.

This is in contrast to most other tissues at rest that use as little as one-fourth of their available oxygen. Because of this high level of oxygen extraction, the increased myocardial oxygen demands during exercise must be met by a proportionate increase in coronary blood flow. During vigorous exercise, coronary blood flow may increase four to six times above the resting level. This is achieved because the increase in myocardial metabolism in exercise has a direct effect on the coronary vessels, causing them to dilate. For example, hypoxia is extremely potent for increasing blood flow through the myocardium. Adenosine, a byproduct of ATP breakdown, is probably also a major mediator in the autoregulation of myocardial blood flow.[3] In addition to local factors, hormones of the sympathetic nervous system are released during exercise to cause coronary dilation. Arterial blood pressure also facilitates coronary blood flow. The increased aortic pressure during exercise forces a proportionately greater quantity of blood into the coronary circulation. The ebb and flow of blood in the coronary vessels fluctuates with each phase of the cardiac cycle. On average, coronary blood flow is about 2.5 times greater during diastole than during systole.

An adequate myocardial oxygen supply is critical because, unlike skeletal muscle, this tissue has a limited ability to generate energy anaerobically. The blood supply to the heart is so profuse that at least one capillary supplies each of the heart's muscle fibers. Impairment in coronary blood flow usually results in chest pains or **angina pectoris.** These pains become pronounced during exercise because the heart's energy requirements increase significantly. The stress of exercise is often used to evaluate the adequacy of myocardial blood flow. A blood clot, or **thrombus,** lodged in a coronary vessels may severely impair normal heart function. Although this form of "heart attack," or more specifically **myocardial infarction,** may be mild, a more complete blockage causes severe damage to the myocardium and could result in death. A more complete discussion of coronary heart disease, stress testing, and the possible role of exercise as preventive medicine is presented in Chapters 30 and 31.

THE RATE-PRESSURE PRODUCT: AN ESTIMATE OF MYOCARDIAL WORK

Myocardial oxygen uptake is determined by interactions between several mechanical factors—most importantly, the development of tension within the myocardium and its contractility, and heart rate. With increases in each of these factors during exercise, myocardial blood flow is adjusted to balance oxygen supply with demand. One commonly used estimate of myocardial workload and resulting oxygen uptake makes use of the product of peak systolic blood pressure (SBP), as measured at the brachial artery, and heart rate (HR). *This index of relative cardiac work, termed the* **double product** *or* **rate-pressure product (RPP),** *is highly related to directly measured myocardial oxygen up-*

take and coronary blood flow in healthy subjects over a wide range of exercise intensities.[33, 41] RPP is computed as follows:

$$RPP = SBP \times HR$$

Changes in heart rate and blood pressure contribute equally to changes in the RPP. Typical values for the RPP range from approximately 6,000 at rest (HR = 50 bpm; SBP = 120 mm Hg) to 40,000 (HR = 200 bpm; SBP = 200 mm Hg) or higher depending on the intensity and mode of exercise. In both resistance training and upper body exercise, the heart rate and blood pressure responses (and hence RPP) are significantly greater than during rhythmic exercise with the lower body. This added myocardial work can pose an unnecessary risk for people with a compromised myocardial oxygen supply such as occurs in coronary heart disease.

The RPP has been used extensively in exercise studies of heart disease patients to provide a physiologic correlate to the onset of angina and electrocardiographic abnormalities. Once this is established, various clinical, surgical, or exercise interventions can be evaluated to determine their effect on cardiac performance. The well-documented lowering of exercise heart rate and systolic blood pressure (hence the myocardial oxygen requirement) with training helps explain the improved exercise capacity of cardiac patients with regular exercise. Furthermore, several research studies have shown that prolonged and intense aerobic training results in a higher RPP achieved by cardiac patients.[13, 24] In nine patients followed over a 7-year training period, the RPP increased by 11.5% before the appearance of ischemic symptoms.[49] These findings are important because they provide indirect evidence for an improved level of myocardial oxygenation, perhaps due to greater coronary vascularization or reduced obstruction as part of the training adaptation.

MYOCARDIAL METABOLISM

As with all tissue, the heart uses the chemical energy stored in food to generate the ATP to power its work. The heart, however, relies almost totally on energy released in aerobic reactions. The human myocardium has a threefold higher oxidative capacity than skeletal muscle.[28] Myocardial fibers have the greatest mitochondrial concentration of all tissues and are highly adapted for lipid catabolism as a primary source of ATP resynthesis.[56]

Figure 15.11 shows the substrate use by the heart at rest and during moderate and heavy exercise. Glucose, fatty acids, and the lactic acid formed in skeletal muscle during glycolysis provide the energy for proper myocardial functioning. At rest, these three substrates are used to synthesize ATP with the primary source of energy derived from the breakdown of free fatty acids.[22] In essence, the heart uses for energy whatever substrate it "sees" on a physiologic level—so during heavy exercise, when the efflux of lactic acid from skeletal muscle into the blood increases signifi-

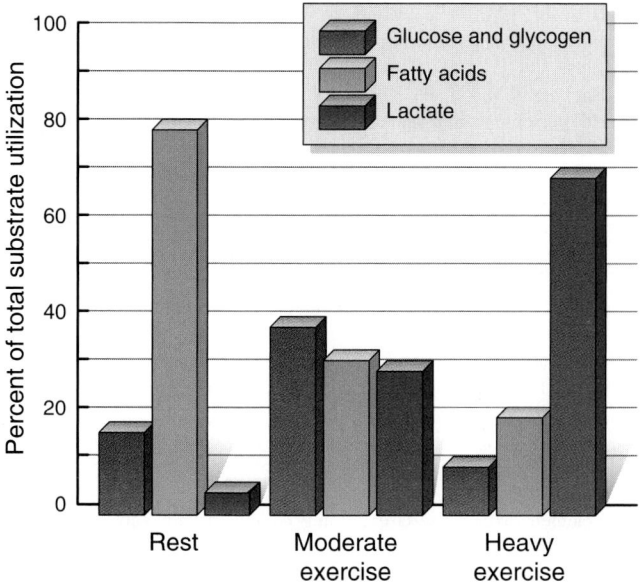

FIGURE 15.11

Generalized pattern of substrate utilization by the myocardium at rest and in relation to exercise intensity.

cantly, the heart derives its major energy from the oxidation of circulating lactate. In more moderate exercise, both lipids and carbohydrates are used in about equal amounts. During prolonged submaximal activity (not illustrated) such as distance running, skiing, or swimming, the myocardial metabolism of free fatty acids rises to almost 70% of the total energy requirement. This metabolic pattern is similar for trained and untrained individuals, although the contribution of lipids to the total energy requirement is consider-ably greater among trained endurance athletes. This difference provides another illustration of the "carbohydrate sparing effect" of training that also occurs in skeletal muscle.

■ SUMMARY ■

1. The striated fibers of the myocardium are interconnected so that portions of the heart contract in a unified manner. Functionally, the heart may be viewed as two separate pumps: one pump receives blood from the body and pumps it to the lungs for aeration (pulmonary circulation), whereas the other receives oxygenated blood from the lungs and pumps it throughout the systemic circulation.

2. Pressure changes created during the cardiac cycle act on the heart's valves to provide a one-way flow of blood into the vascular circuit.

3. The surge of blood with the contraction of the ventricles (and subsequent runoff of blood during relaxation) creates pressure changes within the arterial vessels. The systolic pressure, or highest pressure generated during the cardiac cycle, occurs during ventricular contraction. The diastolic pressure is the lowest pressure reached before the next ventricular contraction.

4. The dense capillary network provides a large and effective surface for exchange between the blood and tissues. These minute-diameter vessels have an autoregulatory capacity to adjust blood flow in response to the tissue's metabolic activity.

5. Nerves and hormones act on the smooth muscle layer of the venous walls, causing them to constrict or stiffen. This alteration in venous tone has a profound effect on the distribution of total blood volume.

6. Compression and relaxation of the veins by the action of skeletal muscles impart considerable energy to facilitate venous return. This provides additional justification for the use of active recovery following vigorous exercise.

7. Hypertension imposes a chronic stress on cardiovascular function. Regular aerobic training can cause modest reductions in systolic and diastolic blood pressure at rest and during submaximal exercise.

8. Systolic blood pressure increases in proportion to oxygen uptake and blood flow during graded exercise, whereas the diastolic pressure remains relatively unchanged or increases slightly. At the same relative and absolute work loads, systolic pressures are greater with arm compared to leg exercise.

9. After exercising, blood pressure falls to below the pre-exercise levels and may remain lower for up to 12 hours.

10. During isometric, free-weight, and hydraulic resistance exercise, peak systolic and diastolic blood pressures mirror the hypertensive state and may pose a risk to individuals with existing hypertension or heart disease. Regular training with resistance exercise blunts this hypertensive response.

11. At rest, approximately 80% of the oxygen flowing through the coronary arteries is extracted by the myocardium. This high extraction means that the increased myocardial oxygen demands in exercise can only be met by a proportionate increase in coronary blood flow.

12. Because the myocardium is essentially aerobic tissue, it must continually be supplied with oxygen. Impairment of coronary blood flow causes anginal pains, and blockage of a coronary artery (myocardial infarction) rapidly causes irreversible damage to the heart muscle.

13. The product of heart rate and systolic blood pressure, termed the rate-pressure product (RPP), provides a convenient estimate of the workload on the myocardium. This index is used in heart disease patients to study the effects of exercise training on cardiac performance.

14. The substrates used by the heart for energy are glucose, fatty acids, and circulating lactate. The percentage utilization of these substrates varies with the severity and duration of exercise.

■ REFERENCES ■

1. American College of Sports Medicine. Position stand. Physical activity, physical fitness, and hypertension. *Med. Sci. Sports Exerc.*, 25:i-x, 1993.

2. Baglivo, H.P., et al.: Effect of moderate physical training on left ventricular mass in mild hypertensive persons. *Hypertension*, 15(Suppl. I):1-153, 1990.

3. Berne, R.M.: The role of adenosine in the regulation of coronary blood flow. *Circ. Res.*, 47:807, 1980.

4. Blair, S.N., et al.: Physical fitness and all-cause mortality: a prospective study of healthy men and women. *JAMA*, 262:2395, 1989,

5. Blomqvist, C.G., et al.: Similarity of the hemodynamic responses to static and dynamic exercise of small muscle groups. *Circ. Res.*, 1:87, 1982.

6. Brown, S.P., et al.: Blood pressure, hemodynamic, and thermal responses after cycling exercise. *J. Appl. Physiol.*, 75:240, 1993.

7. Choquette, G., and Ferguson, R.J.: Blood pressure reduction in "borderline" hypertensives following physical training. *Can. Med. Assoc. J.*, 108:699, 1973.

8. Coconie, C.C., et al.: Effect of exercise training on blood pressure in 70- to 79-yr-old men and women. *Med. Sci. Sports Exerc.*, 23:505, 1991.

9. Collander, E.B., et al.: Blood pressure in resistance-trained athletes. *Can. J. Appl. Sports Sci.*, 13:31, 1988.

10. Dimsdale, J.E., et al.: Postexercise peril: plasma catecholamines and exercise. *JAMA*, 251:630, 1987.

11. Donaldson, M.C.: Varicose veins in active people. *Phys. Sportsmed.*, 18:46, 1990.

12. Duncan, J.J., et al.: The effects of aerobic exercise on plasma catecholamines and blood pressure in patients with mild hypertension. *JAMA*, 254:2609, 1985.

13. Ehsani, A.A., et al.: Improvement of left ventricular contractile function by exercise training in patients with coronary artery disease. *Circulation*, 74:350, 1986.

14. Fagard, R.H., and Tipton, C.M.: Physical activity, fitness, and hypertension. In *Physical Activity, Fitness, and Health*. Edited by C. Bouchard, et al. Champaign, IL, Human Kinetics, 1994.

15. Fagard, R.H., et al.: The effect of gender on aerobic power and exercise hemodynamics in hypertensive adults. *Med. Sci. Sports Exerc.*, 27:29, 1995.

16. Fleck, S.J.: Cardiovascular adaptations to resistance training. *Med. Sci. Sports Exerc.*, 20:S146, 1988.

17. Fleck, S.J., and Dean, L.S.: Resistance training experience and the pressor response during resistance training. *J. Appl. Physiol.*, 63:116, 1987.

17a. Franklin, B.S., et al.: Cardiac demands of heavy snow shoveling. *JAMA*, 273:880, 1995.

18. Freedson, P.F., et al.: Intra-arterial blood pressure during free weight and hydraulic resistive exercise. *Med. Sci. Sports Exerc.*, 16:131, 1984.

19. Fregly, M.J.: Effect of an exercise regimen on development of hypertension in rats. *J. Appl. Physiol.*, 56:381, 1984.

20. Friedman, D.B., et al.: Cardiovascular response to voluntary and non-voluntary static exercise in humans. *J. Appl. Physiol.*, 73:1982, 1992.

21. Gaffney, F.A., et al.: Cardiovascular and metabolic responses to static contraction in man. *Acta Physiol. Scand.*, 138:249, 1990.

22. Gertz, E.W., et al.: Myocardial substrate utilization during exercise in humans: dual carbon-labeled carbohydrate isotope experiments. *J. Clin. Invest.*, 82:2017, 1988.

23. Hagberg, J.M., et al.: Effect of exercise training on the blood pressure and hemodynamics of adolescent hypertensives. *Am. J. Cardiol.*, 52:763, 1981.

24. Hagberg, J.M., et al.: Effect of 12 months of intense exercise training on stroke volume in patients with coronary artery disease. *Circulation*, 67:1194, 1983.

25. Hagberg, J.M., et al.: Effect of weight training on blood pressure and hemodynamics in hypertensive adolescents. *J. Pediatr.*, 104:147, 1984.

26. Hagberg, J.M., et al.: Effects of exercise training on 60- to 69 yr old persons with essential hypertension. *Am. J. Cardiol.*, 64:348, 1989.

27. Hill, D.W., and Butler, S.D.: Haemodynamic responses to weight lifting exercise. *Sports Med.*, 12:1, 1991.

28. Jansson, E., and Sylven, E.: Myoglobin in human heart and skeletal muscle in relation to oxidative potential as estimated by citrate synthase. *Clin. Physiol.*, 1:596, 1981.

29. Kaplan, M.N.: *Clinical Hypertension.* 5th Ed. Baltimore, Williams & Wilkins, 1990.

30. Kasch, F.W., and Boyer, L.J.: Changes in maximum work capacity resulting from six months training in patients with ischemic heart disease. *Med. Sci. Sports Exerc.*, 1:156, 1969.

31. Kaufman, F.L., et al.: Effect of exercise on recovery blood pressure in normotensive and hypertensive subjects. *Med. Sci. Sports Exerc.*, 19:17, 1987.

32. Kelemen, M.H.: Exercise training combined with antihypertensive drug therapy: effects on lipids, blood pressure, and left ventricular mass. *JAMA*, 263:2766, 1990.

33. Kitamura, K., et al.: Hemodynamic correlates of myocardial oxygen consumption during upright exercise. *J. Appl. Physiol.*, 32:516, 1972.

34. Kiyonaga, A., et al.: Blood pressure and hormonal response to aerobic exercise. *Hypertension*, 17:125, 1985.

35. Le Marr, J.D., et al: Cardiorespiratory responses to inversion. *Phys. Sportsmed.*, 11:51, 1983.

36. MacDougall, J.D., et al.: Arterial blood pressure response to heavy resistance exercise. *J. Appl. Physiol.*, 58:785, 1985.

37. McCartney, N., et al.: Weight-training induced attenuation of the circulatory response of older males to weight lifting. *J. Appl. Physiol.*, 74:1056, 1993.

38. Miles, D.S.: Cardiovascular responses to upper body exercise in normals and cardiac patients. *Med. Sci. Sports Exerc.*, 21:S126, 1989.

39. Mitchell, J.H., and Raven, P.B.: Cardiovascular adaptation to physical activity. In *Physical Activity, Fitness, and Health*. Edited by C. Bouchard, et al. Champaign, IL, Human Kinetics, 1994.

40. Nelson, L., et al.: Effect of changing levels of physical activity on blood pressure and haemodynamics in essential hypertension. *Lancet*, 2:473, 1986.

41. Nelson, R.R., et al.: Hemodynamic predictors of myocardial oxygen consumption during static and dynamic exercise. *Circulation*, 50:1179, 1974.

42. O'Conner, P.J., et al.: State anxiety and ambulatory blood pressure following resistance exercise in females. *Med. Sci. Sports Exerc.*, 25:516, 1993.

43. Paffenbarger, R.S., Jr., et al.: Physical activity and hypertension: an epidemiological view. *Ann. Med.*, 23:19, 1991.

44. Pearson, A.C., et al.: Left ventricular diastolic function in weight lifters. *Am. J. Cardiol.*, 58:1254, 1986.

45. Pendergast, D.R.: Cardiovascular, respiratory, and metabolic responses to upper body exercise. *Med. Sci. Sports Exerc.*, 21:S121, 1989.

46. Pescatello, L.S., et al.: Short-term effect of dynamic exercise on arterial blood pressure. *Circulation*, 83:1557, 1991.

47. Raglin, J.S., and Morgan, W.P.: Influence of exercise and quiet rest on state anxiety and blood pressure. *Med. Sci. Sports Exerc.*, 19:456, 1987.

48. Report on Secretary's Task Force on Black and Minority Health. U.S. Dept. of Health and Human Services Publication 0-174-719. Washington, D.C., Government Printing Office, August 1985.

49. Rogers, M.A., et al.: The effects of 7 years of intense exercise training on patients with coronary artery disease. *J. Am. Coll. Cardiol.*, 10:321, 1987.

50. Seals, D.R., and Hagberg, J.M.: The effect of exercise training on human hypertension. *Med. Sci. Sports Exerc.,* 16:207, 1984.

51. Seals, D.R., et al.: Increased cardiovascular response to static contraction of larger muscle groups. *J. Appl. Physiol.,* 54:434, 1983.

52. Smith, M.L., et al.: Effect of muscle tension on the cardiovascular responses to lower body negative pressure in man. *Med. Sci. Sports Exerc.,* 19:436, 1987.

53. The Fifth Report of the Joint National Committee on Detection, Evaluation, and Treatment of High Blood Pressure (JNC V). *Arch. Intern. Med.,* 153:154, 1993.

54. Toner, M.M., et al.: Cardiovascular adjustment to exercise distributed between the upper and lower body. *Med. Sci. Sports Exerc.,* 22:773, 1990.

55. Urata, H., et al.: Antihypertensive and volume-depleting effects of mild exercise on essential hypertension. *Hypertension,* 9:245, 1987.

56. Vary, T.C., et al.: Control of energy metabolism of heart muscle. *Annu. Rev. Physiol.,* 43:419, 1981.

57. Wiley, R.L., et al.: Isometric exercise training lowers resting blood pressure. *Med. Sci. Sports Exerc.,* 24:749, 1992.

Robinson, S.: Experimental studies of physical fitness in relation to age. *Arbeitsphysiologie* **10:18, 1938.**

Robinson's classic research, a comprehensive cross-sectional study, documented the relationship of aging to physiologic responses during rest and submaximal and maximal exercise in 93 healthy, nonathletic males ranging in age from 6 to 91 years. The variables included resting and exercise metabolic rate ($\dot{V}o_2$), lung volumes, heart rate (HR), arterial blood pressure, submaximal treadmill walking performance at 5.6 km · h^{-1} at an 8.6% incline for 15 minutes, and a maximal-effort treadmill run resulting in "exhaustion" within 2 to 5 minutes.

The top figure illustrates a decline of nearly 20% in maximal HR (HRmax) between young boys and older men. The younger individuals showed a more variable HR response to exercise; they displayed a more rapid HR acceleration at the start of exercise; and their HR returned more rapidly to baseline values in recovery than older subjects. As illustrated in the middle figure, the $\dot{V}o_2$ peak increased between the ages of 8 to 12 years, declined markedly for the next few years, then increased further until about age 17, and decreased steadily thereafter. Interestingly, Robinson suggested that the decrease in $\dot{V}o_2$ peak with age was probably related to decreases in general physical activity, and not necessarily "true" aging. Thus, as early as 1938, a sedentary lifestyle had been identified as having deleterious effects on cardiovascular function. The bottom figure shows pulmonary ventilation relative to body mass ($\dot{V}_E \cdot kg^{-1} \cdot min^{-1}$), respiration rate (breaths · min^{-1}), and the tidal air (volume) expressed as a percentage of the vital capacity (TA × 100 ÷ VC) during maximal exercise. Measures of ventilatory function and respiration declined with increasing age, and older men used a greater fraction of their vital capacity as tidal air than did younger men. Moreover, boys increased their ventilation over resting values principally by increasing breathing frequency, whereas the increase in adults occurred by increasing both breathing rate and tidal volume.

This pioneering cross-sectional study demonstrated an age- and sedentary lifestyle–related decline in cardiovascular and pulmonary variables during rest and submaximal and maximal exercise. Subsequent research has indicated that a large component of the decline in functional capacity with aging coincides with lifestyle characteristics rather than chronological aging per se.

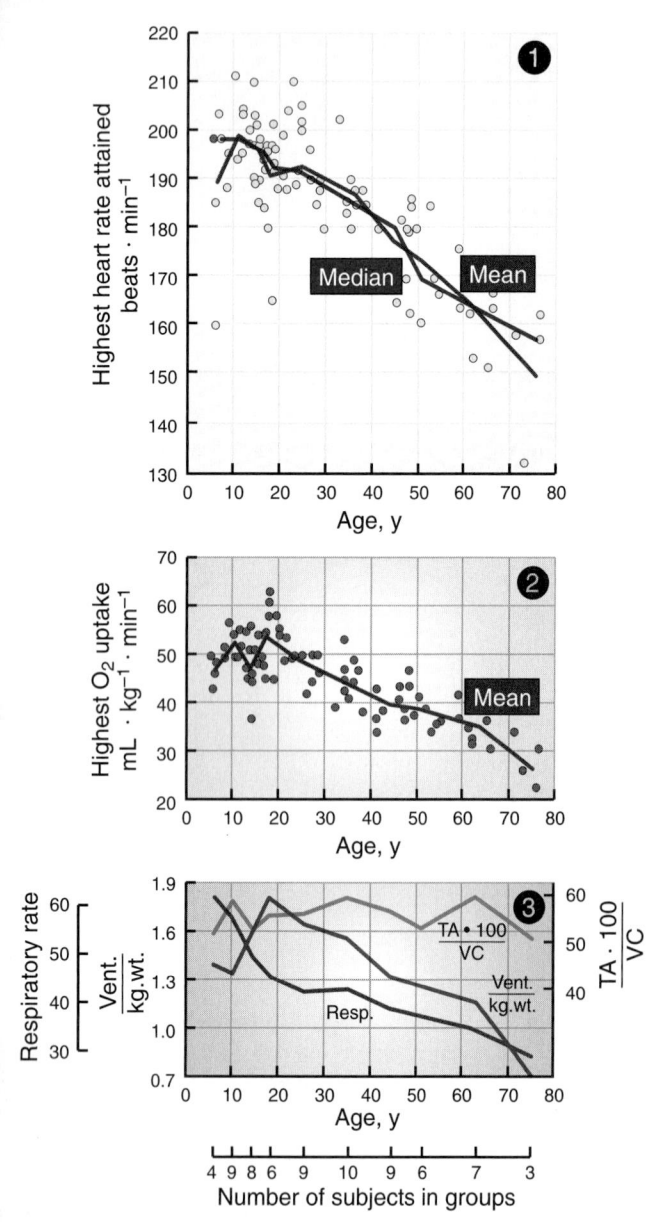

Top, Plot of resting heart rate (beats per minute) as a function of age. *Middle,* Peak (highest) oxygen uptake as a function of age. *Bottom,* Pulmonary ventilation, respiratory rate, and tidal volume as functions of age.

Cardiovascular Regulation and Integration

The vascular system has an exceptional capacity for expansion. The capacity of the vessels of the skin, viscera, and skeletal muscles to conduct blood exceeds by three to four times the pumping capacity of the normal heart.[16] Consequently, complex mechanisms continually interact to maintain a dynamic balance between systemic blood pressure and blood flow to various tissues under diverse conditions. Nerves and chemicals regulate the speed of the pumping heart and the internal opening of the blood vessels. This exquisite cardiovascular regulation provides rapid control of the heart as well as the effective distribution of blood throughout the body. When a person is resting comfortably, for example, approximately 5% of the 5 L of blood pumped by the heart each minute goes to the skin. This is in contrast to when a person exercises in a hot, humid environment, when as much as 20% of the total blood flow is diverted to the body's surface for the purpose of heat dissipation. This "shunting" of blood with appropriate maintenance of blood pressure can occur only within a closed vascular system that has the capability for the immediate redistribution of blood depending on the body's metabolic and physiologic needs.[17]

INTRINSIC REGULATION OF HEART RATE

Cardiac muscle is unique because it can maintain its own rhythm. If left to this inherent rhythm, the heart would beat steadily between 70 and 90 times each minute. Situated within the posterior wall of the right atrium is a small (3-mm-wide and 1-cm-long) mass of specialized muscle tissue called the **sinoatrial node** or **S-A node.** This node spontaneously depolarizes and repolarizes to provide the innate stimulus to the heart. For this reason, the S-A node is referred to as the **"pacemaker."** The normal route for the transmission of the impulse within the myocardium is shown in Figure 16.1 (top).

THE HEART'S ELECTRICAL ACTIVITY

Electrochemical rhythms originating at the S-A node spread across the atria to another small knot of tissue called the **atrioventricular node** or **A-V node.** The timing of the appearance of the impulse once it is propagated from the S-A node is listed in Figure 16.1 (bottom). Note that the impulse is delayed about 0.10 second within the atria to provide sufficient time for the atria to contract and force blood into the ventricles.

The A-V node gives rise to the 1-cm-long **A-V bundle,** also called the **bundle of His** after the German physician Wilhelm His, Jr., who described this tissue in 1893. The A-V bundle transmits the impulse rapidly through the ventricles over specialized conducting fibers referred to as the **Purkinje system** (named after the Bohemian anatomist and physiologist Johannes Von Purkinje, 1787-1869). These fibers form distinct right and left bundle branches that penetrate the right and left ventricles. They transmit the impulse about 6 times faster than the transmission speed of normal ventricular muscle fibers. Each ventricular cell is stimulated within approximately 0.06 second from the passage of the impulse into the ventricles; this permits a unified and simultaneous subsequent contraction of the entire musculature of both ventricles. The transmission of the cardiac impulse can be summarized as follows:

S-A node → Atria → A-V node →
A-V bundle (Purkinje fibers) → Ventricles

The Electrocardiogram (ECG). Like all nerve and muscle tissue, the outer surface of the myocardial cells is electrically more positive than the inside. Polarity is reversed just before contraction, when the heart is stimulated, and the cell's inside becomes more positive than the outside. During the diastolic phase of the cardiac cycle, the membranes repolarize to reestablish the resting membrane potential.

The electrical activity around the myocardium creates an electrical field throughout the body. Because the salty body fluids provide an excellent conducting medium, the sequence of electrical events before and during each cardiac cycle can be detected as voltage changes by electrodes placed on the skin's surface. The graphic record of the heart's electrical activity is called the **electrocardiogram** or simply **ECG.** A characteristic, normal electrocardiogram is presented in Figure 16.2. The **P wave** represents the depolarization of the atria. It lasts approximately 0.15 second and heralds atrial contraction. The P wave is then followed by the relatively large **QRS complex,** which reflects the electrical changes caused by the depolarization of the ventricles;

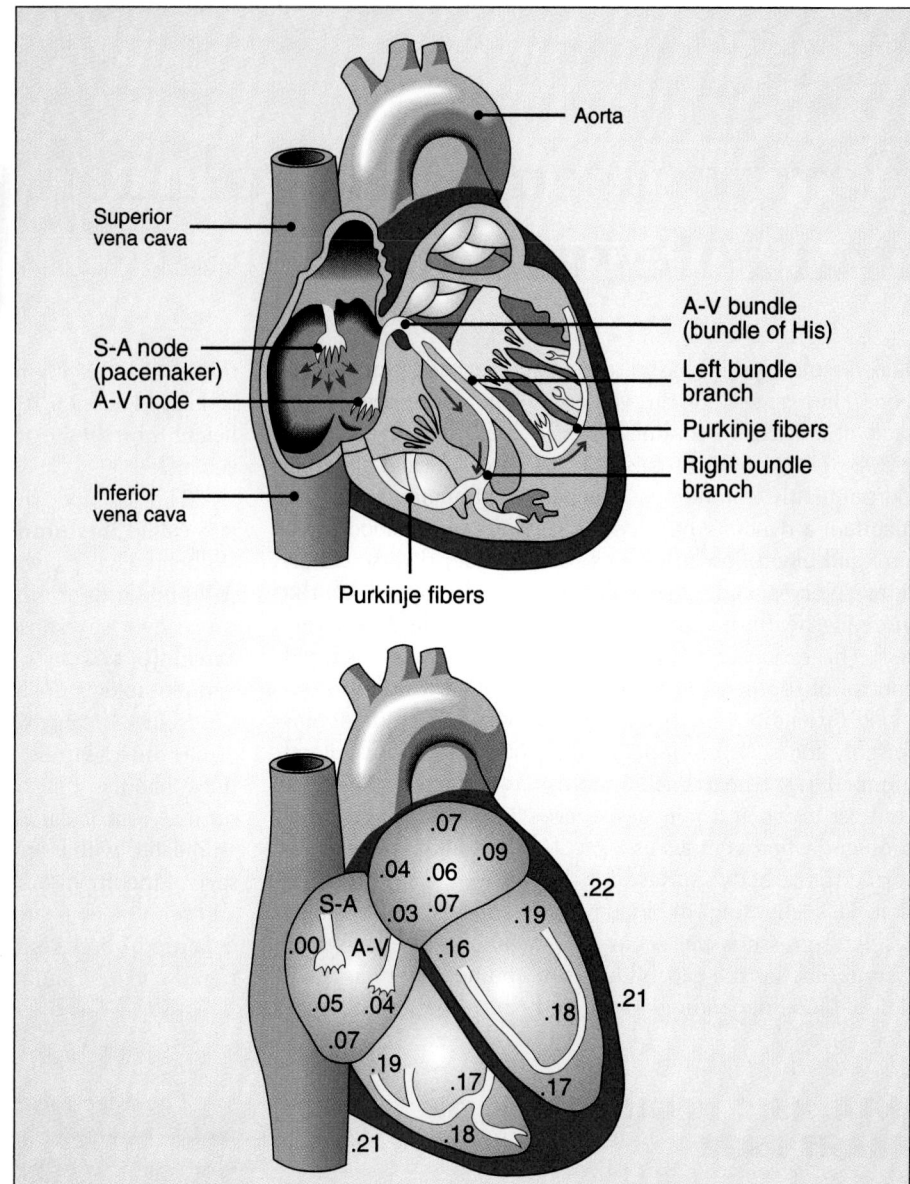

FIGURE 16.1

Top, The normal route for excitation and conduction of the cardiac impulse. This impulse originates at the S-A node and then travels to the A-V node. The impulse is then propagated throughout the ventricular mass. *Bottom,* Time sequence (in seconds) for the transmission of the electrical impulse from the S-A node throughout the myocardium.

at this point, the ventricles contract. Atrial repolarization that follows the P wave produces a wave so small that it usually is obscured by the large QRS complex. The **T wave** represents repolarization of the ventricles. This occurs during ventricular diastole. The heart's relatively long period of depolarization of approximately 0.20 to 0.30 second is required before it can receive another impulse and contract again. This rest or brief "time out" **refractory period** serves an important function because it provides sufficient time for ventricular filling between beats.

The electrocardiogram serves useful purposes for the cardiologist and exercise specialist. It provides an effective means for monitoring heart rate objectively during exercise. Radiotelemetry makes it possible to transmit the ECG while the person is free to perform various types of exercise, including football, weight lifting, basketball, ice hockey, danc-

ing, and even swimming. As discussed in Chapter 30, electrocardiography is a vital diagnostic tool for uncovering abnormalities in heart function, especially those related to cardiac rhythm, electrical conduction, myocardial oxygen supply, and actual tissue damage.

EXTRINSIC REGULATION OF THE HEART AND CIRCULATION

Heart rate can change rapidly through the action of nerves that go directly to the heart and chemicals that circulate in the blood. These **extrinsic controls** of cardiac function cause the heart to speed up in "anticipation," even before the start of exercise and then rapidly adjust to the intensity of physical effort. To a large extent, extrinsic regulation results in heart rates that may be as slow as 25 to 30 beats per minute under normal ambulatory conditions in some highly trained, healthy endurance athletes[2] and exceed 200 beats per minute during maximum exercise.

Figure 16.3 illustrates the various neural mechanisms for cardiovascular regulation before and during exercise. Continual input from the brain and peripheral nervous system impinge upon the cardiovascular control center in the **ventrolateral medulla.** This neural control regulates the output of blood from the heart and its preferential distribution to tissues in need throughout the body.

SYMPATHETIC AND PARASYMPATHETIC NEURAL INPUT

Neural influences are superimposed on the inherent rhythm of the myocardium. These influences originate in the cardiovascular center and are transmitted through the **sympa-**

thetic and **parasympathetic** components of the autonomic nervous system. The distribution of sympathetic and parasympathetic nerve fibers within the myocardium is illustrated in Figure 16.4. The atria are supplied with large numbers of sympathetic and parasympathetic neurons, whereas the ventricles receive sympathetic fibers almost exclusively.

Sympathetic Influence. Stimulation of the sympathetic cardioaccelerator nerves releases the **catecholamines** epinephrine and norepinephrine. These neural hormones act to accelerate the depolarization of the S-A node and cause the heart to beat faster. This acceleration in heart rate is termed **tachycardia.** The catecholamines also increase myocardial contractility, which augments the quantity of blood pumped from the heart with each beat. It is estimated that maximum sympathetic stimulation nearly doubles the force of ventricular contraction. Epinephrine released from the medullary portion of the adrenal glands in

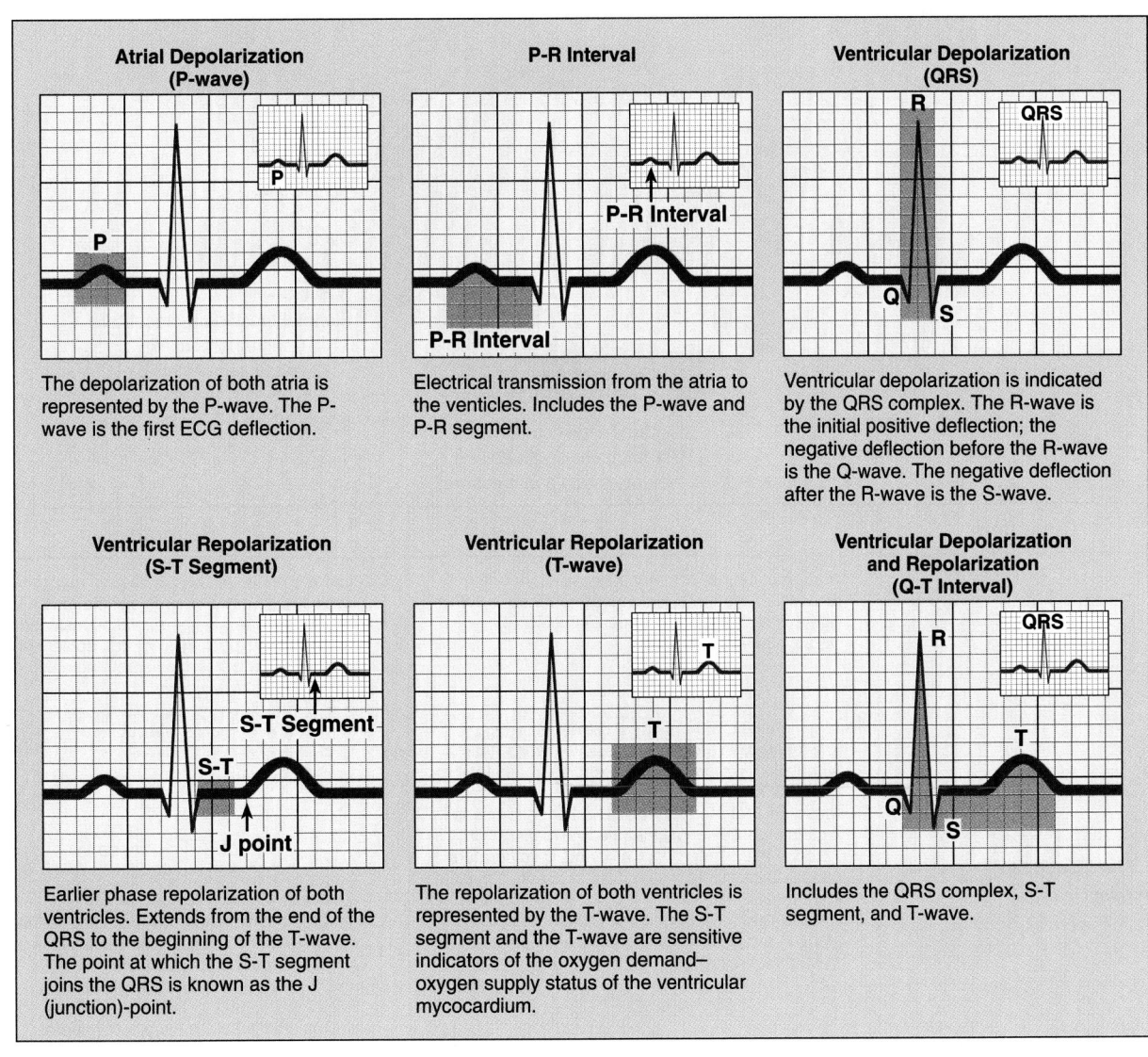

FIGURE 16.2
The different phases of the normal electrocardiogram (ECG) from atrial depolarization (*upper left*) to the repolarization of the ventricles (*lower right*).

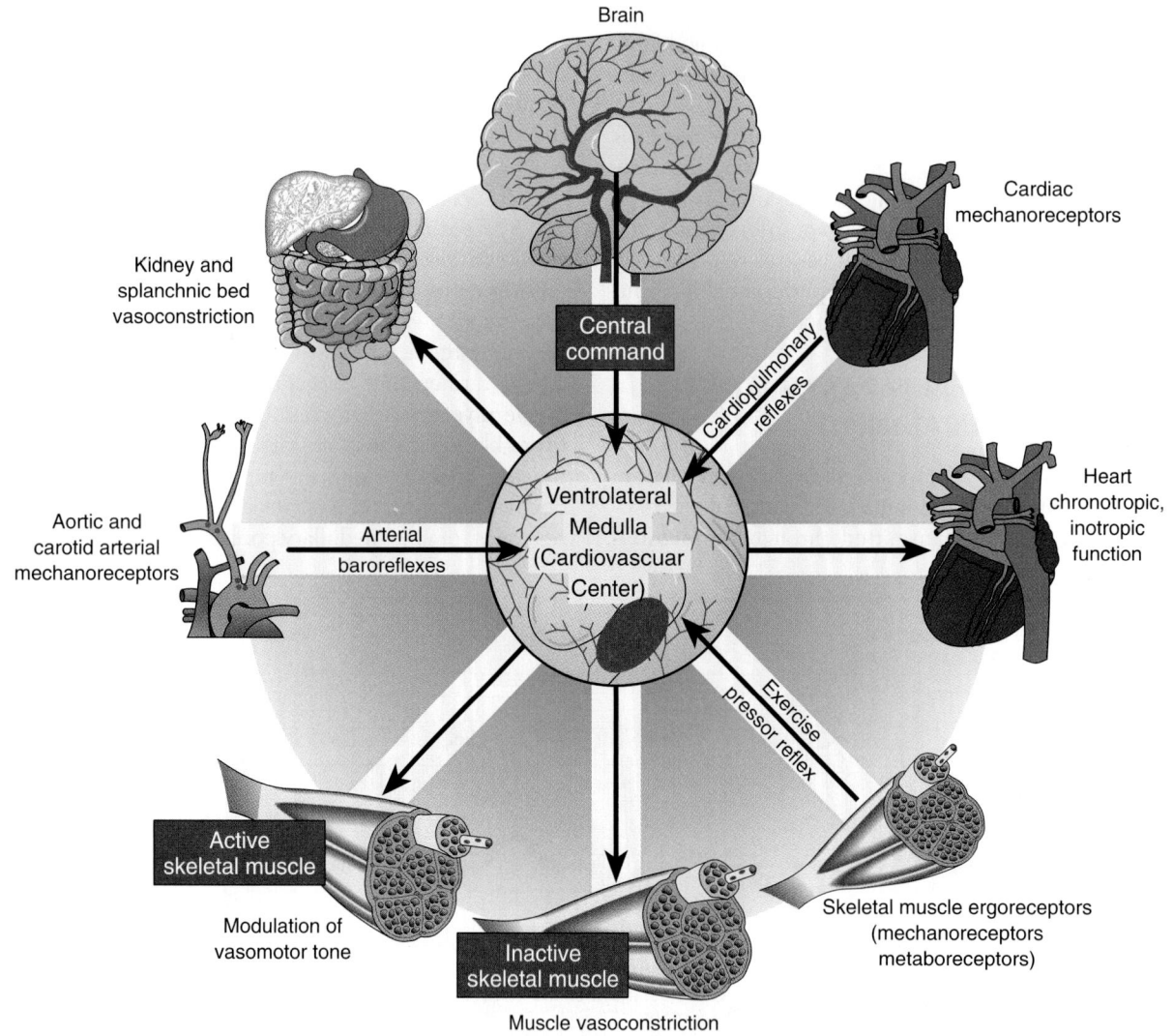

Condition	Activator	Response
Preexercise "anticipatory" response	Activation of central command from motor cortex and higher area of brain causes increase in sympathetic outflow and reciprocal inhibition of parasympathetic activity.	Acceleration of heart rate; increased myocardial contractility; vasodilation in skeletal and heart muscle (cholinergic fibers); vasoconstriction in other areas, especially skin, gut, spleen, liver, and kidneys (adrenergic fibers); increase in arterial blood pressure.
Exercise	Parasympathetic withdrawal at onset and during low-intensity exercise; progressive sympathetic stimulation in more intense exercise; reflex feedback from peripheral mechanical and chemical receptors that monitor muscle action; alterations in local metabolic conditions due to hypoxia, ↓pH, ↑Pco_2, ↑ADP, ↑Mg^{2+}, ↑Ca^{2+}, and ↑temperature cause autoregulatory vasodilation in active muscle.	Further dilation of muscle vasculature.
	Continued sympathetic adrenergic outflow in conjunction with epinephrine and norepinephrine from the adrenal medullae.	Concomitant constriction of vasculature in inactive tissues to maintain adequate perfusion pressure throughout arterial system. Venous vessels stiffen to reduce their capacity. This venoconstriction facilitates venous return and maintains the central blood volume.

FIGURE 16.3

A schematic representation of the neural regulation of the cardiovascular system during exercise. (Modified from Mitchell, J.H., and Raven, P.B.: Cardiovascular adaptation to physical activity. In *Physical Activity, Fitness, and Health*. Edited by C. Bouchard, et al. Champaign, IL, Human Kinetics, 1994.)

response to a general sympathetic activation also produces a similar but slower-acting effect on cardiac function.

In addition to its potent effect on the myocardium, sympathetic stimulation profoundly affects blood flow throughout the body. A schematic view of the distribution of sympathetic outflow is presented in Figure 16.5. These nerve fibers end in the smooth muscle layers of small arteries, arterioles, and precapillary sphincters. Norepinephrine acts as a general vasoconstrictor and is released by specific sympathetic nerve endings. These sympathetic constrictor fibers are called **adrenergic fibers.** Other sympathetic neurons in skeletal and heart muscle release acetylcholine; these are the **cholinergic fibers,** and their action is vasodilation. Thus, the sympathetic nervous system consists of both adrenergic constrictor and cholinergic dilator fibers. The adrenergic constrictor nerves are constantly active; consequently, some blood vessels always are in a state of constriction, or **vasomotor tone.** Dilation of blood vessels under the influence of adrenergic neurons is due more to a reduction in vasomotor tone than to an increase in the action of either cholinergic sympathetic or parasympathetic dilator fibers (see following section). In addition, whatever sympathetically activated vasoconstriction is present in active tissue is rapidly overridden by the powerful vasodilation induced by the by-products of local metabolism (see Local Factors, p. 293).[24]

Parasympathetic Influence. The cell bodies of the parasympathetic nervous system are located in the brain stem and sacral portion of the spinal cord. When stimulated, these neurons release the neurohormone **acetylcholine,** which retards the rate of sinus discharge to slow the heart. This slowing of heart rate is termed **bradycardia.** The effect is largely mediated through the action of the pair of **vagus nerves,** the cell bodies of which originate in the cardioinhibitory center in the medulla. The vagus nerves are the only cranial nerves that leave the head and neck region and descend into the thorax and abdominal regions. The vagus nerves carry approximately 80% of parasympathetic fibers. Vagal stimulation has no effect on myocardial contractility. Aside from affecting heart function, parasympathetic nerve fibers leave the brain stem and spinal cord to affect a variety of areas in the body. As with sympathetic activity, parasympathetic stimulation causes excitation in certain tissues (ciliary muscle of iris, gallbladder and bile ducts, bronchi, coronary arteries) and inhibition in others (gut sphincters, intestinal peristalsis, skin vasculature).

At the onset of and during low to moderate levels of exercise intensity, the increase in heart rate occurs by removal of parasympathetic stimulation. During more strenuous exercise, heart rate acceleration occurs by direct activation of the sympathetic cardioaccelerator nerves; the magnitude of acceleration increases in direct proportion to the intensity and duration of effort.[12, 22]

Training Effects. *Exercise training creates an imbalance between the tonic activity of the sympathetic accelerator and parasympathetic depressor neurons in favor of greater vagal dominance. This is mediated primarily by an*

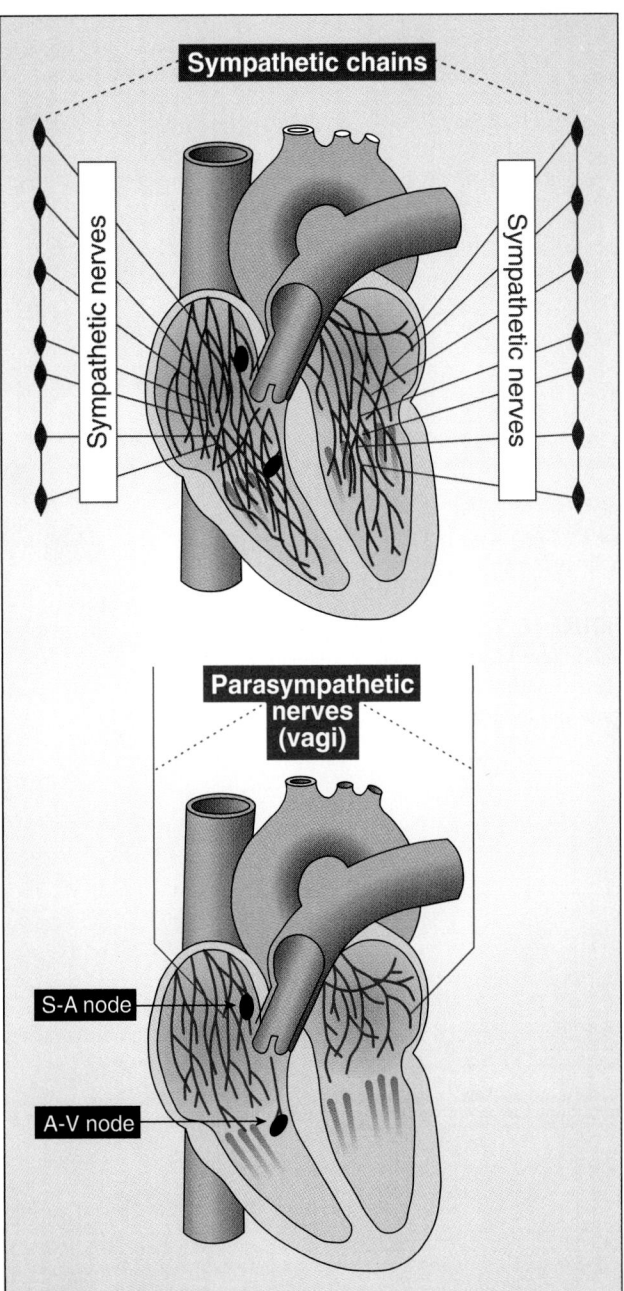

FIGURE 16.4

Distribution of sympathetic and parasympathetic nerve fibers to the myocardium. The endings of the sympathetic nerve fibers secrete the neurohormone epinephrine. These fibers are plentiful in the S-A and A-V nodes and in the muscle of the atria and ventricles. The parasympathetic nerve endings secrete acetylcholine. These fibers are concentrated in the atria, including the S-A and A-V nodes.

increase in parasympathetic activity and perhaps a decrease in sympathetic discharge.[8, 26] In addition, training also may decrease the intrinsic rate of firing of the S-A nodal pacemaker tissue.[7, 19, 20] These adaptations following aerobic training account for the significant resting bradycardia often observed in highly conditioned endurance athletes or in sedentary individuals who engage in aerobic training.

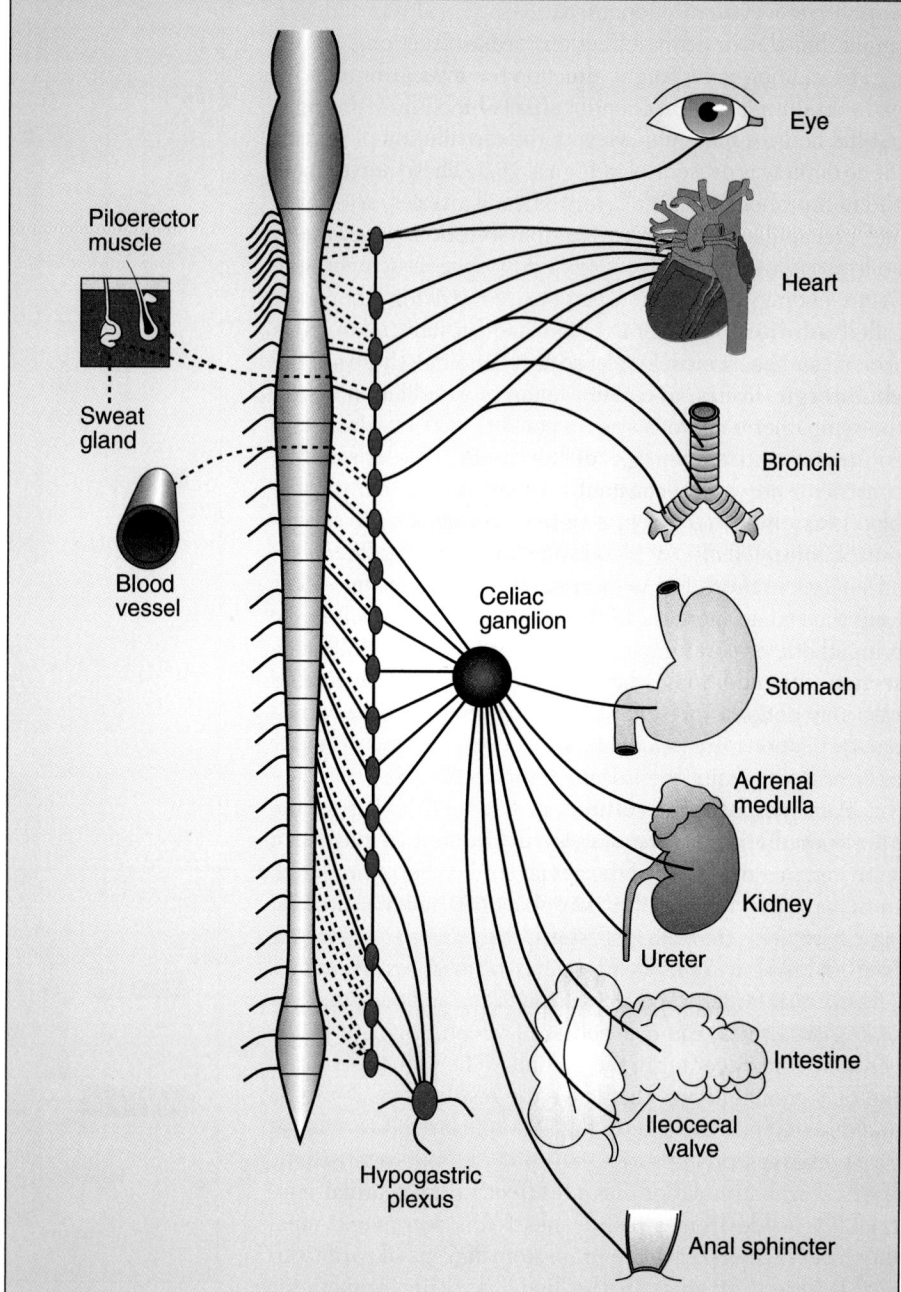

FIGURE 16.5
Schematic view of vascular regulation via sympathetic outflow to various organs and tissues.

INPUT FROM HIGHER CENTERS: A CENTRAL COMMAND

The activity of the medulla is modulated by direct action of neural impulses originating in the brain's higher somatomotor centers. It is these centers that recruit the musculature required for physical activity. Impulses from this "feed forward" **central command** system pass via small afferent nerves through the cardiovascular center in the medulla. This provides the coordinated and rapid response of both the heart and blood vessels to optimize tissue perfusion and maintain central blood pressure in relation to motor cortex involvement. This applies not only during exercise but also during the pre-exercise anticipatory period.[17] A greater stimulation of the medullary center is provided as a larger muscle mass is recruited in more strenuous exercise. *The central command provides the greatest control over heart rate during exercise.*[6, 13, 30a]

The extent of influence of the central command on heart rate is clearly illustrated in the anticipatory response to exercise demonstrated in Figure 16.6. The heart rate of trained sprint runners was measured by telemetry at rest, at the starting commands, and during 60-, 220-, and 440-yard races. Heart rate averaged 148 beats per minute at the starting commands in anticipation of the 60-yard sprint; this represented 74% of the total heart rate adjustment to the run.

The magnitude of the anticipatory heart rate was greatest in the short sprint events and successively lower before the longer sprints. This pattern of anticipatory heart rate was also demonstrated in events of longer duration. For example, the anticipatory heart rates of four athletes trained for the 880-yard run averaged 122 beats per minute, whereas the heart rates averaged 118 beats during the starting commands of the 1-mile run and 108 beats during the 2-mile run. A high level of neural outflow in anticipation of exercise would be desirable before intense activity of short duration (such as sprinting) to provide the rapid mobilization of bodily reserves. On the other hand, this mechanism for "revving the body's engine" might be wasteful before distance events.

In essence, the heart is "turned on" in exercise by a decrease in parasympathetic and an increase in sympathetic neural activity triggered largely by stimulating input from the central command in the brain. More than likely, considerable accelerator input also is provided by the activation of receptors in active joints and muscles as the exercise begins (see following section).[15] Even in the so-called "nonsprint" events, heart rate was approximately 180 beats per minute within 30 seconds of 1- and 2-mile runs. Further increases in heart rate were gradual, and several plateaus were reached during the run. Almost identical results were reported for heart rates measured by telemetry during competitive swimming events; only the maximum exercise heart rates were lower during swimming.[11]

The involvement of central command in cardiovascular regulation also explains how variations in one's emotional state significantly affect cardiovascular responses and make it difficult to obtain "true" resting values for heart rate and blood pressure.

PERIPHERAL INPUT

The cardiovascular center also receives reflex sensory input from peripheral receptors in blood vessels, joints, and muscles. These receptors monitor the physical and chemical state of active muscle. Afferent impulses from the mechanoreceptors and chemoreceptors provide rapid feedback that modifies either vagal (parasympathetic) or sympathetic outflow to bring about the appropriate cardiovascular response to physical activity.[12, 17, 18, 28] This reflex neural input from active muscle (termed the **exercise pressor reflex**), in conjunction with outflow from the motor areas of the central command, assess the nature and intensity of the exercise as well as the quantity of muscle recruited. Input from the mechanoreceptors is particularly important feedback for the central nervous system's regulation of blood flow and blood pressure during dynamic exercise.[29] Pressure-sensitive receptors known as **baroreceptors** are located in the aortic arch and carotid sinus, and cardiopulmonary mechanoreceptors are present in the left ventricle, right atrium, and large veins. These receptors tonically inhibit sympathetic outflow from the cardiovascular center and respond to changes in arterial blood pressure.[21] As blood pressure increases, the stretch of the arterial vessels activates the baroreceptors to bring about a reflex slowing of the heart and a compensatory dilation of the peripheral vasculature. This causes blood pressure to decrease toward more normal levels. To some degree, this feedback mechanism is overridden, or its threshold and/or sensitivity is reset, during physical activity so blood pressure can be effectively modulated but at the higher levels observed during exercise. More than likely, the baroreceptors also act as a brake to prevent abnormally high blood pressure levels during exercise.

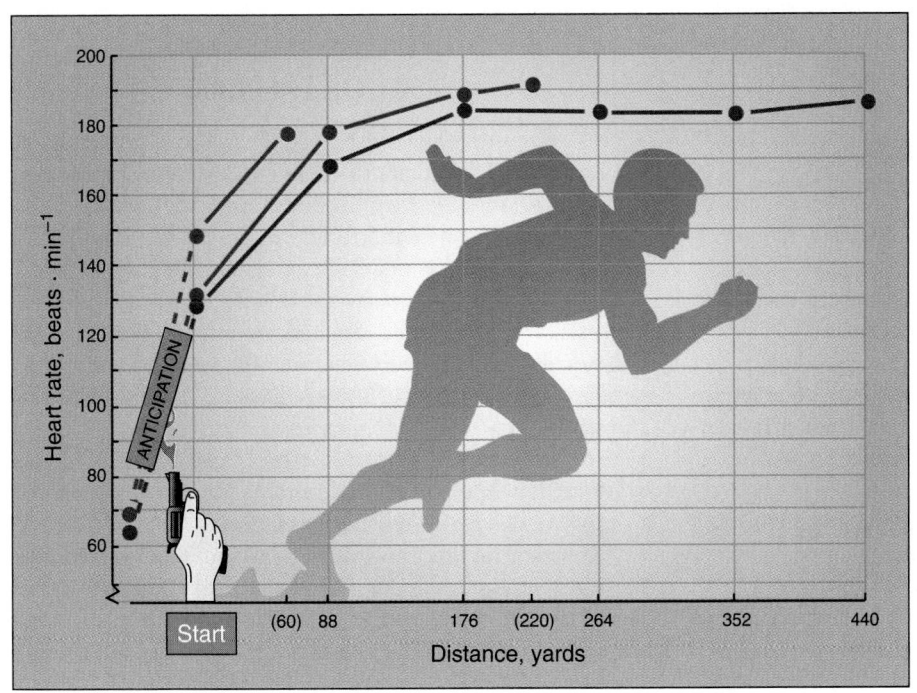

FIGURE 16.6
Heart rate response of sprint-trained runners. The largest increase in anticipatory heart rate (heart rate immediately before exercising) occurred in the short sprint events and became successively smaller before the longer sprints. (From McArdle, W.D., et al.: Telemetered cardiac response to selected running events. *J. Appl. Physiol.*, 23: 566, 1967.)

Carotid Artery Palpation. In some individuals, strong external pressure against the carotid artery produces a slowing effect on the heart rate. This effect probably is mediated by direct stimulation of the baroreceptors that are located at the bifurcation of the carotid artery. Of interest to exercise specialists has been the potential for bradycardia produced by **carotid artery palpation,** because this method is used commonly for determining pulse rate in response to exercise. An accurate measure of heart rate is important for training when specific "target" heart rates are assigned to regulate training intensity (see Chapter 21). If the procedure to monitor the heart rate consistently gave low values (as could occur with carotid artery palpation), the person would be pushed to a higher work level. This method certainly would be undesirable in exercise prescription for cardiac patients.

Research in the late 1970s showed that carotid artery palpation significantly slowed the postexercise heart rate and occasionally produced electrocardiographic abnormalities.[30] Several later reports showed, rather convincingly, that in both healthy adults and cardiac patients, carotid artery palpation caused little or no alteration in heart rate at rest or during exercise and recovery.[4, 14, 23] Palpation of the carotid artery is an appropriate technique to gauge heart rate in healthy people. However, various forms of vascular disease do affect the sensitivity of the carotid sinus. Under such conditions, palpation could give a falsely low reading for the heart rate. When this is a concern, an excellent substitute method is to determine pulse rate at the radial artery (thumb side of wrist) or temporal artery (side of head at temple) because even firm palpation of these vessels causes little or no change in heart rate.

Local Factors. The by-products of energy metabolism provide an autoregulatory mechanism within the muscle itself to augment perfusion during physical activity. This local control of circulation is discussed in the following section.

DISTRIBUTION OF BLOOD

If fully dilated, the body's blood vessels could hold approximately 20 L of blood, even though the actual total blood volume is only approximately 5 L. Thus, a fine regulation of vascular dilation and constriction is required to maintain blood flow and blood pressure, particularly during exercise. The capacity of large portions of the vasculature to either constrict or dilate provides a rapid redistribution of blood to meet the tissue's metabolic requirements while maintaining an appropriate blood pressure throughout the vascular circuit.

PHYSICAL FACTORS THAT AFFECT BLOOD FLOW

Blood flows through the vascular circuit in general accord with the physical laws of hydrodynamics as applied to rigid, cylindrical vessels. Because blood is not a homogeneous fluid and the blood vessels are not rigid tubes, these relationships are true mainly in a qualitative sense. The volume of flow in any vessel is:

- Directly proportional to the pressure gradient between the two ends of the vessels and **not** to the absolute pressure within the vessel.
- Inversely related to the resistance encountered to the flow.

Resistance, or the force impeding blood flow, is caused by friction between the blood and the internal vascular wall. The resistance is determined by three factors: the thickness or **viscosity** of the blood, the **length** of the conducting tube, and most importantly, the **radius** of the blood vessel. The general relationship between pressure differential, resistance, and flow can be expressed by an equation referred to as **Poiseuille's law:**

$$\text{Flow} = \text{Pressure gradient} \times \text{Vessel radius}^4 \div \text{Vessel length} \times \text{Viscosity}$$

In the body, the length of the transport vessel remains constant and the blood viscosity remains relatively constant under most circumstances. The most important factor affecting blood flow is the radius of the conducting tube and the resistance to flow changes with the vessel's radius raised to the fourth power. For example, if vessel radius is reduced by one-half, flow through it decreases by 16 times. Conversely, doubling the vessel's radius increases the volume 16-fold. If the pressure differential within the vascular circuit were to remain constant, a considerable alteration in blood flow would be achieved with only a small change in vessel radius. *In a physiologic sense, the simple constriction and dilation of the smaller blood vessels provide the crucial mechanisms for regulating regional blood flow.*

EFFECT OF EXERCISE

Increased energy expenditure usually requires rapid adjustments in blood flow that affect the entire cardiovascular system. For example, nerves and local metabolites act on the smooth muscle bands of arteriole walls, causing them to alter their internal diameter almost instantaneously. In addition, stimulation of nerves to the venous capacitance vessels causes them to "stiffen." Such **venoconstriction** permits large quantities of blood to move from peripheral veins into the central circulation. *This capability of large portions of the vasculature to either constrict or dilate provides a rapid redistribution of blood to meet the tissue's metabolic requirements while maintaining an adequate blood pressure throughout the entire vascular system.*

During exercise, the vascular portion of active muscles increases considerably by the dilation of local arterioles. Concurrently, other vessels that can temporarily compromise their blood supply constrict or "shut down." Kidney function vividly illustrates this regulatory mechanism for adjusting regional blood flow. Renal blood flow at rest is normally approximately 1,100 mL per minute and represents approximately 20% of the cardiac output. During maximal exercise, renal blood flow is reduced to only approximately 250 mL per minute or 1% of the total exercise blood flow. This large, temporary reduction in blood flow is also observed in tissues of the splanchnic region during strenuous exercise.[17]

Local Factors. At rest, only one of every 30 to 40 capillaries in muscle tissue is actually open.[31] The opening of dormant capillaries in exercise serves three important functions:

- It provides a significant increase in muscle blood flow.
- Because more channels open, a larger volume can be delivered with only a minimal increase in the velocity of flow.
- The enhanced vascularization increases the effective surface for exchange between the blood and the muscle fibers.

Local factors related to the level of tissue metabolism act directly on the smooth muscle bands of the small arterioles and precapillary sphincters to cause vasodilation. The response is rapid and finely adjusted to the muscle's force output and metabolic needs.[1a] A decrease in a tissue's oxygen supply produces a potent local stimulus for vasodilation in skeletal and cardiac muscle. Furthermore, local increases in temperature, carbon dioxide, acidity, adenosine, and ions such as magnesium and potassium as well as the production of nitric oxide by the vascular endothelium lining of blood vessels enhance regional blood flow.[16, 23a] These **autoregulatory mechanisms** for blood flow make sense from a physiologic standpoint because they reflect elevated tissue metabolism and an increased need for oxygen. Local regulation is so powerful that it provides adequate regional blood flow even in patients in whom the nerves to the blood vessels have been surgically removed.

By-products of the metabolism of active muscle act directly on the local sensory chemoreceptors and provide important autoregulatory control of blood supply. This stimulation provides the peripheral neural reflex input for medullary control of the heart and vasculature.

Hormonal Factors. In addition to their effect on the smooth muscle walls of the arterial vasculature, sympathetic nerves terminate in the medullary portion of the adrenal glands. In response to sympathetic activation, this glandular tissue secretes large quantities of epinephrine and a smaller amount of norepinephrine into the blood. These hormones act as chemical messengers to bring about a generalized constrictor response, except in the blood vessels of the heart and skeletal muscles. During exercise, this hormonal control of regional blood flow is relatively minor compared to the more local, rapid, and powerful sympathetic neural drive.

INTEGRATED RESPONSE IN EXERCISE

Cardiovascular changes immediately before and at the onset of exercise are initiated from the neural command center above the medullary region. This feed-forward input suppresses parasympathetic activation and augments sympathetic outflow to increase heart rate and myocardial contractility. At the same time, predictable alterations in regional blood flow occur that are proportional to the exercise severity. These adjustments of dilation and constriction optimize blood flow to areas in need while maintaining blood pressure throughout the arterial system. As exercise continues, reflex feedback to the medulla from peripheral mechanical and chemical receptors in active tissue provides an appraisal of local metabolic activity and circulatory needs. Local metabolic factors also act directly on the blood vessels to cause dilation of resistance vessels in the active muscles. This reduced peripheral resistance permits the active areas to accommodate greater blood flow. Additional centrally mediated constrictor adjustments occur in the vasculature of less active tissues (skin, kidneys, splanchnic region, and inactive muscle); thus, an adequate perfusion pressure is maintained even with the large dilation of the muscle's vasculature. This constrictor action continues to provide the appropriate redistribution of blood to meet the metabolic requirements of working muscles.

Factors that affect venous return are equally as important as those that regulate arterial blood flow. The action of the muscle and ventilatory pumps, and the stiffening of the veins themselves (probably mediated by sympathetic activity), immediately increase the return of blood to the right ventricle. As cardiac output increases, venous tone also increases proportionally in both active and nonactive muscles.[24] With these adjustments, a balance is maintained between cardiac output and venous return. The factors that affect venous blood flow are particularly important in upright exercise, in which gravity tends to counter the normally low venous pressure in the extremities.

EXERCISING AFTER CARDIAC TRANSPLANTATION: A "SLUGGISH" CIRCULATORY RESPONSE

Cardiac transplantation, also called **orthotopic transplantation,** provides a vivid illustration of the role of extrinsic neural control of heart rate during exercise. This medical procedure, performed for severe and progressive left ventricular dysfunction, involves removing the recipient's diseased heart and connecting the donor heart to the remaining great vessels and atria. As a result, neural innervation of the myocardium is eliminated, although hormonal feedback from the adrenal medulla remains intact. In selected patients, a "piggyback" transplant is performed: the donor heart is placed in the recipient's chest without removing the recipient's heart. Regardless of the form of transplantation, recovery is generally complicated (e.g., rejection of the donor heart, infection), including recurrent hospitalization and prolonged medical care. In 1990, the 5-year survival rate for the 12,000 reported transplant patients was 72%.[10] Following successful transplantation, patients generally report a favorable quality of life, and approximately 50% of patients return to work. In general, however, the cardiac transplant patient has a significantly impaired exercise capacity and diminished physiological and hemodynamic function.[3, 5]

The acute response to exercise for transplant patients can be classified as abnormal. Limited cardiac output and oxygen uptake capacities are exhibited during exercise; resting heart rate is elevated and left ventricular ejection is significantly reduced. As shown in Figure 16.7, much of this circulatory "sluggishness" is the result of the denervated heart's inability to rapidly and significantly accelerate in response to increasing exercise demands.[1, 27] In normal individuals, stroke volume increases to approximately 40 to 50% of aerobic capacity and then plateaus; further increases in cardiac output are mainly due to heart rate increases. In transplant patients, on the other hand, there is an absence of a plateau in stroke volume during graded exercise. Consequently, in these patients, increases in stroke volume are an important mechanism for increasing cardiac output in more intense exercise.[9]

The available (although limited) data show that transplant patients can respond positively to aerobic exercise training with significant improvements in aerobic capacity.[1] The guidelines for training the transplant patient are essentially the same as for any postcardiac surgery patient. The exception is that training heart rate guidelines (see Chapter 21) are not applicable because of the delayed and blunted heart rate response of the denervated transplanted organ. Furthermore, because the transplanted heart has no connections to the nervous system, a patient with advanced coronary artery disease in the transplanted heart does not experience the painful warnings of exercise-induced angina pectoris.

■ SUMMARY ■

1. The cardiovascular system provides rapid regulation of heart rate and the effective distribution of blood in the vascular circuit. This is accomplished while maintaining blood pressure in response to the body's metabolic and physiologic needs.
2. The cardiac rhythm is initiated at the S-A node. The impulse then travels across the atria to the A-V node, where it is delayed and then rapidly spreads across the large ventricular mass. The atria and ventricles contract effectively with this normal conduction pattern to provide the impetus for blood flow.
3. The electrocardiogram provides a record of the sequence of the heart's electrical events during the cardiac cycle. This is important for detecting various abnormalities in heart function at rest and during exercise.
4. The sympathetic catecholamines, epinephrine and norepinephrine, act to accelerate the heart rate and increase myocardial contractility. The parasympathetic neurotransmitter, acetylcholine, acts through the vagus nerve to slow the heart.

FIGURE 16.7

Heart rate response of patient during graded exercise before and after orthotopic cardiac transplantation. Note the elevated resting heart rate and the delayed and blunted increase in exercise heart rate after transplantation. (From Squirers, R.W.: Exercise training after cardiac transplantation. *Med. Sci. Sports Exerc.*, 23:686, 1991.)

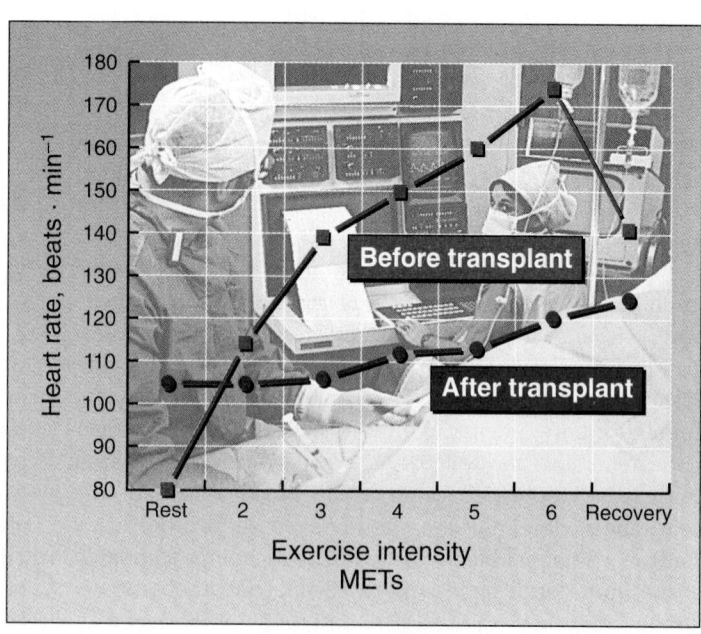

5. The heart is "turned on" in the transition from rest to exercise by an increase in sympathetic and a decrease in parasympathetic activity integrated with input from the central command in the brain.

6. A large part of the heart rate adjustment to exercise is due to cortical influence in anticipation before and during the initial stage of physical activity.

7. Reflex sensory input from peripheral receptors in blood vessels, joints, and muscles provide the cardiovascular center with a continual "update" on the physical and chemical state of active muscle.

8. Neural and hormonal extrinsic factors modify the heart's inherent rhythm. This enables it to speed up rapidly in anticipation of exercise and to increase to 200 beats per minute or higher in maximum exercise.

9. Palpation of the carotid artery is generally an appropriate means for determining the actual heart rate during and immediately after exercise.

10. Nerves, hormones, and local metabolic factors act on the smooth muscle bands in various blood vessels. This causes them to alter their internal diameter to regulate blood flow in response to the demands of metabolism. The flow of blood in the vascular circuit changes with the vessels' radius raised to the fourth power, in general accord with Poiseuille's law. Adrenergic sympathetic fibers release norepinephrine, which causes vasoconstriction; cholinergic sympathetic neurons secrete acetylcholine, which brings about vasodilation.

11. The ability of tissues such as the kidneys and splanchnic region to dramatically compromise their blood flow provides the rapid redistribution of blood to more active tissues during exercise. This augments blood flow to the muscles while at the same maintaining adequate blood pressure throughout the vascular system.

12. Patients undergoing successful orthotopic transplantation demonstrate a "sluggish" cardiovascular response to exercise. This is largely the result of the denervated heart's inability to rapidly and significantly accelerate in response to the demands of exercise.

■ REFERENCES ■

1. Badenhop, D.T.: The therapeutic role of exercise in patients with orthotopic heart transplant. *Med. Sci. Sports Exerc.*, 27:975, 1995.

1a. Bevegård, B.S., and Shepherd, J.T.: Regulation of the circulation during exercise in man. *Physiol. Rev.*, 47:178, 1967.

2. Bjornstad, H., et al.: Ambulatory electrocardiographic findings in top athletes, athletic students and control subjects. *Cardiology*, 84: 42, 1994.

3. Brubaker, P.H., et al.: Relationship of lactate and ventilatory thresholds in cardiac transplant patients. *Med. Sci. Sports Exerc.*, 25:191, 1993.

4. Couldry, W.C., et al.: Carotid vs. radial pulse counts. *Phys. Sportsmed.*, 10:67, 1982.

5. Degre, S.G., et al.: Cardiorespiratory response to early exercise testing after orthotopic cardiac transplantation. *Am. J. Cardiol.*, 60:926, 1987.

6. Innes, J.A., et al: Central command influences cardiorespiratory response to dynamic exercise in humans with unilateral weakness. *J. Physiol. (Lond.)*, 448:551, 1992.

7. Katona, P.G., et al.: Sympathetic and parasympathetic cardiac control in athletes and non-athletes at rest. *J. Appl. Physiol.*, 52:1652, 1982.

8. Kenney, W.L.: Parasympathetic control of resting heart rate: relationship to aerobic power. *Med. Sci. Sports Exerc.*, 17:451, 1985.

9. Keteyain, S.J., et al.: Cardiovascular responses to submaximal arm and leg exercise in cardiac transplant patients. *Med. Sci. Sports Exerc.*, 26:420, 1994.

10. Kriett, J.M., and Kaye, M.P.: The registry of the international society for heart transplantation: seventh official report—1990. *J. Heart Transplant.*, 9:323, 1990.

11. Magel, J.R., et al.: Telemetered heart rate response to selected competitive swimming events. *J. Appl. Physiol.*, 26:764, 1969.

12. Nóbrega, A.C.L., and Araújo, C.G.S.: Heart rate transient at the onset of active and passive dynamic exercise. *Med. Sci. Sports Exerc.*, 25:37, 1993.

13. Nóbrega, A.C.L., et al.: Cardiovascular responses to active and passive cycling movements. *Med. Sci. Sports Exerc.*, 26:709, 1994.

14. Oldridge, N.B., et al.: Carotid palpation, coronary heart disease, and exercise rehabilitation. *Med. Sci. Sports Exerc.*, 13:6, 1981.

15. Petro, J.K., et al.: Instantaneous cardiac acceleration in a man induced by voluntary muscle contractions. *J. Appl. Physiol.*, 29:794, 1970.

16. Rowell, L.B.: General principles of vascular control. In *Human Circulation: Regulation During Physical Stress*. New York, Oxford University Press, 1986.

17. Rowell, L.B.: *Human Cardiovascular Control*. Cary, NC, Oxford University Press, 1994.

18. Rowell, L.B., and O'Leary, D.S.: Reflex control of the circulation during exercise: chemoreflexes and mechanoreflexes. *J. Appl. Physiol.*, 69:407, 1990.

19. Schaefer, M.E., et al.: Adrenergic responsiveness and intrinsic sinoartial automaticity of exercise-trained rats. *Med. Sci. Sports Exerc.*, 24:887, 1992.

20. Scheuer, J., and Tipton, C.M.: Cardiovascular adaptations to physical training. *Annu. Rev. Physiol.*, 39:221, 1977.

21. Seals, D.R., and Victor, R.G.: Regulation of muscle sympathetic nerve activity during exercise in humans. *Exerc. Sport Sci. Rev.*, 19:313, 1991.

22. Seals, D.R., et al.: Exercise and aging: autonomic control of the circulation. *Med. Sci. Sports Exerc.*, 26:568, 1994.

23. Sedlock, D.A., et al.: Accuracy of subject-palpated carotid pulse after exercise. *Phys. Sportsmed.*, 11:106, 1983.

23a. Shen, W., et al.: Nitric oxide production and NO synthase gene expression contribute to vascular regulation during exercise. *Med. Sci. Sports Exerc.*, 27:1125, 1995.

24. Shepherd, J.T.: Behavior of resistance and capacity vessels in human limbs during exercise. *Circ. Res.*, 20(Suppl. I):70, 1967.

25. Shepherd, J.T., et al.: Static (isometric) exercise. Retrospection and introspection. *Circ. Res.*, 48(Suppl. I):179, 1981.

26. Smith, M.L., et al.: Exercise training bradycardia: the role of autonomic balance. *Med. Sci. Sports Exerc.*, 21:44, 1989.

27. Squirers, R.W.: Exercise training after cardiac transplantation. *Med. Sci. Sports Exerc.*, 23:686, 1991.

28. Stebbins, C.L., et al.: Reflex effect of skeletal muscle mechanoreceptor stimulation on the cardiovascular system. *J. Appl. Physiol.*, 65:1539, 1988.

29. Strange, S., et al.: Neural control of cardiovascular responses and of ventilation during dynamic exercise in man. *J. Physiol. (Lond.)*, 70:693, 1993.

30. White, J.R.: EKG changes using carotid artery for heart rate monitoring. *Med. Sci. Sports Exerc.*, 9:88, 1977.

30a. Williamson, J.W., et al.: Instantaneous heart rate increase with dynamic exercise: central command and muscle-heart reflex contributions. *J. Appl. Physiol.*, 78:1273, 1995.

31. Zweifach, B.J.: The microcirculation of the blood. *Sci. Am.*, Jan. 1959.

Coyle, E.F., et al.: Time course of loss of adaptations after stopping prolonged intense endurance training. *J. Appl. Physiol.* 57:1857, 1984.

There is considerable research effort on understanding the effects of varying types of exercise training on physiologic and metabolic function. Much less attention has focused on understanding what happens with discontinuance of such training. A clearer picture of the "detraining" process would

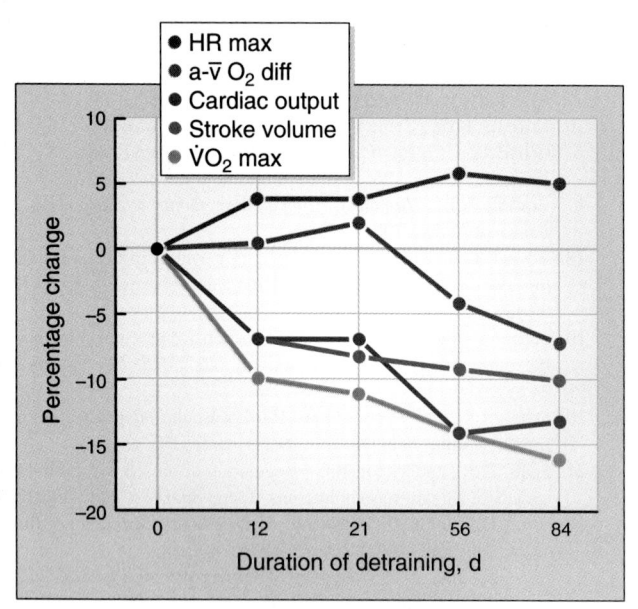

Average changes in maximum heart rate (HRmax), stroke volume, arteriovenous oxygen differences (a-$\bar{v}$ O$_2$ diff), cardiac output, and $\dot{V}o_2$max over 84 days of detraining.

shed light on understanding the body's adaptive process and provide insight into the effects of sedentary living.

Coyle and colleagues studied detraining in seven (six male and one female) highly trained, competitive or recreational runners or cyclists. Prior to discontinuing training, subjects trained for 10 to 12 months a minimum of 5 days per week for approximately 60 minutes daily at an exercise intensity corresponding to 70 to 80% $\dot{V}o_2$max. A group of sedentary subjects (N = 7) served as a

control group. Testing included muscle biopsies obtained on the last day of training and on days 12, 21, 56, and 84 during detraining. Physiological and cardiovascular testing included $\dot{V}o_2$ and cardiac output (CO), heart rate (HR), stroke volume (SV), and arteriovenous oxygen difference (a-$\bar{v}$ O$_2$ diff) performed during 15 minutes of exercise at 75% of $\dot{V}o_2$max and at $\dot{V}o_2$max. The muscle biopsy included the left gastrocnemius for the runners and the vastus lateralis for the cyclists.

Except for the exercise performed during testing, the subjects limited their physical activity to the minimal level required in their sedentary jobs. According to the researchers, the subjects walked less than 500 m a day at a slow pace. The figure shows the average changes in physiological variables at each test period. When training ceased, the $\dot{V}o_2$max declined in all subjects and declined 7% below training levels after 12 days, 14% after 56 days, and 16% by day 84. CO, SV, HR, and a-$\bar{v}$ O$_2$ diff exhibited declines similar to the $\dot{V}o_2$max. Stroke volume decreased by 11% during the first 12 days and stabilized at 86% of the trained value by day 56. No further decrease occurred during the final 4 weeks; the decrease in SVmax was partly compensated for by the increase in HRmax during detraining. Thus, COmax declined by only 8% during the initial 3 weeks of detraining, with a total decrease of 10% over the entire 84-day period.

Impressive detraining changes were noted in the muscle biopsy data. For example, citrate synthase and succinate dehydrogenase (SDH), major enzymes of aerobic respiration, declined roughly in parallel, reaching their lowest levels at day 56. However, detraining did not affect myoglobin and muscle capillarization. Because capillary density did not change with detraining, the researchers attributed the decreased oxygen extraction (maximum a-$\bar{v}$ O$_2$ diff) to reduced mitochondrial capacity reflected in reduced levels of citrate synthase and SDH levels.

This study confirmed that both a decrease in maximum SV (central factor) and in a-$\bar{v}$ O$_2$ diff (peripheral factor) contributed to the decrease in $\dot{V}o_2$max during detraining. The results thus support the age-old dictum, "use it or lose it."

Functional Capacity of the Cardiovascular System

CARDIAC OUTPUT

Cardiac output refers to the amount of blood pumped by the heart, usually during a 1-minute period. The maximal value for cardiac output reflects the functional capacity of the circulation to meet the demands of physical activity. Output from the heart, as with any pump, depends on its rate of pumping (**heart rate**) and the quantity of blood ejected with each stroke (**stroke volume**). Cardiac output is computed according to the following equation:

$$\text{Cardiac output} = \text{Heart rate} \times \text{Stroke volume}$$

MEASURING CARDIAC OUTPUT

Output from a hose, pump, or faucet is easily determined; one need only open the valve and collect and measure the volume of fluid ejected over a given time period. For obvious reasons, this technique does not apply in animals or humans. In addition, an occurrence such as an invasive "opening" of the main output vessel in a closed circulatory system would dramatically alter normal output. With advances in biomedical engineering, however, electromagnetic and ultrasonic flowmeters surgically implanted around a main artery in the vascular circuit measure flow through the intact vessel. This technique, usually limited to animal research, has little application for use in a typical exercise setting with healthy humans. Three common methods assess cardiac output in humans: the direct Fick, indicator dilution, and CO_2 rebreathing methods.

Direct Fick Method. The output of fluid from a pump in a closed circuit can be determined from any change in concentration of a substance between the output and input of the pump, and from the total quantity of that substance taken up (or given off) by the fluid in a given time period. For cardiovascular dynamics, calculating cardiac output requires knowledge of the average difference between the oxygen content of arterial and mixed venous blood (a-$\bar{v}$ O_2 difference) and oxygen uptake during 1 minute. The question then becomes: how much blood must have circulated during the minute to account for the observed oxygen uptake, given the observed a-$\bar{v}$ O_2 difference? The formula that expresses the relationship between cardiac output, oxygen uptake, and a-$\bar{v}$ O_2 difference em-

bodies the principle set forth by the German physician Adolph Fick in 1870 and is termed the **Fick equation.**

$$\begin{array}{c}\text{Cardiac}\\ \text{output}\\ (\text{mL} \cdot \text{min}^{-1})\end{array} = \frac{O_2 \text{ consumption } (\text{mL} \cdot \text{min}^{-1})}{\text{a-}\bar{v} \ O_2 \text{ difference } (\text{mL per 100 mL blood})} \times 100$$

Figure 17.1 illustrates the Fick principle for determining cardiac output. In this example, 250 mL of oxygen is consumed during 1 minute at rest, and the a-$\bar{v}$ O_2 difference during this time averages 5 mL of oxygen per 100 mL of blood. By substituting these values in the Fick equation, the cardiac output is determined as follows:

$$\begin{array}{c}\text{Cardiac}\\ \text{output}\\ (\text{mL} \cdot \text{min}^{-1})\end{array} = \frac{250 \text{ mL } O_2}{5 \text{ mL } O_2} \times 100 = \frac{5000 \text{ mL}}{\text{blood}}$$

Although the Fick principle is straightforward, the actual method of cardiac output measurement is complex and usually is limited to a clinical setting, in which the benefits of measurement exceed any potential risk. Measuring oxygen uptake involves the methods of open-circuit spirometry summarized in Chapter 8. The more difficult task is obtaining the a-$\bar{v}$ O_2 difference. A representative sample of arterial blood can be obtained from any convenient systemic artery, such as the femoral, radial, or brachial artery. Although these arteries are easily located, the actual arterial puncture can be traumatic to the patient. Sampling of **mixed venous blood** presents additional difficulties, because the blood in each vein only reflects the metabolic activity of the specific area it drains. To accurately estimate the average oxygen content of all venous blood, it is necessary to sample from an anatomic "mixing chamber" such as the right atrium, the right ventricle, or—most accurately—the pulmonary artery. This is achieved by threading a small flexible tube (catheter) through the antecubital vein in the arm and into the superior vena cava that leads into the right heart. A sample of arterial and mixed venous blood is then obtained during the same period of measurement as the oxygen uptake.

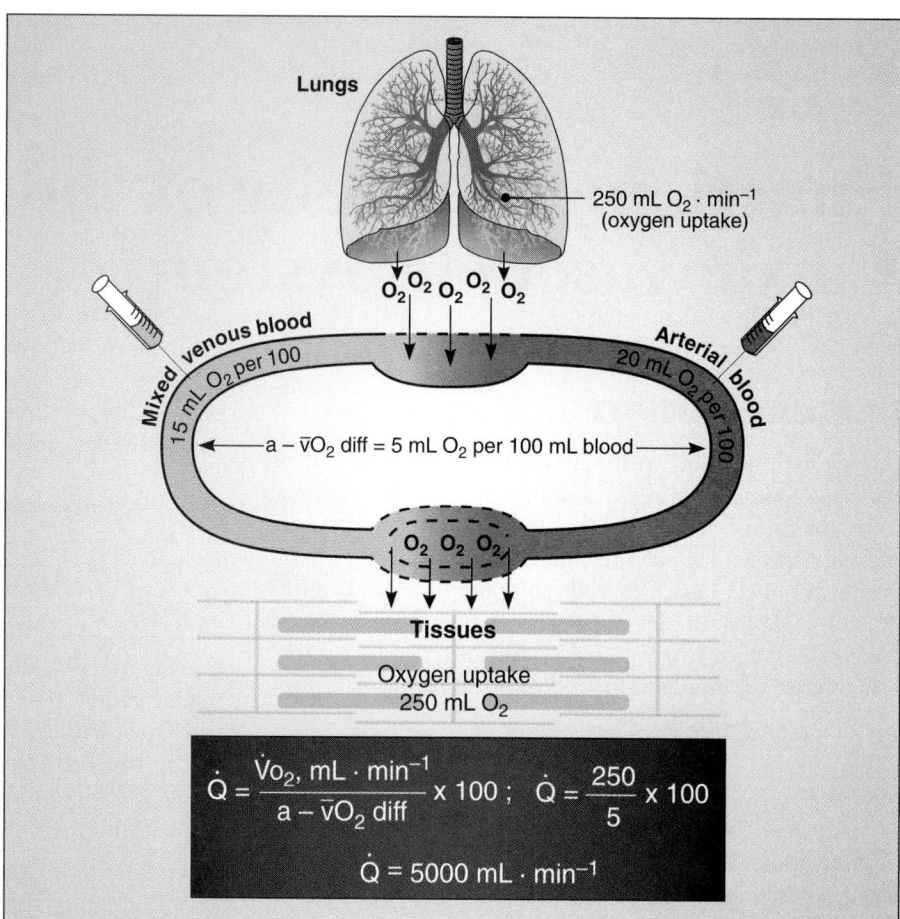

FIGURE 17.1

Application of the Fick principle for measuring cardiac output ($\dot{Q}$).

The direct Fick method has been used in numerous studies of cardiovascular dynamics under a variety of experimental conditions. This method generally serves as the criterion standard to validate other techniques for cardiac output measurement. The main criticism of the method is that by its very nature of being **invasive** to the body, cardiovascular dynamics may be altered during the measurement period. Although the obtained value for cardiac output may be accurate, it may not reflect the person's "normal" cardiovascular response to a particular situation.

Indicator Dilution Method. The indicator dilution method involves venous and arterial punctures but does not require cardiac catheterization. A known quantity of an inert dye (such as indocyanine green) or radioactive substance is injected into a large vein. The indicator material remains in the vascular stream, usually bound to plasma proteins or to red blood cells. It then becomes mixed as the blood travels to the lungs and back to the heart before being ejected into the systemic circuit. Arterial blood samples are continually measured with a radioactive counter or photosensitive device. The area under the dilution-concentration curve obtained by repetitive sampling indicates the average concentration of indicator material as blood is pumped from the heart. From the dilution of a known quantity of dye in an unknown quantity of blood, the cardiac output is calculated as follows:

$$\text{Cardiac output} = \frac{\text{Quantity of dye injected}}{\text{Average concentration dye in blood for duration of curve} \times \text{Duration of curve}}$$

CO$_2$ Rebreathing Method. Cardiac output also can be determined from values of carbon dioxide substituted in the Fick equation. Carbon dioxide production is determined by open-circuit spirometry as used for oxygen uptake measurement in the direct Fick method. By using a rapid carbon dioxide gas analyzer and making certain reasonable assumptions, it is possible to obtain valid estimates of mixed venous and arterial carbon dioxide levels. The technique is noninvasive or "bloodless," and requires a breath-by-breath analysis of carbon dioxide.[3]

After venous and arterial carbon dioxide concentrations are estimated, cardiac output is calculated in accordance with the Fick principle as follows:

$$\text{Cardiac output} = \frac{\text{Carbon dioxide production}}{\bar{\text{v}}\text{-a CO}_2 \text{ difference}} \times 100$$

The CO_2 rebreathing method has obvious advantages over the direct Fick and indicator dilution methods. It is bloodless, involves minimal interference with the subject, and does not require close medical supervision. Because this method is noninvasive, it may provide more accurate estimates of the "real" cardiovascular dynamics during exercise than would be obtained by more invasive techniques. One limitation of the CO_2 rebreathing method is that subjects are required to exercise at a steady metabolic rate, which may restrict the use of this method during maximal and "supermaximal" exercise and during the transition from rest to steady-rate exercise.

CARDIAC OUTPUT AT REST

Cardiac output varies considerably in an individual at rest. It is affected by emotional conditions that alter cortical outflow (central command) to the cardioaccelerator nerves as well as to nerves that act on the arterial resistance and venous capacitance vessels. On the average, however, the entire blood volume of approximately 5 L for a typical male adult is pumped from the left ventricle each minute. A 5-L cardiac output at rest is the average for both trained and untrained individuals.

Untrained. In the average sedentary person, a 5-L cardiac output is usually sustained with a heart rate of approximately 70 beats per minute. Substituting this heart rate value in the cardiac output equation, the calculated stroke volume of the heart equals 71 mL per beat. Stroke volume and cardiac output for women usually average approximately 25% below values for men; in women, the average stroke volume is 50 to 60 mL per beat at rest. This "gender difference" is essentially due to the smaller body size of the average woman.

Endurance Athletes. Endurance training causes the sinus node of the heart to come under greater influence of acetylcholine, the parasympathetic hormone that has a slowing effect on heart rate. At the same time, there is probably a concomitant reduction in resting sympathetic activity. This training adaptation partially explains the relatively low resting heart rates of many endurance athletes. Heart rates in endurance athletes generally average approximately 50 beats per minute at rest, although heart rates below 30 beats per minute have been reported for apparently healthy athletes. Because the resting cardiac output of endurance-trained athletes also averages 5 L per minute, blood is circulated with the proportionately larger stroke volume of

100 mL per beat. Average values for cardiac output, heart rate, and stroke volume of endurance-trained and untrained men at rest are summarized as follows:

	Rest				
	Cardiac output	=	**Heart rate**	×	**Stroke volume**
Untrained:	5000 mL	=	70 beats · min⁻¹	×	71 mL
Trained:	5000 mL	=	50 beats · min⁻¹	×	100 mL

Although these calculations are straightforward, the underlying physiologic mechanisms for the different response patterns are not fully understood. It is not clear whether the bradycardia that occurs with endurance training "causes" a larger stroke volume or vice versa, because the myocardium itself may respond more forcefully in response to regular aerobic exercise. Two factors are probably operative with training:

- Endurance training increases vagal tone, which slows the heart.
- Factors associated with training, such as enhanced blood volume, as well as inherent myocardial factors contribute to a more forceful stroke with each contraction.

CARDIAC OUTPUT DURING EXERCISE

Blood flow increases in proportion to exercise intensity. Cardiac output undergoes a rapid increase in progressing from rest to steady-rate exercise. This is followed by a gradual rise until a plateau is reached. At this point, blood flow is sufficient to meet the metabolic requirements of exercise.

In relatively sedentary, college-aged males, cardiac output during maximal exercise increases four times above the resting level to an average maximum of 20 to 22 L of blood per minute. Maximum heart rate for these young adults usually averages 195 beats per minute. Consequently, the stroke volume is generally between 103 and 113 mL of blood per beat. In contrast, world-class endurance athletes have maximum cardiac outputs of 35 to 40 L per minute. This is even more impressive when one considers that the trained person may have a slightly lower maximum heart rate than the sedentary person of similar age.[35, 42] *Thus, the endurance athlete achieves a large maximal cardiac output solely as the result of a large stroke volume.* For example, the cardiac output of an Olympic medal winner in cross-country skiing increased to 40 L per minute (almost eight times above rest) in maximum exercise; the stroke volume was 210 mL per beat. This is nearly twice the volume of blood pumped per beat in comparison to the maximum stroke volume of a sedentary person of similar age. As a point of comparison between species, note that cardiac outputs of 600 L · min⁻¹ (with an accompanying 150 mL · kg⁻¹ · min⁻¹ $\dot{V}O_2$max) have been reported in thoroughbred racehorses.[18a, 62]

The functional capacity of the heart during maximum exercise in endurance-trained and untrained men is summarized as follows:

	Maximum Exercise					
	Cardiac output	=	Heart rate	×	Stroke volume	
Untrained:	22,000 mL	=	195 beats · min⁻¹	×	113 mL	
Trained:	35,000 mL	=	195 beats · min⁻¹	×	179 mL	

STROKE VOLUME IN EXERCISE: TRAINING EFFECTS

The stroke volume response for two groups of men during upright exercise of increasing intensity is illustrated in Figure 17.2. One group of six endurance athletes had trained for several years; the other group consisted of three sedentary college students. The students' exercise responses were evaluated before and after a 55-day training program designed to improve aerobic fitness.[50]

From these data, several important conclusions can be drawn:

- The heart of an endurance athlete has a considerably larger stroke volume during rest and exercise than that of an untrained person of the same age.
- In both trained and untrained individuals, the greatest increase in stroke volume during upright exercise occurs during the transition from rest to moderate exercise. As exercise becomes more intense, only small increases in stroke volume occur.
- Maximum stroke volume is generally reached at 40 to 50% of the maximal oxygen uptake; this usually represents a heart rate of 110 to 120 beats per minute in young adults. (Endurance training appears to blunt the small decrease in stroke volume that is often observed during heavy exercise. This suggests that even at rapid heart rates there is still adequate time for the ventricles of the trained heart to fill during diastole, so there is no diminution in the stroke volume during heavy exercise.[19,58])
- In the untrained, only a small increase in stroke volume occurs during the transition from rest to exercise. The major increase in cardiac output for these individuals is brought about by an acceleration in heart rate. In trained endurance athletes, **both** heart rate and stroke volume increase to augment cardiac output; the increase in an athlete's stroke volume is generally approximately 60% above resting values.
- In previously sedentary individuals, 8 weeks of aerobic training substantially increases stroke volume, but these values are still well below those observed for elite athletes. It has yet to be determined to what degree this difference reflects prolonged training, genetics, or a combination of both.

Stroke Volume and $\dot{V}O_2$max. The importance of stroke volume in differentiating people who have high and low values for $\dot{V}O_2$max is amplified in Table 17.1.

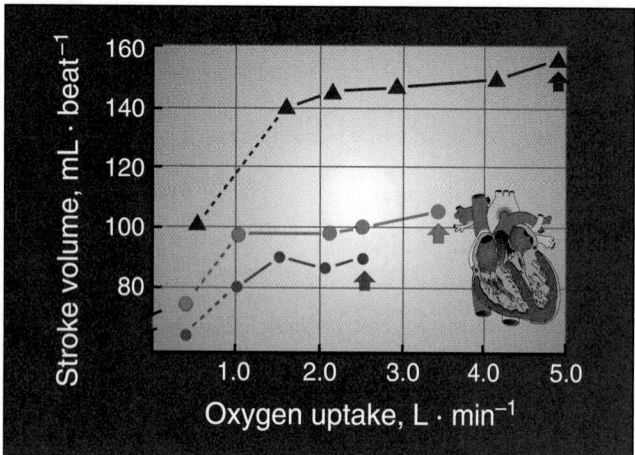

FIGURE 17.2
Stroke volume in relation to oxygen uptake during upright exercise in endurance athletes (▲) and sedentary college students before (●) and after (●) 55 days of aerobic training (↑ = maximal values). (From Saltin, B.: Physiological effects of physical conditioning. *Med. Sci. Sports*, 1:50, 1969.)

TABLE 17.1
MAXIMAL VALUES FOR OXYGEN UPTAKE, HEART RATE, STROKE VOLUME, AND CARDIAC OUTPUT IN THREE GROUPS WITH VERY LOW, NORMAL, AND HIGH AEROBIC CAPACITIES

Group	$\dot{V}O_2$max (L · min⁻¹)	Max Heart Rate (beats · min⁻¹)	Max Stroke Volume (mL)	Max Cardiac Output (L · min⁻¹)
Mitral stenosis	1.6	190	50	9.5
Sedentary	3.2	200	100	20.0
Athlete	5.2	190	160	30.4

Modified from Rowell, L.B.: Circulation. *Med. Sci. Sports*, 1:15, 1969.

TABLE 17.2
THE EFFECT OF BODY POSITION ON CARDIAC OUTPUT, STROKE VOLUME, AND HEART RATE AT REST AND DURING EXERCISE IN WELL-TRAINED ATHLETES

	Rest		Moderate Exercise		Strenuous Exercise	
	Supine	Upright	Supine	Upright	Supine	Upright
Cardiac output, L · min^{-1}	9.2	6.6	19.0	16.9	26.3	24.5
Stroke volume, mL	141	103	163	149	164	155
Heart rate, beats · min^{-1}	65	64	115	112	160	159
Oxygen uptake, mL · min^{-1}	345	384	1769	1864	3364	3387

Data from Bevegård, S., et al.: Circulatory studies in well-trained athletes at rest and during heavy exercise, with special reference to stroke volume and the influence of body position. *Acta Physiol. Scand.*, 57:26, 1963.

These data were obtained from three groups: athletes, healthy but sedentary men, and patients who had mitral stenosis, a valvular disease of the heart that results in inadequate emptying of the left ventricle.[7] The differences in $\dot{V}O_2$max among groups are closely related to differences in maximal stroke volume. Patients with mitral stenosis had an aerobic capacity and maximum stroke volume that was half that of the sedentary subjects. This relationship was also apparent in comparisons of healthy subjects; the $\dot{V}O_2$max of athletes was 62% larger than the sedentary individuals, and the stroke volume was 60% larger in the athletes. Because the maximal heart rate of both groups was similar, the difference in maximal cardiac output (and $\dot{V}O_2$max) was almost entirely due to differences in stroke volume.

STROKE VOLUME: SYSTOLIC EMPTYING VERSUS DIASTOLIC FILLING

Essentially, two physiologic mechanisms influence the heart's stroke volume. The first mechanism is intrinsic to the myocardium and involves enhanced cardiac filling in diastole followed by a more forceful contraction. The second mechanism is governed by neurohormonal influence. It involves normal ventricular filling with a subsequent forceful ejection that brings about greater emptying during systole. *Both factors probably contribute to the increase in the heart's stroke volume during exercise.* Also, training adaptations that reduce resistance to the flow of blood in the peripheral tissues will augment the stroke volume of the heart.[59]

Enhanced Diastolic Filling. Any factor that increases venous return or slows the heart causes greater ventricular filling, or **preload,** during the diastolic phase of the cardiac cycle. This increase in **end-diastolic volume** stretches the myocardial fibers and causes a powerful ejection stroke as the heart contracts. As a result, the normal stroke volume is expelled, along with the additional blood that entered the ventricles and stretched the myocardium.

The relationship between contractile force and the resting length of the heart's muscle fibers was first described by two physiologists, Otto Frank (1895) and E.H. Starling (1915). The enhanced contractility probably results from a more optimum arrangement of the sarcomere's myofilaments as the muscle fiber is stretched. This phenomenon, which always operates during the cardiac cycle and applies to all of the heart's chambers, has been termed **Starling's law of the heart.** For years, it was taught that the Frank-Starling mechanism provided the "modus operandi" for **all** increases in stroke volume during exercise. Physiologists believed that the venous return in exercise caused a greater cardiac filling and that this preload stretched the ventricles in diastole, causing them to respond with a more forceful ejection. It is likely that this is the pattern of response for stroke volume during transition from rest to exercise or as a person moves from the upright to the recumbent position. Enhanced diastolic filling probably occurs in activities such as swimming, in which the body's horizontal position optimizes blood flow into the heart.

From the data presented in Table 17.2, it is clear that body position has a significant effect on circulatory dynamics.[5] Cardiac output and stroke volume are highest and most stable in the horizontal position. In this position, the stroke volume is nearly maximum at rest and increases only slightly during exercise. In contrast, the force of gravity in the upright position acts to counter the return flow of blood to the heart, resulting in a diminished stroke volume and cardiac output. During upright exercise of increasing intensity, however, stroke volume increases and approaches the maximum stroke volume observed in the supine position.

Greater Systolic Emptying. In most forms of upright exercise, the heart does not fill to an extent that would cause the significant increase in cardiac volume observed in the recumbent position. Although research findings are not always consistent on this topic, it is more than likely that during graded upright exercise, progressive increases in stroke volume occur through the **combined effect** of an enhanced diastolic filling and a more complete emptying during systole. This greater systolic ejection occurs despite the increased resistance to blood flow provided by systolic blood pressure, or afterload.[44]

A greater systolic ejection with or without an accompanying increase in end-diastolic volume is possible because the heart contains a **functional residual volume** of blood. At rest in the upright position, approximately 40% of the total end-diastolic blood volume remains in the left ventricle after a contraction; this amounts to between 50 and 70 mL of blood. Myocardial contractile force is enhanced during exercise by the action of catecholamines, which augments stroke power to facilitate the systolic emptying of the heart.

Training Effects. The large stroke volume of the trained endurance athlete during exercise primarily results from an enlarged ventricular chamber (**eccentric hypertrophy**), which is associated with a chronic increased filling of the heart. This increased preload in trained individuals has been attributed to an expanded plasma volume that increases rapidly and remains elevated in response to aerobic training regardless of age.[6, 9] It is also likely that training brings about an increase in the compliance of the left ventricle, thereby increasing its ability to accept blood in the diastolic phase of the cardiac cycle.[19, 30, 31, 38] It remains unknown whether endurance training enhances the innate contractile state of the myocardium. If such a training adaptation does take place, the heart's capability to achieve a large stroke volume would also be augmented.

HEART RATE DURING EXERCISE: TRAINING EFFECTS

The large stroke volume of topflight endurance athletes and the increases in stroke volume of sedentary subjects following aerobic training are accompanied by a proportionate **heart rate reduction** during submaximal exercise. It is common for the submaximal heart rate for a standard exercise task to be lowered by 12 to 15 beats per minute as a result of aerobic training.

The relationship between heart rate and oxygen uptake in graded exercise is shown in Figure 17.3. As illustrated in Figure 17.2 for stroke volume, comparisons are made between athletes and sedentary students before and after training. The lines relating heart rate and oxygen uptake are essentially linear for both groups throughout the major portion of the exercise range. Whereas the untrained students' heart rates accelerated rapidly as exercise severity increased, the heart rates of the athletes accelerated to a much lesser extent; that is, the slope or rate of change of the lines differed considerably. Consequently, an athlete (or trained student) who has good cardiovascular response to exercise will do more intense exercise and achieve a higher oxygen uptake before reaching a particular submaximal heart rate than a sedentary student. At an oxygen uptake of 2.0 L per minute, the heart rates of the athletes averaged 70 beats per minute lower than the sedentary students. After 55 days of training, this difference in submaximal heart rate was reduced to about 40 beats

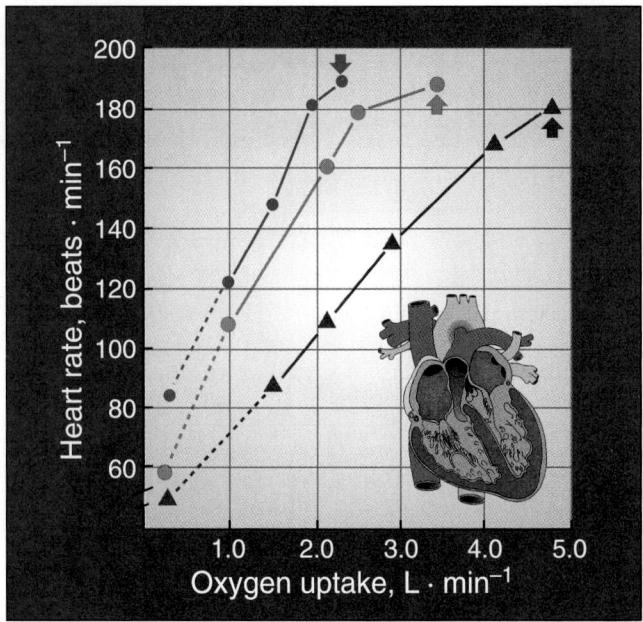

FIGURE 17.3
Heart rate in relation to oxygen uptake during upright exercise in endurance athletes (▲) and sedentary college students before (●) and after (●) 55 days of aerobic training (↑ = maximal values). (From Saltin, B.: Physiological effects of physical conditioning. *Med. Sci. Sports,* 1:50, 1969.)

per minute. In each instance, the cardiac output was about the same—*the difference was the stroke volume.*

DISTRIBUTION OF CARDIAC OUTPUT

Blood flow to the various tissues is generally proportional to their metabolic activity. Blood flow to the kidneys, skin, and splanchnic areas, however, can also vary with the metabolic demands of muscle during physical activity.

BLOOD FLOW AT REST

At rest in a comfortable environment, the 5-L cardiac output is generally distributed in the proportions shown in Figure 17.4A. Approximately one-fifth of the cardiac output is directed to muscle tissue, whereas the major portion of blood flows to the digestive tract, liver, spleen, brain, and kidneys.

BLOOD FLOW DURING EXERCISE

Figure 17.4B shows the percentage distribution of the cardiac output during light, moderate, and strenuous exercise. *Although regional blood flow during physical activity varies considerably depending on environmental conditions, level of fatigue, and the type of exercise, the major portion of the exercise cardiac output is diverted to the working muscles.* At rest, approximately 4 to 7 mL of blood is delivered each minute to every 100 g of muscle. This flow increases steadily in graded exercise, and at maximum exertion, it may be as high as 50 to 75 mL per 100 g of tissue. Actually, the increased flow of blood within active muscle is highly regulated, in that the greatest flow is delivered to the oxidative portions of the muscle at the expense of those areas with high glycolytic capacity.[28] Thus, peak values in a limited amount of active muscle may reach 300 to 400 mL · 100 g^{-1} · min^{-1}.[47] During maximal "big muscle" exercise such as running and cycling, the flow of blood to muscle represents approximately 84% of the total cardiac output.

Redistribution of Blood. The increase in muscle blood flow during exercise is largely due to an increased car-

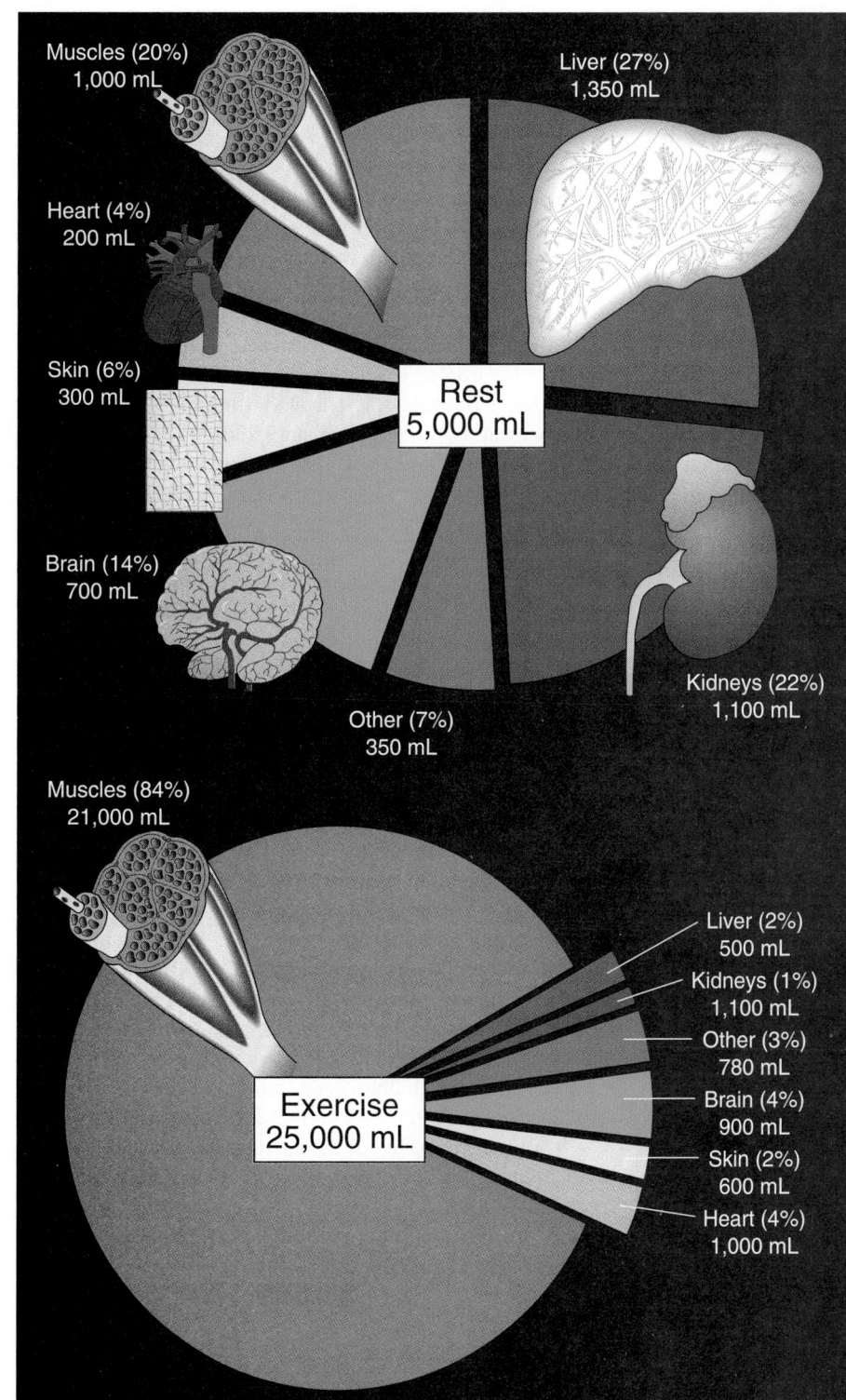

A

Muscles (20%)
1,000 mL

Liver (27%)
1,350 mL

Heart (4%)
200 mL

Skin (6%)
300 mL

Rest
5,000 mL

Brain (14%)
700 mL

Kidneys (22%)
1,100 mL

Other (7%)
350 mL

B

Muscles (84%)
21,000 mL

Exercise
25,000 mL

Liver (2%)
500 mL

Kidneys (1%)
1,100 mL

Other (3%)
780 mL

Brain (4%)
900 mL

Skin (2%)
600 mL

Heart (4%)
1,000 mL

FIGURE 17.4

Relative distribution of cardiac output at rest (**A**) and during strenuous endurance exercise (**B**). The number in parentheses indicates percent of total cardiac output. Note that despite the large mass of muscle, this tissue at rest receives about the same amount of blood as the much smaller kidneys. In strenuous exercise, however, approximately 84% of the cardiac output is diverted to the active muscles.

diac output. Blood flow to muscle, however, is disproportionately large in relation to other tissues. Owing to neural and hormonal vascular regulation and local metabolic conditions, blood is routed through active muscles from areas that can temporarily tolerate a reduction in normal blood flow. This **shunting of blood** from specific tissues occurs primarily during heavy exercise. For example, blood flow to the skin increases during light and moderate exercise so the metabolic heat generated in muscle can be dissipated at the skin's surface. During near-maximal effort, however, this tissue temporarily restricts its blood flow, even if the exercise is performed in a hot environment.[47] The kidneys and splanchnic tissues use only 10 to 25% of the oxygen available in the blood supply. Consequently, a considerable reduction in blood flow to these tissues can be tolerated before oxygen demand exceeds supply and function is compromised.[41] In some instances, renal blood flow is reduced by as much as four-fifths this organ's blood supply at rest. The energy needs of the tissues with reduced blood flow are maintained by increased extraction of oxygen from the available blood supply. A substantial reduction in blood flow to the visceral organs can be sustained for more than 1 hour during heavy exercise. Redistribution of blood away from these tissues during exercise can "free" as much as 600 mL of oxygen each minute for use by the working muscles.[47] Prolonged reduction in blood flow to the liver and kidneys, however, may have its consequences; this may contribute to fatigue, which is a common occurrence during prolonged submaximal exercise.

Blood Flow to the Heart and Brain. Some tissues cannot compromise their blood supply (Fig. 17.4). The myocardium normally uses approximately 75% of the oxygen in the blood flowing through the coronary circulation at rest. With this limited margin of reserve, the increased myocardial oxygen needs during exercise are met mainly by an increase in coronary blood flow. Thus, a four- to fivefold increase in myocardial work during exercise is accompanied by a similar increase in coronary circulation; this amounts to about 1 L of blood per minute during maximum exercise. Cerebral blood flow also increases during exercise by approximately 25 to 30% compared to the flow during rest.[22, 60]

CARDIAC OUTPUT AND OXYGEN TRANSPORT

AT REST

Arterial blood carries approximately 200 mL of oxygen per liter for a person with a normal level of hemoglobin (see Chapter 13). If the cardiac output each minute at rest is 5 L, potentially 1,000 mL of oxygen is available to the body (5 L blood × 200 mL O_2). Because the resting oxygen uptake averages only 250 mL per minute, 750 mL of oxygen returns unused to the heart. This is not an unnecessary waste of cardiac output. On the contrary, the extra oxygen that is circulated above the resting needs represents oxygen in reserve—a margin of safety that can be released immediately if there is a sudden increase in a tissue's metabolic needs.

DURING EXERCISE

A healthy, young adult with a maximum heart rate of 200 beats per minute and a stroke volume of 80 mL (0.8 L) per beat generates a maximum cardiac output of 16 L per minute (200 × 0.8 L). Even during maximum exercise, the saturation of hemoglobin with oxygen is nearly complete for this person, so each liter of arterial blood carries about 200 mL of oxygen. Consequently, 3,200 mL of oxygen is circulated each minute via a 16-L cardiac output (16 L × 200 mL $O_2 \cdot L^{-1}$). If all of the oxygen could be extracted from this cardiac output as it traveled through the body, the $\dot{V}O_2max$ could be no greater than 3,200 mL. However, even though the oxygen needs of certain tissues, such as the brain and skin, do not increase greatly with exercise, these tissues require a rich supply of blood.

Based on the preceding example, if the heart's stroke volume is increased from 80 to 200 mL per beat while the maximum heart rate remained unchanged at 200 beats per minute, maximum cardiac output would be dramatically increased to 40 L of blood per minute. This represents an increase in the quantity of oxygen circulated each minute during exercise of approximately 2.5 times (from 3,200 to 8,000 mL). *An increase in maximum cardiac output clearly results in a proportionate increase in the capacity to circulate oxygen. Within limits, this has a profound impact on the capacity for aerobic metabolism.*

Close Association Between Maximum Cardiac Output and $\dot{V}O_2max$. The relationship between maximum cardiac output and the capacity for achieving a high level of aerobic metabolism is shown in Figure 17.5. Included are values for the sedentary person as well as the elite endurance athlete. The relationship is unmistakable—a low aerobic capacity is closely associated with a low maximum cardiac output, whereas the ability to generate a 5- or 6-L $\dot{V}O_2max$ is always accompanied by a 30- to 40-L cardiac output.

The important role of cardiac output in sustaining aerobic metabolism is further illustrated in Figure 17.6. In both trained athletes and students, the cardiac output increases **linearly** with oxygen uptake throughout the major portion of the work range.[a]

---

[a]This linear relationship between cardiac output and oxygen uptake in graded exercise is also noted in children and adolescents. In these young people, the added cost of exercise as body mass increases with growth is closely matched by an increase in the heart's stroke volume with a proportionate increase in cardiac output.[12]

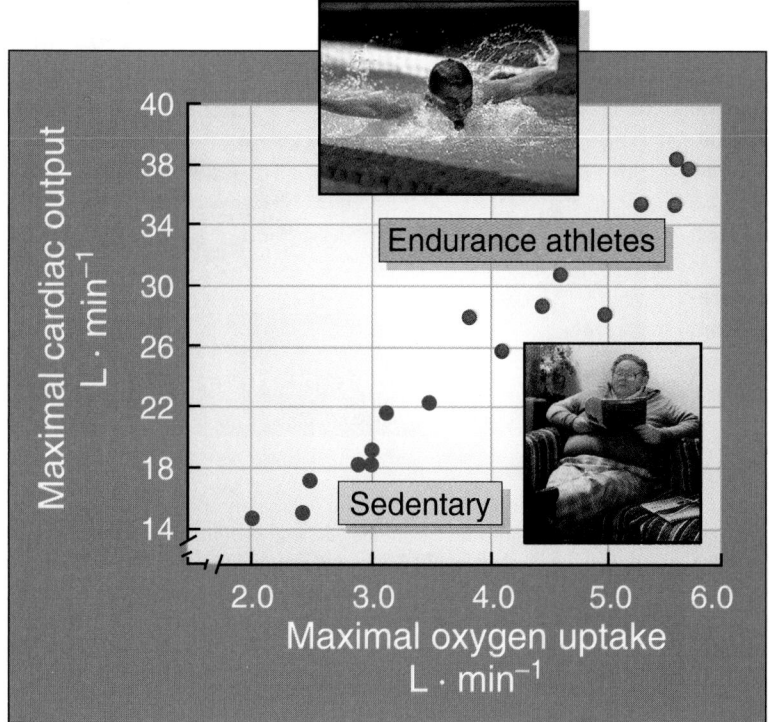

FIGURE 17.5

Relationship between maximal cardiac output and maximal oxygen uptake in trained and untrained individuals. The maximal cardiac output relates to the $\dot{V}O_2$max in a ratio of approximately 6:1. (Top photo courtesy of John Urbanchek, Varsity Men's Swimming Coach, University of Michigan.)

Each 1-L increase in oxygen uptake above rest is generally accompanied by a 5- to 6-L increase in blood flow; this relationship is basically the same regardless of the type of exercise performed. Over a wide range of dynamic exercises, there is a close linkage between cardiac output and oxygen uptake.[32] *The distinguishing feature for both preadolescents and adult endurance athletes is their high level of oxygen uptake and cardiac output capacity.*[50, 57] The 35% increase in $\dot{V}O_2$max noted in Figure 17.5 for the students after 55 days of training was accompanied by an almost proportionate increase in maximum cardiac output.

Differences in Cardiac Output Between Men and Women. The cardiac output response during graded exercise is similar between boys and girls and men and women. Both teenage and adult females, however, have a 5 to 10% **larger** cardiac output at any level of **submaximal** oxygen uptake than males.[2, 55] This apparent sex difference in cardiac output is most likely due to the 10% lower concentration of hemoglobin in women compared to men. This small decrease in the blood's oxygen-carrying capacity is compensated for by a proportionate increase in cardiac output in submaximal exercise.

Training and Submaximal Cardiac Output. Several early reports demonstrated that training, although improving the maximal cardiac output, reduced the minute volume of the heart during moderate exercise.[1, 21] In one study, the average cardiac output of young men after 16 weeks of training was reduced by between 1.1 and 1.5 L per minute at pre-established levels of submaximal oxygen uptake.[16] As expected, the maximal cardiac output increased 8% from 22.4 to 24.2 L per minute. With a reduction in sub-

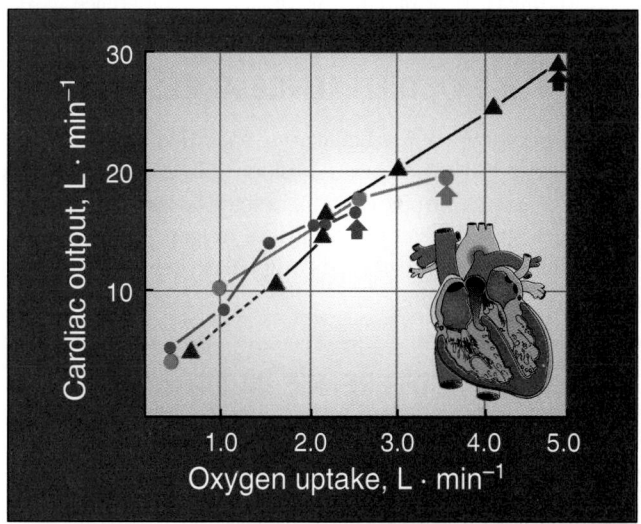

FIGURE 17.6

Cardiac output in relation to oxygen uptake during upright exercise in endurance athletes (▲) and sedentary college students before (●) and after (●) 55 days of aerobic training (⬆ = maximal values). (From Saltin, B.: Physiological effects of physical conditioning. *Med. Sci. Sports,* 1:50, 1969.)

maximal cardiac output, the exercise oxygen requirement is met by a corresponding increase in oxygen extraction in the active muscles. This is presumably the result of a more effective distribution of the cardiac output, coupled with an enhanced ability of the trained muscles to generate adenosine triphosphate (ATP) aerobically at a lower tissue P_{O_2}.

EXTRACTION OF OXYGEN: THE a-v̄ O₂ DIFFERENCE

If blood flow was the only means of increasing a tissue's oxygen supply, then cardiac output would have to increase from 5 L per minute at rest to 100 L during maximum exercise to achieve a 20-fold increase in oxygen uptake—an increase in oxygen uptake that is not uncommon among trained men and women. Fortunately, such a large cardiac output is unnecessary during exercise, because hemoglobin can release a considerable quantity of its "reserve" oxygen from the blood perfusing the active tissues. Consequently, two mechanisms are available to increase the level of oxygen uptake:

- Increase the total quantity of blood pumped by the heart (i.e., increase cardiac output).
- Make greater use of the relatively large quantity of oxygen already carried by the blood (i.e., expand the a-v̄ O₂ difference).

The important relationship between cardiac output, a-v̄ O₂ difference, and aerobic capacity is summarized by rearranging the Fick equation as follows:

Maximal oxygen uptake =
Maximal cardiac output × maximal a-v̄ O₂ difference

a-v̄ O₂ DIFFERENCE AT REST

At rest, an average of 5 mL of oxygen from the 20 mL of oxygen in each 100 mL of arterial blood (50 mL per liter) is used as it passes through the tissue capillaries. This represents an a-v̄ O₂ difference of 5 mL of oxygen. Thus, 15 mL of oxygen, or 75% of the blood's original oxygen load, still remains bound to hemoglobin.

a-v̄ O₂ DIFFERENCE IN EXERCISE

A comparison of the relationship between oxygen extraction (a-v̄ O₂ difference) and exercise intensity for the trained athletes and untrained students is illustrated in Figure 17.7. For the students, a-v̄ O₂ difference increased steadily during light and moderate exercise and reached a maximum of 15 mL of oxygen per 100 mL of blood. Following 55 days of training, the students' maximum oxygen extraction increased about 11% to 17 mL of oxygen. This meant that approximately 85% of the oxygen was extracted from arterial blood during heavy exercise. Actually, even more oxygen is extracted from the active muscles because the value for a-v̄ O₂ difference reflects an **average** based on calculations from mixed venous blood. It is important to note that this blood is returning from tissues in which oxygen use during exercise is not nearly as high as that of active muscle. The posttraining value for the maximal a-v̄ O₂ difference for the students is identical to that achieved by

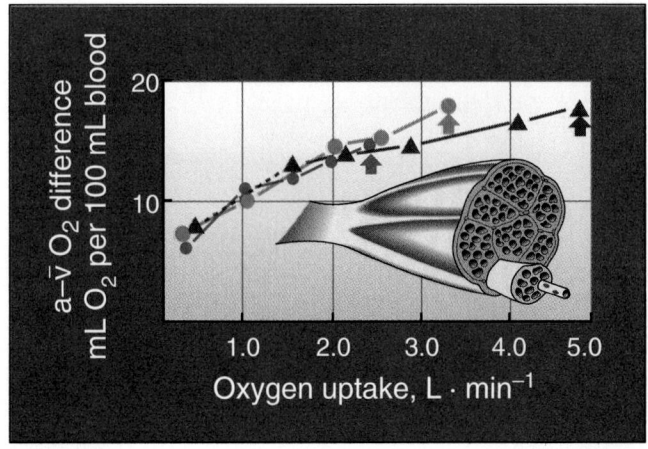

FIGURE 17.7
The a-v̄ O₂ difference in relation to oxygen uptake during upright exercise in endurance athletes (▲) and sedentary college students before (●) and after (●) 55 days of aerobic training (⬆ = maximal values). (From Saltin, B.: Physiological effects of physical conditioning. *Med. Sci. Sports*, 1:50, 1969.)

the endurance athletes. Obviously, the rather large difference in V̇O₂max that still exists between the athletes and students is due to the lower cardiac output capacity of the students.

In Heart Disease. In patients with advanced coronary artery disease, the heart muscle often has an impaired capacity to perform work or to improve with regular exercise. As a result, training adaptations are negligible in maximal stroke volume and cardiac output. For these patients, however, improvements in exercise tolerance and aerobic capacity are still possible because regular exercise increases the skeletal muscles' ability to receive and use oxygen. This contributes to expanding the a-v̄ O₂ difference and enables the patients to exercise at higher levels or at a particular submaximal level with a lower cardiac output.[14] A lower submaximal exercise cardiac output also reduces the workload of the heart; this is of great benefit to patients who suffer from exertional angina.

FACTORS THAT AFFECT a-v̄ O₂ DIFFERENCE IN EXERCISE

The maximal a-v̄ O₂ difference attained during exercise is influenced by the body's capacity to divert a large portion of the cardiac output to working muscles. As mentioned previously, certain tissues can temporarily compromise their blood supply considerably during exercise for purposes of shunting blood to increase the oxygen available for muscle metabolism. This redirection of the central circulation is facilitated by exercise training.[41]

The microcirculation of skeletal muscle is enhanced with aerobic training.[10, 26, 51] Muscle biopsies from the quadriceps femoris show a significantly larger ratio of capillaries to muscle fibers in trained than in sedentary men. An increase in the capillary-to-fiber ratio is a positive adaptation that provides a greater interface for the exchange of nutrients and metabolic gases during exercise. Another important factor determining the capacity for oxygen extraction is the ability of individual muscle cells to generate energy aerobically. Endurance training improves the metabolic capacity of the trained muscle. More specifically, the mitochondria enlarge and even increase in number, as does the quantity of enzymes for aerobic energy transfer.[23, 25] All of the local improvements within the trained muscle ultimately result in an enhanced capacity for the aerobic production of ATP.[68]

CARDIOVASCULAR ADJUSTMENTS TO UPPER BODY EXERCISE

Maximal Oxygen Uptake. *The highest oxygen uptake achieved during exercise with the arms is generally 20 to 30% lower than leg exercise.*[36, 52] Similarly, the maximal values for heart rate and pulmonary ventilation are significantly lower with arm exercise.[34, 66] These differences in maximal physiologic response are probably due to the relatively smaller muscle mass of the upper body used in arm ergometry.[52]

Submaximal Oxygen Uptake. During submaximal exercise, the response pattern for oxygen uptake between upper and lower body exercise is reversed.[20, 43, 63] Figure 17.8 shows that for any level of submaximal exercise, the oxygen uptake is higher when exercising the arms compared to the legs. The difference is small during light exercise but becomes progressively larger as the intensity of effort increases. This response has been attributed to a lower mechanical efficiency in upper body exercise owing to the additional cost of static muscle actions in this form of work (without contributing to the external work accomplished) as well as to the recruitment of extra musculature to stabilize the torso during many activities with the arms.[7, 54]

Physiologic Response. *For any level of submaximal oxygen uptake or percent of* $\dot{V}O_2max$, *the physiologic strain is greater in upper- compared to lower-body exercise.*[52,64] More specifically, heart rate, pulmonary ventilation, and perception of effort are generally higher when the arms are used in comparison to exercise with the legs. This was also the case for blood pressure in comparisons of arm and leg exercise (refer to Chapter 15). Even when the arm position is varied either at, above, or below heart level, the differences in physiologic strain are not reduced between arm and leg work.[11]

The elevated heart rate response in submaximal arm compared to leg exercise is probably the result of a larger input to the medullary control center from the central command in the brain (feed-forward stimulation) as well as an increased feedback stimulation to the medulla from peripheral receptors in active tissue. With upper body exercise, a greater strain (i.e., force per unit muscle, greater percentage of maximum, and increased metabolic by-products) is placed on the relatively smaller upper body musculature for any level of submaximal exercise. This augments peripheral feedback to the medulla, and there is an increase in heart rate (and blood pressure). More than likely, the lower maximum heart rates in upper body exercise are the result of the activation of a significantly smaller muscle mass than during maximal exercise with the legs. This causes a reduced input to the medullary control center from the motor cortex, as well as less peripheral feedback from the smaller upper-body muscle mass.

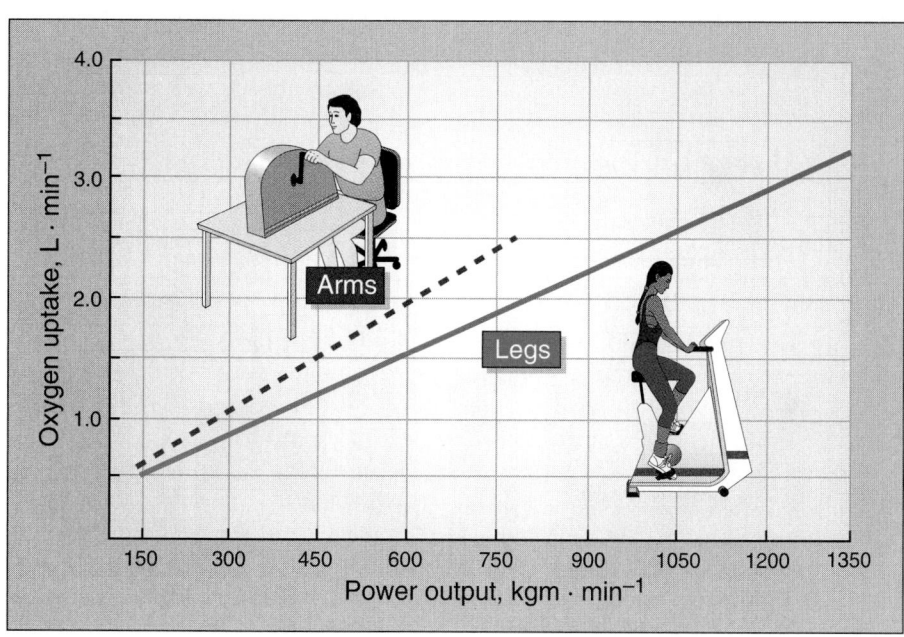

FIGURE 17.8

Arm exercise requires a greater oxygen uptake compared to leg exercise at any submaximal power output throughout the comparison range. The largest differences occur during heavy exercise. Data represent averages for men and women. (From Laboratory of Applied Physiology, Queens College, Flushing, NY.)

Implications. By understanding the differences in physiologic response between arm and leg exercise, the physician and exercise specialist can formulate prudent exercise programs using both forms of work. *The important point is that greater metabolic and physiologic strain accompanies a standard submaximal exercise load (power output or oxygen uptake) with the arms.* For this reason, exercise prescriptions based on running and bicycling **cannot** be applied to arm exercise. Furthermore, because the correlation between $\dot{V}o_2$max in arm and leg exercise is often low, it is not possible to accurately predict capacity for arm exercise from a test using the legs and vice versa.[18, 29] This further substantiates the concept of specificity for aerobic fitness.

CARDIAC HYPERTROPHY AND THE "ATHLETE'S HEART"

A *moderate increase in heart size is often observed in males and females in response to exercise training, regardless of age.* This **cardiac hypertrophy** can be viewed as a fundamental biologic adaptation of muscle to an increased work load. In such situations, a greater synthesis of cellular protein occurs with a concomitant reduction in protein breakdown. Accelerated protein synthesis is due largely to an increase in the trained muscle's content of RNA. Individual myofibrils thicken; at the same time, the number of these contractile filaments increases.

In sedentary men, the average heart volume is approximately 800 mL. In athletes, this volume increases in relation to the aerobic nature of the sport, so that for endurance athletes, the average heart volume is approximately 25% larger than for those who are sedentary. It has yet to be determined to what degree the relatively large heart volumes of some endurance athletes reflect genetic endowment or training adaptations, or both. It does appear, however, that

the duration of training affects cardiac size and structure. Several studies have reported no changes in cardiac dimensions with short-term training, even though there was significant improvement in both $\dot{V}o_2$max and submaximal exercise heart response.[45, 61] When left ventricular size increases with endurance training, this enlargement is not a permanent adaptation. Instead, heart size returns toward pretraining levels when there is a reduction in training intensity with apparently no deleterious effects.[13, 24] The general trend for cardiac enlargement (as reflected by left ventricular mass) in the untrained and various athletic groups is depicted in Figure 17.9.

Considerable cardiac enlargement also occurs in certain diseases. In hypertension, for example, the heart must chronically work against an excessive resistance to blood flow. As a result, the heart muscle is stretched and, in accordance with the Frank-Starling mechanism, generates compensatory force to overcome the added resistance (afterload) to systolic ejection. In addition to ventricular dilation, the individual muscle cells hypertrophy to adjust to the increased myocardial work imposed by the hypertensive state.[4] As untreated hypertension progresses, the myocardial fibers are eventually stretched beyond their optimal length, and the dilated heart weakens and eventually fails. To the pathologist, this "hypertrophied" heart is enlarged, distended, and functionally inadequate to deliver even enough blood to meet minimal resting requirements.

SPECIFIC NATURE OF TRAINING HYPERTROPHY

The ultrasonic technique of **echocardiography** uses sound waves to "map" the dimensions of the myocardium itself and the volume of its chambers. Echocardiography has been used to evaluate the structural characteristics of the hearts

FIGURE 17.9
General trend for cardiac enlargement (left ventricular mass) among the untrained and various groups of male and, where applicable, female athletes.

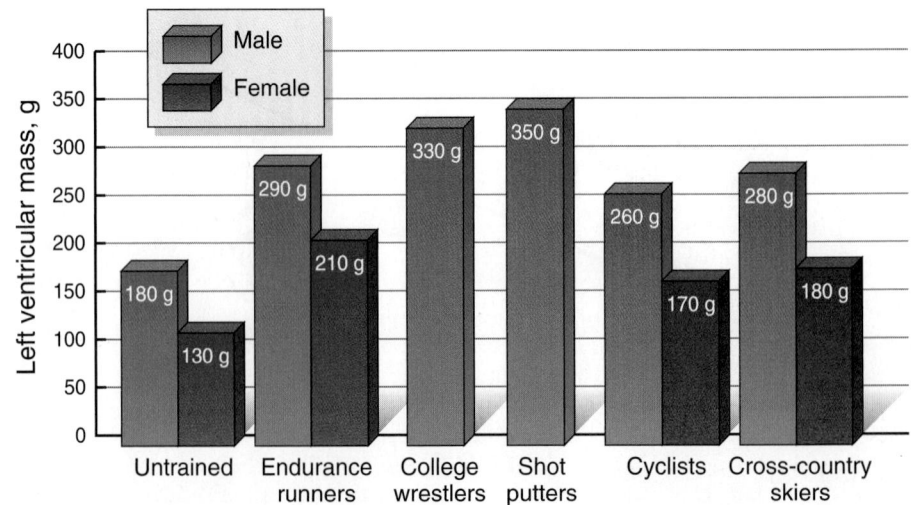

TABLE 17.3
COMPARATIVE AVERAGE CARDIAC DIMENSIONS IN COLLEGE ATHLETES, WORLD-CLASS ATHLETES, AND NORMAL SUBJECTS

Dimension[a]	College Runners (N = 15)	College Swimmers (N = 15)	World Class Runners (N = 10)	College Wrestlers (N = 12)	World Class Shot Putters (N = 4)	Normals (N = 16)
LVID	54	51	48–59[b]	48	43–52[b]	46
LVV, mL	160	181	154	110	122	101
SV, mL	116	—[c]	113	75	68	—[c]
LV wall, mm	11.3	10.6	10.8	13.7	13.8	10.3
Septum, mm	10.9	10.7	10.9	13.0	13.5	10.3
LV mass, g	302	308	283	330	348	211

From Morganroth, J., et al.: Comparative left ventricular dimensions in trained athletes. *Ann. Intern. Med.*, 82:521, 1975.
[a]LVID, left ventricular internal dimension at end diastole; LVV, left ventricular volume; SV, stroke volume; LV wall, posterobasal left ventricular wall thickness; Septum, ventricular septal thickness; LV mass, left ventricular mass.
[b]Range.
[c]Values not reported.

of athletes and to determine whether different patterns of enlargement are associated with different forms of training.[8, 40]

Male competitive swimmers, long-distance runners, wrestlers, and shot putters were studied during their competitive seasons and compared to untrained college men. The swimmers and runners were considered representative of athletes participating in "isotonic" or endurance events; the wrestlers and shot putters represented "isometric" or resistance-trained athletes. It is clear from the results in Table 17.3 that the structural characteristics of the hearts of apparently healthy athletes differ considerably from those of normal individuals. Also, the pattern of these differences is related to the nature of the exercise training. For example, in the swimmers, left ventricular volume was 181 mL and mass was 308 g and in the wrestlers, the left ventricular volume was 110 mL and mass was 330 g; the nonathletic controls averaged 101 mL for ventricular volume and 211 g for ventricular mass. Ventricular wall thickness was enlarged for the resistance-trained athletes but within normal range for the endurance athletes.

An enlarged ventricular cavity (associated with end-diastolic volume) with normal wall thickness also has been observed for other groups of male and female athletes.[37, 46, 48] As discussed on page 302, this intraventricular enlargement, or eccentric hypertrophy, could be brought about by the increase in central blood volume that occurs within several days of endurance training.[33] This, coupled with a decrease in heart rate and an increase in myocardial compliance, would dilate the left ventricular cavity in a manner similar to water being added to a rubber balloon. In contrast, the athletes involved in resistance training have the largest

intraventricular septum, ventricular wall thickness, and ventricular mass with little difference in ventricular cavity dimensions compared to sedentary people.[17, 30, 40] This specific enlargement, termed **concentric hypertrophy,** which does not appear to be caused by use of anabolic steroids, generally falls within the normal range when ventricular mass is expressed in relation to body size, especially fat-free body mass.[17, 49]

It is now apparent that the structural and dimensional differences among the hearts of athletes reflect specific training demands.[15, 56] For example, the training overload for endurance athletes often requires the maintenance of a relatively large cardiac output with relatively modest increases in blood pressure for many hours each week. As shown in Table 17.3, the myocardial internal dimensions with this type of training allow the development of a large stroke volume while optimizing the heart's mechanical performance. On the other hand, athletes who engage in straining, resistance exercise are not subjected to a volume overload but rather to acute episodes of elevated arterial pressure caused by the high force generated by a rather limited mass of skeletal muscle. This added load on the left ventricle is compensated for by an increase in ventricular wall thickness, with little effect on the size of the ventricular cavity. More than likely, considerable variability exists among individuals in terms of the structural response of the heart to different forms of training. When changes do occur, the implications are unknown for myocardial blood supply and long-term cardiovascular health. *However, there is no compelling scientific evidence that a normal heart can be harmed by specific forms of arduous exercise training.*

FUNCTIONAL VERSUS PATHOLOGIC HYPERTROPHY

Cardiac hypertrophy in response to chronic pathologic states such as hypertension has sometimes been confused with the moderate compensatory growth of the myocardium and enlargement of the left ventricular cavity with endurance training. Although the stress of exercise requires that myocardial fibers generate increased tension, which is a critical requirement for initiating compensatory hypertrophy, the application of this overload differs considerably from that of the chronic pressure overload imposed by vascular disease. During exercise training, the myocardial overload is only temporary, so there is a "recuperative" time during nonexercise periods. Also, if compensatory heart growth does occur with training, it is not accompanied by a dilation and weakening of the left ventricle, a frequent response to chronic hypertension. Whereas the hearts of elite athletes are usually larger than the hearts of their untrained counterparts, heart size is generally within the upper range of normal limits in relation to various measures of body size or to the increase in end-diastolic volume. The "athlete's heart" is not a dysfunctional organ. To the contrary, for the endurance athlete, its functional capacity is superior in terms of stroke volume and maximum cardiac output.[39]

OTHER TRAINING ADAPTATIONS

Aerobic exercise training may stimulate an increase in both coronary blood flow and capillary exchange capacity. This may be the result of a structural remodeling that improves the vascularization of the myocardium, particularly at the level of the arteriole, as well as a more effective control of vascular resistance and blood distribution within the heart muscle.[27, 65, 67] In addition, several experiments have reported an increase in mitochondrial mass and cellular concentration of respiratory enzymes in the hearts of endurance-trained animals.[53] The significance of these vascular and cellular adaptations to the functional capacity of the heart during exercise is unknown because it is not believed that the healthy, untrained heart suffers from an oxygen lack during maximum exercise. Such training changes may enable myocardial tissue to better tolerate and recover from transient episodes of ischemia and to function at a lower percentage of its total oxidative capacity during exercise.[58a] In addition, myocardial training adaptations may provide some protection from the degenerative process of heart disease.

■ SUMMARY ■

1. Cardiac output reflects the functional capacity of the circulatory system. The two factors determining the heart's output capacity are heart rate and stroke volume. The relationship between these two components is as follows: Cardiac output = Heart rate × Stroke volume

2. Several invasive and noninvasive methods are used to measure cardiac output. Each has its specific advantages and disadvantages for use with humans during exercise.

3. Cardiac output increases in proportion to the severity of exercise, starting from approximately 5 L per minute at rest to a maximum of 20 to 25 L per minute in college-aged men and 35 to 40 L per minute in elite male endurance athletes. These differences in maximum cardiac output are due entirely to the large stroke volumes of the athletes.

4. During upright exercise, stroke volume becomes larger during the transition from rest to light exercise; maximum values are reached at about 45% of $\dot{V}O_2$max. Thereafter, cardiac output is increased by increases in heart rate.

5. Increases in stroke volume during upright exercise are generally the result of an interaction between a greater filling of the ventricles during diastole and a more complete systolic emptying. Systolic ejection is augmented by sympathetic hormones that increase stroke power during systole.

6. A linear relationship exists between heart rate and oxygen uptake in trained and untrained individuals throughout most of the exercise range. In endurance training, this line shifts significantly to the right due to improvements in the heart's stroke volume. Consequently, heart rate becomes reduced at any submaximal exercise level.

7. Blood flow to specific tissues is generally regulated in proportion to metabolic activity, which causes most of the exercise cardiac output to be diverted to the active muscles. In addition, a significant quantity of blood is shunted to the muscles from the kidneys and splanchnic regions, in which blood supply can be compromised temporarily, often for prolonged periods.

8. The maximal oxygen uptake is determined by the maximum cardiac output and the maximum a-$\bar{v}$ O_2 difference. Large cardiac outputs clearly differentiate endurance athletes from their untrained counterparts. The ability to generate a large a-$\bar{v}$ O_2 difference also is enhanced with training.

9. Aerobic capacity is generally approximately 25% lower in maximal arm compared to leg exercise. For any level of submaximal exercise, however, the physiologic strain is greater in upper-body exercise.

10. Cardiac hypertrophy is a fundamental adaptation to the increased workload imposed by exercise training. It results in a stronger heart, which can generate a large stroke volume.

11. The pattern of structural and dimensional changes in the left ventricle appears to vary with specific forms of exercise training. There is no scientific evidence that a normal heart is harmed by exercise training.

■ REFERENCES ■

1. Andrew, G.M., et al.: Effect of athletic training on exercise cardiac output. *J. Appl. Physiol.*, 21:503, 1966.
2. Bar-Or, O., et al.: Cardiac output of 10- to 13-year old boys and girls during submaximal exercise. *J. Appl. Physiol.*, 30:219, 1971.
3. Beekman, R.H., et al.: Validity of CO_2-rebreathing cardiac output during rest and exercise in young adults. *Med. Sci. Sports Exerc.*, 16:306, 1984.
4. Bennet, D.H., et al.: Echocardiographic left ventricular dimensions in pressure and volume overload. Their use in assessing aortic stenosis. *Br. Heart J.*, 37:971, 1975.
5. Bevegård, S., et al.: Circulatory studies in well-trained athletes at rest and during heavy exercise, with special reference to stroke volume and the influence of body position. *Acta Physiol. Scand.*, 57:26, 1963.
6. Carroll, J.F., et al.: Effect of training on blood volume and plasma hormone concentrations in the elderly. *Med. Sci. Sports Exerc.*, 27:79, 1995.
7. Clausen, J., and Trap-Jensen, J.: Heart rate and arterial blood pressure during exercise in patients with angina pectoris. *Circulation*, 53:436, 1976.
8. Cohen, J.L., and Segal, K.R.: Left ventricular hypertrophy in athletes: an exercise echocardiographic study. *Med. Sci. Sports Exerc.*, 17:695, 1985.
9. Convertino, V.A.: Blood volume: its adaptation to endurance training. *Med. Sci. Sports Exerc.*, 23:1338, 1991.
10. Coyle, E.F., et al.: Time course of loss of adaptations after stopping prolonged intense endurance training. *J. Appl. Physiol.*, 57:1857, 1984.
11. Cummins, T.D., and Gladden, L.B.: Responses to submaximal and maximal arm cycling above, at, and below heart level. *Med. Sci. Sports Exerc.*, 15:295, 1983.
12. Cunningham, D.A., et al.: Development of cardiorespiratory function in circumpubertal boys: a longitudinal study. *J. Appl. Physiol.*, 56:302, 1984.
13. Dickhuth, H.H., et al.: The long-term involution of physiological cardiomegaly and cardiac hypertrophy. *Med. Sci. Sports Exerc.*, 21:244, 1989.
14. Dressendorfer, R., et al.: Therapeutic effects of exercise training in angina patients. In *Physical Conditioning and Cardiomuscular Rehabilitation*. Edited by L. Cohen, et al. New York, John Wiley and Sons, 1981.
15. Effron, M.B.: Effects of resistive training on left ventricular function. *Med. Sci. Sports Exerc.*, 21:694, 1989.
16. Ekblom, B., et al.: Effect of training on circulatory response to exercise. *J. Appl. Physiol.*, 24:518, 1968.
17. Fleck, S.J., et al.: Magnetic resonance imaging determination of left ventricular mass: junior Olympic weightlifters. *Med. Sci. Sports Exerc.*, 25:522, 1993.
18. Franklin, B.A., et al.: Aerobic requirements of arm ergometry: implications for exercise testing and training. *Phys. Sportsmed.*, 11:81, 1983.
18a. Gauvreau, G.M., et al.: Comparison of aerobic capacity between racing standardbred horses. *J. Appl. Physiol.*, 78:1447, 1995.
19. Gledhill, N., et al.: Endurance athletes' stroke volume does not plateau: major advantage is diastolic function. *Med. Sci. Sports Exerc.*, 26:1116, 1994.
20. Hagerman, F.C.: A comparison of energy expenditure during rowing and cycling ergometry. *Med. Sci. Sports Exerc.*, 20:479, 1988.
21. Hanson, J.S., et al.: Long-term physical training and cardiovascular dynamics in middle-aged men. *Circulation*, 38:783, 1968.
22. Herlhoz, K., et al.: Regional cerebral blood flow in man at rest and during exercise. *J. Neurol.*, 234:9, 1987.
23. Hickson, R.C.: Skeletal muscle cytochrome c and myoglobin, endurance, and frequency of training. *J. Appl. Physiol.*, 51:746, 1981.
24. Hickson, R.C., et al.: Reduced training intensities and loss of aerobic power, endurance, and cardiac growth. *J. Appl. Physiol.*, 58:492, 1985.
25. Holloszy, J.O., and Coyle, E.F.: Adaptations of skeletal muscle to endurance training and their metabolic consequences. *J. Appl. Physiol.*, 56:831, 1984.

26. Lash, J.M., et al.: Exercise training effects on collateral and microvascular resistance in rat model of arterial insufficiency. *Am. J. Physiol.*, 28:H125, 1995.
27. Laughlin, M.H., et al.: Vascular transport capacity of hindlimb muscles of exercise-trained rats. *J. Appl. Physiol.*, 62:438, 1987.
28. Laughlin, M.H., et al.: Physical activity and the microcirculation in cardiac and skeletal muscle. In *Physical Activity, Fitness, and Health*. Edited by C. Bouchard, et al. Champaign, IL, Human Kinetics, 1994.
29. Lazarus, B., et al.: Comparison of the reproducibility of arm and leg exercise tests in men with angina pectoria. *Am. J. Cardiol.*, 47:1074, 1981.
30. Levine, B.D., et al.: Left ventricular pressure-volume and Frank-Starling relations in endurance athletes: implications for orthostatic tolerance and exercise performance. *Circulation*, 84:1016, 1991.
31. Levy, W.C., et al.: Endurance exercise training augments diastolic filling at rest and during exercise in healthy young and older men. *Circulation*, 88:116, 1993.
32. Lewis, S.F., et al: Cardiovascular responses to exercise as a function of absolute and relative work load. *J. Appl. Physiol.*, 54:1314, 1983.
33. Luetkemeier, M.J., and Thomas, E.L.: Hypervolemia and cycling time trial performance. *Med. Sci. Sports Exerc.*, 26:503, 1994.
34. Magel, J.R., et al.: Metabolic and cardiovascular adjustment to arm training. *J. Appl. Physiol.*, 45:75, 1978.
35. McArdle, W.D., et al.: Specificity of run training on $\dot{V}o_2$max and heart rate changes during running and swimming. *Med. Sci. Sports Exerc.*, 10:16, 1978.
36. Miles, D.S., et al.: Cardiovascular responses to upper body exercise in normals and cardiac patients. *Med. Sci. Sports Exerc.*, 21:S126, 1989.
37. Milliken, M.C., et al.: Left ventricular mass by magnetic resonance imaging in male endurance athletes. *Am. J. Cardiol.*, 62:301, 1988.
38. Mitchell, J.H., and Raven, P.B.: Cardiovascular adaptation to physical activity. In *Physical Activity, Fitness, and Health*. Edited by C. Bouchard, et al. Champaign, IL, Human Kinetics, 1994.
39. Mitchell, J.H., et al.: How to recognize "athletes heart." *Phys. Sportsmed.*, 20(8):87, 1992.
40. Morganroth, J., et al.: Comparative left ventricular dimensions in trained athletes. *Ann. Intern. Med.*, 82:521, 1975.
41. Musch, T.I., et al.: Training effects on regional blood flow response to maximal exercise in foxhounds. *J. Appl. Physiol.*, 62:1724, 1987.
42. Pechar, G.S., et al.: Specificity of cardio-respiratory adaptation to bicycle and treadmill training. *J. Appl. Physiol.*, 36:753, 1974.
43. Pendergast, D.R.: Cardiovascular, respiratory, and metabolic responses to upper body exercise. *Med. Sci. Sports Exerc.*, 21:S121, 1989.
44. Poliner, L.R., et al.: Left ventricular performance in normal subjects: a comparison of the responses to exercise in upright and supine positions. *Circulation*, 62:528, 1980.
45. Ricci, G., et al.: Left ventricular size following endurance, sprint, and strength training. *Med. Sci. Sports Exerc.*, 14:344, 1982.
46. Riley-Hagen, M., et al.: Left ventricular dimensions and mass using magnetic resonance imaging in female endurance athletes. *Am. J. Cardiol.*, 69:1067, 1992.
47. Rowell, L.B.: *Human Cardiovascular Control*. Cary, NC, Oxford University Press, 1994.
48. Rubal, J.B., et al.: Echocardiographic examination of woman softball champions. *Med. Sci. Sports. Exerc.*, 13:176, 1981.
49. Salke, R.C., et al.: Left ventricular size and function in body builders using anabolic steroids. *Med. Sci. Sports Exerc.*, 17:701, 1985.
50. Saltin, B.: Physiological effects of physical conditioning. *Med. Sci. Sports Exerc.*, 1:50, 1969.
51. Saltin, B., et al.: Fiber types and metabolic potentials of skeletal muscles in sedentary men and endurance runners. *Ann. N. Y. Acad. Sci.*, 301:3, 1977.
52. Sawka, M.N.: Physiology of upper body exercise. *Exerc. Sport Sci. Rev.*, 14:175, 1986.
53. Scheuer, J., and Tipton, C.M.: Cardiovascular adaptations to training. *Annu. Rev. Physiol.*, 39:221, 1977.

54. Schwade, J., et al.: A comparison of the response to arm and leg work in patients with ischemic heart disease. *Am. Heart J.,* 94:203, 1977.

55. Seely, J.E., et al.: Heart and lung function at rest and during exercise in adolescence. *J. Appl. Physiol.,* 36:34, 1974.

56. Snoeckx, L.H.E.H., et al.: Echocardiographic dimensions in athletes in relation to their training programs. *Med. Sci. Sports Exerc.,* 14:428, 1982.

57. Soto, K.I., et al.: Cardiac output in preadolescent competitive swimmers and in untrained normal children. *J. Sports Med. Phys. Fitness,* 23:291, 1983.

58. Spina, R.J., et al.: Exercise training prevents decline in stroke volume during exercise in young healthy subjects. *J. Appl. Physiol.,* 72:2458, 1992.

58a. Stranes, J.W., and Bowles, D.K.: Role of exercise in the cause and prevention of cardiac dysfunction. *Exerc. Sport. Sci. Rev.,* 23:349, 1995.

59. Tate, C.A., et al.: Mechanism for the responses of cardiac muscle to physical activity in old age. *Med. Sci. Sports Exerc.,* 26:561, 1994.

60. Thomas, S.N., et al.: Cerebral blood flow during submaximal and maximal dynamic exercise in humans. *J. Appl. Physiol.,* 67:744, 1989.

61. Thompson, P.D., et al.: Cardiac dimensions and performance after either arm or leg endurance training. *Med. Sci. Sports Exerc.,* 13:303, 1981.

62. Thorston, J., et al.: Effects of training and detraining on oxygen uptake, cardiac output, blood gas tensions, pH, and lactate concentrations during and after exercise in the horse. In *Equine Exercise Physiology.* Edited by D.H. Snow, et al. Cambridge, Granta Editions, 1983.

63. Toner, M.M., et al.: Cardiorespiratory responses to exercise distributed between the upper and lower body. *J. Appl. Physiol.,* 54:1403, 1983.

64. Toner, M.M., et al.: Cardiovascular adjustment to exercise distributed between the upper and lower body. *Med. Sci. Sports Exerc.,* 22:773, 1990.

65. Underwood, F.B., et al.: Altered control of calcium in coronary smooth muscle cells by exercise training. *Med. Sci. Sports Exerc.,* 26:1230, 1994.

66. Vokac, Z., et al.: Oxygen uptake/heart rate relationship in leg and arm exercise, sitting and standing. *J. Appl. Physiol.,* 39:54, 1975.

67. Wang, J., et al.: Chronic exercise enhances endothelium-mediated dilation of epicardial coronary artery in conscious dogs. *Circ. Res.,* 73:829, 1993.

68. Wilson, D.F.: Energy metabolism in muscle approaching maximal rates of oxygen utilization. *Med. Sci. Sports Exerc.,* 27:54, 1995.

Gollnick, P.D., et al.: Effect of training on enzyme activity and fiber composition of human skeletal muscle. *J. Appl. Physiol.* 34:107, 1973.

The muscle biopsy technique in human research permitted analysis of possible differences in muscle structure and function between trained and untrained individuals. Prior research showed high oxidative capacity in the muscles of successful endurance athletes, a finding consistent with reports on the effects of aerobic training on skeletal muscle. The experiment by Gollnick and colleagues was one of the first to determine how a muscle's oxidative capacity and fiber distribution changed with strenuous training.

The effects of 5 months of aerobic exercise training was evaluated for changes in succinate dehydrogenase (SDH, "aerobic" enzyme) and phosphofructokinase (PFK, "anaerobic" enzyme) activity and fiber composition in the skeletal muscle of six men. Measurements included $\dot{V}o_2$max, muscle fiber type and fiber areas, the distribution of aerobic and anaerobic capacity (reflected by cellular enzyme activity), and glycogen concentration in the slow-twitch (ST) and fast-twitch (FT) muscle fibers before and after training. Subjects trained by pedaling a cycle ergometer for 1 hour daily, 4 days per week for 5 months at a workload initially requiring 75% of $\dot{V}o_2$max. After training, subjects could exercise at 85 to 90% of $\dot{V}o_2$max.

The results displayed in the figure show that $\dot{V}o_2$max increased 13% with training, whereas the average SDH activity in the vastus lateralis increased by 95%. The smallest pre-and post-SDH training increase was 40%, while the largest increase equaled 256%. The average PFK increased 117%, with a similar change occurring in all subjects.

The training program did not alter the percentage distribution of ST and FT muscle fibers. Fiber composition was identical before and after training in four of the six subjects. In the other two subjects, there were only about 9% more ST fibers following training (considered normal variation for this sampling procedure). The ST fiber area before training averaged 5495 μm^2 compared to 6638 μm^2 for the FT fibers. After training, the ST fibers occupied an area of 6778 μm^2, while the FT fiber area equaled 6139 μm^2. The ratio of ST to FT fiber areas increased from 0.82 to 1.11 with training. The relatively small increase in $\dot{V}o_2$max compared to the large change in oxidative potential of the trained skeletal muscle supported the idea that a muscle's aerobic capacity did not limit total body $\dot{V}o_2$max.

These results demonstrated an impressive adaptability of skeletal muscle to vigorous physical training. They also demonstrated that the muscle fiber type distribution in an adult remained largely unaltered by training. However, training-induced changes in total area of fiber type probably occurred.

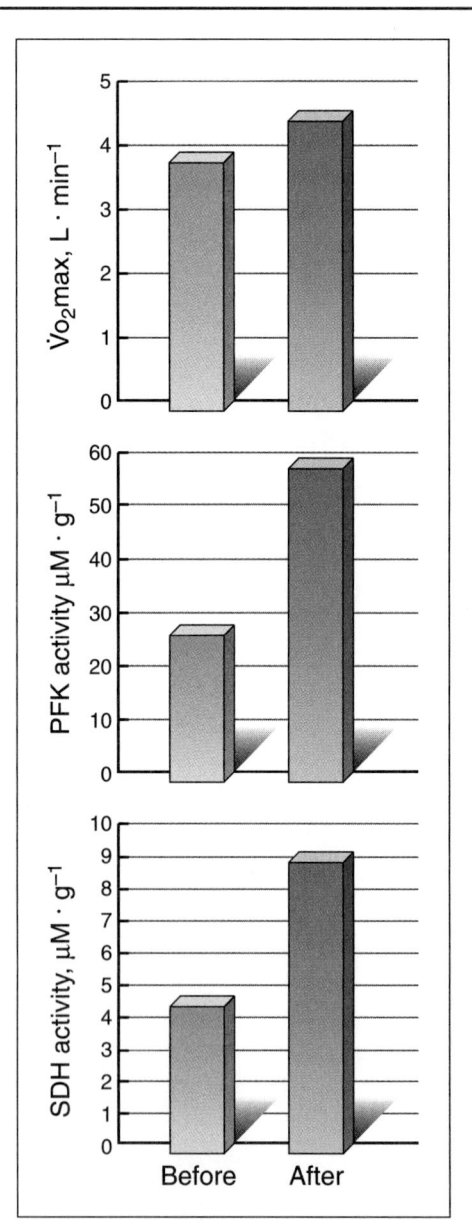

Changes in $\dot{V}o_2$max (*top*), PFK activity (*middle*), and SDH activity (*bottom*) before and after endurance training.

Skeletal Muscle: Structure and Function

Human movement depends on the conversion of the chemical energy of adenosine triphosphate (ATP) into mechanical energy through the action of skeletal muscles. Muscle forces acting on the body's bony lever system cause one or more bones to move about their joint axis; this enables a person to propel an object, move the body itself, or do both simultaneously. The following sections present the architectural organization of skeletal muscle and focus on its gross and microscopic structures. The discussion centers on the sequence of chemical and mechanical events in muscle action and relaxation, as well as the differences in muscle fiber characteristics among sedentary and elite performers in diverse sports.

GROSS STRUCTURE OF SKELETAL MUSCLE

Each of the body's more than 660 skeletal muscles contains various wrappings of fibrous connective tissue. Figure 18.1 is an illustration of the cross section of a muscle that consists of thousands of cylindrical muscle cells called **fibers.** These long, slender multinucleated fibers (whose number is probably largely fixed by the second trimester of fetal development) lie parallel to each other; the force of action is directed along the long axis of the fiber. Individual fiber length varies from a few millimeters in the muscles of the eye to more than 100 mm in the large muscles of the leg.

LEVELS OF ORGANIZATION

Each muscle fiber is wrapped and separated from its neighboring fibers by a fine layer of connective tissue called the **endomysium.** Another layer of connective tissue, the **perimysium,** surrounds a bundle of up to 150 fibers called a **fasciculus.** Surrounding the entire muscle is a fascia of fibrous connective tissue known as the **epimysium.** This protective sheath is tapered at its distal end as it blends into and joins the intramuscular tissue sheaths to form the dense, strong connective tissue of the **tendons.** The tendons connect both ends of the muscle to the outermost covering of the skeleton (the **periosteum**).

The tissues of the tendon are intermeshed with the collagenous fibers within the bone. This forms a powerful link between muscle and bone that is difficult to separate except during severe stress, when it can be severed or literally pulled away from the bone. When the tendon is attached at the end of a long bone, the bone adapts by enlarging at that end to produce a more stable union. Depending on bone size, this overgrowth is called a tubercle, tuberosity, or trochanter.

The force of muscle action is transmitted directly from the muscle's connective tissue harness to the tendons, which then pull on the bones at their points of attachment. The force exerted on the tendinous attachments under various conditions of muscular exertion ranges from approximately 20 to 50 newtons (433 to 1082 lb) per cm^2 of cross-sectional area. The region at which the tendon joins a relatively stable skeletal part, generally at the proximal or fixed end of the lever system or nearest the body's midline, is the **origin** of the muscle; the point of distal attachment to the moving bone is the **insertion.** The bottom portion of Figure 18.1 illustrates the ultrastructural details of a tendon. About 70% of the tendon's dry mass is made up of the protein collagen.

Beneath the endomysium and surrounding each muscle fiber is the **sarcolemma.** This thin, elastic membrane encloses the fiber's cellular contents. It is composed of a plasma membrane (plasmalemma) and a basement membrane. The plasma membrane is a bilayer lipid structure whose main function is to conduct the electrochemical wave of depolarization over the surface of the muscle fiber. This membrane also has the property of insulating one fiber from another during the depolarization process. The basement membrane contains proteins and strands of collagen fibrils that permit the fiber to fuse with the collagenous fibers in the outer covering of the tendon. Between the basement membrane and the plasma membrane are **satellite cells,** which serve an important function in regenerative cellular growth and recovery from injury. The fiber's aqueous protoplasm, or **sarcoplasm,** contains enzymes, lipid and glycogen particles, the nuclei (approximately 250 per millimeter fiber length), the mitochondria, and various other specialized organelles. Embedded within the sarcoplasm is an extensive interconnecting longitudinal network of tubular channels and vesicles known as the **sarcoplasmic reticulum.** This highly specialized system provides the cell with structural integrity and also allows the wave of depolarization to spread rapidly

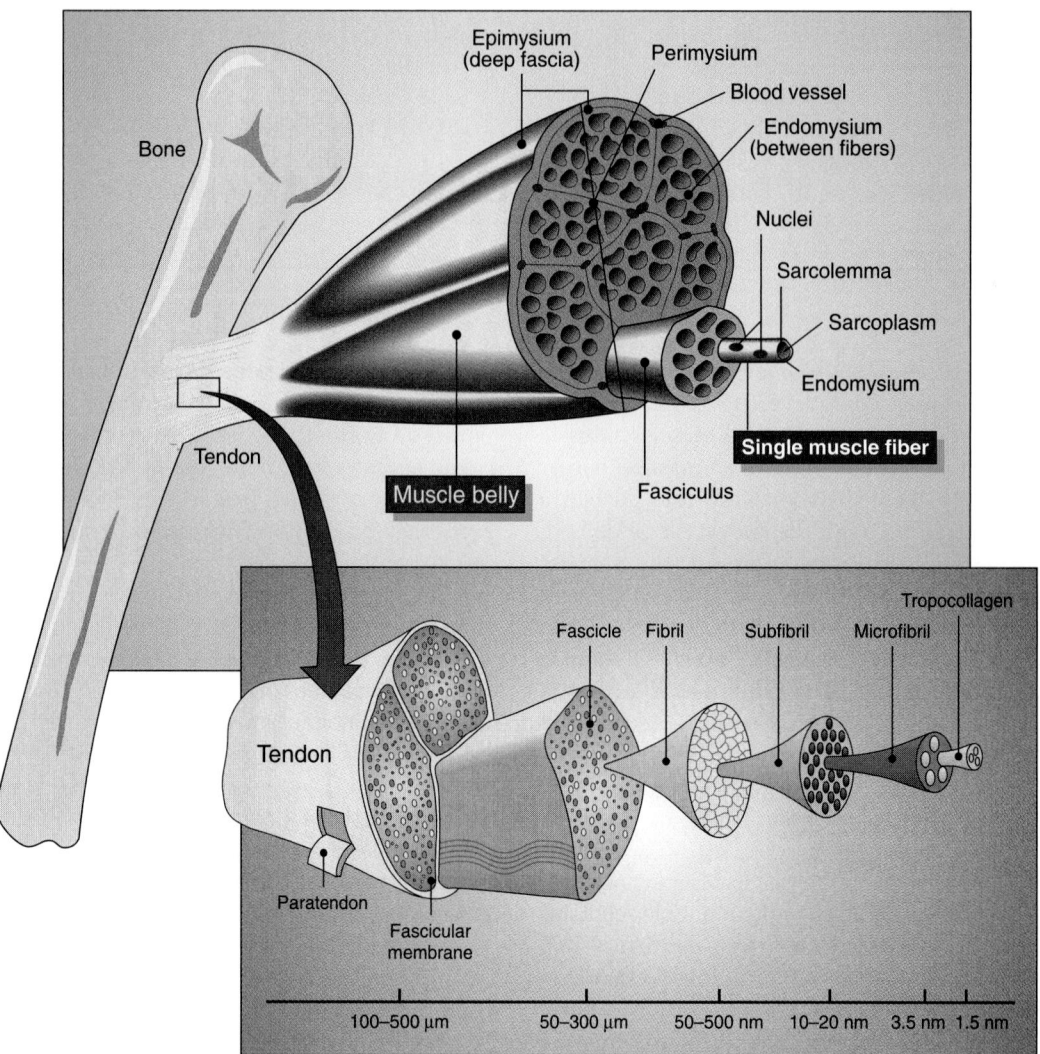

FIGURE 18.1

Cross section of a skeletal muscle and the arrangement of its connective tissue wrappings. The individual fibers are covered by the endomysium. Groups of fibers called fasciculi are surrounded by the perimysium, and the entire muscle is wrapped in a sheath of connective tissue, the epimysium. The sarcolemma is a thin, elastic membrane that covers the surface of each muscle fiber. The insert photo displays the details of tendon structure. The microfibril is formed from five parallel tropocollagen molecules that unite to form fibrils and then collagen fibers. A bundle of fibers is enclosed in an endotendon, and a group of these, known as a fascicle, is surrounded by an epitendon sheath. The fascicles then combine into a tendon that is surrounded by its own sheath, called a paratendon. (Muscle cross section from Sobotta, J., and Hammersen, F.: *Histology. Color Atlas of Microscopic Anatomy.* 3rd ed. Baltimore, Urban & Schwarzenberg, 1992; Tendon insert modified from Kastelic, J., et al.: The multicomposite structure of tendon. *Connect. Tiss. Res.,* 6:11, 1978.)

from the fiber's outer surface to its inner environment to initiate muscle action.

CHEMICAL COMPOSITION

Approximately 75% of skeletal muscle is water, and 20% is protein. The remaining 5% is made up of inorganic salts and other substances, including high-energy phosphates; urea; lactic acid; the minerals calcium, magnesium, and phosphorus; various enzymes; ions of sodium, potassium, and chloride; amino acids; lipids; and carbohydrates. The most abundant of the muscle proteins are **myosin** (approximately 60% of muscle protein), **actin,** and **tropomyosin.** Also, about 700 mg of the conjugated protein **myoglobin** is incorporated into each 100 g of muscle tissue. The specifics of myoglobin function are discussed in Chapter 13.

BLOOD SUPPLY

During exercise that requires an oxygen uptake of 4.0 L per minute, the muscle's oxygen uptake increases nearly 70 times, to approximately 11 mL per 100 g per minute (or a total of 3400 mL per minute). To accommodate this oxygen requirement, the local vascular bed channels large quantities of blood through the active tissues. In rhythmic activities such as running, swimming, or cycling, the blood flow fluctuates; it decreases during the muscle's action phase and increases during the relaxation phase. This provides a "milking action" that facilitates blood flow through the muscles and helps propel the blood back to the heart. Complementing this pulsatile flow is the rapid dilation of previously dormant capillaries. Consequently, between 200 and 500 capillaries may be delivering blood to each square millimeter of active muscle cross section, with as many as four capillaries in direct contact with each fiber.

Straining muscular activities present a somewhat different picture for muscle blood flow.[22] When a muscle generates approximately 60% of its force-generating capacity, local blood flow is occluded due to the elevated intramuscular pressure. When this occurs, energy for continued effort at near-maximal force production is generated from the intramuscular high-energy phosphates and through the anaerobic reactions of glycolysis.

Capillarization of Muscle. One factor that is often proposed for improved exercise capacity with endurance training is an increase in the capillary density of the trained muscles. Aside from its role in delivering oxygen, nutrients, and hormones, the capillary microcirculation also provides the means for removing heat and metabolic by-products from active tissues. All of these functions are enhanced by a greater capillary density.

Endurance training favorably modifies the capillarization of skeletal muscle.[2, 10] In one study using the electron microscope, the number of capillaries per muscle (as well as the capillaries per square millimeter of muscle tissue) averaged about 40% greater in endurance athletes than in untrained counterparts. This was almost identical to the 41% difference in maximal oxygen uptake between the two groups. Reports also indicate a positive relationship between $\dot{V}O_2$max and the average number of muscle capillaries.[51] An enhanced vascularization on the capillary level would be particularly beneficial during exercise requiring a high level of steady-rate aerobic metabolism. The stimulus for capillary development with training may be the actual vascular stretch and shear stress on the vessel walls caused by the increased blood flow in aerobic exercise.[39]

ULTRASTRUCTURE OF SKELETAL MUSCLE

The microscopic anatomy or ultrastructure of skeletal muscle has been revealed with the aid of electron microscopy, x-ray crystallography, and histochemical staining and techniques of helium-neon laser diffraction. The different levels of subcellular organization within a skeletal muscle fiber are shown in Figure 18.2. Each fiber is composed of smaller functional units that lie parallel to the long axis of the fiber. These **fibrils** or **myofibrils** are approximately 1 μm (1 μm = 1/1000 mm) in diameter and are composed of even smaller subunits (the **filaments** or **myofilaments**) that lie parallel

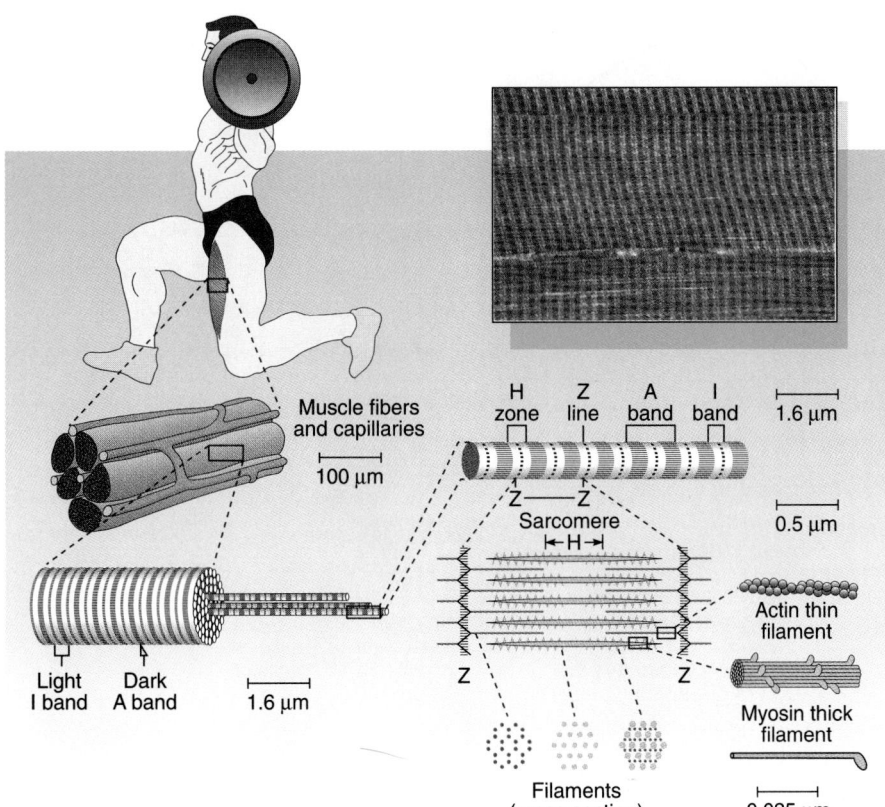

FIGURE 18.2

Microscopic organization of skeletal muscle. The whole muscle is composed of individual fibers; these fibers are made up of myofibrils, of which the actin and myosin protein filaments are a significant part. (This represents a microscopic view ×205,000 magnification.) The insert figure displays a microscopic view of skeletal muscle fibers with prominent cross striations. (Insert graph from Sobotta, J., and Hammersen, F.: *Histology. Color Atlas of Microscopic Anatomy.* 3rd ed. Baltimore, Urban & Schwarzenberg, 1992.)

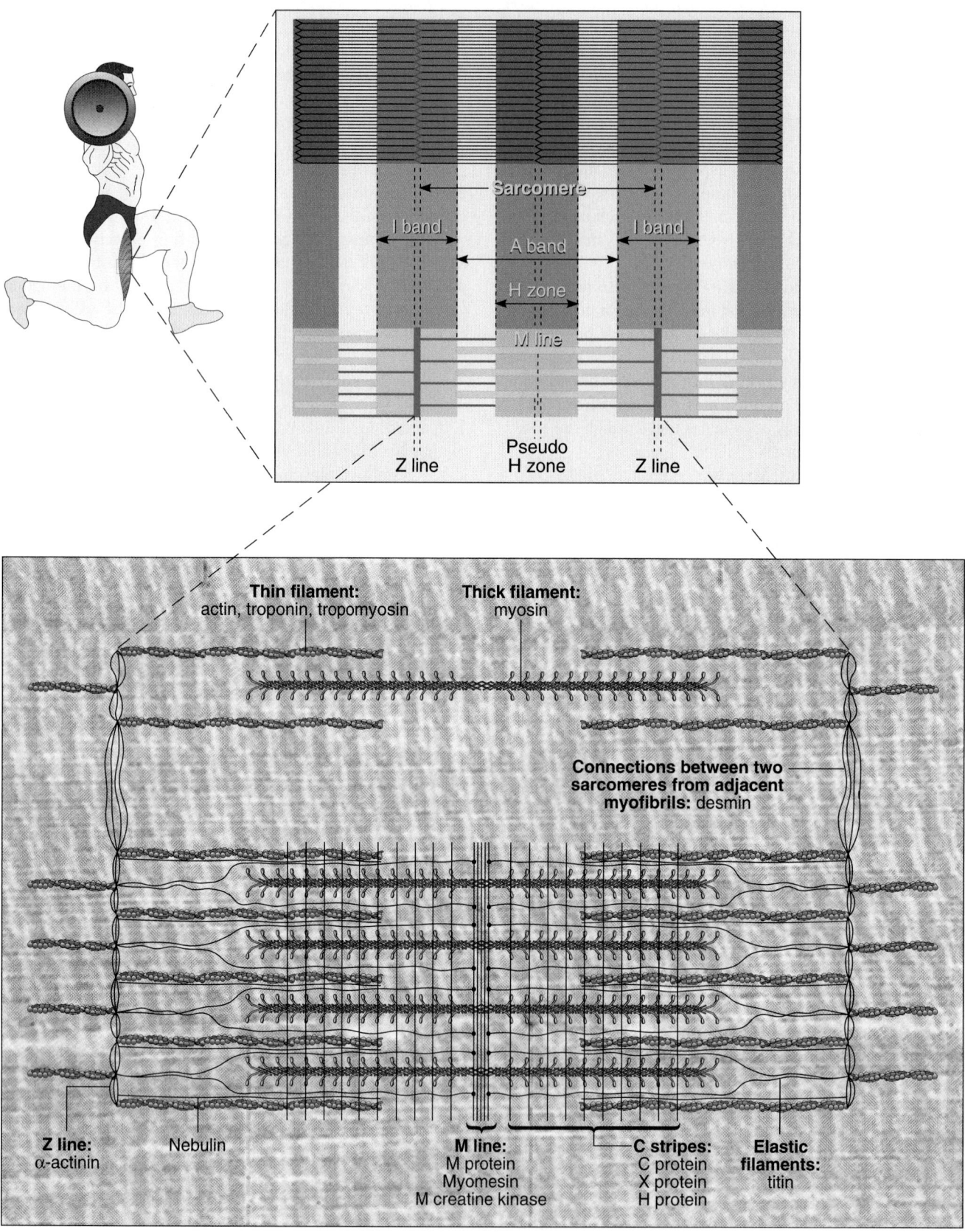

FIGURE 18.3

Top, Structural position of the filaments in a sarcomere. A sarcomere is bounded at both ends by the Z line. *Bottom,* Detailed view of sarcomere including the proteins listed in Table 18.1.

TABLE 18.1
TWELVE PROTEINS ASSOCIATED WITH THE MUSCLE FIBER'S SARCOMERE AND THEIR PROPOSED FUNCTIONS

Structure	Protein	Function
Thin filament	Actin	The main protein of actin that interacts with myosin during excitation-contraction coupling.
	Tropomyosin	Transduces the conformational change of the troponin complex to actin.
	Troponin	Binds Ca^{2+} and affects tropomyosin. Represents the "switch" that transforms the Ca^{2+} signal into a molecular signal that induces crossbridge cycling.
	Nebulin	Present next to actin and believed to control the number of actin monomers joined to each other in a thin filament.
Thick filament	Myosin	Splits ATP and is responsible for the "power stroke" of the myosin head.
C stripes	C protein	Holds the myosin thick filaments in a regular array. May hold the H protein of adjacent thick filaments at an even distance during force generation. May also control the number of myosin molecules in a thick filament.
M line	M protein	Helps hold thick filaments in a regular array.
	Myomesin	Provides a strong anchoring point for the protein titin.
	M-CK	Provides ATP from creatine phosphate; located proximal to the myosin heads.
Z line	Alpha actinin	Holds the thin filaments in place spatially.
	Desmin	Forms the connection between adjacent Z lines from different myofibrils. This protein helps to keep the sarcomeres in register so they maintain their striated appearance.
Elastic filament	Titin	Helps keep the thick filament centered between two Z lines during contraction; believed to control the number of myosin molecules contained in the thick filament.

to the long axis of the myofibril. The myofilaments consist mainly of two proteins, **actin** and **myosin,** which account for about 85% of the myofibrillar complex. Six other proteins that have either a structural function or that significantly affect the interaction of protein filaments during muscle action have also been identified. These are (*a*) **tropomyosin,** located along the actin filaments (5%); (*b*) **troponin,** located in the actin filaments (3%); (*c*) *α*-**actinin,** distributed in the region of the Z band (7%); (*d*) *β*-actinin, found in the actin filaments (1%); (*e*) **M protein,** identified in the region of the M lines within the sarcomere (less than 1%); and (*f*) **C protein** (less than 1%), which is believed to contribute to the structural integrity of the sarcomere.

THE SARCOMERE

At low magnification, the alternating light and dark bands along the length of the muscle fiber give it a characteristic **striated** appearance. The structural details of this cross-striation pattern within a myofibril are illustrated in Figure 18.3. The lighter area is referred to as the "I band," and the darker zone is termed the "A band." The "Z line" bisects the I band and adheres to the sarcolemma to give stability to the entire structure.[a] *The repeating unit between*

two Z lines is called the **sarcomere.** *This structural entity is the functional unit of a muscle fiber.* The actin and myosin filaments within the sarcomere are primarily involved in the mechanical process of muscle action. One sarcomere adjacent to another is said to be arranged in series; the filaments are arranged in a parallel configuration within a given fiber. In its resting state, the length of each sarcomere is approximately 2.5 μm. Thus, for a myofibril with a length of 15 mm, there would be about 6000 sarcomeres joined end to end.

The position of the thin actin and thicker myosin proteins in the sarcomere results in an interdigitating overlap of the two filaments. The center of the A band contains the "H zone," a region of lower optical density caused by the absence of actin filaments in this area. The central portion of the H zone is bisected by the "M line," which delineates the sarcomere's center. The M line consists of the protein structures that support the arrangement of the myosin filaments. A detailed view of a sarcomere is shown at the bottom of Figure 18.3, and the specific proteins identified within a sarcomere are listed in Table 18.1.

    Alignment of Sarcomeres in a Muscle Fiber. The arrangement of the individual fibers varies in relation to the long axis of the muscle (determined as an imaginary line drawn through the origin and insertion, or the fiber angle

---

[a]The bands are named for their optical properties. When polarized light passes through the I band, its velocity is the same in all directions (isotropic). Light passing through the A band does not scatter equally (anisotropic). The letter Z is from the German "zwischenscheibe," which means "between"; the letter M ("mittelscheibe") means middle; and the letter H ("hellerscheibe") means clear disc or zone.

FIGURE 18.4

Top, Effect of pennation on force development in a fusiform muscle in which there is no angle of pennation ($\theta = 0°$) and when $\theta = 30°$. At this extreme angle of pennation, there is a loss of 13% of each fiber's force generating capacity on the tendon solely due to muscle mechanics. However, the effect of angle of pennation alters the number of fibers that can be packed into a given volume of muscle. This is an important concept because it illustrates that whereas muscle mass and the contractile machinery are related in a proportional way within a muscle, it does not follow that muscle mass per se relates to an equivalent tension output in comparisons among different muscle groups. (Modified from Lieber, R.L.: *Skeletal Muscle Structure and Function.* Baltimore, Williams & Wilkins, 1992.) *Bottom,* Illustration of unipennate, bipennate, and multipennate muscle groups.

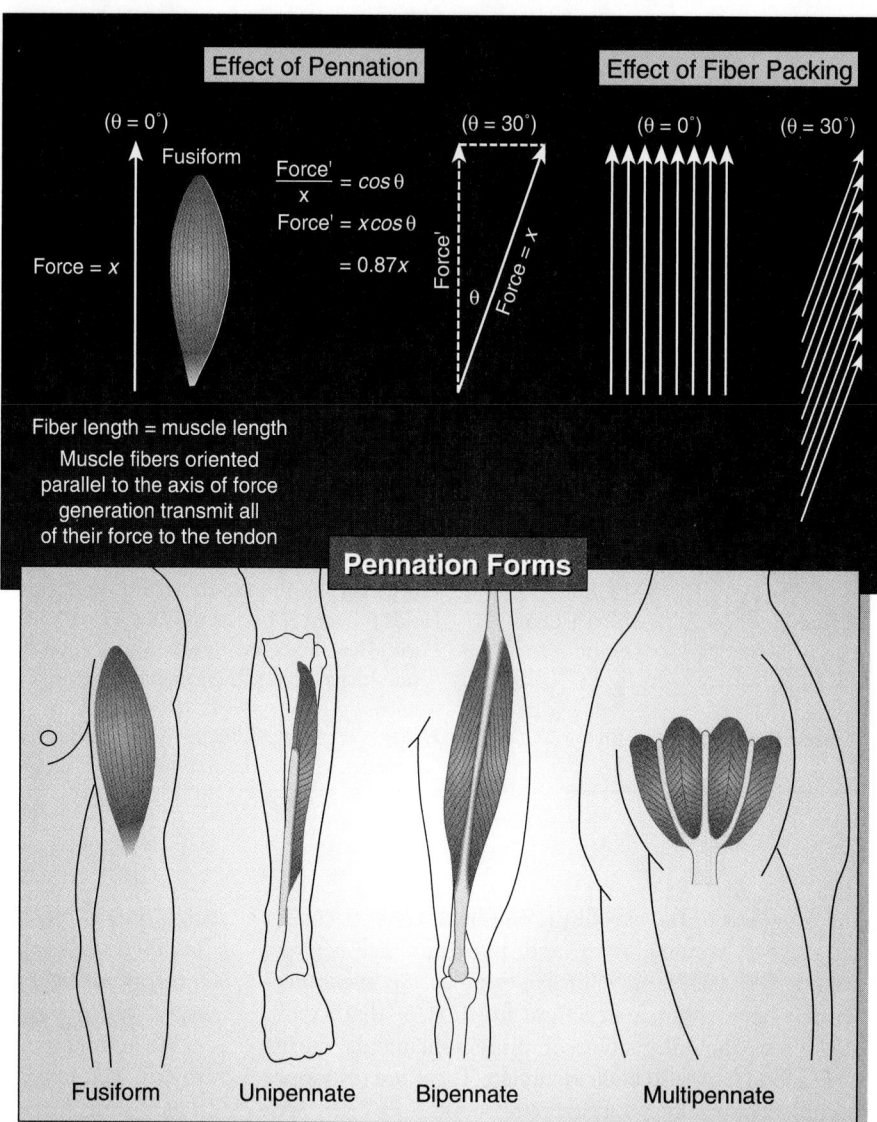

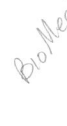

relative to the force-generating axis). This difference in sarcomere alignment plays an important role in a muscle's overall capacity to generate force. If the fibers run parallel to the muscle's long axis (for example, biceps brachii), the fibers are said to be **fusiform** or spindle-shaped, because they taper at the tendinous attachment. In contrast, a muscle can be **pennate** or fan-shaped because the fasciculi (bundles of fibers) lie at a pennation angle that varies up to 30°.[40] In the soleus muscle, for example, the pennation angle is approximately 25°, whereas for the vastus medialis, the pennation angle is 5°, and there is no angle of pennation for the sartorius muscle. It is noteworthy that the degree of pennation directly affects how many sarcomeres are present per cross-sectional area in a particular fiber. In a fusiform fiber (no pennation), the cross-sectional area of the fiber

represents the true anatomical cross section. In pennate muscle, on the other hand, the cross-sectional area is larger because more sarcomeres can be "packed" into a given volume of muscle. The term physiological cross-sectional area (PCSA) refers to the sum of the cross-sectional areas of all of the fibers within a particular muscle.[b] At an unusually large pennation angle of 30°, there would be only a 13% loss in an individual fiber's force capacity for a huge increase in total fiber packing ability.[40] Thus, pennation per se allows for packing a large number of fibers into a smaller cross-sectional area. This effect of pennation on fiber packing and force-generating capacity is illustrated in Figure 18.4.

The fibers in a fusiform muscle are oriented parallel to the long axis of the muscle (Fig. 18.4, *bottom left*). *This arrangement facilitates a rapid rate of muscle shortening. A*

---

[b]PCSA (cm²) = Muscle mass (g) · cos θ/muscle density (g · cm⁻³) · fiber length (cm). In this equation, muscle density = 1.056 g · cm⁻³, and θ represents the surface pennation angle.

unipennate fiber arrangement, (Fig. 18.4, *bottom*), in which the muscle fibers lie at an oblique angle to the tendon, causes a larger effective cross-sectional area than in the fusiform muscle. Muscles with greater pennation, although slower in contractile velocity, are capable of greater force production than fusiform muscles (other things being equal) because of the greater number of sarcomeres contributing to the muscle action.[49] A bipennate muscle has two sets of fibers that lie obliquely on both sides of a common tendon (for example, gastrocnemius and rectus femoris muscles), whereas a multipennate muscle has more than two sets of fibers that converge at different angles on a common tendon (for example, deltoid). Pennate muscle fibers are generally shorter than fusiform muscles, but they possess a greater number of individual fibers. Because of their shorter individual lengths, pennate muscles are not able to produce as great a range of motion as fusiform muscles.

Fiber Length to Muscle Length Ratio. The ratio of individual fiber length to a muscle's total length usually varies between 0.2 and 0.6. This indicates that even in the longest muscles (for example, muscles of the upper and lower limbs), the individual fibers are still shorter than the muscle's overall length.[40] This is illustrated in Figure 18.5 for four muscles of the lower limbs. On average, the quadriceps muscles have pennation angles that average 4.6°, PCSAs of approximately 21.7 cm², and a fiber length that averages 68 mm. This is in contrast to the biceps femoris (hamstring) muscle, which has relatively long fibers (111 mm) and intermediate PCSAs (11.7 cm²). In terms of force generation, the quadriceps muscles have approximately 50% greater capacity than the hamstrings, which are designed for a faster shortening velocity. This suggests that the hamstrings would be susceptible to tearing if a rapid imbalance in force output between the quadriceps and the hamstring muscles should occur during sprint forward running.

The generalized muscle force–muscle length and muscle force–muscle velocity relationships for a fusiform and pennate muscle with the same quantity of contractile protein and identical muscle fiber type are shown in Figure 18.5 (*bottom*). In this hypothetical example, the muscle force–muscle length curve for the fusiform muscle shows that it would have a longer working range and lower maximum force output due to the longer individual fibers and smaller PCSA. The opposite occurs for the pennate muscle, with its shorter fibers and larger PCSA. In this case, force output capacity is about twice as large. For the muscle force–muscle velocity curve, the fusiform muscle with longer fibers would have a higher contractile velocity but lower maximum force output.

ACTIN-MYOSIN ORIENTATION

Thousands of myosin filaments lie along the actin filaments in a muscle fiber. The actin-myosin orientation within a sarcomere at resting length is illustrated in Figure 18.6A; the hexagonal arrangement of myosin and actin filaments are shown in Figure 18.6B. A thick myosin filament (150 angstroms [Å] in diameter and 1.5 μm long) is bordered by six thinner filaments, each about 50 Å in diameter and 1 μm long. This substructure of muscle is extremely impressive. For example, a myofibril that is 1 μm in diameter contains approximately 450 thick filaments in the center of the sarcomere and 900 thin filaments at each end of the sarcomere. A single muscle fiber that is 100 μm in diameter and 1 cm long contains approximately 8000 myofibrils; each myofibril consists of 4500 sarcomeres. This results in a total of 16 billion thick filaments and 64 billion thin filaments in a single fiber.[58]

The spatial orientation of the various components of the contractile filaments is illustrated in Figure 18.7. Projections or "crossbridges" spiral around the myosin filament in the region at which the actin and myosin filaments overlap. These crossbridges are repeated at intervals of approximately 450 Å along the filament. Their globular "lollipop-like" heads extend perpendicularly to latch onto the thinner strands of actin; this makes the structural and functional link between the myofilaments.

Tropomyosin and troponin are two other important constituents of the actin helix structure. These proteins regulate the make-and-break contacts between the myofilaments during muscle action. Tropomyosin is distributed along the length of the actin filament in a groove formed by the double helix. Tropomyosin is believed to inhibit actin and myosin interaction, or coupling, thus preventing a permanent bonding of these filaments. Troponin, which is embedded at fairly regular intervals along the actin strands, has a high affinity for calcium ions (Ca^{2+}). This mineral plays a crucial role in muscle action and fatigue.[35, 44] For example, it is the action of Ca^{2+} and troponin that triggers the myofibrils to interact and slide past each other. When the fiber is stimulated, the troponin molecules undergo a conformational change that in some way "tugs" on the tropomyosin protein strand. This moves the tropomyosin deeper into the groove between the two actin strands. This "uncovers" the active sites of the actin and allows muscle action to proceed.

The M line consists of transversely and longitudinally oriented proteins that serve to maintain the proper orientation of the myosin filament within a sarcomere. As can be observed in Figure 18.7, the perpendicularly oriented M bridges connect with six adjacent thick (myosin) filaments in a hexagonal pattern.

INTRACELLULAR TUBULE SYSTEMS

The tubule system within a muscle fiber is illustrated in Figure 18.8. An extensive network of interconnecting tubular channels, the sarcoplasmic reticulum, lies parallel to the myofibrils. The lateral end of each tubule terminates in a saclike vesicle that stores Ca^{2+}. Another network of tubules, known as the transverse tubule system or **T-tubule system,** runs perpendicular to the myofibril. The T tubules are situ-

FIGURE 18.5

Top, Muscle architectural properties in the lower limb. The quadriceps and plantar flexor are designed for high force production because of their low fiber length (FL)–muscle length (ML) ratios and relatively large cross-sectional areas. The hamstring and dorsiflexor muscles, on the other hand, generally are designed for high contractile velocity because of their relatively high fiber length–muscle length ratios and long muscle fibers. *Bottom,* Hypothetical pennate (short fibers) and fusiform (long fibers) muscles of the same length and same amount of contractile machinery. The muscle force–muscle length curve *(A)* shows that the fusiform muscle has a longer working range and lower maximum force output compared to the pennate muscle. This is because for a given change in muscle length, the individual sarcomeres lengthen less, with the change in muscle length being distributed over more sarcomeres. The greater force output is due to a greater physiological cross-sectional area (PCSA) (bottom inset, *left*). The muscle force–muscle velocity curve *(B)* shows that the fusiform muscle with longer fibers (bottom inset, *right*) has a higher contractile velocity but a lower maximum force output. (Modified from Lieber, R.L.: *Skeletal Muscle Structure and Function.* Baltimore, Williams & Wilkins, 1992.)

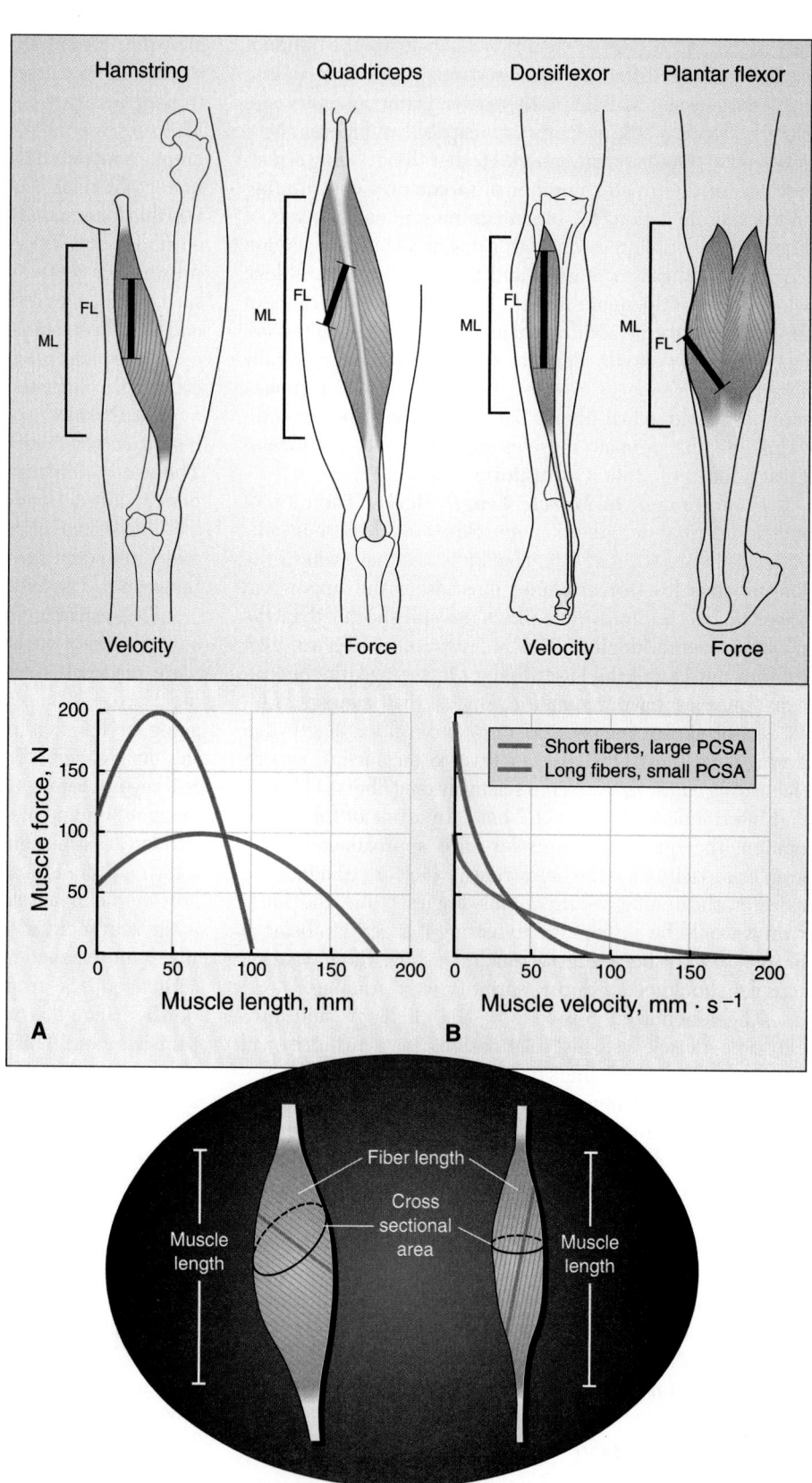

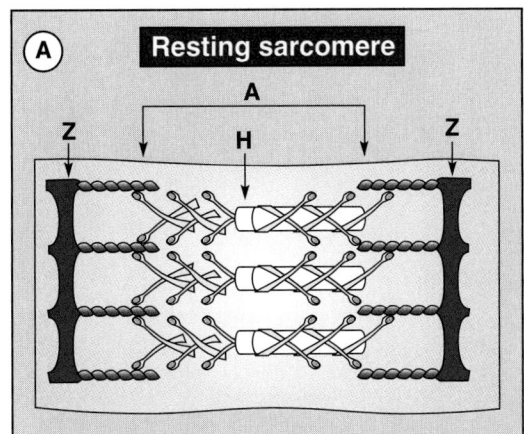

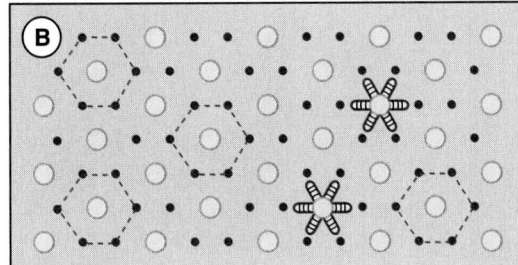

FIGURE 18.6

A, Ultrastructure of actin-myosin orientation within a resting sarcomere. **B,** Representation of electron micrograph through a cross section of myofibrils in a single muscle fiber. Note the hexagonal orientation of the smaller actin and larger myosin filaments, as well as crossbridges that extend from a thick to thin filament.

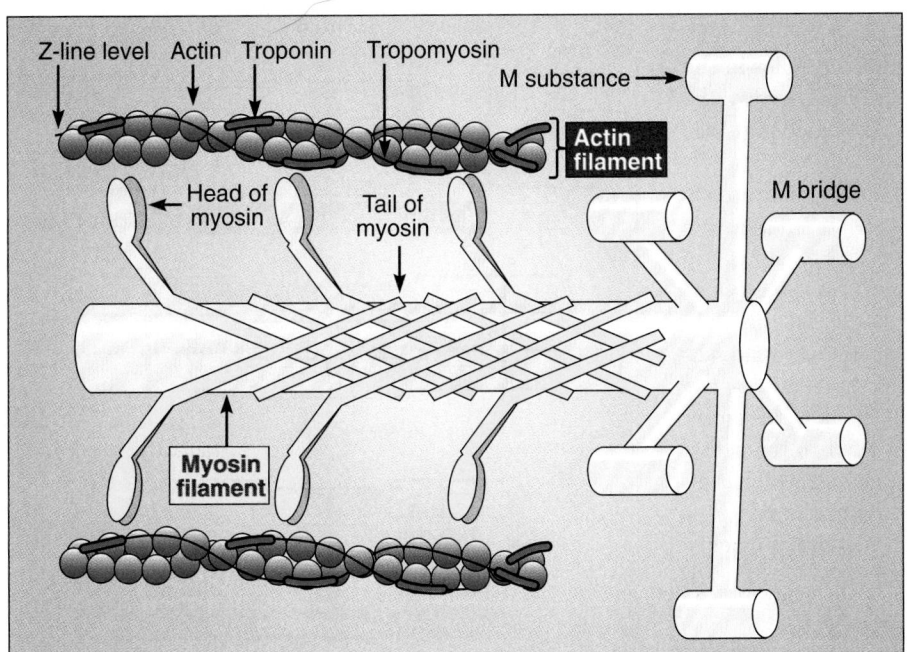

FIGURE 18.7

Details of the thick and thin protein filaments, including tropomyosin, troponin, and the M line. The myosin ATPase is located on the globular heads of the myosin; this "active" head frees the energy from ATP to be used in muscle action.

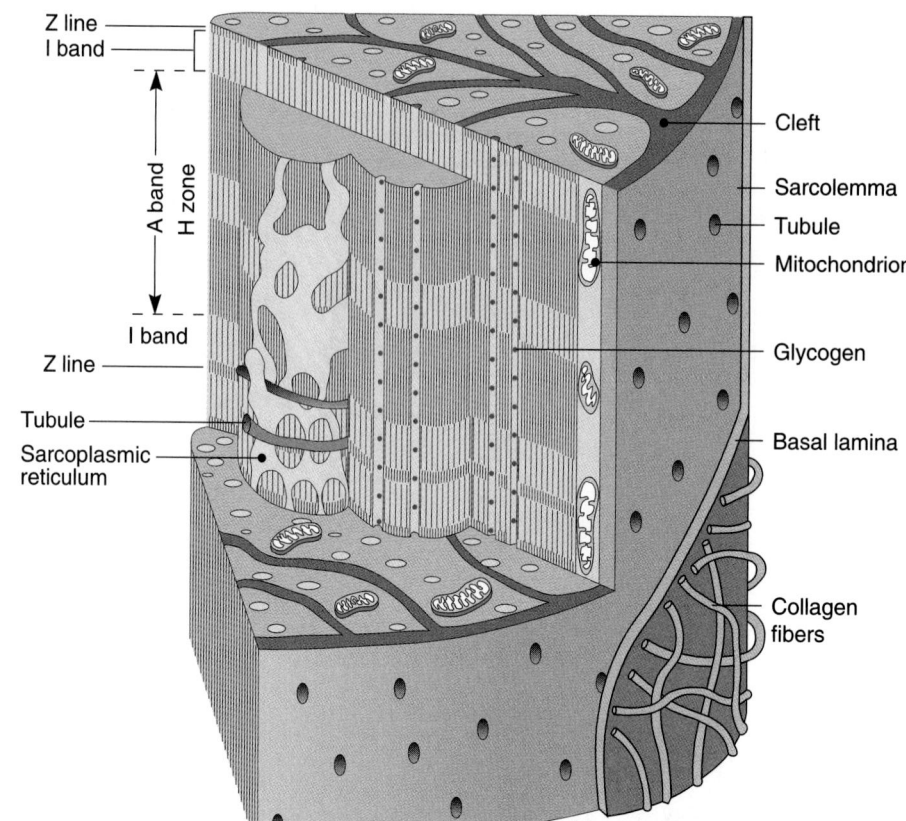

FIGURE 18.8
Three-dimensional view of sarcoplasmic reticulum and T-tubule system within the muscle fiber.

ated between the most lateral portion of two sarcoplasmic channels; the vesicles of these structures abut the T tubule. This repeating pattern of two vesicles and T tubules in the region of each Z line is known as a **triad.** There are two triads in each sarcomere, and the pattern is repeated regularly throughout the length of the myofibril.

The T tubules pass through the fiber and open externally from the inside of the muscle cell. *The triad and T-tubule system function as a microtransportation network to spread the action potential (a wave of depolarization) from the fiber's outer membrane inward to the deep regions of the cell.* During this process, calcium ions are released from the triad sacs and diffuse a short distance, presumably to "activate" the actin filaments. Muscle action is initiated when the crossbridges of the myosin filaments are attracted to the active sites on the actin filaments. When electrical excitation ceases, there is a decrease in Ca^{2+} concentration in the cytoplasm; this is associated with the relaxation of the muscle.

CHEMICAL AND MECHANICAL EVENTS DURING MUSCLE ACTION AND RELAXATION

The electron microscope and x-ray diffraction have helped unravel many secrets of cellular structure, contributing to reasonable hypotheses concerning the chemical and mechanical events in muscle action and relaxation. Although

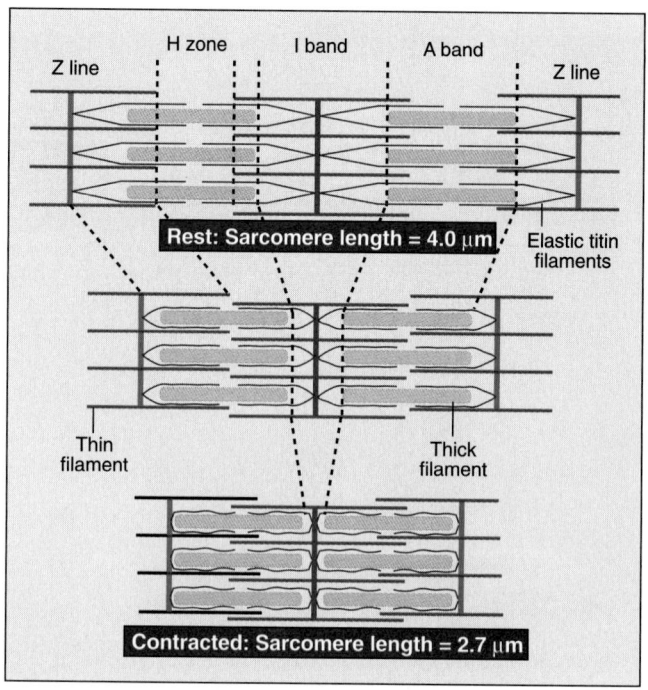

FIGURE 18.9
Structural rearrangement of actin and myosin filaments at rest (sarcomere length = 4.0 μm) and during muscle shortening (contracted sarcomere length = 2.7 μm). At rest, the protein elastic filament (titin) links the M lines of the thick filaments to the Z lines and keeps the myosin filaments centered within the sarcomere.

many gaps remain, there is considerable evidence to support a **sliding-filament theory** of muscle function. Although this theory was proposed nearly 40 years ago to explain the molecular movements that underlie muscle action, the model still fits nicely with the details of muscle ultrastructure and function that are continually being uncovered.

SLIDING-FILAMENT THEORY

The sliding-filament theory proposes that a muscle shortens or lengthens because the thick and thin filaments slide past each other without actually changing length. The molecular motor to drive this shortening process is the action of the myosin crossbridges, which cyclically bind or attach, rotate, and detach from the actin filaments with energy provided by ATP hydrolysis. This causes a major change in the relative size of the various zones and bands within a sarcomere, and produces a force at the Z bands. As illustrated in Figure 18.9, the thin actin filaments slide past the myosin myofilaments and move into the region of the A band during shortening (and move out during relaxation). The major struc-

tural rearrangement during shortening, therefore, occurs in the region of the I band, which decreases markedly as the Z bands are pulled toward the center of each sarcomere. There is no change in the width of the A band, although the H zone can disappear when the actin filaments are in contact at the center of the sarcomere. In a static action, force is generated while the fiber's length remains unchanged, and the relative spacing of I and A bands stays constant; in this situation, the same molecular groups repeatedly react. In an eccentric action in which force is generated while the muscle fiber lengthens, the A band widens.

Mechanical Action of the Crossbridges. Myosin plays both an enzymatic and structural role in muscle action. The globular head of the myosin crossbridge contains an actin-activated ATPase in its actin binding site and provides the mechanical power stroke for the actin and myosin filaments to slide past each other through the hydrolysis of ATP.[26, 48] The cyclic oscillating to-and-fro nature of the crossbridges, which move in a manner somewhat similar to the action of oars in water, is shown schematically in Figure 18.10. Unlike oars, however, the crossbridges all do not move in a

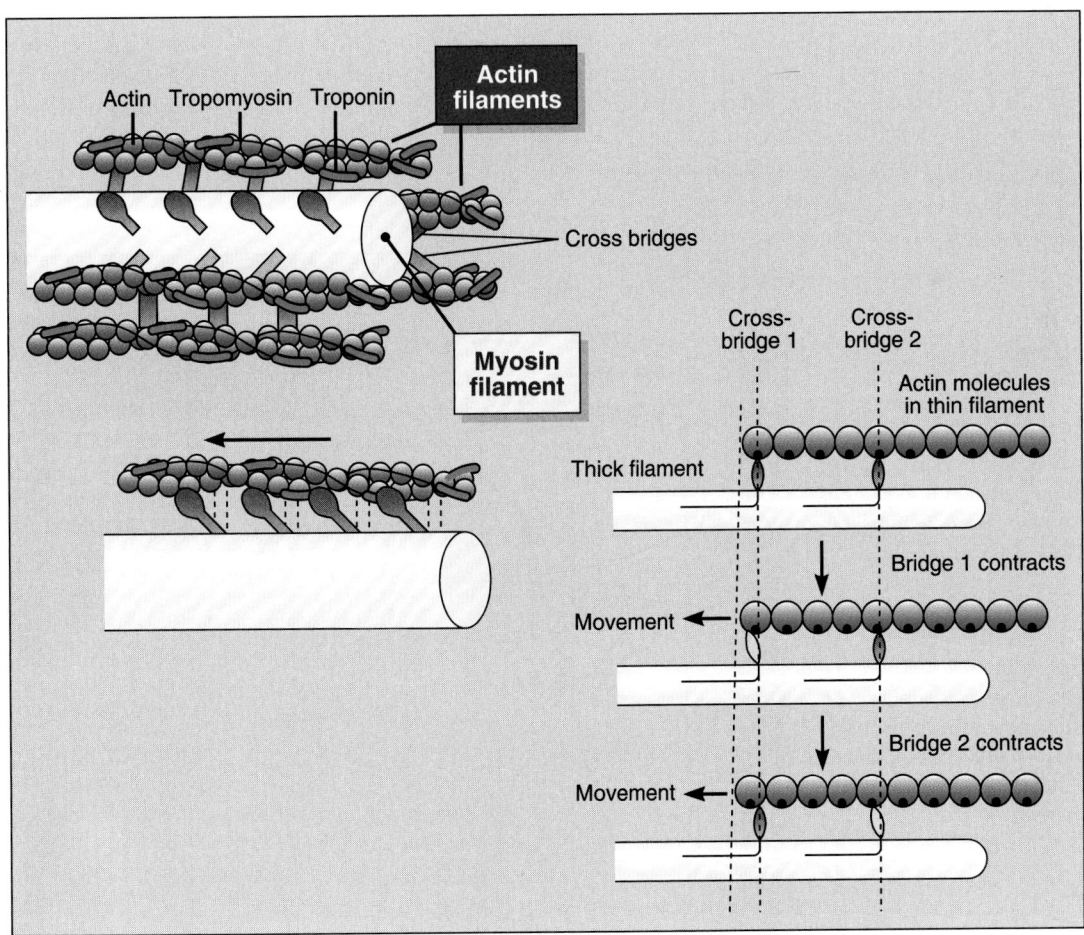

FIGURE 18.10
Relative positioning of actin and myosin filaments during the oscillation movement of the crossbridges. The action of each crossbridge contributes a small displacement of movement. For clarity, one of the actin strands is omitted from the left side of the figure.

synchronous manner. If they did, the resulting muscle action would be a series of jerky movements instead of finely graded movements and force outputs. During muscle shortening, each crossbridge undergoes many repeated but independent cycles of asynchronous movement.

At any one time, only about 50% of the crossbridges are in contact with the actin filaments to form the protein complex **actomyosin,** which has contractile properties; the other crossbridges are at some other position in their vibrating cycle. As illustrated in Figure 18.10 (*right*), each crossbridge action contributes to only a small longitudinal displacement in terms of the total sliding action of the filaments. This process has been likened to the action of a person climbing a rope. The arms and legs represent the crossbridges. Climbing is accomplished by first reaching with the arms, then grabbing, pulling, and breaking contact, and then repeating this process over and over throughout the climb as the person traverses from point A to point B and so on.

Sarcomere Length–Isometric Tension Curve in an Isolated Fiber. The interactions between actin and myosin during isometric tension development in an isolated skeletal muscle preparation are displayed in Figure 18.11. This "length-tension curve" was obtained approximately 40 years ago by British and Swedish researchers who electrically stimulated a single frog muscle fiber (8 mm long and 75 μm in diameter) and then plotted maximum tension output at selected muscle sarcomere lengths.[17, 25] The length of the sarcomere (horizontal axis) ranged from 1.6 μm at maximum overlap of the actin filaments (ap-

proximately 70% of maximum tension) to 3.6 μm when no tension was present. Note that the crest of the upward curve for tension occurred at a sarcomere length between 2.0 and 2.2 μm; this length for maximal tension is the region of maximum interaction between the actin and myosin filaments. Interestingly, the difference of 0.2 μm at this part of the curve is precisely the width of the region in which there is no change in actin-myosin interaction. As the sarcomere is stretched beyond 2.2 μm in length, the curve shifts downward as peak tension output declines. This occurs because of less overlap between the actin and myosin filaments. With less overlap there is less crossbridge interaction and, therefore, less active tension development. The capacity to develop tension is lost at the maximum point of stretch of 3.65 μm (maximum length of the actin filament is 2.0 μm, and maximum length of myosin is 1.65 μm). At the sarcomere length of 3.65 μm, there cannot be any crossbridge interaction.

Sarcomere Length–Isometric Tension Curve in Human Muscle Fibers in Vivo. An elegant procedure has determined the range over which human sarcomeres operate on their length-tension curve for sarcomeres in the intact human muscle during different angles of wrist position for patients undergoing surgery to correct chronic lateral epicondylitis or "tennis elbow."[41] This provided the unique opportunity to compare the length-tension characteristics of an animal preparation (Fig. 18.11) to that of human muscle in vivo. The use of the intraoperative helium-neon laser during surgery to quantify sarcomere length is depicted in Figure

FIGURE 18.11

Relationship between tension and sarcomere length in skeletal muscle during an isometric muscle action. Optimal sarcomere length (i.e., the greatest interaction between actin and myosin filaments) occurs between 2.0 and 2.25 μm. Tension output decreases steadily as sarcomere length increases beyond the optimal length. Note the amount of overlap in the actin and myosin filaments at various regions of the tension-length curve and how tension output changes at different sarcomere lengths.

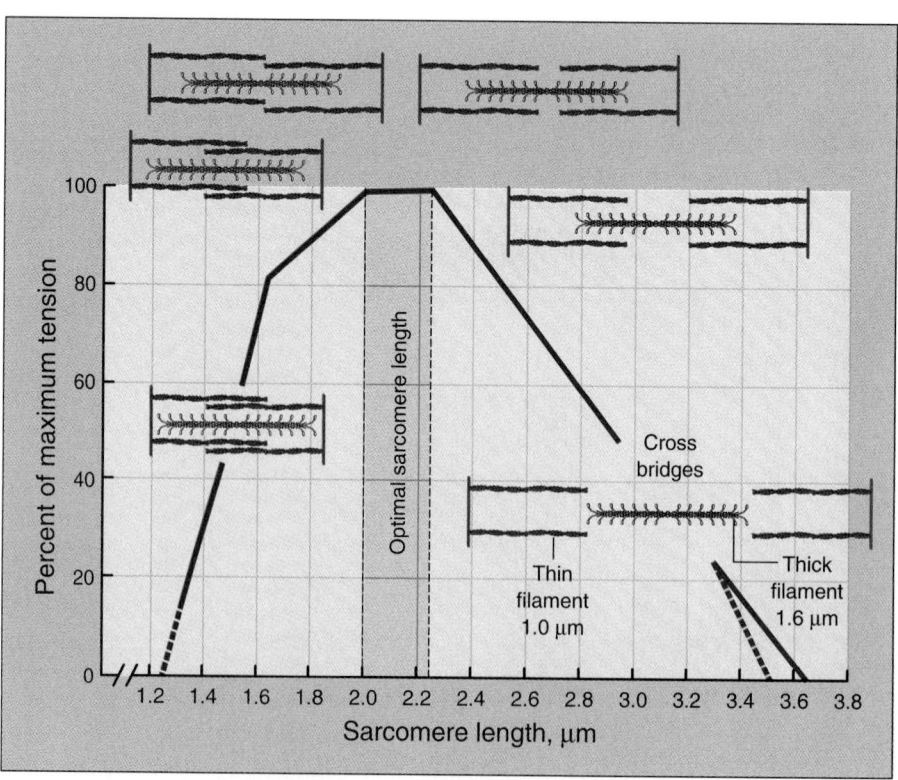

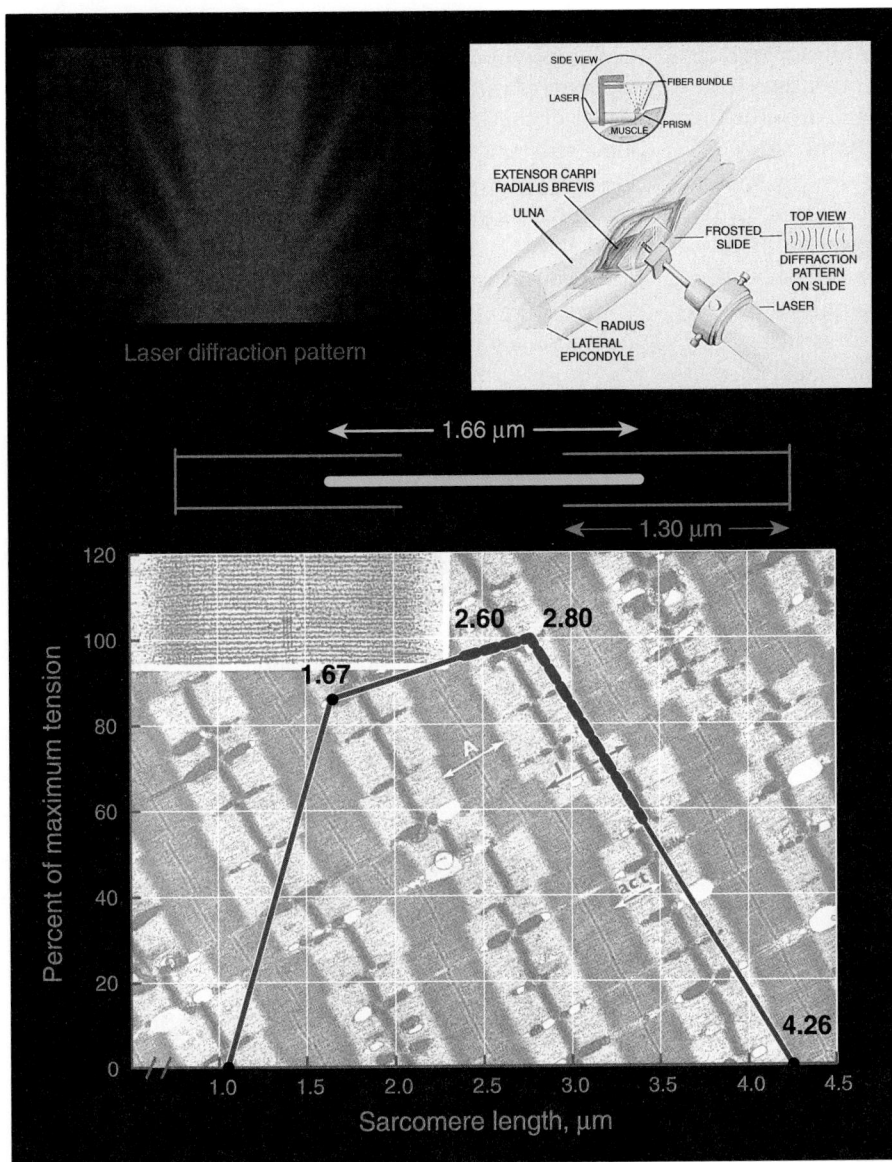

FIGURE 18.12

Changes in the length-tension curve for sarcomeres in vivo during human wrist flexion and extension. The insert at the top illustrates the helium-neon laser procedure (and a view of the illumination prism) that was used during the surgery. The electron micrograph depicted behind the length-tension curve shows the actin and myosin filaments and the A and I bands from biopsy samples of the extensor carpi radialis brevis muscle (ECRB) that were used to verify the sarcomere lengths. The thickened blue portion of a hypothetical length-tension curve represents sarcomere length change during wrist flexion (causing a sarcomere length increase) and wrist extension (causing a sarcomere length decrease). The numbers over the curve represent the inflection points based on the measured filament lengths. (Modified from Lieber, R.L., et al.: In vivo measurement of human wrist extensor muscle sarcomere length changes. *J. Neurophysiol.*, 71:874, 1994. Illustration of experimental pro-cedure, including the example of the laser diffraction pattern and electron micrograph courtesy of Dr. R.L. Lieber, Professor of Orthopaedics and Bioengineering, Muscle Physiology Laboratory, University of California and Veterans Administration Medical Centers, San Diego, CA.)

18.12 (*top right*). The laser was positioned beneath the lateral end of the extensor carpi radialis brevis muscle (ECRB) to obtain sarcomere lengths at three different wrist positions: full flexion to cause sarcomere length to increase, neutral, and full extension to cause a decrease in sarcomere length. An example of the laser diffraction pattern used in computing sarcomere length is shown in Figure 18.12 (*top left*). Muscle biopsies were also taken from the same muscle to verify the laser determinations. An electron micrograph from a biopsy sample is displayed behind the length-tension curve. In this experiment, the length of the actin filaments was 1.30 μm and that of the myosin filaments was 1.66 μm. The thicker blue portion for the plateau and downward part of the curve shows the operating range of the ECRB sarcomeres during both passive (2.6 to 3.4 μm) and active (2.44 to 3.33 μm) muscle contraction. An important finding is the relative position of the sarcomere lengths measured in vivo at a given tension output superimposed on the length-tension curve of the isolated human muscle.

Link Between Actin, Myosin, and ATP. The interaction and movement of the protein filaments during muscle action necessitate that the myosin crossbridges continually undergo oscillatory movements by combining, detaching, and recombining to new sites (or the same sites in a static action) along the actin strands. The detachment of the myosin crossbridges from the actin filament is brought about when the ATP molecule is joined to the actomyosin complex. This chemical reaction enables the myosin crossbridge to return to its original state so it is available to bind a new active site on the actin. The dissociation of actomyosin occurs as follows:

$$\text{Actomyosin} + \text{ATP} \rightarrow \text{Actin} + \text{Myosin-ATP}$$

The transduction of energy from ATP hydrolysis into mechanical force occurs during the formation of the end products, ADP and inorganic phosphate. One of the reacting sites on the globular head of the myosin crossbridge binds to the reactive site on the actin. The other myosin active site acts as an actin-activated enzyme, **myofibrillar adenosinetriphosphatase (myosin ATPase).** This enzyme splits ATP so that its energy can be used for muscle action. The rate of ATP splitting is relatively slow if myosin and actin remain apart; when they join, however, the reactive rate of myosin ATPase increases considerably. It is believed that energy released from ATP splitting somehow activates the crossbridges, causing them to oscillate. This energy transfer process causes a conformational change in the shape of the globular head of the myosin crossbridge so it interacts with the appropriate actin molecule.

The elongated, pear-shaped myosin is not rigid. Before a muscle action, the myosin head literally bends around the energy-carrying ATP molecule and becomes cocked, almost like a spring. The myosin then interacts with the adjacent actin filament, splits a phosphate from ATP, and releases its stored mechanical energy as it straightens. This forces the sliding motion that makes the muscle generate tension.[47, 48] The actin and myosin filaments can slide past each other at a speed of up to 15 μm $\cdot$ s^{-1}.[8]

EXCITATION-CONTRACTION COUPLING

Excitation-contraction coupling *is the physiologic mechanism whereby an electrical discharge at the muscle initiates the chemical events at the cell surface that lead to the release of intracellular Ca^{2+} and ultimately cause a muscle action.* Intracellular Ca^{2+} is intimately involved in regulating a muscle cell's level of contractile and metabolic activity.[35] The nonactive muscle fiber's Ca^{2+} concentration is relatively low compared to the extracellular fluid bathing the cell. When the fiber is stimulated, there is an immediate, small increase in intracellular Ca^{2+}, which precedes the initiation of muscle action. This increase in Ca^{2+} is initiated by the action potential at the transverse tubules that causes Ca^{2+} release from the lateral sacs of the sarcoplasmic reticulum. The inhibitory action of troponin that prevents actin-myosin interaction is rapidly removed when Ca^{2+} binds with this and other proteins in the actin filaments. In a sense, the muscle is "turned on" for action.

Actin + Myosin ATPase → Actomyosin ATPase

When the active sites on actin and myosin are joined, myosin ATPase is activated, which then splits ATP. The energy generated in this process causes movement of the myosin crossbridges, and the muscle generates tension.

Actomyosin ATPase → Actomyosin + ADP + P + Energy

The crossbridges uncouple from actin when ATP binds to the myosin bridge. Coupling and uncoupling continue as long as the Ca^{2+} concentration remains at a sufficient level to inhibit the troponin-tropomyosin system. When neural stimulation is removed, Ca^{2+} moves back into the lateral sacs of the sarcoplasmic reticulum. This restores the inhibitory action of the troponin-tropomyosin, and actin and myosin remain separated as long as ATP is present. (In rigor mortis, the muscles become stiff and rigid soon after death. This occurs because ATP is no longer available in the muscle cells. Without ATP, the myosin crossbridges and actin remain attached and cannot pull apart.) The interaction between the actin and myosin filaments, Ca^{2+}, and ATP in both a relaxed and shortened muscle fiber is illustrated in Figure 18.13.

In isolated muscle preparations, there is evidence that following a twitch stimulation, there is a threefold greater rise in both the Ca^{2+} concentration and the action potential in type II (fast-twitch) compared to type I (slow-twitch) muscle fibers.[50] This may make it possible for the faster transport of Ca^{2+} through the sarcoplasmic reticulum and ultimately to the actomyosin contractile proteins in the type II fibers. During this excitation-contraction coupling, there is a series of electrochemical events that occur within the membranes at the site of "excitation." The common pathway for precisely delivering the chemical signals to the contractile proteins depends to a large extent on ion channel regulators. These structures act as selective "gates" or

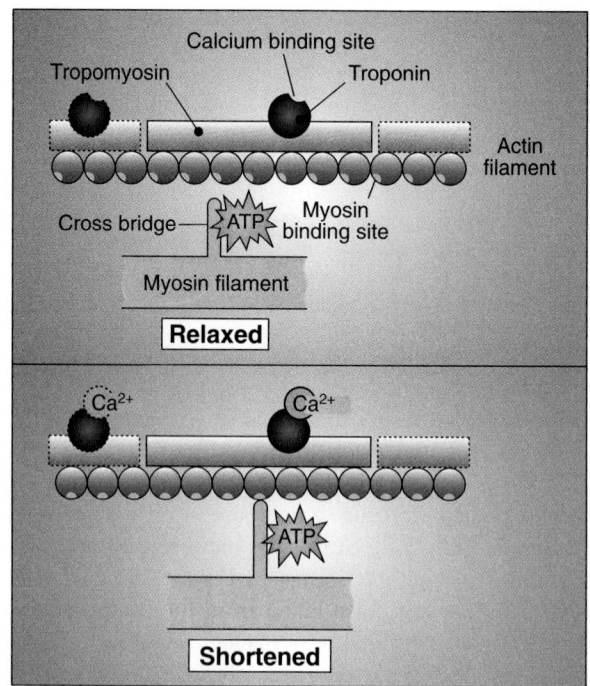

FIGURE 18.13

Interaction between the actin-myosin filaments, Ca^{2+}, and ATP in relaxed and shortened muscle. In the relaxed state, troponin and tropomyosin interact with actin, preventing the coupling of the myosin crossbridge to actin. During muscle action, the crossbridge couples with actin as a result of the binding of Ca^{2+} with troponin-tropomyosin.

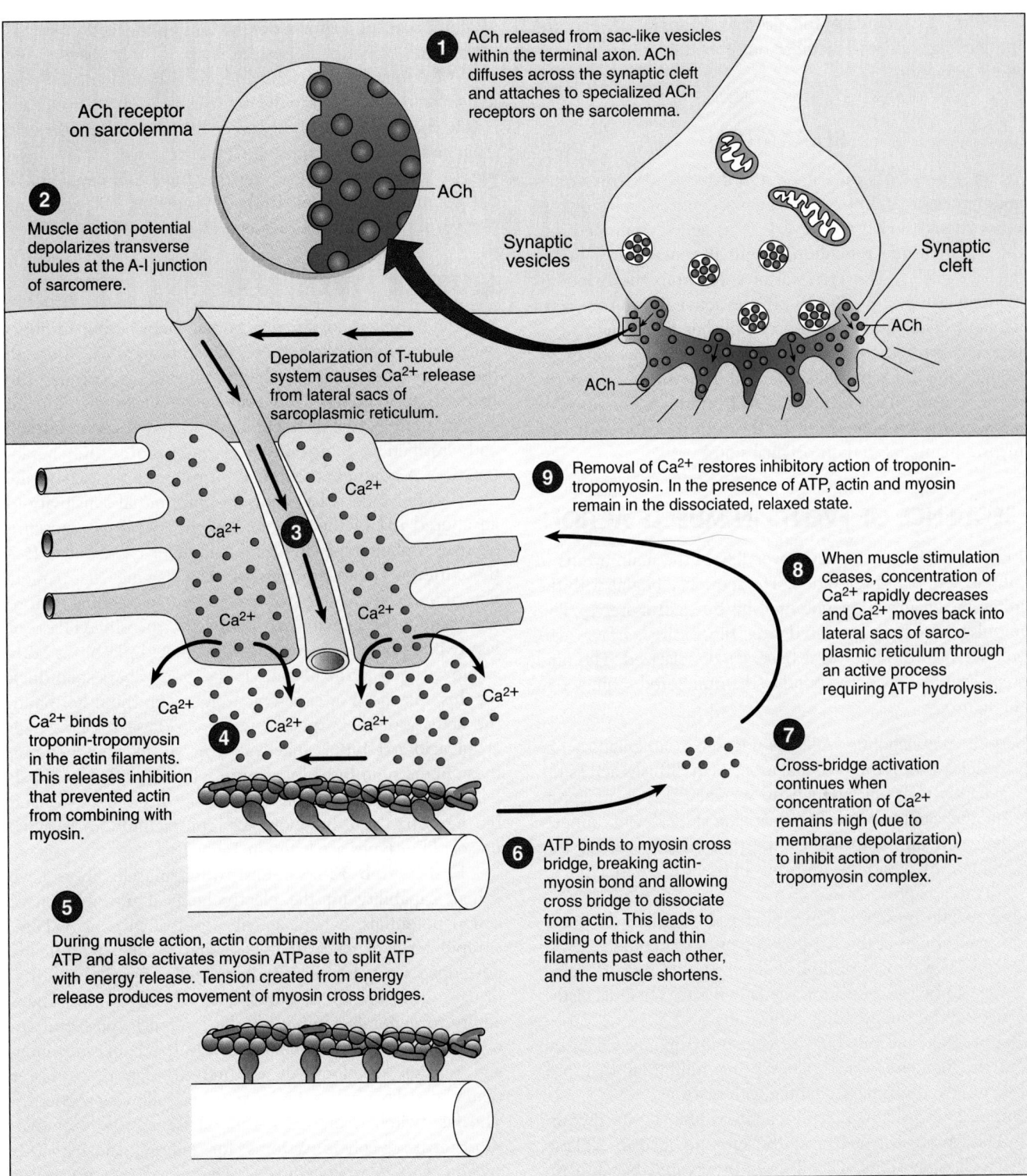

① ACh released from sac-like vesicles within the terminal axon. ACh diffuses across the synaptic cleft and attaches to specialized ACh receptors on the sarcolemma.

ACh receptor on sarcolemma

ACh

② Muscle action potential depolarizes transverse tubules at the A-I junction of sarcomere.

Synaptic vesicles

Synaptic cleft

ACh

ACh

Depolarization of T-tubule system causes Ca^{2+} release from lateral sacs of sarcoplasmic reticulum.

Ca^{2+}

Ca^{2+}

③

Ca^{2+}

Ca^{2+}

⑨ Removal of Ca^{2+} restores inhibitory action of troponin-tropomyosin. In the presence of ATP, actin and myosin remain in the dissociated, relaxed state.

⑧ When muscle stimulation ceases, concentration of Ca^{2+} rapidly decreases and Ca^{2+} moves back into lateral sacs of sarcoplasmic reticulum through an active process requiring ATP hydrolysis.

Ca^{2+}

Ca^{2+}

Ca^{2+}

④ Ca^{2+} binds to troponin-tropomyosin in the actin filaments. This releases inhibition that prevented actin from combining with myosin.

⑦ Cross-bridge activation continues when concentration of Ca^{2+} remains high (due to membrane depolarization) to inhibit action of troponin-tropomyosin complex.

⑥ ATP binds to myosin cross bridge, breaking actin-myosin bond and allowing cross bridge to dissociate from actin. This leads to sliding of thick and thin filaments past each other, and the muscle shortens.

⑤ During muscle action, actin combines with myosin-ATP and also activates myosin ATPase to split ATP with energy release. Tension created from energy release produces movement of myosin cross bridges.

FIGURE 18.14

Schematic view of the main events in muscle action and relaxation. The numbers correspond to the sequence of nine steps outlined in the text. The neuromuscular junction, where the electrochemical signal "jumps" across the 0.05-μm cleft between neuron and muscle fiber, is aided by the neurotransmitter substance acetylcholine (ACh) released from saclike vesicles within the terminal axon. After ACh binds to its receptor on the other side of the cleft, it is rapidly cleaved off and rendered nonfunctional before being retrieved through the postsynaptic membrane. The electrical impulse, traveling at a velocity of about 1 m · s^{-1} or more, starts on its way through the muscle fiber's tubule system to eventually reach the inner "machinery" of the myofibrils.

"sensors" to modulate the passage of ions between the intracellular and extracellular fluids before actual myofilament activation.

RELAXATION

When a muscle is no longer stimulated, Ca^{2+} flow ceases and troponin is free once again to inhibit actin-myosin interaction. During recovery, Ca^{2+} is actively pumped into the sarcoplasmic reticulum, where it concentrates in the lateral vesicles. The retrieval of Ca^{2+} from the troponin-tropomyosin proteins "turns off" the active sites on the actin filament. This deactivation accomplishes two things: (a) it prevents any mechanical link between the myosin crossbridges and the actin filaments, and (b) it inhibits the activity of myosin ATPase to curtail ATP splitting. The muscle's relaxation is brought about by the return of the actin and myosin filaments to their original state.

SEQUENCE OF EVENTS IN MUSCLE ACTION

Figure 18.14 is a schematic overview of the main events in muscle action and relaxation. The sequence begins with the initiation of an action potential by the motor nerve. This impulse is then propagated over the entire surface (sarcolemma) of the fiber as it becomes depolarized. The nine steps listed below correspond to the numbered sequence in the figure.

Step 1: Acetylcholine (ACh) is released from small saclike vesicles within the terminal axon. ACh diffuses across the synaptic cleft and attaches to specialized ACh receptors on the sarcolemma. There is almost perfect symmetry between the "imprint" of the presynaptic vesicles that contain ACh and the "imprint" of the postsynaptic receptors that capture ACh.

Step 2: The muscle action potential depolarizes the transverse tubules at the A-I junction of the sarcomere.

Step 3: The depolarization of the T tubule system causes Ca^{2+} to be released from the lateral sacs (terminal cisternae) of the sarcoplasmic reticulum.

Step 4: Calcium ions bind to troponin-tropomyosin in the actin filaments. This releases the inhibition that prevented actin from combining with myosin.

Step 5: During muscle action, actin combines with myosin-ATP. Actin also activates the enzyme myosin ATPase, which then splits ATP. Tension is created because the energy from this reaction produces movement of the myosin crossbridge.

Step 6: ATP binds to the myosin crossbridge. This breaks the actin-myosin bond and allows the crossbridge to dissociate from actin. This leads to a relative movement or sliding of the thick and thin filaments past each other, and the muscle shortens.

Step 7: Crossbridge activation continues as long as the concentration of Ca^{2+} remains high enough (due to membrane depolarization) to inhibit the action of the troponin-tropomyosin system.

Step 8: When the muscle is no longer stimulated, the concentration of Ca^{2+} rapidly decreases as Ca^{2+} moves back into the lateral sacs of the sarcoplasmic reticulum through an active process requiring ATP hydrolysis.

Step 9: The removal of Ca^{2+} restores the inhibitory action of troponin-tropomyosin. In the presence of ATP, actin and myosin remain in the dissociated, relaxed state.

MUSCLE FIBER TYPE

Skeletal muscle is not simply a homogeneous group of fibers with similar metabolic and contractile properties. Although there has been considerable discussion concerning the method, terminology, and criteria for classifying human skeletal muscle, **two** distinct fiber types have been identified and classified by their **contractile** and **metabolic** characteristics.[3] A common technique for establishing the specific muscle fiber type is based on the differential sensitivity to an altered pH of the enzyme myosin ATPase (a measure of myosin phenotype) in each of the fiber types.[35, 37, 45] It is the different characteristics of this enzyme that largely determine the velocity of sarcomere shortening. More specifically, the activity of the specific myosin ATPase of fast-twitch fibers is inactivated with an acid pH but is fairly stable with pH in the alkaline range; these fibers stain **dark** for this enzyme. For slow-twitch fibers, on the other hand, the activity of their specific myosin ATPase remains high at an acid pH but is inactivated in an alkaline medium; these fibers stain **light** for myosin ATPase. Different classification schemes based on morphology, histochemistry and biochemistry, and function and contractility for skeletal muscle fiber types are listed in Table 18.2.

Fast-Twitch Fibers. Fast-twitch muscle fibers have a high capability for the electrochemical transmission of action potentials, a high activity level of myosin ATPase, a rapid level of calcium release and uptake by a highly developed sarcoplasmic reticulum, and a high rate of crossbridge turnover, all of which are related to this fiber's ability to generate energy rapidly for quick, powerful actions. The fast twitch fiber's intrinsic speed of shortening and tension development is three to five times faster than fibers classified as slow-twitch (see following section).[21] The fast-twitch fibers often rely on their well-developed, short-term glycolytic systems for energy transfer. *This explains how these fibers are activated in short-term, sprint activities as well as in other forceful muscle actions that depend almost entirely on anaerobic metabolism for energy.*[24, 33] Activation of the fast-twitch fibers is also important in the stop-and-go or change-of-pace sports such as basketball, soccer, lacrosse, or field hockey. These activities at times require rapid energy that is only supplied by the anaerobic metabolic pathways.

Slow-Twitch Fibers. Slow-twitch fibers generate energy for ATP resynthesis predominantly through the aerobic

TABLE 18.2
CLASSIFICATION SCHEMES OF SKELETAL MUSCLE FIBER TYPES

Characteristic		Fiber Type	
Electrical activity pattern	Phasic		Tonic
	High frequency		Low frequency
Morphology	**FTb**	**FTa**	**ST**
Color	White	White/red	Red
Fiber diameter	Large	Intermediate	Small
Capillaries/mm^2	Low	Intermediate	High
Mitochondrial volume	Low	Intermediate	High
Histochemistry	**IIB**	**IIA**	**I**
Biochemistry	**FG**	**FOG**	**SO**
Myosin ATPase	High	High	Low
Calcium-handling capacity	High	Medium/high	Low
Glycolytic capacity	High	High	Low
Oxidative capacity	Low	Medium/high	High
Function	**FF**	**FR**	**S**
Contractility	**FT**	**FT**	**ST**
Speed of contraction	Fast	Fast	Slow
Speed of relaxation	Fast	Fast	Slow
Fatigability	High	Moderate/High	Low
Force capacity	High	Intermediate	Low

From Kraus, W E.: Skeletal muscle adaptation to chronic low-frequency motor nerve stimulation *Exerc. Sport Sci. Rev.*, 22:313, 1994.
Abbreviations: FT, fast twitch; FG, fast, glycolytic; FOG, fast, oxidative, glycolytic; SO, slow, oxidative; FF, Fast-contracting, fast-fatigue; FR, fast-contracting, fatigue-resistant; S, slow-contracting.

system for energy transfer. They are distinguished by a relatively low activity level of myosin ATPase, slower calcium-handling ability and speed of shortening, and a glycolytic capacity that is less well developed than their fast-twitch counterparts. Slow-twitch fibers also contain relatively large and numerous mitochondria. *It is this concentration of mitochondria (and accompanying iron-containing cytochromes) combined with high myoglobin levels that give the slow-twitch fiber its characteristic red pigmentation.* Accompanying this enhanced metabolic machinery is a high concentration of mitochondrial enzymes that is required to sustain aerobic metabolism.[19, 20, 23, 29] *Thus, slow-twitch fibers are fatigue-resistant and well suited for prolonged aerobic exercise.* These fibers have been labeled **SO fibers** to describe their slow speed of shortening and their great reliance on oxidative metabolism. Unlike the fast-twitch fibers, which fatigue readily, the SO fibers (more precisely, motor units) are adapted for prolonged work and are selectively recruited in aerobic activities.[32] Studies of muscle glycogen depletion patterns indicate that in prolonged exercise there is almost exclusive reliance on the slow-twitch muscle fibers. Even after up to 12 hours of exercise, the limited glycogen that remains in muscle is found mostly in the "unused" fast-twitch fibers.[52] It is also apparent that the capacity for blood flow through muscle is determined by differences in the oxidative capacity of the two fiber types; the slow-twitch fibers receive the largest portion of blood.[38, 39, 54]

Many researchers classify slow-twitch fibers as **type I**, whereas the fast-twitch fibers (and proposed subdivisions) are categorized as **type II**. *Both types of muscle fibers are activated when a person exercises at near-maximum aerobic and anaerobic levels, as in middle-distance running or swimming or in sports such as basketball, field hockey, or soccer, which require a blend of a high level of aerobic and anaerobic energy transfer.*[24, 51]

Fast-Twitch Subdivisions. Fast-twitch muscle fibers are further classified into subdivisions. The **type IIa** fiber is considered intermediate, in that its fast shortening speed is combined with a moderately well-developed capacity for both aerobic (high level of the aerobic enzyme succinic dehydrogenase or SDH) and anaerobic (high level of the anaerobic enzyme phosphofructokinase or PFK) energy transfer. These are the fast-oxidative-glycolytic or FOG fibers. Another subdivision, the **type IIb** fiber, possesses the greatest anaerobic potential and is the "true" fast-glycolytic or FG fiber. The **type IIc** fiber is normally a rare and undifferentiated fiber that may be involved in reinnervation or motor unit transformation.[36]

Species Differences: A Brief Comparative Look.
Throughout the animal kingdom, there are examples of extraordinary feats of muscular strength, power, and endurance that make the athletic feats of humans pale by comparison. The world's fastest humans can run for up to 200 meters at an average velocity of 10.4 m · s⁻¹ (23.3 mph; 1994 World Record pace). The greyhound dog, in contrast, can cover 60% more distance at a velocity of 16.6 m · s⁻¹. For the world's best endurance athletes, their increase in aerobic metabolism during sustained muscular effort is about 25 times greater than the resting requirement. Other animal species, however, have adapted their muscle machines over millions of years to perform extraordinary feats of metabolism and performance. Consider the hummingbird, a super athlete of the avian species that can sustain a wing beat frequency of 80 Hz with an ATP turnover rate of 500 μmol of ATP per gram of muscle per minute (500 times greater than at rest). This is the highest metabolic rate in the vertebrate world, and it is accomplished from the resting state to full wing activity in less than 15 ms! Intuitively, it might at first seem that the hummingbird has an advanced, complicated chemical system to fuel a multifaceted network of muscle fiber types. Some might argue that this would be necessary to keep the fiber machinery operational with a fuel supply that overcomes the anaerobic component of metabolism characteristic of the human response during "all-out" effort. This, however, is not the case.

In contrast to having multiple fiber types and their intermediates, the hummingbird's flight muscles have a simple architecture consisting only of fast-twitch oxidative (FOG) fibers. Instead of heterogeneity, there is homogeneity of the internal machinery (muscle cells nearly identical in structure) with tremendous up-regulation of aerobic functions. For example, compared to the human muscle fiber, there is a fivefold to sevenfold greater mitochondrial volume density. Capillaries literally wrap around each muscle fiber, and there is a large expansion in the volume of sarcoplasmic reticulum, a higher-than-normal surface area of mitochondrial cristae, a reduced diameter of individual fibers (to increase diffusion rates), and high concentrations per gram of muscle of key aerobic enzymes (for example, hexokinase, malate dehydrogenase, creatine phosphokinase, citrate synthase, protein kinase). Even lipid droplets are stored next to mitochondria for immediate uptake as aerobic fuel along with glucose. To accentuate these remarkable aerobic adaptations, there is no capability for anaerobic metabolism within the FOG fibers.

Other species in the animal and insect world also show a remarkable adaptation in muscle function to the tasks required for survival.[12] Homogeneity in cellular architecture and function is present in the fast-twitch muscle fibers of sprint fish (for example, pike and white tuna), in which there is tremendous up-regulation, emphasizing glycolytic and high-energy phosphate-mediated power performance with a corresponding blunting of the aerobic processes.

Consider the muscle fiber type of the cicada, an insect with skeletal muscles that can resonate for indefinite periods an at extremely high frequency (up to 550 Hz).[31] In this case, the muscle is adapted for sound rather than power output, and the homogeneous muscle architecture has adapted by having unusually large and numerous mitochondrial and sarcoplasmic reticular components. Another interesting adaptation in muscle machinery occurs in the electric eel, in which the muscle cell has adapted to discharge an electric current by up-regulating metabolism to an extent that there is a 2000-fold increase in ATP use to generate an electric charge within 300 ms.[9] The study of comparative physiology not only gives one an appreciation for the diversity of function and adaptation between various species in relation to specific needs, but it also provides insight for understanding the unique aspects of human physiology and metabolism.

DIFFERENCES BETWEEN ATHLETIC GROUPS

Several observations have been made concerning muscle fiber type and the possible influence of specific training on fiber composition and metabolic capacity. Men, women, and children possess, on average, 45 to 55% slow-twitch fibers in their arm and leg muscles.[6, 16] Of the fast-twitch fibers, there are probably equal percentages of the type IIa and type IIb subdivisions. Although there are no sex differences in fiber distribution, the variation can be large among individuals. Generally, the trend in one's muscle fiber type distribution is consistent among the body's major muscle groups.

Certain patterns of muscle fiber distribution are readily apparent among highly proficient athletes.[55] Successful endurance athletes generally demonstrate a predominance of slow-twitch fibers in the muscles activated in their specific sport. For successful sprint athletes, the fast-twitch muscle fiber predominates.[7] This is illustrated in Figure 18.15 for top Scandinavian competitors who represent different sports. Athletic groups with the highest aerobic and endurance capacities, such as distance runners and cross-country skiers, have the highest percentage of slow-twitch fibers, often as high as 90 to 95% in the leg's gastrocnemius muscle. Weight lifters, ice hockey players, and sprinters, on the other hand, tend to have more fast-twitch fibers and a relatively lower aerobic capacity. As might be expected, men and women who perform in middle-distance events have an approximately equal percentage of the two types of muscle fibers. This distribution also occurs in power athletes such as throwers, jumpers, and high jumpers.[15]

These relatively clear-cut distinctions between exercise performance and muscle fiber composition are for elite athletes who have achieved prominence in a specific sport category. A person's fiber composition, however, is clearly not the sole determinant of performance. Several researchers have shown that for a particular group, either

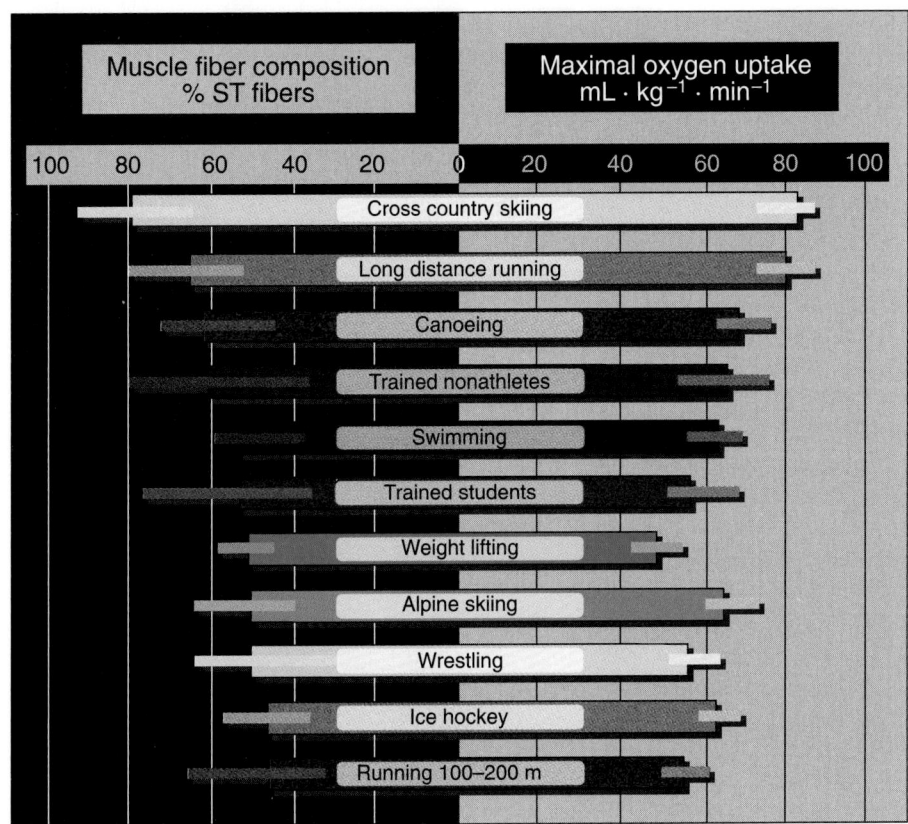

FIGURE 18.15

Muscle fiber composition (% slow-twitch fibers, *left side*) and maximal oxygen uptake (*right side*) in athletes representing different sports. The outer, lightly shaded bars denote the range. (From Bergh, U., et al.: Maximal oxygen uptake and muscle fiber types in trained and untrained humans. *Med. Sci. Sports,* 10:151, 1978.)

trained or untrained, knowledge of a person's predominant muscle fiber type is of limited value in predicting exercise performance.[11, 36] This is not surprising, because performance capacity is the end result of the blending of many physiologic, biochemical, neurological, and biomechanical "support systems" and is not determined by a single factor such as muscle fiber type.[34]

In terms of muscle size, endurance athletes exhibit slow-twitch fibers of relatively normal size.[18] Weight lifters and other power athletes, on the other hand, show a definite enlargement, especially in the fast-twitch muscle fibers.[56, 57] These fibers may be 45% larger than those of endurance athletes or of sedentary people of the same age.[18] This is because power and strength training induces a definite enlargement of the fiber's contractile apparatus—specifically the actin and myosin filaments and the total glycogen content.[42, 43] The principal sex difference in muscle composition is the occurrence of generally larger muscle fibers in male athletes.

CAN MUSCLE FIBER TYPE BE CHANGED?

To determine whether the fiber composition characteristics of specific athletic groups are the result of training or natural endowment (that is, to ascertain whether a person's fiber composition can be changed), six men participated in a 5-month program of aerobic bicycle training.[23] Muscle biopsies from the lateral portion of the quadriceps before and after training indicated no change in fiber composition, although all men improved considerably in exercise capacity and aerobic power. Similar observations were reported for the fiber composition of subjects after either endurance or sprint training programs.[52] These data are often used to support the argument that a fast-twitch fiber before training will still be a fast-twitch fiber after training, with the same holding true for the slow-twitch fibers.

Additional studies with humans and animals, however, suggest the possibility of changes in the biochemical-physiologic properties of muscle fibers with a progressive transformation in fiber type during training.[1, 4, 24, 46] In one study of 18 weeks of "aerobic" training followed by 11 weeks of "anaerobic" training in four athletes, the anaerobic training caused an increase in the percentage of type IIc fibers and a decrease in the percentage of type I fibers; the opposite was observed in the aerobic phase of the training sequence.[30] Similarly, a 23% increase in the percentage of fast-twitch fibers and a commensurate decrease in slow-twitch fiber percentage was shown after only 6 weeks of sprint training.[28] These findings suggest that specific training (and perhaps inactivity) may induce an **actual conversion** of type I to type II fibers (or vice versa).[53, 55] More research is required before definitive statements can be made concerning the fixed nature of a muscle's fiber composition. *The characteristics of fiber-type distribu-*

TABLE 18.3
EFFECTS OF SPECIFIC FORMS OF TRAINING ON SKELETAL MUSCLE

Muscle Factor	Slow-Twitch Fibers		Fast-Twitch Fibers	
	Type of Training			
	Strength	Endurance	Strength	Endurance
Percent composition	0 or ?	0 or ?	0 or ?	0 or ?
Size	+	0 or +	+ +	0
Contractile property	0	0	0	0
Oxidative capacity	0	+ +	0	+
Anaerobic capacity	? or +	0	? or +	0
Glycogen content	0	+ +	0	+ +
Fat oxidation	0	+ +	0	+
Capillary density	?	+	?	? or +
Blood flow during work	?	? or +	?	?

0 = no change; ? = unknown; + = moderate increase; + + large increase.
Modified from Gollnick, P. D., and Sembrowich, W. L.: Adaptations in human skeletal muscle as a result of training. In *Exercise in Cardiovascular Health and Disease*. Edited by E. A. Amsterdam, et al. New York, Yorke Medical Books, 1977.

tion are determined largely by genetic code; the major direction of a muscle's fiber composition is probably fixed before birth or early in life. It does appear, however, that some transformation is possible in muscle fiber type with chronic and specific types of physical activities.

METABOLIC ADAPTATIONS ARE REAL AND SIGNIFICANT

It is likely that a particular fiber distribution is "required" for success at elite levels of sport performance. Although the relatively fixed nature of muscle fiber type suggests an obvious genetic predisposition for exceptional performance, it is well documented that specific training significantly enhances the metabolic power of both fiber types in men and women regardless of age.[5, 14, 29] Enhancement of the oxidative capacity of fast-twitch fibers with endurance training brings them to a level at which they are almost as well equipped for oxidative metabolism as the slow-twitch fibers of untrained subjects.[13, 30]

Age is no barrier to the training adaptations of muscle fibers. If the training stimulus is adequate, the skeletal muscles of older men and women adapt (fiber size, capillarization, glycolytic and respiratory enzymes) to both endurance and resistance training exercise in a manner similar to younger people.[14] Endurance-trained men and women show some conversion of the type IIb fiber to the more aerobic type IIa fiber.[13, 14] This is accompanied by the well-documented increase in mitochondrial size and number and a corresponding increase in the total quantity of the

enzymes of the Krebs cycle and electron transport.[27] Only the specifically trained muscles (more precisely, muscle fibers) adapt to exercise; this explains why highly trained athletes who switch to a sport requiring different muscle groups feel "untrained" for the new activity. Within this framework, swimmers or canoeists (with well-developed upper body musculature) will not necessarily transfer their upper body "fitness" to a running sport that relies predominantly on well-developed lower body musculature.

The changes that occur in skeletal muscle with specific training modalities are summarized in Table 18.3. Generally, both fiber types are recruited in physical activity; however, certain activities require activation of a much greater proportion of one fiber type over another.

▪ SUMMARY ▪

1. Skeletal muscle is encased in various wrappings of connective tissue that blend into and join the tendinous attachment to bone. This harness enables muscles to act on the bony levers to transform the chemical energy of ATP into the mechanical energy of motion.
2. Seventy-five percent of skeletal muscle is water, 20% is protein, and the remainder consists of inorganic salts, enzymes, pigments, lipids, and carbohydrates.
3. During vigorous exercise, the muscle's oxygen uptake increases up to 70 times above the resting level. Supporting this metabolic requirement are immediate adjustments and longer-term training adaptations that increase the size or the local vascular bed.

4. The sarcomere is the functional unit of the muscle fiber. It contains the contractile proteins actin and myosin. In an average muscle fiber, there are 4500 sarcomeres and a total of 16 billion thick (myosin) and 64 billion thin (actin) filaments.

5. Myosin projections or "crossbridges" provide the structural links between the thick and thin contractile filaments. Two myofibrillar proteins, tropomyosin and troponin, regulate the make-and-break contacts between the filaments during a muscle action. Tropomyosin inhibits actin and myosin interaction; troponin with Ca^{2+} triggers the myofibrils to interact and slide past each other.

6. The triad and T-tubule system serve as a microtransportation network for spreading the action potential from the fiber's outer membrane inward to deep regions of the cell. Muscle action occurs when Ca^{2+} activates actin, causing the myosin crossbridges to attach to active sites on the actin filaments. Relaxation occurs when Ca^{2+} concentration decreases.

7. The sliding filament theory proposes that a muscle shortens or lengthens because the protein filaments slide past each other without changing length. Excitation-contraction coupling is the mechanism by which electrochemical and mechanical events are linked to achieve muscle action.

8. The two types of muscle fibers can be classified by their contractile and metabolic characteristic. These are (a) fast-twitch fibers, in which energy is predominantly generated anaerobically for quick, powerful actions (these are labeled FG fibers to signify their fast speed of shortening and high glycolytic properties); and (b) slow-twitch fibers, which shorten at a relatively slow speed and generate energy predominantly via aerobic metabolism (these are called SO fibers to denote their slow shortening speed and reliance on oxidative metabolism). Also present is an intermediate, fast-oxidative-glycolytic (FOG) fiber.

9. The percentage distribution of fiber type differs significantly among people. This distribution is largely determined by genetic code, although some modification may take place with specific forms of training.

10. With appropriate training, fast-twitch and slow-twitch muscle fibers can markedly improve their metabolic capacity.

■ REFERENCES ■

1. Aitken, J.C., et al.: The effects of high intensity training upon respiratory gas exchanges during fixed term maximal incremental exercise in man. *Eur. J. Appl. Physiol.*, 58:717, 1989.

2. Andersen, P., and Henrickson, J.: Capillary supply of the quadriceps femoris muscle of man: adaptive response to exercise. *J. Physiol. (Lond.)*, 270:677, 1977.

3. Armstrong, R.B.: Muscle fiber recruitment patterns and their metabolic correlates. In *Exercise, Nutrition, and Energy Metabolism*. Edited by E.S. Horton and R.L. Terjung. New York, Macmillan, 1988.

4. Baldwin, K.M., et al.: Biochemical properties of overloaded fast-twitch skeletal muscle. *J. Appl. Physiol.*, 52:457, 1982.

5. Baumann, H., et al.: Exercise training induces transitions of myosin isoform subunits within histochemically typed human muscle fibers. *Pflugers Arch.*, 409:349, 1987.

6. Bell, R.D., et al.: Muscle fiber types and morphometric analysis of skeletal muscle in six-year-old children. *Med. Sci. Sports,* 12:28, 1980.

7. Bergh, U., et al.: Maximal oxygen uptake and muscle fiber types in trained and untrained humans. *Med. Sci. Sports,* 10:151, 1978.

8. Billeter, R., and Hoppeler, H.: Muscular basis of strength. In *Strength and Power in Sport.* Edited by P. Komi. London, Blackwell Scientific Publications, 1992.

9. Blum, H., et al.: Coupled in vivo activity of the membrane band Na^+K^+ ATPase in resting and stimulated electric organ of the electric fish *Narcine brasiliensis. J. Biol. Chem.*, 266:1054, 1991.

10. Brodal, P., et al.: Capillary supply of skeletal muscle fibers in untrained and endurance trained men. *Acta Physiol. Scand.*, 440(Suppl.):1, 1976.

11. Campbell, C.J., et al.: Muscle fiber composition and performance capacities of women. *Med. Sci. Sports,* 11:260, 1979.

12. Casey, T.M., et al.: Allometric scaling of muscle performance and metabolism: insects. *Adv. Biosci.*, 84:152, 1992.

13. Chi, M.M.-Y., et al.: Effects of detraining on enzymes of energy metabolism in individual human muscle fibers. *Am. J. Physiol.*, 244 (Cell Physiol. 13):276, 1983.

14. Coggan, A.R., et al.: Skeletal muscle adaptations to endurance training in 60- to 70-yr old men and women. *J. Appl. Physiol.*, 72:1780, 1992.

15. Costill, D.L., et al.: Skeletal muscle enzyme and fiber composition in male and female track athletes. *J. Appl. Physiol.*, 40:149, 1976.

16. Dudley, G.A., et al.: Muscle fiber composition and blood ammonia levels after intense exercise in humans. *J. Appl. Physiol.*, 54:582, 1983.

17. Edman, K.A.P.: The relation between sarcomere length and active tension in isolated semitendinosus fibers of the dog. *J. Physiol. (Lond.)*, 183:407, 1966.

18. Edström, L., and Ekblom, B.: Differences in sizes of red and white muscle fibers in vastus lateralis of musculus quadriceps of normal individuals and athletes: relation to physical performance. *Scand. J. Clin. Lab. Invest.*, 30:175, 1972.

19. Essen, B., et al.: Metabolic characteristics of fiber types in human skeletal muscles. *Acta Physiol. Scand.*, 95:153, 1975.

20. Faulkner, J.A., et al.: Contractile properties of isolated human muscle preparation. *Clin. Sci.*, 57:20, 1979.

21. Fitts, R.H., et al.: Effect of swim exercise training on human muscle fiber function. *J. Appl. Physiol.*, 66:465, 1989.

22. Gaffney, F.A.: Cardiovascular and metabolic responses to static contraction in man. *Acta Physiol. Scand.*, 138:249, 1990.

23. Gollnick, P.D.: Effects of training on enzyme activity and fiber composition of human skeletal muscle. *J. Appl. Physiol.*, 34:107, 1973.

24. Gollnick, P.D., et al.: Fiber number and size in overloaded chicken anterior latissimus dorsi muscle. *J. Appl. Physiol.*, 54:1292, 1983.

25. Gordon, A.M., et al.: The variation in isometric tension with sarcomere length in vertebrate muscle fibers. *J. Physiol. (Lond.)*, 184:170, 1966.

26. Hochachka, P.W.: *Muscles as Molecular and Metabolic Machines.* Boca Raton, FL, CRC Press, 1994.

27. Holloszy, J.O., and Coyle, E. F.: Adaptations of skeletal muscle to endurance training and their metabolic consequences. *J. Appl. Physiol.*, 56:831, 1984.

28. Jacobs, I.: Sprint training effects on muscle myoglobin, enzymes, fiber types, and blood lactate. *Med. Sci. Sports Exerc.*, 19:368, 1987.

29. Jansson, E., and Kaijser, L.: Muscle adaptation to extreme endurance training in man. *Acta Physiol. Scand.*, 100:315, 1977.

30. Jansson, E., et al.: Changes in muscle fiber type distribution in man after physical training. *Acta Physiol. Scand.*, 104:235, 1978.

31. Josephson, R.K., and Young, D.: A synchronous insect muscle with an operating frequency greater than 500 Hz. *J. Exp. Biol.*, 118:185, 1985.

32. Karlsson, J., and Jacobs, I: Onset of blood lactate accumulation during muscular exercise as a threshold concept. I. Theoretical considerations. *Int. J. Sports Med.,* 3:190, 1982.

33. Karlsson, J.B., et al.: LDH isozymes in skeletal muscles of endurance and strength trained athletes. *Acta Physiol. Scand.,* 93:150, 1975.

34. Klausen, K., et al.: Adaptative changes in work capacity, skeletal muscle capillarization and enzyme levels during training and detraining. *Acta Physiol. Scand.,* 113:9, 1981.

35. Klug, G.A., and Tibbits, G.F.: The effects of activity on calcium-mediated events in striated muscle. *Exerc. Sport Sci. Rev.,* 16:1, 1988.

36. Komi, P.V., and Karlsson, J.: Skeletal muscle fiber types, enzyme activities and physical performance in young males and females. *Acta Physiol. Scand.,* 103:210, 1978.

37. Kraus, W.E., et al.: Skeletal muscle adaptation to chronic low-frequency motor nerve stimulation. *Exerc. Sport Sci. Rev.,* 22:313, 1994.

38. Laughlin, M.H., et al.: Vascular transport capacity of hindlimb muscles of exercise-trained rats. *J. Appl. Physiol.,* 62:438, 1987.

39. Laughlin, M.H., et al.: Physical activity and the microcirculation in cardiac and skeletal muscle. In *Physical Activity, Fitness, and Health.* Edited by C. Bouchard, et al. Champaign, IL, Human Kinetics, 1994.

40. Lieber, R.L.: *Skeletal Muscle Structure and Function.* Baltimore, Williams & Wilkins, 1992.

41. Lieber, R.L., et al.: In vivo measurement of human wrist extensor muscle sarcomere length changes. *J. Neurophysiol.,* 71:874, 1994.

42. MacDougall, J.D., et al.: Biochemical adaptation of human skeletal muscle to heavy resistance training and immobilization. *J. Appl. Physiol.,* 43:700, 1977.

43. MacDougall, J.D., et al.: Mitrochondrial volume density in human skeletal muscle following heavy resistance training. *Med. Sci. Sports,* 11:164, 1979.

44. Macintosh, B.R.: Skeletal muscle staircase response with fatigue or dantroline sodium. *Med. Sci. Sports Exerc.,* 23:56,1991.

45. Pette, D., and Staron, R. S.: Cellular and molecular diversities of mammalian skeletal muscle fibers. *Rev. Physiol. Biochem. Pharmacol.,* 116:1, 1990.

46. Pette, Q., and Vrbova, G.: Invited review: neural control of phenotypic expression in mammalian muscle fiber. *Muscle Nerve,* 8:676, 1985.

47. Rayment, I., et al.: Three-dimensional structure of myosin subfragment-1: a molecular motor. *Science,* 261(July 2):50, 1993.

48. Rayment, I., et al.: Structure of the actin-myosin complex and its implications for muscle contraction. *Science,* 261(July 2):58, 1993.

49. Roy, R.R., and Edgerton, V.R.: Skeletal muscle architecture and performance. In *Strength and Power in Sport.* Edited by P. V. Komi. Boston, Blackwell Scientific, 1992.

50. Rugg, J.C.: *Calcium in Muscle Activation. A Comparative Approach.* Berlin, Springer-Verlag, 1986.

51. Saltin, B., and Gollnick, P.D.: Skeletal muscle adaptability: significance for metabolism. In: *Handbook of Physiology. Skeletal Muscle.* Bethesda, MD, American Physiological Society, 1983.

52. Saltin, B., et al.: Fiber types and metabolic potentials of skeletal muscles in sedentary man and endurance runners. *Ann. N. Y. Acad. Sci.,* 301:3, 1977.

53. Simoneau, J.-A., et al.: Human skeletal muscle fiber type alteration with high-intensity intermittent training. *Eur. J. Appl. Physiol.,* 54:240, 1985.

54. Terjung, R.L., and Engbretson, B.M.: Blood flow to different rat skeletal muscle fiber type sections during isometric contractions in situ. *Med. Sci. Sports Exerc.,* 20:S124, 1988.

55. Tesch, P.A., and Karlsson, J.: Muscle fiber type and size in trained and untrained muscles of elite athletes. *J. Appl. Physiol.,* 59:1716, 1985.

56. Tesch, P.A., and Larsson, L.: Muscle hypertrophy in body builders. *Eur. J. Appl. Physiol.,* 49:301, 1982.

57. Thorstensson, A.: Muscle strength, fiber types and enzyme activities in man. *Acta Physiol. Scand.* 443(Suppl.):1, 1976.

58. Vander, A.J., et al.: *Human Physiology: The Mechanisms of Body Function.* 6th ed. New York, McGraw-Hill, 1993.

Merton, P.A.: Voluntary strength and fatigue. *J. Physiol. (Lond.)* 123:553, 1954.

Since the turn of the century, scientists have attempted to explain why repeated maximal muscle actions result in fatigue and associated decreased tension output. The debate over the site of fatigue focuses on the existence of either a central or a peripheral mechanism. "Central mechanism" refers

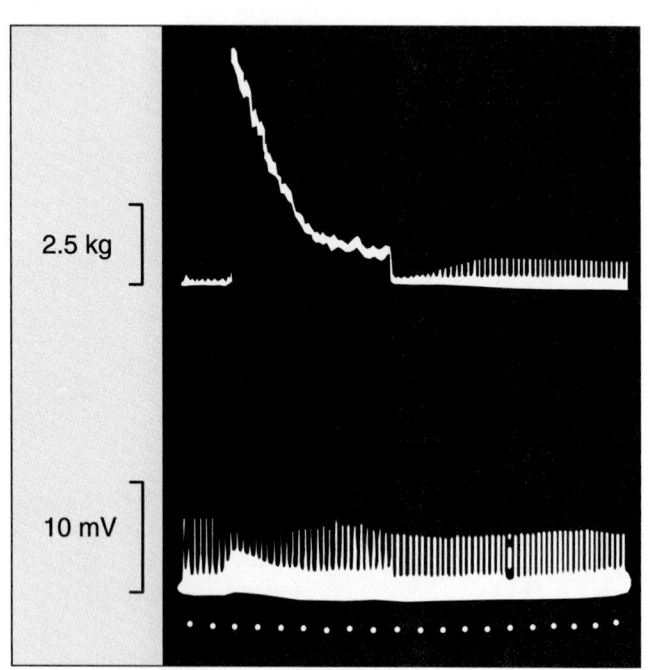

Top, Fatigue curve for skeletal muscle during the sustained isometric maximal voluntary contraction. *Bottom,* Action potentials in response to repeated nerve stimulation during the contraction period.

to a site proximal to the motor neuron (that is, mainly in the brain); a "peripheral mechanism" would involve the motor units (that is, the anterior motor neurons, the peripheral nerves, the motor endplates, and the muscle fibers). Merton reasoned that one way to distinguish between central and peripheral mechanisms was to induce fatigue in a muscle group using maximal voluntary contractions (MVC) and then, when signs of fatigue became apparent, to directly stimulate the motor

unit electrically. If the "extra" localized stimulation did not result in increased force production (that is, no change in the fatigue pattern) it would indicate a purely peripheral site of fatigue. In contrast, if muscle tension increased (that is, the pattern of fatigue decreased) this would support a hypothesis for a central site of muscular fatigue.

Merton's experiments (performed mainly on himself) used an apparatus for measuring the muscle tension output of the isolated adductor pollicis, a muscle producing thumb adduction. The upper arm remained fixed in a flexed position with the hand rotated outward and stabilized in a grasping position. The arm and hand rested in a splint-type device to allow only thumb abduction/adduction movement. This particular hand and arm position enabled isolation and recording of muscle tension either by voluntary muscle action or by electrical stimulation of the ulnar nerve.

The results showed that muscle tension at fatigue could not be altered by specific motor nerve stimulation. Subjects performed maximal sustained isometric actions to total fatigue, and a series of single twitches (evoked by stimulation of the ulnar nerve) was delivered at intervals of about 12 seconds preceding and following fatigue. The top tracing in the figure shows the fatigue curve for the muscles during the sustained isometric MVC. Tension declined linearly, reaching half its initial value in 1 minute. The lower tracing shows the corresponding action potentials in response to the repeated nerve stimulation. No return occurred in muscle tension (that is, the pattern of fatigue remained unaltered by stimulating the motor nerve electrically). Merton reasoned that some part of the peripheral apparatus directly affected the fatigue observed during MVC, because fatigue induced by MVC could not be altered by direct nerve stimulation. Because nerve stimulation did not diminish the amplitude of the action potential during fatigue (lower tracing), the site of fatigue must have resided in the muscle fiber itself, rather than being caused by neuromuscular block. Merton's classic experiments established the first strong support for the role of peripheral neuromuscular factors in the fatigue process.

Neural Control of Human Movement

The effective application of force in relatively complex, learned movements such as a tennis serve, shot put, or golf swing depends on a series of coordinated neuromuscular patterns and not just on the strength of the muscle groups recruited for the activity. Such movements are regulated by neural control mechanisms linked together by pathways in the nervous system. This neural circuitry in the brain and spinal cord, as well as in the body's periphery, is somewhat analogous to a modern computer network, although the integrative and organizational structure of the nervous system is far more advanced and specialized. In response to changing internal and external stimuli, millions of bits of sensory input are automatically synchronized for rapid processing by the central neural control mechanisms. The input is properly organized, routed, and transmitted at high speed to the effector organs, the skeletal muscles.

In the following sections, a general outline describing the neural control of human movement is presented. This outline includes:

- Structural organization for motor control.
- Neuromuscular transmission.
- Motor unit function and activation.
- Sensory input from muscle activity.

ORGANIZATION OF THE NEUROMOTOR SYSTEM

The human nervous system consists of two major parts: (a) the **central nervous system** consists of the brain and spinal cord, and (b) the **peripheral nervous system** contains the nerves that transmit information to and from the central nervous system. An overview of these two subdivisions of the human nervous system is presented in Figure 19.1.

CENTRAL NERVOUS SYSTEM—THE BRAIN

As illustrated in Figure 19.2, the brain can be categorized into six main areas: the **medulla oblongata, pons, midbrain, cerebellum, diencephalon,** and **telencephalon.** The origin of each of the 12 pairs of cranial nerves is in one of these anatomic areas. The four lobes of the cerebral cortex and the sensory areas are depicted in Figure 19.2 (*bottom*). As a frame of reference, there are roughly 10 million sensory (afferent) neurons, 50 billion central neurons, and 500,000 motor (efferent) neurons. Therefore, the ratio is about 20:1 between the sensory and motor circuits.

Brain Stem. The medulla, pons, and midbrain make up the **brain stem.** The medulla, located immediately above the spinal cord, extends into the pons and serves as a bridge between the two hemispheres of the cerebellum. The midbrain, only 1.5 cm long, is attached to the cerebellum and forms a connection between the pons and the cerebral hemispheres. The midbrain contains parts of the extrapyramidal motor system, specifically the red nucleus and substantia. The **reticular formation** integrates various incoming and outgoing signals that flow through it. These signals originate from the stretching of sensors in joints and muscles, from pain receptors in the skin, and as visual signals from the eye and auditory impulses from the ear. Once activated, the reticular system produces either an inhibitory or facilitory effect on other neurons.

Cerebellum. The cerebellum, made up of two lateral hemispheres and a central vermis, functions by means of intricate feedback circuits to monitor and coordinate other areas of the brain and spinal cord involved in motor control. The cerebellum receives motor output signals from the central command in the cortex, and sensory information from peripheral receptors in muscles, tendons, joints, and skin, as well as from visual, auditory, and vestibular end organs. *This specialized brain tissue serves as the major comparing, evaluating, and integrating center for postural adjustments, locomotion, maintenance of equilibrium, perceptions of speed of body movement, and other reflex functions related to movement.* In essence, the cerebellum provides the "fine tuning" for all forms of muscular activity.

Diencephalon. The diencephalon, located immediately above the midbrain, is a part of the cerebral hemispheres. The major structures of the diencephalon are the thalamus, hypothalamus, epithalamus, and subthalamus. The **hypothalamus,** situated below the thalamus, regulates functions ranging from metabolism to body temperature. The hypothalamus also influences activity of the autonomic nervous system (see p. 343) and is affected by input from the thalamus and limbic brain system as well as the body's various hormones (see Chapter 20). Hypothalamic activity is influenced by changes in arterial blood pressure and blood gas tensions via peripheral receptors located in the aortic arch and carotid arteries.

Telencephalon. The telencephalon contains the two hemispheres of the **cerebral cortex** as well as the corpus striatum and the medulla. The cerebral cortex makes up about 40% of the total brain weight and is divided into four

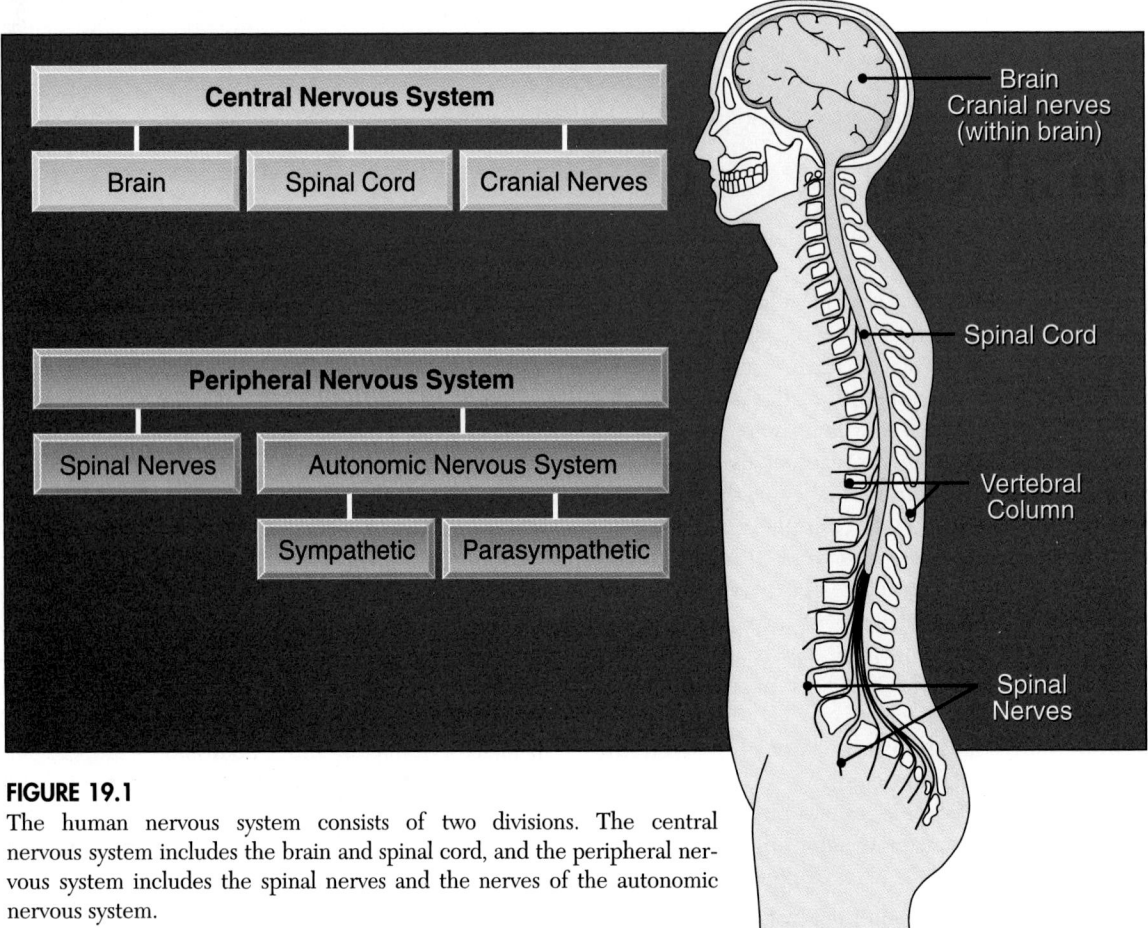

FIGURE 19.1
The human nervous system consists of two divisions. The central nervous system includes the brain and spinal cord, and the peripheral nervous system includes the spinal nerves and the nerves of the autonomic nervous system.

lobes: frontal, temporal, parietal, and occipital. The cortical cells have specialized sensory and motor functions. Beneath each cerebral hemisphere, and in close association with the thalamus, is the basal ganglia, which plays an important role in the control of motor movements.

Limbic System. Various parts of the frontal and temporal lobes of the cerebral cortex, thalamus, and hypothalamus and their neural connections make up the **limbic system.** This configuration of neurons, located around the brain stem, is believed to be involved with emotional behavior and learning.

CENTRAL NERVOUS SYSTEM— THE SPINAL CORD

The spinal cord, illustrated in Figure 19.3, is about 45 cm long and 1 cm in diameter and is encased by 33 vertebrae (7 cervical, 12 thoracic, 5 lumbar, 5 sacral, and 4 coccygeal). When viewed in cross section, the spinal cord has an H-shaped core of gray matter. The limbs of this core are known at the **ventral** (anterior) and **dorsal** (posterior) **horns.** This core contains principally three types of neurons: interneurons, motoneurons, and sensory neurons. The motoneurons

(efferent) are routed through the ventral horn to supply the extrafusal and intrafusal skeletal muscle fibers (see p. 351). Sensory **(afferent)** nerve fibers enter the spinal cord from the periphery by way of the dorsal horn. Surrounding the gray core within the cord itself is an area of white matter that contains the ascending and descending nerve tracts.

Ascending Nerve Tracts. Ascending nerve tracts in the spinal cord forward sensory information from peripheral receptors to the brain for processing. The sensory pathway is typically made up of three neurons. The cell body of the first neuron is in the dorsal root ganglion, from which its axon relays information to the spinal cord. The cell body of the second neuron is in the cord itself, and its axon passes up the spinal cord to the thalamus, which contains the third neuron's cell body. The axon of this third nerve passes up to the central command center in the cerebral cortex.

Sensory Receptors. *Peripheral sensory nerve endings are specialized receptors to detect both conscious and subconscious sensory information.* The "conscious" receptors are sensitive to such input as body position (kinesthesia and proprioception), temperature, and pain, as well as the sensations of light, sound, smell, taste, and touch. There are also receptors to monitor subconscious changes in the body's internal environment; these include **chemoreceptors,** which respond to changes in blood gas tension (P_{O_2}, P_{CO_2}) and pH, and **baroreceptors,** which detect and respond immediately to changes in arterial blood pressure.

Descending Nerve Tracts. Tracts of nerve tissue descend from the brain and terminate at neurons within regions of the spinal cord. The **pyramidal** and **extrapyramidal** tracts are the two major pathways that serve this function.

Pyramidal Tract. Neurons in the pyramidal or corticospinal tract transmit impulses downward through the spinal cord. By means of direct routes and interconnecting neurons in the cord, these nerves eventually excite the **alpha** (α) **motoneurons,** which control skeletal muscle activity.

Extrapyramidal Tract. The extrapyramidal neurons originate in the brain stem and connect at all levels of the spinal cord. These neurons control posture and provide a continual background level of neuromuscular tone. This is in contrast to the discrete muscle movements that occur by stimulation of neurons in the pyramidal tract.

Reticular Formation. The reticular formation is an extensive and intricate neural network running through the core of the brain stem that integrates the spinal cord, cerebral cortex, basal ganglia, and cerebellum. It receives a continuous flow of sensory "data." Once activated, the reticular system produces either an inhibitory or facilitory effect on other neurons. For example, the reticular formation contributes to postural control by regulating the sensitivity of neurons to the antigravity muscles. Excitation of peripheral sensory neurons arouses the reticular nerve cells, which causes excitation in the cerebral cortex, and signals are transmitted back to the reticular system to maintain an appropriate level of cortical arousal and wakefulness. The reticular formation also exerts a powerful influence on vital functions such as cardiovascular and pulmonary regulation.

Superimposed on reticular formation activity are the modulating influences of other feedback networks. For example, with increased neural outflow to the postural mus-

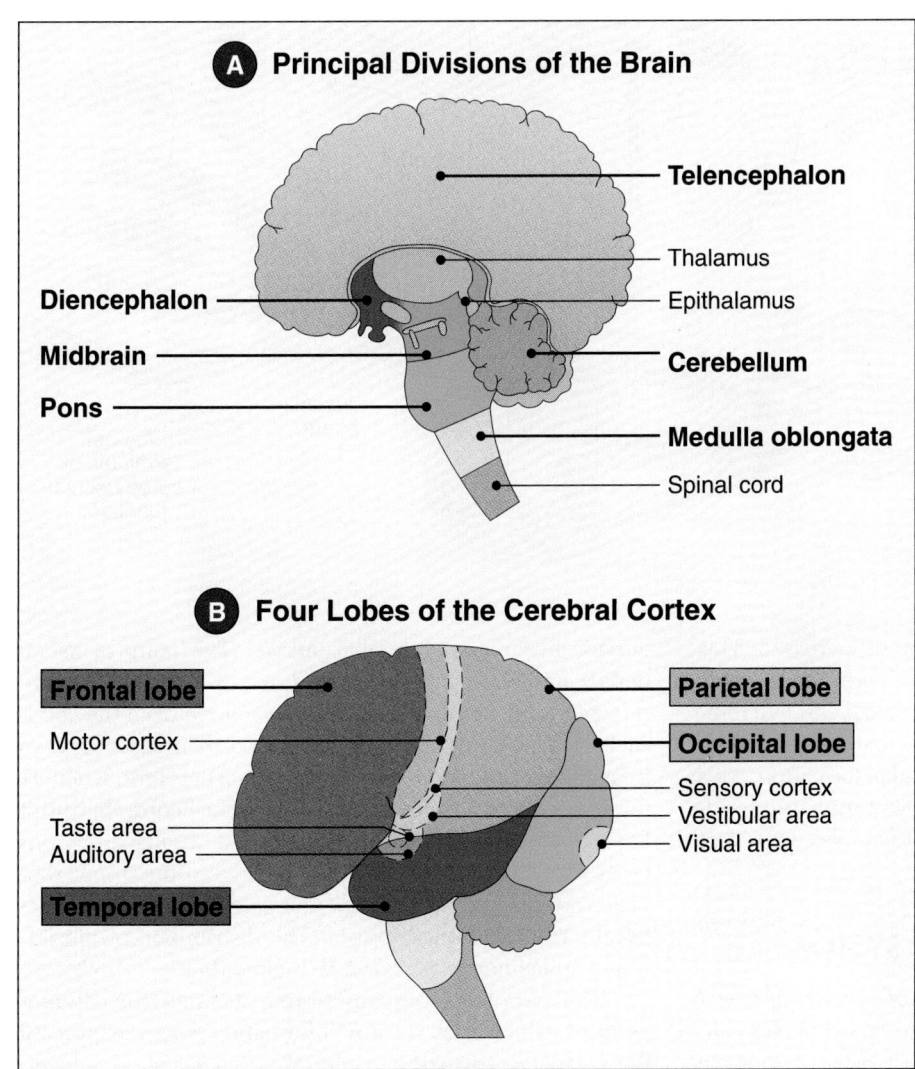

A, Principal Divisions of the Brain

Telencephalon
Thalamus
Diencephalon
Epithalamus
Midbrain
Cerebellum
Pons
Medulla oblongata
Spinal cord

B, Four Lobes of the Cerebral Cortex

Frontal lobe
Parietal lobe
Motor cortex
Occipital lobe
Sensory cortex
Vestibular area
Taste area
Visual area
Auditory area
Temporal lobe

FIGURE 19.2
A, The principal divisions of the brain.
B, The four lobes of the cerebral cortex.

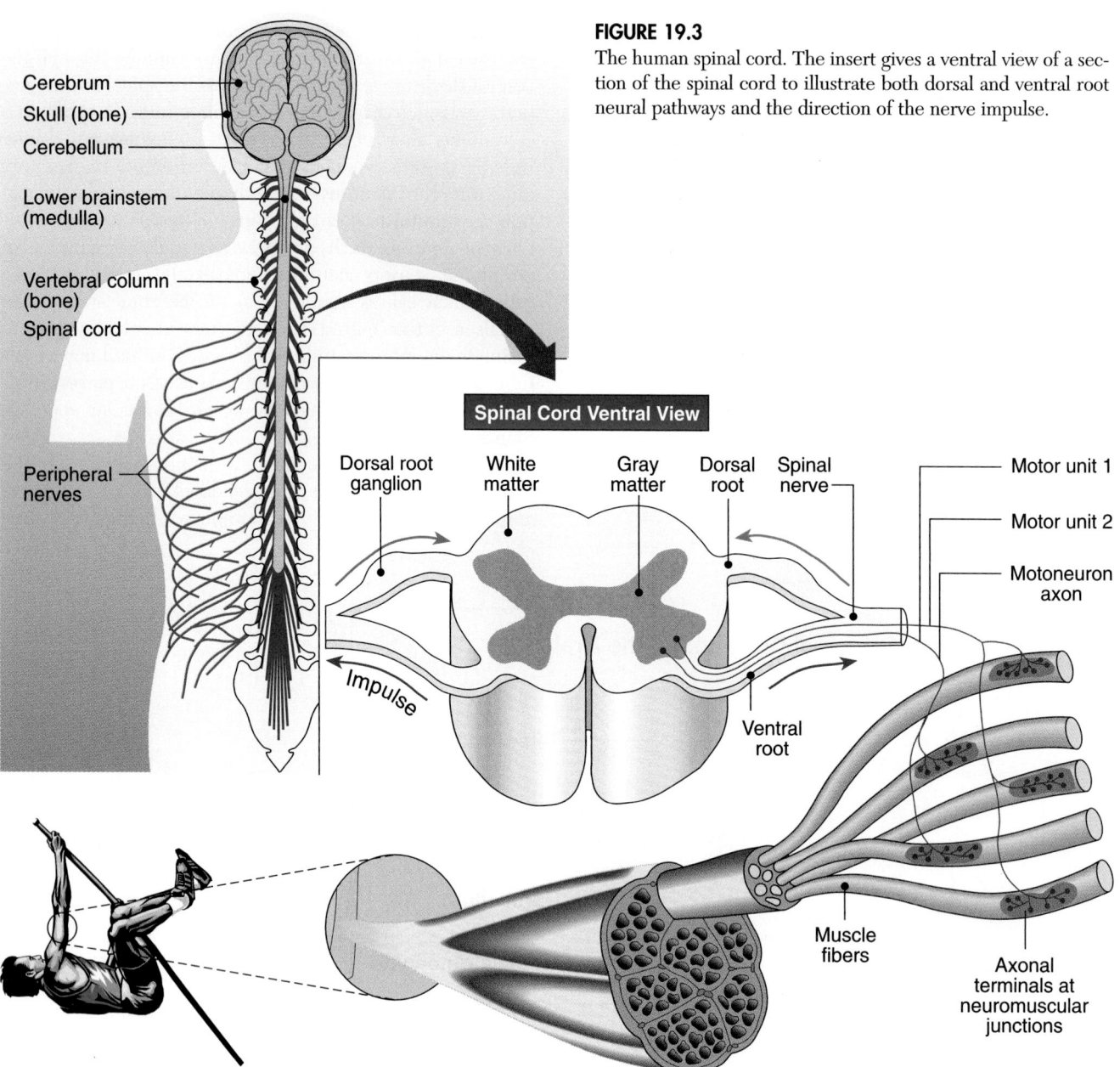

FIGURE 19.3

The human spinal cord. The insert gives a ventral view of a section of the spinal cord to illustrate both dorsal and ventral root neural pathways and the direction of the nerve impulse.

cles, the tension of these muscles becomes increased. This increase in neuromuscular tone also stimulates the muscle's own set of internal sensors, the spindles (see p. 351), to redirect impulses back to the central nervous system to maintain the proper activation level of the reticular formation. This level of integrated response is an example of **multiple feedback control,** which is one of the most complex aspects of nervous system function.

PERIPHERAL NERVOUS SYSTEM

The peripheral nervous system consists of 31 pairs of spinal nerves and 12 pairs of cranial nerves. The spinal nerves consist of eight pairs of cervical nerves, 12 pairs of thoracic nerves, five pairs of lumbar nerves, five pairs of sacral nerves, and one pair of coccygeal nerves. These nerves are referred to by number (e.g., C-1, first nerve from the cervical region). Careful research has traced their exact location by mapping the tissues they innervate. Therefore, when an injury occurs to a specific area of the spinal cord, the result is predictable neurological damage that results in various types of paralysis. For example, damage to the upper thoracic vertebra and the corresponding descending nerve tract usually results in quadriplegia. The distribution of the different spinal nerves is shown in Figure 19.4.

The peripheral nervous system includes the afferent neurons, which relay sensory information from receptors in the periphery **toward** the central nervous system, and efferent neurons, which transmit information **away** from the brain to peripheral tissues. The two types of efferent neurons are known as **somatic** and **autonomic** nerves.

Somatic nerve fibers (also called motoneurons) innervate skeletal muscle. The firing of these neurons is always excitatory in response and causes a muscle action. The autonomic nerves activate smooth muscle (also called involuntary muscle) such as the muscle in the intestines and walls of blood vessels, sweat and salivary glands, cardiac muscle, and some endocrine glands. Activity of these neurons can have either an excitatory or inhibitory effect, depending on the specific neurons activated. Whereas tissues of the heart and viscera display autonomic excitability, conscious control is also possible over these tissues. For example, individuals who practice yoga or meditation can control their heart rate or even blood flow "on command." Such conscious control of the autonomic system can have some application as an alternative treatment in medicine as well as in sport. Competitors in archery and the biathlon, for example, are able to control their cardiovascular activity and respiratory movements so that the normal cycle of breathing and even the pulse rate become temporarily "halted" during the crucial phase of the performance (that is, for several seconds prior to releasing the bowstring or firing the rifle).

Sympathetic and Parasympathetic Nervous System. Based on anatomical and physiological differences, the autonomic nervous system is subdivided into its **sympathetic** and **parasympathetic** components. The fibers of the sympathetic nervous system leave the spinal cord in the thoracic and upper lumbar region. The distribution of sympathetic fibers, while displaying some overlap, supplies the heart, smooth muscle, sweat glands, and viscera. The fibers of the parasympathetic nervous system leave the brain stem and sacral segments of the spinal cord and supply the thorax, abdomen, and pelvic regions.

Regions of the medulla, pons, and diencephalon control the autonomic nervous system. For example, blood pressure, heart rate, and respiration are controlled from fibers that originate in the medullary region of the lower brain stem, whereas body temperature is regulated by nerve fibers of upper hypothalamic origin.

THE REFLEX ARC

The diagram in Figure 19.5 illustrates the neural arrangement for a typical **reflex arc** in one of the 31 spinal cord segments. Sensory input is transmitted from the receptor by afferent neurons that enter the spinal cord through the dor-

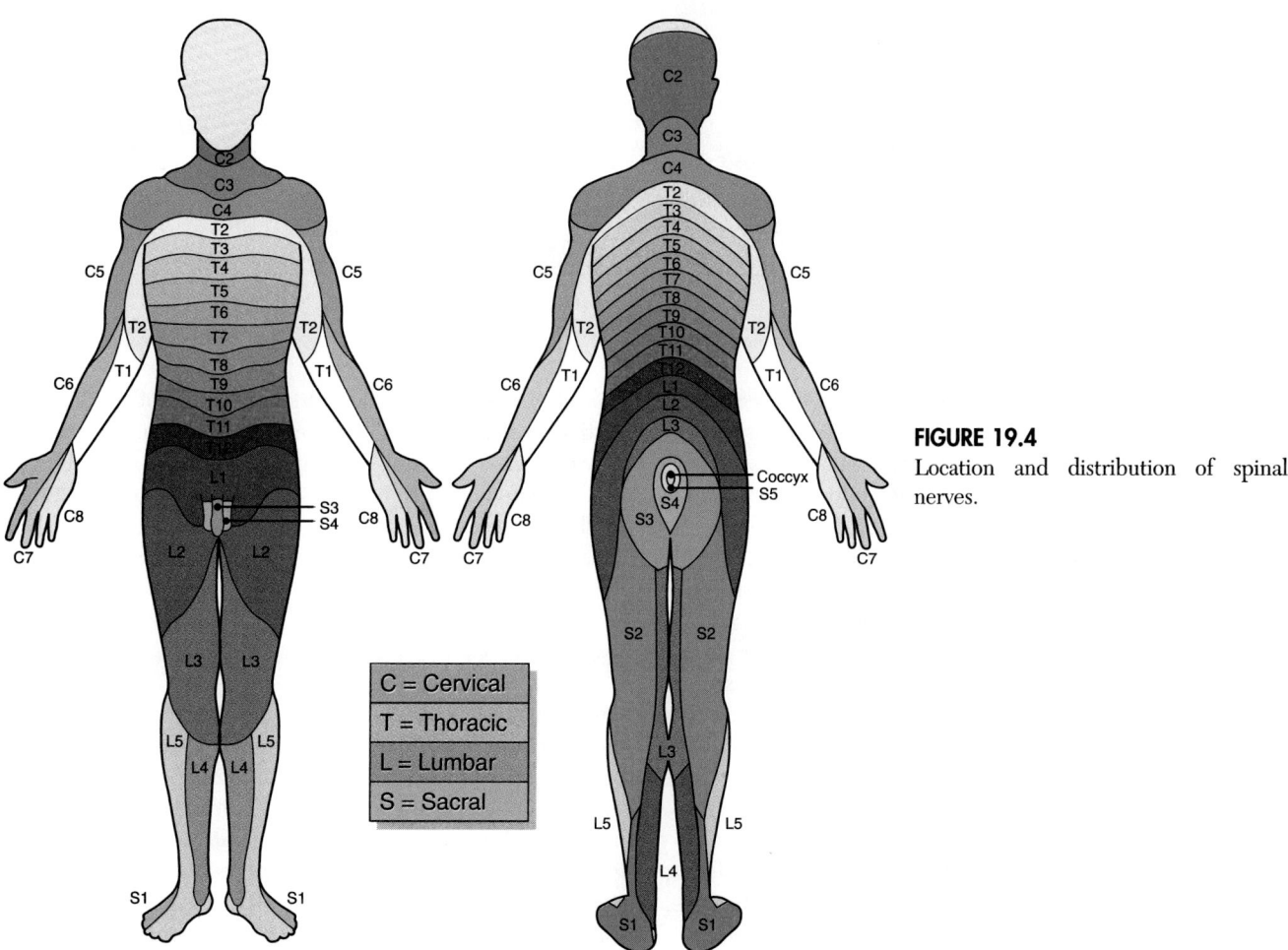

FIGURE 19.4
Location and distribution of spinal nerves.

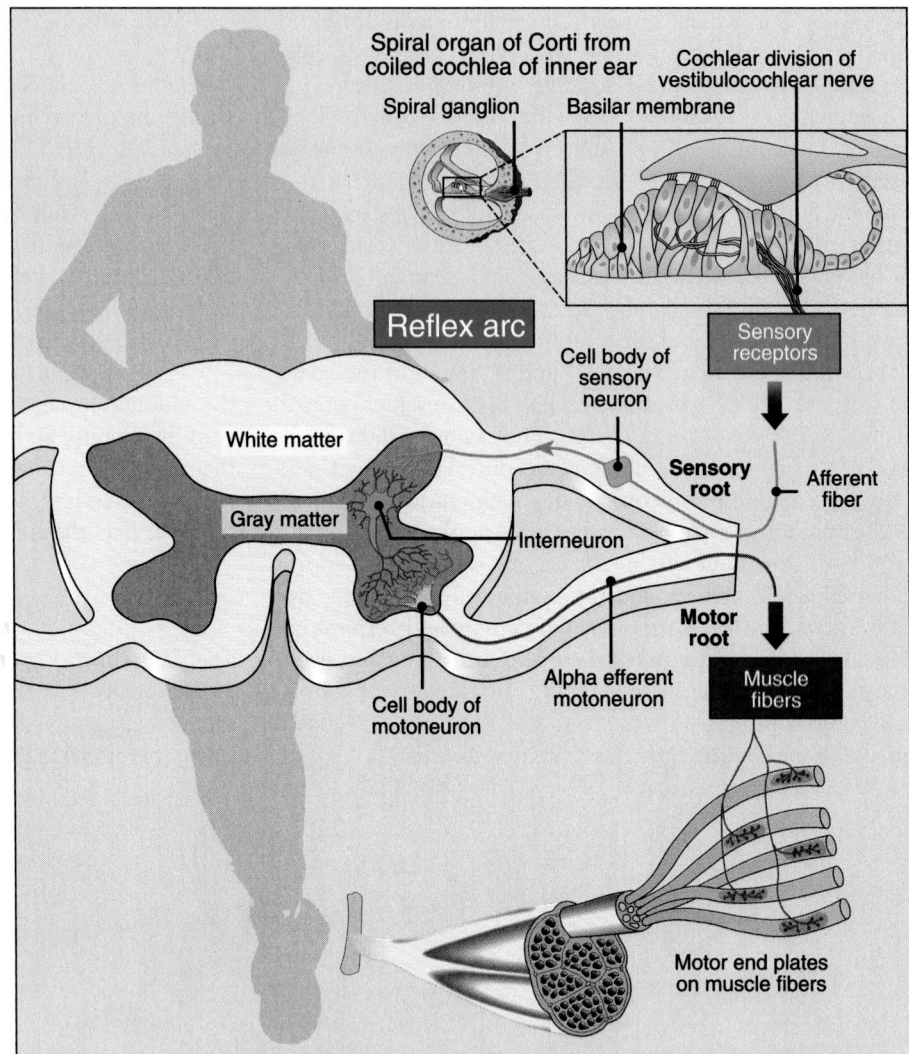

FIGURE 19.5

The reflex arc. The afferent and efferent neurons are shown, in addition to an interneuron in a spinal cord segment. The shaded or gray matter contains the neuron cell bodies; the white matter is made up of longitudinal columns of nerve fibers. Stimulation of a single alpha motoneuron can activate as many as 3000 muscle fibers. The motoneuron and the fibers it innervates are collectively referred to as a motor unit. Only one side of the spinal nerve complex is shown.

sal or sensory root. These neurons interconnect or **synapse** in the cord through **interneurons,** which relay information to various levels of the cord. The impulse then is passed over the **motor root pathway** via anterior motoneurons to the effector organ, the muscles.

The operation of the reflex arc is evident when one unknowingly touches a hot object. Pain receptors in the fingers are stimulated and send sensory information rapidly over afferent fibers to the spinal cord. The efferent motor fibers are then activated to bring about an appropriate muscular response (the hand is rapidly pulled away). Concurrently, the signal is transmitted through interneuron activity up the cord to sensory areas in the brain, where the pain sensation actually is "felt." These various levels of operation for sensory input, processing, and motor output, including the reflex action just described, account for the removal of the hand from the hot object before the pain is actually perceived. Many muscle functions are controlled by reflex actions in the spinal cord and other subconscious areas of the

central nervous system. Hundreds of hours of practicing a particular skill "grooves" the neuromuscular movements so they become automatic, requiring little or no conscious control. Of course, improper practice also can automate a task so the neuromuscular actions are less than optimal. The adage, "practice makes perfect" should be amended to "perfect practice makes perfect."

NERVE SUPPLY TO MUSCLE

One nerve or its terminal branches innervates at least one of the approximately 250 million muscle fibers in the human body. Because there are only about 420,000 motoneurons, this means that a single nerve usually supplies many individual muscle fibers. *The ratio of muscle fibers per motoneuron is generally related to a muscle's particular movement function.* The delicate and precise work of the eye muscles, for example, requires that a neuron control fewer than 10 muscle fibers. For less complex movements of the large muscle groups, a motoneuron may innervate as many as 2000 or 3000 fibers. For muscular activity, the spinal cord is the major processing and distribution center for motor control. The next sections take a closer look at how information processed in the central nervous system is delivered to the muscles to bring about an appropriate motor response.

MOTOR UNIT ANATOMY

The functional unit of movement is the **motor unit;** *this anatomic unit consists of the anterior motoneuron and the specific muscle fibers it innervates.* Although each muscle fiber generally receives input from only one neuron, a mo-

toneuron may innervate many muscle fibers because the terminal end of an axon forms numerous branches. Some motor units contain up to 3,000 muscle fibers, whereas others contain relatively few. For example, the first dorsal interosseous muscle of the finger contains 120 motor units that control 41,000 fibers; the medial gastrocnemius (calf) muscle has 580 motor units and 1,030,000 muscle fibers. The average ratio of muscle fibers per motor unit is, therefore, 340 for the finger muscle and 1,900 for the gastrocnemius muscle.[8]

The Anterior Motoneuron. The anterior motoneuron, illustrated in Figure 19.6, consists of a **cell body, axon,** and **dendrites.** Its unique design enables it to transmit an

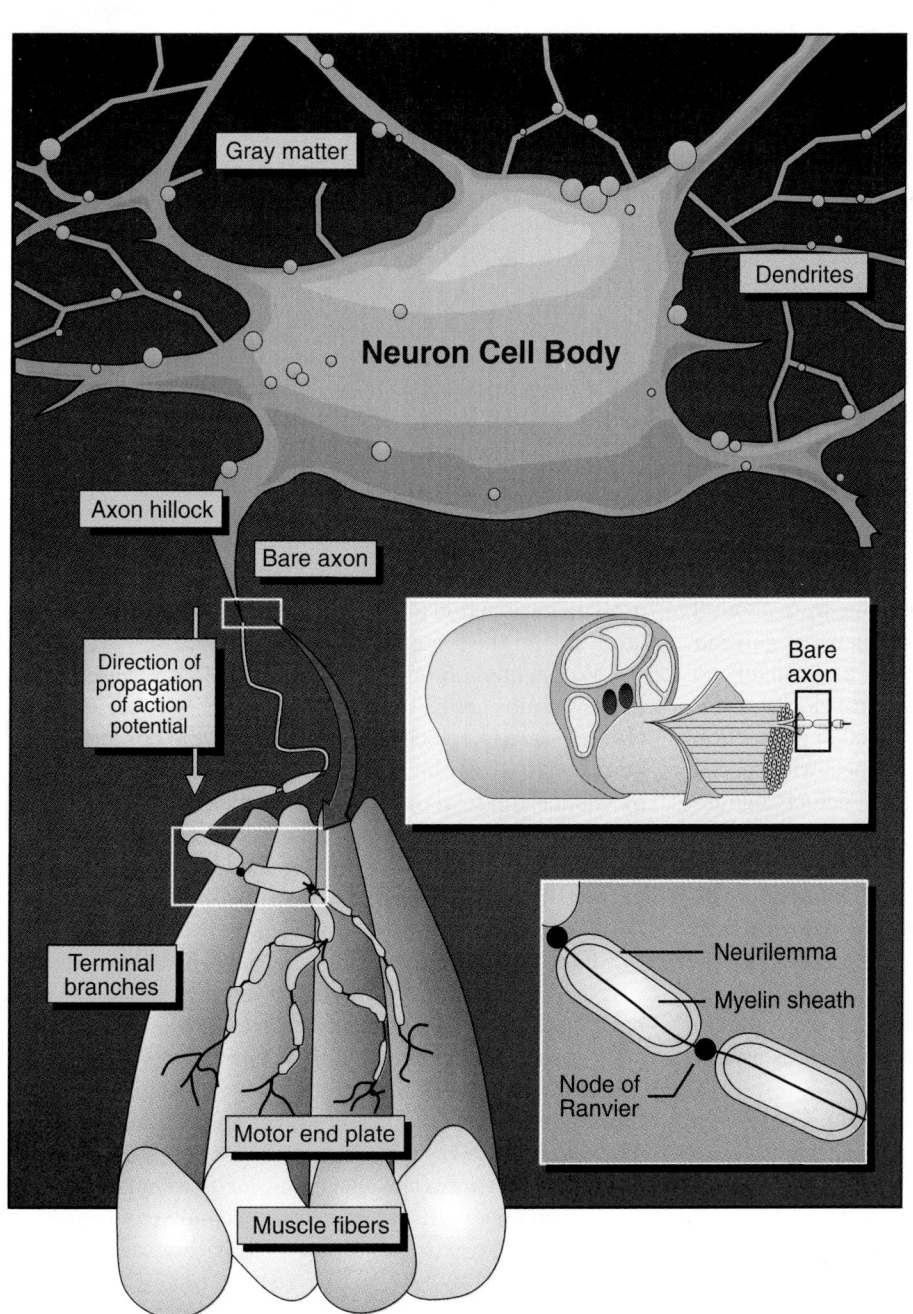

FIGURE 19.6
The anterior motoneuron consists of a cell body, axon, and dendrites. The *top* inset depicts a nerve trunk containing numerous individual nerve fibers, including a bare axon. The *bottom* inset illustrates a node of Ranvier on the bare axon, which permits impulses to "jump" from one node to another as the electrical current travels toward the terminal branches at the motor endplate.

electrochemical impulse from the spinal cord to the muscle. The cell body houses the control center—the structures involved in replication and transmission of the genetic code. This part of the motoneuron is located within the gray matter of the spinal cord. The axon extends from the cord to deliver the impulse to the muscle; the dendrites are the short neural branches that receive impulses through numerous connections and conduct them toward the cell body. Nerve cells conduct impulses in one direction only—down the axon away from the point of stimulation.

The larger nerve fibers are encased in a **myelin sheath,** a lipid-protein membrane that wraps around the axon over most of its length. A specialized cell known as a **Schwann cell** encases the bare axon and then spirals around it, sometimes up to 100 times in the biggest fibers. Myelin forms a large part of this sheath and insulates the axon. A thinner membrane, the **neurilemma,** covers the myelin sheath. The Schwann cells and myelin are interrupted every 1 or 2 millimeters along the axon's length at the **nodes of Ranvier.** Whereas the myelin sheath insulates the axon to the flow of ions, the nodes of Ranvier permit depolarization of the axon to occur. This alternating sequence of myelin sheath and nodes of Ranvier permits impulses to "jump" from node to node (called saltatory conduction) as the electrical current travels toward the terminal branches at the **motor endplate.** This means of conduction is responsible for the higher transmission velocity in myelinated than in unmyelinated fibers. The speed of conduction in a nerve fiber is proportional to its diameter and to the thickness of the myelin sheath. Large, myelinated neurons can conduct an impulse at speeds exceeding 100 m per second (224 mph).

The anterior motoneurons are known also as **type A (α) nerve fibers.** Their diameter is large, ranging from about 8 to 20 μm. Other smaller type A fibers are known as **gamma (γ) efferent motoneurons.** They have a diameter no larger than about 10 μm and a conduction velocity about half that of the larger α fibers. As is discussed in the section on proprioception, the γ efferent fibers connect with special stretch sensors in skeletal muscle that detect minute changes in the length of muscle fibers.

Neuromuscular Junction (Motor Endplate). The interface between the end of a myelinated motoneuron and a muscle fiber is known as the **neuromuscular junction** (NMJ) or **motor endplate.** Its function is to transmit the nerve impulse to the muscle fiber to initiate a muscle action. The details of the neuromuscular junction are illustrated in Figure 19.7. For each skeletal muscle fiber, there is usually only one NMJ.

The NMJ has five common features:[4] (a) presence of a Schwann cell, (b) the terminal section of a neuron that contains the neurotransmitter substance acetylcholine (ACh), (c) a basement membrane that lines the synaptic space, (d) a membrane on the other side of the synaptic space (the postsynaptic membrane) that contains receptors of ACh, and (e) connector microtubules at the postsynaptic membrane that function to transmit the electrical signal to the muscle fiber.

The terminal portion of the axon below the myelin sheath forms several smaller axon branches whose endings are the **presynaptic terminals.** In this region, there are approximately 50 to 70 vesicles that contain ACh per square micrometer.[3, 10] They lie close to but not in contact with the sarcolemma of the muscle fiber. The invaginated region of the **postsynaptic membrane** (also called the **synaptic gutter**) has many infoldings that increase its surface area. The **synaptic cleft** is the region between the synaptic gutter and the presynaptic terminal of the axon. The transmission of the neural impulse takes place in this region.

Excitation. *The process of excitation normally occurs only at the NMJ.* This is facilitated by ACh, the neurotransmitter responsible for changing a basically electrical neural impulse into a chemical stimulus. When an impulse arrives at the NMJ, ACh is released from saclike vesicles within the terminal axons into the synaptic cleft and combines with a transmitter-receptor complex in the postsynaptic membrane. The resulting change in the electrical properties of the postsynaptic membrane elicits an **endplate potential (EPP)** that spreads from the motor endplate to the extrajunctional sarcolemma. This then causes an **action potential** (wave of depolarization) to travel the length of the fiber, enter the T-tubule system, and then travel through the T-tubule system to the inner structures of the muscle fiber. After this occurs, the contractile machinery of the muscle fiber is primed for its major function: contraction. The micrographs at the bottom of Figure 19.7 illustrate the remarkable symmetry between the ACh vesicles at the presynaptic junction (*left side*) and the ACh receptors on the other side of the synaptic cleft (*right side*).

Within about 5 milliseconds after ACh is released from the synaptic vesicles, it is degraded by the enzyme **cholinesterase,** which is concentrated at the borders of the junctional folds at the synaptic cleft. The hydrolysis of ACh by cholinesterase allows the postsynaptic membrane to repolarize. Acetic acid and choline, the end products of cholinesterase action, are resynthesized by the axon to ACh so the entire process can begin again with the arrival of another neural impulse.

Facilitation. When ACh is released from the synaptic vesicles, it excites the postsynaptic membrane of its connecting neuron. This changes the membrane permeability and permits sodium ions to diffuse rapidly into this neuron. An action potential is generated if the change in transmembrane microvoltage (influx of extracellular sodium and efflux of intracellular potassium) is sufficient to reach the **threshold for excitation.** This change in membrane potential at the junction between two neurons, which increases the flow of positive charges to inside the cell, is referred to as the

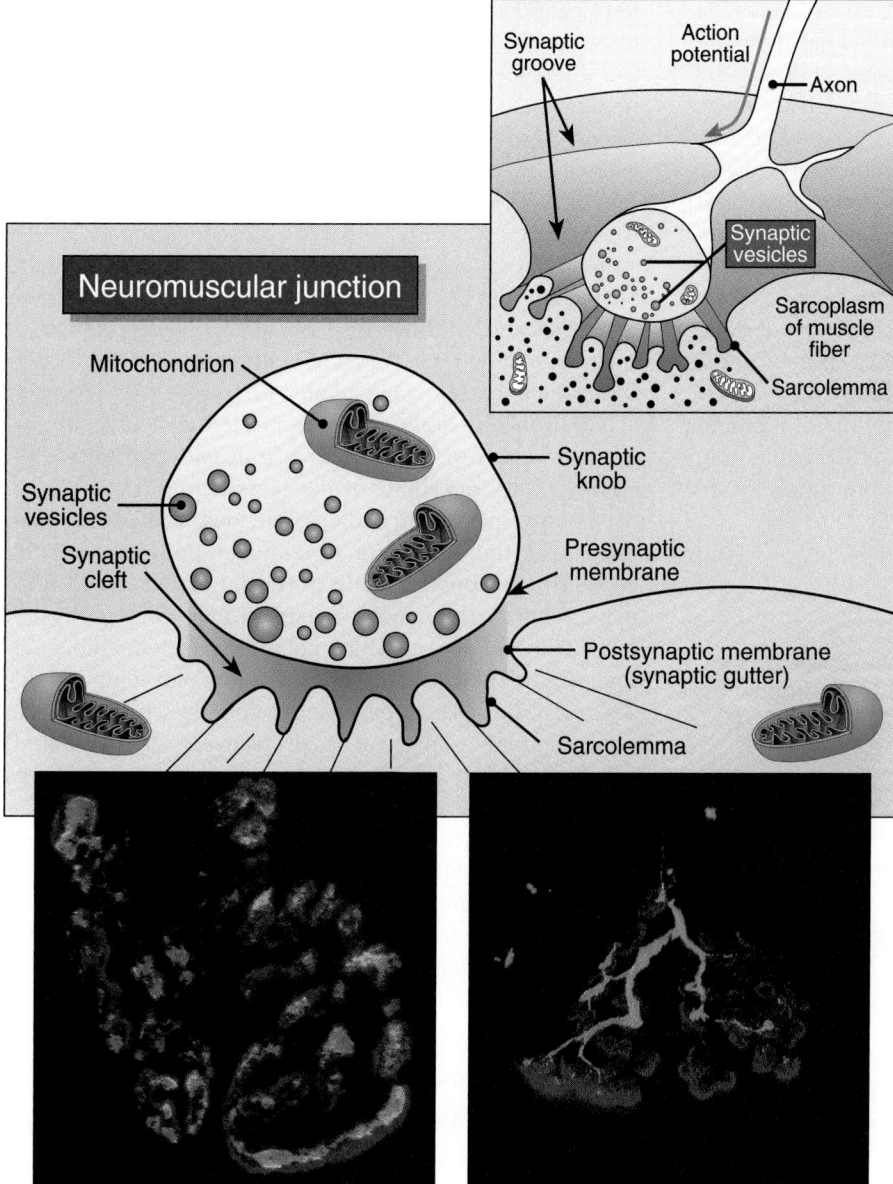

FIGURE 19.7

Microanatomy of the neuromuscular junction. The top insert displays the details of the presynaptic and postsynaptic contact area between the motoneuron and the muscle fiber it innervates. The left micrograph *(bottom)* shows almost perfect symmetry between the "imprint" of the presynaptic vesicles, which contain ACh, and the "imprint" of the postsynaptic receptors, which capture ACh. Green areas indicate ACh vesicles; red staining represents ACh receptors; yellow staining represents zones of colocalization of ACh vesicles and receptors. The right micrograph *(bottom)* illustrates the relationship between presynaptic nerve terminal branches (green) and postsynaptic ACh receptors (red). Magnification × 630. (Micrograph courtesy of Dr. Michael Deschenes, Department of Kinesiology, The College of William and Mary, Williamsburg, VA.)

excitatory postsynaptic potential or **EPSP.** If the EPSP is subthreshold, the neuron does not discharge, but its **resting membrane potential** (usually an electrical potential of −70 mV between the outside and inside of the cell) is lowered and its tendency to "fire" is temporarily increased. The neuron fires when many subthreshold excitatory impulses arrive in rapid succession and the resting membrane potential is lowered to about −50 mV. For neural activity, this condition of repeated subthreshold stimulation is known as **temporal summation.** When different presynaptic terminals on the same neuron are stimulated at the same time, the condition is called **spatial summation.** In this situation, an action potential is initiated as each individual effect is "summed."

Neural facilitation is important under certain exercise conditions. In all-out strength and power activities, for example, the ability to "disinhibit" and maximally activate all motoneurons required for a movement may be crucial to topflight performance.[22] *This enhanced facilitation (disinhibition) could lead to full activation of muscle groups during all-out excitation and probably accounts for the rapid and highly specific strength increases noted during the early stages of strength training.*[14, 15, 18, 23] Neural facilitation also probably accounts for the significant improvements in muscular strength noted during resistance training with only minimal contributions from increases in muscle size.[26] The general response curve for neural factors and muscle size increases during a resistance training program are illustrated in Figure 19.8. The time-course of the response is clear; almost all of the strength improvements at the start of the program occur from neural factors rather than from factors inherent to the muscle. It is noteworthy that neural disinhibition is a phenomenon that affects nerve fibers from the central nervous system rather than modification of electrochemical events at the NMJ. This is because the NMJ does not contain or release inhibitory neurotransmitters.[7] Disinhibition can occur from decreased sensitivity of the cell body of the motoneuron to inhibitory neurotransmitters, there can be less inhibitory neurotransmitter substance transported to the motoneuron at the spinal cord, or a combination of both mechanisms can take place.[4]

Research has considered the effects of physical training on structural changes associated with the NMJ. In one study with rats, endurance training improved the ratio of nerve terminal area to muscle fiber size (by reducing fiber diameter without altering nerve terminal size).[28] In another study with humans, the effects of high-intensity and low-intensity training differentially affected the size of the NMJ.[4] The less intense workouts produced a more expansive NMJ area, whereas higher intensity exercise caused a greater dispersion of synapses. More research is required to further clarify the compensatory effects of exercise training on the structure and function of the NMJ. Central nervous system facilitation and/or disinhibition also is a mechanism to enhance maximal performance by intense concentration or "psyching." The "psychological" influence on strength performance is discussed in Chapter 22.

Inhibition. Some presynaptic terminals set up inhibitory impulses. The inhibitory transmitter substance increases the permeability of the postsynaptic membrane to the efflux of potassium and chloride ions. This produces an increase in the cell's resting membrane potential, creating an **inhibitory postsynaptic potential** or **IPSP.** The IPSP hyperpolarizes the neuron, making it more difficult to fire. If the IPSP is large, no action potential is generated if a motoneuron is subjected to both excitatory and inhibitory influences. The reflex to pull one's hand away when removing a splinter, for example, can usually be overridden (inhibited) so the hand can be steadied to expedite this sometimes painful task.

The exact neurochemical that provokes an IPSP is unknown, although gamma aminobutyric acid (GABA) and the protein glycine are believed to be involved in the inhibitory process. Neural inhibition serves protective functions and reduces the input of "unwanted" stimuli to produce a smooth, purposeful response.

Motor Unit Functional Characteristics

Motor units are composed of fibers of one specific fiber type or a subdivision of a particular fiber type with the same metabolic profile.[19] In addition to anatomic distinctions, Table 19.1 indicates that motor units can be classified based on three physiologic and mechanical properties of the muscle fibers they innervate. These properties include: (*a*) twitch characteristics (force and speed of shortening), (*b*) tension characteristics, and (*c*) fatigability.

TWITCH CHARACTERISTICS

Early experiments in motor unit physiology revealed that motor units developed high, low, or intermediate tension in response to a single electrical impulse. Additionally, the motor units with low force capacity had slow shortening times (and time to peak force) but were fatigue resistant, whereas those with higher force capacity shortened rapidly but were prone to early fatigue. The following characteristics for the three categories of motor units are illustrated in Figure 19.9:

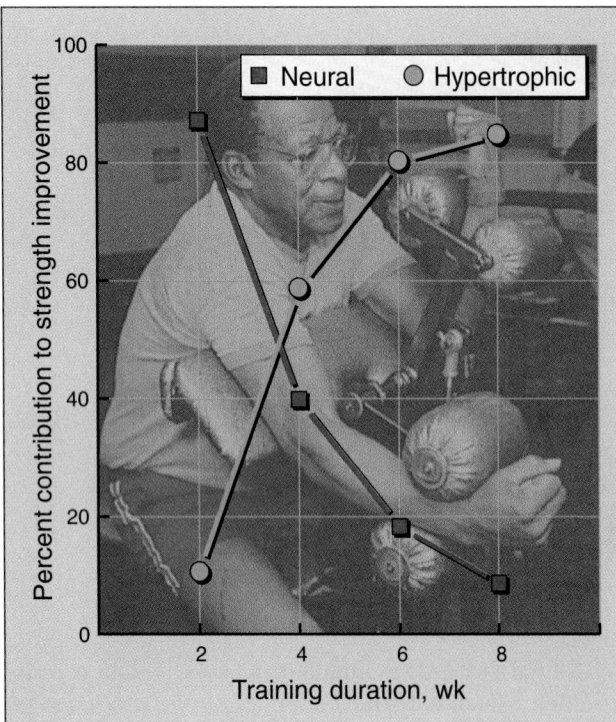

FIGURE 19.8

Generalized response curve for showing gains in muscle strength with resistance training that are due to neural (■) versus muscular (●) factors. During a typical 8-week training period, approximately 90% of the strength gained during the first 2 weeks is from neural factors. In the subsequent 2 weeks, between 40 and 50% of the strength improvement is still related to adaptation within the nervous system. Thereafter, adaptations within the muscle fibers become progressively more important to strength improvement. In experiments of this type, the neural factors are evaluated from integrated electromyographic recordings of the muscle groups being trained.

TABLE 19.1
CHARACTERISTICS AND CORRESPONDENCE BETWEEN MOTOR UNITS AND MUSCLE FIBER TYPES

Motor Unit Designation	Force Production	Contraction Speed	Fatigue Resistance	Sag[a]	Muscle Fiber Type in the Motor Unit
Fast Fatigable (FF)	High	Fast	Low	Yes	Fast Glycolytic (FG)
Fast Fatigue-Resistant (FR)	Moderate	Fast	High	Yes	Fast Oxidative-Glycolytic (FOG)
Slow (S)	Low	Slow	High	No	Slow Oxidative (SO)

Modified from Lieber, R. L.: *Skeletal Muscle Structure and Function: Implications for Rehabilitation and Sports Medicine.* Baltimore, Williams & Wilkins, 1992.

[a]Under repetitive stimuli, some motor units respond smoothly with a systematic increase in tension, while others first increase tension and then decrease or "sag" slightly in response to the same tetanic stimulus. These sag characteristics can be used to classify the different motor units. Only the S motor units do not exhibit sag, which is probably related more to their diminished force generating capabilities than to their fatigue characteristic.

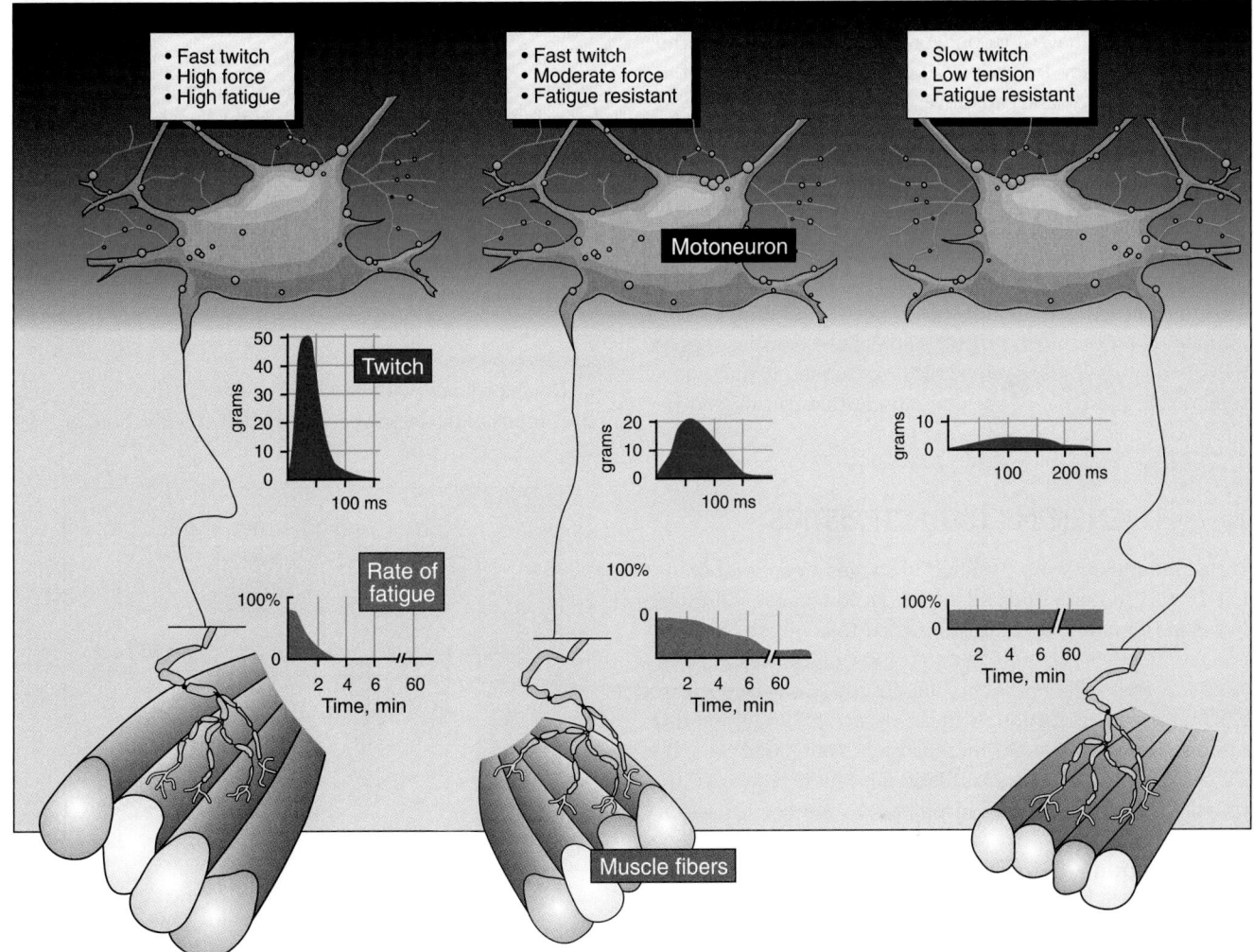

FIGURE 19.9
Speed, force, and fatigue characteristics of motor units. Motoneurons that fire rapidly with short bursts are termed "phasic," whereas those that fire slowly but continuously are considered "tonic."

- Fast twitch, high force, and fast fatigue (type IIb).
- Fast twitch, moderate force, and fatigue resistant (type IIa).
- Slow twitch, low tension, and fatigue resistant (type I).

The two subdivisions of fast-twitch muscle fibers are innervated by relatively large motoneurons with fast conduction velocities. These motor units generally contain between 300 and 500 muscle fibers. The fast-fatigable (FF) and fast-fatigue-resistant (FR) units reach greater peak tension and develop it much faster than slow-twitch (S) motor units, which are innervated by smaller motoneurons with slow conduction velocities. The slower contracting units, however, are more fatigue-resistant than the fast-twitch units. As was discussed in Chapter 18 (refer to p. 334), the particular metabolic characteristics of all muscle fibers can be modified by specific exercise training. *With prolonged aerobic training, for example, fast-twitch muscle fibers can become almost as fatigue resistant as their slow-twitch counterparts.*

There is some evidence that the particular motoneurons themselves have a trophic or stimulating effect on the muscle fibers they innervate in a way that modulates the fibers' properties and adaptive response to stimuli.[11, 12] Innervating fast-twitch muscle fibers with the neuron from a slow-twitch motor unit, for example, eventually alters the twitch characteristics of the fast-contracting fibers. Furthermore, the application of a chronic, low frequency stimulation to intact fast-twitch motor units induces a conversion of the muscle fibers to the slow-twitch type.[16, 20] If this neurotrophic effect is as great as believed, then the myoneural junction takes on much greater significance than just being the site of muscle fiber depolarization. In fact, it suggests a remarkable plasticity of skeletal muscle that can indeed be altered with chronic use.

TENSION CHARACTERISTICS

If the stimulus is strong enough to trigger an action potential in the motoneuron, all of the accompanying muscle fibers in the motor unit are stimulated to contract synchronously. There is no such thing as a strong or weak action from a motor unit—either the impulse is strong enough to elicit an action or it is not. After the neuron is "fired" and the impulse reaches the neuromuscular junctions, all of the motor unit's muscle fibers act at that time. This is known as the principle of **"all-or-none"** in relation to the normal action of skeletal muscle.

Gradation of Force. The force of muscle action is varied from slight to maximal in two ways:

- Increasing the **number** of motor units recruited for the activity.
- Increasing their **frequency** of discharge.

The force generated is considerable if all of a muscle's motor units are activated. Also, if repetitive stimuli reach a muscle before it has relaxed, there is a further increase in the total tension produced. By blending these two factors, recruitment of motor units and the rate of their firing, optimal patterns of neural discharge permit a wide variety of graded muscle actions—from the delicate touch required in eye surgery to the maximal effort in throwing a baseball from deep center field to home plate.

Motor Unit Activity. Few motor units are activated for low-force muscle actions, whereas higher force progressively enlists more motor units. The process of adding more motor units to increase muscle force is known as **motor unit recruitment.** As muscle force increases, motoneurons with progressively larger axons are recruited. This is known as the **size principle,** which provides an anatomic basis for the orderly recruitment of specific motor units to produce a smooth muscle action.

All of the motor units in a muscle do not fire at the same time (Fig. 19.10). If they did, it would be virtually impossible to control muscle force output. Consider the tremendous gradation of forces and speeds that muscles generate. For example, when lifting a barbell, specific muscles act to move the limb at a particular speed under a particular rate of tension development. If the weight is relatively light, it can be lifted at a number of speeds. If a heavier weight is used, however, the speed options decrease accordingly. With a light object such as a pencil, the proper force is generated to lift the pencil regardless of how fast or slow the arm is moved. *From the standpoint of neural control, the fast-twitch and slow-twitch motor units are selectively recruited and modulated in their firing pattern to produce the desired response.*

In accordance with the size principle, the slow-twitch motor units, with the lowest threshold for activation, are se-

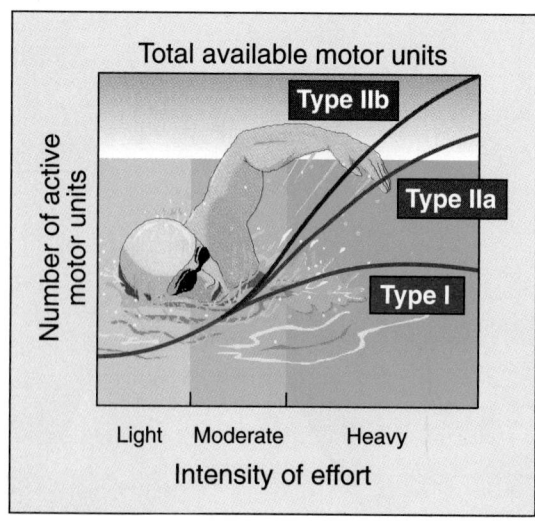

FIGURE 19.10

Recruitment of slow-twitch and fast-twitch muscle fibers (motor units) in relation to the intensity of exercise. As the effort becomes more intense, progressively more fast-twitch fibers are recruited.

lectively recruited during lighter effort. These slow-twitch fibers are activated during sustained activities such as jogging or cycling on a level grade or during slow swimming or slowly lifting a light weight. For more rapid, powerful movements, there is a progressive activation of the more powerful fast-twitch fatigue-resistant (type IIa) fibers up through the fast-twitch fatigable units (type IIb) when peak force is required.[5, 9, 24] More than likely, as a runner or cyclist reaches a hill during a distance race, some fast-twitch units also are activated so that a constant pace can be maintained over varying terrain.

The differential control of the motor unit firing pattern is a major factor that distinguishes not only skilled from unskilled performances but also distinguishes specific athletic groups.[6] For example, weight lifters generally demonstrate a synchronous pattern of motor unit firing (i.e., many motor units are recruited simultaneously during lifting), whereas the firing pattern of endurance athletes is more asynchronous (i.e., some units fire while others recover).[25] As discussed previously, the compositional characteristics of a muscle in terms of its specific motor units (muscle fibers) also contribute to the performance characteristics of various athletes.[2, 27] In addition, the synchronous firing of a muscle's fast-twitch motor units certainly aids the weight lifter in generating force quickly for the desired lift. For the endurance athlete, on the other hand, the asynchronous firing of predominantly slow-twitch, fatigue-resistant units provides a built-in recuperative period to permit performance to continue with minimal fatigue as the various motor units share the burden of exercise.

Neuromuscular Fatigue

Fatigue is defined as the decline in muscle tension capacity with repeated stimulation. Motor unit fatigue is the result of many factors, each of which is related to the specific demands of the exercise that produces it.[1, 17] These factors can interact in a manner that ultimately affects either contraction or excitation or both.

Voluntary muscle actions have four main components. These are as follows, in order of nervous system hierarchy:

- Central nervous system.
- Peripheral nervous system.
- Neuromuscular junction.
- Muscle fiber function.

Fatigue results if the chain of events is interrupted between the central nervous system and the muscle fiber, independent of the reason. For example:

- A significant reduction in the glycogen content of the active muscle fibers is related to fatigue during prolonged submaximal exercise. This "nutrient fatigue" occurs even though sufficient oxygen is available to generate energy through aerobic pathways.

- Muscle fatigue in short-term, maximal exercise is associated with oxygen lack and an increased level of blood and muscle lactic acid. Accompanying this lactate accumulation is a dramatic increase in H^+ concentration in the active muscle, which can dramatically affect the intracellular environment.[21] These alterations in contractile function are related to a depletion of intramuscular high-energy phosphates, an impaired glycolytic energy transfer capacity owing to reduced activity of key enzymes, a disturbance in the tubule system for transmitting the impulse throughout the cell, and ionic imbalances.[13] Certainly a change in Ca^{2+} distribution could alter the activity of the myofilaments and impair muscular performance. This would cause fatigue even though nerve impulses continue to bombard the muscle fiber.

- Fatigue also occurs at the neuromuscular junction when an action potential fails to cross from the motoneuron to the muscle fiber. The precise mechanism for this aspect of "neural fatigue" is unknown.

As muscle function becomes impaired during prolonged submaximal exercise, additional motor-unit recruitment takes place to maintain the required force output for the activity. In all-out exercise, when all motor units are presumably maximally activated, fatigue is accompanied by a decrease in neural activity (as measured by the electromyogram, or EMG). A decrease in neural activity supports the contention that this form of fatigue is caused by a failure in neural or myoneural transmission.

RECEPTORS IN MUSCLES, JOINTS, AND TENDONS: THE PROPRIOCEPTORS

Specialized sensory receptors in the muscles and tendons are sensitive to stretch, tension, and pressure. These end organs, known as **proprioceptors,** rapidly relay information concerning muscular dynamics and limb movement to conscious and subconscious portions of the central nervous system. This enables the progress of any sequence of movements to be continually charted to provide a basis for modifying subsequent motor behavior.

MUSCLE SPINDLES

The **muscle spindles** provide sensory information regarding the changes in the length and tension of muscle fibers. Their main function is to respond to stretch of a muscle and, through reflex action, to initiate a stronger muscle action to reduce this stretch.

Structural Organization. As shown in Figure 19.11, a muscle spindle is fusiform in shape and is aligned in parallel to the regular muscle fibers, or **extrafusal fibers.** Consequently, when the muscle is stretched, the spindle is stretched as well. The number of spindles contained per

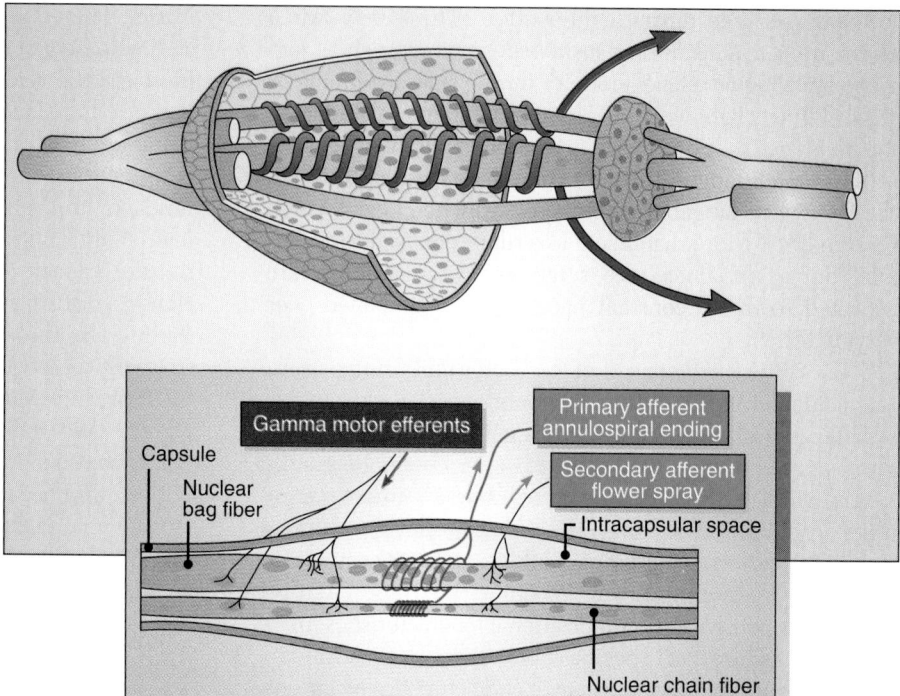

FIGURE 19.11
Structural organization of the muscle spindle. The insert shows an enlarged view of the equatorial region of the spindle.

gram of muscle varies depending on the muscle group. On a relative basis, there are more spindles in muscles involved in complex movements than in those performing gross patterns of movement. The spindle, covered by a sheath of connective tissue, contains two specialized types of muscle fiber called **intrafusal fibers.** One type of intrafusal fiber, the **nuclear bag fiber,** is fairly large, with numerous nuclei centrally packed through its diameter. There are usually two nuclear bag fibers per spindle. The other type of intrafusal fiber, the **nuclear chain fiber,** contains many nuclei along its length. These fibers are attached to the surface of the longer nuclear bag fibers. There usually are four to five chain fibers in each spindle. The ends of the intrafusal fibers contain actin and myosin filaments and are capable of shortening.

Three different types of nerve fibers service the spindles; two are sensory afferent and one is a motor efferent fiber. A primary afferent nerve fiber is entwined about the midregion of the bag fiber. This is the **annulospiral nerve fiber,** which responds directly to the stretch of the spindle; its firing frequency is proportional to the degree of stretch. A second group of smaller, sensory nerve fibers known as **flower-spray endings** makes connections mainly on the chain fibers, although there also are attachments to the bag fibers. These endings are less sensitive to stretch than the annulospiral fibers. Activation of the annulospiral and flower-spray sensors relays impulses through the dorsal root into the cord to cause a reflex activation of the motoneurons to the stretched muscle. This causes the muscle to act more

forcefully and to shorten and, in turn, reduces the stretch stimulus from the spindles.

The third type of spindle nerve fiber has a motor function. These are the thin **gamma efferent fibers** that innervate the contractile, striated ends of the intrafusal fibers. These fibers, activated by higher centers in the brain, provide the mechanism for maintaining optimal sensitivity of the spindle at all muscle lengths. Gamma efferent stimulation activates the intrafusal fibers, thereby regulating their length and sensitivity regardless of the overall length of the muscle itself. This mechanism prepares the spindle for other lengthening actions that may occur, even though the muscle itself already may be shortened. These adjustments in gamma efferent activation enable the spindle to monitor continuously the length of the muscles where they are located.

The Stretch Reflex. The functional significance of the muscle spindle is its ability to detect, respond to, and modulate changes in the length of the extrafusal muscle fibers. This is important in the regulation of movement and the maintenance of posture. Postural muscles are continuously bombarded by neural input; they must maintain their readiness to respond to conscious (voluntary) movements. They must also, however, maintain some degree of constant subconscious activity to counter the pull of gravity in upright posture. To this end, the stretch reflex is a fundamental controlling mechanism.

The stretch reflex has three main components: (*a*) the muscle spindle that responds to stretch, (*b*) an afferent nerve fiber that carries the sensory impulse from the spindle to the spinal cord, and (c) an efferent motoneuron in the spinal cord that activates the stretched muscle fibers.

The neural pathways in the stretch reflex are illustrated in Figure 19.12. In Figure 19.12A, the biceps muscle is activated to maintain the bony lever at a 90° angle while holding a book. If the book is suddenly increased twofold in weight (Fig. 19.12B), the muscle fibers would become stretched. This causes the spindles' sensory endings to direct impulses through the dorsal root into the spinal cord, where they directly activate the motoneurons. The resulting neural impulses (Fig. 19.12C) cause the muscle to act more forcefully and return the limb to its original position. During this reflex process, interneurons within the cord also are activated to facilitate the appropriate motor response. Excitatory impulses are conveyed to muscles (known as **synergistic** muscles) that support the desired movement, while inhibitory impulses flow to the motor units of muscles,

which are **antagonists** of the movement. In this way, the stretch reflex acts as a self-regulating, compensating mechanism; it enables the muscle to adjust automatically to differences in load (and length) without requiring an immediate processing of information through higher centers of the central nervous system.

GOLGI TENDON ORGANS

In contrast to the muscle spindles that lie parallel to the extrafusal muscle fibers, the **Golgi tendon organs** are connected in series to as many as 25 extrafusal fibers within the tendons near the junction of the muscle. These sensory receptors detect differences in the tension generated by active muscle rather than muscle length. As shown in Figure 19.13, the Golgi tendon organs respond as a feedback monitor to discharge impulses under either of two conditions: (a) in response to tension created in the muscle

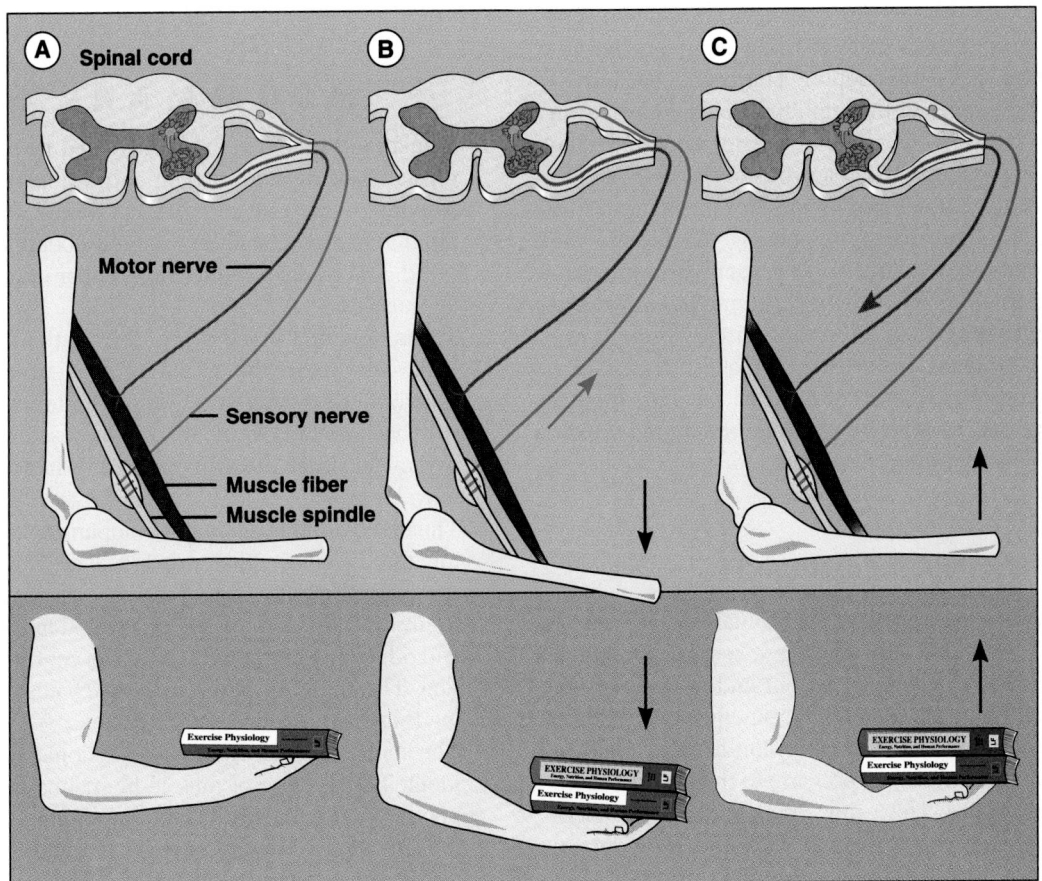

FIGURE 19.12
Schematic representation of the stretch reflex. Because the spindles are arranged in parallel with the extrafusal fibers, they become stretched when these fibers are elongated. The spindle's sensory receptors fire when its intrafusal fibers are stretched. This activation of the spindle's sensory receptors reflexly stimulates the alpha motoneurons and activates the extrafusal muscle fibers, causing them to shorten. This reduces the stretch of the intrafusal fibers and silences the spindle afferents. In the diagram, the stretch reflex acts as a self-regulating mechanism to maintain the relative constancy of limb position.

FIGURE 19.13

The Golgi tendon organ. Excessive tension or stretch on a muscle activates the tendon's Golgi receptors, which brings about a reflex inhibition of the muscles they supply. In this way, the Golgi tendon organ functions as a protective sensory mechanism to detect and subsequently inhibit undue strain within the muscle-tendon structure. The Golgi structure was named after the Italian anatomist Camillo Golgi, who described them in the late 1800s.)

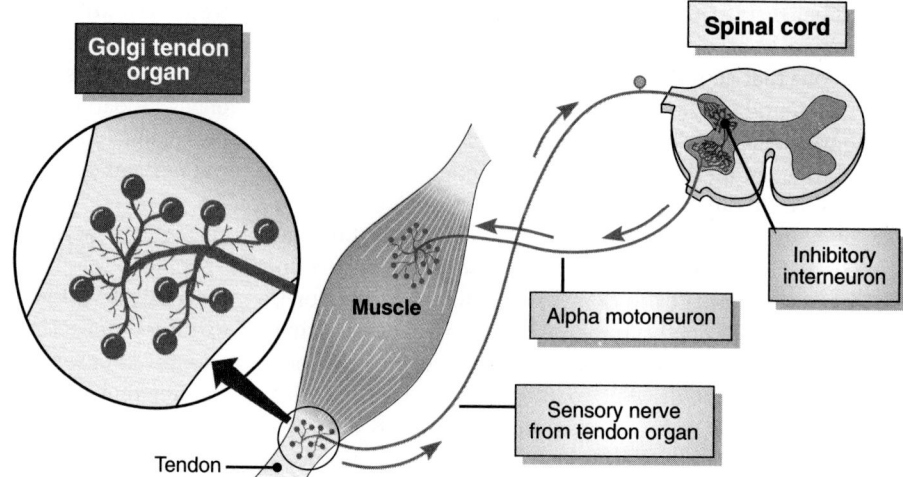

when it shortens and (b) in response to tension when the muscle is stretched passively.

When stimulated by excessive tension, the Golgi receptors conduct their signals rapidly to bring about a **reflex inhibition** of the muscles they supply. This occurs because of the overriding influence of the inhibitory spinal interneuron on the motoneurons supplying the muscle. Therefore, the Golgi tendon organ functions as a protective sensory mechanism or "governor," much as a suppressor mechanism that keeps motorized "go-carts" from moving too fast. If the change in tension is too great, the sensor's discharge increases; this depresses the activity of the motoneurons and reduces the tension generated in the muscle fibers. If the muscle action produces little tension, Golgi receptors are only weakly activated and exert little influence. *The ultimate function of the Golgi tendon organs is to protect the muscle and its connective tissue harness from injury due to an excessive load.*

PACINIAN CORPUSCLES

Pacinian corpuscles are small, ellipsoidal bodies located close to the Golgi tendon organs. These sensory receptors, which are sensitive to quick movement and deep pressure, are embedded in a single, nonmyelinated nerve fiber. Deformation or compression of the onion-like capsule by a mechanical stimulus transmits pressure to the sensory nerve ending within its core. This produces a change in the electric potential of the nerve ending. If this **generator potential** is of sufficient magnitude, a sensory signal is established and propagated down the myelinated axon that leaves the corpuscle.

Pacinian corpuscles are "fast-adapting" mechanical sensors because they discharge a few impulses at the onset of a steady stimulus and then remain electrically silent or may discharge a second volley of impulses when the stimulus is removed. Consequently, they detect **changes** in movement

or pressure, rather than how much movement occurred or how much pressure was applied.

■ SUMMARY ■

1. Human movement is finely regulated by neural control mechanisms located in the central nervous system. In response to internal and external stimuli, bits of sensory input are automatically and rapidly coded, routed, organized, and transmitted to the effector organ, the skeletal muscles.

2. Tracts of neural tissue descend from the brain to influence neurons in the spinal cord. Neurons in the extrapyramidal tract control posture and provide a continual background level of neuromuscular tone; the pyramidal tract neurons provide discrete muscular movement.

3. The cerebellum is the major comparing, evaluating, and integrating center that provides the "fine-tuning" for muscle activity.

4. Many muscle functions are controlled in the spinal cord and other subconscious areas of the central nervous system. The reflex arc is the basic mechanism for processing these "automatic" muscle actions.

5. The motor unit is the basic functional unit of movement. The number of muscle fibers in a motor unit depends on the muscle's movement function. Intricate movement patterns require a small fiber-to-neuron ratio, whereas a single neuron may innervate several thousand muscle fibers for gross movements.

6. The anterior motoneuron (cell body, axon, and dendrites) transmits the electrochemical nerve impulse from the spinal cord to the muscle. The dendrites receive impulses and conduct them toward the cell body, whereas the axon transmits the impulse in one direction only—down the axon to the muscle.

7. The neuromuscular junction (NMJ) is the interface between the motoneuron and the muscle fiber. Acetylcholine (ACh) release at the NMJ provides the chemical stimulus that activates the muscle fiber.

8. The following sequence of events occur between stimulation of a motoneuron and the generation of an action potential: (*a*) the action potential is propagated down the axon, (*b*) calcium channels open at the end of the nerve terminal, (*c*) calcium moves into the nerve terminal, (*d*) ACh is "primed," (*e*) ACh traverses the synapse and binds to ACh receptors on the postsynaptic membrane at the interface of the sarcolemma, and (*f*) an endplate potential is generated and a depolarization spreads through the T-tubular network.

9. Both excitatory and inhibitory impulses continually bombard the synaptic junctions between neurons. These alter a neuron's threshold for excitation by either increasing or decreasing its tendency to "fire." During all-out power exercise, a high degree of neural facilitation (disinhibition) is beneficial because it enables maximal activation of a muscle's motor units.

10. There are three types of motor units, depending on the speed of muscle action, force generated, and fatigability: (*a*) fast twitch, high force, and high fatigue, (*b*) fast twitch, moderate force, and fatigue resistant, and (*c*) slow twitch, low tension, and fatigue resistant.

11. Gradation of muscle force is accomplished through an interaction of factors that regulate the number and type of motor units recruited as well as their frequency of discharge. Light exercise is accomplished through predominant recruitment of slow-twitch motor units, followed by activation of fast-twitch units when a more powerful force is required.

12. Alterations in motor unit recruitment and firing pattern probably explain a large portion of the strength improvement with resistance training, especially during the early stages of training.

13. Special sensory receptors in muscles, tendons, and joints relay information concerning muscular dynamics and limb movement to specific portions of the central nervous system. This provides important sensory feedback during physical activity.

■ REFERENCES ■

1. Asmussen, E.: Muscle fatigue. *Med. Sci. Sports Exerc.*, 25:412, 1993.
2. Bergh, U., et al.: Maximal oxygen uptake and muscle fiber types in trained and untrained humans. *Med. Sci. Sports*, 10:151, 1978.
3. DeCamilli, P., et al.: Synapsin I (protein I), a nerve-terminal-specific phosphoprotein. II. Its specific association with synaptic vesicles demonstrated by immunocytochemistry in agorose-embedded synaptosomes. *J. Cell Biol.*, 96:1355, 1983.
4. Deschenes, M.R., et al.: The neuromuscular junction: structure, function, and its role in the excitation of muscle. *J. Strength Cond. Res.*, 8:103, 1994.
5. Edgerton, V.R.: Mammalian muscle fiber types and their adaptability. *Am. Zoology*, 18:113, 1978.
6. Edgerton, V.R., et al.: The matching of neuronal and muscular physiology. In *Frontiers of Exercise Biology*. Edited by K. T. Borer, et al. Champaign, IL, Human Kinetics, 1991.
7. Engle, A.G.: The neuromuscular junction. In *Myology, Basic and Clinical*. Edited by A.G. Engle and B. Banker. New York, McGraw-Hill, 1986.
8. Feinstein, B., et al.: Morphologic studies of motor units in normal human muscle. *Acta Anat. (Basel)*, 23:127, 1955.
9. Freund, H.J.: Motor unit and muscle activity in voluntary motor control. *Physiol. Rev.*, 63:387, 1983.
10. Gershon, M.D., et al,: Morphology of chemical synapses and patterns of interconnection. In *Principles of Neural Science*. Edited by E.R. Kandel and J.H. Schwartz. New York, Elsevier North Holland, 1985.
11. Gordon, T., and Pattullo, M. C.: Plasticity of muscle fiber and motor unit types. *Exerc. Sport Sci. Rev.*, 21:331, 1993.
12. Gutman, E.: Neurotrophic relations. *Annu. Rev. Physiol.*, 38:177, 1976.
13. Hermansen, L.: Effect of metabolic changes on force generation in skeletal muscle during maximal exercise. In *Human Muscle Fatigue: Physiological Mechanisms*. London, Pitman Medical, 1981.
14. Häkkinen, K., and Komi, P.V.: Electromyographic changes during strength training and detraining. *Med. Sci. Sports Exerc.*, 15:455, 1983.
15. Häkkinen, K., et al.: Effect of combined concentric and eccentric strength training and detraining on force-time, muscle fiber, and metabolic characteristics of leg extensor muscles. *Scand. J. Sports Sci.*, 3:50, 1981.
16. Kraus, W.E., et al.: Skeletal muscle adaptation to chronic low-frequency motor nerve stimulation. *Exerc. Sport Sci. Rev.*, 22:313, 1994.
17. MacLaren, C.P., et al.: A review of metabolic and physiologic factors in fatigue. *Exerc. Sport Sci. Rev.*, 17:29, 1989.
18. Moratini, T., and DeVries, H.: Neural factors versus hypertrophy in the time course of muscle strength gain. *Am. J. Phys. Med.*, 58:115, 1979.
19. Nemete, P., et al.: Comparison of enzyme activities among single muscle fibers within defined motor units. *J. Physiol.*, 311:489, 1985.
20. Pette, D., and Vrbova, G.: Invited review: neural control of phenotypic expression in mammalian muscle fibers. *Muscle Nerve*, 8:676, 1985.
21. Sahlin, K.: Intracellular pH and energy metabolism in skeletal muscle of man. *Acta Physiol. Scand.*, 455(Suppl.):1, 1978.
22. Sale, D.G.: Influence of exercise and training on motor unit activation. In *Exercise and Sport Sciences Reviews*. Vol. 15. Edited by K.B. Pandolf. New York, Macmillan, 1987.
23. Sale, D.G., et al.: Neural adaptation to resistance training. *Med. Sci. Sports Exerc.*, 20:S135, 1988.
24. Spectar, S.A., et al.: Muscle architecture and force-velocity characteristics of cat soleus and medial gastrocnemius: implications for motor control. *J. Neurobiol.*, 44:951, 1980.
25. Stepanov, A.S., and Burlakov, M.L.: Electrophysiological investigation of fatigue in muscular activity. *Sechenov Physiol. J. USSR*, 47:43, 1961.
26. Tesch, P.A., et al.: Effects of strength training on G tolerance. *Aviat. Space Environ. Med.*, 54:691, 1984.
27. Tesch, P.A., and Karlsson, J.: Muscle fiber type and size in trained and untrained muscles of elite athletes. *J. Appl. Physiol.*, 59:1716, 1985.
28. Waerhaug, O., et al.: Different effects of physical training on the morphology of motor nerve terminals in the rat extensor digitorum longus and soleus muscles. *Anat. Embryol.*, 186:125, 1992.

Weltman, A., et al.: Endurance training amplifies the pulsatile release of growth hormone: effects of training intensity. _J. Appl. Physiol._ 72:2188, 1992.

Recent research has focused on growth hormone (GH) responses to a single session of exercise and long-term training. While most investigators report that a period of intense exercise increases the subject's plasma concentration of GH, there is less information on GH levels during long-term exercise training. The dynamics of GH

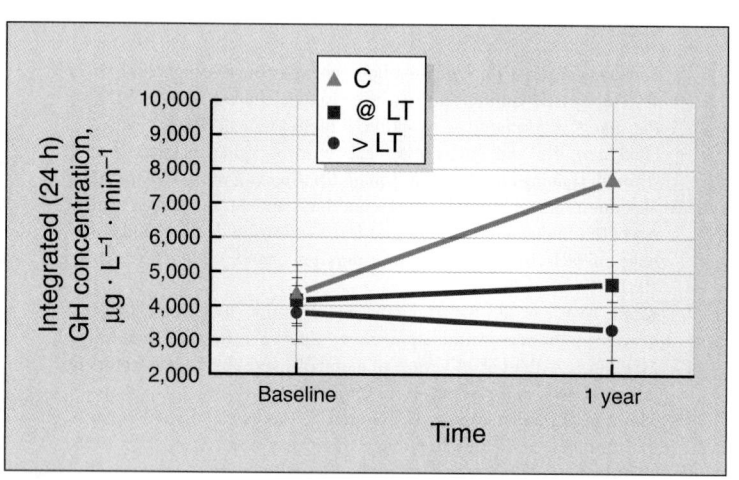

Integrated 24-hour GH concentrations for the control and exercise groups. Note the large (50%) increase in GH concentration for the >LT group compared to the group that trained at LT and the control group.

secretions during exercise training assumes clinical importance because of the causal relationship between GH availability and the maintenance of lean body tissue in aging and obesity and during weight loss.

Weltman and colleagues studied the GH response to a 52-week aerobic run training program in 21 healthy, eumenorrheic women. There were two training groups: one ran at a speed corresponding to their lactate threshold (@LT), and one at a relatively faster speed above their lac-

tate threshold level (>LT). Nontraining subjects served as a control group. Both training groups completed similar weekly mileage. The distance covered during the first week was 5 miles; the weekly mileage gradually increased to 24 miles per week by week 20 and continued at 24 miles per week until week 40. Thereafter, weekly mileage increased by 1.25 miles for three of the weeks. Subjects ran between 35 and 40 miles per week by the end of the study.

The year-long training program increased $\dot{V}o_2$max by 9.9% for the @LT group and by 11.8% for the >LT group. In addition, the @LT group increased exercise $\dot{V}o_2$ at their lactate threshold ($\dot{V}o_2$-LT) by 21.5%, while the >LT group's $\dot{V}o_2$-LT increased by 28%. No changes occurred for the control group. No differences in body mass, percent body fat, or body fat mass emerged among or within groups, although the >LT group showed a trend for reducing percent fat. Both training groups, however, increased their fat-free body mass with training.

The figure presents the effects of the run training program on 24-hour integrated serum GH concentrations. The main finding for the >LT group included a marked increase of 50% in resting GH concentration. For the control group and the @LT group, the integrated 24-hour GH concentrations remained unaffected. The investigators speculated that relatively heavy exercise (like that performed by the >LT group) facilitated GH secretion by causing the release of endogenous opiates and catecholamines while at the same time inhibiting somatostatin release.

This research showed that exercise training augments the pulsatile release of GH at rest by amplitude enhancement, but only when training intensity occurs above the LT. Training at intensities above the LT may be a useful way to increase pulsatile secretion of GH in conditions associated with decreased GH release, as for example in aging and obesity (in which there is often an accompanying loss of fat-free body mass).

The Endocrine System and Exercise

The endocrine system helps integrate and control bodily functions and thus provides stability to the body's internal environment. Hormones produced by endocrine glands affect almost all aspects of human function. They regulate growth, development, and reproduction and augment the body's capability for handling physical and psychological stress. Hormones contribute to the maintenance of internal equilibrium (homeostasis) by modulating electrolyte and acid-base balance and the specific mixture of fuels used to power biologic work. The following sections provide a general overview of various aspects of the endocrine system, its functions at rest and during physical activity, and its response to the chronic demands of exercise training.

ENDOCRINE SYSTEM OVERVIEW

The endocrine glands are quite small compared to other organs in the body; combined, they weigh only approximately 0.5 kg. The major endocrine organs include the pituitary, thyroid, parathyroid, adrenal, pineal, and thymus glands; the locations of these organs are shown in Figure 20.1. Several other body organs contain discrete areas of endocrine tissue that also produce hormones. These include the pancreas, gonads (ovaries and testes), and the hypothalamus, which is also a major organ of the nervous system; consequently, the hypothalamus is considered a **neuroendocrine organ.** Pockets of hormone-producing cells also are found in the walls of the small intestine, stomach, kidneys, and heart, although these organs have little to do with hormone production per se.

ENDOCRINE SYSTEM ORGANIZATION

The endocrine system consists of a host organ (gland), minute quantities of chemical messengers (hormones), and a target or receptor organ. Glands can be classified as either **endocrine** or **exocrine.** Some glands can serve both functions.

Endocrine glands have no ducts and are referred to as "ductless glands." They secrete substances directly into the extracellular spaces around the gland. As shown in Figure 20.2, these hormones then diffuse into the blood for transport throughout the body to fulfill their function for intercellular communication. It is customary to use the term "endocrine" in the same context as "hormone secreting." Exocrine glands, on the other hand, have secretory ducts that carry substances directly to a specific compartment or surface. Almost all exocrine glands are controlled by the nervous system. Examples of exocrine glands include sweat glands and glands of the upper digestive tract.

NATURE OF HORMONES

Hormones are chemical substances synthesized by a specific host gland, secreted into the blood, and carried throughout the body. Hormones generally fall into two distinct "chemical" categories: (*a*) hormones derived from **steroid** compounds and (*b*) hormones that are amino acid or **polypep-**

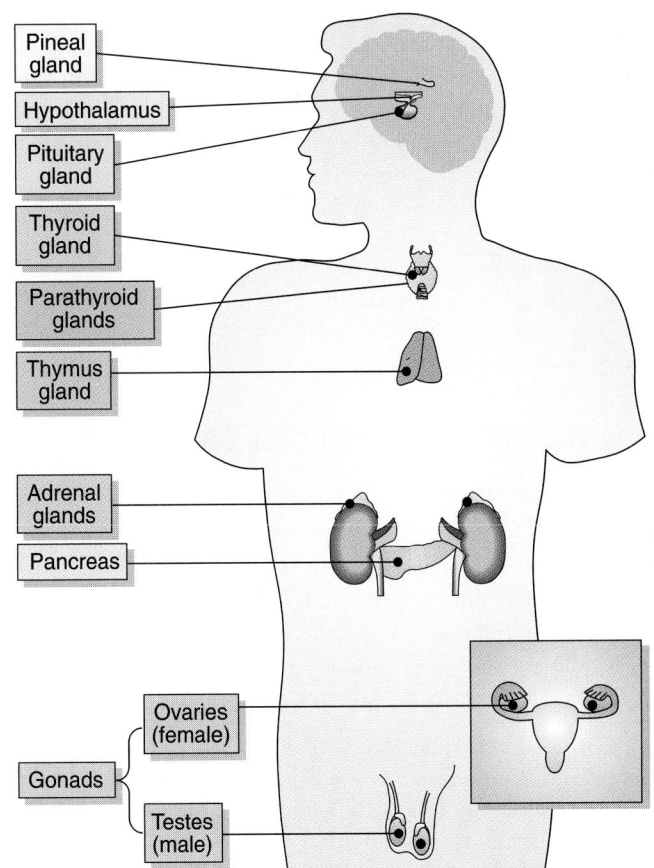

FIGURE 20.1
Location of the hormone-producing endocrine organs.

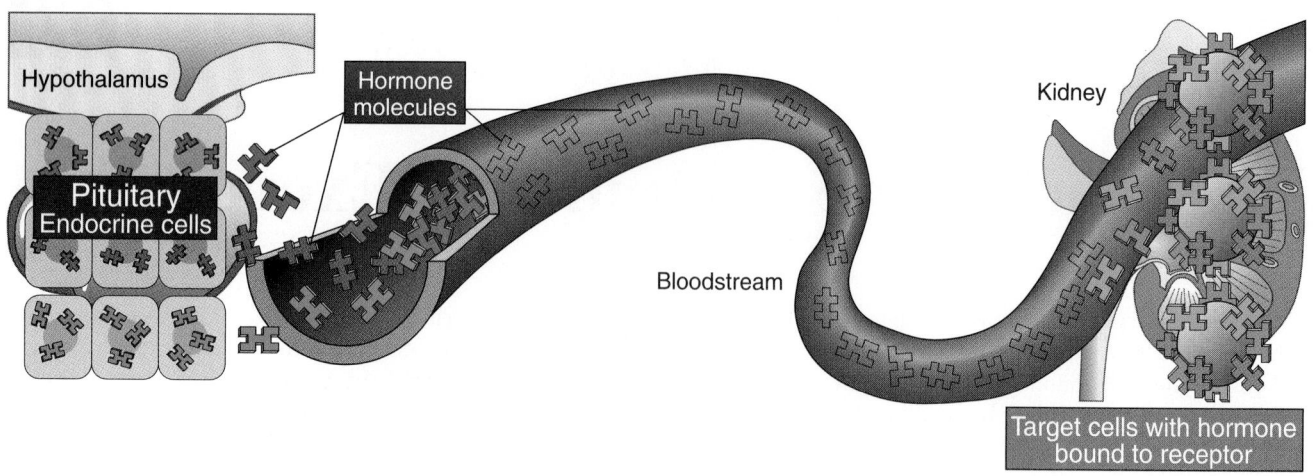

FIGURE 20.2
Hormones secreted from endocrine glands travel in the bloodstream to exert their influence on various tissues throughout the body.

tide derivatives. The steroid hormones are synthesized from circulating cholesterol by the adrenal cortex and the gonads, whereas other glands produce the polypeptide hormones that range in size from small to large proteins.

Eight different hormones produced by organs other than the major endocrine glands are listed in Table 20.1. Of these, **prostaglandins** constitute a third chemical class of hormones; they are biologically active lipids found in the plasma membrane of nearly all cells. Another example is **erythropoietin**, a glycoprotein that stimulates production of red blood cells by the bone marrow.

Although most hormones circulate in the blood as messengers that affect tissues a distance from the specific gland, other hormones, such as the prostaglandins and the gastrointestinal hormone **gastrin**, exert local effects in the areas where they are produced and are metabolized within a limited anatomic region.

HORMONE-TARGET CELL SPECIFICITY

The major function of hormones is to alter the rates of specific cellular reactions of specific "target cells." This is accomplished by:

• Altering the rate of intracellular protein synthesis.
• Changing the rate of enzyme activity.
• Modifying plasma membrane transport.
• Inducing secretory activity.

A target cell's ability to respond to a hormone depends largely on the presence of specific protein receptors on its plasma membrane (up to 10,000 receptors per cell) or in its interior (usually for lipid-soluble steroid hormones that can pass through the plasma membrane) to which that hormone can bind in a complementary way. Receptors for **adreno-corticotropic hormone (ACTH)**, for example, normally

are found only on certain cells of the adrenal cortex. In contrast, receptors for **thyroxine**, the principal hormone that stimulates cellular metabolism, are found on all cells of the body.

Hormone-Receptor Binding. *Hormone-receptor binding is the first step in initiating hormone action.* The extent of a target cell's activation by a hormone depends on three factors: (*a*) blood hormone levels, (*b*) relative number of target cell receptors for that hormone, and (*c*) sensitivity or strength of the union between hormone and receptor. Hormone receptors are dynamic structures that adjust to physiologic demands. More specifically, **upregulation** is the state in which target cells form more receptors in response to increasing hormone levels. In contrast, prolonged exposure to high hormone concentrations can desensitize target cells so they begin to respond less vigorously to hormonal stimulation. This **downregulation** probably also involves a loss of receptors to prevent target cells from over-responding to persistently high hormone levels.

Cyclic AMP: The Intracellular Messenger. The binding of a hormone with its specific receptor in the plasma membrane can alter the target cell's permeability to a particular chemical (for example, the effect of insulin on cellular glucose uptake) or even alter the cell's ability to manufacture intracellular substances, primarily proteins. Such actions ultimately affect the level of cellular function. As shown in Figure 20.3 for the nonsteroid hormones such as epinephrine and glucagon, the binding hormone acts as a "first messenger" to react with the enzyme **adenylate cyclase**, which is present in the plasma membrane. This causes the formation of the compound cyclic 3',5'-adenosine monophosphate (**cyclic AMP**), from an original molecule of ATP. The cyclic AMP then acts as a ubiquitous "second messenger" to activate a specific protein kinase, which then

TABLE 20.1
HORMONES PRODUCED BY ORGANS OTHER THAN THE MAJOR ENDOCRINE ORGANS

Hormone	Composition	Source and Stimulus for Secretion	Target and Outcome
Prostaglandins	20-carbon fatty acid synthesized from arachidonic acid	Source: plasma membrane of different body cells Stimulus: local irritation, different hormones	Target: multiple sites Outcome: controls local hormone response; stimulates arterioles to increase blood pressure; increases uterine contractions, HCl and pepsin secretion in stomach, platelet aggregation, blood clotting, constriction of bronchioles, inflammation, pain, and fever
Gastrin	Peptide	Source: stomach Stimulus: food	Target: stomach Outcome: release of HCl
Enterogastrin	Peptide	Source: duodenum Stimulus: food (especially lipids)	Target: stomach Outcome: inhibits HCl secretion and gastrointestinal motility
Secretin	Peptide	Source: duodenum Stimulus: food	Target: pancreas Outcome: release of bicarbonate-rich juice Target: liver Outcome: release of bile Target: stomach Outcome: inhibits secretion
Cholecystokinin	Peptide	Source: duodenum Stimulus: food	Target: pancreas Outcome: release of bicarbonate-rich juice Target: gallbladder Outcome: expulsion of bile Target: sphincter of Oddi Outcome: relaxes sphincter and allows bile to enter duodenum
Erythropoietin	Glycoprotein	Source: kidneys[a] Stimulus: hypoxia	Target: bone marrow Outcome: production of red blood cells
Active vitamin D$_3$	Steroid	Source: kidney activates vitamin D made by epidermal skin cells Stimulus: parathyroid hormone	Target: intestine Outcome: active transport of dietary Ca^{2+} across intestinal membranes
Atrial natriuretic hormone	Peptide	Source: atrium of heart Stimulus: atrial stretching	Target: kidney Outcome: inhibits Na^+ reabsorption and renin release Target: adrenal cortex Outcome: inhibits secretion of aldosterone

[a]The kidneys release an enzyme that modifies a circulating blood protein to produce erythropoietin.

activates a target enzyme to produce changes in cellular function.

The sequence of reactions set into motion by cyclic AMP depends on three factors: (a) type of target cell, (b) specific protein enzymes it contains, and (c) specific hormone that acts as first messenger. In thyroid cells, for exam-ple, the cyclic AMP generated in response to the binding of thyroid-stimulating hormone promotes the synthesis of the hormone thyroxine. In bone and muscle cells, on the other hand, the cyclic AMP produced by the action of **growth-hormone** binding activates anabolic reactions so amino acids can be synthesized into tissue proteins.

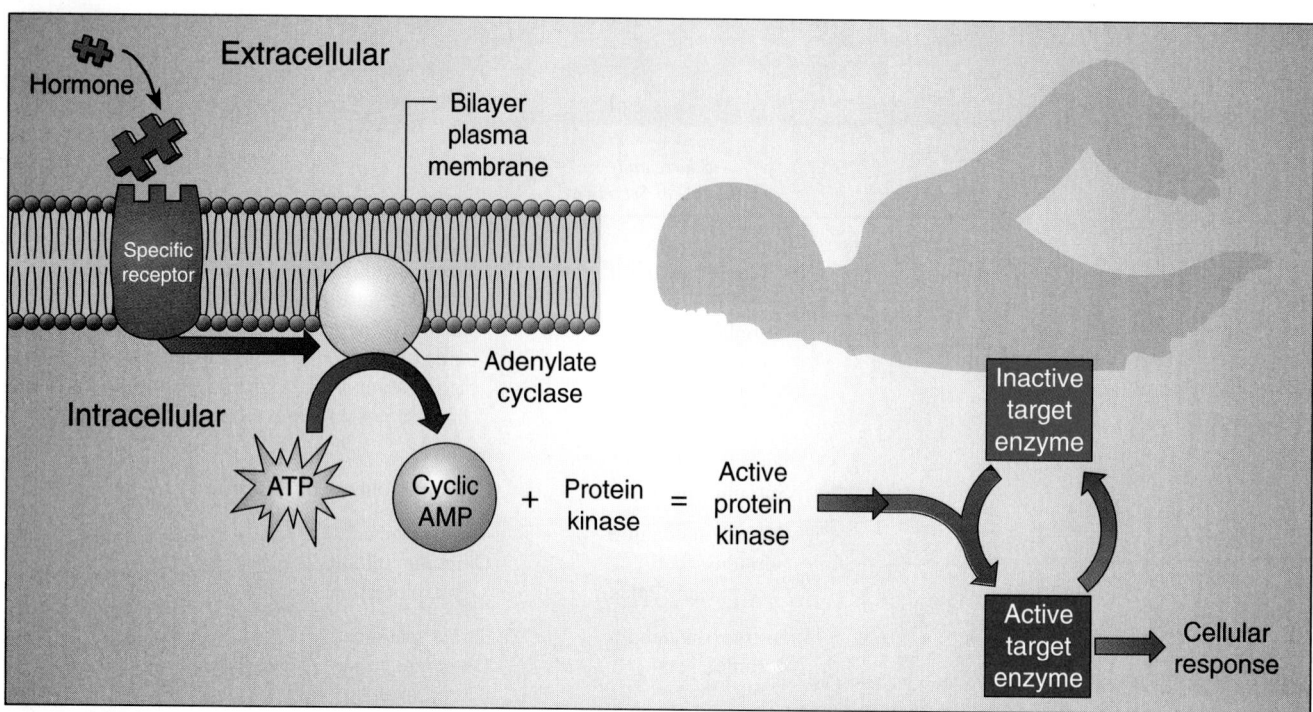

FIGURE 20.3

Action of the nonsteroid hormones. Circulating hormone ("first messenger") binds to a specific receptor in the cell's plasma membrane to trigger the production of cyclic AMP from ATP. This reaction is catalyzed by the enzyme adenylate cyclase. Cyclic AMP then acts as a "second messenger" to activate a protein kinase within the cell, which in turn activates a target enzyme to elicit the cellular response.

Effects on Enzymes. *A major role of hormone action is to alter enzyme activity and enzyme-mediated membrane transport.* Hormones increase enzyme activity in one of three ways:

- Stimulate increased production of the enzyme.
- Combine with the enzyme to alter its shape and ability to act through the process of **allosteric modulation.** This either increases or decreases the enzyme's effectiveness as a catalyst.
- Activate inactive forms of a particular enzyme, thus increasing the total quantity of active enzyme.

In addition to altering enzyme activity, hormones can either facilitate or inhibit the uptake of substances by cells. Insulin, for example, facilitates glucose transport into the cell by combining with extracellular glucose and a glucose carrier within the plasma membrane. In contrast, the hormone epinephrine acts in opposition to inhibit insulin release, thus slowing glucose uptake.

The secondary effects of hormone action can be potent, although often indirect. The release of insulin, for example, increases glucose transport into muscle fibers, which leads to the increased synthesis of muscle glycogen. This influence on glucose uptake is important for fuel homeostasis in exercise. For individuals with insulin insufficiency, the effects of depressed glucose metabolism on exercise performance are debilitating. An inadequate cellular uptake of glucose caused by chronic insulin deficiency increases the level of blood glucose that ultimately spills over into the urine. This condition of insulin insufficiency and/or resistance is called diabetes mellitus and is discussed in more detail on pages 374 to 376.

FACTORS THAT DETERMINE HORMONE LEVELS

Hormone secretion rarely occurs at a constant rate. As with the activity of the nervous system, hormone secretion must be adjusted rapidly to meet the demands of changing bodily functions. For this reason, all protein hormone secretions are pulsatile in nature. Two factors determine the concentration of a particular hormone in the blood: (*a*) the quantity of hormone synthesized in the host gland and (*b*) the amount of hormone released into the blood. Over an extended time, hormone synthesis tends to equal hormone release. For a short period, however, it is possible for hormone release to exceed its synthesis. The plasma concentration of a hormone is referred to as the "secreted amount." In reality, this is actually the sum of both hormone synthesis and release by the host gland, as well as its uptake by receptor tissues and its removal by the liver and kidneys. In most cases, the rate of removal (usually measured in the urine) is equal to the rate of release, although this assumption is not always true.

Endocrine glands are under the control of hormonal, humoral, and neural stimulation.

- **Hormonal Stimulation:** Many hormones influence the secretion of other hormones. For example, the release of most anterior pituitary hormones is regulated by releasing-inhibiting hormones produced by the hypothalamus. Anterior pituitary hormones, in turn, stimulate other endocrine organs to release their hormones into the blood. As the blood levels of hormones produced by the final target glands increase, they provide feedback to inhibit the release of anterior pituitary hormones and, ultimately, their own release.

- **Humoral Stimulation:** Changing levels of certain ions and nutrients in blood, bile, and other body fluids also stimulate hormone release. Such stimuli are referred to as humoral stimuli to distinguish them from hormonal stimuli, which also are fluid-borne chemicals. For example, the release of insulin by the pancreas is prompted by an increase in blood sugar concentration (the humoral agent). Because insulin promotes glucose entry into cells, blood sugar levels soon decline, thus ending the stimulus for insulin release.

- **Neural Stimulation:** Hormone release also is affected by neural activity. For example, the sympathetic nervous system's activation of the adrenal medulla during periods of stress releases the catecholamines, epinephrine, and norepinephrine. In certain cases, the nervous system overrides normal endocrine control to maintain homeostasis. Blood sugar levels are normally maintained within the range of 80 to 120 mg per 100 mL of blood primarily by the action of insulin. During exercise, however, activation of the hypothalamus and sympathetic nervous system blunts the release of insulin. This attenuates a further drop in blood sugar and ensures that nervous tissue and active muscle will have sufficient carbohydrate fuel.

RESTING AND EXERCISE-INDUCED ENDOCRINE SECRETIONS

The different endocrine host organs, specific hormones secreted, control factors, hormone function, effects of hyposecretion and hypersecretion, and the influence of exercise on hormone output are listed in Table 20.2. In the following sections, these hormones will be reviewed, with special emphasis on their response to exercise and physical training.

ANTERIOR PITUITARY HORMONES

The pituitary gland (also called the **hypophysis**), its secretions, and various target glands and their hormone secretions are illustrated in Figure 20.4. Located beneath the base of the brain, the pituitary secretes at least six different polypeptide hormones. Because of its widespread influence, the anterior pituitary gland often was called the "master gland." It is now known, however, that the hypothalamus actually controls anterior pituitary activity; therefore, the hypothalamus should truly have the title "master gland." In addition to the hormones displayed in Figure 20.4, the pituitary also secretes a large molecule called **proopiomelanocortin** or **POMC.** POMC is a large precursor molecule from which other active molecules are split by enzymatic cleavage. POMC is the source of adrenocorticotropic hormone and some of the naturally produced opiates such as **beta-endorphin** (see p. 382).

GROWTH HORMONE

Growth hormone (**GH** or **somatotropin**) has widespread physiologic activity because it promotes cell division and cellular proliferation throughout the body. In the adult, GH facilitates protein synthesis by increasing amino acid transport through plasma membranes, stimulating RNA formation, or activating cellular ribosomes, which increase protein synthesis.[39] GH release also causes a decrease in carbohydrate breakdown and a subsequent mobilization and use of lipids as an energy source.

GH secretion during rest is influenced by a GH-releasing factor that acts directly on the anterior pituitary gland. Each of the primary pituitary hormones has its own hypothalamic releasing hormone, often called a **releasing factor.** These releasing factors are controlled by neural input to the hypothalamus from stimuli such as anxiety, stress, and physical activity. Regardless of training status, women seem to have higher levels of GH at rest compared to men; this difference disappears during prolonged exercise.[18]

GH, Exercise, and Tissue Synthesis. An acute period of physical activity stimulates the release of GH and, with increasing exercise intensity, there is a sharp rise in GH production and total secretion.[7, 37, 39] This would be a beneficial response for muscle, bone, and connective tissue growth, as well as for optimizing the metabolic mixture during exercise. The exact stimulus has not been identified for increased GH production in exercise. Concurrent measurements of circulating lactate, alanine, pyruvate, blood glucose, and body temperature reveal that none of these factors are associated with the pattern of GH secretion.[68] Most probably, **neural factors,** possibly via cholinergic and opioid pathways, control GH secretion during exercise and recovery.[16, 138]

It is not clear how GH and exercise interact to augment protein synthesis (and subsequent muscle hypertrophy), cartilage formation, skeletal growth, and cell proliferation.[19, 87, 98] One hypothesis suggests that exercise directly stimulates GH release, which in turn stimulates anabolic processes.[7] For example, exercise is associated

TABLE 20.2
ENDOCRINE GLANDS AND THEIR SECRETIONS, FUNCTIONS, CONTROL FACTORS, EFFECTS OF HYPOSECRETION AND HYPERSECRETION, AND THE ACUTE EFFECTS OF EXERCISE ON HORMONE OUTPUT

Host Gland	Hormone	Hormone Effects	Control of Hormone Secretion	Effects of Hyposecretion and Hypersecretion	Exercise Effects on Hormone Secretion
Anterior pituitary	Growth hormone (GH; somatotropin)	Stimulates tissue growth; mobilizes fatty acids for energy; inhibits CHO metabolism	Hypothalamic releasing factor (GHRF)	*Hypo-*: dwarfism in children; *Hyper-*: gigantism in children, acromegly in adults	↑ with increasing exercise
	Thyrotropin (TSH)	Stimulates production and release of thyroxine from thyroid gland	Hypothalmic TSH-releasing factor; thyroxine	*Hypo-*: cretinism in children (stunted growth, mental retardation); myxedema in adults (low BMR, constipation, dry skin, puffy eyes, edema, lethargy); *Hyper-*: Graves' disease (autoimmune disease—elevated BMR, weight loss, irregular heartbeat), heart disease	↑ with increasing exercise
	Corticotropin (ACTH)	Stimulates production and release of cortisol, aldosterone, and adrenal hormones	Hypothalamic ACTH-releasing factor; cortisol	*Hypo-*: rarely seen; *Hyper-*: Cushing's disease	Unknown
	Gonadotropic (FSH and LH)	FSH works with LH to stimulate production of estrogen by ovaries, LH works with FSH to stimulate production of estrogen and progesterone by ovaries and testosterone by male testes	Hypothalamic FSH and LH releasing factor; female—estrogen and progesterone; male—testosterone	*Hypo-*: Failure of sexual maturation; *Hyper-*: none	No change
	Prolactin (PRL)	Inhibits testosterone; mobilizes fatty acids	Hypothalamic PRL-inhibiting factor	*Hypo-*: poor milk production in nursing women; *Hyper-*: galactorrhea, cessation of menses in females, impotence in males	↑ with increasing exercise
	Endorphins	Blocks pain; promotes euphoria; affects feeding and female menstrual cycle	Stress—physical/emotional (may be intensity related)	Unknown	↑ with long duration exercise
Posterior pituitary	Vasopressin (ADH)	Controls water excretion by kidneys	Hypothalamic secretory neurons	*Hypo-*: diabetes; *Hyper-*: unknown	↑ with increasing exercise
	Oxytocin	Stimulates muscles in uterus and breast; important in birthing and lactation	Hypothalamic secretory neurons	Unknown	Unknown

TABLE 20.2—continued

Host Gland	Hormone	Hormone Effects	Control of Hormone Secretion	Effects of Hyposecretion and Hypersecretion	Exercise Effects on Hormone Secretion
Adrenal cortex	Cortisol Corticosterone	Promotes use of fatty acids and protein catabolism; conserves blood sugar/insulin antagonist; has anti-inflammatory effects with epinephrine	ACTH; stress	*Hypo-*: Addison's disease (weight loss; glucose and sodium levels drop and potassium levels rise, resulting in hypotension and dehydration); *Hyper-*: Cushing's disease (persistant hyperglycemia, dramatic losses in muscle and bone protein, and water and salt retention leading to hypertension)	↑ in heavy exercise only
	Aldosterone	Promotes retention of sodium, potassium, and water by the kidneys	Angiotensin and plasma potassium concentration; renin	*Hypo-*: Addison's disease; *Hyper-*: aldosteronism (excessive sodium and water retention and accelerated excretion of potassium)	↑ with increasing exercise
Adrenal medulla	Epinephrine Norepinephrine	Facilitates sympathetic activity, increases cardiac output, regulates blood vessels, increases glycogen catabolism and fatty acid release	Stress stimulated hypothalamic sympathetic nerves	*Hypo-*: unimportant; *Hyper-*: hypertension, increased metabolism	Epinephrine, ↑ in heavy exercise Norepinephrine, ↑ with increasing exercise
Thyroid	Thyroxine (T_4) Triiodothyronine (T_3)	Stimulates metabolic rate; regulates cell growth and activity	TSH; whole body metabolism	*Hypo-*: decreased BMR and body temperature, cold intolerance, decreased appetite, weight gain, decreased glucose metabolism, elevated cholesterol, decreased protein synthesis, hypotension, muscle cramps, growth retardation, depressed ovarian function; *Hyper-*: increased BMR, temperature, heat intolerance, increased appetite, weight loss, hypertension, enhanced catabolism of glucose, lipid, and protein, loss of muscle, muscle atrophy, depressed ovarian function.	↑ with increasing exercise

TABLE 20.2—continued

Host Gland	Hormone	Hormone Effects	Control of Hormone Secretion	Effects of Hyposecretion and Hypersecretion	Exercise Effects on Hormone Secretion
Pancreas	Insulin	Promotes CHO transport into cells; increases CHO catabolism and decreases blood glucose; promotes fatty acid and amino acid transport into cells	Plasma glucose levels	*Hypo-*: diabetes; *Hyper-*: hypoglycemia, anxiety, nervousness, weakness	↓ with increasing exercise
	Glucagon	Promotes release of glucose from liver to blood; increases lipid metabolism, reduces amino acid levels	Plasma glucose levels	*Hypo-*: chronic hypoglycemia, low circulating amino acids; *Hyper-*: hyperglycemia	↑ with increasing exercise
Parathyroid	Parathormone	Raises blood calcium; lowers blood phosphate	Plasma calcium concentration	*Hypo-*: hypocalcemia, respiratory paralysis, uncontrolled spasms and convulsions; *Hyper-*: hypercalcemia, extreme leaching of calcium from bones, depression of nervous system activity, muscle weakness, formation of kidney stones	↑ with long-term exercise
Ovaries	Estrogen Progesterone	Controls menstrual cycle; increased fat deposition; promotes female sex characteristics	FSH, LH	*Hypo-*: (estrogen); *Hyper-*: (progesterone) masculinization or virilization	↑ with exercise; depends on menstrual phase
Testes	Testosterone	Controls muscle size; increases RBC; decreases body fat; promotes male sex characteristics		*Hypo-*: feminization; *Hyper-*: masculinization or virilization	↑ with exercise
Kidney	Renin	Simulates aldosterone secretion	Plasma sodium	*Hypo-*: hypertension; *Hyper-*: hypotension	↑ with increasing exercise

directly with a doubling of both GH pulse frequency and amplitude. Furthermore, exercise stimulates the production of endogenous opiates, which facilitate GH release by inhibiting the liver's production of **somatostatin**, a hormone that blunts the release of GH.[8] A proposed plan for classifying the overall metabolic actions of GH is shown in Figure 20.5. For modulating the metabolic mixture during exercise, GH stimulates lipid release from adipose tissue while inhibiting glucose uptake by the cells. This glucose-sparing action helps maintain blood glucose at fairly high levels and contributes to one's ability to sustain prolonged exercise.

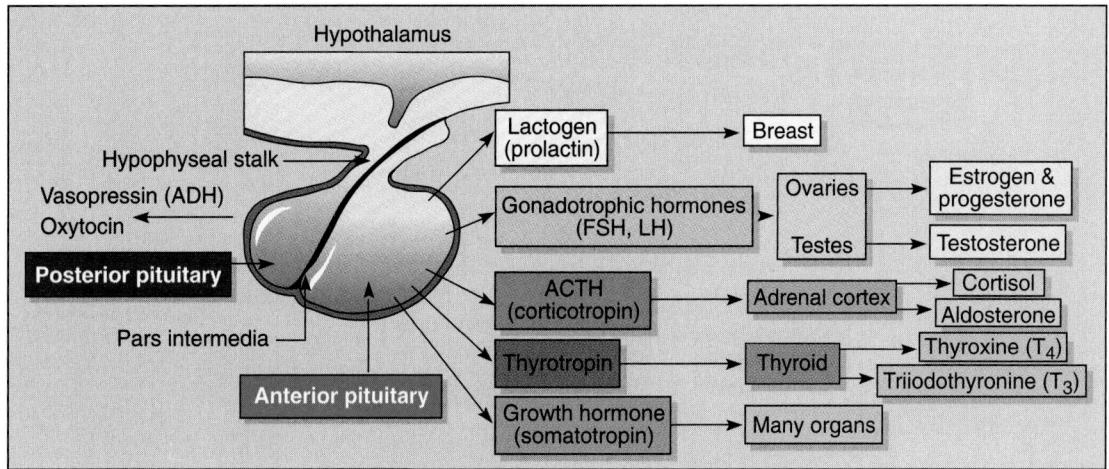

FIGURE 20.4
The pituitary gland and its secretions.

When exercised to exhaustion, both fit and sedentary subjects show similar increases in GH concentration, although sedentary individuals maintain high levels for several hours into recovery. For standard submaximal exercise, the GH response is greater in the sedentary.[125] Because this absolute work level is more taxing on the less fit person, GH release may be related to the relative strenuousness of effort. Researchers often use the term insulin-like growth factors (IGF) to describe the anabolic effects of GH on exercise-induced muscle hypertrophy. The IGF polypeptides (referred to as IGF-I and IGF-II) interact with GH to help carry out its many effects on muscle fibers.[77]

THYROTROPIN

Thyrotropin, sometimes called **thyroid-stimulating hormone (TSH),** controls the amount of hormone secreted by the thyroid gland. TSH also acts to maintain the growth and development of the thyroid gland and to increase the metabolic activity of thyroid cells. Considering the important role of thyroid hormone in regulating cellular metabolism throughout the body, it is not surprising that TSH output from the pituitary increases during exercise, although this effect may not always be consistent.[129]

CORTICOTROPIN

Corticotropin, also known as **adrenocorticotropic hormone (ACTH),** regulates the output of the hormones secreted by the adrenal cortex as TSH controls secretion of the thyroid gland. ACTH acts directly to enhance lipid mobilization from adipose tissue, increase the rate of gluconeogenesis, and stimulate protein catabolism. Owing to difficulty in assay methods and the rapid disappearance of this hormone from the blood, data are scarce concerning the response of ACTH during exercise. Limited data suggest, however, that ACTH concentrations increase with exercise duration if intensity is greater than 25% of aerobic capacity.[39]

PROLACTIN

Prolactin **(PRL)** initiates and supports milk secretion from the mammary glands. PRL levels increase at high intensities of exercise and return toward baseline within 45 minutes during recovery.[17] Owing to its important role in female sexual function, it is possible that repeated exercise-induced PRL release may inhibit the ovaries and contribute to the alterations in the menstrual cycle often observed among athletic women.[6, 11, 94] Increases in PRL are greater in women who run without wearing a bra; the release of this hormone is also enhanced by either fasting or consuming a high-fat diet.[44, 64, 111] There also is evidence that PRL increases in men following a maximal period of exercise.[27]

GONADOTROPIC HORMONES

Gonadotropic hormones stimulate the male and female sex organs to grow and secrete their hormones at a faster rate. The two gonadotropic hormones are **follicle-stimulating hormone (FSH)** and **luteinizing hormone (LH).** In the female, FSH initiates growth of follicles in the ovaries and stimulates the ovaries to secrete estrogen, one type of female sex hormone. LH works with FSH to cause estrogen secretion as well as the rupture of the follicle to allow the

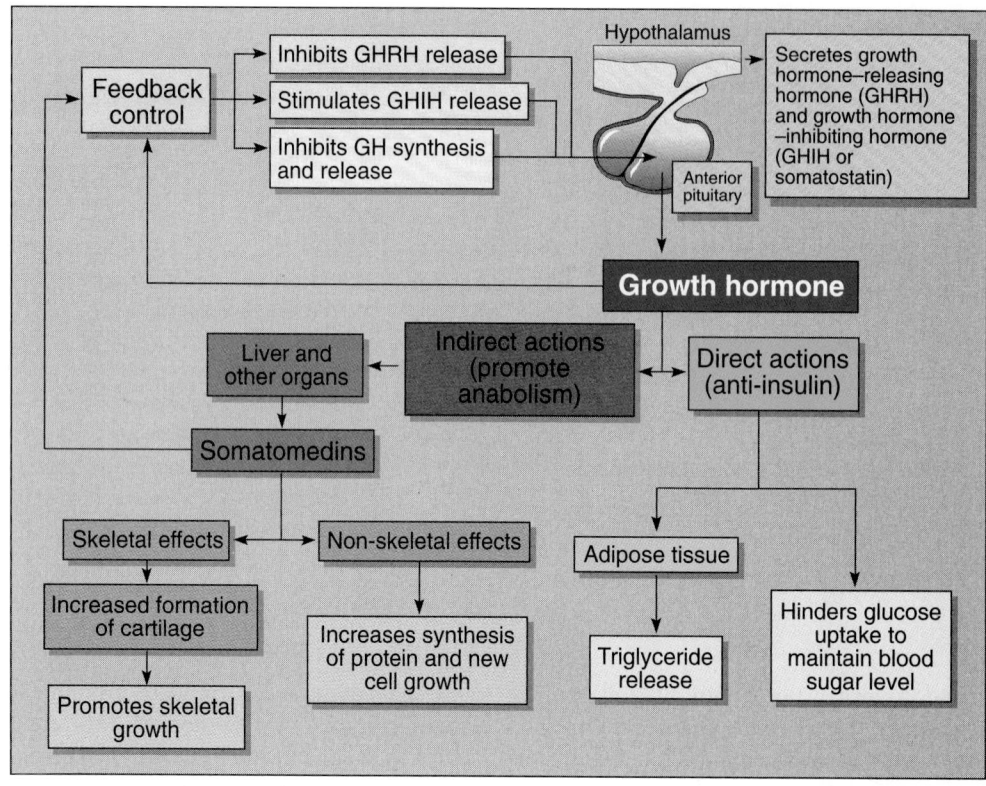

FIGURE 20.5

Overview plan for classifying the actions of growth hormone (GH). GH stimulates the breakdown and release of triglycerides from adipose tissue and hinders glucose uptake by the cells (anti-insulin effect) to maintain a relatively high level of blood glucose. The indirect anabolic effects of GH are mediated through somatomedins. Elevated levels of GH and somatomedins provide feedback to promote GH-inhibiting hormone (GHRH) release and depress the release of GH-releasing hormone (GHRH) by the hypothalamus; this further inhibits GH release by the anterior pituitary.

ovum to pass through the fallopian tube for fertilization. In the male, FSH stimulates growth of the germinal epithelium in the testes to promote sperm development. LH also stimulates the testes to secrete the male hormone testosterone.

Reports of exercise-associated alterations in FSH and LH are inconsistent and are confounded by the nature of gonadotropin release.[25, 52, 131] Because LH is normally released in a pulsatile manner, it is difficult to separate any specific exercise-related change from the normal pattern of pulsatile release. In addition, anxiety can either raise or lower LH levels by the action of norepinephrine, the release of which is augmented by stress.[73] Generally, LH concentration rises even before exercise begins and reaches its peak during recovery.

POSTERIOR PITUITARY HORMONES

The posterior pituitary gland is an outgrowth of the hypothalamus and, in actuality, resembles true neural tissue

(Fig. 20.4). This tissue often is called the **neurohypophysis** and stores two hormones, **antidiuretic hormone (ADH or vasopressin)** and **oxytocin.** This gland does not synthesize its hormones. Instead, they are produced in the hypothalamus and secreted to the neurohypophysis, where they are then released as needed via neural stimulation. The production of ADH and oxytocin would not be dramatically affected if the posterior pituitary was damaged or surgically removed.

The major function of ADH is to control the excretion of water by the kidneys. ADH limits the production of large volumes of urine by stimulating reabsorption of water in the kidney tubules. The role of oxytocin is to initiate the contraction of muscle in the uterus and to stimulate ejection of milk from the breasts during lactation; therefore, oxytocin is important during birthing and nursing.

Exercise is a potent stimulus for ADH secretion.[126, 133] The stimulating effect of exercise on ADH secretion explains the increased water retention by the kidneys during and after severe exercise.[21, 28] An increased ADH production, believed to be stimulated by sweating, would certainly be helpful in aiding the body to conserve fluids, particularly during hot-weather exercise, when dehydration is a real risk. In response to a fluid overload, ADH release is decreased and urine volume is increased proportionately.

THYROID HORMONES

The thyroid gland, located in the neck just below the larynx, is under the influence of TSH produced by the anterior portion of the pituitary gland. The thyroid gland secretes two protein-iodine-bound hormones, **thyroxine (T_4),** and **triiodothyronine (T_3,** the active form of thyroid hormone). T_4 is secreted in greater quantity than T_3; although less abundant, T_3 acts several times faster than T_4. Most receptor cells for T_4 can metabolize T_4 to T_3.

An increase in T_4 secretion raises the metabolic rate of all cells, probably through its stimulating effect on enzyme activity.[142] T_4, for example, can raise the basal metabolic rate (BMR) by as much as four times. Because of this thermogenic effect, deviations in the BMR are often used as an index of thyroid gland abnormality (see Chapter 9). If thyroid activity is abnormally high, a person may lose weight rapidly. With low thyroid production, on the other hand, the person has a blunted BMR and will usually gain weight. *Because fewer than 3% of obese people have abnormal thyroid function, this cannot be used to explain obesity in most individuals.*[4, 15] In terms of nervous system function, T_3 release facilitates neural reflex activity, whereas a decrease in the level of T_4 can cause sluggishness, often inducing people to sleep as many as 10 to 15 hours per day.

Whole body metabolism influences the synthesis of the thyroid hormones. If the metabolic rate falls to some critical value, hypothalamic release of TSH is directly stimulated, thyroid output increases, and the resting metabolic rate becomes elevated. Conversely, increases in metabolic rate tend to reduce TSH production, causing metabolism to slow down. This exquisite "feedback" system is illustrated in Figure 20.6.

During exercise, blood levels of "free T_4" (that is, thyroxine not bound to plasma proteins) increase by approximately 35%.[43, 129] This could be the result of an exercise-induced elevation in core temperature, which alters the protein binding of several hormones, including T_4. Whereas liver concentrations of T_4 increase during exercise, muscle-concentrations remain unchanged.[143] The importance of these transient alterations in thyroid hormone dynamics with exercise is unknown.

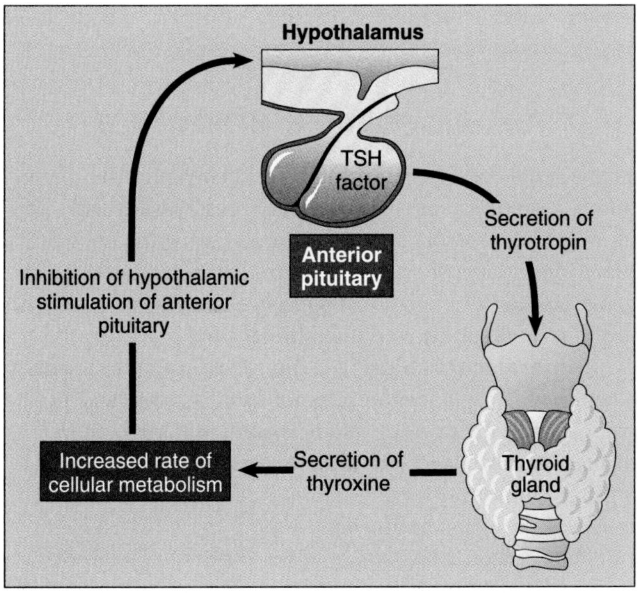

ADRENAL HORMONES

The adrenal glands are flattened, caplike tissues located just above each kidney (Fig. 20.7). There are two distinct parts to the adrenal gland: the **medulla** (inner portion) and the **cortex** (outer portion). Each part secretes different types of hormones; consequently, the cortex and medulla are generally considered to be two distinct glands.

ADRENAL MEDULLA HORMONES

The adrenal medulla is part of the sympathetic nervous system. It acts to prolong and augment sympathetic effects by secreting the two hormones **epinephrine** and **norepinephrine,** collectively called **catecholamines.** The chemical structure of epinephrine and norepinephrine is shown in Figure 20.8. Norepinephrine is a hormone in its own right and is a precursor of epinephrine. It also is considered a neurotransmitter when released by sympathetic nerve endings. Eighty percent of adrenal medulla secretions are in the form of epinephrine, whereas the principal neurotransmitter released from the sympathetic nervous system is norepinephrine. An outflow of neural impulses from the hypothalamus stimulates the adrenal medulla to increase catecholamine release. These hormones then affect the heart, blood vessels, and glands in the same way as direct stimulation by the sympathetic nervous system. A primary function of epinephrine in energy metabolism is to stimulate glycogenolysis in the liver and active muscle and lipolysis in adipose tissue and active muscle; norepinephrine is a powerful stimulator of lipolysis in adipose tissue.[135, 137]

FIGURE 20.6
Feedback system that controls the release of thyroid hormone.

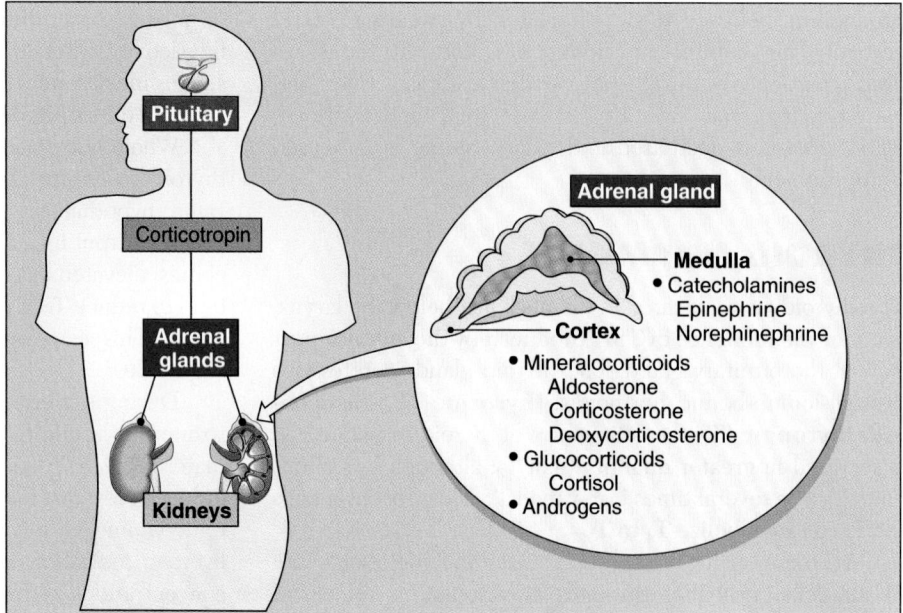

FIGURE 20.7
The adrenal gland and its secretions.

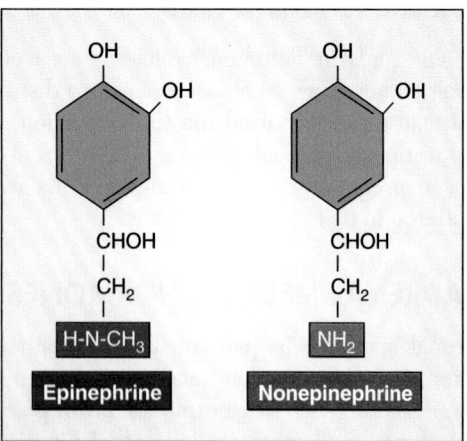

FIGURE 20.8
Chemical structure of the catecholamines epinephrine and norepinephrine. Norepinephrine is a hormone and a precursor of epinephrine. Norepinephrine also is considered to be a neurotransmitter when it is released by sympathetic nerve endings. The structural difference between these hormones is shown by the purple and red shaded boxes.

Because sympathetic nerve endings (including those to the adrenal gland) secrete both epinephrine and norepinephrine, it is appropriate to discuss the "sympathoadrenal" response to exercise and training rather than simply the adrenal gland response. *The sympathoadrenal response to exercise is related to the relative rather than to the absolute intensity of exercise performed.* There is a two- to sixfold increase in norepinephrine levels during light to maximal exercise. More than likely, this secretion is from sympathetic postganglionic nerve endings and is related to the cardiovascular and metabolic adjustments of the active tissues. Epinephrine output from the adrenal medulla increases with exercise, and the magnitude of this increase is related directly to the intensity and duration of effort.[35, 40, 75] There does not appear to be an age-related effect on catecholamine response to exercise if individuals are matched for aerobic fitness.[69] The effects of increased adrenal medulla activity on blood flow distribution, cardiac contractility, and substrate mobilization are all beneficial to the exercise response.[72]

ADRENOCORTICAL HORMONES

The adrenal cortex, stimulated by corticotropin from the pituitary, secretes **adrenocortical (corticosteroid)** hormones. These steroid hormones can be categorized by function into one of three groups: **mineralocorticoids, glucocorticoids,** and **androgens;** each is produced in a different zone or layer of the adrenal cortex.

Mineralocorticoids. As the name suggests, mineralocorticoids regulate the mineral salts, sodium and potassium, in the extracellular fluid spaces. Although there are three mineralocorticoids, **aldosterone** is the most physiologically important and comprises almost 95% of all the mineralocorticoids produced.

The major controlling mechanism for aldosterone release from the adrenal cortex is shown in Figure 20.9. *Aldosterone secretion is essential for controlling total sodium concentration as well as the extracellular fluid volume. It acts by regulating sodium reabsorption in the*

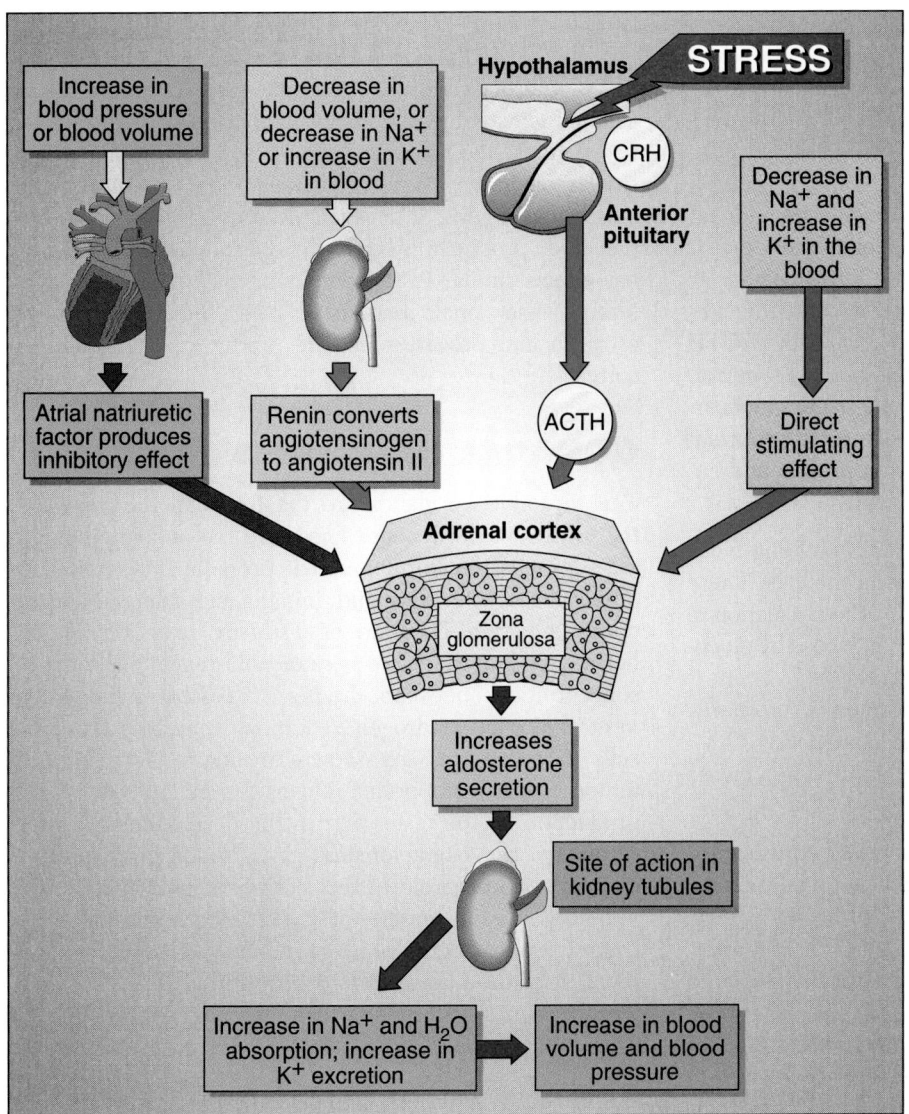

FIGURE 20.9
Major mechanisms that control aldosterone release from the adrenal cortex.

distal tubules of the kidneys.[24, 29] When large quantities of aldosterone are secreted, the sodium ions that enter the tubules are reabsorbed into the blood along with fluid. Consequently, little sodium (and fluid) is voided in the urine. The increase in plasma volume with aldosterone secretion is also accompanied by an increase in cardiac output and arterial blood pressure. In contrast, sodium and water are literally poured into the urine with cessation of aldosterone secretion. Aldosterone also contributes to the maintenance of serum potassium and pH because the kidneys exchange either K^+ or a H^+ for each sodium ion that is reabsorbed. Proper mineral balance is important for nerve transmission and muscle function. Neuromuscular activity would be impossible without the effective regulation and modulation of sodium and potassium exchange.

Renin-Angiotensin Mechanism. During exercise, the increased activity of the sympathetic nervous system constricts blood vessels to the kidneys. This reduces renal blood flow, which stimulates the kidneys to release the hormone **renin** into the blood. Increased renin stimulates the production of still another kidney hormone, **angiotensin,** which stimulates the adrenal cortex to secrete aldosterone.[28, 127] Aldosterone secretion rises progressively during exercise; peak plasma levels reach as high as six times the resting level.[90]

A chronic reduction in renal blood flow at rest, perhaps due to abnormal sympathetic stimulation, will activate the **renin-angiotensin mechanism.** An over-responsiveness of this mechanism is a causative factor in the development of certain forms of hypertension. High blood pressure associated with increased aldosterone production is prevalent in teenage obesity. Teenage hypertension is related to decreases in salt sensitivity (and hence increased water retention) and increased sodium intake and decreased sensitivity to the effects of insulin (hyperinsulinemia).[114] These interrelationships suggest a direct link between obesity as a disease and hypertension.

Glucocorticoids. The glucocorticoids are ideally suited for severe stress situations. Emotional stress or the demands of physical exertion induce the hypothalamus to secrete **corticotropin-releasing factor,** which stimulates the anterior pituitary to release ACTH. In turn, ACTH causes glucocorticoid release by the adrenal cortex. **Cortisol,** also called hydrocortisone, is the major glucocorticoid secreted by the adrenal cortex. The most important function of cortisol relates to its effects on protein and energy metabolism. Cortisol does the following:

- Stimulates the breakdown of protein to its building-block amino acids in all cells of the body except the liver. These "liberated" amino acids are delivered by the circulation to the liver, where they are synthesized to glucose by gluconeogenesis.
- Supports the action of other hormones, primarily glucagon and GH, in the gluconeogenic process.
- Serves as an insulin antagonist by inhibiting glucose uptake and oxidation.

Prolonged, high-serum concentrations of cortisol ultimately lead to excessive protein breakdown, tissue wasting, and a negative nitrogen balance. Cortisol secretion also accelerates lipid mobilization for energy. This is particularly apparent during starvation and exercise. With rapid and large increases in cortisol output, the liver splits the mobilized lipid into its simple ketoacid components. Above-normal ketoacid concentrations in the extracellular fluid can lead to the potentially dangerous condition of **ketosis** (a form of acidosis). Ketosis, stimulated by increased cortisol secretion, is common in individuals who subsist on very low-carbohydrate, low-calorie (ketogenic) weight-loss diets.

There is considerable variability in the cortisol response to exercise, depending on such factors as exercise intensity and duration, fitness level, nutritional status, and even circadian rhythm.[12, 127] Most research indicates that cortisol output increases with exercise intensity.[99] In addition, extremely high cortisol levels have been observed following long-duration exercise such as marathon running.[13, 22, 110] Even during more moderate exercise, plasma cortisol rises if the exercise duration is sufficiently long.[12] Cortisol response to exercise is best studied by observing cortisol turnover; that is, the difference between its production and removal. When this approach is used, the data indicate that highly trained runners are in a state of hypercortisolism that is particularly heightened before competition.[86] Cortisol levels also remain elevated for as long as 2 hours following exercise. These responses are probably related to cortisol's anti-stress functions.

Gonadocorticoids. Although the reproductive organs or gonads are the major producers of the so-called sex steroids, the adrenal cortex produces hormones with similar actions. These gonadocorticoid hormones are mostly androgens. For example, the adrenal cortex is the chief producer of **dehydroepiandrosterone,** which has effects similar to the dominant male hormone testosterone. Also, small amounts of the "female" hormones, estrogen and progesterone, are produced by the adrenal cortex.

GONADAL HORMONES

The reproductive glands are the testes in the male and the ovaries in the female. These are the endocrine glands that produce the hormones that promote the sex-specific physical characteristics and initiate and maintain reproductive function. There are no distinctly "male" or "female" hormones, but there are general differences in hormone concentrations between the sexes. **Testosterone** is the most important androgen secretion from the interstitial cells of the testes. As shown in Figure 20.10, testosterone plays an important role in the initiation of sperm production by the testes and in the development of male secondary sex characteristics. In addition, the anabolic or tissue-building role of this hormone contributes to the sex differences in muscle mass and muscular strength that begin to appear at the onset of puberty. As noted in Chapter 2, it is the conversion of testosterone to estrogen in peripheral tissues that provides the male with significant protection in the maintenance of bone structure throughout life.

The ovaries are the primary source of estrogens, particularly **estradiol** and **progesterone.** The estrogens promote the regulation of ovulation, menstruation, and the physiologic adjustments during pregnancy. Progesterone also contributes specific regulatory input to the female reproductive cycle, uterine smooth muscle action, and lactation.

Plasma testosterone concentration in females, although approximately one-tenth that of males, has been shown to increase with exercise. Exercise also elevates estradiol and progesterone.[65] In untrained males, both resistance exercise and moderate aerobic exercise significantly increase both serum and free testosterone levels after approximately 15 to 20 minutes.[27, 131] Research is unclear regarding the effect of prolonged, strenuous exercise such as marathon running on testosterone levels.[83, 110, 131] The mechanism responsible for the alterations in testosterone levels with this form of exercise remains unknown.

Figure 20.11 shows the pattern of plasma cortisol and testosterone 48 hours before swimming, immediately

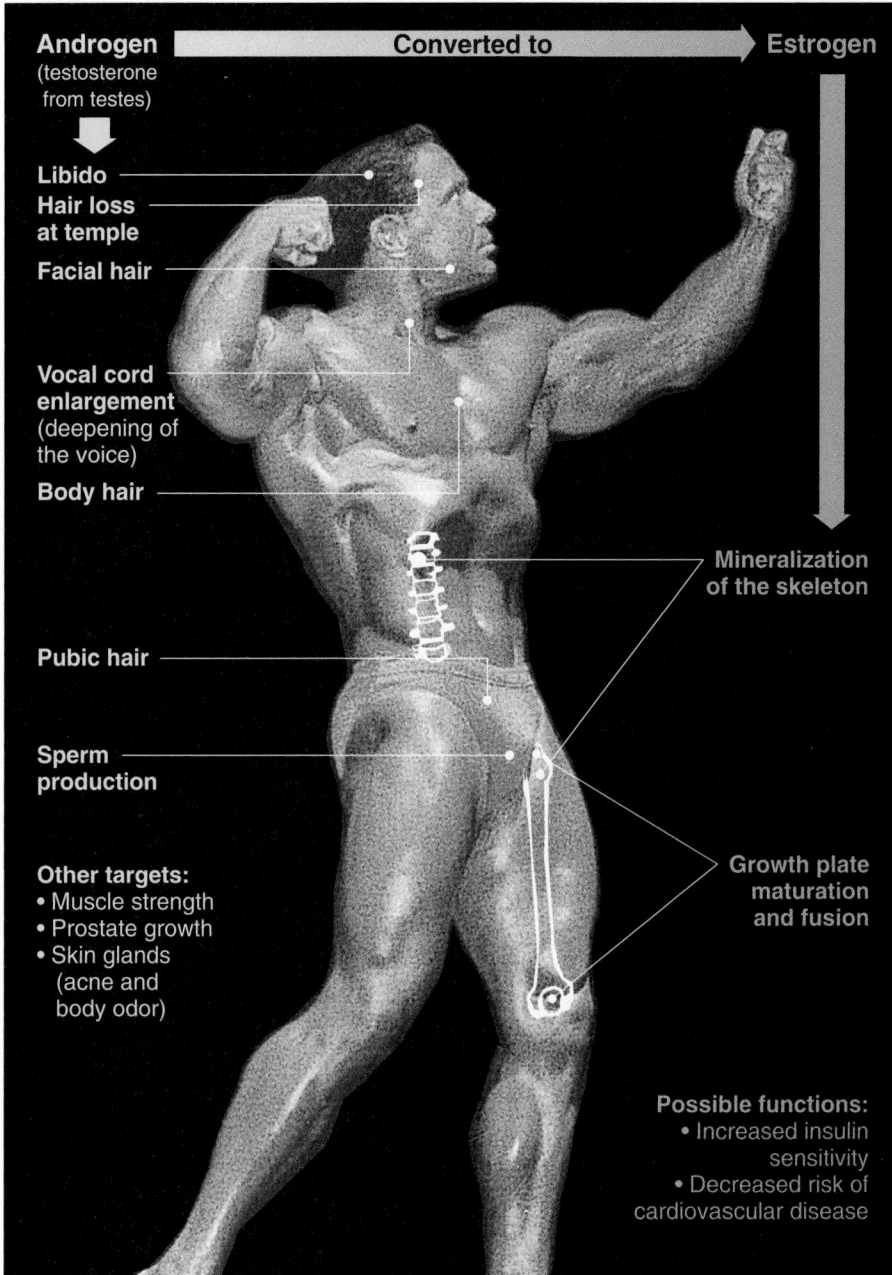

Androgen (testosterone from testes)

Converted to → **Estrogen**

Libido
Hair loss at temple
Facial hair

Vocal cord enlargement (deepening of the voice)

Body hair

Pubic hair

Sperm production

Other targets:
• Muscle strength
• Prostate growth
• Skin glands (acne and body odor)

Mineralization of the skeleton

Growth plate maturation and fusion

Possible functions:
• Increased insulin sensitivity
• Decreased risk of cardiovascular disease

FIGURE 20.10
Androgen's effects in men. By binding with special receptor sites in muscle and various other tissues, androgen (testosterone) greatly contributes to the male secondary sex characteristics and to the sex differences in muscle mass and strength that begin to develop at the onset of puberty. The ability of some androgen to convert to estrogen in peripheral tissues gives the typical male a significant "edge" over the typical female in maintaining bone mass throughout life. (Photo courtesy of Bill Pearl, holder of four Mr. Universe titles.)

following 15×200 m freestyle at the swimmer's competitive velocity with a 20-second rest interval between swims, and 1 hour following the swims. The training period was subdivided into four 6-week periods; training volume was monitored carefully. The insert shows values for swim volume during the four training periods, along with average performance during time trials. The results show clearly that cortisol and testosterone increased significantly after

exercise compared to rest but that baseline values were not attained 1 hour after exercise except for testosterone levels in training periods II and IV. The generalized decrease in cortisol and testosterone concentrations when the swimmers were "peaking" for their championships (period IV) indicates that there is a chronic adaptation for these hormones and not the acute result of excess stress induced by overtraining and subsequent poor performance. This

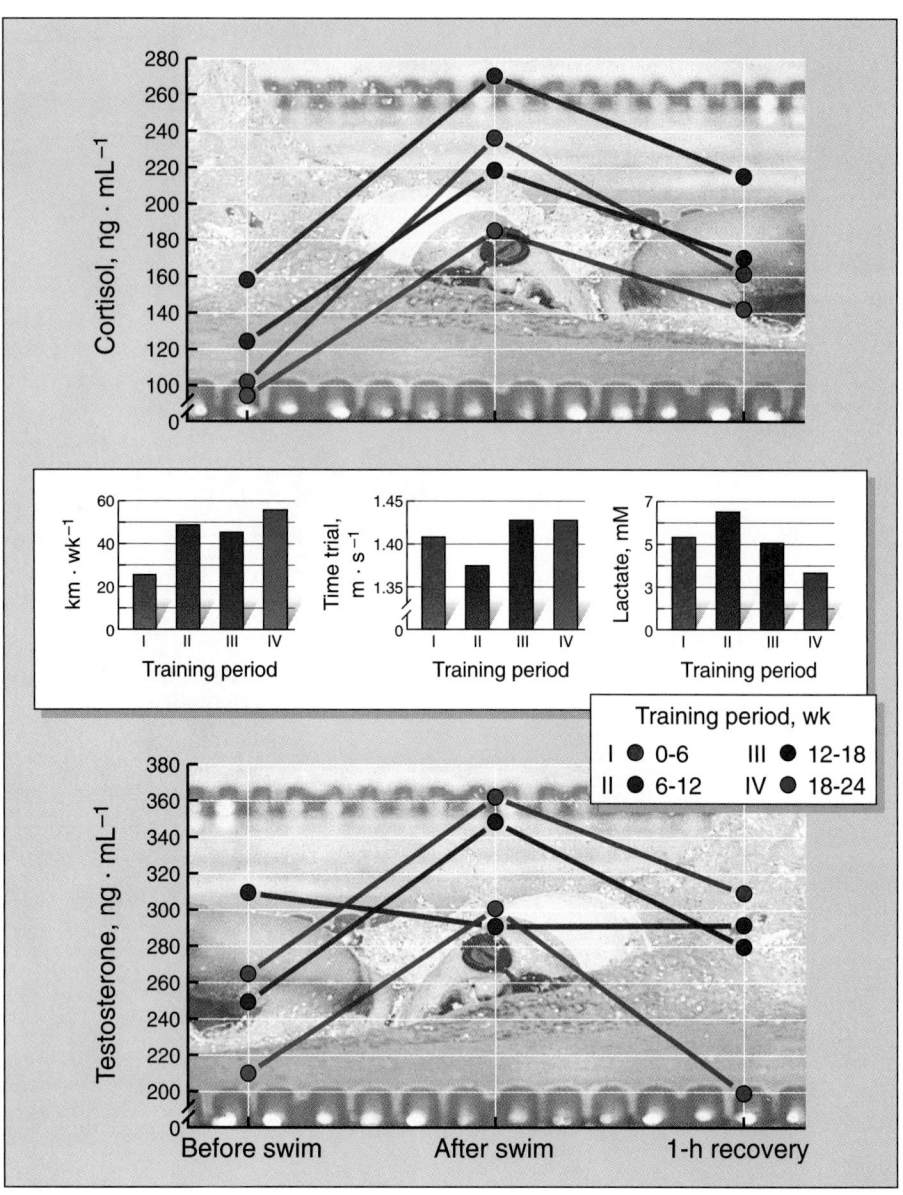

FIGURE 20.11
Pattern of plasma cortisol and testosterone concentration measured at three time intervals (4 hours before swimming, immediately after multiple sprint swims, and after 1-hour recovery) over a 24-week swim training season. The inset shows values for swim volume, time-trial performance, and blood lactate during the four 6-week training periods. (Modified from Bonifazi, M., et al.: Blood levels of cortisol and testosterone before and after swimming exercise during the training season. In *Medicine and Science in Aquatic Sports.* Edited by M. Miyashita, et al. Basel, Karger, 1994.)

might have been inferred from the depressed performance results during period II, which corresponded to a large increase in training volume.

PANCREATIC HORMONES

The pancreas gland, approximately 14 cm long and weighing about 60 g, is situated just below the stomach. It is composed of two different types of tissues, **acini** and **islets of Langerhans** (Fig. 20.12). The islets of Langerhans are endocrine tissues composed of **alpha** cells that secrete glucagon and **beta** cells that secrete insulin. The acini portion of the pancreas is exocrine in function and secretes digestive enzymes.

INSULIN

The major function of insulin is regulation of glucose metabolism in all tissues except the brain. This is accomplished by increasing the rate of glucose transport into muscle and adipose tissue cells. Insulin is the mediator of "facilitated diffusion," whereby glucose in the presence of insulin combines with a glucose carrier (located on the cell's plasma membrane) for transport into the cells. In this way, insulin actually controls the level of glucose metabolism. Any glucose not immediately catabolized for energy is stored as glycogen for later use. Without insulin, only trace amounts of glucose can be transported into cells. Figure 20.13 diagrams the role of insulin in metabolism.

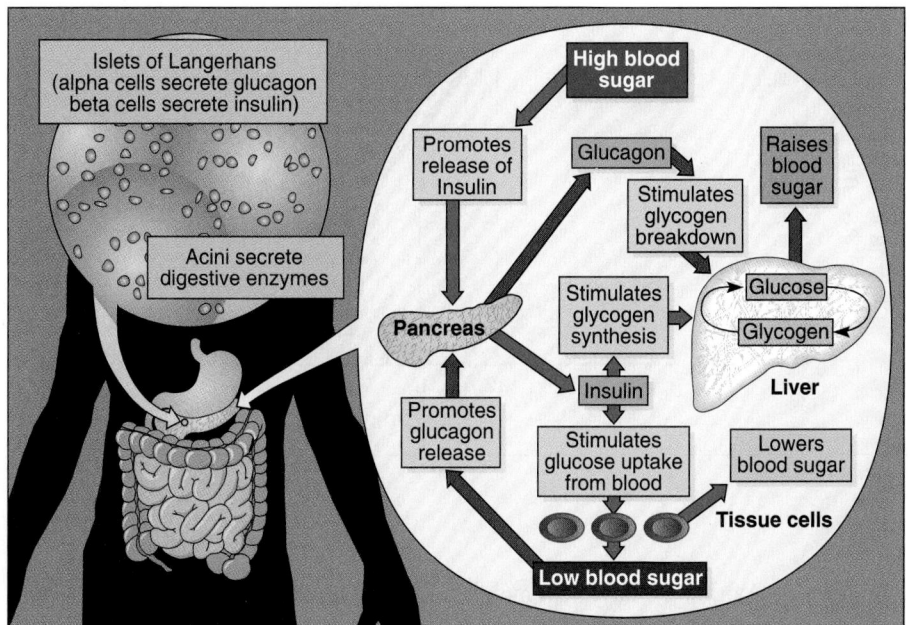

FIGURE 20.12
The pancreas and its secretions.

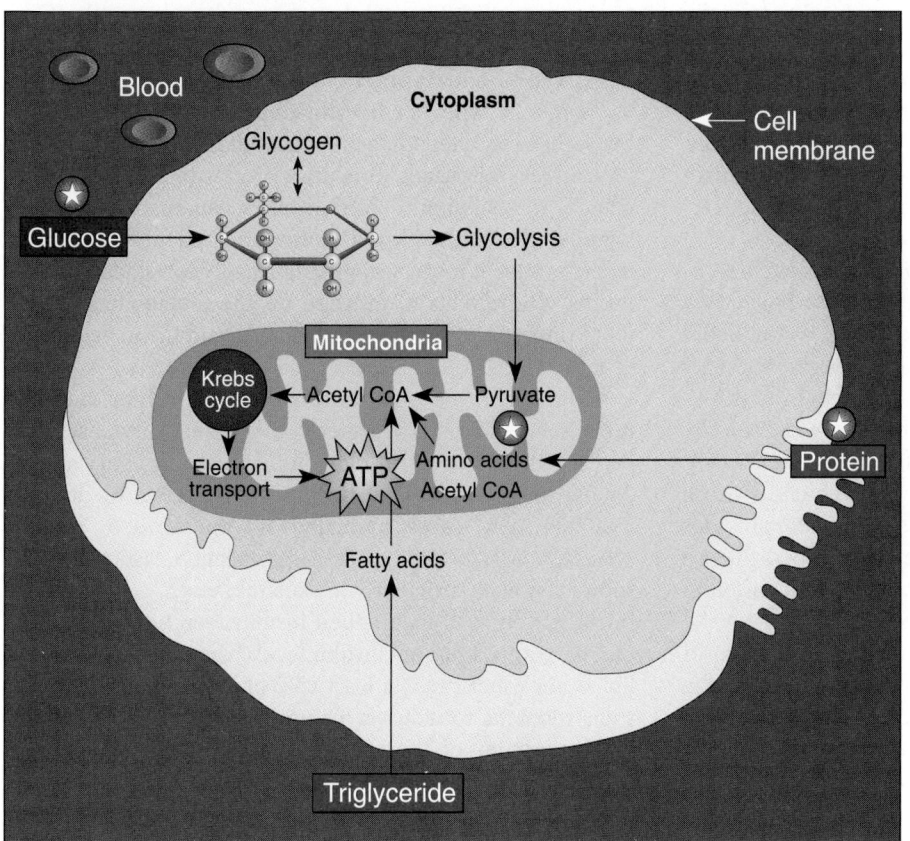

FIGURE 20.13
Primary functions of insulin in the body. The circled stars show the location in metabolism where insulin exerts its influence. The trace element chromium is involved as a cofactor to augment insulin's effects in cellular metabolic factors. However, supplementing with Cr^{3+} as chromium picolinate, combined with 12 weeks of progressive resistance exercise (to increase protein uptake into muscle cells by insulin), does not increase lean body mass or reduce total body fat (densitometry) or site-specific body fat (anthropometry).[52a]

Insulin-mediated glucose uptake by the cells and subsequent glycogen synthesis leads to a decrease in the circulating levels of blood glucose. In essence, insulin exerts a hypoglycemic effect. Conversely, if insulin secretion is insufficient, blood glucose concentration increases and sometimes rises from a normal level of 90 mg · 100 mL^{-1} blood

to a high of 350 mg · 100 mL^{-1}. Unless these high levels of blood glucose are lowered, glucose will eventually spill into the urine.

Insulin also has a pronounced effect on lipid metabolism. As blood glucose levels rise (as normally occurs after a meal), insulin is released, which causes some glucose to be

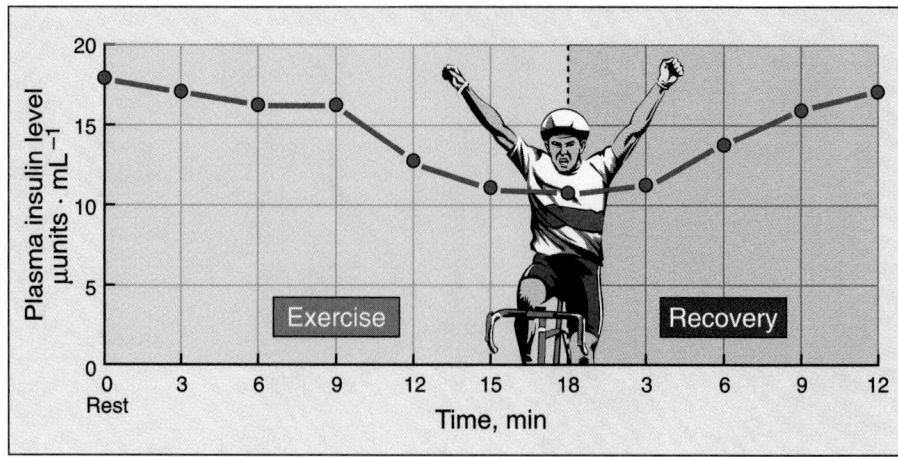

FIGURE 20.14
Generalized response for plasma insulin levels during high-intensity aerobic exercise and in recovery. (From the Applied Physiology Laboratory, University of Michigan, Ann Arbor.)

taken up by fat cells and synthesized to triglyceride. With a well-regulated insulin response, carbohydrates are used preferentially for energy; excess carbohydrate not synthesized to glycogen is converted to and stored as lipid. In the absence of insulin, fatty acids are mobilized and used as the prime energy substrate. Insulin's action also triggers enzyme activity within the cell, which facilitates protein synthesis. This is accomplished by one or all of the following: (*a*) increasing the levels of cellular RNA, (*b*) increasing the rate of amino acid transport through the plasma membrane, and (*c*) increasing the formation of proteins by ribosomes.

Glucose-Insulin Interaction. *Insulin secretion is directly controlled by the level of glucose in the blood that passes through the pancreas.* Insulin secretion is stimulated by increased blood glucose levels. This induces glucose entry into the cells, lowers blood glucose, and removes the stimulus for insulin release. A reduction in blood glucose, on the other hand, causes blood insulin levels to fall dramatically, thus providing a favorable milieu to increase blood glucose levels. This interaction between glucose and insulin provides a feedback mechanism that normally regulates blood glucose within a narrow range. Insulin secretion also is increased in response to rising levels of plasma amino acids.

The levels of plasma insulin decrease as a function of exercise duration (Fig. 20.14). This is most likely due to the inhibitory effect of an increased catecholamine release on the beta cell activity of the pancreas.[42, 137] A lowering of blood glucose with prolonged exercise directly enhances hepatic glucose output and sensitizes the liver to the glucose-releasing effects of the hormones glucagon and epinephrine. This helps to maintain the level of blood glucose. *The catecholamine suppression of insulin is proportional to the intensity of exercise. This exercise-blunting of insulin output helps explain why an over-release of insulin with concentrated pre-exercise glucose feeding is not a concern when consuming glucose during exercise.* During prolonged exercise, there is progressively more energy available from free

fatty acid mobilization in the adipocytes due to reduced insulin output and a decrease in carbohydrate reserves.[137]

Diabetes Mellitus. The syndrome of **diabetes mellitus** consists of different subgroups of disorders with different pathophysiologies. The two largest subgroups are labeled **Type I** and **Type II.**

Type I. Type I or **insulin-dependent diabetes mellitus,** formerly called juvenile-onset diabetes, usually occurs in younger individuals. It is associated with an absolute deficiency of insulin and often of other pancreatic hormones. Compared with the Type II subgroup, patients with Type I diabetes have a more severe abnormality for glucose homeostasis. The effects of exercise on the metabolic state are more pronounced in these individuals, and the management of exercise-related problems is more difficult.

Type II. Type II or **noninsulin-dependent diabetes mellitus (NIDDM),** formerly called maturity-onset diabetes, tends to occur in older individuals. This disease accounts for 80 to 90% of the 14 million cases of diabetes (500,000 new cases annually) in the United States.[81] NIDDM is associated with a significant resistance to insulin's actions (particularly in skeletal muscle), an abnormal but relatively well-maintained insulin secretion, and a normal to elevated plasma insulin level.[49] An estimated 80 million other Americans (at least 25% of the population) are insulin resistant to a lesser extent but have not developed overt symptoms of Type II diabetes. Insulin-resistant means that the body overproduces insulin in response to an increase in blood glucose as occurs from the rapid digestion and absorption of some dietary starches and simple sugars. This could cause more glucose conversion to and storage as body fat. For the insulin-resistant individual, a diet that is high in simple sugars and refined carbohydrates (with a relatively high glycemic index) may actually facilitate an increase in body fat.

As in Type I diabetes, adequate amounts of glucose fail to enter the cells. This causes abnormally high levels of blood glucose that must be filtered by the kidney tubules and voided in the urine. The excessive glucose particles in renal filtrate cause an increased osmotic effect, which also diminishes the reabsorption of water by the kidneys. As a result, the person with diabetes loses large amounts of fluid from the body. With decreased glucose uptake by the cells, the person with diabetes relies heavily on lipid metabolism for energy, which produces an excess of ketoacids and a tendency toward acidosis. In extreme situations, the plasma pH falls to as low as 7.0, eventually resulting in a diabetic coma. Also associated with NIDDM are such medical conditions as arteriosclerosis, small blood vessel and nerve disease, and susceptibility to infection.[66]

Diabetes and Exercise. For persons with diabetes receiving exogenous insulin, hypoglycemia is the most common disturbance in glucose homeostasis during exercise. It is particularly severe in patients who undergo intensive insulin therapy to normalize plasma glucose levels throughout the day. Usually, hypoglycemia occurs during a prolonged session of moderate exercise when hepatic glucose production cannot keep pace with the increased use of glucose by active muscle. Patients with NIDDM often demonstrate a reduced exercise tolerance that is independent of glycemic control. Contributing factors include genetics, lifestyle, excessive body fat, and an overall poor level of physical fitness.

Physical Activity and Risk for NIDDM. *Regular physical activity greatly reduces the chances of developing NIDDM.* More than likely, those at greatest risk (obese, hypertensive, family history, sedentary lifestyle) are the men and women to reap the most benefit from physical activity in the prevention and treatment of NIDDM.[14, 57, 82, 93] This is

illustrated in Figure 20.15 for adult Native Americans of the Pima tribe in Arizona, a group that has 10 to 15 times more NIDDM than the typical U.S. population.[81] These men and women retrospectively rated their participation in various sports and leisure activities at various stages of their lives. Regardless of sex, individuals with diabetes consistently reported less physical activity over their lifetime than those who were disease free. This relationship existed even after accounting for factors of age, body mass, body fat distribution, family history, and current level of physical activity. These retrospective data are remarkably similar to prospective data obtained over a 5-year follow-up of more than 21,000 healthy United States male physicians aged 40 to 85 years (Fig. 20.16).[93] Clearly, those physicians that reported more physical activity, regardless of body mass, had less incidence of NIDDM.

Exercise Benefits For NIDDM

• **Glycemic Control:** Acute exercise causes an abrupt decrease in plasma glucose levels. This improvement in glucose regulation with high-intensity and low-intensity exercise may persist for up to several days[71] and is possibly due to the active muscles' increased insulin sensitivity. Most likely, the long-term improvement in glycemic control with regular exercise is due to the acute effects of each exercise session, rather than to chronic change in tissue function. Interestingly, research shows that the hyperinsulinemic patient (i.e., the one requiring the largest insulin production for glucose regulation) is most likely to benefit from regular exercise.[71, 116, 136] This is consistent

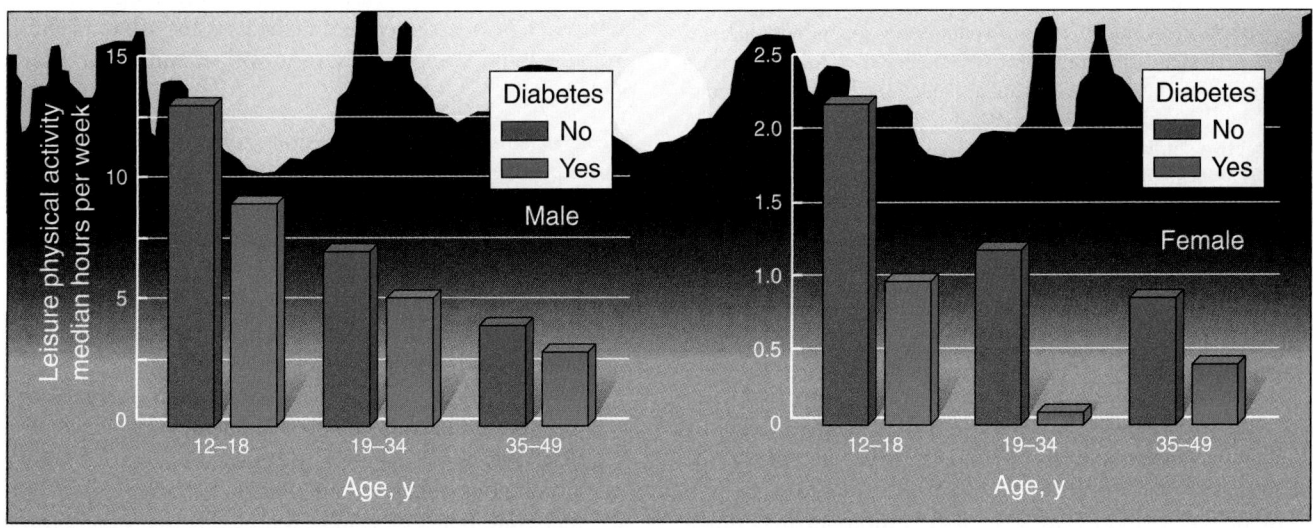

FIGURE 20.15
Reported leisure physical activity over a lifetime in diabetic and nondiabetic Native American men and women of the Pima tribe. (Adapted from Kriska, A.M., et al.: The association of physical activity with obesity, fat distribution and glucose intolerance in Pima Indians. *Diabetologia*, 36:863, 1993.)

A

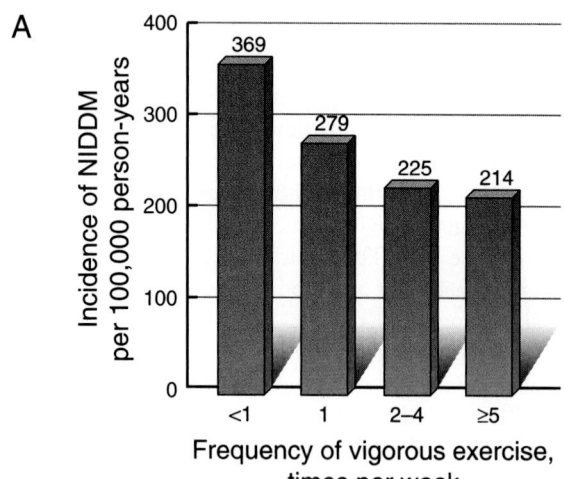

B

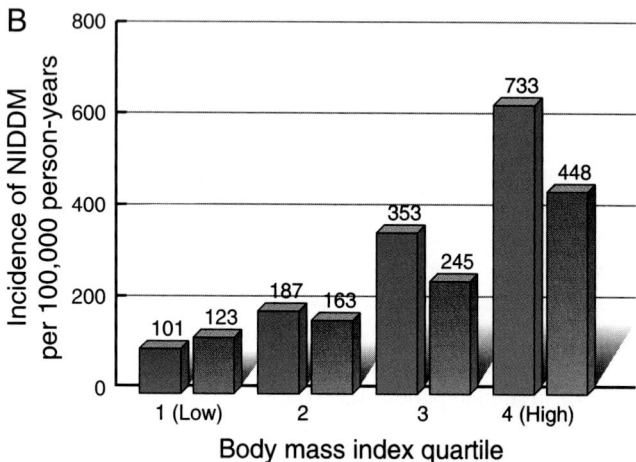

Vigorous exercise less than once per week
Vigorous exercise once a week or more

FIGURE 20.16
Age-adjusted incidence rates of noninsulin-dependent diabetes mellitus (NIDDM) in relation to frequency of vigorous exercise **(A)** and for individuals with similar values for body size as measured by the body mass index **(B)**. (From Manson, J.E., et al.: A prospective study of exercise and incidence of diabetes among US male physicians. *JAMA*, 268:63, 1992.)

with the theory that exercise acts by reversing insulin resistance (i.e., exercise increases insulin sensitivity).

• **Cardiovascular Disease:** The excess morbidity and mortality in NIDDM is attributed to coronary heart disease, stroke, and peripheral vascular disease resulting from accelerated atherosclerosis.[120a] Risk factors for diseases that may improve as a result of regular exercise participation include favorable modifications in hyperinsulinemia, hyperglycemia, plasma lipoproteins, some blood coagulation parameters, and blood pressure.

• **Weight Loss:** Weight loss and the accompanying reduction in body fat and its distribution enhance glucose tol-

erance and insulin sensitivity.[81, 82] The beneficial effects of exercise on weight loss are often underestimated because the changes in body weight with exercise do not always reflect the even more favorable changes in body composition. There are probably no preferential effects of exercise on body composition and weight loss for the diabetic compared with the nondiabetic. Available data indicate that the combination of diet and regular exercise is more effective in reducing body fat in diabetics then either treatment alone.[144]

• **Psychological Profile:** As in nondiabetic persons, increases in exercise capacity in patients with diabetes are associated with decreased anxiety, improved mood and self-esteem, increased sense of well-being and psychological control, and an enhanced quality of life.

• **NIDDM Occurrence:** Regular exercise contributes to delaying and even preventing the onset of insulin resistance and NIDDM in men and women at high risk for developing these problems (Fig. 20.15). These benefits are particularly pronounced among overweight individuals and perhaps all people with abdominal obesity.[56, 82, 92, 93]

Exercise Risks For NIDDM

The potential for complications from exercise should be considered in patients with diabetes. These risks can be minimized if patients are properly screened before starting an exercise program and carefully monitored during exercise. Some potential adverse effects of exercise for the patient with NIDDM are listed in Figure 20.17.

Exercise Guidelines for Type I Diabetes

The following guidelines are useful for individuals with well-controlled, insulin-dependent diabetes who wish to perform prolonged and strenuous exercise with minimal risk of hypoglycemia:[130]

• Ingest 15 to 30 g of carbohydrate for every 30 minutes of intense exercise.

• Consume a snack of carbohydrate soon after exercising.

• Adjust the insulin dose:
  a. Intermediate-acting insulin—decrease the dose by 30 to 35% on the day of exercise.
  b. Intermediate- and short-acting insulin—omit the dose if it normally precedes exercise.
  c. Multiple doses of short-acting insulin—reduce the dose before exercise by 30% and supplement carbohydrate intake.
  d. Continuous subcutaneous insulin infusion—eliminate mealtime bolus or insulin increment that precedes or follows exercise.

• Avoid exercising for 1 hour those muscles into which short-acting insulin was injected.

• Avoid exercising in the late evening.

Potential problems of exercising with NIDDM	
System	**Potential Problem**
Systemic	• Retinal hemorrhage • Increased proteinuria • Acceleration of microvascular lesions
Cardiovascular	• Cadiac arrhythmias • Ischemic heart disease (often silent) • Excessive blood pressure during exercise • Post-exercise orthostatic hypertension
Metabolic	• Increased hyperglycemia • Increased ketosis
Musculoskeletal	• Foot ulcers (in presence of neuropathy) • Orthopedic injury related to neuropathy • Accelerated degenerative joint disease • Eye injuries and retinal hemorrhage

FIGURE 20.17
Potential physical and physiologic problems faced by the noninsulin-dependent diabetic who begins an exercise program.

GLUCAGON

Glucagon, termed the "insulin antagonist" hormone, is secreted from the alpha cells of the islets of Langerhans. In contrast to insulin's effect in lowering blood sugar, glucagon's major function in the body is to stimulate both glycogenolysis and gluconeogenesis by the liver. The glucose generated in this process is then released into the blood. Glucagon exerts its effect by activating the enzyme adenylate cyclase. This stimulates cyclic AMP in the liver cells, which causes the breakdown of liver glycogen to glucose. Glucagon also exerts a stimulating effect on gluconeogenesis by promoting amino acid uptake by the liver.

Similar to insulin, glucagon is controlled by the level of glucose in the blood flowing through the pancreas. When there is a decrease in blood glucose concentration, as occurs in prolonged, high-intensity exercise or food restriction, the alpha cells of the pancreas are stimulated to release glucagon. This causes an almost instantaneous release of glucose from the liver.[36]

Unlike insulin secretion, glucagon release does not appear to be mediated by autonomic nervous stimulation because neither alpha nor beta autonomic receptor blockade influences glucagon secretion in prolonged exercise.[41] Also, there are no sex differences in the glucagon response to exercise when men and women exercise at the same percentage of aerobic capacity.[128] Because glucagon release is considerably delayed following the onset of exercise, it is doubtful that this hormone is important in the early regulation of hepatic glycogenolysis.[3] More than likely, its major role in exercise is to contribute to blood glucose regulation as exercise progresses and existing glycogen reserves become depleted.

OTHER GLANDS AND HORMONES

Other hormones also exert an influence on bodily functions. The liver, for example, secretes the hormone **somatomedin,** which affects the growth of muscle, cartilage, and other tissues. The mucosal lining of the small intestine secretes **secretin, gastrin,** and **cholecystokinin** to promote and coordinate digestive processes. The parathyroid gland secretes **parathormone,** a hormone that promotes calcium absorption by the intestine, kidneys, and bones. This hormone provides for the critical regulation of blood calcium. Limited evidence suggests that prolonged physical activity has a powerful effect in stimulating the release of parathormone, which may contribute to the positive effects of exercise on the maintenance of bone mass.[84] The hypothalamus itself is an important endocrine gland that secretes several stimulating or releasing hormones. For example, hypothalamic release of **somatoliberin** stimulates secretion of somatotropin from the anterior pituitary gland.

EXERCISE TRAINING AND ENDOCRINE FUNCTION

The different hormones and their general response to exercise training are listed in Table 20.3. Because of the complex interactions between endocrine secretions and the nervous system, research is particularly sparse concerning multiple hormone secretions and changes consequent to physical training. *Generally, the magnitude of hormonal response to a standard exercise load declines with endurance training.* For example, when highly trained athletes perform at the same exercise level as sedentary subjects, hormonal responses are lower in the athletes. Much of this response is probably the result of an improved target tissue sensitivity

TABLE 20.3
HORMONES AND THEIR RESPONSES TO ENDURANCE TRAINING

Hormone	*Training Response*
Hypothalamus-Pituitary Hormones	
Growth hormone	No effect on resting values; trained tend to have less dramatic rise during exercise
Thyrotropin	No known training effect
ACTH	Trained have increased exercise values
Prolactin	Some evidence that training lowers resting values
FSH, LH, and	Trained females have depressed values; reduced testosterone in males
Testosterone	(Testosterone levels may increase in males with long-term resistance training)
Posterior Pituitary Hormones	
Vasopressin (ADH)	Some evidence that training results in slight reduction in ADH at a given workload
Oxytocin	No research available
Thyroid Hormones	
Thyroxine (T_4)	Reduced concentration of total T_3 and an increased free thyroxine at rest
Triiodothyronine (T_3)	Increased turnover of T_3 and T_4 during exercise
Adrenal Hormones	
Aldosterone	No significant training adaptation
Cortisol	Trained exhibit slight elevations during exercise
Epinephrine	Decrease in secretion at rest and same exercise intensity after training
Norepinephrine	
Pancreatic Hormones	
Insulin	Training increases sensitivity to insulin; normal decrease in insulin during exercise is greatly reduced in response to training
Glucagon	Smaller increase in glucose levels during exercise at both absolute and relative workloads
Kidney Hormones	
Renin	No apparent training effect
Angiotensin	

and/or responsiveness to a given quantity of hormone.[23, 60, 115] When subjects exercise at the same relative exercise intensity (i.e., the same percentage of maximum and lower absolute load for the untrained), hormonal responses are generally similar regardless of state of training.[113] With maximal exercise, trained subjects have a hormonal response that is either identical or somewhat higher than the response of untrained subjects.

ANTERIOR PITUITARY HORMONES

GH. Because GH stimulates lipolysis and inhibits carbohydrate breakdown, it may be hypothesized that training should enhance GH secretion and conserve carbohydrate. However, this does not appear to be the case. Compared to untrained counterparts, endurance-trained individuals tend to have **less** of a rise in blood levels of GH. This has been attributed to a reduction in psychological stress with exercise as training progresses.[5] The effect of chronic exercise may

be more apparent under nonexercise conditions; aerobic training above the lactate threshold level caused an amplification in the 24-hour pulsatile release of GH during rest.[138]

ACTH. Corticotropin is a potent stimulator of the adrenal cortex and thus increases lipid mobilization for energy. Training appears to increase levels of ACTH during exercise. This would increase the activity of the adrenal gland and result in a greater sparing of glucose. Such a response would certainly be beneficial to long-term exercise performance.

PRL. Long-term exercise training changes in PRL are poorly documented. In one report, the resting PRL levels of male runners were significantly lower compared to sedentary nonrunners.[139]

FSH, LH, and Testosterone. Regular exercise generally depresses reproductive hormone responses in both women and men.[26, 140]

Women. Women with a long history of exercise participation have altered levels of FSH and LH at different times in their menstrual cycles,[10] and such hormonal alterations are usually responsible for menstrual dysfunction. FSH levels, for example, are depressed in chronically trained females throughout an abbreviated anovulatory menstrual cycle, whereas LH and progesterone concentrations are elevated in the follicular phase of the cycle. Several factors other than exercise may alter reproductive function. These include energy drain, weight loss, dietary changes, alterations in the lean-to-fat ratio, the physical and emotional stress of heavy training and competition, and alterations in clearance rates of gonadal steroid hormones.

Men. Endurance training affects pituitary-gonadal function, including levels of testosterone and PRL.[59] The results of comparisons among 46 male runners (average weekly distance = 64 km) and 18 nonrunners matched for age, stature, and body mass are shown in Figure 20.18. The runners had depressed testosterone levels with no significant differences in the levels of LH and FSH compared to the nonrunners. The reduced testosterone concentration (both increased clearance and lower production) in endurance-trained men is similar to and may be the parallel of the sex-steroid reductions observed in women who undergo endurance training and its associated reduction in body fat.[10, 124] Because both LH and FSH are not different between trained and untrained men, an impaired gonadotropin release from the anterior pituitary is not responsible for the reduced testosterone levels in the trained state.

POSTERIOR PITUITARY HORMONES

ADH. There is no difference in ADH levels between trained and untrained individuals following exercise to exhaustion or at the same relative intensity of submaximal exercise.[21, 95] There is some evidence that ADH concentration is reduced during training in response to exercise at the same absolute submaximal exercise intensity.[132]

Oxytocin. We are unaware of research on training-induced changes in this hormone.

THYROID HORMONES

Thyroxine. Training results in a coordinated pituitary-thyroid response that reflects an increased turnover of thyroid hormones. Such increased turnover often is associated with excessive hormonal action, which ultimately leads to hyperthyroidism. There is no evidence, however, that this condition occurs in highly trained individuals.[40] For example, in the trained state, there rarely are aberrant levels of BMR and body temperature. Thus, it appears that the greater T_4 turnover that accompanies physical training occurs through a mechanism that differs from the "normal" dynamics for this hormone. The importance of changes in thyroxine levels in the adaptive process of training has not been established.

Research on women who engage in endurance training has revealed some interesting results regarding thyroid turnover. Changing from a baseline of relatively sedentary living to run training 48 km per week resulted in a mild thyroid impairment as reflected by a decrease in the levels of T_3 and T_4.[11] Increasing training to 80 km per week was associated with a significant increase in the blood level of these hormones. It was suggested that changes in body composition that accompany heavy training might play a role in any exercise-induced change in thyroid function in females. Six months of resistance training in men slightly reduced the concentrations of T_4 and plasma-free T_4, with no change in thyrotropin. The researchers concluded that the small changes were of no clinical or physiologic significance.[104]

ADRENAL HORMONES

Aldosterone. The response of the renin-angiotensin-aldosterone system during exercise is well suited for homeostatic control.[134] These responses are apparently transient, however, because exercise training does not affect resting levels of these hormones or their normal response to exercise.[45]

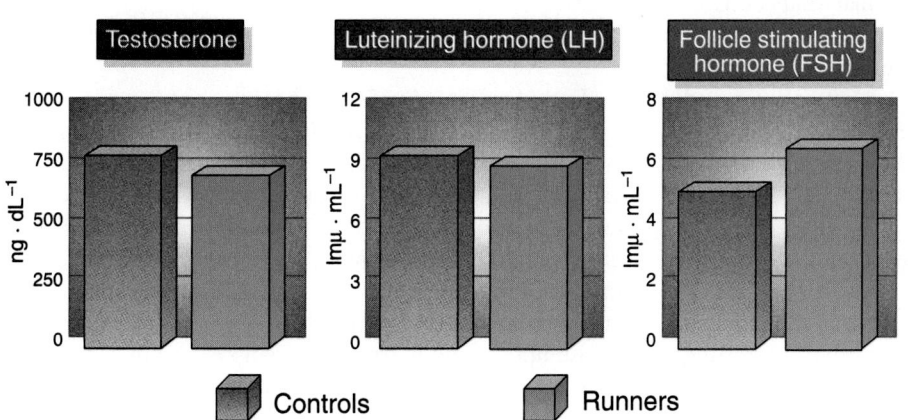

FIGURE 20.18
Comparison of testosterone, LH, and FSH levels between trained runners and untrained controls. There are significantly reduced testosterone levels in runners with no significant difference in LH and FSH compared with controls. (From Wheeler, G.D., et al.: Reduced serum testosterone and prolactin levels in male distance runners. *JAMA*, 252:514, 1984.)

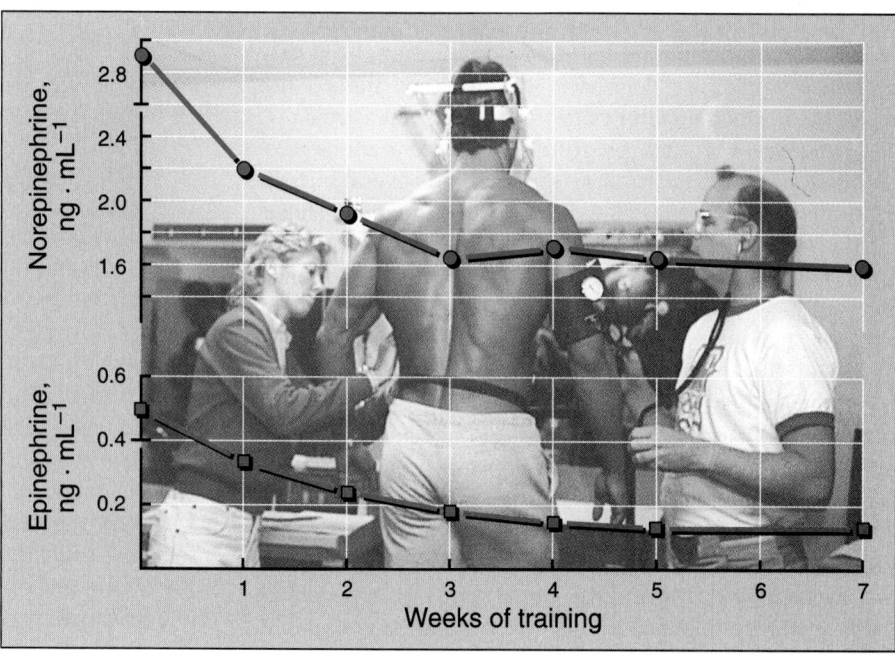

FIGURE 20.19
Week-by-week changes in catecholamines during a 5-minute period of exercise at 243 watts for six male subjects. Training consisted of running and stationary cycling for 6 days per week. Catecholamine levels decreased progressively during training; the most rapid decline was observed during the early phase of training. (From Winder, W.W., et al.: Time course of sympathoadrenal adaptations to endurance exercise training in man. *J. Appl. Physiol.*, 45:370, 1969.)

Cortisol. Plasma cortisol levels tend to increase less in trained compared to sedentary subjects who perform the same absolute level of submaximal exercise.[119] With repeated bouts of high-intensity exercise and correspondingly high cortisol output, adrenal gland enlargement can occur due to both cellular hypertrophy and hyperplasia.[121]

Epinephrine and Norepinephrine. Sympathoadrenal activity (especially for norepinephrine) to a given submaximum workload is lower in trained than in untrained individuals.[33, 51] For equivalent relative exercise intensities, on the other hand, the sympathoadrenal response is similar between trained and untrained individuals. The time course for the reduction in epinephrine and norepinephrine to standard heavy exercise during physical training is illustrated in Figure 20.19. As can be seen, the concentration of both hormones falls dramatically during the first several weeks of training. The appearance of bradycardia and the smaller rise in blood pressure during submaximal exercise with training are probably the most familiar reflections of this sympathoadrenal training response. Such adaptations are favorable because they contribute to a lowering of myocardial oxygen demands during submaximal exercise and perhaps during other forms of stress.[85] It is not clear whether exercise training alters the resting levels of catecholamines.[9, 107]

PANCREATIC HORMONES

Insulin and Glucagon. Studies of training-induced changes in insulin and glucagon reveal several interesting findings. With endurance training, the blood levels of insulin and glucagon are maintained closer to resting values during exercise. *In essence, the trained state requires less insulin at any stage from rest through light to moderate intensities of exercise.* This seemingly blunted hormonal response to exercise training probably is brought about in one of several ways:

- Physical training increases a muscle tissue's sensitivity to insulin.[49, 115] Consequently, less insulin is required to regulate blood glucose after training than before training.[31, 34] This **improved insulin sensitivity** is probably related to the binding capacity of insulin to the receptor sites of individual muscle cells. There also is an increase in the liver's insulin sensitivity.[30]
- The trained person can reduce carbohydrate utilization through a facilitated use of lipid as an energy fuel. In addition, a smaller insulin output is required to clear any excess glucose from the circulation as would occur after a high carbohydrate meal. With the resumption of a sedentary lifestyle, there is a decrease in the muscle's sensitivity to insulin; thus, more insulin is required to regulate a given quantity of blood glucose.[96]

Exercise Training in Diabetes

Type I Diabetes. Despite the clear association between physical training effects and improved insulin sensitivity, the clinical utility of regular exercise for improving glucose control in Type I diabetes has not been clearly demonstrated.[58] Furthermore, some patients with diabetes must be cautious because regular exercise can actually trigger a potentially dangerous dual response—an enhanced glucose uptake and a greater exogenous insulin supply due to the rapid circulation of the injected insulin that accompanies exercise. Such an exacerbated response would actually worsen the imbalance between glucose supply and utilization and could result in serious complications from hypoglycemia.[74] Appropriate precautions and guidelines for physically active individuals with Type I diabetes have been presented on page 376.

Type II Diabetes. Because of obesity, many overweight individuals have a reduced glucose tolerance that results in hyperinsulinemia, a generalized insulin resistance, and eventual development of NIDDM. In this situation, exercise training can reduce resting plasma insulin levels and lower insulin output from the pancreas during a glucose tolerance test, both of which are evidence for improved insulin sensitivity. *Improved insulin sensitivity with exercise training is important "therapy" that can ultimately result in a lowered insulin requirement for those diabetics who are noninsulin-dependent.*

RESISTANCE TRAINING AND ENDOCRINE FUNCTION

Muscle remodeling in resistance training is a complex process involving cell receptor interaction with different hormones and the DNA-mediated production of new contractile proteins. The specific exercise response is initially linked to the configuration of the particular exercise stimulus that involves the order, frequency, rest interval, intensity, volume, and mode of workouts during training. Figure 20.20 is a schematic flow chart of how heavy resistance exercise training might ultimately produce significant improvements in overall muscular size, strength, and power. The factors responsible for the exercise-induced changes in muscle size and function include changes in hepatic and extrahepatic clearance rates, differential rates of secretion of various hormones (and accompanying fluid shifts around the receptor sites), and alterations in how the receptor sites for hormone activation are mediated via neurohumoral control.[76] Considerably more data are needed to piece together how the myriad of factors actually interact to induce cellular and performance adaptations with resistance training.

The two primary hormones involved in resistance training adaptations are testosterone and GH.[75, 79] It appears that testosterone's primary role is to augment the release of GH and to interact with the nervous system. These functions may be more important than any direct anabolic effect of testosterone per se. An exercise session of resistance training generally causes a short-term rise in serum testosterone and a decrease in cortisol levels; the response is greater in men than in women.[79, 117, 122] The magnitude of this response, however, may be no greater than that observed with acute aerobic exercise.[63]

Current beliefs indicate that with resistance training, both testosterone and GH increase in frequency and amplitude of secretion, thereby establishing a more favorable hormonal environment for muscular growth. Sex differences in the long-term response of these hormones to resistance training may ultimately explain any sex differences in the "responsiveness" of muscle strength and muscle size to resistance training.

OPIOID PEPTIDES AND EXERCISE

In the 1970s, scientists studying the pain-relieving effects of opioid peptides (e.g., morphine) on brain function discovered that these substances had neurotransmitter properties

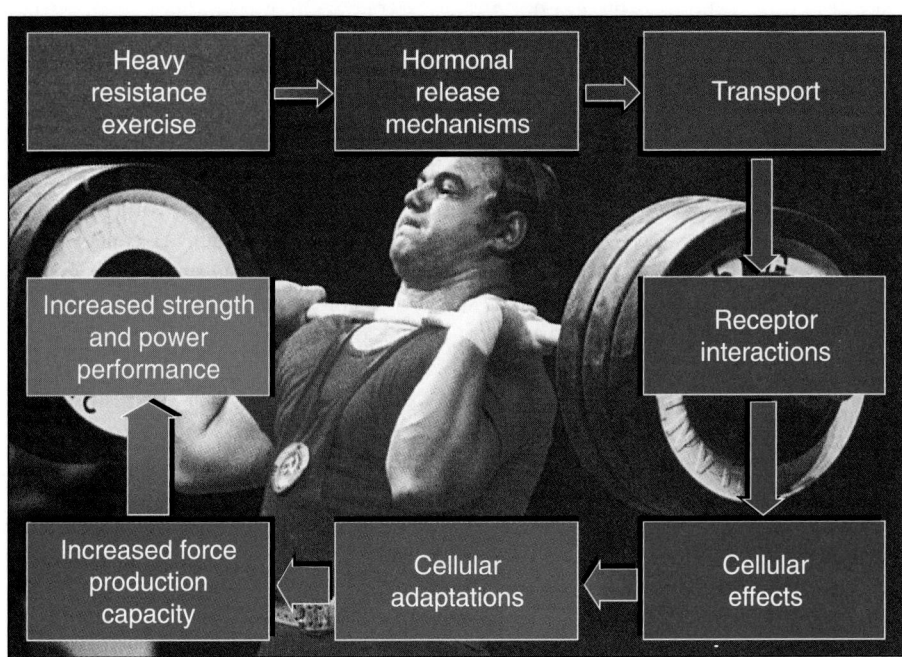

FIGURE 20.20
Schematic model of how heavy resistance exercise training might produce favorable adaptations in muscle structure and performance. (Modified from Kraemer, W.J.: Endocrine responses and adaptations to strength training. In *Strength and Power in Sport.* Edited by P.V. Komi. London, Blackwell Scientific, 1992.)

that probably acted on specific opioid receptor sites in the brain. With this finding came the realization that perhaps the brain itself produced endogenous opioid-like, mood-altering substances.[97]

Evidence for the existence of endogenous substances that behaved as opiates was first provided with the isolation and purification of two opioid pentapeptides, methionine and leucine enkephalin (enkephalin is Greek meaning "in the brain").[48] These opioids are part of a larger proopio-cortin precursor molecule produced in the anterior part of the pituitary gland. Other opioid substances include **β-lipotrophin, β-endorphin,** and more recently, **dynorphin,** the most potent of the opioid peptides.

The effects of the various endogenously produced opioids are widespread, ranging from their function as a neurohormone to that of a neurotransmitter. The endogenous opiates produce a strong inhibition of hormonal release from the posterior pituitary, principally the release of LH and FSH.[48, 75] This regulation may play a key role in menstrual cycle disturbances such as delay in menarche, dysfunctional uterine bleeding, secondary amenorrhea, and inadequacy of the luteal phase.[2] On the other hand, release of GH and PRL are stimulated by the opioid peptides.

Endorphins also have been implicated in the regulation of other hormones, including ACTH, the catecholamines, and cortisol.[94] Serum concentrations of endogenous opioids, primarily β-endorphin and/or β-lipotrophin, generally increase in response to exercise although the response is variable.[32, 46, 78, 91] The elevation of β-endorphin during exercise increases as much as five times the resting level, with even higher values probably occurring in the brain itself.[54, 112] For aerobic exercise, the intensity of exercise is a primary factor in stimulating elevations in plasma β-endorphin.[47] With resistance exercise, β-endorphin release responds differently to various exercise protocols with the protocol of longer duration (lighter resistance, 10-RM) and longer interset rest intervals causing the greatest response.[80]

Although the precise physiologic significance of the exercise response of the various endogenous opioid peptides remains unclear, several important effects must be considered. The most notable postulated opioid effect has been their role in triggering a so-called "exercise high"—a state described by some as euphoria and exhilaration as the duration of moderate to intense aerobic exercise progresses. Endorphin secretion also has been implicated in increased pain tolerance, improved appetite control, and a reduction in anxiety, tension, anger, and confusion—all of which are proposed "psychological" benefits of regular exercise.[97, 146]

The effect of training on endorphin response is controversial, partly because of limited data and partly because of the variations in exercise protocols.[1, 20, 61] In one study, there were no significant changes in β-endorphin response to prolonged exercise following 8 weeks of endurance training. In contrast, another study showed that general physical conditioning augmented the responses of β-endorphins and

β-lipotrophins to exercise.[20] Large increases in endorphin release have been noted with heavy sprint-type training.[78] This suggests that anaerobic factors may affect the pattern of endorphin release.

It is tempting to speculate that with physical training, the individual becomes more sensitive to opioid effects so that it takes less of the hormone to induce a specific effect. In this sense, regular exercise could be viewed as a type of "positive addiction." It also appears that exercise training causes the opiates produced in the body during exercise to be degraded more slowly compared to the pretraining condition.[62] Certainly, this slower rate of disposal would facilitate and prolong an opiate response and possibly augment one's tolerance for extended exercise.

EXERCISE, INFECTIOUS ILLNESS, CANCER, AND IMMUNE RESPONSE

"Don't exercise until you're fatigued or you'll get sick," is a common perception held by many parents, athletes, and coaches that too much heavy exercise makes a person more susceptible to certain illnesses. In contrast, there is also the belief that regular, more moderate exercise makes a person "healthy" and less susceptible to infectious illness such as the common cold.

It was reported as early as 1918 that most of the cases of pneumonia among boys in boarding school occurred in athletes and that respiratory infections seemed to progress toward pneumonia after intense sports training. There also have been reports relating the severity of poliomyelitis to participation in heavy physical activity at a critical time of infection. Although most of this evidence was anecdotal, accumulating epidemiological and clinical data began to indicate that acute, unusually heavy physical activity profoundly affected the dynamics of immune function in a manner that increased one's susceptibility to illness, particularly upper respiratory tract infection.

The immune system is a highly complex and well-regulated grouping of cells, hormones, and interactive modulators that defend the body from invasion from outside microbes (bacterial, viral, and fungal) or any foreign macromolecules and from abnormal cells such as cancer cells. If infection does take place, the immune system aids greatly in blunting the severity of illness and speeding the recovery.

A proposed model depicted in Figure 20.21 is for the interactions between exercise, stress, illness, and the immune system. Within this framework, exercise, stress, and illness are interactive factors, each with its own effect on the body's immune system. For example, exercise can affect susceptibility to illness, and certain illnesses clearly affect exercise capability. Likewise, psychological and other forms of stress, including an acute alteration in one's normal sleep schedule, can influence one's resistance to illness, whereas exercise can positively and negatively moderate the response to stress. Each factor—stress, illness, and

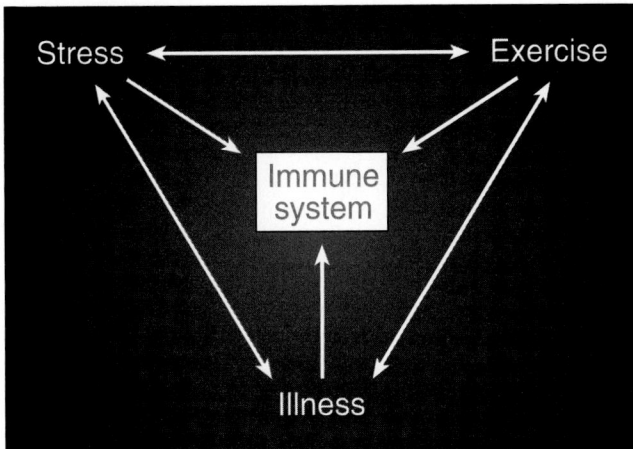

FIGURE 20.21
Theoretical model of the interrelationships between stress, exercise, illness, and the immune system. (From MacKinnon, L.T.: Current challenges and future expectations in exercise immunology: back to the future. *Med. Sci. Sports Exerc.*, 26:191, 1994.)

acute and chronic exercise—has an independent effect on immune status, immune function, and resistance to disease.

UPPER RESPIRATORY TRACT INFECTIONS

The general "J"-shaped model that describes the relationship between an acute period of exercise or unusually heavy training on markers of immune function and/or one's susceptibility to upper respiratory tract infection (URTI) is illustrated in Figure 20.22. As illustrated, light to moderate levels of physical activity may offer some protection against URTI compared to a sedentary lifestyle.[101] In contrast, a period of intense activity such as a marathon or a heavy training session places one at an increased risk of infection within 1 or 2 weeks of the exercise stress.[55, 108] For example, approximately 13% of the participants in a Los Angeles Marathon reported an episode of infectious URTI during the week following the race. For runners of comparable ability who did not compete for reasons other than illness, the infection rate was only approximately 2%.[100]

Acute Exercise Effects

- **Moderate exercise:** *A bout of moderate exercise provides a boost to the level of natural immune function and host defense that lasts for up to several hours into recovery.*[70] Of significance is the increase in **natural killer (NK) cell** activity. These phagocytic lymphocyte subpopulations enhance the cytotoxic capacity of the blood and provide the body's first line of defense against various pathogens. The NK cell does not require prior or specific sensitization to foreign bodies or neoplastic cells. These cells demonstrate spontaneous cytolytic activity that ulti-

mately ruptures and/or inactivates viruses and the metastatic potential of tumor cells.[89, 106, 141]

- **Exhaustive exercise:** *Whereas moderate exercise heightens immune function, a period of exhaustive exercise (and other forms of extreme stress or increased levels of training) has the opposite effect and severely blunts the body's first line of defense against infectious agents.*[50, 65a, 88, 109, 120] This immunodepression of the body in general, as well as the mucosal immune system following severe exercise, may be mediated by the effects of elevated temperature, cytokines, and the various stress-related hormones such as epinephrine, GH, cortisol, and β-endorphins.[67, 106] This certainly supports the wisdom of advising individuals with URTI symptoms to refrain from or at least "go easy" on physical activity to optimize the effectiveness of the normal immune mechanisms in combating the infection.

Effects of Chronic Exercise. *Limited data indicate that regular aerobic exercise training has desirable effects on natural immune function in both young and old individuals.*[89, 106, 118] Those areas of improvement include a significant enhancement in the functional capacity of natural cytotoxic

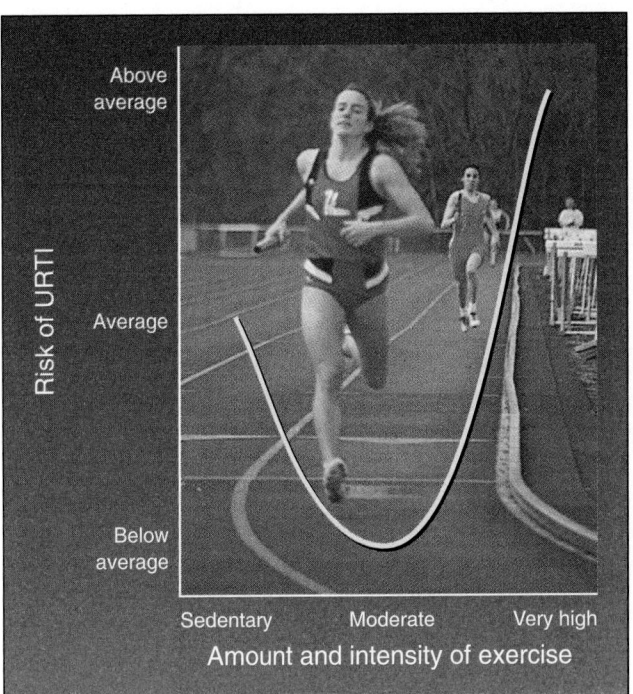

FIGURE 20.22
General model for relationship between an acute period of physical activity and susceptibility to upper respiratory tract infection (UTRI). The inference from this model is that moderate exercise reduces risk of URTI whereas exhaustive competition or training places the participant at increased risk. (From Nieman, D.C.: Exercise, upper respiratory tract infection, and the immune system. *Med. Sci. Sports Exerc.*, 26:128, 1994.)

immune mechanisms such as the antitumor actions of NK cell activity and a blunting in the age-related decrease in T-cell function.[89, 101] It is the cytotoxic **T cells** that directly defend against viral and fungal infections and contribute to the regulation of other immune mechanisms.

Resistance Training. In contrast to aerobic exercise, 9 years of prior resistance exercise training appeared to have no effect on resting NK cell activity or the number of NK cells when comparing experienced weight trainers to sedentary controls.[102] The researchers suggested that resistance training activates monocytes more than aerobic training, releasing prostaglandins that downregulate NK cells following exercise,[105] thus blunting the long-term effect. These same investigators had shown previously that NK cells increase a substantial 225% following an acute period of resistance exercise training.[103] This response is similar to that reported for an acute period of aerobic exercise.[38, 53]

One might ask that if exercise training enhances the level of immune function, why are trained individuals more susceptible to URTI after intense competition? The reason may be explained by what has been termed the "open window hypothesis." This position argues that the highly conditioned athlete, through variations in the level of training or in the stress of actual competition, is exposed to a "non-normal" exercise level that severely depresses natural killer cell function. It is during this period of immunodepression or "open window" that infection is more easily established. In individuals who perform only moderate exercise regularly, the window of opportunity for infection remains "closed" and there is maintenance of the protective benefits of regular exercise.[106]

THE EXERCISE-CANCER CONNECTION

Although findings have not always been consistent, various epidemiological studies have demonstrated a protective association between regular physical activity and risk of cancers of the breast, colon, lung, and prostate (refer to Chapter 31).[83a, 123] One possible mechanism for this protection, other than exercise's beneficial effect on NK cell activity, is the long-term enhancement of other natural immune functions. These include an augmented phagocytic capacity of the monocyte-macrophage lineage as well as a more robust cytotoxic and intracellular killing capacities (T-cell activity) that inhibit tumor growth and destroy cancer cells.[141, 145] Other potential effects of regular exercise on aspects of cancer development include beneficial changes in the body's antioxidant functions, endocrine profiles, prostaglandin metabolism, body composition, and in the case of colon cancer, a beneficial increase in intestinal transit time (total or segmental) with exercise. More research will certainly be forthcoming in these important and exciting areas as new technologies develop and more effort is devoted to these multidisciplinary fields of investigation.

■ SUMMARY ■

1. The endocrine system consists of a host organ, a transmitted substance called a hormone, and a target or receptor organ. Hormones are either steroids or amino acid (polypeptide) derivatives.

2. The major function of hormones is to alter the rate of cellular reactions. This function is achieved through hormones that act at specific receptor sites by either enhancing or inhibiting enzyme function.

3. Blood hormone concentration is determined by the quantity of hormone synthesized, the amount released, the amount taken up by the target organ, and the rate of hormone removal from the blood.

4. The anterior pituitary is responsible for the secretion of at least six hormones, including PRL, the gonadotropic hormones FSH and LH, corticotropin, TSH, and GH.

5. GH promotes cell division and cellular proliferation; TSH controls the amount of hormone secreted by the thyroid gland; ACTH regulates the output of the hormones secreted by the adrenal cortex; PRL is important in reproduction and in the development of secondary sex characteristics of females; FSH and LH stimulate the ovaries to secrete estrogen in females and sperm in males.

6. The posterior pituitary secretes the hormone ADH, which controls water excretion by the kidneys. It also secretes oxytocin, which is an important hormone in birthing and lactation.

7. TSH has a stimulating effect on the metabolic rate of all cells and increases the breakdown of carbohydrate and lipid in energy metabolism.

8. The inner (medulla) and outer (cortex) portions of the adrenal gland secrete two different types of hormones. The medulla secretes the catecholamines epinephrine and norepinephrine. The adrenal cortex secretes mineralocorticoids, which regulate extracellular sodium and potassium levels, glucocorticoids, which stimulate gluconeogenesis and serve as an insulin antagonist, and androgens, which control male secondary sex characteristics.

9. The gonads are the testes in the male and the ovaries in the female. These glands produce testosterone in the testes and estrogens (estradiol and progesterone) in the ovaries.

10. Moderate levels of aerobic exercise and resistance training increase testosterone levels in untrained males. For females, plasma levels of testosterone and estrogens are elevated during exercise.

11. Insulin is secreted by the beta cells of the islets of Langerhans of the pancreas. The main function of insulin is to increase the rate of glucose transport into cells and thereby control blood sugar levels and the body's rate of carbohydrate metabolism. Lack of insulin, or a decreased sensitivity or increased resistance to this hormone, results in the serious medical condition of di-

abetes mellitus. The alpha cells of the pancreas secrete glucagon, an insulin antagonist that acts to raise the level of blood sugar.

12. Exercise training has differential effects on resting and exercise-induced hormone production and release. Trained persons generally show elevated hormone response during exercise for ACTH and cortisol, depressed values for GH, PRL, FSH, LH, testosterone, ADH, thyroxine, catecholamines and insulin, and no training response for aldosterone, renin, and angiotensin.

13. Exercise-induced elevation of β-endorphins and associated opioid-like hormones has been associated with euphoria, increased pain tolerance, the "exercise high," and altered menstrual function.

14. Unusually heavy physical activity may affect the dynamics of immune function in a manner that increases one's susceptibility to upper respiratory tract infection (URTI). Moderate activity, on the other hand, may protect against URTI.

15. Regular exercise appears to have a desirable effect on natural immune function. This may protect not only against URTI but a variety of cancers.

■ REFERENCES ■

1. Aforzo, G.A., et al.: In vivo opioid receptor occupation in the rat brain following exercise. *Med. Sci. Sports Exerc.*, 18:380, 1986.
2. Baker, E.R.: Menstrual dysfunction and hormonal status in athletic women: a review. *Fertil. Steril.*, 36:391, 1981.
3. Bjorkman, O., et al.: Influence of hypoglucagonemia on splanchnic glucose output during leg exercise in man. *Clin. Physiol.*, 1:43, 1981.
4. Björntrop, P., et al.: Physical training in human hyperplastic obesity. IV. Effects on the hormonal system. *Metabolism*, 26:319, 1977.
5. Bloom, S.R., et al.: Differences in the metabolic and hormonal responses to exercise between racing cyclists and untrained individuals. *J. Physiol. (Lond.)*, 258:1, 1976.
6. Bonen, A., et al.: Effects of exercise and training on menstrual cycle hormones. *Aust. J. Sports Med.*, 10:39, 1978.
7. Borer, K.T.: Exercise-induced facilitation of pulsatile growth hormone (GH) secretion and somatic growth. In *Hormones and Sport*. Vol. 55. Edited by Z. Laron and A.D. Rogol. New York, Raven Press, 1989.
8. Borer, K.T., and Pearson, W.: Adrenergic restraint of somatostatin action promotes pulsatile growth hormone secretion in hamsters (Abstract). Program of the 68th Annual Meeting of the Endocrine Society. Cornell University, New York, 1986.
9. Bove, A.A., et al.: Increased conjugated dopamine in plasma after exercise training. *J. Lab. Clin. Med.*, 104:77, 1984.
10. Boyden, T.W., et al.: Prolactin responses, menstrual cycles and body composition of women runners. *J. Clin. Endocrinol. Metab.*, 58:711, 1982.
11. Boyden, T.W., et al.: Thyroidal changes associated with endurance training in women. *Med. Sci. Sports Exerc.*, 16:234, 1984.
12. Brandenberger, G., and Follenius, M.: Influence of timing and intensity of muscular exercise on temporal patterns of plasma cortisol levels. *J. Clin. Endocrinol. Metab.*, 54:592, 1982.
13. Brandenberger, G.: Cortisol responses to exercise and other interactions with diurnal secretory peaks. In *Exercise Endocrinology*. Edited by F. Fotherby and S. B. Pal. Berlin, Walter de Gruyter, 1985.
14. Braun, B., et al.: Effects of exercise intensity on insulin sensitivity in women with non-insulin-dependent diabetes mellitus. *J. Appl. Physiol.*, 78:300, 1995.
15. Bray, G.: *The Obese Patient. Major Problems in Internal Medicine.* Vol. 9. Philadelphia, W. B. Saunders, 1976.
16. Brillon, D., et al.: Cholinergic but not serotonergic mediation of exercise-induced growth hormone secretion. *Endocr. Res.*, 12:137, 1986.
17. Brisson, D., et al.: Exercise-induced dissociation of the blood prolactin response in young women according to their sports habits. *Horm. Metab. Res.*, 12:201, 1980.
18. Bunt, J.C., et al.: Sex and training differences in human growth hormone levels during prolonged exercise. *J. Appl. Physiol.*, 61:1796, 1986.
19. Cappa, M.R., et al.: Modification of somatostatinergic tone induced by physical exercise. In *Hormones in Sport*. Vol. 55. Edited by Z. Laron and A.D. Rogol. New York, Raven Press, 1989.
20. Carr, D.B., et al.: Physical conditioning facilitates exercise induced secretion of beta-endorphins and beta-lipotrophin in women. *N. Engl. J. Med.*, 305:560, 1981.
21. Convertino, V.A., et al.: Exercise induced hypervolemia: role of plasma albumin, renin and vasopressin. *J. Appl. Physiol.*, 48:665, 1980.
22. Cook, N.J., et al.: Changes in adrenal and testicular activity monitored by salivary sampling in males throughout marathon runs. *J. Appl. Physiol.*, 55:634, 1986.
23. Crampes, F., et al.: Effect of physical training in humans on the response of isolated fat cells to epinephrine. *J. Appl. Physiol.*, 61:25, 1991.
24. Criswell, D., et al.: Fluid replacement beverages and maintenance of plasma volume during exercise: Role of aldosterone and vasopressin. *Eur. J. Appl. Physiol.*, 65:445, 1992.
25. Cumming, D.C., and Rebar, R. W.: Exercise and reproductive function in women. *Prog. Clin. Biol. Res.*, 117:113, 1983.
26. Cumming, D.C., et al.: Defects in pulsatile LH release in normally menstruating runners. *J. Clin. Endocrinol. Metab.*, 60:810, 1985.
27. Cumming, D.C., et al.: Reproductive hormone increases in response to acute exercise in men. *Med. Sci. Sports Exerc.*, 18:369, 1986.
28. De Souza, M.J., et al.: Menstrual status and plasma vasopressin, renin activity, aldosterone and exercise responses. *J. Appl. Physiol.*, 67:736, 1989.
29. DeSousa, M.J., et al.: Menstrual status and plasma vasopressin, renin activity, aldosterone, and exercise response. *J. Appl. Physiol.*, 68:520, 1990.
30. Devlin, J.T., et al.: Enhanced peripheral and splanchnic insulin sensitivity in NIDDM men after a single bout of exercise. *Diabetes*, 36:434, 1987.
31. Dolkas, C.B., et al.: Effect of body weight gain on insulin sensitivity after retirement from exercise training. *J. Appl. Physiol.*, 68:520, 1990.
32. Donevan, R.H., and Andrew, G.M.: Plasma β-endorphin immunoreactivity during graded cycle ergometry. *Med. Sci. Sports Exerc.*, 19:229, 1987.
33. Duncan, J.J., et al.: The effects of aerobic exercise on plasma catecholamines and blood pressure in patients with mild hypertension. *JAMA*, 254:2609, 1985.
34. Farrell, P.A.: Decreased insulin response to sustained hyperglycemia in exercise trained rats. *Med. Sci. Sports Exerc.*, 22:469, 1988.
35. Farrell, P.A., et al.: Enkephalins, catecholamines, and psychological mood alterations: effects of prolonged exercise. *Med. Sci. Sports Exerc.*, 19:347, 1987.
36. Felig, P., et al.: Plasma glucagon levels in exercising man. *N. Engl. J. Med.*, 287:184, 1972.
37. Friedmann, B., and Kindermann, W.: Energy metabolism and regulatory hormones in women and men during continuous exercise. *Eur. J. Appl. Physiol.*, 59:1, 1989.
38. Gabriel, H.A., et al.: Circulating leukocyte and lymphocyte subpopulations before and after intensive endurance exercise to exhaustion. *J. Appl. Physiol.*, 63:449, 1991.
39. Galbo, H.: *Hormonal and Metabolic Adaptation to Exercise.* New York, G. T. Verlag, 1983.

40. Galbo, H.: Exercise physiology: Humoral function. *Sport Sci. Rev.*, 1:65,1992.

41. Galbo, H., et al.: Glucagon and plasma catecholamine responses to graded and prolonged exercise in man. *J. Appl. Physiol.*, 38:70, 1975.

42. Galbo, H., et al.: Catecholamines and pancreatic hormones during autonomic blockade in exercising man. *Acta Physiol. Scand.*, 101:428, 1977.

43. Galbo, H., et al.: Thyroid and testicular hormone response to graded and prolonged exercise in man. *Eur. J. Appl. Physiol.*, 36:101, 1977.

44. Galbo, H., et al.: The effect of fasting on the hormonal response to graded exercise. *J. Clin. Endocrinol. Metab.*, 52:1106, 1981.

45. Geyssant, A., et al.: Plasma vasopressin, renin activity, and aldosterone: effects of exercise and training. *Eur. J. Appl. Physiol.*, 46:21, 1980.

46. Goldfarb, A.H., et al.: Serum β-endorphin levels during a graded exercise test to exhaustion. *Med. Sci. Sports Exerc.*, 19:78, 1987.

47. Goldfarb, A.H., et al.: Beta-endorphin time course response to intensity of exercise: effect of training status. *Int. J. Sports Med.*, 12:264, 1991.

48. Grossman, A., and Sutton, J.R.: Endorphins: What are they? How are they measured? What is their role in exercise? *Med. Sci. Sports Exerc.*, 17:74, 1985.

49. Gudat, V., et al.: Physical activity, fitness, and non-insulin-dependent (Type II) diabetes mellitus. In *Physical Activity, Fitness, and Health*. Edited by C. Bouchard, et al. Champaign, IL, Human Kinetics, 1994.

50. Hag, A., et al.: Changes in peripheral blood lymphocyte subsets associated with marathon running. *Med. Sci. Sports Exerc.*, 25:186, 1993.

51. Haggendal, L., et al.: Arterial noradrenaline concentration during exercise in relation to the relative work levels. *Scand. J. Clin. Lab. Invest.*, 26:337, 1970.

52. Hale, R.W., et al.: A marathon: the immediate effect on female runners' luteinizing hormone, follicle-stimulating hormone, prolactin, testosterone, and cortisol levels. *Am. J. Obstet. Gynecol.*, 146:550, 1983.

52a. Hallmark, M.A., et al.: Effects of chromium and resistive training on muscle strength and body composition. *Med. Sci. Sports Exerc.*, 28:139, 1996.

53. Hansen, J.B., et al.: Biphasic changes in leukocytes induced by strenuous exercise. *Eur. J. Appl. Physiol.*, 62:157, 1991.

54. Harbor, V.J., and Sutton, J.R.: Endorphins and exercise. *Sports Med.*, 1:154, 1984.

55. Heath, G.W., et al.: Exercise and the incidence of upper respiratory tract infections. *Med. Sci. Sports Exerc.*, 23:152, 1991.

56. Helmrich, S.P., et al.: Physical activity and reduced occurrence of Non-insulin dependent diabetes mellitus. *N. Engl. J. Med.*, 325:147, 1991.

57. Helmrich, S.P., et al.: Prevention of non-insulin-dependent diabetes mellitus with physical activity. *Med. Sci. Sports Exerc.*, 26:824, 1994.

58. Holm, G., and Stromblad, G.: Type I diabetes and physical exercise. *Acta Med. Scand.*, 671(Suppl.):95, 1983.

59. Houmard, J.A., et al.: Testosterone, cortisol, and creatine kinase levels in male distance runners during reduced training. *Int. J. Sports Med.*, 11:41, 1990.

60. Houmard, J.A., et al.: Elevated skeletal muscle glucose transporter levels in exercise-trained middle-aged men. *Am. J. Physiol.*, 261:E437, 1991.

61. Howlett, T.A., et al.: Release of beta-endorphin and met-enkephalin during exercise in normal women: response to training. *Br. Med. J.*, 288:1950, 1984.

62. Jaskowski, M.A., et al.: Enkephalin metabolism: effect of acute exercise stress and cardiovascular fitness. *Med. Sci. Sports Exerc.*, 21:154, 1989.

63. Jensen, J., et al.: Comparison of changes in testosterone after strength and endurance exercise in well trained men. *Eur. J. Appl. Physiol.*, 63:467, 1991.

64. Johannessen, A., et al.: Prolactin, growth hormone, thyrotropin, 3,5,3-triiodothyronine, and thyroxine response to exercise after fat and carbohydrate enriched diet. *J. Clin. Endocrinol. Metab.*, 52:56, 1981.

65. Jurkowski, J., et al.: Ovarian hormone response to exercise. *J. Appl. Physiol.*, 44:109, 1978.

65a. Kajuura, J.S., et al.: Immune responses to changes in training intensity and volume in runners. *Med. Sci. Sports Exerc.*, 27:1111, 1995.

66. Kannel, W.B., and McGee, D.L.: Diabetes and cardiovascular risk factors: the Framingham study. *Circulation*, 59:8, 1979.

67. Kappel, M., et al.: Evidence that the effect of physical exercise on NK cell activity is mediated by epinephrine. *J. Appl. Physiol.*, 70:2530, 1991.

68. Karagiorgos, A., et al.: Growth hormone response to continuous and intermittent exercise. *Med. Sci. Sports*, 11:302, 1979.

69. Kastello, G.M., et al.: Young and old subjects matched for aerobic capacity have similar noradrenergic responses to exercise. *J. Appl. Physiol.*, 74:49, 1993.

70. Keast, D., et al.: Exercise and the immune response. *Sports Med.*, 5:248, 1988.

71. King, D.S., et al.: Time course for exercise-induced alterations in insulin action and glucose tolerance in middle aged people. *J. Appl. Physiol.*, 78:17, 1995.

72. Kjaer, M.: Regulation of hormonal and metabolic responses during exercise in humans. *Exerc. Sport Sci. Rev.*, 20:161, 1992.

73. Knobil, E.: The neuroendocrine control of the menstrual cycle. *Recent Prog. Horm. Res.*, 36:53, 1980.

74. Koivisto, V.A., and Felig, P.: Effects of leg exercise on insulin absorption in diabetic patients. *N. Engl. J. Med.*, 298:79, 1978.

75. Kraemer, W.J.: Endocrine responses and adaptations to strength training. In *Encyclopedia of Sports Medicine: Strength and Power.* Edited by P.V. Komi. London, Blackwell Scientific, 1992.

76. Kraemer, W.J.: Endocrine responses and adaptations to strength training. In *Strength and Power in Sport.* Edited by P. V. Komi. London, Blackwell Scientific Publications, 1993.

77. Kraemer, W.J.: Hormonal mechanisms related to the expression of muscular strength and power. In *Strength and Power in Sport.* Edited by P. V. Komi. London, Blackwell Scientific Publications, 1993.

78. Kraemer, W.J., et al.: Training responses of plasma beta-endorphin, adrenocorticotropin, and cortisol. *Med. Sci. Sports Exerc.*, 21:146, 1989.

79. Kraemer, W.J., et al.: Endogenous anabolic hormonal and growth factor responses to heavy resistance exercise in males and females. *Int. J. Sports Med.*, 12:228,1991.

80. Kraemer, W.J., et al.: Effects of different heavy-resistance exercise protocols on plasma β-endorphin concentrations. *J. Appl. Physiol.*, 74:450, 1993.

81. Kriska, A.M., et al.: The association of physical activity with obesity, fat distribution and glucose intolerance in Pima Indians. *Diabetologia*, 36:863, 1993.

82. Kriska, A.M., et al.: The potential role of physical activity in the prevention of non-insulin-dependent diabetes mellitus: the epidemiological evidence. *Exerc. Sport Sci. Rev.*, 22(1):21, 1994.

83. Kuoppasalmi, K., et al.: Plasma cortisol, androstenedione, testosterone and luteinizing hormone in running exercise of different intensities. *Scand. J. Clin. Lab. Invest.*, 40:403, 1980.

83a. Lee, I.-M.: Physical activity, fitness and cancer. In *Physical Activity, Fitness, and Health*. Edited by C. Bouchard, et al. Champaign, IL, Human Kinetics, 1994.

84. Ljunghall, S., et al.: Increase in serum parathyroid hormone levels after prolonged physical exercise. *Med. Sci. Sports Exerc.*, 20:122, 1988.

85. Lockette, W., et al.: Endurance training and human α_2-adrenergic receptors on platelets. *Med. Sci. Sports Exerc.*, 19:7, 1987.

86. Luger, A., et al.: Acute hypothalamic-pituitary-adrenal responses to the stress of treadmill exercise: physiologic adaptations to physical training. *N. Engl. J. Med.*, 316:1309, 1987.

87. MacIntyre, J.G.: Growth hormone and athletes. *Sports Med.*, 4:129, 1987.

88. Mackinnon, L.T., and Jenkins, D.G.: Decreased salivary immunoglobins after intense interval exercise before and after training. *Med. Sci. Sports Exerc.*, 25:678, 1993.

89. MacNeil, B., and Hoffman-Goetz, L.: Chronic exercise enhances *in vivo* and *in vitro* cytotoxic mechanisms of natural immunity in mice. *J. Appl. Physiol.*, 74:388, 1993.

90. Maher, J.T., et al.: Aldosterone dynamics during graded exercise at sea level and high altitude. *J. Appl. Physiol.*, 39:18, 1975.

91. Mahler, D.A., et al.: β-endorphin activity and hypercapnic ventilatory responsiveness after marathon running. *J. Appl. Physiol.*, 66:2431, 1989.

92. Manson, J.D., et al.: Physical activity and incidence of non-insulin dependent diabetes mellitus in women. *Lancet*, 338:774, 1991.

93. Manson, J.E., et al.: A prospective study of exercise and incidence of diabetes among US male physicians. *JAMA*, 268:63, 1992.

94. McArthur, J.W.: Endorphins and exercise in females: possible connection with reproductive dysfunction. *Med. Sci. Sports Exerc.*, 17:82, 1985.

95. Melin, B., et al.: Plasma AVD, neurophysin, renin activity and aldosterone during submaximal exercise performed until exhaustion in trained and untrained men. *Eur. J. Appl. Physiol.*, 44:141, 1980.

96. Mikines, K.J., et al.: Seven days of bed rest decreases insulin action on glucose uptake in leg and whole body. *J. Appl. Physiol.*, 70:1245, 1991.

97. Morgan, W.P.: Affective beneficence of vigorous physical activity. *Med. Sci. Sports Exerc.*, 17:94, 1985.

98. Naveri, H., et al.: Metabolic and hormonal changes in moderate and intense long-term running exercises. *Int. J. Sports Med.*, 6:276, 1985.

99. Newmark, S.R., et al.: Adrenalcortical response to marathon running. *J. Clin. Endocrinol. Metab.*, 42:393, 1976.

100. Nieman, D.C.: Physical activity, fitness, and infection. In *Physical Activity, Fitness, and Health*. Edited by C. Bouchard, et al. Champaign, IL, Human Kinetics, 1994.

101. Nieman, D.C., et al.: Physical activity and immune function in elderly women. *Med. Sci. Sports Exerc.*, 25:823, 1993.

102. Nieman, D.C., et al.: Natural killer cell cytotoxic activity in weight trainers and sedentary controls. *J. Strength Cond. Res.*, 8:251, 1994.

103. Nieman, D.C., et al.: The acute immune response to exhaustive resistance exercise. *Int. J. Sports Med.*, 16:322, 1995.

104. Pakarinen, A., et al.: Serum thyroid hormones, thyrotropin and thyroxine binding globulin during prolonged strength training. *Eur. J. Appl. Physiol.*, 57:394, 1988.

105. Pedersen, B.K.: Influence of physical activity on the cellular immune system: mechanism of action. *Int. J. Sports Med.*, 12(Suppl. 1):S23, 1991.

106. Pedersen, B.K., and Ullum, H.: NK cell response to physical activity: possible mechanism of action. *Med. Sci. Sports Exerc.*, 26:140, 1994.

107. Peronnet, F., et al.: Plasma norepinephrine response to exercise before and after training in humans. *J. Appl. Physiol.*, 51:812, 1992.

108. Peters, E.M., et al.: Vitamin C supplementation reduces the incidence of postrace symptoms of upper-respiratory-tract infection in ultramarathon runners. *Am. J. Clin. Nutr.*, 57:170, 1993.

109. Pizza, F.X., et al.: Run training versus cross-training: effect of increased training on circulating leukocyte subsets. *Med. Sci. Sports Exerc.*, 27:355, 1995.

110. Ponjee, G.A.E., et al.: Androgen turnover during marathon running. *Med. Sci. Sports Exerc.*, 26:1274, 1994.

111. Prior, J.C., et al.: Prolactin changes with exercise vary with breast motion: Analysis of running versus cycling. *Fertil. Steril.*, 36:268, 1981.

112. Rahkila, P., et al.: Response of plasma endorphins to running exercises in male and female endurance athletes. *Med. Sci. Sports Exerc.*, 19:451, 1987.

113. Richter, E.A., and Sutton, J.R.: Hormonal adaptation to physical activity. In *Physical Activity, Fitness, and Health*. Edited by C. Bouchard, et al. Champaign, Il, Human Kinetics, 1994.

114. Rocchini, A.P., et al.: The effects of weight loss on the sensitivity of blood pressure to sodium in obese adolescents. *N. Engl. J. Med.*, 321:580, 1989.

115. Rodnick, K., et al.: Improved insulin action in muscle, liver and adipose tissue in physically trained human subjects. *Am. J. Physiol.*, 253:E489, 1987.

116. Schneider, S.H., et al.: Exercise and NIDDM. Technical report. *Diabetes Care*, 15(Suppl. 2):50, 1992.

117. Schwab, R., et al.: Acute effects of different intensities of weight lifting on serum testosterone. *Med. Sci. Sports Exerc.*, 25:1381, 1993.

118. Shephard, R.J., and Shek, P.N.: Exercise, aging and immune function. *Int. J. Sports Med.*, 16:1, 1995.

119. Shephard, R.J., and Sidney, K.H.: Effects of physical exercise on plasma growth hormone and cortisol levels in human subjects. In *Exercise and Sport Sciences Reviews*. Vol. 3. Edited by J.H. Wilmore. New York, Academic Press, 1975.

120. Shephard, R.J., et al.: The impact of exercise on the immune system: NK cells, interleukins 1 and 2, and related responses. *Exerc. Sport Sci. Rev.*, 23:215, 1995.

120a. Solomon, C.: Diabetes mellitus and risk of cardiovascular disease in women. *Med. Sci. Sports Exerc.*, 28:15, 1996.

121. Song, M.K., et al.: The mode of adrenal gland enlargement in the rat in response to exercise training. *Pflugers Arch.*, 339:59, 1973.

122. Staron, R.S., et al.: Skeletal muscle adaptations during the early phase of heavy-resistance training in men and women. *J. Appl. Physiol.*, 76:1247, 1994.

123. Sternfeld, B.: Cancer and the protective effect of physical activity: the epidemiological evidence. *Med. Sci. Sports Exerc.*, 24:1195, 1992.

124. Strauss, R.H., et al.: Weight loss in amateur wrestlers and its effects on serum testosterone levels. *JAMA*, 254:3337, 1985.

125. Sutton, J.R., et al.: The hormonal response to physical exercise. *Aust. Ann. Med.*, 18:84, 1969.

126. Sutton, J.R., et al.: Plasma vasopressin, catecholamines and lactate during exhaustive exercise at extreme simulated altitude: "Operation Everest II." *Can. J. Appl. Sports Sci.*, 11:43P, 1986.

127. Sutton, J.R., and Farrell, P.: Endocrine responses to prolonged exercise. In *Exercise Science and Sports Medicine*. Vol. 1. Edited by D.R. Lamb and R. Murray. Indianapolis, Benchmark Press, 1988.

128. Tarnopolsky, L., et al.: Gender differences in hormonal and metabolic responses to prolonged exercise in males and females. *J. Appl. Physiol.*, 68:650, 1990.

129. Terjung, R., and Tipton, C.M.: Plasma thyroxine and thyroid-stimulating hormone levels during submaximal exercise in humans. *Am. J. Physiol.*, 220:1840, 1971.

130. Vitug, A., et al.: Exercise and Type I diabetes mellitus. In *Exercise and Sport Sciences Reviews*. Vol. 16. Edited by K.B. Pandolf. New York, Macmillan, 1988.

131. Vogel, R.B., et al.: Increase of free and total testosterone during submaximal exercise in normal males. *Med. Sci. Sports Exerc.*, 17:119, 1985.

132. Wade, C.E.: Response, regulation, and actions of vasopressin during exercise: a review. *Med. Sci. Sports Exerc.*, 16:506, 1984.

133. Wade, C.E., and Claybaugh, J.R.: Plasma renin activity, vasopressin concentration, and urinary excretory responses to exercise in men. *J. Appl. Physiol.*, 49:930, 1980.

134. Wade, C.E., et al.: Plasma aldosterone and renal function in runners during a 20-day road race. *Eur. J. Appl. Physiol.*, 54:456, 1985.

135. Wahrenberg, H., et al.: Acute adaptation in adrenergic control of lipolysis during physical exercise in humans. *Am. J. Physiol.*, 253:E383, 1987.

136. Wallberg-Henriksson, H.: Exercise and diabetes mellitus. *Exer. Sport Sci. Rev.*, 20:339, 1992.

137. Wasserman, D.H., et al.: Hepatic fuel metabolism during muscular work: Role and regulation. *Am. J. Physiol.*, 260:E811, 1991.

138. Weltman, A., et al.: Endurance training amplifies the pulsatile release of growth hormone: effects of training intensity. *J. Appl. Physiol.,* 72:2188, 1992.

139. Wheeler, G.D.: Reduced serum testosterone and prolactin levels in male distance runners. *JAMA,* 252:514, 1984.

140. Wheeler, G.D.: Endurance training decreases serum testosterone levels in men without change in luteinizing hormone pulsatile release. *J. Clin. Endocrinol. Metab.,* 72:422, 1991.

141. Whiteside, T.L., and Herberman, R.B.: Short analytical review: the role of natural killer cells in human diseases. *Clin. Immunol. Immunopathol.,* 53:1, 1989.

142. Winder, W.W.: Time course of the T_3- and T_4-induced increase in rat soleus muscle mitochondria. *Am. J. Physiol.,* 5:C132, 1979.

143. Winder, W.W., and Heninger, V.: Effect of exercise on tissue levels of thyroid hormones in the rat. *Am. J. Physiol.,* 221:1139, 1971.

144. Wing, R.R., et al.: Exercise in a behavioral weight control programme for obese patients with type II (non-insulin-dependent) diabetes. *Diabetologia,* 31:902, 1988.

145. Woods, J.A., and Davis, J.M.: Exercise, monocyte/macrophage function, and cancer. *Med. Sci. Sports Exerc.,* 26:147, 1994.

146. Yates, A., et al.: Running—an analogue of anorexia. *N. Engl. J. Med.,* 308:251, 1983.

PART 2

APPLIED
EXERCISE
PHYSIOLOGY

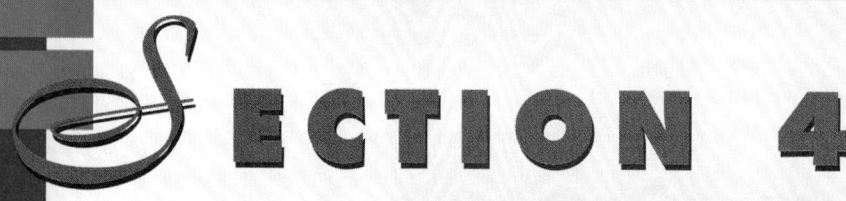

SECTION 4

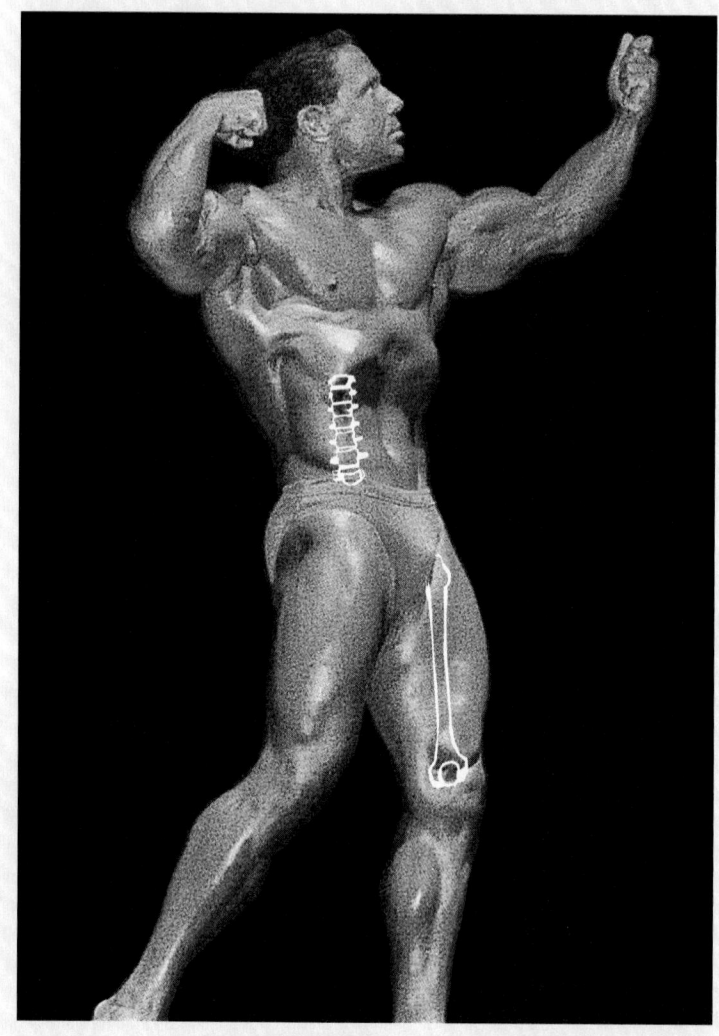

"AN ENHANCED LEVEL OF

NEURAL FACILITATION PROBABLY

ACCOUNTS FOR THE RAPID AND

SIGNIFICANT STRENGTH

INCREASE EARLY IN TRAINING."

Enhancement of Energy Capacity

Exercise training in many cases is more art than science. The success of different conditioning programs often is based on individual achievements or won-lost records rather than on scientific inquiry and discovery. Too often, coaches place considerable emphasis on developing aerobic capacity and devote little time to vigorous anaerobic conditioning. While sports such as basketball and soccer do require relatively steady, high-level releases of aerobic energy, certain crucial game situations demand all-out effort. The athlete having a poor anaerobic energy-transfer capacity may not perform at full potential. Training the anaerobic capacity of endurance athletes, on the other hand, would be wasteful because the contribution of anaerobic energy transfer is minimal to successful performance. Instead, endurance activities demand both a well-conditioned heart and vascular system capable of circulating large quantities of blood and a high capacity within the muscle cells to generate ATP aerobically. At the other extreme, one's capacity for aerobic metabolism contributes little to overall success in sprint activities and sports such as volleyball and football. Here, performance depends largely on muscular strength and explosive power output during which energy is generated primarily from reactions that do not utilize oxygen.

Developing an appropriate program of training to achieve optimum exercise performance requires a clear understanding of energy transfer and the effects of specific training on the systems of energy delivery and utilization. In Chapters 21 and 22, we discuss the basis of training for aerobic and anaerobic power and muscular strength, the physiologic consequences of such training, and the important factors that affect training success. In Chapter 23, we take a closer look at special aids that purport to augment the training response or significantly enhance human exercise performance.

Pechar, G.S., et. al.: Specificity of cardiorespiratory adaptation to bicycle and treadmill training. *J. Appl. Physiol.* 36:753, 1974.

In the early 1970s, little quantitative information existed about the general or specific physiological adaptations to different modes of exercise training. Some researchers focused on determining the effectiveness of various training modes to enhance sport-specific performance and developing testing protocols to assess the magnitude of the training adaptation. The study by Pechar and coworkers directly evaluated the specificity of cardiorespiratory adaptations to bicycle ergometer (BE) and treadmill (TM) training. This was done by comparing the magnitude of aerobic training effects by the use of BE and TM test procedures.

Sixty college-aged men (average age, 20.4 years; body mass, 73.1 kg; stature, 177.2 cm) participated in either TM training (N = 20), BE training (N = 20), or a no-training control group (N = 20). To equalize training intensity, subjects exercised on the TM or BE for 20 minutes daily (four 5-minute periods), 3 days weekly for 8 weeks at an exercise heart rate of 85% of maximal heart rate (HRmax) determined during the initial BE or TM $\dot{V}O_2$max test. The TM training group ran at a speed of 6 mph. By adjusting TM evaluation or frictional resistance for BE training, work rate could be maintained at 85% of HRmax on each apparatus. Assessment of $\dot{V}O_2$max occurred before and after training by use of discontinuous TM and BE test procedures for all groups, with test order (bike-treadmill or treadmill-bike) randomly assigned.

Prior to training, no significant between-group difference existed in $\dot{V}O_2$max. Pre-training BE $\dot{V}O_2$max averaged 12.1% lower than $\dot{V}O_2$max measured on the TM. For the TM training group, $\dot{V}O_2$max after training significantly increased 6.9% on the BE test, and 6.8% on the TM test. In contrast, $\dot{V}O_2$max for the BE training group increased 7.8% on the BE test but only 2.6% on the TM test. For both training groups, HRmax and R were significantly lower on both apparatus after training. No significant changes occurred for the control group. The results indicated an interaction between the specific form of aerobic training and the method for assessing $\dot{V}O_2$max (refer to the figure). For the TM group, improvement in $\dot{V}O_2$max after 8 weeks of training occurred independently of the method of $\dot{V}O_2$max measurement. Improvements in $\dot{V}O_2$max for the BE group, however, differed significantly depending on the method of assessing aerobic capacity. Although the BE training group improved in TM and BE $\dot{V}O_2$max, BE $\dot{V}O_2$max (same mode of exercise as training) improved significantly more compared to improvements in TM $\dot{V}O_2$max (different mode of exercise than training). In fact, if only TM testing had evaluated changes in $\dot{V}O_2$max, the researchers would have concluded that run training produced *greater* changes in aerobic capacity than bicycle training. Training-specific measurements produced equivalency from both forms of training.

The researchers hypothesized that changes in local metabolic and circulatory factors accounted for the specific training improvements in $\dot{V}O_2$max resulting from cycling training. In addition, although 85% of HRmax equated work intensity for the BE and TM groups, the central cardiorespiratory response might have been less during cycling training because of a lower stroke volume in this form of exercise. The researchers concluded that the mode of exercise used to assess changes in cardiorespiratory function resulting from training plays an important role when evaluating the quantitative effects of such training. Furthermore, a specificity of the adaptation to aerobic training may be linked to the muscle mass activated in training. Subsequent research has supported and expanded the concept of aerobic training specificity.

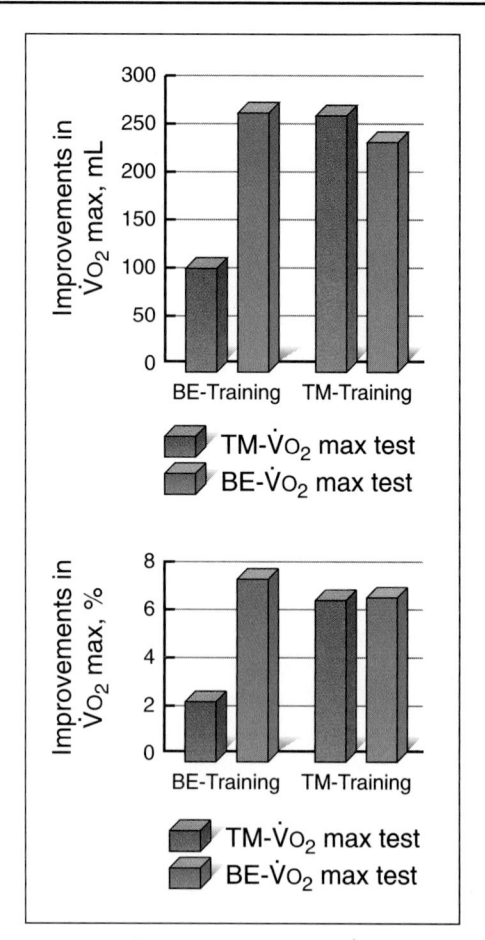

Interaction between the improvements resulting from a specific mode of aerobic training and the mode of exercise to assess $\dot{V}O_2$max.

Training for Anaerobic and Aerobic Power

Throughout this book we have stressed that different activities, depending on their durations and intensities, require the activation of specific energy systems. This is illustrated in Figure 21.1, in which exercise is broadly classified in terms of its duration and the predominant energy pathways. We realize that it is difficult to place certain activities into one category. For example, as a person increases in aerobic fitness, an activity previously classified as anaerobic might be reclassified as aerobic. In many cases, all three energy-transfer systems—the ATP-CP system, the glycolytic or lactic acid system, and the aerobic system—operate at different times during exercise. Their relative contributions to the energy continuum directly relate to the duration and intensity (power output) of the specific activity.

Brief power activities lasting up to about 6 seconds rely almost exclusively on "immediate" energy generated from the breakdown of the stored intramuscular high-energy phosphates, ATP and CP. Consequently, power athletes such as sprinters, shot-putters, and pole vaulters must gear their training toward improving the capacity of this energy-transfer system. As all-out exercise progresses to 60-seconds duration and power output decreases somewhat, the major portion of energy is still generated through anaerobic pathways. These metabolic reactions, however, involve the short-term energy system of glycolysis and subsequent lactic acid formation. As exercise intensity diminishes somewhat and duration extends to 2 to 4 minutes, reliance on energy from phosphate stores and anaerobic glycolysis decreases, and the aerobic production of ATP becomes increasingly more important. Prolonged exercise progresses on a "pay-as-you-go" basis, with more than 99% of the energy requirement being generated by aerobic metabolism. Clearly, an efficient training program is one that allocates a proportionate commitment to proper training of the specific energy systems involved in the activity. In the sections that follow, we discuss anaerobic and aerobic conditioning, with special emphasis on principles, methods, and short- and long-term training adaptations. *The approach to physiologic conditioning is basically the same for men and women within a broad age range: both respond and adapt to training in essentially the same manner.*

PRINCIPLES OF TRAINING

The major objective in training is to facilitate biologic adaptations that improve performance in specific tasks. These adaptations require adherence to carefully planned workout programs, with attention focused on factors such as frequency and length of workouts; type of training; speed, intensity, duration, and repetition of the activity; rest intervals; and appropriate competition. Although these factors vary depending on the performance goal, several principles of physiologic conditioning are common to the performance classifications illustrated in Figure 21.1.

OVERLOAD PRINCIPLE

An exercise **overload** *specific to the activity must be applied to enhance physiologic improvement and bring about a training response.* Exercising at a level of intensity higher than is normally performed can induce a variety of highly specific training adaptations that enable the body to function more efficiently. Achieving the appropriate overload for each person requires manipulating combinations of training **frequency, intensity,** and **duration,** with specific consideration given to the **mode** of exercise.

The concept of individualized and progressive overload applies to athletes, sedentary people, the disabled, and even cardiac patients. An increasing number in this latter group have used an appropriately formulated exercise rehabilitation program to walk, jog, and eventually run and even complete marathons![52] As will be discussed in Chapter 30, the level of overload required to bring about the significant health-related benefits of regular exercise is considerably less than that required to improve fitness.[4, 20]

SPECIFICITY PRINCIPLE

When applied to training, specificity refers to adaptations in the metabolic and physiologic systems depending on the type of overload imposed. A specific exercise stress, such as strength-power training, induces specific adaptations, in this case strength-power adaptations, and a specific aero-

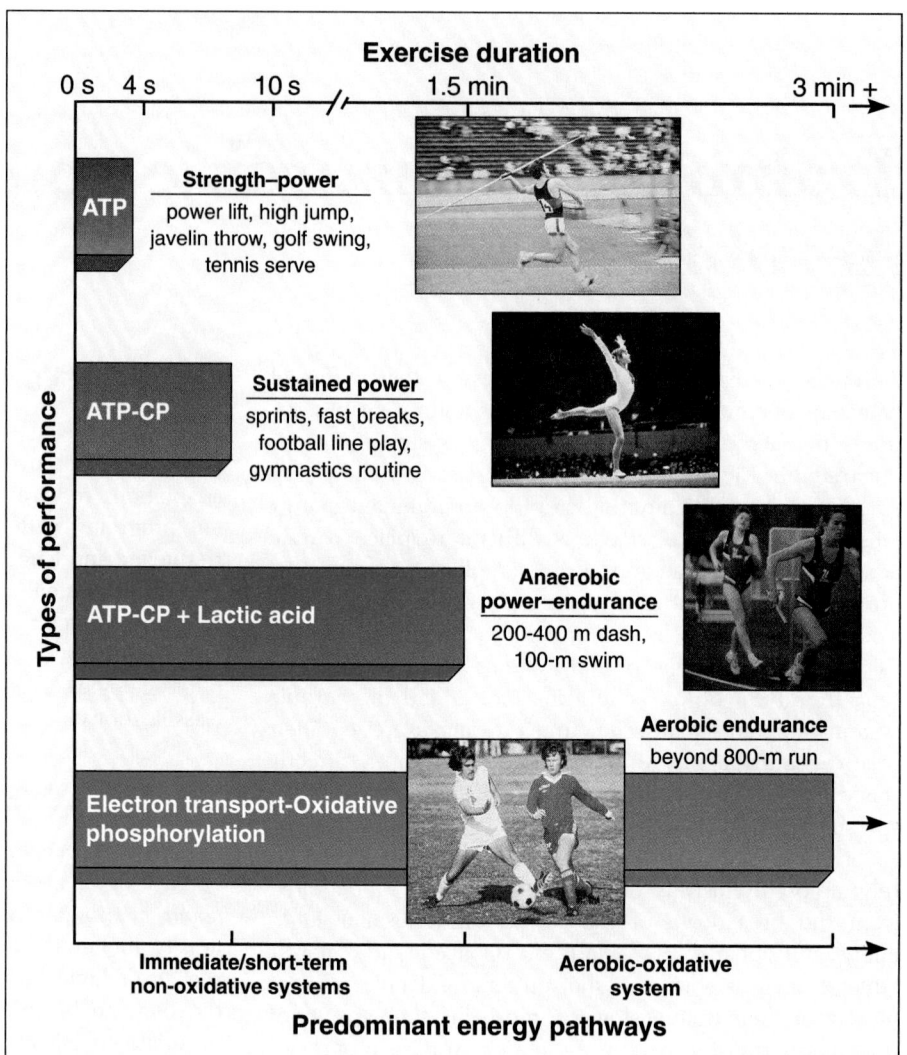

FIGURE 21.1

Classification of physical activity based on the duration of all-out exercise and the corresponding predominant intracellular energy pathways.

bic or cardiovascular exercise elicits specific endurance-training adaptations, with only a limited interchange of benefits derived between muscular strength and aerobic training.[36, 43, 46, 100] The specificity principle goes beyond this, however, because aerobic fitness for swimming,[66] bicycling,[79, 105] running,[69] or arm exercise[59] is most effectively improved by training the specific muscles involved in the desired performance. *Simply stated, specific exercise elicits specific adaptations, creating specific training effects.*

Specificity of $\dot{V}O_2max$

Table 21.1 gives the results of a study in one of our laboratories designed to investigate the specificity of endurance swim training on improvements in aerobic capacity.[66] Fifteen men trained 1 hour per day, 3 days per week, for 10 weeks. For all subjects, measurements were made of

$\dot{V}O_2max$ during treadmill running and swimming before and after training. Because vigorous training exercise such as swimming elicits a general overload to the central circulation, we had expected at least some improvement, or "transfer," in aerobic power from swimming to running. This was not the case, however, as almost total specificity accompanied the improvement in $\dot{V}O_2max$ with swim training. If only treadmill running had been used to evaluate swim training effects, we would have mistakenly concluded that there was no training effect!

Based on available research, it is reasonable to advise that during training for specific aerobic activities such as cycling, swimming, rowing, or running, the overload must both engage the appropriate muscles required by the activity and induce an exercise stress on the central cardiovascular system.[25, 32, 79] Little improvement is observed when aerobic capacity is measured during a dissimilar exercise, yet improvements are significant when the test exercise is the same exercise used in training.[27, 54, 67, 69] Thus, one can appreciate how difficult it is to be in "good shape" for diverse forms of aerobic exercise. It also is noteworthy from the data presented in Table 21.1 that although swimming $\dot{V}O_2$max improved 11% with swim training, the maximum work time increased 34% during the swim test. Improvements in $\dot{V}O_2$max probably reach a peak in training, and, thereafter, improvements in performance are supported by other mechanisms only partly related to the capacity of the oxygen transport system. These adaptations most likely take place in the active musculature rather than being related to central circulatory factors.

Whereas the improvement in aerobic fitness with training is highly specific, improvements in cardiac function (for example, ventricular contractility) are rather general in nature. Training studies indicate that improved heart function induced by one form of exercise also is observed when the untrained limb is exercised.[98] This finding indicates that the heart muscle per se can be conditioned during a variety of "big-muscle" exercise modes.

Specificity of Local Changes

In endurance training, the overload of specific muscle groups enhances work performance and aerobic power by facilitating both oxygen transport and utilization at the local level of the trained muscles.[32, 43, 84] The oxidative capacity of the vastus lateralis muscle, for example, is greater in well-trained cyclists than in endurance runners and improves significantly following training on a bicycle ergometer.[30, 31] Such adaptations would certainly increase the capacity of the trained muscles to generate ATP aerobically. The specificity of aerobic improvement may also result from greater regional blood flow in active tissues because of either (a) an increased microcirculation, (b) a more effective distribution of cardiac output, or (c) the combined effect of both factors. Regardless of the mechanism, such adaptations would occur only in the specifically trained muscles, and the benefits only would be manifested when these muscles were activated.

INDIVIDUAL DIFFERENCES PRINCIPLE

Many factors contribute to individual variation in training response. For example, a person's relative fitness level is important at the start of training. It is unrealistic to expect different people who start an exercise program together to be at the same "state" of training at the same time. Consequently, it is counterproductive to insist that all athletes on the same team (or even in the same event) train the same way or at the same relative or absolute work rate. It also is unrealistic to expect that all individuals will respond to a given training stimulus in precisely the same manner.

TABLE 21.1
EFFECTS OF 10 WEEKS OF INTERVAL SWIM TRAINING ON CHANGES IN $\dot{V}O_2$max AND ENDURANCE PERFORMANCE AS MEASURED DURING RUNNING AND SWIMMING

Subjects	Measure	Running Test			Swimming Test		
		Pre-Training	Post-Training	% Change	Pre-Training	Post-Training	% Change
Swim Training							
	$\dot{V}O_2$max						
	L · min^{-1}	4.05	4.11	+1.5	3.44	3.82	+11.0
	mL · kg^{-1} · min^{-1}	54.9	55.7	+1.5	46.6	51.8	+11.0
	Max work time,						
	min	19.6	20.5	+4.6	11.9	15.9	+34.0
Nontraining Controls							
	$\dot{V}O_2$max						
	L · min^{-1}	4.12	4.18	+1.5	3.51	3.40	+3.1
	mL · kg^{-1} · min^{-1}	55.1	55.5	+0.7	46.8	45.0	−3.8
	Max work time,						
	min	20.7	19.7	−4.8	11.5	11.5	0

From Magel, J.R., et al.: Specificity of swim training on maximum oxygen uptake. *J. Appl. Physiol.*, 38:151, 1975.

FIGURE 21.2

Individual differences in telemetered heart rate response, during a 60-minute basketball game, in two forwards. For Player A *(red line)*, the heart rate averaged 174 beats · min⁻¹, and for Player B *(blue line)*, the heart rate averaged 163 beats · min⁻¹. Heart rate was monitored simultaneously for both players using miniature telemetry transmitters taped on the players' backs at the pants line. (Data from F. Katch, Department of Exercise Science, University of Massachusetts, Amherst.)

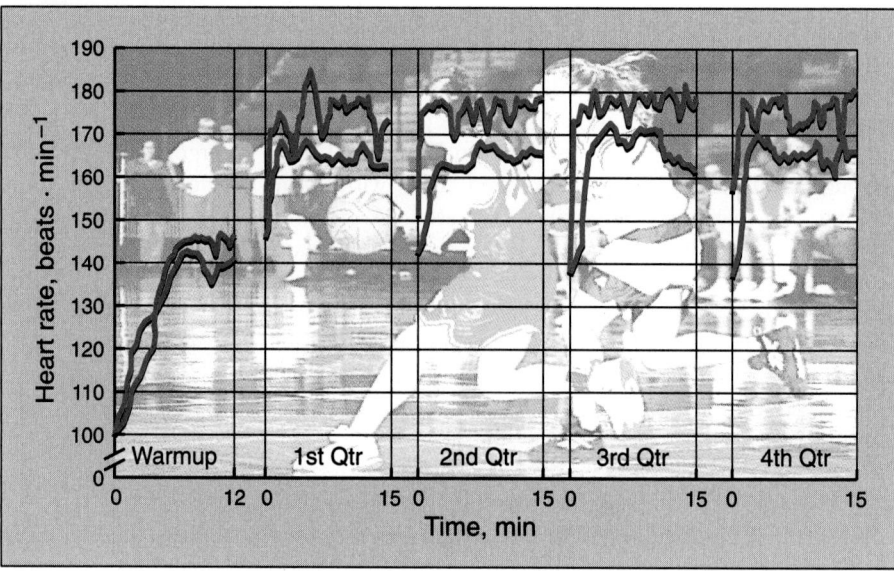

Figure 21.2 displays the heart rate curves during a warm-up and four consecutive 15-minute quarters of a basketball game in two college varsity forwards. The heart rate for player A (red line) averaged 174 beats per minute during each of the four quarters, although the range in heart rate was about 22 beats and did not exceed 180 beats per minute at any time. For player B (blue line), the heart rate response pattern was similar except that the curve for heart rate averaged 163 beats per minute during the game. This difference in the magnitude of heart rate response during the hour-long game illustrates that two individuals can perform at an approximately equivalent intensity but at a 6.3% different level of cardiovascular strain as reflected by the exercise heart rate. *Training benefits are optimized when programs are planned to meet the individual needs and capacities of the participants.* As discussed in Chapter 11, genetic factors clearly interact to influence the training response.

REVERSIBILITY PRINCIPLE

Detraining occurs rapidly when a person terminates participation in an exercise program. After only 1 or 2 weeks of detraining, significant reductions in both metabolic and exercise capacity can result, and many of the training improvements are lost within several months. Table 21.2 shows the biologic consequences of various durations of short-term (3 weeks or less) and long-term (3 to 12 weeks) detraining in aerobically trained individuals. The data represent average responses reported in the literature. The research of one group is particularly interesting.[87] In five subjects confined to bed for 20 consecutive days, $\dot{V}O_2max$ decreased by 25%. This decrease accompanied a similar decrement in maximal stroke volume and cardiac output, which had the effect of decreasing aerobic capacity by an average of 1% each day. Additionally, the number of capillaries within trained muscle decreases between 14 and 25% within 3 weeks after training ceased.[86]

The important point is that even among highly trained athletes, the beneficial effects of many years of prior exercise training are transient and reversible.[10, 15, 76] For this reason, most athletes begin a reconditioning program several months prior to the start of the competitive season or maintain some moderate level of off-season, sport-specific exercise to blunt the rate of decline in physiologic and metabolic functions during deconditioning.[77]

PHYSIOLOGIC CONSEQUENCES OF TRAINING

Many of the biologic changes that accompany training have been presented in other sections throughout this book. We summarize below the various training adaptations outlined in Table 21.3.

ANAEROBIC SYSTEM CHANGES

Figure 21.3 summarizes the metabolic adaptations in **anaerobic function** that accompany strenuous physical training. Consistent with the concept of training specificity, activities that demand a high level of anaerobic metabolism bring about specific changes in the immediate and short-term energy systems, without a concomitant increase in aerobic functions. The changes that occur with sprint and power-type training include:

TABLE 21.2
CHANGES IN PHYSIOLOGIC AND METABOLIC VALUES RESULTING FROM VARIOUS DURATIONS OF DETRAINING[a]

Variable	Trained	Detrained	Change, % Short Term Detraining[b]	Change, % Longer Term Detraining[c]
$\dot{V}O_2$max, mL $\cdot$ kg^{-1} $\cdot$ min^{-1}	62.2	57.3	−8	
	62.1	50.8		−18
$\dot{V}O_2$max, L $\cdot$ min^{-1}	4.45	4.16	−7	
Cardiac output, L $\cdot$ min^{-1}	27.8	25.5	−8	
	27.8	25.2		−10
Stroke volume, mL $\cdot$ beat^{-1}	155	139	−10	
	148	129		−13
Heart rate, beats $\cdot$ min^{-1}	186	193	4	
	187	197		5
Oxygen pulse, mL $\cdot$ beat^{-1}	12.7	10.9		−14
Sum 3-min recovery HR	190	237		25
Plasma volume, L	2.91	2.56	−12	
a-$\bar{v}O_2$ diff, mL $\cdot$ (100 mL)$^{-1}$	15.1	15.4	−2 (NS)	
	15.1	14.1		−7
CP, mmol $\cdot$ (g wet wt)$^{-1}$	17.9	13.0		−27
ATP, mmol $\cdot$ (g wet wt)$^{-1}$	5.97	5.08		−15
Glycogen, mmol $\cdot$ (g wet wt)$^{-1}$	113.9	57.4		−50
Capillary density, cap $\cdot$ mm^{-2}	511	476	−7	
	464	476		−2 (NS)
Oxidative enzyme capacity			−29	−32
Myoglobin, mg $\cdot$ (g protein)$^{-1}$	43.3	41.0	−5 (NS)	
	43.3	40.7		−6
Insulin (rest)			17–120	
Norepinephrine/epinephrine (rest)			No change	
Norepinephrine/epinephrine (exercise)				65–100
Blood lactate			88	
Lactate threshold			−7	−18
Exercise lipolysis			−52	
Muscle glycogen synthesis			−29	−40
Time to fatigue, min			−10	
Swim power, W				−14
Elbow extension strength, ft $\cdot$ lb	39.0	25.5		−35

[a]Data represent an average computed from individual studies as cited in the following sources: McArdle, W.D., et al.: *Essentials of Exercise Physiology*. Philadelphia, Lea & Febiger, 1993 (Table 12.2, 5 citations) and Wilber, R.L., and Moffatt, R.J.: Physiological and biochemical consequences of detraining in aerobically trained individuals. *J. Strength Cond. Res.*, 8:110, 1994. (101 citations). Note that a + change for heart rate represents a decline in functional capacity. Omitted values for trained and detrained excluded in original sources.
[b]Short term = 3 wk or less in primarily aerobically trained individuals. NS = not statistically significant
[c]Longer term = 3 to 12 wk in primarily aerobically trained individuals

- *Increases in resting levels of anaerobic substrates.*[64] As determined from muscle biopsies taken before and after resistance training (Table 21.4), a 28% improvement in muscular strength was accompanied by significant increases in the trained muscle's resting levels of ATP, CP, free creatine, and glycogen.

- *Increases in the quantity and activity of key enzymes that control the anaerobic phase of glucose breakdown.*[47, 99] These changes are not of the magnitude observed for oxidative enzymes during aerobic training. The most dramatic increases in anaerobic enzyme function and fiber size occur in the fast-twitch muscle fibers.

TABLE 21.3
TYPICAL METABOLIC AND PHYSIOLOGIC VALUES FOR HEALTHY TRAINED AND UNTRAINED MEN[a]

Variable	Untrained	Trained	Percent Difference[b]
Glycogen, mmol · (g wet muscle)$^{-1}$	85.0	120	41
Number of mitochondria, mmol^3	0.59	1.20	103
Mitochondrial volume, % muscle cell	2.15	8.00	272
Resting ATP, mmol · (g wet muscle)$^{-1}$	3.0	6.0	100
Resting CP, mmol · (g wet muscle)$^{-1}$	11.0	18.0	64
Resting creatine, mmol · (g wet muscle)$^{-1}$	10.7	14.5	35
Glycolytic enzymes			
Phosphofructokinase, mmol · (g wet muscle)$^{-1}$	50.0	50.0	0
Phosphorylase, mmol · (g wet muscle)$^{-1}$	4–6	6–9	60
Aerobic enzymes			
Succinate dehydrogenase, mmol · (kg wet muscle)$^{-1}$	5–10	15–20	133
Max lactic acid, mmol · (kg wet muscle)$^{-1}$	110	150	36
Muscle fibers			
Fast twitch, %	50	20–30	−50
Slow twitch, %	50	60	20
Max stroke volume, mL · beat^{-1}	120	180	50
Max cardiac output, L · min^{-1}	20	30–40	75
Resting heart rate, beats · min^{-1}	70	40	−43
Max heart rate, beats · min^{-1}	190	180	−5
Max a-$\bar{v}O_2$ diff, mL · 100 mL^{-1}	14.5	16.0	10
$\dot{V}O_2$max, mL · kg^{-1} · min^{-1}	30–40	65–80	107
Heart volume, L	7.5	9.5	27
Blood volume, L	4.7	6.0	28
$\dot{V}_E$max, L · min^{-1}	110	190	73
Percent body fat	15	11	−27

[a]In some cases, approximate values are used. In all cases, the trained values represent data from endurance athletes. Caution is advised in assuming that the percent differences between trained and untrained are necessarily the results of training because genetic differences between individuals probably exert a strong influence on many of these factors.
[b]Computed as the percent that the value for the trained differs from the corresponding value for the untrained.

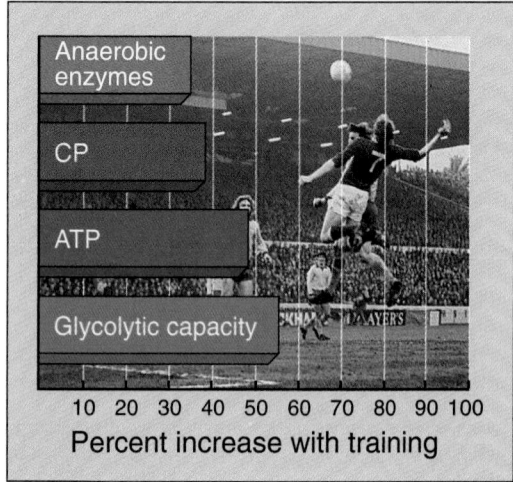

FIGURE 21.3
Potential for increases in the anaerobic energy metabolism of skeletal muscle with heavy physical training.

• *Increases in the capacity for generating high levels of blood lactate during all-out exercise.*[29, 47] An enhanced lactate-producing capacity is probably a result of increased levels of glycogen and glycolytic enzymes and improved motivation and "pain" tolerance to fatiguing exercise.

AEROBIC SYSTEM CHANGES

Aerobic overload training is associated with adaptations in a variety of functional capacities related to oxygen transport and utilization. *If the training stimulus is adequate, the majority of these responses are independent of sex and age.*[11, 50, 103] In addition, many of these training-induced aerobic adaptations can occur in coronary heart disease patients undergoing high-intensity aerobic training.[33] The most notable adaptations accompanying aerobic training include those discussed below.

TABLE 21.4
CHANGES IN RESTING CONCENTRATIONS OF CP, CREATINE, ATP, AND GLYCOGEN FOLLOWING 5 MONTHS OF HEAVY-RESISTANCE WEIGHT TRAINING IN NINE MALE SUBJECTS

Variable[a]	Control	Post-Training	Percent Difference[b]
CP	17.07	17.94	+5.1
Creatine	10.74	14.52	+35.2
ATP	5.07	5.97	+17.8
Glycogen	86.28	113.90	+32.0

From MacDougall, J.D., et al.: Biochemical adaptation of human skeletal muscle to heavy resistance training and immobilization. *J. Appl. Physiol.*, 43:700, 1977.
[a]All values are expressed in mmol per gram of wet muscle.
[b]All percent differences are statistically significant.

Metabolic Adaptations

There is an improved respiratory control in skeletal muscle with aerobic training. This is the result of adaptations in:

- *Metabolic machinery:* Mitochondria from trained skeletal muscle are **larger** and **more numerous** compared to those of less active muscle fibers.
- *Enzymes:* Associated with the increased structural machinery for cellular respiration is a greatly **increased** capacity to generate ATP aerobically through oxidative phosphorylation. This increased capacity is reflected in a nearly two-fold increase in the level of aerobic system enzymes.[42] This is not the result of an increase in enzymatic activity per unit of mitochondrial protein, but rather the direct result of an increase in the total amount of mitochondrial material. These changes are probably important factors in increasing a person's ability to sustain a high percentage of aerobic capacity during prolonged exercise without significant lactate buildup.[19, 89]
- *Lipid metabolism:* As illustrated in Figure 21.4, an **increase** in the trained muscle's capacity to mobilize, deliver, and oxidize lipid accompanies submaximal exercise.[12, 83] This more lively lipolysis results from greater blood flow within trained muscle and enhanced quantity of lipid-mobilizing and lipid-metabolizing enzymes. At any submaximal exercise level, a trained person uses more fatty acid for energy than an untrained counterpart.[12a] This factor is beneficial to endurance athletes because it allows them to conserve the carbohydrate stores so important during prolonged exercise. Furthermore, any improvement in fatty acid β-oxidation and Krebs cycle production of ATP with aerobic training may aid in maintaining cellular integrity and a high level of function. This would contribute significantly to enhanced endurance, independent of one's glycogen reserves or aerobic capacity.

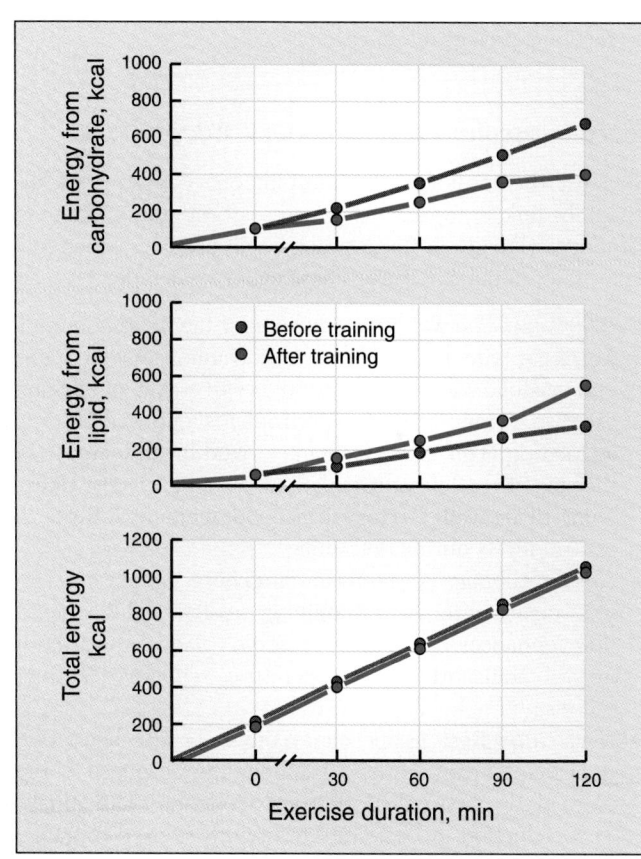

FIGURE 21.4

Training enhances the ability to catabolize lipid. During constant-load, prolonged exercise, the energy derived from lipid oxidation is significantly increased following aerobic training, with a corresponding decrease in carbohydrate breakdown. This carbohydrate-sparing adaptation may result from a release of fatty acids from adipose tissue depots (augmented by a reduced level of blood lactate) and an increased amount of intramuscular lipid in the endurance-trained muscle. (From Hurley, B.F., et al.: Muscle triglyceride utilization during exercise: effect of training. *J. Appl. Physiol.*, 5:62, 1986.)

- *Carbohydrate metabolism:* Trained muscle exhibits a **greater** capacity to oxidize carbohydrate.[42] Consequently, large quantities of pyruvate move through the aerobic energy pathways. This effect is consistent with the increased oxidative capacity of the mitochondria and increased glycogen storage within the trained muscles.
- *Muscle fiber type:* Aerobic training elicits metabolic adaptations in each type of muscle fiber. The basic fiber type probably does not "change" to any great extent, but, rather, all fibers maximize their already-existing aerobic potentials.
- *Muscle fiber size:* There is **selective hypertrophy** of different muscle fiber types to specific overload training. Highly trained endurance athletes have slow-twitch fibers that are larger than the fast-twitch fibers in the same muscle. Conversely, in athletes trained in anaerobic-power activities, fast-twitch fibers occupy more of the cross-sectional area of the muscle.

Cardiovascular and Pulmonary Adaptations

Because the cardiovascular and pulmonary systems are intimately linked to aerobic processes, endurance training produces changes in these systems that are both functional and dimensional in nature. These changes include:

- *Heart size:* The weight and volume of the heart generally **increase** with long-term aerobic training, with greater end diastolic volumes being noted both at rest and during exercise. A mild cardiac hypertrophy is a normal training adaptation. This effect is characterized by an increase in the size of the left ventricular cavity and a modest thickening of its walls.[73] This cardiac enlargement returns to control levels during detraining.[41]
- *Plasma volume:* A significant **increase** in plasma volume occurs after 3 to 5 training sessions. This adaptation enhances circulatory reserve, augmenting both oxygen transport and temperature regulation during exercise.[13, 63]
- *Heart rate:* Resting and submaximal exercise heart rate **decrease** during aerobic training, the response being particularly apparent in previously sedentary individuals. This reduction in heart rate frequently is used to gauge the magnitude of training improvement.
- *Stroke volume:* Training causes the heart's stroke volume to **increase** both at rest and during exercise. Generally, this change results from an increase in internal ventricular volume and possibly an enhanced ventricular contractility.[93] Regardless of age, enhanced left ventricular systolic performance accompanies endurance training.[21]
- *Cardiac output: An **increase** in maximum cardiac output is the most significant change in cardiovascular*

function with aerobic training. Because the maximal heart rate may even decrease slightly with training, the increased cardiac output capacity results directly from an improved stroke volume. A large cardiac output is the major factor distinguishing champion endurance athletes from other well-trained athletes and from untrained individuals.
- *Oxygen extraction:* Training elicits a significant **increase** in the quantity of oxygen extracted from the circulating blood.[67, 85] This increase in arteriovenous oxygen (a-$\bar{v}$ O_2) difference results from more effective distribution of the cardiac output to active muscles as well as an enhanced capacity of the trained muscle fibers to extract and use oxygen. Among older men and women, the role of the a-$\bar{v}$ O_2 difference may be more important in contributing to improved aerobic capacity with training than it is among younger counterparts.[55, 88, 90]
- *Blood flow and distribution:* A trained person performs **submaximal** exercise with **lower** cardiac output than an untrained person. This is probably the result of specific local changes that occur with training. As the muscle's ability to deliver, extract, and use oxygen increases, less regional blood flow is required to meet the active tissue's oxygen needs.
- Aerobic training causes a large **increase** in total muscle blood flow during **maximal** exercise because of (a) a larger maximal cardiac output, (b) the redistribution of blood to muscle from nonactive areas that can temporarily compromise their blood flow in response to an all-out effort, and (c) increases in the cross-sectional areas of the large and small arteries and veins, as well as an increase in microcirculation (by about 10%) per gram of muscle.[57, 73]
- *Blood pressure:* Regular aerobic training tends to **reduce** systolic and diastolic blood pressure both at rest and during submaximal exercise. The largest reduction occurs in systolic pressure and is most apparent in hypertensive subjects.
- *Pulmonary function:* Increased breathing volumes accompany improvements in $\dot{V}O_2$max. Higher maximum ventilation results from **increases** in tidal volume and breathing frequency. During submaximal exercise, trained subjects ventilate **less** than they do before training. This adaptation is helpful in prolonged exercise because improved ventilatory economy means more oxygen availability to the active muscles.

Other Adaptations

- *Body composition changes:* For the person who is obese or borderline obese, regular endurance exercise leads to a reduction in body mass and fat. Increases in lean body mass often accompany a program of resistance training. When exercise is used alone or combined with an adjusted diet, more of the weight lost is fat weight compared to weight lost as a result of dieting only because exercise has a conserving effect on the body's lean tissue.[6, 97]

- *Body heat transfer:* Well-hydrated, trained individuals exercise more comfortably in hot environments because of larger blood volumes and more responsive thermoregulatory mechanisms.[68, 75] These men and women dissipate heat faster and more economically. As a result, metabolic heat generated by exercise poses less of a potential detriment to exercise performance and safety.

- *Performance changes:* Enhanced exercise performance usually accompanies the physiologic adaptations elicited by training. For example, Figure 21.5 depicts the results of cycling exercise performed for 40 to 60 minutes, 4 days per week for 10 weeks, and at an intensity of 85% of $\dot{V}O_2$max. The performance test consisted of an attempt to maintain a constant work rate of 265 watts for 8 minutes. Following training, drop-off in power output during the prescribed 8-minute bout of exercise was significantly less than in the pre-training trials.

- *Psychological benefits:* As illustrated in Table 21.5, regular exercise, regardless of age, has the potential to favorably modify the psychological state of men and women.[56, 70] These potential modifications include a reduction in state anxiety; decreased level of mild to moderate depression; reduction in neuroticism; and improved mood, self-esteem, self-concept, and general perception of personal worth.

PRACTICAL IMPLICATIONS

A schema is proposed to summarize adaptive changes in active muscle that accompany a change in $\dot{V}O_2$max with endurance training. As shown in Figure 21.6, aerobic capacity increases about 15 to 30% over the first 3 months of intensive training and may rise by as much as 50% over a 2-year period. When training stops, the aerobic capacity decreases toward the pretraining level. The effect is even more impressive for the aerobic enzymes of the Krebs cycle and the electron-transport chain. These enzymes, which facilitate carbohydrate and lipid breakdown, increase rapidly and substantially throughout the training period in both fiber types and subdivisions. Conversely, a large portion of this metabolic adaptation is lost within a few weeks after training ceases.[10, 15, 53] The number of muscle capillaries increases throughout training.[8, 85] This adaptation in blood supply is probably lost at a relatively slow rate when training stops.

Intensive training lasting longer than 6 months also causes an increase in the mitochondrial respiratory capacity of the trained muscles. This "local" metabolic improvement greatly exceeds the improvement in the

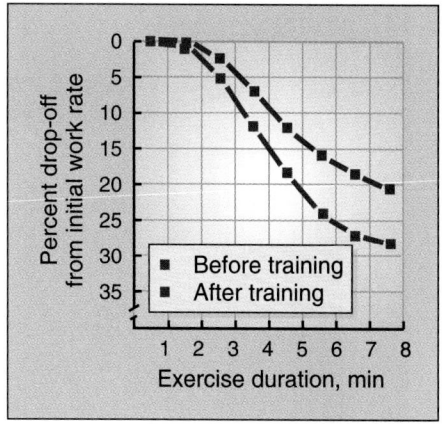

FIGURE 21.5
Percent drop-off from initial exercise intensity before and after 10 weeks of endurance cycling training. (From Applied Physiology Laboratory, University of Michigan, Ann Arbor.)

**TABLE 21.5
POTENTIAL PSYCHOLOGICAL BENEFITS OF REGULAR EXERCISE**

- Reduction in state anxiety, i.e., the level of anxiety at the time of measurement
- Decrease in mild to moderate depression
- Reduction in neuroticism (long-term exercise)
- Adjunct to professional treatment of severe depression
- Improvement in mood, self-esteem, and self-concept
- Reduction in the various indices of stress

body's capacity to circulate, deliver, and use oxygen (as demonstrated by the increase in $\dot{V}O_2$max) during intense aerobic exercise. In this phase of training, however, a muscle's lactate level (lower production or greater removal rate[19]) may be much lower than observed during similar submaximal exercise before training. *These cellular adjustments probably account for a trained person being able to perform steady-rate exercise at a larger percentage of $\dot{V}O_2$max.* To a large extent, endurance for sustained exercise may be more closely related to the oxidative capacity of mitochondria within specific muscles than to whole body oxygen uptake as reflected by the $\dot{V}O_2$max. In addition, the local metabolic and circulatory adaptations that accompany long-term training contribute to the lowered rates of glycogen utilization and concomitant increases in lipid catabolism during submaximal exercise.[12, 72] This glycogen-sparing effect becomes important during prolonged strenuous exercise.

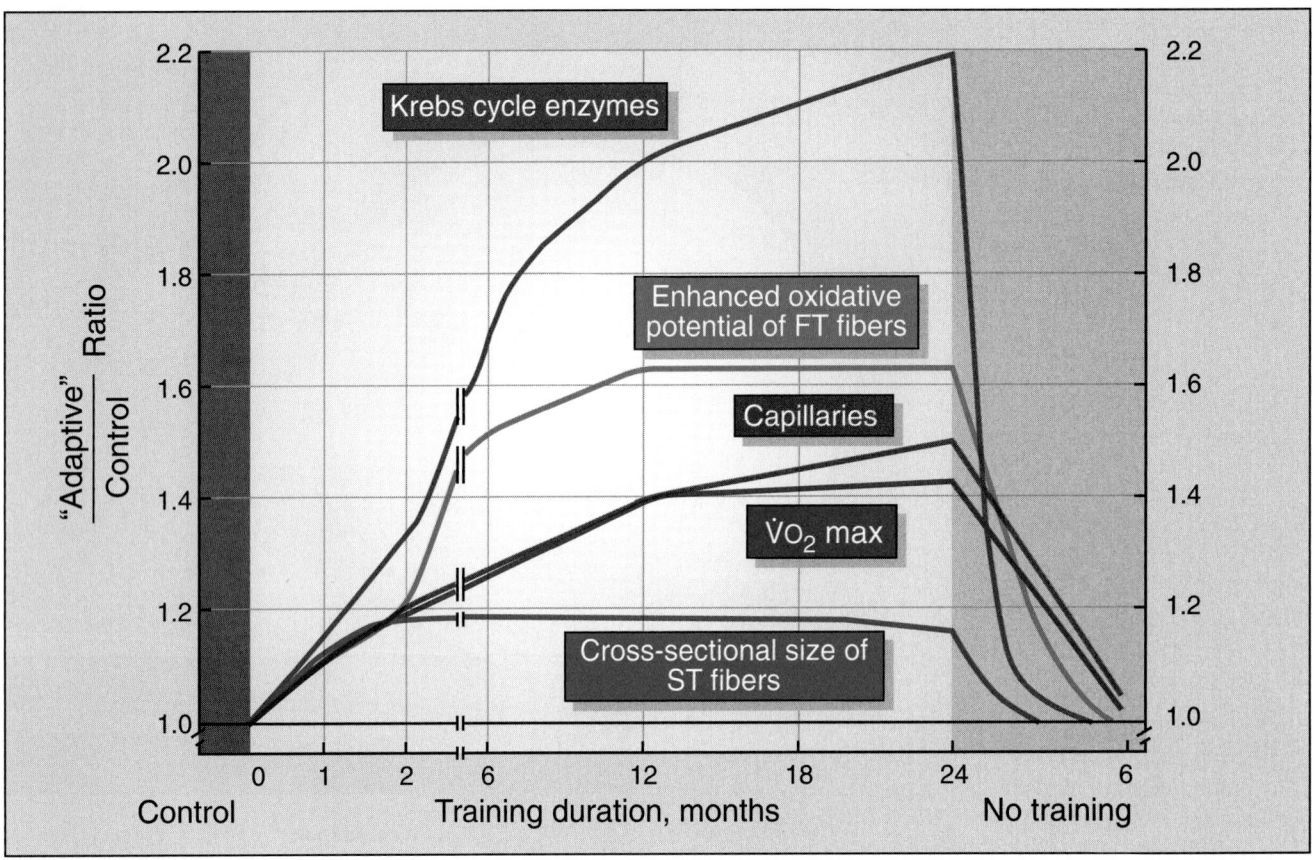

FIGURE 21.6

A generalized summary of adaptations in aerobic capacity and trained musculature with endurance training based on longitudinal and cross-sectional studies of humans. (Modified from Saltin, B., et al.: Fiber types and metabolic potentials of skeletal muscles in sedentary man and endurance runners. *Ann. N.Y. Acad. Sci.,* 301:3, 1977.)

FACTORS THAT AFFECT THE AEROBIC TRAINING RESPONSE

Four factors significantly influence the aerobic training response:

- Initial level of aerobic fitness,
- Intensity of training,
- Frequency of training, and
- Duration of training.

INITIAL LEVEL OF AEROBIC FITNESS

The response to training depends on one's initial fitness level. Someone who rates low at the start will have room for considerable improvement. If capacity is already high, the magnitude of improvement is relatively small. In studies of sedentary, middle-aged men with heart disease, for example, $\dot{V}O_2max$ improved by 50%, while the same type of training in normally active, healthy adults elicited only a 10 to 15% improvement.[80] Of course, a 5% improvement

in aerobic capacity is just as critical to an elite athlete as a 40% increase is to a sedentary person. *As a general guideline, expected aerobic fitness improvements of 5 to 25% will result from systematic programs of endurance training.* Some of this improvement occurs within the first week of training.[39]

EXERCISE INTENSITY

Training-induced physiologic changes depend primarily on the intensity of the overload. There are at least seven ways to express exercise intensity:

- As calories expended per unit time (for example, 9 kcal · min^{-1} or 37.8 kJ · min^{-1}).
- As a particular absolute exercise level or power output (for example, 180 kg-m · min^{-1} or 29.4 W).
- As a particular relative metabolic level expressed as a percentage of $\dot{V}O_2max$ (for example, 85% $\dot{V}O_2max$).
- As a level of exercise below, at, or above the lactate threshold (for example, 4 mmol lactate).

- As a particular exercise heart rate or percentage of maximum heart rate (for example, 180 beats per minute or 80% HRmax).
- As multiples of resting metabolic rate (for example, 6 METs).
- As some rating of perceived exertion (for example, RPE = 14).

An example of an absolute training intensity would be to have all individuals exercise at the same power output or energy expenditure, for example 200 watts on the bicycle ergometer or 300 kcal over a 30-minute exercise session. When everyone performs the same level of exercise, however, the task may pose a considerable stress to one person yet fall short of the training threshold intensity of another, more fit, person. For this reason, the exercise training level is usually based on the **relative stress** placed on a person's physiologic systems. Consequently, exercise intensity is assigned as some percentage of maximum function, for example $\dot{V}O_2$max, maximum heart rate (HRmax), or maximum working capacity. The general practice for establishing aerobic training intensity is direct measurement or estimation of the person's $\dot{V}O_2$max or HRmax, followed by assignation of an exercise level that corresponds to some percentage of these maximums.

Although establishing training intensity from measures of oxygen uptake is reasonably accurate, it is impractical without sophisticated equipment. An effective alternative is to use **heart rate** to classify exercise for relative intensity and then establish the training protocol. This practice is possible because the percent $\dot{V}O_2$max and percent HRmax are related in a predictable way regardless of gender, fitness level, or age. Selected values for percent $\dot{V}O_2$max and corresponding percentages of HRmax obtained from several sources are presented in Table 21.6.[1, 2, 61, 96] The error in estimating percent $\dot{V}O_2$max from percent HRmax, or vice versa, is about ± 8%. Because of this

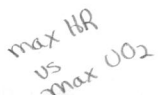

TABLE 21.6
RELATIONSHIP BETWEEN PERCENT MAXIMUM HEART RATE AND PERCENT $\dot{V}O_2$max

Percent HRmax	Percent $\dot{V}O_2$max
50	28
60	40
70	58
80	70
90	83
100	100

intrinsic relationship, it is only necessary to monitor heart rate to estimate the exercise stress or percent $\dot{V}O_2$max. The relationship between percent HRmax and percent $\dot{V}O_2$max is essentially the same for arm or leg exercises among healthy subjects, normal weight and obese groups, cardiac patients, and people with spinal cord injuries.[25, 34, 44, 71] *The important point is that HRmax is significantly lower in arm compared to leg exercises, and this difference must be considered when formulating the exercise prescription for different exercise modes* (refer to p. 405).

Train at a Percentage of HRmax

As a general rule, aerobic capacity improves if exercise is sufficiently intense to increase heart rate to about 70% of maximum. During leg exercise such as cycling, walking, or running, this increase is equivalent to about 55% of the $\dot{V}O_2$max or, for college-aged men and women, to a heart rate of 130 to 140 beats per minute.

An alternative and equally effective method for establishing the training threshold is to have the subject exercise at a heart rate that is about 60% of the difference between resting and maximum.[51] This rate is calculated as follows:

$$HR_{threshold} = HR_{rest} + 0.60 \, (HR_{max} - HR_{rest})$$

This approach to determining the threshold training heart rate tends to give a somewhat higher value compared to computing the heart rate simply as 70% of *HRmax*.

Clearly, exercise need not be strenuous to obtain positive training adaptations. An exercise heart rate of 70% maximum represents moderate exercise with little or no discomfort. This training level, frequently referred to as **"conversational exercise,"** is sufficiently intense to stimulate a training effect yet not so strenuous that it limits a person from talking during the workout. It is unnecessary to exercise above this heart rate to improve physiologic capacity.

Figure 21.7 illustrates that as aerobic fitness improves, the exercise heart rate is reduced at a given oxygen uptake. It is common for submaximal heart rate to be lowered 10 to 20 beats per minute as a result of aerobic training. To keep pace with physiologic improvement, the exercise level must be increased periodically to attain the desired heart rate. A person who began training by walking would have to walk more briskly; walking would gradually give way to jogging for periods of the workout; and eventually, continuous running would be required to achieve the same relative strenuousness or exercise at the desired heart rate. If the progression in exercise intensity is not matched to training improvements, the exercise program becomes a "maintenance" program for aerobic fitness without further improvements.[39, 41]

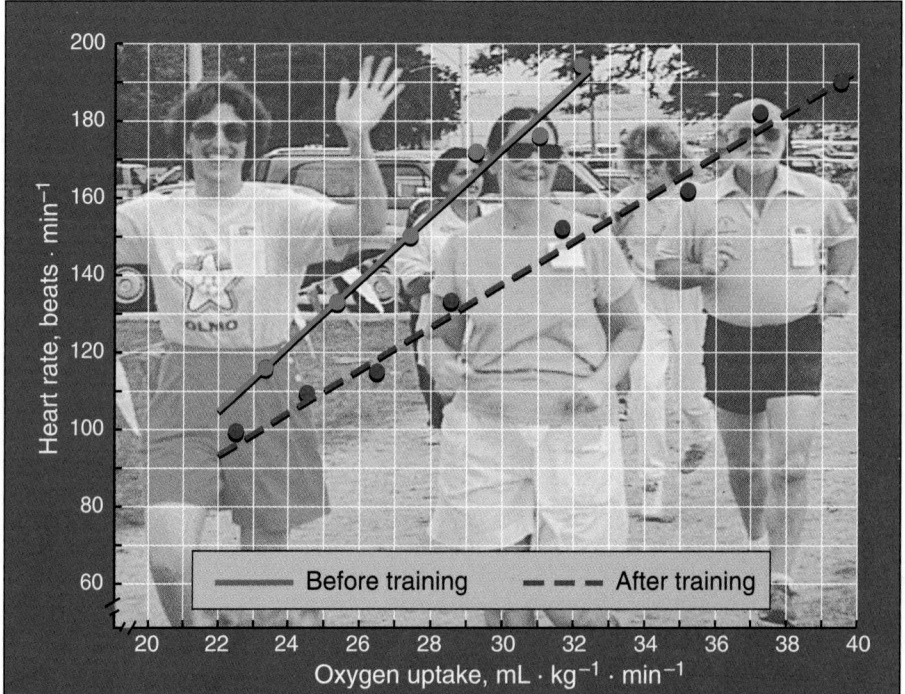

FIGURE 21.7
Improvements in heart rate response with aerobic training in relation to oxygen uptake. A significant reduction in exercise heart rate with training usually reflects an enhanced stroke volume of the heart.

Is Strenuous Training More Effective?

Generally, the greater the relative training intensity above threshold, the greater the training improvement will be. However, this only is true within certain limits. Although there may be a minimal "threshold" intensity below which a training effect does not occur, there may also be a "ceiling" above which no further gains are realized. More fit men and women generally must achieve higher threshold levels to stimulate a training response. The ceiling for training intensity is unknown, although 85% $\dot{V}O_2$max (corresponding to 90% HRmax) is considered an upper limit. At present, no definitive research is available to either prove or disprove this notion. An important point is that regardless of the exercise level selected, more is not necessarily better. Excessive exercise increases the chance for injury to bones, joints, and muscles.[49]

The "Training-Sensitive Zone"

Maximum exercise heart rate usually can be determined immediately after 2 to 4 minutes of all-out effort during a specific form of exercise. This level of exercise, however, requires considerable motivation and certainly is not advisable for adults without medical clearance, particularly individuals predisposed to coronary heart disease. Consequently, people should consider themselves "average" and use the **age-predicted maximum heart rates** presented in Figure 21.8.

Although people of a particular age possess varying HRmax values, the loss in accuracy resulting from individual variation (generally, ± 10 beats per minute is the standard deviation for any age-predicted HRmax) is usually of little significance in establishing an effective training program for healthy people. *Maximum heart rate is established as 220 minus the person's age in years, with values being independent of race or sex in children and adults.*[48, 60] (Note: This decrease in maximum heart rate with age is probably the result of a reduced sympathetic output from the medulla and possibly changes in the inherent characteristics of the S-A node.[85]) Although this formula represents a convenient "rule of thumb," it is only an estimate. Within normal variation, about 95% (± 2 standard deviations) of 40-year-old men and women have a maximum heart rate between 160 and 200 beats per minute. Figure 21.8 also depicts the "training-sensitive zone" in relation to age. Conditioning of the aerobic systems should occur as long as the exercise heart rate is maintained within this zone.

A 40-year-old woman (or man) wishing to train at moderate intensity but still achieve the threshold level would select a training heart rate equal to 70% of age-predicted HRmax, that is, a target exercise heart rate of 126 beats per minute (0.70 × 180). Then, by trial and error (using progressive increments of light to moderate exercise), the person could arrive at a walking, jogging, or cycling exercise level that produces this target heart rate. If the person wishes to increase training intensity to 85% of maximum, the exercise intensity must be increased to produce a heart rate of 153 beats per minute (0.85 × 180).

Running versus swimming and other forms of upper body exercise. *An adjustment must be made in estimating HRmax if swimming or other forms of upper body exercise are used for training.*[25] Maximum heart rate during these exercise modes averages about 13 beats per minute lower than that in running for both trained and untrained men and women.[66, 69, 101] This difference is probably the result of a smaller feedforward stimulation from the motor cortex to the medulla as well as less feedback stimulation from the smaller active upper body muscle mass. In swimming, the horizontal body position and cooling effect of the water also may contribute to a lower HRmax.

To establish the appropriate exercise intensity for swimming and upper body exercise, the difference of 13 beats per minute noted above should be subtracted from the age-predicted HRmax given in Figure 21.8. Consequently, a 30-year-old person wishing to swim at 70% HRmax would select a swimming speed that produces a heart rate of 124 beats per minute [(0.70) × (190 − 13)]. This more accurately represents the appropriate threshold training heart rate for swimming. If this is not done, a prescription of upper body exercise based on a percentage of the HRmax during leg exercise results in an **overestimation** of the appropriate threshold training heart rate.

Is Less Intense Training Effective?

The recommendation of using 70% HRmax as a training threshold for aerobic improvement should be viewed as a **general guideline** for establishing an effective, yet comfortable exercise level. This lower limit may depend on the participant's initial exercise capacity and current state of training. In addition, older and less fit men and women may have training thresholds closer to 60% of HRmax, which corresponds to about 45% $\dot{V}O_2$max.[26] Although 20 to 30 minutes of continuous exercise at the 70% level will stimulate a training effect, exercise at the lower intensity of 60% for 45 minutes also will prove beneficial. *Generally, a lower exercise intensity can be offset by a longer exercise duration.*

Train at a Perception of Effort

In addition to oxygen uptake, heart rate, and blood lactate as indicators of exercise intensity, one also can use the **rating of perceived exertion (RPE)**.[5, 18, 95] Using this approach, the exerciser rates on a numerical scale (Borg scale, after the researcher who developed this scaling system) how he or she feels in relation to the level of exertion. The exercise levels that correspond to higher levels of energy expenditure and physiologic strain result in higher RPE ratings. For example, an RPE of 13 or 14

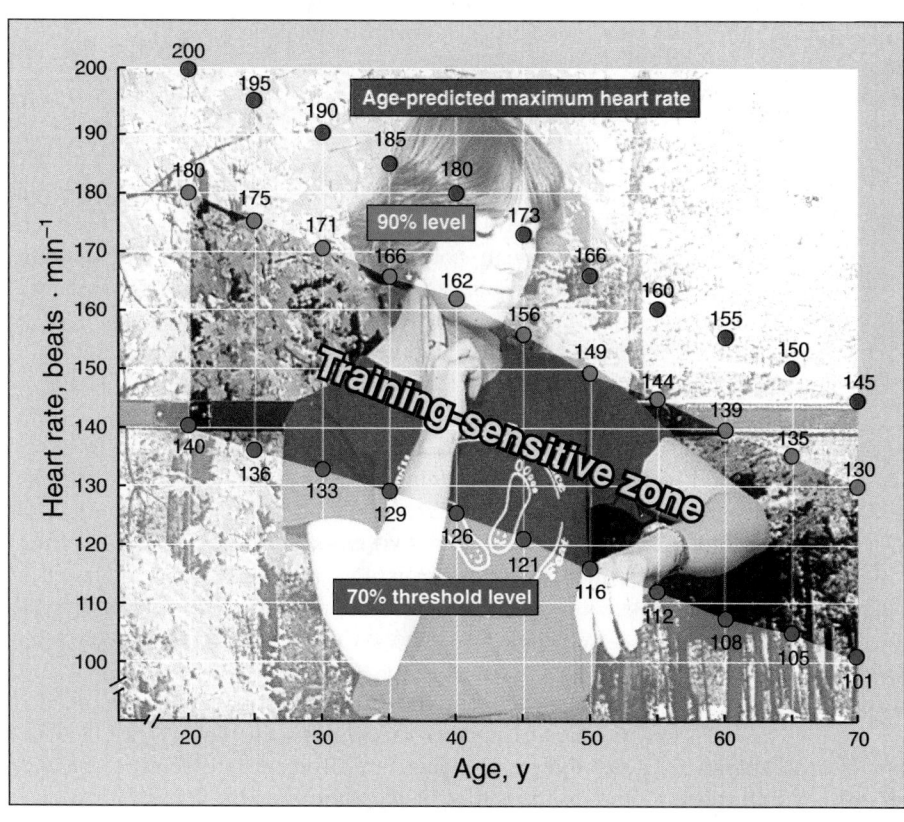

FIGURE 21.8

Maximal heart rates and the training-sensitive zone for use in aerobic training of men and women of different ages.

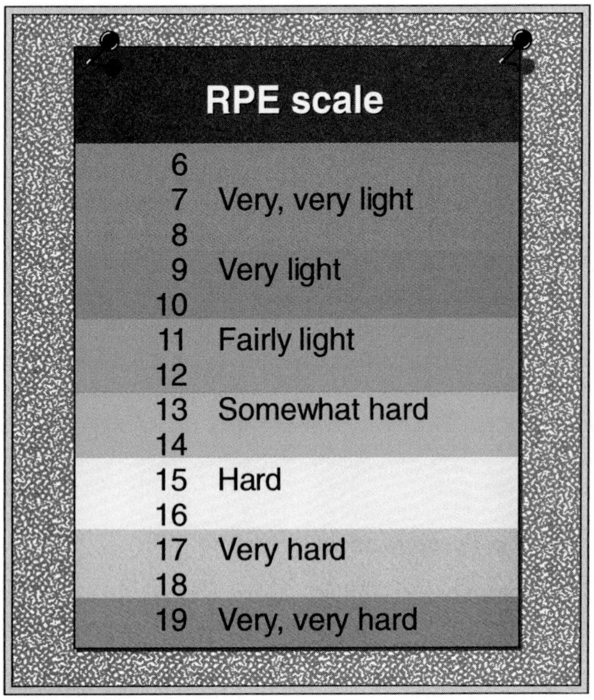

RPE scale

6	
7	Very, very light
8	
9	Very light
10	
11	Fairly light
12	
13	Somewhat hard
14	
15	Hard
16	
17	Very hard
18	
19	Very, very hard

FIGURE 21.9

The Borg scale used in obtaining the rating of perceived exertion (RPE) during exercise. (From Borg, G.A.: Psychological basis of physical exertion. *Med. Sci. Sports Exerc.*, 14:377, 1982.)

(exercise that feels "somewhat hard"), as illustrated in Figure 21.9, coincides with an exercise heart rate of about 70% HRmax; an RPE of 11.0 corresponds to exercise at the lactate threshold for both trained and untrained subjects.[91] Individuals can quickly learn to exercise at a specific RPE that coincides nicely with the more objective physiologic measures of exercise intensity. In this sense, the axiom "listen to your body" is apropos.

Train at the Lactate Threshold

It is also effective to set training at or slightly above the level of exercise that represents one's lactate threshold, with the higher level of exercise being most effective.[3, 104] This exercise level can be determined by plotting exercise intensity (for example, running speed) in relation to blood lactate level, as illustrated in Figure 21.10. In this example, the running speed at which blood lactate reached the 4 mmol level (the point of onset of blood lactate accumulation or OBLA) was the recommended training intensity. Periodic re-evaluation of the blood lactate–exercise intensity relationship is required to continually upgrade the level of exercise as improvements occur in aerobic fitness.

One difference between the percent HRmax and lactate threshold methods for setting the training intensity

lies in the physiologic system being overloaded.[72] More than likely, the heart rate method will establish a level of exercise stress for central circulation (for example, stroke volume, cardiac output), whereas adjustments to lactate threshold are dictated by the capability of the periphery (local vasculature and active muscles) to sustain steady-rate aerobic metabolism.

TRAINING DURATION

A threshold duration per workout has **not** been identified for optimal aerobic improvement. This threshold probably depends on the interaction of many factors including the total work accomplished (duration or training volume), exercise intensity, training frequency, and initial fitness level. Whereas 3- to 5-minute periods of daily exercise produce training effects in some poorly conditioned people, 20- to 30-minute exercise sessions achieve more optimal results (yet are still practical in terms of time) if the intensity is at least 70% HRmax. At higher-intensity training, significant improvements will occur during a 10-minute workout. Conversely, 60 minutes of continuous exercise may be required to produce a training effect when exercise intensity is below the threshold heart rate.

As for training volume, more is not necessarily better. In a study of collegiate swimmers, one group trained for 1.5 hours daily while another group performed two 1.5-hour exercise sessions daily.[14] Despite one group exercising at twice the daily exercise volume of the other, no differences in swimming power, endurance, or performance time improvements were observed between groups.

TRAINING FREQUENCY

Is it better to work out 2 or 5 days a week if duration and intensity are the same for each training session? Unfortunately, a precise answer is unavailable to this question. Although some investigators report that training frequency is an important factor in eliciting cardiovascular improvements others maintain that this factor is considerably less important than either exercise intensity or duration.[17, 81] Studies using interval training (refer to Interval Training section) showed that training 2 days per week resulted in $\dot{V}O_2$max changes similar to those observed when training 5 days per week.[23] In other studies for which total exercise volume was held constant, there were no differences in $\dot{V}O_2$max improvements when training frequency was 2 versus 4 or 3 versus 5 days per week.[92] As was the case with training duration, more frequent training is beneficial if the training is performed at a lower intensity.

It seems that the extra investment of time needed to increase training frequency may not always be that profitable in inducing improvements in physiologic function. On the other hand, when exercise is used for weight

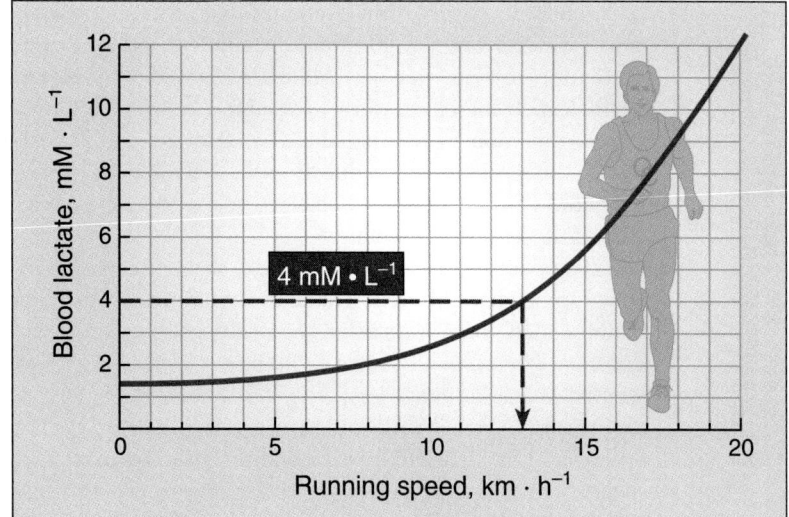

FIGURE 21.10
Blood lactate level in relation to running speed for one subject. At a lactate level of 4.0 mM · L⁻¹, the corresponding running speed was approximately 13 km · hr⁻¹. This running speed then became the subject's initial training intensity.

loss, strong consideration should be given to exercising on a daily basis, because this exercise frequency represents a considerable caloric expenditure compared to training only a few days a week. *To effect a meaningful weight loss through exercise, it is recommended that each exercise session last at least 60 minutes and be of sufficient intensity to expend at least 300 kcal.* Training fewer than 2 days per week generally does not produce meaningful changes in anaerobic or aerobic capacity or body composition.[1]

Typical aerobic exercise training programs are conducted 3 days per week with a rest day usually spaced between two of the workout days. A reasonable question, however, is whether training could occur on consecutive days and still produce equally effective results? In an experiment concerned with this exact question, improvements in V̇o₂max were nearly identical regardless of the sequence of the 3-day-per-week training schedule.[74] This finding suggests that perhaps the stimulus for aerobic training is closely tied to the intensity **and** total work accomplished and **not** to the sequence of training.

EXERCISE MODE

If exercise intensity, duration, and frequency are held constant, training improvements are similar, regardless of training mode—as long as the exercise involves relatively large muscle groups and improvement is evaluated in the exercise mode used during the training. Bicycling, walking, running, rowing, swimming, in-line skating, rope skipping, bench-stepping, stair climbing, and simulated arm-leg climbing are all excellent activities for stressing the aerobic system.[7, 62, 78, 80, 102] Of course, based on the specificity concept, the magnitude of training changes may vary considerably depending on the **mode of testing.** Individuals trained

on a bicycle show greater improvements when tested on the bicycle than on the treadmill.[79] Likewise, individuals that train by swimming show the greatest improvements when measured during an upper body exercise.[27, 66]

How Long Does It Take Before Improvements Are Noted?

The answer to this question depends on the specific biologic systems affected. Adaptations in aerobic fitness occur rapidly, and significant improvements are often noted within several weeks.[38] Figure 21.11 shows absolute and percentage improvements in V̇o₂max for subjects who trained 6 days per week for 10 weeks. Training consisted of 30 minutes of bicycling 3 days per week combined with running for up to 40 minutes on alternate days. As illustrated, aerobic capacity improved continuously from week to week. This suggests that training improvements in previously sedentary people occur rapidly and continue in a relatively steady fashion. Of course, these adaptive responses eventually begin to level off as subjects approach their "genetically predisposed" maximums. The exact time it takes until this leveling off is unknown, particularly for those who undergo high-intensity training. This time no doubt varies depending on the particular physiologic and metabolic systems affected.

More exercise is not necessarily better. This is true not only for aerobic improvement, but also because the number of running injuries increases dramatically with large increases in training volume.[94] For both men and women, the only variable consistently associated with running injuries has been the number of miles run per week.[82] In preadolescent children, running excessive distances may place undue strain on the articular cartilage. This type of strain could injure the bone's growth

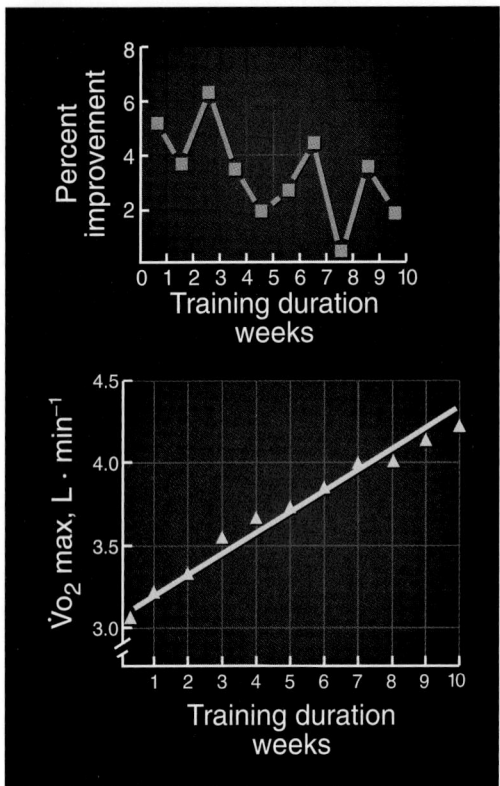

FIGURE 21.11

Continuous improvements in $\dot{V}O_2$max over 10 weeks of high-intensity aerobic training. (From Hickson, R.C., et al.: Linear increases in aerobic power induced by a program of endurance exercise. *J. Appl. Physiol.*, 42:373, 1977.)

plate (epiphysis) and have subsequent adverse effects on growth.[9]

MAINTENANCE OF AEROBIC FITNESS

Another important question concerns the optimal frequency, duration, and intensity of exercise required to maintain aerobic improvements attained through training. In one study, healthy young adults achieved a 25% improvement in $\dot{V}O_2$max after 10 weeks of interval training by bicycling and running for 40 minutes, 6 days a week.[37] They were then placed into one of two groups that continued to exercise for an additional 15 weeks at the same intensity and duration but at a reduced **frequency** of either 4 or 2 days a week. For both groups, the gains in aerobic capacity were maintained despite as much as a two-thirds reduction in training frequency.

The effect of reduced training duration on the maintenance of improved aerobic fitness has been similarly studied.[40] Following the same protocol outlined above for the initial 10 weeks of training, the subjects continued to maintain the intensity and frequency of training for an

additional 15 weeks, but they reduced training **duration** from the original 40-minute sessions to either 26- or 13-minute sessions per day. Almost all of the $\dot{V}O_2$max and performance increases were maintained despite this two-thirds reduction in training duration. However, if the **intensity** of training was reduced and frequency and duration held constant, even a one-third reduction in intensity caused the $\dot{V}O_2$max to decline.[41]

It appears that improvements in aerobic capacity involve somewhat different training requirements than its maintenance. *If intensity is held constant, the frequency and duration of exercise required to maintain a certain level of aerobic fitness is much less than that required for its improvement.* A small drop off in exercise intensity, on the other hand, is associated with a reduction in $\dot{V}O_2$max. This suggests strongly that training intensity plays a principal role in maintaining the increase in aerobic power achieved through training.

Fitness components other than $\dot{V}O_2$max may more readily suffer adverse effects from a reduction in exercise training volume. In a recent study, well-trained endurance athletes who normally trained from 6 to 10 hours a week reduced their weekly training to one 35-minute session and showed no decrease in $\dot{V}O_2$max over 4 weeks.[65] However, their endurance capacities at 75% of $\dot{V}O_2$max were significantly reduced, which was associated with reduced pre-exercise glycogen stores and a diminished level of lipid oxidation. *Such findings indicate that the factors that affect training and detraining adaptations cannot be adequately evaluated through the use of a single measure such as $\dot{V}O_2$max.*

METHODS OF TRAINING

Each year, improvements in performance are noted in almost all athletic activities. These advances are generally attributed to increased opportunities for participation: individuals with "natural endowment" are more likely to be exposed to particular sports. Also contributing to superior performances are improved nutrition and health care, better athletic equipment, and more systematic and scientific approaches to athletic training and conditioning.

In the following sections, general guidelines for anaerobic and aerobic training are presented, with particular emphasis on three general training classifications: (*a*) **interval training,** (*b*) **continuous training,** and (*c*) **fartlek training**.

ANAEROBIC TRAINING

As demonstrated in Figure 21.1, the capacity to perform all-out exercise for brief periods of time (up to 60 seconds) largely depends on ATP generated by the immediate and short-term anaerobic energy systems.

The Intramuscular High-Energy Phosphates

Sports such as football, weightlifting, and various other brief sprint activities rely almost exclusively on energy derived from the ATP and CP that comprise the muscle's high-energy phosphates. This phosphate pool can be overloaded by engaging specific muscles in repeated **maximum** bursts of effort for 5- to 10-second durations. Because the intramuscular high-energy phosphates supply energy for such intense, intermittent exercise, only small amounts of lactic acid are produced and recovery is rapid (alactic recovery oxygen uptake). Thus, a subsequent exercise bout can begin after about a 30-second rest period. This use of brief, all-out exercise periods interspersed with recovery represents a specific application of interval training to anaerobic conditioning.

In training to enhance ATP-CP energy transfer capacity, the activities selected must engage the specific muscles at the movement speed and power output for which the athlete desires improved anaerobic power. Not only does this enhance the metabolic capacity of the specifically trained muscle fibers, but it also facilitates recruitment (and modulation in firing sequence) of the appropriate motor units used in the actual movement.

Lactic Acid–Generating Capacity

As the duration of all-out effort extends beyond 10 seconds, dependence on anaerobic energy from the intramuscular phosphates decreases while the magnitude of anaerobic energy generated in glycolysis increases. To improve the capacity for energy transfer by the short-term lactic acid energy system, training must overload this aspect of energy metabolism.

Anaerobic training is both physiologically and psychologically taxing and requires considerable motivation. Repeated bouts of up to 1 minute of maximum exercise, such as running, swimming, or cycling, stopped about 30 seconds before subjective feelings of exhaustion cause blood lactate to increase to near-maximum levels. Each exercise bout should be repeated after 3 to 5 minutes of recovery. This repetition of exercise causes a "lactate stacking," which results in higher lactate levels than if just one bout of all-out effort were performed to the point of exhaustion.[35] Of course, as with all training, it is crucial to exercise the specific muscle groups that require this enhanced anaerobic capacity. A backstroke swimmer should train by swimming the backstroke, a cyclist should bicycle, and basketball, hockey, or soccer players should rapidly perform various movements and direction changes similar to those required by the demands of their sports.

The time necessary for recovery can be considerable when exercise involves a significant anaerobic component. For this reason, anaerobic power training should occur at the end of the conditioning session. Otherwise, fatigue would carry over and perhaps hinder one's ability to perform subsequent aerobic training.

AEROBIC TRAINING

Figure 21.12 indicates two important factors in formulating an aerobic training program. For one thing, the training must provide a sufficient cardiovascular overload to stimulate increases in stroke volume and cardiac output. This central circulatory overload should be accomplished by exercising the sport-specific muscle groups to enhance their local

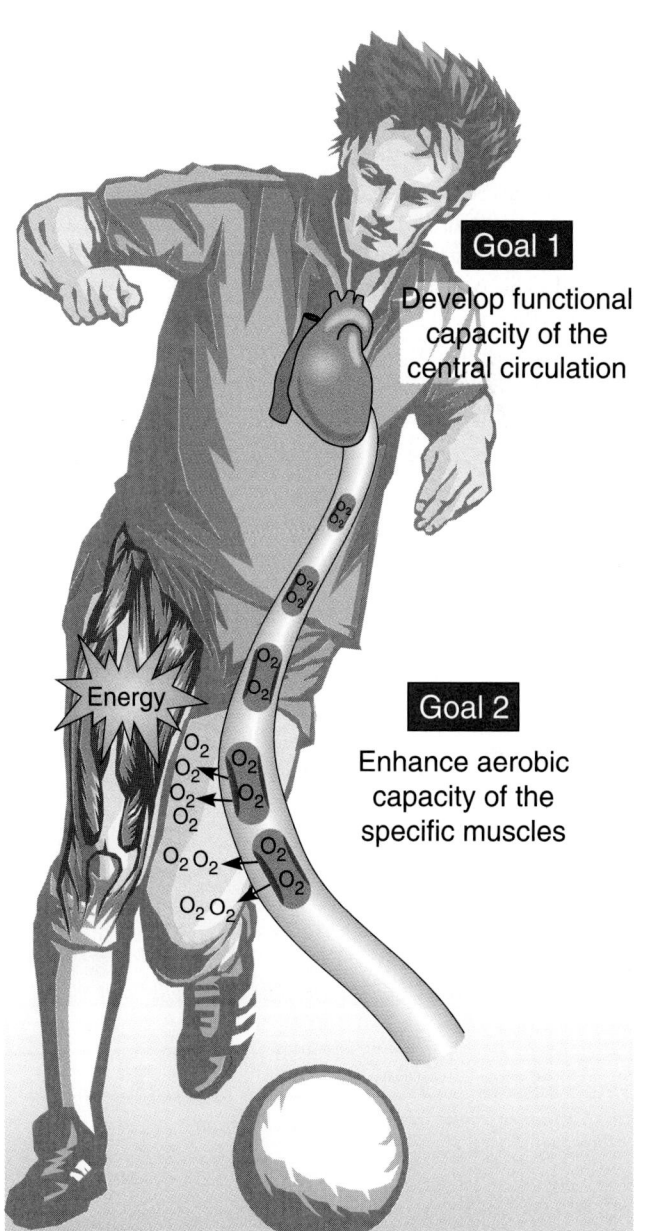

Goal 1
Develop functional capacity of the central circulation

Goal 2
Enhance aerobic capacity of the specific muscles

FIGURE 21.12

The two major goals of aerobic training: (*Goal 1*) develop the capacity of the central circulation to deliver oxygen, and (*Goal 2*) enhance the capacity of the local musculature to supply and process oxygen.

circulation and "metabolic machinery." This consideration essentially embodies the specificity principle as applied to aerobic training. Simply stated, runners should run, cyclists should bicycle, rowers should row, and swimmers should swim.

Relatively brief bouts of repeated exercise (interval training), as well as continuous, long-duration efforts (continuous training), enhance aerobic capacity, provided the exercise is sufficiently intense to overload the aerobic system. Interval training, continuous training, and fartlek training are three common methods for improving aerobic fitness.

Interval Training

With the correct spacing of exercise and rest periods, an extraordinary amount of high-intensity exercise, normally not possible if the exercise were done continuously, can be performed. The repeated exercise bouts (with rest periods or **relief intervals**) can vary from a few seconds to several minutes or more depending on the desired training outcome.[16, 23, 24] The interval training prescription is based on the following considerations:

• Intensity of exercise,
• Duration of exercise interval,
• Length of recovery, and
• Number of repetitions of the exercise-recovery interval.

The ability to perform a considerable volume of high-intensity exercise during an interval training workout is illustrated in the following example. Few people can maintain a 4-minute-mile pace for longer than 1 minute, let alone complete a mile within 4 minutes. If running intervals,

however, were limited to only 10 seconds, followed by 30 seconds of recovery, it would not be exceedingly difficult to maintain these exercise-rest intervals and complete the mile in 4 minutes of actual running. Although this does not parallel a world-class performance, the point is that a significant quantity of normally exhausting exercise can be achieved given the proper spacing of rest and exercise intervals.

Rationale for Interval Training. Interval training has a sound basis in physiology and energy metabolism. In the example of a continuous run at a 4-minute-mile pace, a large portion of energy would be supplied through anaerobic glycolysis. Within a minute or two, lactic acid levels would rise precipitously and the runner would become exhausted. During interval training, on the other hand, repeated exercise bouts of about 10 seconds' duration would permit a severe load to be imposed without an appreciable buildup of lactic acid because the primary energy source for such brief exercise is the high-energy phosphates. Fatigue incurred during the predominantly "alactic" exercise interval would be minor and recovery would be rapid. The exercise interval could then begin after only a brief rest period.

In interval training, as in other forms of physiologic conditioning, the intensity of exercise should be geared to the particular energy systems to be trained. A practical method for determining the appropriate exercise and recovery intervals is presented in Table 21.7.

• **Exercise interval**—Generally 1.5 to 5.0 seconds is **added** to the exerciser's "best time" for training distances between 55 and 220 yd for running and 15 and 55 yd for swimming.[24, 106] If a person can run 60 yd from a

---

TABLE 21.7
GUIDELINES FOR DETERMINING INTERVAL-TRAINING EXERCISE RATES FOR RUNNING AND SWIMMING DIFFERENT DISTANCES

Interval Training Distances (yards)		Work Rate for Each Exercise Interval or Repeat	
Run	Swim		
55	15	1.5	seconds *slower* than best
110	25	3.0	times from a running (or swimming) start
220	55	5.0	for each distance
440	110		1 to 4 seconds *faster* than the average run or 110-yard swim times recorded during a mile run or 440-yard swim
660–1320	165–320		3 to 4 seconds *slower* than the average run or 100-yard swim times recorded during a mile run or 440-yard swim

From Fox, E.L., and Mathews, D.K.: *Interval Training*. Philadelphia, W.B. Saunders, 1974.

running start in 8 seconds, the training time for each repeat would therefore be 8 + 1.5, or 9.5 seconds. For an interval training distance of 110 yd, 3 seconds is added, and for a distance of 220 yd, 5 seconds is added to the best running times. This particular application of interval training is suited to training of the ATP-CP energy system.

- For training distances of 440 yd running or 110 yd swimming, the exercise rate is determined by **subtracting** 1 to 4 seconds from the best 440-yd part of a mile run or 110-yd part of a 440-yd swim. If a person runs a 7-minute mile (averaging 105 seconds per 440 yd), the interval time for each 440-yd repeat would be between 104 seconds (105 − 1) and 101 seconds (105 − 4). For training intervals beyond 440 yd, 3 to 4 seconds is **added** for each 440-yd portion of the interval distance. In running an interval of 880 yd, the 7-minute miler would thus run each interval at about 216 seconds [(105 + 3) × (2) = 216].

- **Relief interval**—The relief interval can be either passive (rest-relief) or active (work-relief). The recommended duration of relief usually is expressed as a ratio of exercise duration to recovery duration. *The ratio of 1 to 3 is generally recommended for training the immediate energy system.* Thus, for a sprinter who runs 10-second intervals, the relief interval is usually about 30 seconds. *For training the short-term energy system of glycolysis, the relief interval is twice as long as the exercise interval, or a ratio of 1 to 2.* These specific work-to-relief ratios for anaerobic training supposedly ensure sufficient restoration of intramuscular phosphates and/or sufficient lactic acid removal to allow the next exercise bout to continue with minimal or no fatigue.

- *For training the long-term aerobic energy system, the work-recovery interval ratio is usually 1:1 or 1:1.5.* During a 60- to 90-second exercise interval, for example, oxygen uptake increases rapidly to a high level, but this increase is insufficient to meet the energy requirements of the exercise. The recommended recovery interval is such that the succeeding exercise interval begins before recovery is complete (in other words, before the return of baseline or resting oxygen uptake). This ensures that cardiovascular and aerobic metabolic stress reach near peak levels with repeated but relatively short exercise intervals. The duration of the rest interval is not as crucial with longer periods of intermittent exercise because there is sufficient time for adjustments in metabolic and circulatory parameters.

Continuous Training

Continuous or **long slow distance (LSD)** training involves steady-paced, prolonged exercise at either moderate or high aerobic intensity and performed at 60 to 80% of the $\dot{V}O_2max$. The exact pace can vary, but it must at

least meet threshold intensity to ensure physiologic adaptation. The method to establish this threshold so that the person might exercise in the "training-sensitive zone" was outlined previously (p. 404). Continuous training for an hour or longer is popular among joggers and other fitness enthusiasts as well as among competitive endurance athletes such as triathletes and cross-country skiers. For example, some elite distance runners train twice a day and run between 100 and 150 miles each week in preparing for competition. In one report, a man training for the 52.5 mile ultramarathon ran twice per day, 20 miles in the morning and 13 miles in the evening, and interspersed these runs with occasional 30- to 60-mile nonstop runs at a 7- to 8-minute per mile pace. Following this schedule, he ran more than 800 miles each month and totaled 9600 miles for the year! The precise effects and benefits of such considerable training are unknown.

By nature, continuous exercise training is submaximal and, therefore, can be performed for a considerable time in relative comfort. Because of the potential hazards of high-intensity interval training in coronary-prone individuals (as well as the considerable motivation required for such strenuous exercise), continuous training is particularly suitable for those just beginning an exercise program or those wishing to accumulate a considerable expenditure of calories for purposes of weight loss. When applied in athletic training, continuous training really is "over-distance" training, with most athletes training two to five times the actual distances of their competitive events.

One of the advantages of continuous training for endurance athletes is that it permits exercising at nearly the same intensity as actual competition. Because the recruitment of appropriate motor units depends on the exercise intensity, continuous training may be best suited to the endurance athlete in terms of adaptations at the cellular level.[22, 28] This is in contrast to interval training, which may place a disproportionate stress on the fast-twitch muscle fibers; these are **not** the fibers predominantly recruited in endurance competition.

Fartlek Training

Fartlek is a Swedish word meaning "speed play." This training method, introduced to the United States in the 1940s, is a relatively "unscientific" adaptation of interval and continuous training and is well suited to exercise out-of-doors and over natural terrain. In this system, alternate running is done at both fast and slow speeds on both a level and hilly course.

In contrast to the precise exercise prescription in interval training, fartlek training does not require systematic manipulation of the exercise and relief intervals. Instead, the performer determines the training schema based on "how it feels" at the time. If used properly, this method can overload one or all of the energy systems. Although lacking the systematic and quantified approaches of interval and continuous training, fartlek training is ideally suited to general conditioning and off-season training and to maintaining a certain "freedom" and variety in workouts.

Insufficient evidence is available to declare the superiority of any specific training method for improving aerobic capacity. Each training procedure results in success. The various methods can probably be used interchangeably and certainly should be used to modify training and achieve a more psychologically pleasing exercise program.

OVERTRAINING: TOO MUCH OF A GOOD THING

With heavy and prolonged regular training, especially in endurance sports, certain athletes experience the syndrome of overtraining, or "staleness". As a result, normal exercise performance deteriorates because the individual experiences increasing difficulty recovering from a workout.[58] The overtrained condition is more than just a short-term inability to train as hard as usual or a slight dip in competition-level performance; rather, it involves a more chronic fatigue experienced during both exercise workouts and subsequent recovery periods. It also is associated with sustained poor exercise performance, frequent infections, and a general malaise and loss of interest in high-level training. Injuries also are more frequent in the overtrained state. Although the specific symptoms of overtraining are highly individualized, those outlined in Table 21.8 generally represent the most common ones. Little is known about the etiology of this syndrome, although neuroendocrine alterations that affect the sympathetic nervous system,[45] as well as alterations in immune function probably are involved. Generally, these symptoms will persist unless the athlete rests, with complete recovery requiring weeks or even months.

TABLE 21.8
THE OVERTRAINING SYNDROME: SYMPTOMS OF STALENESS

- Unexplained and persistant poor performance
- Disturbed mood states characterized by general fatigue, depression, and irritability
- Elevated resting pulse, painful muscles, and an increased susceptibility to upper respiratory infections and gastrointestinal disturbances
- Insominia
- Weight loss
- Overuse injuries

■ SUMMARY ■

1. Physical activities can be classified in terms of the specific system of energy transfer they predominantly activate. An effective training program includes a commitment to training the appropriate energy system or systems for improving a desired function.

2. Proper physical conditioning based on sound principles produces optimum improvements. Of crucial importance are the overload, specificity of exercise, individual differences, and reversibility principles.

3. Exercise training brings about specific metabolic and physiologic adaptations, which involve subtle cellular as well as gross physiologic changes. Anaerobic training increases resting levels of anaerobic substrates and key glycolytic enzymes. These increases usually are accompanied by concomitant increases in all-out exercise performance. Aerobic training changes include increases in mitochondrial size and number as well as changes in the activity of aerobic enzymes, increased capillarization of the trained muscle, and enhanced oxidation of lipids and carbohydrates. These adaptations are geared to a greater aerobic production of ATP.

4. Aerobic training induces functional and dimensional changes in the cardiovascular system. These changes include decreases in resting and submaximal exercise heart rate, enhanced stroke volume and cardiac output, and an expanded $a\text{-}\bar{v}\,O_2$ difference.

5. Major factors that affect training improvement are initial fitness level; frequency, intensity, and duration of exercise; and type (mode) of training. Of these, intensity is most crucial.

6. Training intensity can be applied either on an absolute basis in terms of exercise load or relative to a person's physiologic response. It is practical and effective to set exercise intensity to a percent of a person's HRmax. Training levels that correspond to between 70 and 90% of HRmax are most desirable for inducing aerobic fitness changes.

7. Training duration and intensity are intimately related in their effects on training response. Generally, 30-minute exercise sessions are practical and effective for exercise duration. Extending the duration can compensate somewhat for a reduced exercise intensity.

8. The minimum frequency for aerobic training is probably about 2 to 3 days per week. Optimal frequency levels have not been established.

9. If intensity, duration, and frequency are held constant, training improvements are similar, regardless of training mode, as long as large muscle groups are exercised and evaluated in the training activity.

10. The frequency and duration of training required to maintain an improved level of aerobic fitness is much less than that required to improve it. Even small decreases in exercise intensity, however, cause a loss in $\dot{V}O_2$max.

11. Interval, continuous, and fartlek training can effectively improve the capacity of the different systems of energy transfer. Interval training seems to be most desirable for improving the immediate and short-term anaerobic energy systems.
12. Aerobic training must be geared to enhancing both cardiovascular function and metabolic capacity of the specific muscles. Peripheral adaptations in muscle may profoundly enhance endurance performance.
13. Heavy and prolonged endurance training can lead to the syndrome of overtraining, or staleness. This syndrome is associated with chronic fatigue, poor exercise performance, frequent infections, and a general loss of interest in training. These symptoms generally persist until the athlete takes adequate time off from training, possibly several days to months.

■ REFERENCES ■

1. American College of Sports Medicine: *Guidelines for Exercise, Testing and Prescription*. 4th ed., Philadelphia, Lea & Febiger, 1991.
2. Åstrand, P.O., and Rodahl, K.: *Textbook of Work Physiology*. 3rd ed., New York, McGraw-Hill, 1986.
3. Belman, M.J., and Gaesser, G.A.: Exercise training below and above the lactate threshold in the elderly. *Med. Sci. Sports Exerc.*, 23:562, 1991.
4. Blair, S.N., et al.: Physical fitness and all-cause mortality: a prospective study of healthy men and women. *JAMA*, 262:2395, 1989.
5. Borg, G.A.: Psychological basis of physical exertion. *Med. Sci. Sports Exerc.*, 14:377, 1982.
6. Bouchard, C., et al.: Long-term exercise training with constant energy intake. I: Effect on body composition and selected metabolic variables. *Int. J. Obesity*, 14:57, 1990.
7. Brahler, C.J., and Blank, S.E.: VersaClimbing elicits higher V̇o₂max than does treadmill running or rowing ergometry. *Med. Sci. Sports Exerc.*, 27:249, 1995.
8. Brodahl, P., et al.: Capillary supply of skeletal muscle fibers in untrained and endurance-trained men. *Am J. Physiol.*, 232:705, 1977.
9. Caine, D.J., and Lindner, D.J.: Growth plate injury: a threat to young distance runners. *Phys. Sportsmed.*, 12:119, 1984.
10. Chi, M.-Y., et al.: Effects of detraining on enzymes of energy metabolism in individual human muscle fibers. *Am. J. Physiol.*, 244 (Cell Physiol. 13):276, 1983.
11. Coggan, A.R., et al.: Skeletal muscle adaptations to endurance training in 60- to 70-yr-old men and women. *J. Appl. Physiol.*, 72:1780, 1992.
12. Coggan, A.R., et al.: Isotopic estimation of CO₂ production during exercise before and after endurance training. *J. Appl. Physiol.*, 75:70, 1993.
12a. Coggan, A.R., et al.: Glucose kinetics during high-intensity exercise in endurance-trained and untrained humans. *J. Appl. Physiol.*, 78:1203, 1995.
13. Convertino, V.A.: Blood volume: its adaptation to endurance training. *Med. Sci. Sports Exerc.*, 23:1338, 1991.
14. Costill, D.L., et al.: Adaptations to swimming training: influence of training volume. *Med. Sci. Sports Exerc.*, 23:371, 1991.
15. Coyle, E.F., et al.: Time course of loss of adaptations after stopping prolonged intense endurance training. *J. Appl. Physiol.*, 57:1857, 1984.
16. Daniels, J., and Scardinia, N.: Interval training and performance. *Sports Med.*, 1:327, 1984.
17. Davies, C.T.M., and Knibbs, A.V.: The training stimulus: the effects of intensity, duration and frequency of effort on maximum aerobic power output. *Int. Z. Angew. Physiol.*, 29:299, 1971.
18. Dishman, R.K.: Prescribing exercise intensity for healthy adults using perceived exertion. *Med. Sci. Sports Exerc.*, 26:1087, 1994.
19. Donovan, C.M., and Brooks, G.A.: Endurance training affects lactate clearance, not lactate production. *Am. J. Physiol.*, 244 (Endocrinol. Metab. 7):83, 1983.
20. Duncan, J.J., et al.: Women walking for health and fitness: how much is enough? *JAMA*, 266:3295, 1992.
21. Ehsani, A.A., et al.: Exercise training improves left ventricular systolic function in older men. *Circulation*, 83:96, 1991.
22. Fouriner, M., et al.: Skeletal muscle adaptation in adolescent boys: sprint and endurance training and detraining. *Med. Sci. Sports Exerc.*, 14:453, 1982.
23. Fox, E.L., et al.: Intensity and distance of interval training programs and changes in aerobic power. *Med. Sci. Sports*, 5:18, 1973.
24. Fox, E.L., et al.: Frequency and duration of interval training programs and changes in aerobic power. *J. Appl. Physiol.*, 38:481, 1975.
25. Franklin, B.A.: Aerobic exercise training programs for the upper body. *Med. Sci. Sports Exerc.*, 21:S141, 1989.
26. Gaesser, G.A., and Rich, G.A.: Effects of high- and low-intensity exercises on aerobic capacity and blood lipids. *Med. Sci. Sports Exerc.*, 16:269, 1984.
27. Gergley, T.J., et al.: Specificity of arm training on aerobic power during swimming and running. *Med. Sci. Sports Exerc.*, 16:349, 1984.
28. Gillespie, A.C.: Enzyme adaptations in rat skeletal muscle after two intensities of treadmill training. *Med. Sci. Sports Exerc.*, 14:461, 1982.
29. Gollnick, P., and Hermansen, L.: Biochemical adaptation to exercise: anaerobic metabolism. In *Exercise and Sport Sciences Reviews*. Vol. 1., J. Wilmore (Ed.), New York, Academic Press, 1973.
30. Gollnick, P., et al.: Enzyme activity and fiber composition in skeletal muscle of untrained men. *J. Appl. Physiol.*, 33:312, 1972.
31. Gollnick, P., et al.: Effects of training on enzyme activity and fiber composition of human skeletal muscle. *J. Appl. Physiol.*, 34:107, 1973.
32. Gregg, S.G., et al.: Interactive effects of anemia and muscle oxidative capacity on exercise endurance. *J. Appl. Physiol.*, 67:765, 1989.
33. Hagberg, J.M.: Physiologic adaptations to prolonged high-intensity exercise training in patients with coronary artery disease, *Med. Sci. Sports Exerc.*, 23:661, 1991.
34. Hellerstein, H.K., and Franklin, B.A.: Exercise testing and prescription. In *Rehabilitation of the Coronary Patient*. N.K. Wenger and H.K. Hellerstein (Eds.), New York, Wiley, 1978.
35. Hermansen, L.: Lactate production during exercise. In *Muscle Metabolism During Exercise*. B. Pernow and B. Saltin (Eds.), New York, Plenum Press, 1971.
36. Hickson, R.C.: Interference of strength development by simultaneously training for strength and endurance. *Eur. J. Appl. Physiol.*, 45:255, 1980.
37. Hickson, R.C., and Rosenkoetter, M.A.: Reduced training frequencies and maintenance of aerobic power. *Med. Sci. Sports Exerc.*, 13:13, 1981.
38. Hickson, R.C., et al.: Linear increases in aerobic power induced by a strenuous program of endurance exercise. *J. Appl. Physiol.*, 42:373, 1977.
39. Hickson, R.C., et al.: Time course of the adaptive responses of aerobic power and heart rate to training. *Med. Sci. Sports Exerc.*, 13:17, 1981.
40. Hickson, R.C., et al.: Reduced training duration effects on aerobic power, endurance, and cardiac growth. *J. Appl. Physiol.*, 53:255, 1982.
41. Hickson, R.C., et al.: Reduced training intensities and loss of aerobic power, endurance, and cardiac growth. *J. Appl. Physiol.*, 58:492, 1985.
42. Holloszy, J.O.: Metabolic consequences of endurance exercise training. In *Exercise, Nutrition, and Energy Metabolism*. E.S. Horton, and R.L. Terjung (Eds.), New York, Macmillan, 1988.

43. Holloszy, J.O., and Coyle, E.F.: Adaptations of skeletal muscle to endurance exercise and their metabolic consequences. *J. Appl. Physiol.*, 56:831, 1984.

44. Hooker, S.P., et al.: Oxygen uptake and heart rate relationship in persons with spinal cord injury. *Med. Sci. Sports Exerc.*, 25:1115, 1993.

45. Hooper, S.L., et al.: Markers for monitoring overtraining and recovery. *Med. Sci. Sports Exerc.*, 27:106, 1995.

46. Hurley, B.F., et al.: Effects of high intensity strength training on cardiovascular function. *Med. Sci. Sports Exerc.*, 16:483, 1984.

47. Jacobs, I.: Sprint training effects on muscle myoglobin, enzymes, fiber types, and blood lactate. *Med. Sci. Sports Exerc.*, 19:368, 1987.

48. James, F., et al.: Responses of normal children and young adults to controlled bicycle exercise. *Circulation*, 61:902, 1980.

49. Jones, B.H., et al.: Epidemiology of injuries associated with physical training among young men in the army. *Med. Sci. Sports Exerc.*, 25:197, 1993.

50. Joyner, M.J.: Physiological limiting factors and distance running: influence of gender and age on record performances. *Exerc. Sport Sci. Rev.*, 21:103, 1993.

51. Karvonen, M.J., et al.: The effects of training on heart rate. A longitudinal study. *Ann. Med. Exp. Biol. Fenn.*, 35:305, 1957.

52. Kavanagh, T., et al.: Characteristics of postcoronary marathon runners. *Ann. N.Y. Acad. Sci.*, 301:455, 1977.

53. Klausen, K., et al.: Adaptative changes in work capacity, skeletal muscle capillarization, and enzyme levels during training and detraining. *Acta Physiol. Scand.*, 113:9, 1981.

54. Kohrt, W.M., et al.: Longitudinal assessment of responses of triathletes to swimming, cycling, and running. *Med. Sci. Sports Exerc.*, 21:569, 1989.

54a. Koplan, J.P., et al.: The natural history of exercise: a 10-yr follow-up of a cohort of runners. *Med. Sci. Sports Exerc.*, 27:1180, 1995.

55. Lakatta, E.G.: Cardiovascular regulatory mechanisms in advanced age. *Physiol. Rev.*, 73:413, 1993.

56. Landers, D.M., and Petruzzewllo, S.J.: Physical activity, fitness, and anxiety. In *Physical Activity, Fitness, and Health*. Bouchard, C., et al. (Eds.), Champaign, Ill., Human Kinetics, 1994.

57. Lash, J.M., et al.: Exercise training effects on collaterol and microvascular resistance in rat model of arterial insufficiency. *Am. J. Physiol.*, 28:H125, 1995.

58. Lehmann, M., et al.: Overtraining in endurance athletes: a brief review. *Med. Sci. Sports Exerc.*, 25:854, 1993.

59. Loftin, M., et al.: Effect of arm training on central and peripheral circulatory function. *Med. Sci. Sports Exerc.*, 20:136, 1988.

60. Londeree, B.R., and Moeschberger, M.L.: Effect of age and other factors on maximal heart rate. *Res. Q. Exerc. Sport*, 53:297, 1982.

61. Londeree, B.R., et al.: %VO_{2max} regressions for six modes of exercise. *Med. Sci. Sports Exerc.*, 458, 1995.

62. Loy, S.F., et al.: Effects of stairclimbing on $\dot{V}O_2$max and quadriceps strength in middle-aged females. *Med. Sci. Sports Exerc.*, 26:241, 1994.

63. Luetkemeier, M.J., and Thomas, E.L.: Hypervolemia and cycling time trial performance. *Med. Sci. Sports Exerc.*, 26:503, 1994.

64. MacDougall, J.D., et al.: Biochemical adaptation of human skeletal muscle to heavy resistance training and immobilization. *J. Appl. Physiol.*, 43:700, 1977.

65. Madsen, K., et al.: Effects of detraining on endurance capacity and metabolic changes during prolonged endurance exercise. *J. Appl. Physiol.*, 75:1444, 1993.

66. Magel, J.R., et al.: Specificity of swim training on maximum oxygen uptake. *J. Appl. Physiol.*, 38:151, 1975.

67. Magel, J.R., et al.: Metabolic and cardiovascular adjustment to arm training. *J. Appl. Physiol.*, 45:75, 1978.

68. Maughan, R.F.: Fluid and electrolyte loss and replacement in exercise. In *Foods, Nutrition and Sports Performance.*. Williams, C, and Devlin, J.T. (Eds.). London, E. & F. Spoon, 1992.

69. McArdle, W.D., et al.: Specificity of run training on VO_2max and heart rate changes during running and swimming. *Med. Sci. Sports*, 10:16, 1978.

70. McAuley E.: Physical activity and psychosocial outcomes. In *Physical Activity, Fitness, and Health*. Bouchard, C., et al. (Eds.). Champaign, IL, Human Kinetics, 1994.

71. Miller, W.C., et al.: Predicting max HR and HR-$\dot{V}O_2$ relationship for exercise prescription in obesity. *Med. Sci. Sports Exerc.*, 25:1077, 1993.

72. Minotti, J.R., et al.: Training-induced skeletal muscle adaptations are independent of systemic adaptations. *J. Appl. Physiol.*, 68:289, 1990.

73. Mitchell, J.H., and Raven, P.B.: Cardiovascular adaptation to physical activity. In *Physical Activity, Fitness, and Health*. Bouchard, C., et al. (Eds.). Champaign, IL, Human Kinetics, 1994.

74. Moffatt, R.: Placement of tri-weekly training sessions: importance regarding enhancement of aerobic capacity. *Res. Q.*, 48:583, 1977.

75. Montain, S.J., and Coyle, E.F.: Fluid ingestion during exercise increases skin blood flow independent of increases in blood volume. *J. Appl. Physiol.*, 73:903, 1992.

76. Murase, Y., et al.: Longitudinal study of aerobic power in superior junior athletes. *Med. Sci. Sports Exerc.*, 13:180, 1981.

77. Neufer, P.D., et al.: Effect of reduced training on muscular strength and endurance in competitive swimmers. *Med. Sci. Sports Exerc.*, 19:486, 1987.

78. Olson, M.S., et al.: The cardiovascular and metabolic effects of bench stepping exercise in females. *Med. Sci. Sports Exerc.*, 23:1311, 1991.

79. Pechar, G.S., et al.: Specificity of cardiorespiratory adaptation to bicycle and treadmill training. *J. Appl. Physiol.*, 36:753, 1974.

80. Pollock, M.L., et al.: Effects of mode of training on cardiovascular function and body composition of adult men. *Med. Sci. Sports*, 7:139, 1975.

81. Pollock, M.L., et al.: Effects of frequency and duration of training on attrition and incidence of injury. *Med. Sci. Sports*, 9:31, 1977.

82. Powell, K.E., et al.: An epidemiological perspective on the causes of running injuries. *Phys. Sportsmed.*, 14:100, 1986.

83. Riviere, D., et al.: Lipolytic response of fat cells to catecholamines in sedentary and exercise-trained women. *J. Appl. Physiol.*, 66:330, 1989.

84. Roca, J., et al.: Evidence for tissue diffusion limitation of VO_2max in normal humans. *J. Appl. Physiol.*, 67:291, 1989.

85. Rowell, L.B.: *Human Cardiovascular Control*. Cary, N.C., Oxford University Press, 1994.

86. Saltin, B., and Rowell, L.B.: Functional adaptations to physical activity and inactivity. *Fed. Proc.*, 39:1506, 1980.

87. Saltin, B., et al.: Response to exercise after bed rest and after training. *Circulation*, 38(Suppl. 7), 1968.

88. Seals, D.R., et al.: Endurance training in older men and women. I. Cardiovascular responses to exercise. *J. Appl. Physiol.*, 57:1024, 1984.

89. Seals, D.R., et al.: Endurance training in older men and women. II. Blood lactate response to submaximal exercise. *J. Appl. Physiol.*, 57:1030, 1984.

90. Seals, D.R., et al.: Exercise and aging: autonomic control of the circulation. *Med. Sci. Sports Exerc.*, 26:568, 1994.

91. Seip, R.L., et al.: Perceptual responses and blood lactate concentration: effect of training state. *Med. Sci. Sports Exerc.*, 23:80, 1991.

92. Sidney, K. H., et al.: *Training: Scientific Basis and Application*. Taylor, A.W. (Ed.). Springfield, IL, Charles C Thomas, 1972.

93. Spina, R.J., et al.: Exercise training improves left ventricular contractile response to β-adrenergic agonist. *J. Appl. Physiol.*, 72:307, 1992.

94. Stanish, W.D.: Overuse injuries in athletes; a perspective. *Med. Sci. Sports Exerc.*, 16:1, 1984.

95. Steed, J., et al.: Rating of perceived exertion and blood lactate concentration during submaximal running. *Med. Sci. Sports Exerc.*, 26:797, 1994.

96. Swain, D.P., et al.: Target heart rates for the development of cardiorespiratory fitness. *Med. Sci. Sports Exerc.*, 26:112, 1994.

97. Tanaka, K., et al.: Assessment of exercise-induced alterations in body composition of patients with coronary heart disease. *Eur. J. Appl. Physiol.*, 66:323, 1993.

98. Thompson, P.D., et al.: Cardiac dimensions and performance after either arm or leg endurance training. *Med. Sci. Sports Exerc.*, 13:303, 1981.

99. Thorstensson, A., et al.: Enzyme activities and muscle strength after sprint training in man. *Acta Physiol. Scand.*, 94:313, 1975.

100. Thorstensson, A., et al.: Effect of strengh training on enzyme activities and fiber characteristics in human skeletal muscle. *Acta Physiol. Scand.*, 96:392, 1976.

101. Vander, L.B., et al.: Cardiorespiratory responses to arm and leg ergometry in women. *Phys. Sportsmed.*, 12:101, 1984.

102. Wallick, M.E., et al.: Physiological responses to in-line skating compared to treadmill running. *Med. Sci. Sports Exerc.*, 27:242, 1995.

103. Wanger, P.D.: Muscle O_2 transport and O_2 dependent control of metabolism. *Med. Sci. Sports Exerc.*, 27:47, 1995.

104. Weltman, A., et al.: Exercise training at and above lactate threshold in previously untrained women. *Int. J. Sports Med.*, 13:257, 1992.

105. Wilmore, J., et al.: Physiological alterations consequent to 20-week conditioning programs of bicycling, tennis, and jogging. *Med. Sci. Sports*, 12:1, 1980.

106. Wilt, F.: Training for competitive running. In *Exercise Physiology*. Falls, H. (Ed.). New York, Academic Press, 1968.

DeLorme, T.L.: Restoration of muscle power by heavy-resistance exercises. *J. Bone Joint Surg.* **27:645, 1945.**

The accepted principle for muscle rehabilitation from injury prior to DeLorme's classic research involved low-resistance, high-repetition exercises (so-called "endurance-building" exercises). Examples included stationary cycling, lifting light sand-

Based on observations of 300 patients, the majority of whom required lower-extremity rehabilitation, DeLorme developed a new training "system" called "progressive resistance exercises" or PRE. Within the PRE system, DeLorme introduced the concepts of one-repetition maximum (1-RM strength) and 10-RM for setting and adjusting the increasing resistance, maximal sets and repetitions, and muscle training specificity. For rehabilitation, DeLorme recommended that patients perform 70 to 100 repetitions (7 to 10 sets of an exercise, 10 repetitions each set). Initially, PRE workouts began with a weight considerably less than 10-RM so subjects could complete the 10 repetitions during the final set. In this way, when the person achieved the 10-RM, total repetitions would equal 70 to 100. For example, if 10-RM for the first week equaled 20 lb, then beginning the first set with 2.5 lb and increasing 1.5 lb after each 10-repetition set would produce a total of 80 repetitions when performing the final 10-RM with 20 lb.

DeLorme advocated exercising once daily, 5 days per week, with workouts lasting no longer than 30 minutes. The patient exerted maximal power only once a week. Attainment of 1-RM required maximal weight lifted for one repetition. DeLorme believed that the exercises should be performed *"smoothly, rhythmically, and without haste, but not so slowly that the mere holding of the weight would tire the patient. Sudden motions should be avoided, and a momentary pause at the end of each repetition was advocated."*

Determination of the weekly 1-RM required continually adjusting the weight to progressively maintain 10-RM level during training. The figure illustrates the changes in one patient undergoing rehabilitation from a femur fracture. Note the 8% gain in thigh girth and the 40-lb (70%) increase in quadriceps muscle strength accomplished in 35 days.

The DeLorme paper was the first publication in the modern strength literature advocating the concept of training *"specificity."* DeLorme argued that power-building and endurance exercises *"were two entirely different types, each one producing its own results, and each being wholly incapable of producing the results obtained by the other."* Fifty years of subsequent research validated the specificity concept for strength improvement, including almost every claim made by DeLorme about the beneficial effects of PRE.

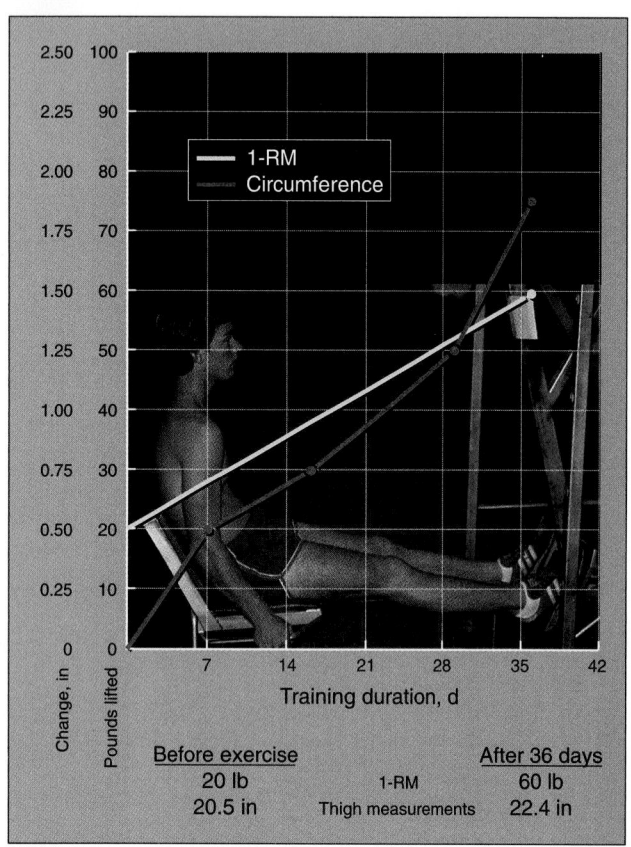

Before exercise		After 36 days
20 lb	1-RM	60 lb
20.5 in	Thigh measurements	22.4 in

Time course for 1-RM *(yellow line)* and changes in thigh girth *(red line)* for one subject during 35 days of progressive resistance exercises.

bags or weights by use of pulleys, and stair climbing. The prevailing theory to restore atrophied, weak, or "neglected" muscle relied on developing muscular endurance and not muscle strength and power. DeLorme challenged the classic concept by advocating heavy resistance exercise. He reasoned that a proportionality existed between the rate and extent of muscle hypertrophy and the load resisting muscle action. DeLorme predicted that a person's strength would return faster with heavy-resistance than with low-resistance exercise.

Muscular Strength: Training Muscles to Become Stronger

In America in the early 1840s, weightlifting began as a spectator sport, and was practiced by "strongmen" who showcased their prowess in traveling carnivals and sideshows. By the mid-1880s, measuring muscular strength became more comonplace, and as pointed out in the Introduction, the practice had found its way into the military during the Civil War for purposes of evaluation, and was used in physical education programs in many colleges and universities. In fact, in 1897 at a meeting of College Gymnasium Directors (Dr. D.A. Sargent, Chairman from Harvard University), strength test contests were established where at least 50 members of a college competed to determine overall body strength based on measures of back, leg, arm, and chest strength evaluated using several of the devices depicted in Figure 9 of the Introduction. (The first 5 colleges to rank in the 1898–1899 contest were Harvard, Columbia, Amherst, University of Minnesota, and Dickinson.) After the turn of the century, strength assessment became commonplace, and by the mid-1900s, "weightlifting" exercises were used predominantly by physical culture specialists, body builders, competitive weight lifters, field event athletes, and some wrestlers. Most other athletes, however, refrained from weightlifting for fear that such exercises would slow them down and increase muscle size to the point where they would lose joint flexibility and become **musclebound.** This myth was dispelled by subsequent research in the late 1950s and early 1960s that showed that muscle-strengthening exercises did not reduce movement speed or flexibility. The opposite was usually the case because elite weight lifters and body builders demonstrated exceptional joint flexibility and were certainly not limited in general movement speed. In longitudinal experiments with untrained healthy subjects, heavy-resistance exercises have increased both speed and power of muscular effort. Certainly, these effects would not be detrimental to sports performance.

In the sections that follow, we explore the underlying rationale of resistance training and the process and physiologic adjustments that occur as muscles are trained to become stronger. The discussion centers on various ways of measuring muscle strength, strength differences between men and women, and various resistance training programs to increase strength.

MEASUREMENT OF MUSCLE STRENGTH

Muscle strength, or, more precisely, *the maximum force or tension generated by a muscle (or muscle groups)*, is generally measured using one of four methods:

- Tensiometry
- Dynamometry
- One-repetition maximum, or 1-RM
- Computer-assisted force and power output determinations

CABLE TENSIOMETRY

Figure 22.1A shows a **cable tensiometer** and its use for measuring muscle force of the knee extensors. As the force on the cable increases, the riser over which the cable passes is depressed. This deflects the pointer and indicates the subject's strength score. This instrument measures the muscle force of a static, or isometric, muscle action, during which there is little or no change in the muscle's external length. This application of the tensiometer differs considerably from its original use in the early 1900s for measuring the tension of the steel cables linking the upper and lower wings of early airplanes.

The tensiometer is lightweight, portable, and easy to use and has the advantage of versatility for recording force measurements at virtually all angles in the range of motion (ROM) of a specific joint. Measurements of the static force of all the major muscle groups can be accomplished using cable tension strength-test batteries.[22, 23] These excellent tests evaluate strength impairment in muscles weakened from disease or injury. The muscle can be evaluated at a specific joint angle, which can be objectively reproduced on repeated measurements to determine the strength status prior to and following a resistance training program. Because more than one muscle group usually is activated in a particular movement, the tensiometer can be applied at many stages over the full movement. This method often gives a clearer picture of "strength" (or weakness) than relying solely on standard weightlifting tests.

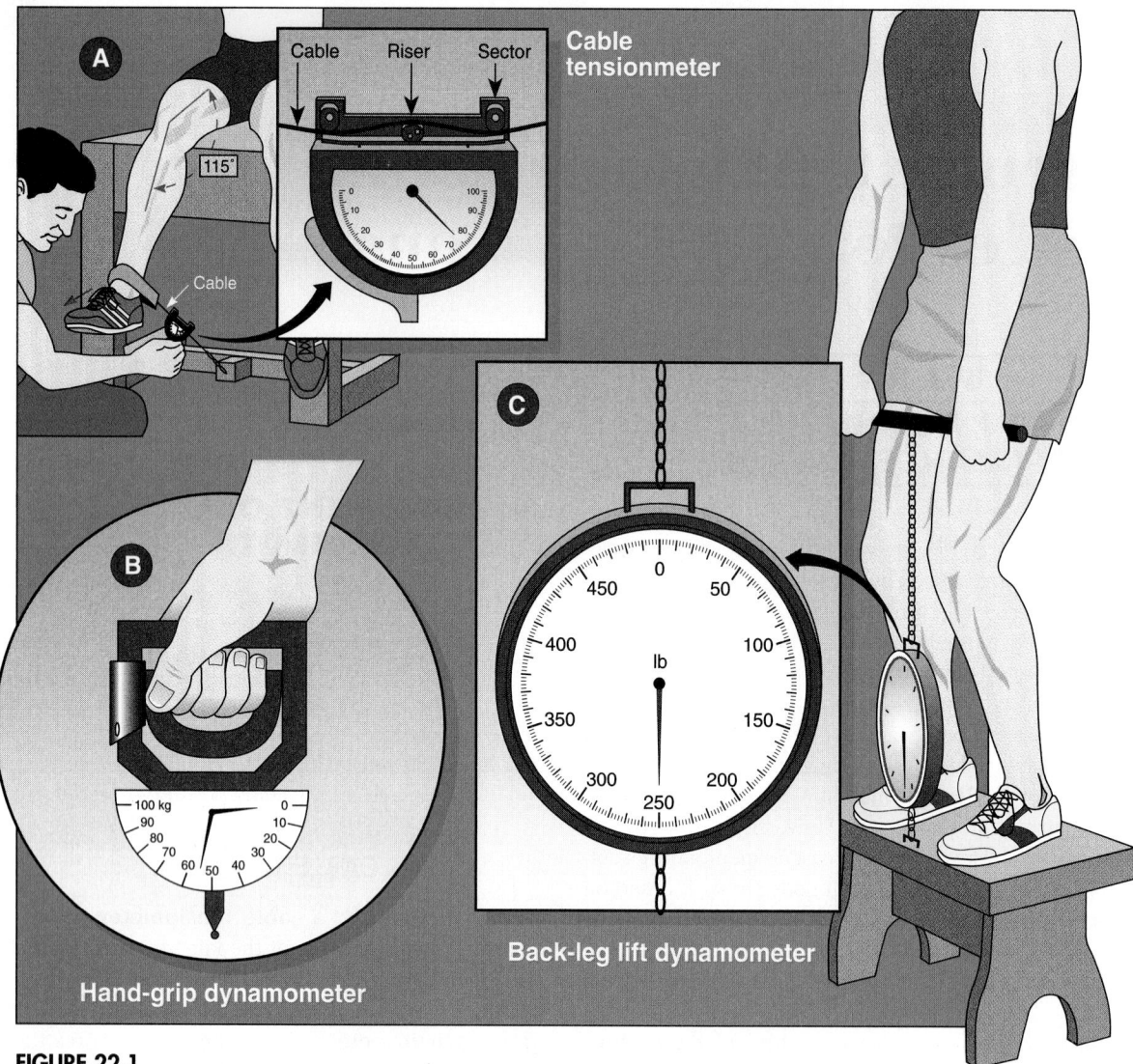

FIGURE 22.1
Measurement of static strength using (**A**) a cable tensiometer, (**B**) a hand-grip dynamometer, and (**C**) a back-leg lift dynamometer.

DYNAMOMETRY

Figures 22.1*B* and *C* illustrate hand-grip and back-lift **dynamometers** used for static strength measurement. Both devices operate on the principle of compression. An external force applied to the dynamometer compresses a steel spring and moves a pointer. Knowing the force required to move the pointer a particular distance, one can determine exactly how much external force has been applied to the dynamometer.

ONE-REPETITION MAXIMUM (1-RM)

A dynamic method for measuring muscular strength makes use of the **one-repetition maximum,** or **1-RM,** method. The 1-RM refers to the maximum amount of weight lifted **one time** with correct form during a standard weightlifting exercise. To test 1-RM for any particular muscle group, a suitable starting weight is selected close to, but below, the person's maximum lifting capacity. If one repetition is completed, weight is added to the exercise device until the maximum lift capacity is achieved. Depending on the muscle group evaluated, the weight increments usually range between 1 and 5 kg. Suitable rest intervals ranging from 1 to 5 minutes usually are sufficient before attempting a lift at the next heavier weight.

Estimate the 1-RM. Because it may be undesirable or impractical to perform an actual 1-RM measure with certain populations such as preadolescents, the elderly, hypertensives, or cardiac patients, the 1-RM can be estimated with submaximal effort by using one of the two equations shown below. Equations are given for both untrained and trained subjects because resistance training alters the relationship between a submaximal performance (7- to 10-RM) and a maximal performance (1-RM). Generally, the weight that can be lifted for a 7- to 10-RM represents about 68% of the 1-RM score for the untrained person and about 79% of the new 1-RM score after training.[14]

Untrained:

1-RM, kg = 1.554 (7- to 10-RM weight, kg) − 5.181

Trained:

1-RM, kg = 1.172 (7- to 10-RM weight, kg) + 7.704

COMPUTER-ASSISTED, ELECTROMECHANICAL, AND ISOKINETIC METHODS

Microprocessor technology makes it possible to rapidly quantify the forces, torques, and accelerations and velocities of body segments in various movement patterns. Force platforms can measure the external application of muscle force by a limb as in jumping. Other electromechanical devices measure the forces generated during all phases of an exercise movement, such as in cycling, or during movements that primarily utilize the arms (supine bench press) or legs (leg press).[69]

An **isokinetic dynamometer** is an electromechanical accommodating resistance instrument containing a speed-controlling mechanism that accelerates to a preset constant velocity only when force is applied. Once this speed is attained, the isokinetic loading mechanism adjusts automatically to provide a counterforce to the variations in force generated by the muscle as movement continues throughout the "strength curve." *Thus, maximum force (or any percentage of maximum effort) can be applied during all phases of the movement at a preestablished velocity of limb movement.* This allows training to be performed under either high-velocity (low-resistance) or low-velocity (high-resistance) conditions. A load cell within the dynamometer continuously monitors the immediate level of applied force (and matching resistance). An electronic integrator placed in series with a recorder (or monitor) provides a read-out of the average or peak force generated during any time period. The voltage output from the integrator can be interfaced directly with a computer to provide almost instantaneous read-outs of whatever performance score—for example, force, torque, or work—is desired.

The interface of computer technology with mechanical devices provides the exercise scientist with valuable data for evaluating, testing, and training muscles. This technology, however, is not accepted universally by many who still consider a maximum lift (1-RM) the best criterion of overall muscular strength. The counter-argument of such an assumption is that the dynamics of muscle strength involve considerably more than just the final outcome of a 1-RM. Even if two people have a 1-RM score of 100 kg, for example, the force-time curves could be quite dissimilar. Such differences in force dynamics (such as time to peak tension) may reflect an entirely different underlying neuromuscular physiology. Figure 22.2 illustrates the differences in results from conventional 1-RM testing (*top*), where the force score represents the total amount of weight lifted, and testing using a force curve (*bottom*) obtained from a microprocessor-controlled resistance device, where the magnitude of the force applied is presented in relation to the duration of force application. Table 22.1 lists the units of measurement for various expressions of muscular performance during linear and angular motions.

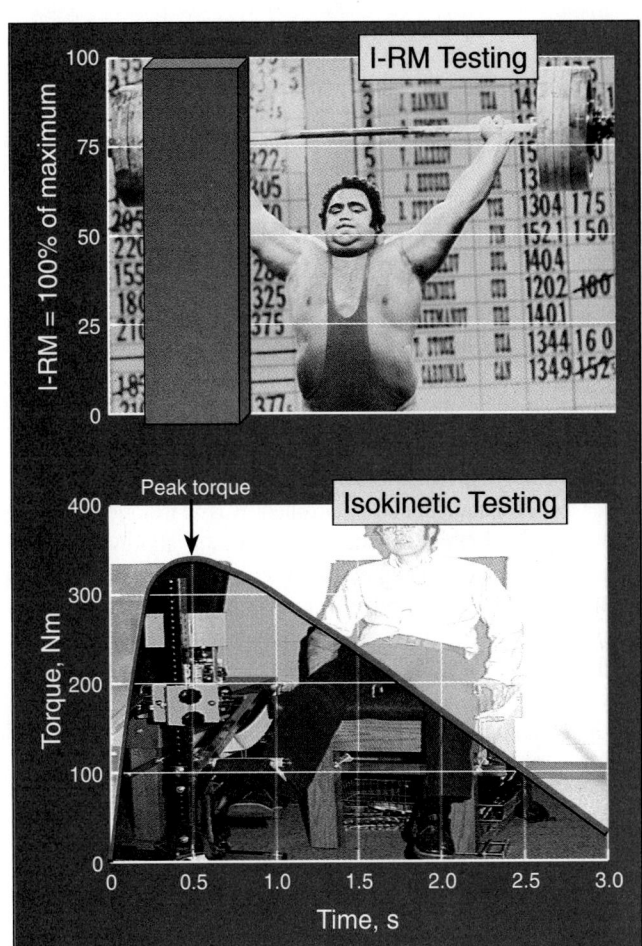

FIGURE 22.2

Top, Conventional 1-RM testing. The greatest weight lifted constitutes the 1-RM. If 106 kg constitutes the maximum weight lifted, then 106 kg equals the 1-RM. *Bottom,* Force curve obtained during an isokinetic test performed at an angular velocity of $30° \cdot s^{-1}$ over a 3-second time interval. Peak torque in this example equals 342 N · m. Average torque is computed as the force-time integral or impulse divided by time. In this example, impulse equals 602 N · m · s^{-1} and average torque equals 200.7 N · m. Work equals the product of average torque × distance moved (90° or 1.57 radians). Using the data for average torque and distance, work equals 174 N · m × 157 radians = 273 N · m, or 273 joules (J). Power is calculated as work per unit time, or 273 J ÷ 3.0 s = 91 W.

TABLE 22.1
INTERNATIONAL SYSTEM OF UNITS (SI) FOR VARIOUS EXPRESSIONS OF MUSCULAR STRENGTH AND POWER DURING LINEAR AND ANGULAR MOTIONS[a]

Linear Motion		*Angular Motion*	
Quantity	*Unit*	*Quantity*	*Unit*
Force	Newton, N	Torque, T	Newton meter, N · m
Velocity, v	Meters per second, m · s^{-1}	Velocity, w	Radians per second, rad · s^{-1}
Mass	Kilogram, kg	Moment of inertia, I or J	Kilogram meter squared, kg · m^2
Acceleration, a	Meters per second squared, m · s^{-2}	Acceleration, a	Radians per second squared, rad · s^{-2}
Displacement, d	Meter, m	Displacement, θ	Radian, rad
Time, t	Second, s	Time, t	Second, s

[a]Appendix A provides additional information about SI units, including interconversions

CATEGORIES OF RESISTANCE TRAINING EQUIPMENT

There are currently three categories of resistance exercise equipment used to train muscles. The first category includes the more standard-type weightlifting equipment such as free weights and barbells, which control for neither speed of movement nor level of resistance through the full ROM. Within the second category, two subdivisions exist: one subdivision provides for a constant speed, controlled by true isokinetic equipment, and variable resistance; the other subdivision also provides for a constant speed and variable resistance by means of a hydraulic device, but the individual controls the movement speed. In the third category, movement speed is variable and resistance is constant; this category includes some cam devices and concentric-eccentric devices. There currently is no machine whereby muscles exert force under conditions of true constant speed and true constant resistance.

STRENGTH TESTING CONSIDERATIONS

The following considerations are important when individuals are tested for muscle strength, whether by cable tensiometry, dynamometry, 1-RM, or computer-assisted methods. It is essential that all subjects be tested under the same conditions so that fair comparisons can be made among them.

- Give standardized instructions prior to testing.
- If a warm-up is given, ensure that it is of uniform duration and intensity.
- Provide the subject with adequate practice prior to the actual test to minimize a "learning" component that could compromise initial results. (This topic is discussed following this section.)
- Take care to ensure that the angle of measurement on the limb or the test device is consistent among subjects.

- Determine a minimum number of trials (repetitions) beforehand to establish a criterion score. For example, if five repetitions of a test are administered, what score should be used as the individual's strength score? Is the highest score best, or should an average be used? There is no clear answer on this point, which depends on the nature of the test. In most cases, however, an average of several trials will provide a more representative score of a person's strength or power performance than a single trial. Stated another way, a single score is usually less reliable (reproducible) than an average of several scores. Researchers have reported high test-retest reliability in repeated measurements of maximal effort muscle actions when administering multiple repetitions of bench press and squat 1-RM and bidirectional hydraulic exercise on the same and different days.[68, 93]
- Select tests known for having high score reproducibility. This is a crucial aspect of testing but often overlooked. If a test is developed without determining the variability of the subject's responses, the resultant test scores may not truly reflect an individual's performance (or change in performance when evaluating a strength-improvement protocol). Unreliability of measurement per se can mask the individual's true performance on the test.
- Be prepared to consider individual differences in such factors as body size and composition when evaluating strength scores between individuals and groups. For example, is it fair to compare the "strength" of a 120-kg defensive lineman with the "strength" of a 62-kg distance runner? Unfortunately, there is no clear-cut answer to this dilemma, but in the next section, we do present some alternatives.

Learning Factors in Assessing Muscular Strength

In Chapter 19, we emphasized that the initial gains in muscular strength could be attributed in large measure to neural factors instead of muscular hypertrophy or hyperplasia. Figure 22.3 presents repetition-by-repetition performance improvements in maximal effort (1-RM) muscle actions at an angular velocity of $5° \cdot s^{-1}$ during a supine bench press and standing squat. One-RM was measured with a single maximal effort using a computerized dynamometer. The amount of improvement averaged 11.4% between 1-RM attempt 1 and 5 and 2.1% between the last two attempts. The improvement in performance between the last two 1-RMs was not statistically significant (it was significant between 1-RMs 1, 2, and 3 versus 1-RMs 4 and 5). This means that at least three attempts are required before a plateau can be achieved in the 1-RM score. The results were unchanged with 3-, 4-, or 5-minute rest intervals between maximal attempts. This is consistent with research showing that only 1-minute intervals between 1-RM lifts were satisfactory for achieving the maximum lift.[169]

The important point is that had only one or two attempts been used to represent the 1-RM, then the "true" 1-RM would have been underestimated by as much as 11%. If the 1-RM testing preceded a 15-week strength-development program, then gains in strength attributable to strength training really would have included the 11% strength improvement resulting only from testing! If only two attempts had been given to assess 1-RM on the pretest, then the two trials on the post-test would have in reality been equivalent to attempts 3 and 4 of the pretest, had they been administered.

SEX DIFFERENCES IN MUSCLE STRENGTH

Several approaches have been used to determine whether true "sex differences" exist in muscle strength. Strength has been evaluated (*a*) in relation to the muscle's cross-sectional area, (*b*) on an absolute basis as total force exerted, and (*c*) as relative strength in relation to body mass or fat-free body mass.

STRENGTH IN RELATION TO MUSCLE CROSS SECTION

Human skeletal muscle can generate approximately 16 to 30 newtons (N) of force per square centimeter of muscle cross section regardless of sex. *In the body, however, this force-output capacity varies depending on the arrangement of the bony levers and muscle architecture* (refer to Chapter 18). If a value of 30 N is used as the specific amount to represent force capacity per square centimeter of muscle tissue, then a muscle with a cross-sectional area of 5.0 cm² would be able to develop a maximal force of 150 N. If all of the muscles in the body were to be maximally activated at the same time (and the force generated applied in the same direction), the resulting force would equal 168 kN. This estimation is based on an assumed muscle total cross section of 0.56 m².[38]

Figure 22.4 presents a comparison of the arm flexor strength of men and women in relation to the muscle's cross-sectional area. Clearly, the greatest absolute force is exerted by individuals with the largest muscle cross sections. The linear relationship between strength and muscle size, however, indicates little difference in arm flexor strength for the same size muscle in men and women. This is further demonstrated in the insert graph, where the strength of men and women is expressed per unit area of muscle cross section.[77] The footnote on the bottom of page 422 discusses

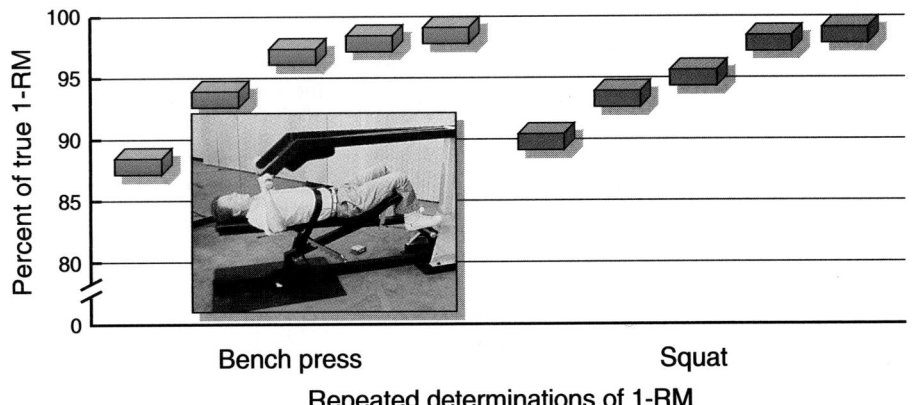

FIGURE 22.3

Five repeated determinations of 1-RM for the supine bench press and standing squat using an electromechanical dynamometer. The lever arm on the dynamometer connects to a potentiometer and force transducer with analog/digital (A/D) interface to a microcomputer for on-line data acquisition at an A/D sampling rate of 16,000 Hz. A monitor provides audio and visual feedback to the subject on range of motion and performance. Strong verbal encouragement was provided on each attempt. To avoid an excessive Valsalva maneuver, subjects exhaled immediately as they completed the movement. (Photo courtesy of Ariel Dynamics, Inc., San Diego, CA.)

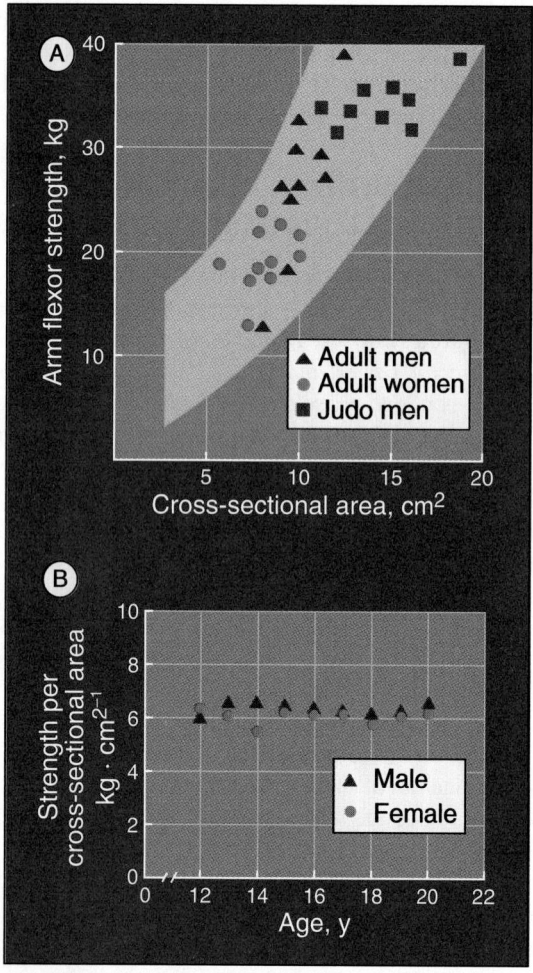

FIGURE 22.4

A, Variability of upper arm flexion strength of men and women in relation to the flexor muscle's cross-sectional area. **B,** Strength per unit muscle cross-sectional area in males and females aged 12 to 20 years. (From Ikai, M., and Fukunaga, T.: Calculation of muscle strength per unit cross-sectional area of human muscle by means of ultrasonic measurements. *Arbeitsphysiologie*, 26:26, 1968.)

the method for computing the muscle + bone cross-sectional area and volume of a limb based on anthropometric measures.[a]

ABSOLUTE MUSCLE STRENGTH

When strength is compared on an absolute score basis (that is, total force in pounds or kilograms), men are usually considerably stronger than women for all muscle groups tested. These strength differences are particularly apparent in comparisons of upper body strength, where women are about 50% weaker than men; in lower body strength, women are about 30% weaker.[62, 112] This sex characterization for strength is true regardless of the device used to measure strength and is generally attributed to the sex-related difference in the distribution of lean body mass.[19, 110] Exceptions are some strength-trained female track-and-field athletes and body builders who significantly increase the strength of specific muscle groups through resistance exercises.

Sex Differences in Weightlifting Championships

A unique set of data is available on sex differences in weightlifting, where men and women participate in the same weightlifting categories based on identical body mass. Figure 22.5 displays the percent differences in the maximal amount of weight lifted in the combined snatch and clean-and-jerk lifts during National Championship competition. In these comparisons, there is no "equating" or "adjusting" of performance scores based on sex differences in body composition. There are six weight categories ranging from 52 kg to 82.5 kg. In general, the smallest difference between men and women is noted in the lighter weight categories, with the sex effect most pronounced in the heavier weight category. Women of 75 and 82.5 kg body mass achieve only about 60% of the maximal weight lifted by their male counterparts. The differences in this comparison are more pronounced than in other experiments where men and women were initially matched for body composition.

RELATIVE MUSCLE STRENGTH

Traditionally, to compare the performance of different individuals, a ratio score is created by dividing the strength score by a reference measurement such as body mass, fat-free body mass, muscle cross section, limb volume, or girth. For example, when men and women are compared for strength using a ratio score based on body mass or fat-free body mass, the large absolute strength differences between sexes are reduced considerably, if not eliminated.[19, 175] Such findings support the argument that there are no differences in the "quality" of muscle between sexes and that the observed difference in absolute muscle strength is simply related to the quantity of muscle mass. Men and women did not differ significantly in either upper or lower body strength when sex differences were "corrected" using the traditional ratio method, which incorporates

[a]The muscle + bone cross-sectional area for the upper arm at the level of the biceps (MCSA-Bi) is calculated as π (r − [BiFF + TrFF]/4)^2, where r is the radius of the upper arm calculated from biceps girth, BiFF is biceps fatfold, and TrFF is triceps fatfold. Muscle + bone cross-sectional area for the lower limb at the thigh (MCSA-Thi) is estimated as π (r − [ThFF]/2)^2, where r is radius of the thigh and ThFF is thigh fatfold. The following equation is used to estimate the volume of a limb from girth measurements: volume = $\pi h/3$ (R^2/2π + r^2/2π + Rr), where h is the length of the upper arm or thigh in cm, R is the upper arm or thigh girth, and r is the elbow or knee girth. It also is possible to predict MCSA based on a regression equation validated by magnetic resonance imaging.[72] MCSA at the midthigh for the quadriceps in men = 1.99 (X$_1$) − 0.24 (X$_2$) − 34.4, where X$_1$ = midthigh girth (cm) and X$_2$ = thigh fatfold at the girth level.

lean body mass, local girth, and estimated local fat content.[62]

We must point out, however, that this statistical method of equating for sex differences in body size may not truly "equalize" women and men in terms of the underlying physiology. Ratio method scoring only presumes to eradicate apparent sex differences. As was the case for aerobic capacity discussed in Chapter 11, one fair way to evaluate sex differences in a criterion trait such as muscular strength (or aerobic capacity) is to compare men and women who do **not** differ in body size variables such as body mass or fat-free body mass or to control for these variables through appropriate statistical techniques. This method precludes the need to create a ratio score because the men and women are of equal body size and composition. With this approach, five measures of muscular strength were assessed for men and women using concentric (shortening) muscle actions for the bench press and squat (1-RM) and isokinetic dynamometry for assessing maximum force during knee flexion and extension and seated shoulder presses for men and women.[88] Figure 22.6 shows that when men and women were matched for body mass, the sex differences were larger in the sedentary group (44.0% for the shoulders and 25.1% for knee flexion) than in the trained group (33.0% for the bench press and 10.7% for knee flexion). The percentage differences were reduced (but not at all eliminated) for both groups when they were matched for fat-free body mass. The largest sex differences in the sedentary group resulted from the shoulder press (39.4%) and bench press (31.2%); the corresponding sex differences for the trained group were 30.6% (shoulder press) and 35.4% (bench press).

These results and those of other researchers[175] differ markedly from prior studies that have used the traditional approach of attempting to equate sexes by generating a ratio score to express strength performance. Ratio scores do support the argument that few sex differences exist in muscle quality, at least as reflected by force output capacity. In contrast, when men and women are matched before testing for body size and composition and training status, the results reveal that males are still "stronger," especially in measures of upper body strength, but also in lower body strength as assessed with a weight-stack simulated power clean lift.[116] In this study of military personnel (2,061 males, 1,301 females), mean lift capacity was 51% greater in males than females, even with a mathematical adjustment (regression, ratio, or exponential) in the strength score based on individual differences among subjects in fat-free body mass.

Allometric Scaling

Allometric scaling is a mathematical procedure for establishing a proper relationship between a body size variable (usually stature, body mass, or fat-free body mass) and some other variable of interest such as muscular strength, aerobic capacity, jumping height, or running speed. Allometric scaling is based on three assumptions: (a) the relationship is curvilinear between the two variables in question (for example, body mass and strength), (b) the slope of the relationship passes through the origin (someone with zero mass has no muscular strength), and (c) the form of the equation is $Y = bX^a$, where Y is the outcome variable (strength), X is the scaling variable (body mass), b is a constant multiplier, and a is a constant exponent. With allometric scaling, the object is to solve for the exponent a. When the value of a is known, then the new outcome variable no longer is influenced by individual differences in the scaling factor (in this case, body mass). Stated in another way, allometric scaling permits a variable of interest to be free of confounding effects that are inherently related to the variable in question. When the basic allometric scaling equation in (c) above is transformed into a log-linear model, it becomes possible to solve for the exponent a. This is done by taking the log of both sides of the equation in (c) and substituting values for the outcome variable (muscular strength) and body mass in kilograms. The equation is log strength = (a) log body mass + log(b). Linear regression then is applied to solve for the value of a by entering the log (strength) and log (body mass) into the regression. For muscular strength, the exponent b usually is 0.67, but the value may be slightly higher or lower depending on the particular data set. Recent

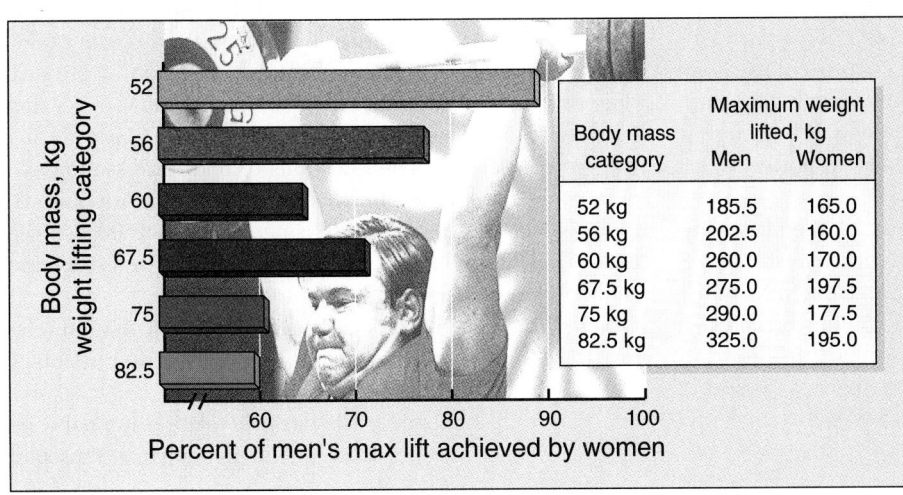

Body mass category	Maximum weight lifted, kg	
	Men	Women
52 kg	185.5	165.0
56 kg	202.5	160.0
60 kg	260.0	170.0
67.5 kg	275.0	197.5
75 kg	290.0	177.5
82.5 kg	325.0	195.0

FIGURE 22.5

World records in weightlifting between men and women in the same body mass categories. The insert presents the absolute weight lifted by the men and women for each body mass category. (Weightlifting data from U.S. Weightlifting Federation National Championships. Blaine, MN, April 26–28, 1991.)

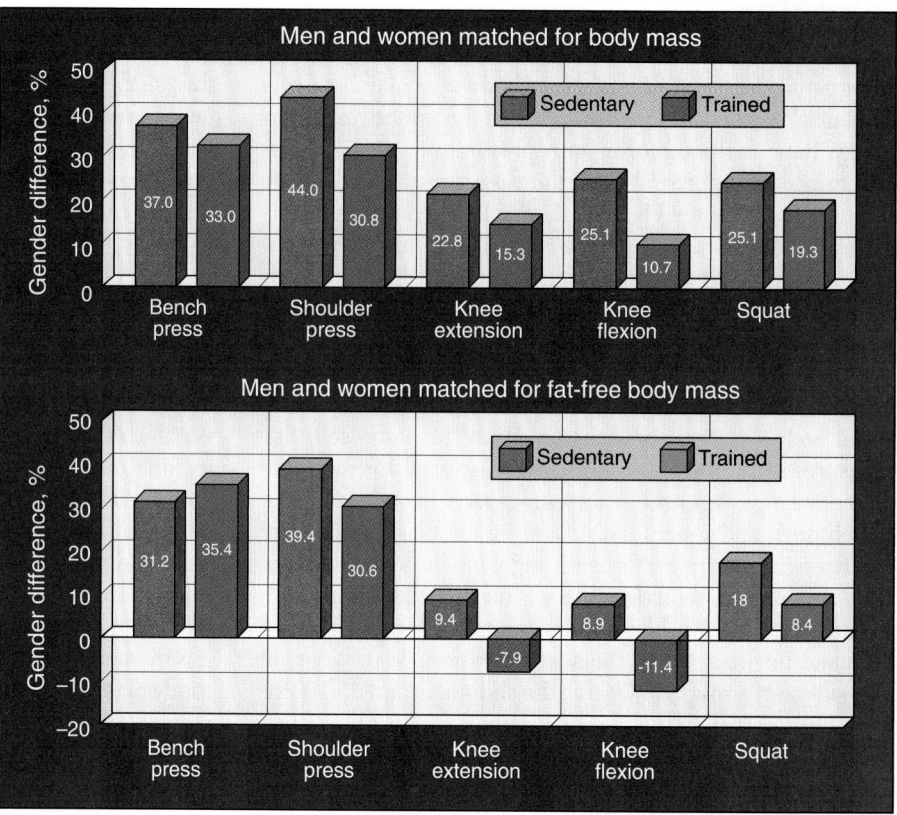

FIGURE 22.6

Men and women matched for body mass (*top*) and fat-free body mass (*bottom*) for five measures of muscle strength. Above the zero line is the percent that the values for men exceed the values for women. (Data courtesy of Keller, B.: The influence of body size variables on gender differences in strength and maximum aerobic capacity. Unpublished doctoral dissertation, University of Massachusetts, Amherst, 1989.)

data for grip strength of college-age men and women reported body mass$^{0.51}$ as the appropriate scaling factor, but this study did not scale by fat-free body mass that might have given a scaling value closer to body mass$^{0.67}$. *If the relationship were linear between muscular strength and body mass, the value of b would be 1.0, and it would be justifiable to express strength per unit body mass without a correction.* However, this is not the case, and muscular strength should instead be expressed per unit body mass raised to an appropriate exponent that has been determined for the particular data set.

Applying allometry to an outcome variable such as muscular strength permits comparisons among individuals or groups who exhibit large individual differences in a particular body size variable. As stated, this comparison is free of confounding effects that are inherently related to the variable in question. For example, how is one to compare or evaluate the maximum strength of two individuals who vary widely in body size? If one competitor weighs 100 kg and is 190 cm tall, and the other weighs 70 kg and is shorter by 12 cm (with strength scores of 125 kg for the taller, heavier person and 110 kg for the shorter, lighter person), then how can both individuals be "equated" in terms of muscular strength? An obvious approach is simply to divide the strength score by body mass, resulting in a ratio score of 1.250 for the heavier person (125 kg lifted ÷ 100 kg body mass) and 1.571 for the other competitor. In this system, the latter person would be deemed "stronger." In effect, the heavier person actually is penalized because the divisor in the ratio is a larger score.

But is this procedure really fair? This is further complicated because the difference in stature has not been considered (stature is strongly related to body mass); nor has the difference in total muscle mass (either fat-free body mass or lean body mass). If one is interested in knowing who is the strongest person, then the resulting outcome variable (in this example, muscular strength) must be properly scaled to remove the confounding influence of the body size variable.

Because the absolute strength of a muscle is related to its cross-sectional area, and because there usually are many muscles involved in generating the maximum force in a particular movement, is it better to express strength per unit cross-sectional area of the different muscles? Unfortunately, there is no simple answer either to this question or to the ones raised previously. More complications arise when exercise performance scores are potentially affected by physical dimensional characteristics between males and females and between individuals of different ages (particularly during the growth period). The questions of body size scaling and outcome variables have been considered by anthropologists, biologists, and other scientists since the mid-1600s, so the idea of scaling biological variables is steeped in history and is discussed in the contemporary literature.[7, 53, 128, 151, 160] Other studies also have dealt with allometric scaling in relation to variables commonly measured in exercise physiology studies.[11, 12, 85, 86, 113, 164, 165, 166, 174]

Figure 22.7 illustrates the intrinsic relationship between body mass and several different expressions of muscular

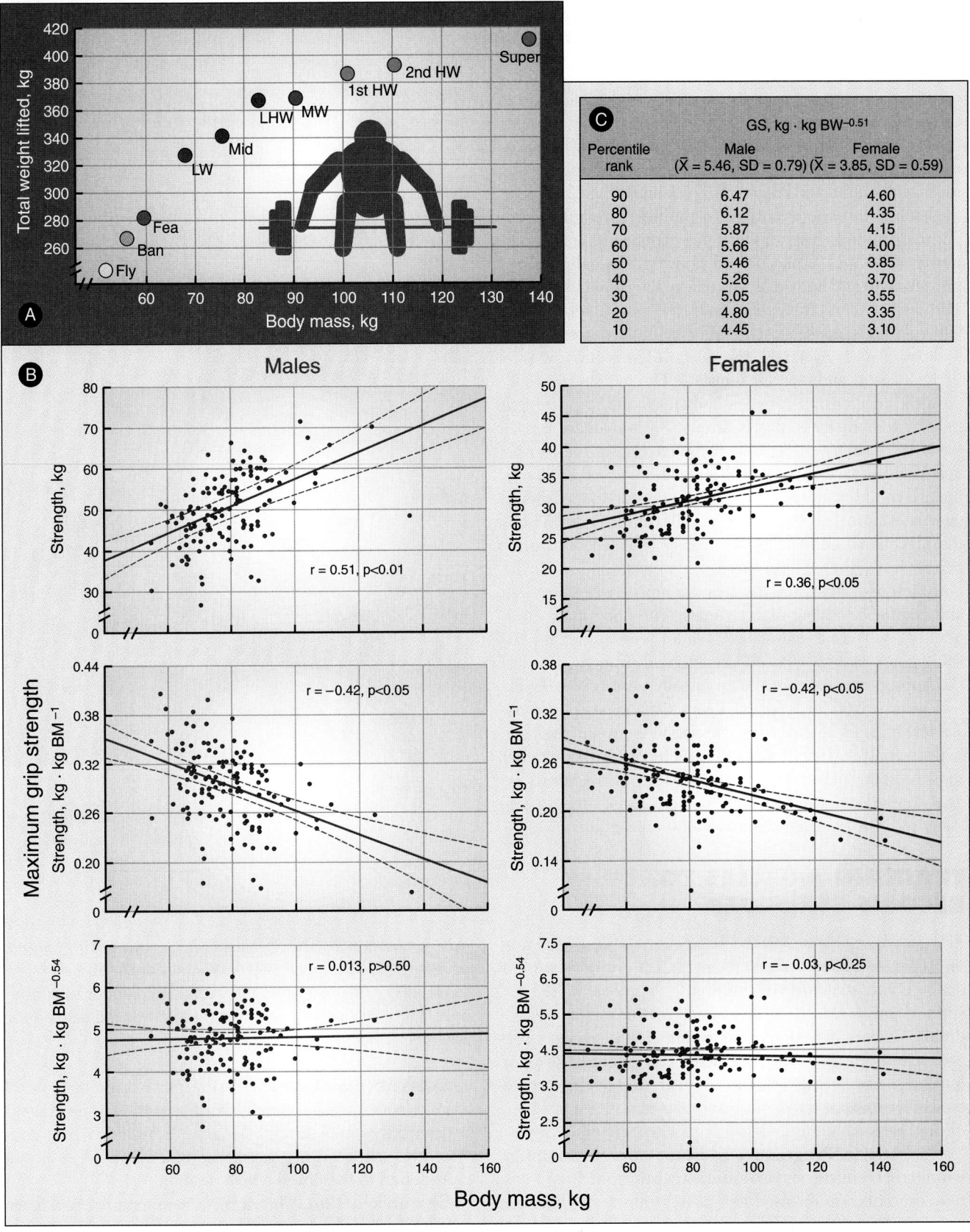

FIGURE 22.7

A, Total weight lifted in two events as a function of body mass in Olympic weight lifters (1980 Olympic Games). Each point represents the body mass of the top six weight lifters in each weight category. The various categories are as follows: *Fly,* flyweight; *Ban,* bantamweight; *Fea,* featherweight; *LW,* lightweight; *Mid,* middleweight; *LHW,* light-heavyweight; *MW,* middle-heavyweight; *1stHW,* 1st heavyweight; *2ndHW,* 2nd heavyweight; and *Super,* superheavyweight. (Modified from data of Lathan and cited by Titel, K., and Wutscherk, H.: *Strength and Power in Sport.* P.V. Komi (Ed.), Oxford, Blackwell Scientific Publications, 1993.) **B,** Maximal absolute grip strength, relative strength, and strength allometrically scaled in relation to body mass in 100 men and 105 women of college age. **C,** Percentile norms for grip strength. (Data from reference 166; courtesy of Dr. Paul Vanderburgh, Department of Exercise Science, University of Dayton, Dayton, OH.)

strength. The top curve plots the total weight lifted versus body mass for Olympic weight lifters. Each point represents the body mass of the top weight lifters in each body mass category. The important point is that the relationship between total weight lifted and body mass is not linear but curvilinear, thus supporting the idea that weightlifting strength is proportional to body mass raised to the exponent 0.7. The bottom three curves depict the relationship between maximal grip strength and body mass in college-age men and women. The first of these curves illustrates the simple relationship between body mass and strength without a correction for body size. As is expected, the relationship is positive ($r = 0.51$ for males and 0.33 for females). The middle curve depicts the relationship between body mass and grip strength indexed to body mass (that is, strength ÷ body mass, kg). In this case, dividing strength by body mass penalized heavier males and females ($r = -0.43$ for males and -0.38 for females). If body mass is not a confounding variable, it should correlate approximately zero ($r = 0.00$) with strength. This is the ideal situation because no penalty is levied on heavier people (who also might have a higher percent body fat). The bottom curve illustrates the relationship between strength and allometric scaling of body mass. The body mass exponent is $a = 0.54$ for males and 0.475 for females, and the resulting correlations between strength and strength raised to the appropriate exponent is essentially zero ($r = 0.08$ for males and -0.06 for females), thus satisfying one of the basic tenets of allometry: the correlation between the new scaled variable (strength) and the scaling factor (body mass) must be zero. The insert table presents percentile norms for grip strength adjusted to body mass$^{0.51}$ (grip strength per kilogram$^{0.51}$) for college-age males and females.

TRAINING MUSCLES TO BECOME STRONGER

As a general rule, a muscle worked close to its force-generating capacity will increase in strength. The overload can be applied with standard weightlifting equipment, pulleys or springs, immovable bars, or a variety of isokinetic and hydraulic devices. The important point is that strength improvements are generally governed by the intensity (level of tension placed on muscle) of overload and not by the specific type of exercise used to apply that overload. Certain methods of exercise lend themselves to a precise and systematic overload application. **Progressive resistance weight training, isometric training,** and **isokinetic training** are three common exercise systems used for training muscles to become stronger. These systems rely on the three types of muscle actions illustrated in Figure 22.8A to C.

DIFFERENT FORMS OF MUSCLE ACTION

Neural stimulation of a muscle causes the contractile elements to attempt to shorten along the cells' longitudinal

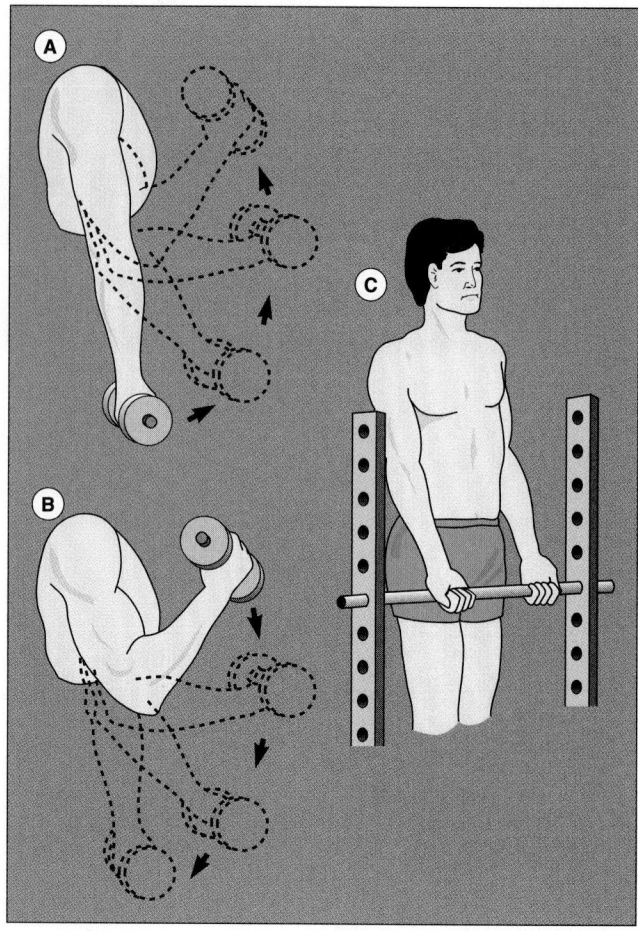

FIGURE 22.8
Muscle force generated during **(A)** concentric (shortening), **(B)** eccentric (lengthening), and **(C)** isometric (static) muscle actions.

axis. If there is no change in muscle length during muscle activation, the action is said to be isometric, or **static.** When movement of the skeleton takes place, the action is considered to be **dynamic.** Concentric and eccentric actions are two types of dynamic activity.

- **Concentric action.** This is the most common type of muscle action. The muscle shortens, and joint movement occurs as tension develops. Figure 22.8A illustrates a concentric action during the raising of a dumbbell from the extended to the flexed elbow position.
- **Eccentric action.** This occurs when external resistance exceeds muscle force and the muscle lengthens while developing tension, as illustrated in Figure 22.8B. The weight is slowly lowered against the force of gravity. The muscle fibers (more specifically, the sarcomeres) of the upper arm muscles lengthen in an eccentric action to prevent the weight from crashing to the floor. In weightlifting, muscles frequently act eccentrically as

the weight is returned slowly to the starting position to begin the next concentric (shortening) action. During this recovery phase of resistance exercise, eccentric muscle action can add significantly to the total work of the exercise repetition. *The combination of concentric and eccentric muscle actions augments the effectiveness of the exercise in terms of enhanced muscle strength and fiber size.*[35, 58, 117a, 177] Data also suggest that the strength gains with training are better preserved when training is discontinued if the overload training also includes eccentric muscle actions.[26]

- **Isometric action.** This occurs when a muscle generates force and attempts to shorten but cannot overcome the external resistance. As a result, no external work is performed. Considerable muscular force can be generated, however, during an isometric (static) action even though there is no noticeable lengthening or shortening of the muscle and no joint movement. Figure 22.8C illustrates an isometric muscle action.

Both concentric and eccentric muscle actions are commonly referred to as isotonic because in both cases, movement occurs. The term *isotonic* is derived from the Greek word *isotonos* (*iso* meaning the same or equal, *tonos* meaning tension or strain). Actually, this term is imprecise when applied to most dynamic muscle actions that involve movement because the muscle's effective force-generating capacity varies as the joint angle changes; thus, maximum force output is not uniform throughout the ROM.

RESISTANCE TRAINING FOR CHILDREN

Relatively little is known concerning the benefits and possible risks of resistance training in pre-adolescents. Because the skeletal system is in the formative stage for this age group, obvious concern arises as to the potential for injury (epiphyseal fractures, ruptured intervertebral discs, lower back bony disruptions) from heavy muscle overload in growing children. Furthermore, because a child's hormonal profile is still developing, especially for the tissue-building hormone testosterone, one might question whether resistance training could even induce significant strength improvements in children.

The available evidence indicates that closely supervised resistance training programs that employ concentric muscle actions with high repetitions and relatively low resistance can significantly improve the muscle strength of children with no adverse effect on bone, muscle, or connective tissue.[126, 138, 170] More than likely, these strength gains are primarily the result of the learning and enhancing of neuromuscular activation rather than an increase in muscle size.[118] Certainly, more studies are warranted before definitive statements can be made regarding the benefit-to-risk ratio and long-term effect on growth and development of regular and more stressful muscle overloads on children.

PROGRESSIVE RESISTANCE WEIGHT TRAINING

Probably the most popular form of resistance training involves weightlifting. With this method, exercises are designed to strengthen specific muscles by causing them to overcome a fixed resistance, usually in the form of a barbell, dumbbell, or weight plates on a pulley- or cam-type machine.

Progressive Resistance Exercise (PRE)

The technique of **progressive resistance exercise,** or **PRE,** is a practical application of the overload principle and forms the basis of most resistance training programs.

Working in a rehabilitation setting after World War II, researchers devised a method of weight training to improve the strength capacity of previously injured limbs[32] (see Focus on Research, p. 416). Their method involved three sets of exercises—each set consisting of 10 repetitions done consecutively without resting. The first set was done with one-half of the maximum weight that could be lifted 10 times, or ½ 10-RM; the second set was done with ¾ 10-RM, and the final 10-RM set was done with maximum weight. As patients trained, the exercised limbs became stronger, so it was necessary to increase periodically the 10-RM resistance to maintain continued strength improvements. Similar improvements occurred even when the progression of exercise intensity was reversed so that the 10-RM was performed as the first set.

Variations of PRE. Variations of PRE for weight training have been studied to determine the optimal number of sets and repetitions and the frequency and relative intensity of training required to improve muscular strength. The findings can be summarized generally as follows:

- Performing an exercise between 3-RM and 12-RM provides the most effective number of repetitions for increasing muscular strength.
- PRE training once weekly with 1-RM for one set increases strength significantly after week 1 of training and continues to increase strength each week thereafter up to at least week 6.
- No particular sequence of PRE training with different percentages of 10-RM is most effective for strength improvement, as long as one set of 10-RM is performed each training session.
- Performing one set of an exercise is less effective for increasing strength than performing two or three sets, and there is some indication that performing three sets is more effective than performing two sets.
- The optimum number of training days per week using PRE is unknown. Significant strength increases have occurred with as little as training 1 day weekly for beginners.
- When PRE training includes a variety of different exercises, training 4 or 5 days per week may be less effective than

FIGURE 22.9

Top, The periodization concept subdivides a macrocycle (usually a 1-year time period) into distinct phases or mesocycles. These, in turn, usually are separated into weekly microcycles. While modifications can be made to the general plan, the mesocycles usually include a preparation phase, a first transition phase, a competition phase, and a second transition, or recovery, phase. *Bottom,* Example of periodization for an elite athlete (discus thrower) preparing for top-level competition. Competitions were scheduled throughout the yearly training program, with the goal of achieving peak performance at the end of the macrocycle. A major objective in structuring the intensity, duration, and frequency of strength-power workouts is to avoid overtraining (staleness), minimize the potential for injury, and reduce the monotony of training, while achieving peak performance during competitions (represented as filled circles).

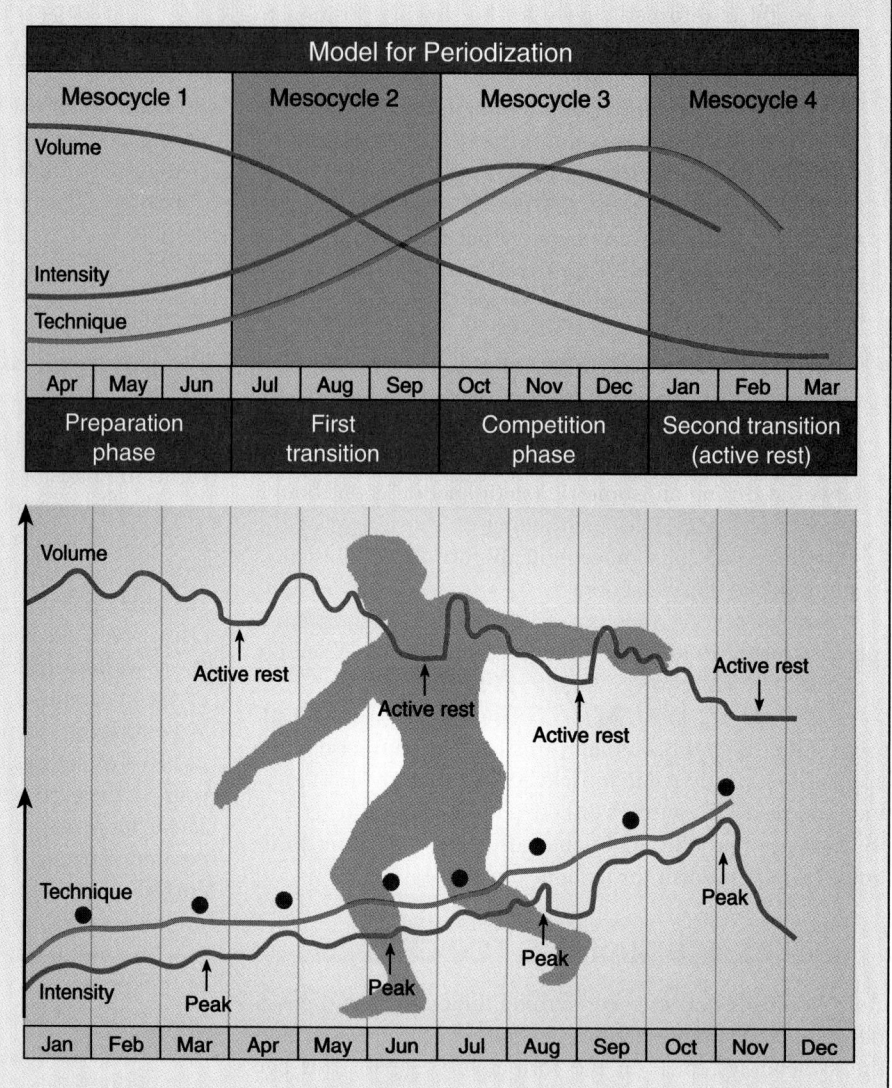

training 2 or 3 times per week. Daily training of the same muscle group may prevent sufficient recuperation between training sessions. This possibly could retard progress in neuromuscular adaptation and strength development.

• For a given resistance or load, a fast rate of movement may generate a better strength improvement than lifting at a slower rate. Furthermore, neither free weights (barbells, weight plates, or dumbbells) nor the diverse array of resistance exercise machines are inherently superior in terms of developing muscle strength.[59, 67]

Periodization. The concept of strength training periodization was first revealed in 1972 by a Russian scientist[108] and has been incorporated into the training regimens of both novice and champion athletes.[46, 136] The idea of periodization is to subdivide a specific resistance training period, such as a year (macrocycle), into smaller periods or phases (mesocycles), with each mesocycle again separated into weekly microcycles. The purpose of fractionating the macrocycle into

component parts is to manipulate training intensity, volume, frequency, sets, repetitions, and rest periods (to prevent overtraining) and alter the variety of workouts. It is hoped that this will reduce any negative effects from overtraining or "staleness" and culminate in "peak" performance at the time of competition.[167] The top part of Figure 22.9 depicts the basic design of periodization, and a typical mesocycle with four distinct phases. The goal of periodization as competition gets closer is to gradually decrease training volume while at the same time increasing training intensity.

• **Preparation phase.** Specific strength development is emphasized with *high-volume* (3 to 5 sets of 8 to 12 reps) and *low-intensity* workouts (50 to 80% of 1-RM plus flexibility and aerobic and anaerobic training).

• **First transition phase.** Specific strength development is emphasized with *moderate-volume* (3 to 5 sets of 5 to 6 reps) and *moderate-intensity* workouts (80 to 90% of 1-RM plus flexibility and interval aerobic training).

- **Competition phase.** Specific strength development is emphasized with *low-volume, high-intensity* workouts (3 to 5 sets of 2 to 4 reps at 90 to 95% of 1-RM), plus short periods of interval training that emphasize sport-specific exercises. During this phase, the participant peaks for competition.
- **Second transition phase (recuperation period).** This phase could emphasize recreational activities, low-intensity, nontaxing workouts incorporating different exercise modes. The periodization cycle can now be repeated in preparation for the next competition.

Periodization involves an inverse relation between training volume and training intensity through the competition phase, and then a decrease in both of these aspects during the second transition or recuperation period. Note the increase in the amount of time devoted to technique training as competition approaches, with training volume at the lowest point of the cycle.

The bottom part of Figure 22.9 shows how training volume and intensity can be varied within a mesocycle for an athlete engaging in a particular sport, in this case a discus thrower preparing for international competition. This example included eight competitions, and volume and intensity were varied throughout the macrocycle. Note the decrease in training intensity and volume during the transition or recovery cycles. Throughout the year of training, there also was considerable emphasis on sport skill and training techniques.

Generally, periodization is sport-specific; principles of training specificity are operative as coaches design the athlete's training based on the sport's particular strength, power, and endurance requirements. Also incorporated into the training is a detailed analysis of the metabolic and technical requirements of the sport. While the concept of periodization makes intuitive sense, and numerous studies have determined an optimum mix of training requirements, few if any studies can be considered "conclusive" because of difficulty in controlling for differences in training intensity, training volume, and participants' fitness capacities. Thus, as an alternative to evaluating the efficacy of particular macrocycles, shorter mesocycles have been evaluated to determine the best combination of training factors for optimizing improvements in particular aspects of performance. In one study, in which training volume and intensity were equated among three different approaches to periodization (linear periodization, undulating periodization, and a nonperiodized time interval), there were no significant differences in muscular strength (1-RM squat and bench press) or vertical jump following training.[8] The results indicated that each method of training was equally effective as reflected by approximately equal gains in strength (25% squat, 13.1% bench press) and power (7.6% vertical jump) among the groups. Had training volume and intensity not been equated, any significant differences could have favored one or more of the groups as reported in other studies.[117, 171]

Considerably more research is needed in the area of periodization, particularly as it relates to fitness status, sex, and sports preferences. Studies must equate and then manipulate different training loads and intensities and evaluate additional factors such as biomechanics and motor control in the actual sport skill, changes in segmental and whole-body composition, biochemical and ultrastructural tissue adaptations, and transfer of newly acquired strength to subsequent measures of performance.

Practical Recommendations for Initiating a Weight-Training Program

Maximum lifts should be avoided in the beginning stages of a weight-training program. Excessive resistance contributes little to strength development and greatly increases the chances of muscle or joint injury. *A load that is equal to 60 to 80% of a muscle's force-generating capacity is sufficient to increase strength.* Such a load generally permits the completion of about ten repetitions of a particular exercise. Using a lighter resistance (and thus more repetitions) is prudent when beginning a weight-training program. Experience has shown that novices should initially attempt to complete 12 to 15 repetitions. This regimen will not place an excessive strain on the musculoskeletal system during the early phase of the program. A heavier weight should be used if 12 repetitions feels too easy. The weight is too heavy if the exerciser cannot do 12 repetitions. This is a trial-and-error process and may take several exercise sessions before a proper starting weight is selected. After a week or two of training, when the muscles have adapted and the correct movements are learned, the number of repetitions can be reduced to between six and eight. More weight is added each time this target number of repetitions is reached. This program represents progressive resistance training: as the muscles become stronger, the weight is adjusted and a heavier load is attempted. In general, the exercise sequence should proceed from larger to smaller muscle groups to prevent an inability to perform big-muscle exercise caused by the premature fatigue of the small group required for the movement.

The Lower Back

Many orthopedists consider muscular weakness, particularly in the abdominal region, and poor joint flexibility in the back and legs primary factors related to **low back pain syndrome.** Both muscle-strengthening and joint flexibility exercises are commonly prescribed for prevention of and rehabilitation from chronic low back strain.[66] Even continuing normal daily activities within the limits dictated by pain tolerance leads to a more rapid recovery from an episode of acute back pain than bed rest; in fact, maintaining normal physical activity has led to a more rapid recovery than the use of specific back-mobilizing exercises performed after the onset of pain.[102]

The proper application of resistance training provides an excellent means for strengthening the abdomen and lumbar extensor muscles of the lower back through their full ranges of motion.[42, 125] These muscles provide the necessary support and protection for the spine. A considerable strain is imposed on the lower spine if exercises are performed improperly, with a heavy load and the hips thrust forward and back in an arched position. Pressing and curling exercises, for example, if performed with excessive hyperextension of the back, create unusually high shearing stress on the lumbar vertebrae. This spinal pressure can trigger an episode of low back pain. Proper execution of an exercise should not be sacrificed to lift a heavier load or "squeeze out" an additional repetition. The extra weight lifted through improper technique will not facilitate muscle strengthening, and it may precipitate an injury resulting from improper body alignment or unwarranted muscle substitution.

Wearing a weightlifting belt during heavy lifts (squats, dead lifts, clean-and-jerk maneuvers) significantly reduces intra-abdominal pressure compared to not wearing such a belt.[56] A belt may reduce the potentially injurious compressive forces on spinal discs during heavy lifting such as most Olympic and power lifting events. Researchers concluded that a belt should always be worn for near-maximal or maximal lifts and that someone who normally trains wearing a belt should be extremely cautious about lifting without one. A further recommendation is that at least some resistance training be done without a belt to help strengthen the deep abdominal muscles and develop the proper pattern of muscle recruitment needed to generate high intra-abdominal pressures when a belt is not worn.

Resistance Training Plus Aerobic Training Often Equals Less Strength Improvement

Concurrent maintenance of both resistance and aerobic training programs blunts the magnitude of muscular strength and power improvement.[34, 60, 63, 70, 92a] This may partly explain why power athletes and body builders often refrain from endurance activities while participating in resistance training. It is possible that the added energy (and perhaps protein) demands of such heavy endurance training may impose a limit on muscle growth and responsiveness to resistance training. Such findings, however, should not deter those who desire a well-rounded conditioning program offering the specific fitness and health benefits available from both forms of exercise training.

ISOMETRIC STRENGTH TRAINING

Research in Germany during the mid-1950s showed that an increase in isometric strength of about 5% weekly could be achieved by performing daily a single, maximum isometric muscle action of only 1-second duration or a 6-second action at two-thirds maximum.[61] Repeating this action 5 to 10 times daily produced greater increases in isometric strength.

Limitations of Isometric Exercise

Although isometric exercise is effective for providing muscle overload and improving strength, it may be of limited use for sports training. For one thing, the isometric method makes it difficult to evaluate progress in training: because there is no movement, it is impractical to measure force output during training or determine whether a person's strength is actually improving. Also, the development of isometric strength is highly **specific;** thus, a muscle trained isometrically demonstrates improved strength mainly when the muscle acts isometrically and particularly at the joint angle and body position in which the strength was developed.[89, 97]

If isometric training is used to develop "strengths" in a particular movement, it probably is necessary to train at many points through the range of motion. This can become time consuming, particularly given the availability of conventional dynamic activities such as weight training and isokinetic and hydraulic methods.

Benefits of Isometric Exercise

The isometric method does seem to provide benefits during muscle testing and rehabilitation. Specific muscle weakness can be detected using isometric techniques, and strengthening exercises can be performed at the appropriate joint angle to optimize the muscle overload.

WHICH ARE BETTER, STATIC OR DYNAMIC METHODS?

Both static and dynamic training methods produce significant increases in muscle strength. The resistance training method selected is determined by the individual's specific needs and governed by the specificity of the training response.[111a]

Specificity of the Training Response

The isometrically trained muscle is stronger when measured isometrically, whereas the dynamically-trained muscle is stronger when evaluated during resistance activities requiring movement. Angle-specific isometric training responses are frequently observed if any strength developed at or near one joint angle is transferred to other angles or body positions. This occurs even when the same muscles are involved.[89, 169] In dynamic exercise, muscles trained through movement over a particular limited range of motion demonstrate the greatest strength improvement when measured in that ROM.[52] This specificity of the response to resistance training is understandable because strength improvement is related to a blend of adaptations that occur both in the muscle fiber itself and in the neural organization and excitability for a particular pattern of voluntary movement.[101, 133, 147, 176] Likewise, maximal muscle effort depends not only on local factors such as muscle fiber type and muscle cross-section, but also on neural factors that determine the effective recruitment and synchronization for firing of the appropriate motor units.[74, 111, 124, 132]

A 3-month study of young adult men and women emphasized the highly specific nature of adaptations to resistance training.[33] One group trained the adductor pollicus muscle isometrically with ten daily muscle actions of 5-seconds duration and at a frequency of one per minute. The other group trained the same muscle dynamically with ten daily ten-repetition bouts of weight movement at one-third maximal strength. The untrained muscle served as the control. To eliminate any training influences resulting from psychological factors and central nervous system adaptations, the trained muscle was evaluated with a supermaximal electrical stimulation applied to the motor nerve. Results indicated that both groups improved in maximal force capacity and peak rate of force development with training. The improvement in maximal force for the isometrically trained group, however, was nearly twice that of the group that trained dynamically. Conversely, improvement in the speed of force development was about 70% greater in the group that trained with dynamic muscle actions. Such findings provide strong evidence that resistance training per se is not all-inclusive for adaptations in muscle structure and function. Rather, improvements in the contractile properties (maximal force, velocity of shortening, and rate of tension development) of the muscle itself can vary in a manner that is highly specific to the type of muscle action used in training. Consequently, although it is true that both static and dynamic training methods produce significant strength increases, no one system can really be considered "superior" to the other. The crucial consideration is the intended purpose of the newly acquired strength.

Practical Implications. The complex interaction between the nervous and muscular systems provides some explanation for the observation that the leg muscles, when strengthened in an activity like squats or deep knee bends, do not usually show improved force capability when used in another leg movement such as jumping. Low relationships have been demonstrated between dynamic measures of leg extension force at any speed and vertical jumping height.[71] Also, a muscle group strengthened by weight training does not demonstrate an equal improvement in force capacity when measured isometrically. Consequently, strengthening muscles for use in a specific activity such as golf, rowing, swimming, or football requires more than just identifying and overloading the muscles involved in the movement. It requires that training be specific to the exact movements for which the improved strength is desired. Training the muscles of the legs to become stronger through weightlifting does not necessarily mean that the performance of all subsequent leg movements will improve. There is often little transfer of newly acquired strength to other types of movements even when the same muscles are involved.[30, 33] This is clearly demonstrated in a study in which a 227% increase in leg extension strength occurred through a standard program of weight training. When peak torque of the same leg extensors

was evaluated with an isokinetic dynamometer, however, there was only a 10 to 17% improvement![45] *To improve a specific physical performance through resistance training, the muscles must be trained in movements as close as possible to the movement or actual skill that is to be improved.* This coordination can be accomplished with supplemental resistance training that uses modified sports equipment without disrupting the mechanics of the particular performance.

Supplemental Resistance Training with Modified Sports Equipment

Conventional resistance training utilizes external resistance in the form of barbells, dumbbells, weight plates on pulley and cam machines, or other types of resistance machines. Not so common is training with supplemental sports equipment by augmenting the equipment to make it heavier than normal to provide a muscular overload.[107] It also is possible to train with a lighter-than-normal implement in an attempt to develop fast-firing motor units needed for high-velocity or speed training.[137, 141] Figure 22.10 displays the results from two similar studies during which heavier- (6 oz) and lighter- (4 oz) than-normal-weight (5 oz) baseballs were used for a 10-week baseball pitching training program. The object was to determine the effects of training with underweighted and overweighted baseballs on pitching velocity.

In Study 1 (Fig. 22.10 A), 30 high school pitchers were randomly assigned to train with up to a 20% increase or decrease in the weight of a normal 5-oz baseball (maximum of 6 oz and minimum of 4 oz). The baseballs were increased or decreased in weight by one-fourth ounce every 2 weeks for 10 week. Both groups threw a total of 1,500 pitches during the thrice-weekly sessions. Each training session began with stretching and warm-up throwing for 10 minutes with a standard-weight ball. During the next 10 minutes, each subject threw 20 pitches with a standard-weight ball, 20 pitches with an overweight (or underweight) baseball, and then 10 pitches with the standard-weight ball. A control group trained with the two experimental groups but used only the standard-weight baseball. Pitching velocity was determined by electromagnetic radiation radar validated by two high-speed video cameras interfaced to a computerized video analysis system. Pitching velocity before and after the supplemental training was determined by averaging ten consecutive pitches with a regulation baseball. While all three groups improved significantly in throwing velocity (gain for group throwing overweighted baseball = 3.74 mph, gain for group throwing underweighted baseball = 4.72 mph, gain for controls = 0.88 mph), the two experimental groups improved throwing velocity significantly more than the control group. This improved pitching velocity could be attributed to supplemental training because there was no other form of resistance training during the study period.

Study 2 (Fig. 22.10 *B*) was a repeat of Study 1 but with a larger sample size (15 high school pitchers and 60 college pitchers in each training group). Both of the experi-

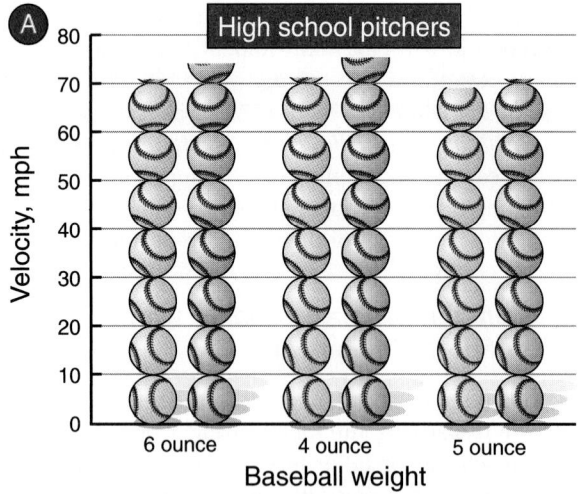

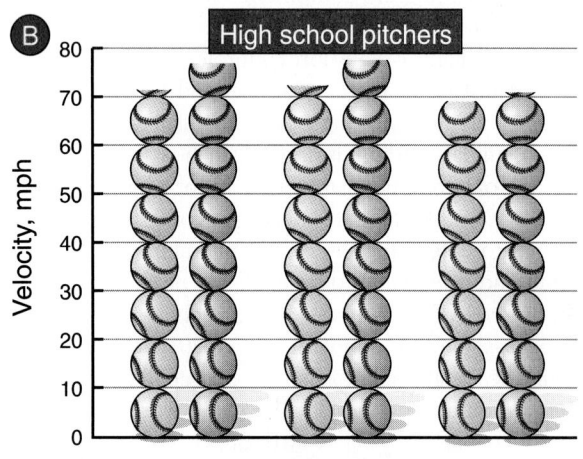

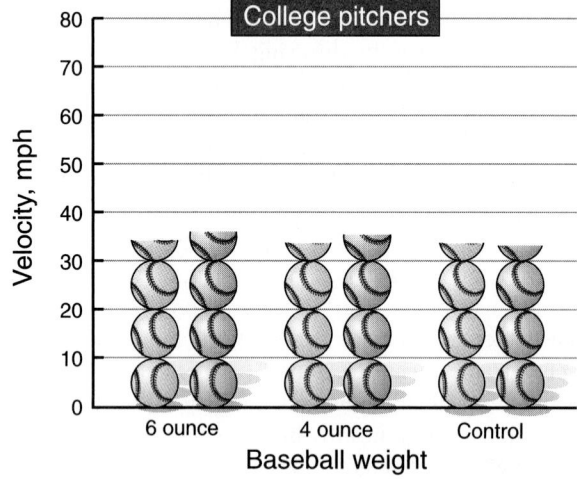

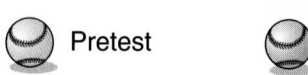

mental groups trained with underweight (4-oz) and overweight (6-oz) baseballs to determine if there was a synergistic effect of both types of supplemental training. In this study, ball velocity was determined from 15 consecutive throws with a standard-weight baseball. One group trained with all three weighted baseballs (6, 5, and 4 oz) for 10 weeks. The second group trained first with the 5- and then 6-oz baseballs for the first 5 weeks and then switched to pitching with the 5- followed by the 4-oz baseballs for the second 5-week period. The control group only trained with a 5-oz baseball. All three groups threw the same number of total pitches (1,980 excluding 50 warmup throws with a regulation baseball before each training session). The high school pitchers and college pitchers in the experimental groups significantly improved throwing velocity, by approximately 2.0 mph, compared to the control subjects.

Considered together, the results of both studies reinforce the concept of specificity with supplemental training that mimics actual performance (in this case, pitching) when using sports equipment that has been modified but does not alter the general movement mechanics and pattern (including ROM) of the selected activity. For baseball pitching, which has a significant skill component, it seems that the nervous system is able to incorporate the seemingly minor alteration in overload (±1 oz) and translate the training adaptations to enhanced performance under conditions utilizing standard equipment. Improved performance also occurred for supplemental training (100 swings per day, 3 times per week) for 6 weeks with a lighter or heavier baseball bat.[137]

Specificity Not Always Observed

Even though the results of most training studies support the concept of specificity, the exceptions are often overlooked.[82, 90, 120] In one study, subjects in a free-weight (FW) training group trained three times a week for 12 weeks using eccentric and concentric muscle actions; a second group trained using concentric actions only with hydraulic resistance (HY); and a control group did not train.[69] Training with FW and HY included five sets of supine bench presses and upright squats at an intensity of 1- to 6-RM plus five supplementary exercises at 5- to 10-RM, for a total of 20 sets per session for approximately 50 minutes. Testing before and after training included the 1-RM bench press and squat performed with concentric and eccentric muscle actions and without prestretch (concentric only) and using standard FW testing procedures.

Figure 22.11 (*top*) shows that the FW group made large increases in concentric squat strength (+35%), but these in-

FIGURE 22.10

A, Effects in high school pitchers of training three times per week for 10 weeks with heavier (6-oz) and lighter (4-oz) baseballs on pitching velocity with standard 5-oz balls. (Data from DeRenne, C., et al.: Effects of weighted implement training on throwing velocity. *J. Appl. Sport Sci. Res.,* 4:16, 1990.) **B,** Combined effects of 10 weeks of training three times weekly with heavier (6-oz) and lighter (4-oz) baseballs on throwing velocity in high school and college pitchers. In these studies, a control group trained only with standard 5-oz baseballs. (Data from DeRenne, C., et al.: Effects of under- and overweighted implement training on pitching velocity. *J. Strength Cond. Res.,* 8:247, 1994.)

creases were not significantly different from those of the group that trained using only concentric muscle actions (+39%). When squat strength was assessed with eccentric and concentric actions (*bottom*), both groups improved about 30%. Although the specificity principle in resistance training may encompass joint angle or muscle length specificity, velocity specificity, and task or movement pattern specificity,[83, 152] the principle may not be totally applicable to the type of muscle action or test mode.[81, 120, 121] It is likely that resistance training with free weights and hydraulic devices was not distinct enough in terms of muscle action to elicit highly specific training adaptations. Unlike isokinetic and hydraulic routines, FW exercise includes both eccentric and concentric actions. During an exercise that incorporates both eccentric and concentric muscle actions, the limiting factor in overcoming resistance is the concentric and not the eccentric muscle force. Thus, despite differences between the muscle actions used for free-weight and hydraulic exercise, FW- and HY-trained subjects may still have used the same training stimulus via the concentric load. It is, therefore, a distinct possibility that any form of concentric or combined concentric plus eccentric resistance training should result in comparable gains in muscle strength as long as similar movement patterns and velocities are employed for training and testing.[105]

ISOKINETIC RESISTANCE TRAINING

Isokinetic resistance training attempts to combine the features of both isometrics and weight training to provide muscle overload at a preset constant speed while the muscle mobilizes its force-generating capacity throughout the full ROM. Any effort during the exercise encounters an opposing force relative to that applied; this represents the **accommodating resistance exercise,** which is accomplished with the aid of a mechanical device. Theoretically, isokinetic-type training makes it possible to activate the largest number of motor units and consistently overload muscles at their force output capacities during movement, even at the relatively "weaker" joint angles.

Isokinetics Versus Standard Weightlifting

An important distinction can be made between a muscle overloaded isokinetically and one overloaded with a stan-

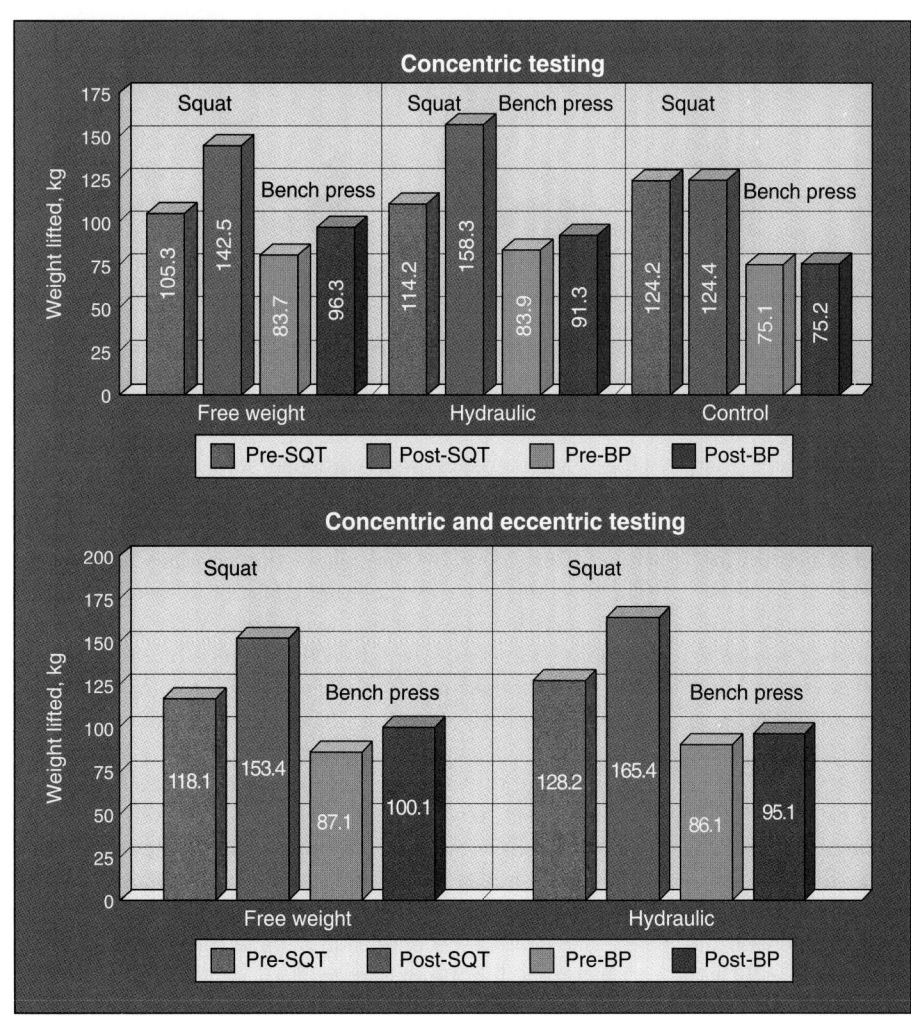

FIGURE 22.11

Effects of 12 weeks of resistance training with concentric resistance (*top*) and combined concentric + eccentric resistance (*bottom*) on pre- and post-test squat (*SQT*) and bench press (*BP*) muscle actions. (From Hortobágyi, T., and Katch, F.I.: Role of concentric force in limiting improvement in muscular strength. *J. Appl. Physiol.*, 68:650, 1990.)

FIGURE 22.12

The force-generating capacity of a muscle or muscle group varies in relation to joint angle throughout the range of motion in both flexion and extension. Work and power can be computed in performing such dynamic movements. For rotational work, the mathematical equation is work = torque × angular displacement, where torque is the product of a force acting on the object and the perpendicular distance from the line of action of the force to the point about which the object rotates; the angular displacement is the angle through which the object rotates. To compute rotational power, power = work/time = (torque × angular displacement)/time; rewriting the equation, power = torque × (angular displacement/time), and power = torque × angular velocity. Using SI units, torque is expressed in newton meters, and angular displacement is expressed in radians (angles in degrees are converted to radians by dividing by 57.3 deg/rad). The SI unit for work done in rotating an object is joules, and power is expressed in watts (joules/second). Work and power are related as follows: work = force × distance, and power = work/time = (force × distance)/time. Rewriting the last expression, power = force × distance/time, and power = force × velocity. (Equations from Harmon, E. The measurement of human mechanical power. In Maud, P.J., and Foster, C. [Eds], *Physiological Assessment of Human Fitness*, Champaign, IL, Human Kinetics, 1995:88–89.)

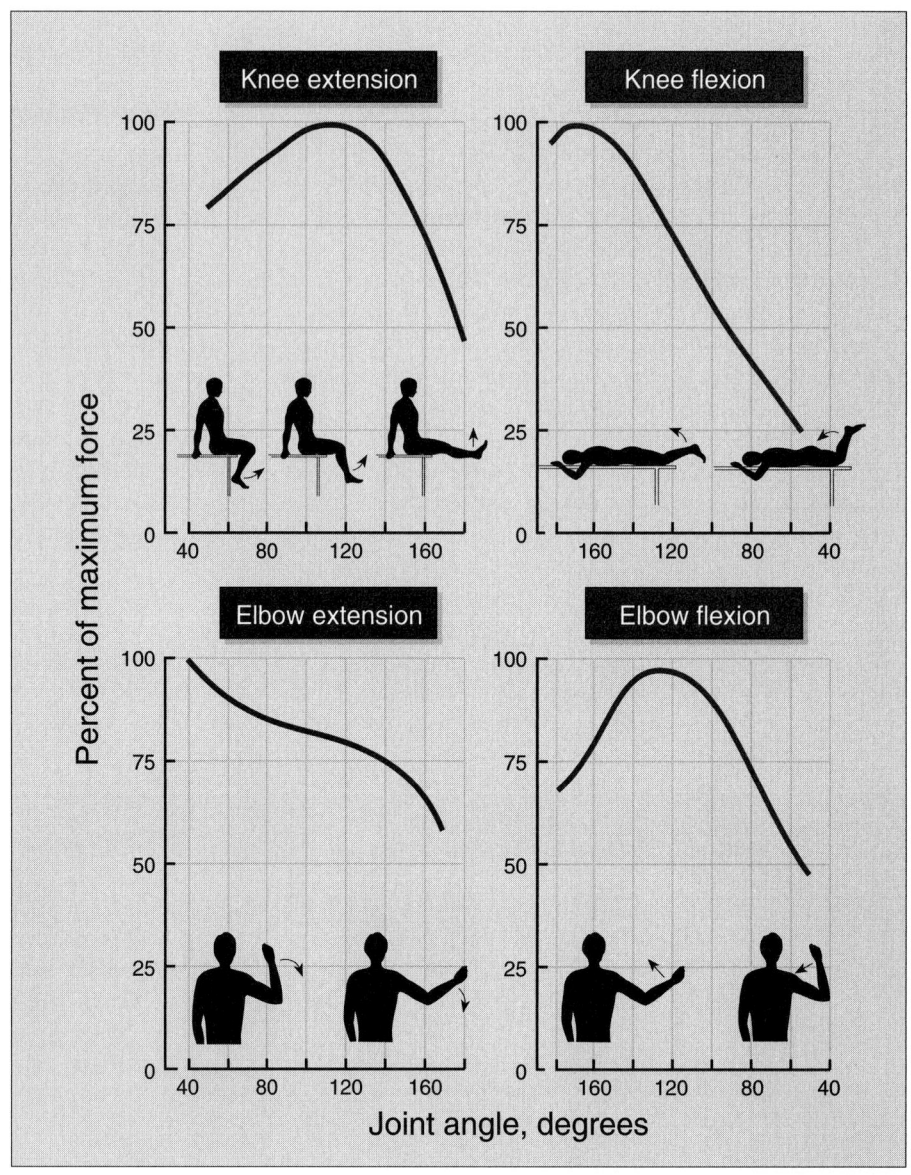

dard weight-lifting exercise. Figure 22.12 illustrates that the capacity of a muscle or muscle group varies in relation to the bony lever configuration (joint angle) as the joint moves through the ROM. During weight training, the resistance is usually fixed at the greatest load that allows completion of the movement for the desired number of repetitions. *Consequently, the resistance can be no greater than the maximum strength of the weakest muscle (or joint position) in the ROM. Otherwise, the movement would not be completed.* Weight lifters frequently refer to this point in the ROM as the "sticking point."

A main limitation of weightlifting exercise is that the force generated by the muscles is not maximum through all phases of the movement. To help overcome this problem, manufacturers have devised **variable resistance** training equipment that utilizes an irregularly shaped metal cam or other device to adjust the resistance in accordance with the

lever characteristics of a particular joint movement. This equipment still represents a classic mode of weightlifting, except that the relative resistance offered to the muscle is, in theory, fairly constant throughout the full range of motion. The machine, however, does not control the speed of movement, and the design of the mechanical device to achieve a variable resistance is based on the average physical dimensions of a population. It is difficult to adjust for individual variations in body structure. Furthermore, there is little evidence that such cam devices actually compensate fully for differences in mechanics and force applications at all phases of the particular movement on a given piece of exercise equipment.[55] This is not the case with an isokinetically loaded muscle. The desired speed of movement occurs almost instantaneously when force is applied, and the muscle is able to generate peak power output throughout the range of motion at a controlled shortening velocity.

Figure 22.13 presents a generalized two-dimensional view of torque development in relation to angular velocity at two specific joint angles during eccentric and concentric muscle actions. This type of analysis permits a more comprehensive evaluation of muscular force-generating capability compared to measurement at only one joint angle or using standard 1-RM measures.

Experiments with Isokinetic Exercise and Training

Experiments using isokinetic exercise have explored the force-velocity relationships in various movements in relation to the muscle's fiber-type composition. Figure 22.14 displays the progressive decline in peak torque output with increasing angular velocity of the knee extensor muscles in two groups who differed in sports training and muscle fiber type. In the experiments, which involved movement at 180° per second, the decrement in maximal torque was about 55% of the maximal isometric $(0° \cdot s^{-1})$ force. However, the two curves in Figure 22.13 can be distinguished in terms of peak torque depending on the group's muscle fiber composition. At zero velocity, peak force was the same for athletes with relatively high (power athletes) or low (endurance athletes)

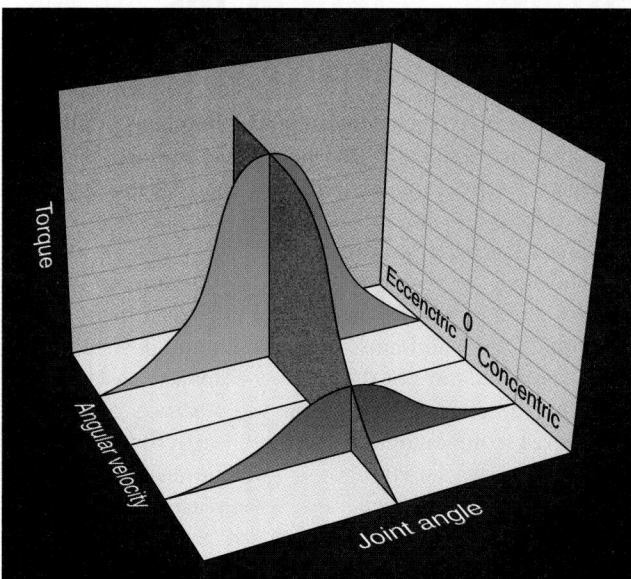

FIGURE 22.13

Two-dimensional curve of maximal torque versus joint angle derived from measurement at two angular velocities. The height of the line of intersection of the red (torque) and blue (angular velocity) curves represents the maximal torque at this particular combination of angular velocity and joint angle. Maximal torque at the other angular velocity (green curve) and joint angle is also reflected as the height of the intersection of the red and green curves. (Two-dimensional curve analysis courtesy of Dr. E. Harmon, research physiologist and Director of Biomechanics Research, U.S. Army Research Institute of Environmental Medicine, Natick, MA.)

percentages of fast-twitch muscle fibers; this indicated that both fast- and slow-twitch motor units were activated in maximal isometric knee extension. *As movement velocity increased, greater torque per unit body mass was achieved by individuals with higher percentages of fast-twitch fibers.* This suggests that a high percentage of fast-twitch fibers is desirable for power activities in which success is largely influenced by one's capacity to generate torque at rapid velocities of movement.[29, 158]

Fast- Versus Slow-Speed Isokinetic Training

Research has compared strength and power improvement with isokinetic training at slow and fast limb speeds. These studies have provided further support for the principle of specificity as applied to both exercise performance and the training response. For example, several studies support the contention that gains in "strength" from slow-speed isokinetic training are highly specific to the angular velocity of the movement used in the training. Exercising at fast speeds, on the other hand, facilitates a more general improvement: increases in power output were noted at both fast and slow speeds of movement, although the greatest improvement was noted at the fast angular velocity used in training.[122] Muscle hypertrophy occurred only during fast-speed training and only in the fast-contracting type II muscle fibers.[30] This hypertrophy possibly accounts for the more general strength improvement with fast-speed training. Furthermore, recent data indicate that greater power increases and hypertrophy of type II fibers occur during training with concentric muscle actions than during eccentric training at equivalent relative power levels.[101a]

The fundamental basis for isokinetic training is attractive because muscles can be overloaded through a full range of motion and at a variety of muscle shortening velocities. However, this concept is limited in practical application because the most rapid speed of movement using an isokinetic dynamometer is about $400° \cdot s^{-1}$. Even movement at this relatively "fast" speed does not approach the movement speeds during many sports activities such as baseball pitching, for which the velocity of upper limb extension exceeds $2000° \cdot s^{-1}$ in professional pitchers; interestingly, the hip rotators move at the relatively "slow" velocity of $600° \cdot s^{-1}$.[18] Also, the present generation of isokinetic dynamometers cannot provide overload of eccentric muscle actions that are important for limb deceleration and "braking" control in normal movements.

PLYOMETRIC TRAINING

Some athletes in sports requiring specific powerful movements—football, volleyball, sprinting, and basketball—use a special form of exercise training drill termed **plyometrics,** or explosive jump training. In plyometric exercise, various jumps in place or rebound jumping (drop-jumping from a

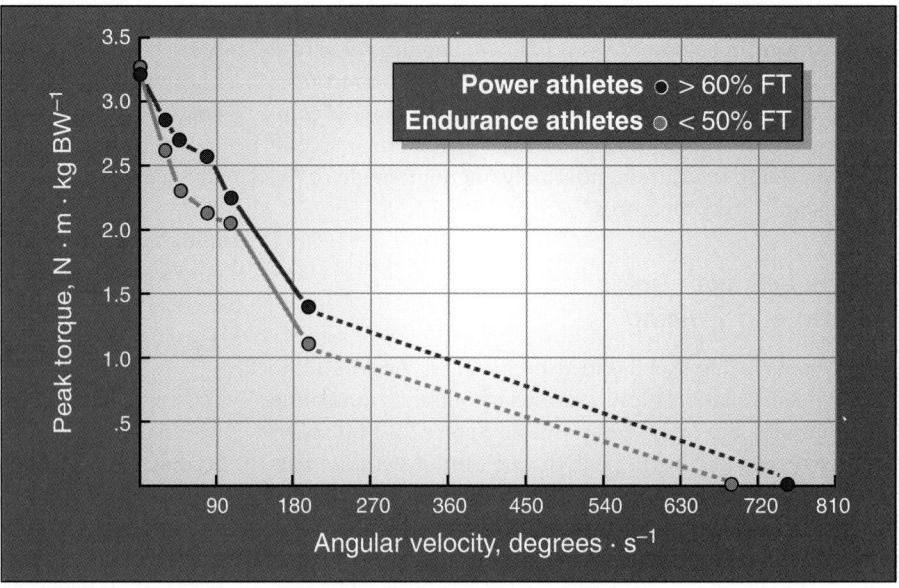

FIGURE 22.14

Peak torque generated per unit body mass in relation to angular velocity of joint movement in two groups of athletes with different muscle fiber-type compositions. The torque-velocity curves were extrapolated (dashed line) to the approximated maximal velocity for knee extension. (From Thorstensson, A.: Muscle strength, fiber types, and enzyme activities in man. *Acta Physiol. Scand., Suppl.* 443, 1976.)

height) are structured to make use of the inherent stretch-recoil characteristics of skeletal muscle and its modulation via the stretch or myotatic reflex. In plyometric exercise (as in many sport situations), overload is applied to skeletal muscle in a manner that rapidly stretches the muscle (eccentric or stretch phase) immediately prior to the concentric or shortening phase of action. This rapid lengthening phase in the **stretch-shortening cycle** probably facilitates subsequently a more powerful movement believed to enhance the speed-power benefits of this form of training.[75]

Practical Application of Plyometrics

A plyometric drill utilizes one's body mass and the force of gravity to provide the all-important rapid prestretch, or "cocking," phase to "activate" the muscle's natural elastic recoil elements. This action then augments the subsequent concentric muscle action in the opposite direction. An example of a natural form of plyometric movement is an eccentric prestretch of the quadriceps muscle group brought on by rapidly lowering and dropping the arms to the side prior to vertical jumping. Specific plyometric drills for the lower body include a standing jump, multiple jumps, repetitive jumping in place, depth-jumps or drop-jumping from a height of about 1 m, single- and double-leg jumps, and various modifications. The belief is that repetitions of these exercises will provide the proper neuromuscular training for enhancing the power performance of specific muscles.[21]

Testimonials abound to the benefits of plyometric training, but carefully controlled evaluation of both the benefits and possible orthopedic risks of such exercise is lacking.[13] Concern for musculoskeletal injury is partly based on the estimation that activities such as drop jumping may generate an external load on the skeleton equivalent to between seven and ten times the body mass.[2, 95] More research is required to quantify the appropriate role, if any, of plyometric drills in a total strength-power training program.

PHYSICAL TESTING IN THE OCCUPATIONAL SETTING: THE ROLE OF SPECIFICITY

A comprehensive discussion of the development of physical tests and professionally and legally defensible validation strategies for pre-employment selection of candidates for occupations requiring some level of physical ability or physical fitness has been presented.[79]

The high degree of specificity in the various components of physical performance and physiologic function such as aerobic fitness and muscular strength and power, as well as the specific nature of the training response, casts serious doubt on the assumption that broad constructs of physical fitness exist to any significant extent. Clearly, there is no one measure of muscular strength and no one measure of aerobic fitness: an individual possesses an array of muscular "strengths" and "powers." Often, these expressions of physiologic function and performance are poorly related to each other, if at all. Likewise, a person has diverse capabilities for expressing aerobic function, depending on the muscle mass used to perform the activity. Certainly, within the occupational setting, the use of a 12-minute run test to infer aerobic capacity for firefighting or lumbering (both requiring significant upper body aerobic function) or the use of static-grip or leg-strength tests to evaluate the diverse dynamic strengths and powers required in such occupations is physiologically naive in light of current knowledge in exercise physiology.

Measurements applied in the occupational setting should most closely resemble the actual requirements of the job, not only in terms of specific tasks but also in a manner that faithfully reflects the intensity, duration, and pace (that is, physiologic demands) of the job. If such "content testing" is not possible, it is imperative to substantiate alternative testing based on proper validation studies.

ELECTROMYOGRAPHY DURING MAXIMAL BALLISTIC MUSCLE ACTIONS

The electromyography (EMG) signal provides a convenient means for studying the intricacies of neuromuscular physiology during various types of muscle action. The EMG is influenced by both the quality and quantity of electrical activity generated by muscle. In isometric actions, for example, the EMG signal is proportional to the muscle force generated. In dynamic actions, the situation is more complex because of the changing force-torque characteristics during different phases of the range of motion. In rapid, ballistic-type movements, the EMG is characterized by alternating bursts of electrical activity in the agonist and antagonistic muscles. The EMG pattern in this situation is triphasic in nature: the first burst of electrical activity occurs in the agonist, followed by signals from the antagonist (during the time the agonist is electrically silent), and then another burst of activity in the agonist. Each phase of the EMG is associated with certain aspects of the muscle action. The first burst of the agonist creates the propulsive force that sets the limb in motion, the antagonist's first burst stops the limb, and the agonist's second burst is required for the final positioning of the limb. In our studies of professional baseball pitchers and champion body builders, there were striking differences between the groups in triphasic EMG patterns during maximal-speed, unloaded arm flexion. Figure 22.15 displays a comparison using the integrated EMG signal. For the 19 pitchers, the second burst occurs sooner (probably a protective mechanism to slow the

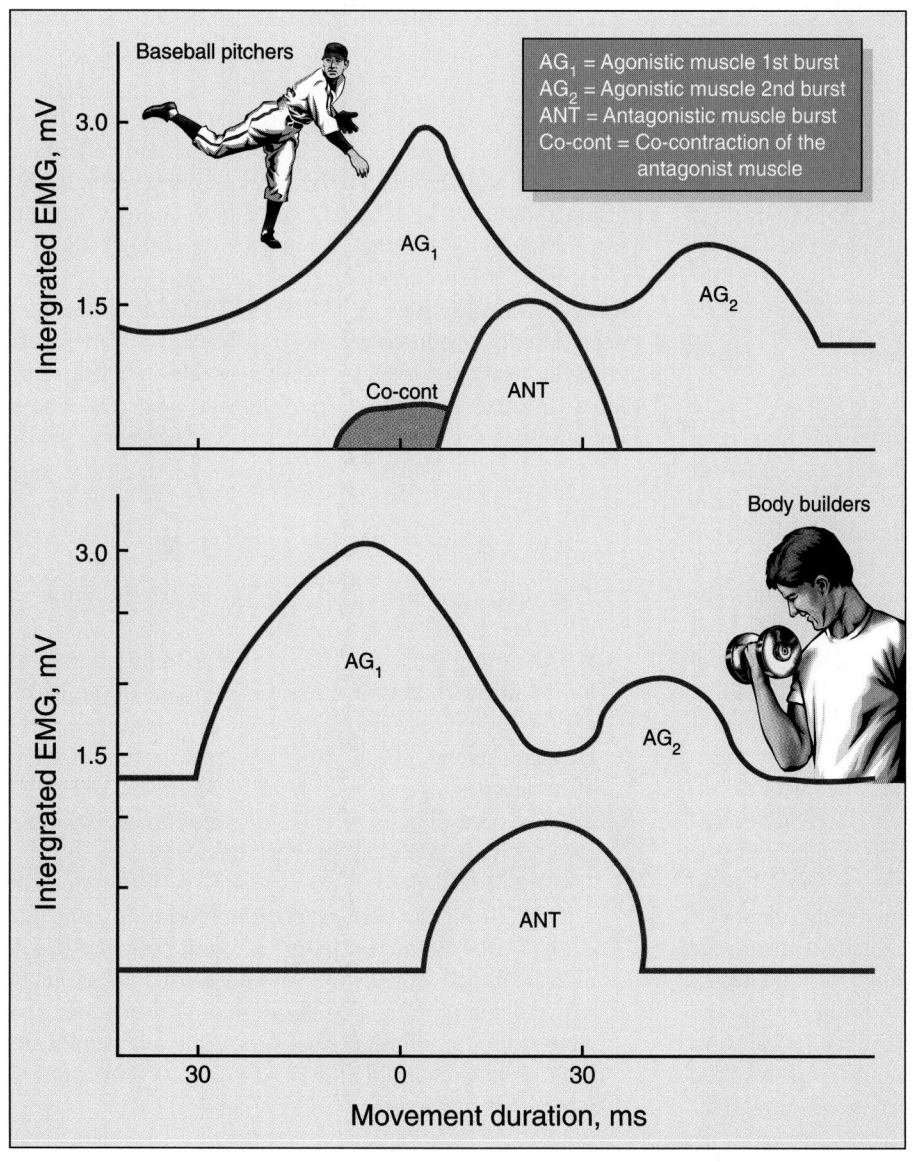

FIGURE 22.15

Comparison of the triphasic EMG pattern during rapid arm flexion in professional baseball pitchers and champion body builders. (Data Courtesy of Dr. Pierre Lagasse, Human Motor Performance Research Laboratory, Laval University, Quebec City, Quebec, Canada.)

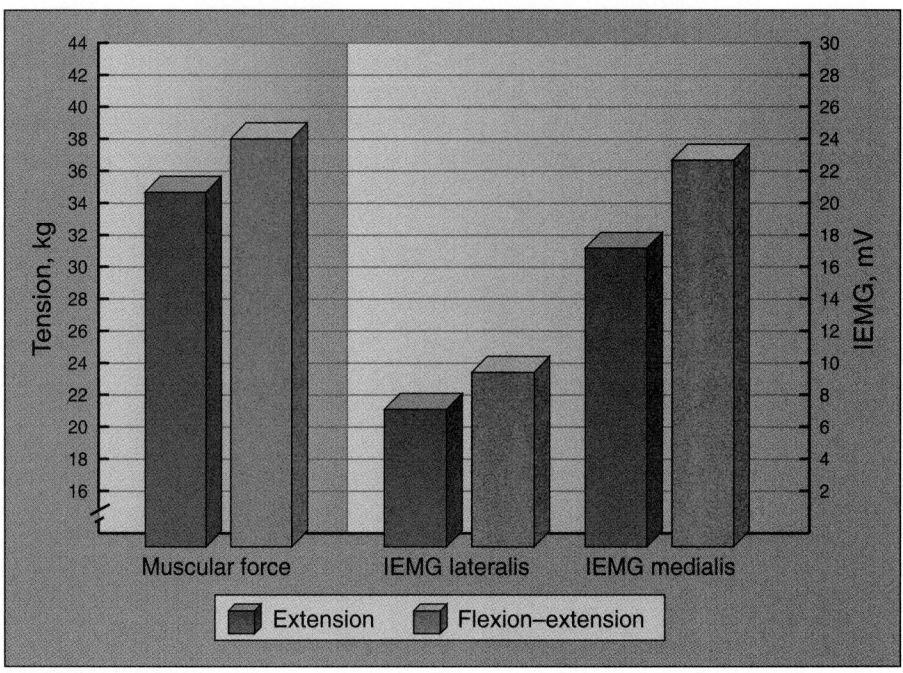

FIGURE 22.16

Maximal knee extension force (kg) and integrated EMG (IEMG) activity (mV) during knee extension and knee extension preceded by knee flexion. (From Lagasse, P., et al.: Neuromuscular facilitation of muscle tension output by reciprocal muscle work. *Annals of the French-Canadian Association for the Advancement of Sciences*, 50:222, 1983.)

extremely fast limb speed), and the amplitude is less than for the body builders. For the 11 elite body builders, the first agonistic burst occurs rapidly, and there is a distinct "delay" before the antagonist fires. This is probably related to training adaptations due to differences in limb acceleration that result from many years of specific training.

EMG During Concentric Bidirectional Muscle Work

A series of experiments has demonstrated the benefit of bidirectional (reciprocal) concentric muscle exercise over conventional, unidirectional concentric muscle actions.[94] There were two treatment conditions: (*a*) from a fully flexed right knee position, subjects executed a maximal knee extension while seated in an exercise device that permitted a concentric-only muscle action; (*b*) from a fully extended knee position, the leg was flexed through the full range of motion and then extended to the original starting position. All actions during flexion and extension were performed at maximal speed. Figure 22.16 indicates the results for maximal tension output (determined by strain gauge with simultaneous recordings of joint displacement) and integrated EMG from the vastus lateralis and vastus medialis during the two treatment conditions. When the maximal flexion movement preceded extension, tension output increased significantly, by 11.4%, and the EMG activity from the quadriceps increased by 31.2% (vastus medialis) and 42.9% (vastus lateralis). The augmentation of tension output and greater EMG activity during the concentric reciprocal work compared to unidirectional, concentric-only work resulted from the recruitment of a large number of motor units. This

was likely caused by the facilitatory neuromuscular effects of the muscle proprioceptors. If the right and left limbs were flexed and then extended in alternating fashion, the tension output and EMG activity of both limbs was even greater than single-limb activation because of the facilitative influence of the double reciprocal muscle actions. An appropriate term for such facilitatory effects during bidirectional, double concentric actions is **quadruple neuromuscular facilitation,** or **QNF** (term suggested by Professor Pierre Lagasse, Human Motor Performance Research Laboratory, Laval University, Quebec City, Canada).[130]

■ SUMMARY ■

1. The most common methods for measuring muscular strength are (*a*) tensiometry, (*b*) dynamometry, (*c*) 1-RM testing with weights, and (*d*) computer-assisted force and work-output determinations including isokinetic-type measurements.

2. Human skeletal muscle can generate a maximum force of about 30 N per square centimeter of muscle cross section, regardless of sex. On an absolute basis, however, men are generally stronger than women.

3. The traditional method to evaluate sex differences in muscle strength involves creating a ratio score for strength (for example, strength per unit body size [body mass, lean body mass, limb volume, girth]). When body size and composition are considered in this manner, the large strength differences between men and women are often reduced considerably, and in some cases, women score higher than men.

4. Allometric scaling is a mathematical procedure for establishing a proper relationship between a body size variable such as stature, body mass, or fat-free body mass and some other variable of interest such as muscular strength or aerobic capacity. Allometry eliminates the confounding effects of factors inherently related to the variable in question and permits comparisons among individuals or groups that exhibit large individual differences in particular body size variables.

5. Muscles become stronger in response to overload training. Overload is created by either increasing the resistance (load), increasing the speed of muscle action, or through a combination of both load and speed increases.

6. A load of between 60 and 80% of a muscle's force-generating capacity usually represents a sufficient overload to produce strength gains.

7. The three major systems for developing muscle strength are progressive resistance weight training, isometrics, and isokinetic-type training. Each system results in strength gains that are highly specific to the type of training. Isokinetic training, because of the possibility for generating maximum force throughout the full range of joint motion at different angular velocities of limb movement, offers a unique method of resistance training.

8. Based on limited data, closely supervised resistance training programs using relatively moderate levels of concentric muscle action significantly improve the strength of children with no adverse effect on bone or muscle.

9. Periodization is a training approach that divides a distinct period of resistance training (macrocycle) into smaller training cycles called mesocycles; these, in turn, are subdivided into weekly microcycles. This compartmentalization of training attempts to minimize overtraining effects. It also attempts to vary the training focus over the long term so that peak performance coincides with the time of competition. Emphasis is placed not only on varying the training overload during a training cycle but on adapting the training to the sport/skill-specific nature of the desired performance improvement.

10. The magnitude of strength improvement is somewhat blunted if strength and aerobic training are performed concurrently.

11. Plyometric training drills attempt to utilize the inherent stretch-recoil characteristics of the neuromuscular system to facilitate the development of muscle power. A determination of both the risks and benefits of such training awaits further research.

12. The high degree of specificity of physiologic and performance measures, as well as their responses to training, casts doubt on the wisdom of using general fitness measures to infer one's ability to perform specific tasks or occupations.

13. EMG activity during rapid, ballistic movements can be characterized by a distinct triphasic pattern, which may differ among individuals depending on prior athletic training and methods of strength acquisition.

14. Muscle force output and EMG activity are augmented during concentric, bidirectional muscle actions compared to unilateral actions because of neuromuscular facilitation and subsequent recruitment of additional motor units.

PART 2
ADAPTATIONS WITH RESISTANCE TRAINING

Figure 22.17 displays six factors that have an impact on the development and maintenance of muscle mass. Without a doubt, genetics provides the governing frame of reference that modulates the effect of each of the other factors on the ultimate outcome of increased muscle mass and strength. Muscle activity contributes little to tissue growth without

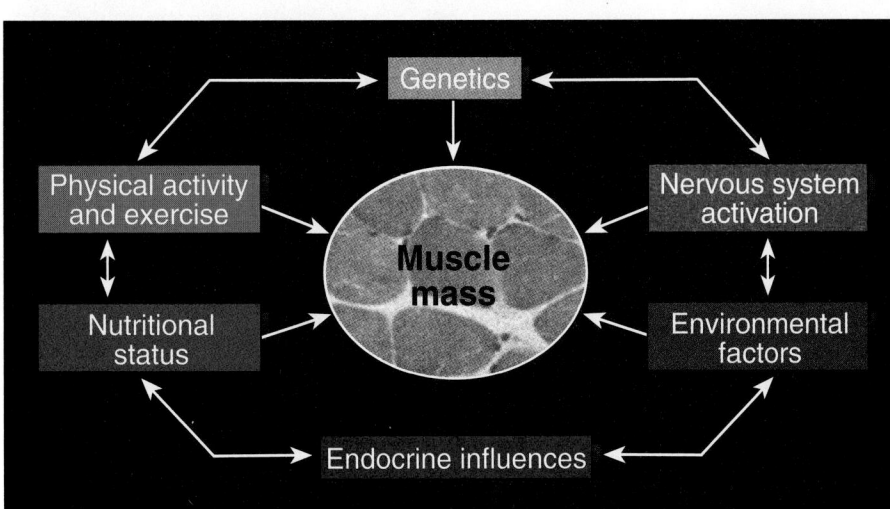

FIGURE 22.17

Six factors that have an impact on the development and maintenance of the body's muscle mass.

appropriate nutrition to provide essential building blocks. Similarly, specific hormones and patterns of nervous system innervation are crucial for patterning the appropriate training response. Without tension overload, however, each of the other factors is relatively ineffective in producing the desired training response.

FACTORS THAT MODIFY THE EXPRESSION OF HUMAN STRENGTH

As illustrated in Figure 22.18, factors broadly characterized as psychological (neural) and muscular influence the expression of human strength. Many of these factors are modified by a program of resistance training, whereas others appear to be training-resistant. The latter are probably determined by natural endowment or established early in life.

PSYCHOLOGICAL-NEURAL FACTORS

An enhanced level of neural facilitation probably accounts for the rapid and significant strength increase early in training, which is not necessarily associated with an increase in muscle size and cross-sectional area.[37, 124, 131, 147] These neural adaptations with resistance training may be the result of:

- More efficient neural recruitment patterns,
- Increased central nervous system activation,
- Improved synchronization of motor units,

- Lowering of neural inhibitory reflexes, or
- Inhibition of Golgi tendon organs.

A unique series of experiments illustrates the importance of psychological factors in the expression of human muscular strength.[78] Arm strength was measured for the following circumstances: under normal conditions; immediately after a loud noise; while the subject screamed loudly at the time of exertion; under the influence of alcohol and amphetamines, or "pep pills"; and under hypnosis when they were told they would be considerably stronger than usual and should have no fear of injury. Each of the alterations generally increased strength above normal levels. The greatest increments were observed under hypnosis, the most "mental" of all treatments!

The investigators speculated that strength improvements under the various experimental treatments resulted from temporary modifications in central nervous system function. It was argued that most people normally operate at a level of neural inhibition, perhaps via protective reflex mechanisms, that prevents them from expressing their true strength capacities. These capacities are largely established by muscle cross section and fiber type and by the mechanical arrangement of bone and muscle. Neuromuscular inhibition could result from unpleasant past experiences with exercise, an overly protective home environment, or fear of injury. Regardless of the reason, the person is usually unable to express maximum strength capability. During the excitement of intense competition or under the influence of disinhibitory drugs or hypnotic suggestion,

FIGURE 22.18
The relative roles of neural and muscular adaptations in resistance training. Note that neural adaptations predominate in the early phase of training (this phase also encompasses most training studies). With longer-term training, improvement becomes limited by the extent of muscular adaptation, most notably hypertrophy; hence, the temptation is to use anabolic steroids when it becomes difficult to induce continual hypertrophy by training alone. (From Sale, D.G.: Neural adaptation to resistance training. *Med. Sci. Sports Exerc.*, 20:135, 1988.)

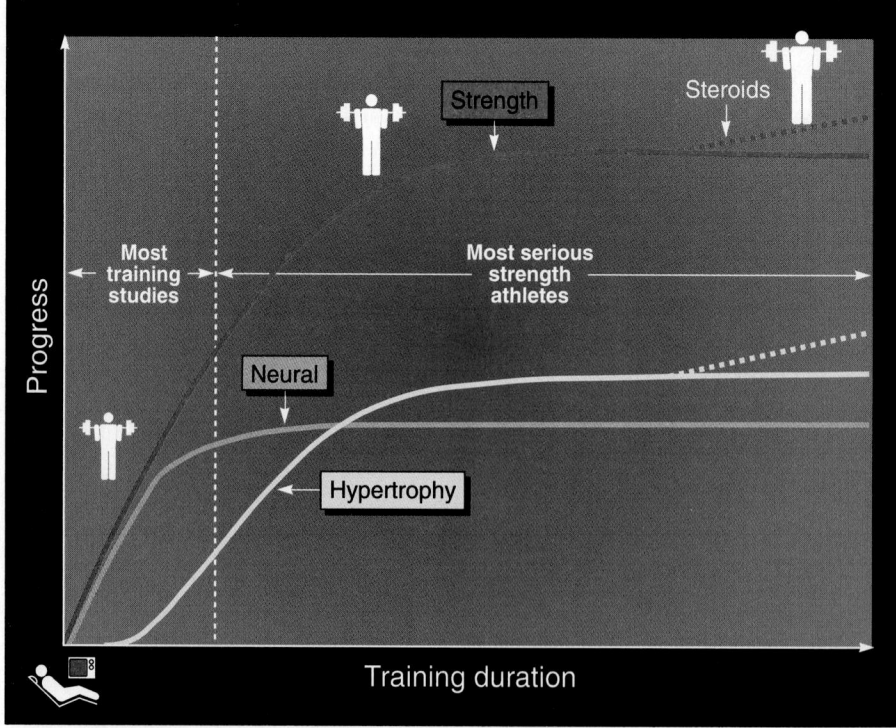

a supermaximal performance can be achieved because inhibition is greatly reduced and motoneurons are optimally recruited.

Highly trained athletes in many sports create an almost self-hypnotic state by intensely concentrating or "psyching" prior to competition. This enhanced arousal level and accompanying disinhibition (or neural facilitation) could lead to the full activation of muscle groups.[76] This also may account for the so-called "unexplainable" feats of strength during emergency situations.

MUSCULAR FACTORS

Although psychological inhibition and learning factors greatly modify one's ability to express muscle strength in the early phase of training, ultimate strength limitation is determined by anatomic and physiologic factors within the joint-muscle itself. These factors, listed in Table 22.2, are not immutable; they can be modified with appropriate resistance exercise, and some modifications occur early in training for both men and women.[147] The changes in resistance-trained muscles are generally limited to adaptations in the contractile structures and usually are accompanied by substantial increases in muscular force and muscular power through a given range of movement. For muscular power, there is an inherent relationship between a muscle's power production and its speed of contraction. The data in Figure 22.19 reveal

TABLE 22.2
PHYSIOLOGIC ADAPTATIONS THAT OCCUR IN RESPONSE TO RESISTANCE TRAINING

System/Variable	Response
Muscle Fibers	
Number	Equivocal
Size	Increase
Type	Unknown
Capillary Density	
In body builders	No change
In power lifters	Decrease
Mitochondrial	
Volume	Decrease
Density	Decrease
Twitch Contraction Time Enzymes	Decrease
Creatine phosphokinase	Increase
Myokinase	Increase
Enzymes of Glycolysis	
Phosphofructokinase	Increase
Lactate dehydrogenase	No change
Aerobic Metabolism Enzymes	
Carbohydrate	Increase
Triglyceride	Not known
Intramuscular Fuel Stores	
Adenosine triphosphate	Increase
Phosphocreatine	Increase
Glycogen	Increase
Triglycerides	Not known
V̇o₂max	
Circuit resistance training	Increase
Heavy resistance training	No change
Connective Tissue	
Ligament strength	Increase
Tendon strength	Increase
Collagen content of muscle	No change
Bone	
Mineral content	Increase
Cross-sectional area	No change

Modified from Fleck, S.J., and Kramer, W.J.: Resistance training: physiological responses and adaptations (Part 2 of 4). *Phys. Sportsmed.*, 16:108, 1988.

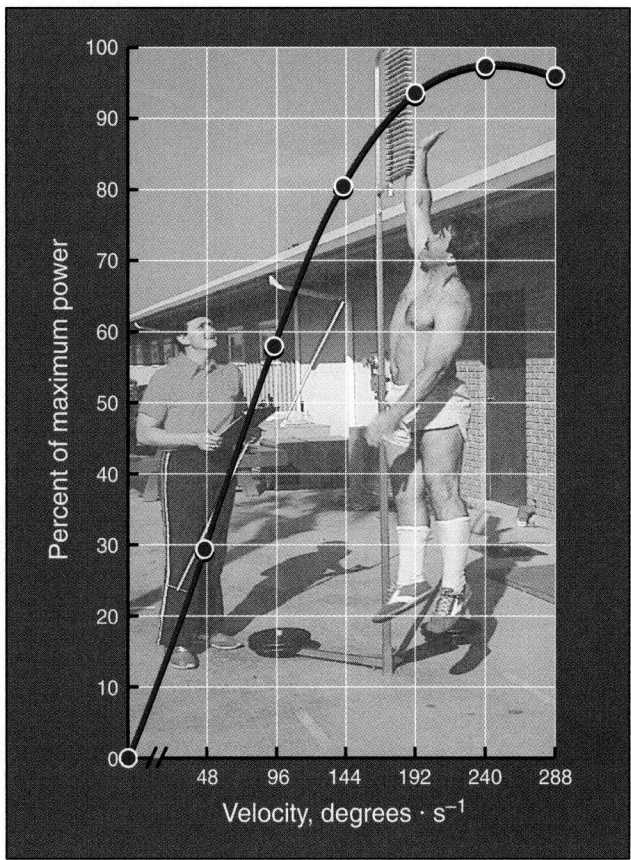

FIGURE 22.19
Muscle power (knee extensors) in relation to muscle contraction speed. (Data from Perrine, J.J., and Edgerton, V.R.: Muscle force-velocity and power-velocity relationships under isokinetic loading. *Med. Sci. Sports*, 10:159, 1978.)

that approximately sixty percent of the knee extensors' maximum power is generated at a movement speed of 100 degrees per second, and that total power further increases with increasing speed of contraction. Work output (force × distance), in contrast to power output, declines with increasing velocity of movement (speed of contraction).

Muscle Hypertrophy

*An increase in muscular tension (force) is the primary requirement for initiating skeletal muscle growth, or **hypertrophy**, with exercise training.* Increases in muscle size through increased protein synthesis during resistance training is a fundamental biologic adaptation to an increased workload in men and women regardless of age.[20, 40, 41] As discussed in the preceding section, an increase in muscle size is not necessarily a prerequisite for improving strength and power with training because important neurological factors significantly affect the expression

of human strength. The later, slower strength improvements generally coincide with noticeable alterations in muscle architecture.

Muscle growth in response to overload training results primarily from an enlargement of individual muscle fibers.[5, 76] The fast-twitch muscle fibers of weight lifters, for example, are about 45% larger than those of healthy sedentary people and endurance athletes.[36] The process of hypertrophy is directly related to the synthesis of cellular components, particularly the protein filaments that constitute the contractile elements. This growth may involve the repeated actual injury of muscle fibers (especially with eccentric actions) followed by an overcompensation of protein synthesis, resulting in a net anabolic effect.[5] The cell's myofibrils thicken and increase in number, and additional sarcomeres are formed by accelerated protein synthesis and corresponding decreases in protein breakdown.[4, 37] Significant increases are also noted in local stores of ATP, CP, and glycogen.[99] Undoubtedly, these intramuscular anaerobic energy

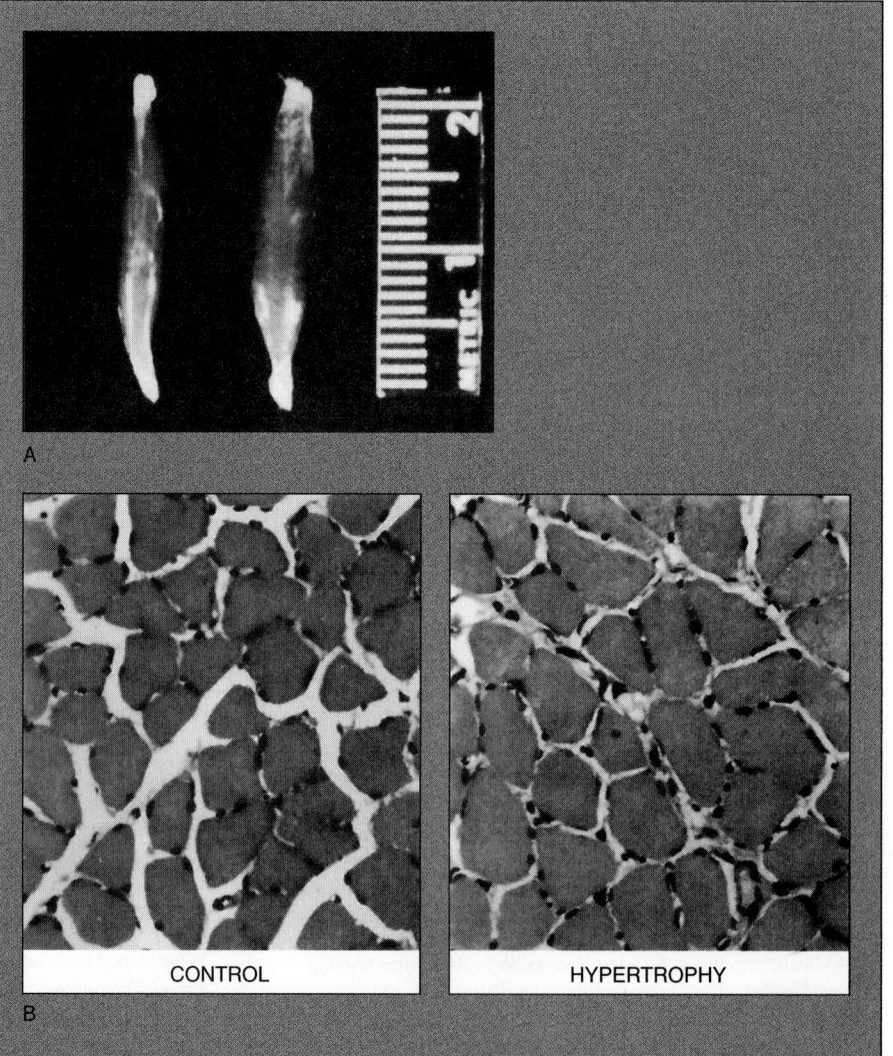

FIGURE 22.20

A, Control and hypertrophied rat soleus muscle. **B,** Cross sections of control and hypertrophied muscles shown in **A.** The average diameter for 50 fibers of the hypertrophied muscle was 24 to 34% greater than in the controls; the average number of nuclei in the hypertrophied muscle was 40 to 52% greater than in the controls. (From Goldberg, A.L., et al.: Mechanism of work-induced hypertrophy of skeletal muscle. *Med. Sci. Sports,* 3:185, 1975.)

CONTROL

HYPERTROPHY

stores contribute to the rapid rate of energy transfer required for resistance training. Body build also may play a role in explaining individual differences in responsiveness to resistance training. The greatest increases in muscle mass occur in individuals with the largest relative fat-free mass (fat-free mass corrected for stature and body fat) at the start of training.[163]

The change in muscle fiber size that accompanies exercise-induced hypertrophy is displayed in Figure 22.20. The top figure compares the exercised and unexercised soleus muscle of a rat. The hypertrophied muscle is on the right. The bottom figures are typical cross sections of untrained and hypertrophied muscles. Not only is the average diameter of the hypertrophied muscle larger by about 30%, but there is also a 46% increase in the number of nuclei present within the cells. These compensatory changes with intense muscular overload are related to a marked increase in DNA synthesis and a proliferation of connective tissue cells and small, mononucleated satellite cells located under the basement membrane adjacent to the muscle fibers.[48] This proliferation thickens and strengthens the muscle's connective tissue harness and improves the structural and functional integrity of both tendons and ligaments.[144, 150, 162] These adaptations may provide some protection from joint and muscle injury, which offers justification for using resistance exercise in preventive and rehabilitative programs.

Total contractile protein and energy-generating compounds increase with regular resistance exercise without parallel increases in capillarization, total volume of mitochondria, or mitochondrial enzymes within the trained muscle fibers.[135, 153, 156] Thus, the ratio of mitochondrial volume and/or enzyme concentration to myofibrillar (contractile protein) volume is actually **reduced** in resistance-trained muscle.[3] Although this training response probably does not hinder performance in strength and power activities because of the anaerobic nature of such efforts, it probably does hinder endurance performance by reducing the fiber's aerobic capacity per unit of muscle mass.

Even the Very Elderly Respond. Physiologic and performance adaptations to resistance training take place in both men and women and are independent of the effects of aging.[20, 25, 40, 139, 178] The remarkable plasticity of human skeletal muscle among the elderly was clearly demonstrated for five healthy men who averaged about 68 years of age (Figure 22.21).[127] These men trained for 12 weeks using heavy-resistance, isokinetic, and free-weight exercises. With training, muscle volume and cross-sectional area of the biceps brachii and brachialis increased by 13.9 and 26.0%, respectively, while hypertrophy increased by 37.2% in the type II muscle fibers. These cellular changes were accompanied by average increases of 46.0% in peak torque and 28.6% in total work output.

Such training responses are equally impressive in the very elderly. In a recent study, 100 nursing home residents used high-intensity resistance training over a 10-week period.[41] In the 63 women and 37 men who participated, muscle strength increased an average of 113%. This increase was associated with an improved level of function as reflected by an 11.8% increase in normal gait velocity and a 28.4% improvement in stair-climbing speed. These performance improvements were accompanied by a 2.7% increase in thigh muscle cross-sectional area. These women and men averaged 87.1 years in age!

Muscle Hyperplasia: Are New Muscle Fibers Made?

A question frequently raised is whether the actual number of muscle cells increases (**hyperplasia**) with training. If this does take place, to what extent does it contribute to muscle enlargement in humans? Researchers have reported that overload training of skeletal muscle in various animal species causes the development of some new muscle fibers from **satellite cells** (those cells between the basement layer and plasma membrane),[5, 134] or through a process of **longitudinal splitting**.[5, 50, 65] Under conditions of stress, neuromuscular disease, and muscle injury, the normally dormant satellite cells can develop into new muscle fibers. With longitudinal splitting, a relatively large hypertrophied muscle fiber splits into two or more smaller individual daughter cells through a process of lateral budding. These fibers function more efficiently than the large single fiber from which they were formed.[6]

One of the problems encountered with animal research is generalizing the findings to humans. For example, the massive cellular hypertrophy observed in humans with resistance training does not occur in many animal species. Thus, for these animals, muscle fiber proliferation may be an important compensatory adjustment to overload. Whether this takes place in humans is currently an area of debate, but some supportive evidence for its occurrence exists. For example, autopsy data from young, healthy men who died accidentally indicate that actual muscle fiber counts of the larger and stronger leg (leg opposite the dominant hand) contained 10% more muscle fibers than the smaller leg.[140] Cross-sectional studies of body builders with relatively large limb circumferences and muscle masses have failed to show that these athletes possessed a significant hypertrophy of individual muscle fibers.[100, 101, 155] While it is possible that some athletes inherit an initially large number of small muscle fibers, the findings from these body builders certainly leave open the possibility of hyperplasia in humans with certain forms of resistance training. Muscle fibers may adapt differently to the high-volume, high-intensity training used by body builders than they would to the typical low-repetition, heavy-load system favored by strength and power athletes. *Even if hyperplasia is replicated in other human studies (and even if the response is a positive adjustment), the*

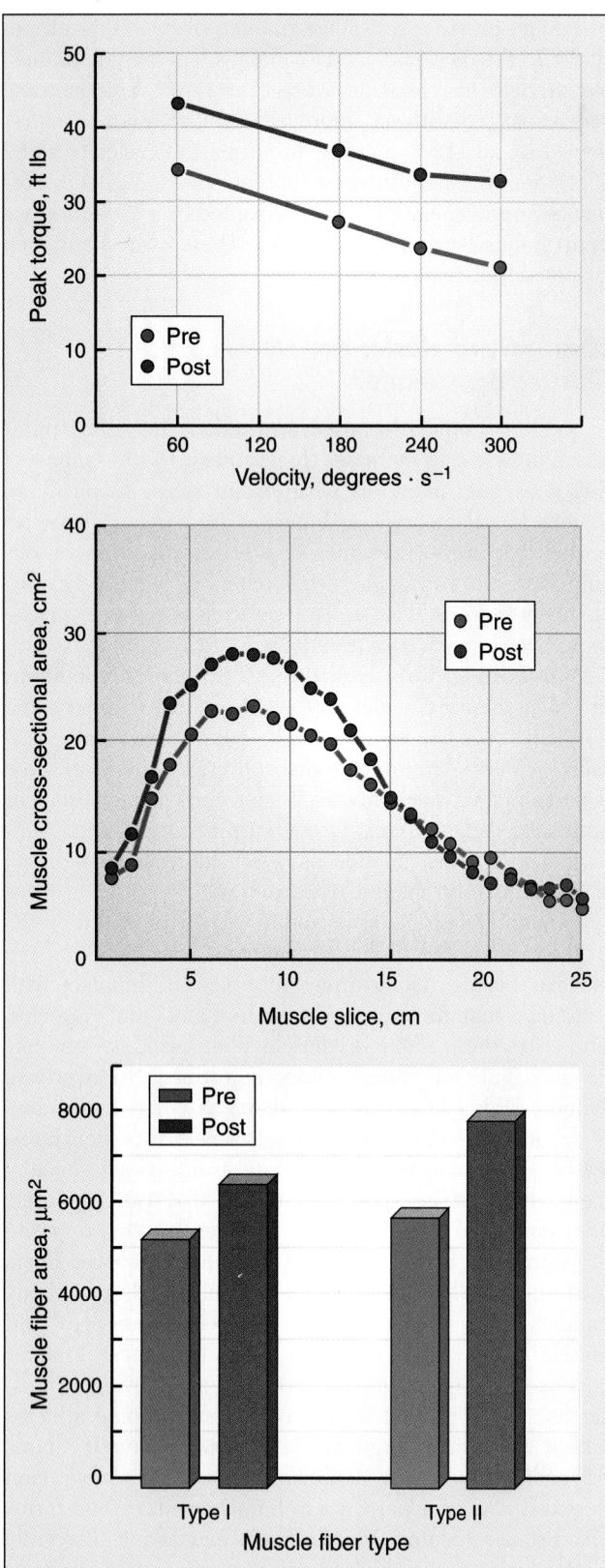

greatest contribution to muscular size from overload training is made by the enlargement of existing individual muscle fibers.[5, 101]

Changes in Muscle Fiber-Type Composition

The effects of 8 weeks of progressive resistance exercise on muscle fiber size and composition were evaluated for the leg extensor muscles of 14 men who performed three sets of 6-RM leg squats three times per week.[157] Biopsies were taken from the vastus lateralis muscle before and after training. The results for muscle fiber type were clear: there was no change with resistance training in the percentage distribution of fast- and slow-twitch muscle fibers as indicated by the activity level of myofibrillar ATPase. This finding was consistent with previous short-term studies using both resistance and endurance-type training and suggests that several months of resistance training in adults does not alter the basic fiber composition of skeletal muscle.[49] It is still open to question, however, as to whether specific training early in life or for the prolonged periods engaged in by Olympic-caliber athletes can actually cause a change in the inherent twitch (speed of shortening) characteristics of muscle fibers. Although research indicates the possibility of progressive fiber-type transformation with prolonged, specific training (refer to Chapter 18), the current position is that the predominant muscle fiber distribution is established early in life and largely determined by genetic factors.

Although the inherent muscle fiber type probably does not change dramatically with training, the metabolic characteristics of specific fibers and fiber subdivisions can undergo change in men and women within 4 to 8 weeks of resistance training. One of the more prominent and rapid adaptations is a decrease in the percentage of type IIb and corresponding increase in type IIa fibers.[1, 58, 147] This is then followed by the slower process of muscle hypertrophy. Furthermore, in the resistance training experiment described in the beginning of this section, there were significant increases in the volume of fast-twitch fibers in the leg extensor muscles.[157] This increase is clearly illustrated in Figure 22.22 for the relative areas of the fast- and slow-twitch muscle fibers, which are shown for each subject before and after training. Progressive resistance training, particularly as performed among power and Olympic-type lifters, produced a significant hypertrophy, predominantly of the fast-twitch fibers.[154, 156] This makes sense within the framework of exercise specificity because the fast-twitch motor units are re-

FIGURE 22.21

The plasticity of aging muscle. Data are from 5 men of about 68 years of age prior to (○) and following (◉) 12 weeks of heavy-resistance training. *Top,* Peak torque of elbow flexors. *Middle,* Plot of flexor cross-sectional area computed from MRI scans from proximal (right) to distal (left) end of muscle. *Bottom,* Average type I and type II fiber areas. (From Roman, W.J., et al.: Adaptations in the elbow flexors of elderly males after heavy-resistance training. *J. Appl. Physiol.,* 74:750, 1993.)

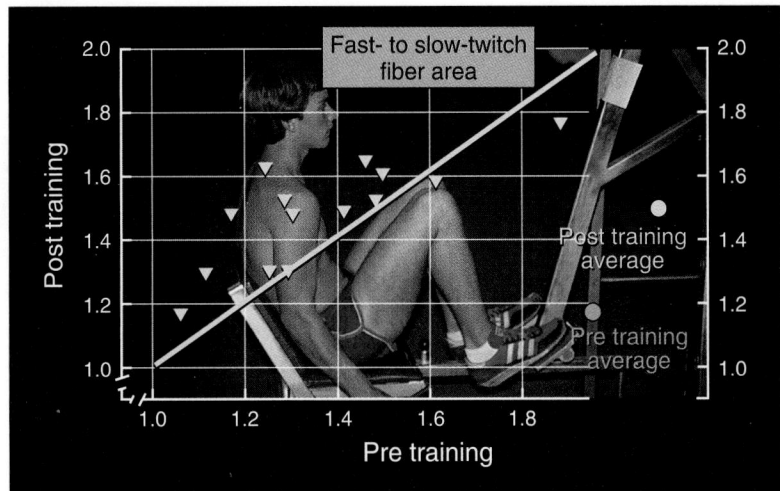

FIGURE 22.22

Individual changes for 14 men in the ratio of the area of fast- to slow-twitch muscle fibers following 8 weeks of resistance training. Orange circle on right indicates average pretraining FT:ST area ratio; yellow circle represents the post-training average. (From Thorstensson, A.: Muscle strength, fiber types, and enzyme activities in man. *Acta Physiol. Scand.,* Suppl. 443, 1976.)

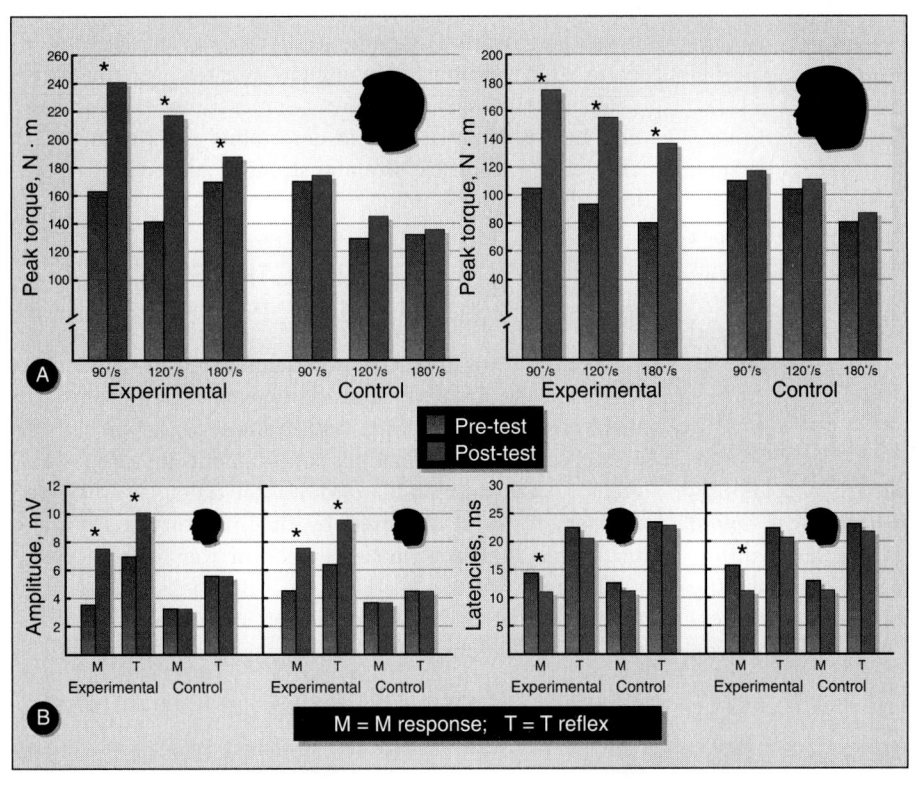

FIGURE 22.23

Effects of slow-speed resistance training on neuromuscular factors in men and women. **A,** Changes in peak torque ($N \cdot m$) measured concentrically at three movement velocities. **B,** Changes in the amplitude and latency of the vastus medialis (*M*) response and patellar tendon (*T*) reflex. The stars indicate significant differences between pre- and post-training values. (From Roy, M.A., et al.: Changes in alphamotoneuron excitability following isokinetic training in sedentary males and females. *Can. J. Appl. Sport Sci.,* 9:20P, 1984.)

cruited in near-maximal, low-volume, high-resistance exercise that involves powerful muscle actions and requires anaerobic energy transfer.

NEUROMUSCULAR FACTORS

Previous sections have presented evidence that neural factors play an important role in the expression of muscle strength. Less well researched are the changes in neuromuscular control resulting from resistance training. One study focused on the effects of strength training on the adaptations of neuromuscular patterning.[129] Relatively slow-speed, isokinetic training was studied in sedentary men and women to determine its effect on the latencies and amplitudes of the muscle (M) and patellar tendon reflex (T) responses that accompany improved torque output. The T reflex was elicited by percussion of the patellar tendon and measured by EMG surface electrodes placed over the vastus medialis. The M response was measured by stimulation of 1-ms pulses at 0.2 Hz frequency of the femoral nerve. For training, subjects performed two sets of 15 concentric knee extensions at an angular velocity of 90° per second 5 days per week for 10 weeks. The top part of Figure 22.23 displays the improvements in peak torque output measured at three movement velocities (90°, 120°, and 180° · s⁻¹). These improvements ranged from 48 to 54% for males and 67 to 70% for females, while values were unchanged for a non-training control group. The bottom part of the figure demonstrates that for men and women, the T-reflex latencies were unaltered as a result of training. However, the M-response latencies decreased significantly for all subjects, while the amplitude of the M response increased approximately twofold. These neural and muscular changes that accompanied the substantial increases in maximal torque were attributed to an enhanced alpha motor neuron excitability (which facilitated motor unit recruitment) and an improvement in the elastic properties of the specifically trained muscles.

COMPARATIVE TRAINING RESPONSES OF MEN AND WOMEN

In today's society, women are successfully participating in all sports and physical activities. Until recently, one area that women had generally shied away from was resistance training. Many women feared that such exercise would develop overly enlarged muscles similar to those observed for men engaged in heavy weightlifting programs. This inhibition was unfortunate because both men and women often lack sufficient strength to successfully perform activities such as tennis, golf, skiing, dance, and gymnastics as well as physically demanding occupational tasks such as firefighting and heavy construction work.

MUSCULAR STRENGTH AND HYPERTROPHY

The basic sex difference in response to resistance training appears to be the absolute amount of muscle hypertrophy. Researchers have speculated that this is a result of differences in hormonal levels between the sexes, especially the 20- to 30-times higher testosterone level in men, which exerts a strong anabolic effect. It should be noted, however, that testosterone levels are on a continuum between men and women, with some females normally possessing high concentrations of this hormone.

Experiments using computed axial tomography (CAT) scans to directly evaluate muscle cross-sectional area suggest that the hypertrophic response to resistance training is similar for men and women. Absolute changes in size are certainly greater for men (because the initial muscle mass of the male is greater), but the enlargement of muscle on a percentage basis is the same between sexes.[31, 117a] Substantial muscular hypertrophy in females with long-term resistance training also has been suggested in comparisons between elite male and female body builders.[4, 145, 146] More research is needed before definitive statements can be made concerning possible sex differences in resistance training responses. The limited data from relatively short-term studies do suggest that women can utilize conventional resistance training exercise without developing overly large muscles. However, longer-term differences in hormonal responses to resistance training (such as increased testosterone and decreased cortisol for men) may be important factors in determining any ultimate sex differences in muscle size and strength adaptations to prolonged resistance training.[92, 178]

IS MUSCLE STRENGTH RELATED TO BONE DENSITY?

Laboratory experiments have documented differences in maximum flexion and extension dynamic strength in postmenopausal women with and without osteoporosis.[80, 149] Osteoporosis was defined as bone mineral density (BMD) greater than one standard deviation below age-adjusted normal levels as measured by dual-photon absorptiometry in the lumbar spine and neck of the femur. Muscle strength was measured during a 5-RM bench press, a lat pull, and knee and shoulder flexion and extension concentric muscle actions at three velocities using a hydraulic dy-

FIGURE 22.24

Comparison of chest press extension and flexion strength in age- and weight-matched postmenopausal women with normal and low bone mineral densities (BMD). Women with low BMDs scored significantly lower on each measure of muscular strength than the reference group. (From Stock, J.L., et al.: Dynamic muscle strength is decreased in postmenopausal women with low bone density. *J. Bone Min. Res.*, 2:338, 1987; Janey, C., et al.: Maximum muscular strength differs in postmenopausal women with and without osteoporosis. *Med. Sci. Sports Exerc.*, 19:S61, 1987.)

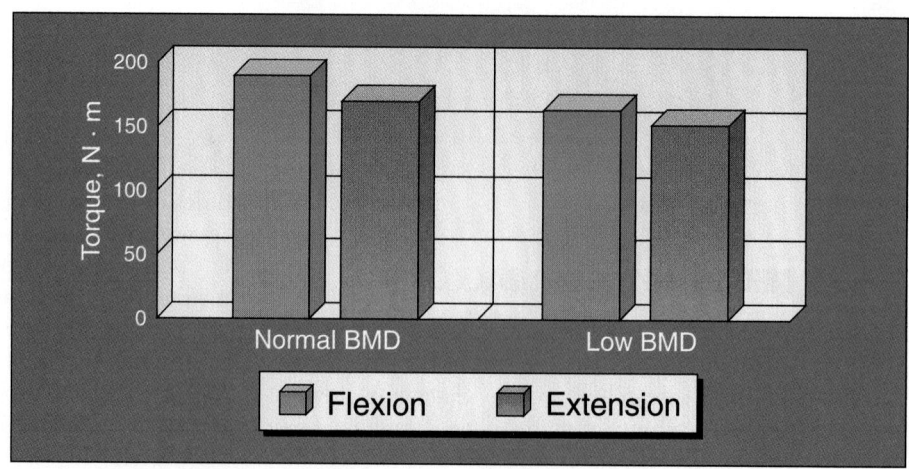

namometer. Figure 22.24 displays the results for chest flexion and extension strength in the two groups of women. The results were unequivocal: in 11 of 12 test comparisons for flexion, the women with normal BMD were about 20% stronger; in the extension tests, 4 of 12 comparisons were significantly higher, by 13%, in women without osteoporosis than in their counterparts with osteoporosis. These results demonstrate that differences in maximum dynamic strength among postmenopausal women may serve a clinically useful role in screening for osteoporosis. Recent data complement these findings and indicate that regional lean tissue mass (which often reflects muscular strength) is also a significant predictor of bone mineral density.[115]

DETRAINING

Limited data are available concerning the loss of muscle strength and associated factors with the cessation of resistance training. In one study of male power lifters, a 2-week detraining period caused a 12% loss in isokinetic eccentric muscle strength and a 6.4% reduction in the type II muscle fibers. No change was noted in type I fiber area.[71] Upon discontinuing a short period of resistance training in previously sedentary men, the improvements in muscular strength return to baseline values within several weeks. This relatively rapid strength loss has been attributed to a reversal of the neuromuscular and hormonal adaptations that occur as a result of training.[26] The encouraging news is that strength gains can be maintained even if training frequency is reduced to only one or two training sessions per week.[51]

METABOLIC STRESS OF RESISTANCE TRAINING

Although the various traditional resistance training methods are effective in enhancing a muscle's force-generating capacity, these exercises provide only minimal stimuli to improve aerobic capacity and reduce body fat and have little effect in improving one's blood-lipid profile and other heart disease risk factors.[63, 91, 104] In terms of cardiovascular function, a program of high-intensity, variable-resistance (Nautilus®) strength training produced no improvement in $\dot{V}O_2$max or submaximal exercise heart rate and stroke volume.[73] This lack of improvement is probably due to the relatively low "whole body" metabolic demand of standard resistance training exercises. For example, data obtained on young men during maximal isometric and 8- to 10-RM weightlifting exercises indicate that such exercise would be classified as only light to moderate in terms of heart rate response (generally less than 130 beats per minute) and oxygen uptake (about 3 to 4 METs).[109]

Undoubtedly, localized stress on specific muscles is considerable during resistance training. Owing to the brief activation period and relatively small muscle mass usually activated, however, the cardiovascular and aerobic metabolic demands are small compared to those of vigorous walking or running, swimming, cycling, or any other activity requiring the sustained use of a large muscle mass. Although a person may spend an hour or more completing a strength training workout, the total time spent in actual exercise is relatively small, usually no more than 6 or 7 minutes per hour! Clearly, traditional resistance training exercise should not make up the major portion of a program designed for cardiovascular improvement and weight control.

CIRCUIT RESISTANCE TRAINING

The caloric cost of exercise can be increased to bring about improvements in more than one aspect of fitness by modifying the standard approach to resistance training.[54, 172, 173] This approach, called **circuit resistance training,** or **CRT,** de-emphasizes the brief intervals of heavy-local muscle overload, providing for a more general conditioning to improve body composition, muscle strength and endurance, and cardiovascular fitness.[9, 84, 106] With this approach, a person lifts a weight between 40 and 55% of the 1-RM. The weight is then lifted as many times as possible for 30 seconds. After a 15-second rest, the participant moves to the next resistance exercise station and so on to complete the circuit. Between 8 and 15 exercise stations are usually used. (A modification that appears to result in similar energy expenditures during CRT is to employ exercise-to-rest ratios of 1:1 with either 15- or 30-second exercise periods.[10]) The circuit is repeated several times to allow for 30 to 50 minutes of continuous exercise. As strength increases, a new 1-RM is determined and the weight lifted is increased accordingly at each station.

This modification of standard resistance training is an attractive alternative for those desiring a generalized conditioning program. Medically supervised programs of CRT also have been effective for coronary-prone, cardiac, and spinal-cord-injured patients who desire a well-rounded fitness program using resistance exercises.[27, 87, 143] It also may provide supplemental off-season conditioning for athletes involved in sports that require high levels of strength, power, and muscular endurance.

Specificity of Aerobic Improvement. CRT is generally believed to be less effective for improving aerobic fitness than bicycle or run training.[47] CRT usually involves substantial upper body exercise, but the assessment of aerobic benefits of such training has utilized treadmill or bicycle tests that predominantly activate the lower body musculature. In one study, the effects of CRT on aerobic capacity were assessed using both treadmill running and arm-crank ergometry tests.[57] In keeping with the training specificity principle, aerobic capacity increased 7.8% with treadmill testing but 21.1% with arm cranking. These findings were particularly impressive because they were obtained without negative effects in a group of borderline hypertensives. CRT

TABLE 22.3
COMPARISON OF ENERGY EXPENDITURE FOR DIFFERENT MODES OF RESISTANCE EXERCISE[a]

Mode	Sex	kJ · min⁻¹	kcal · min⁻¹
Nautilus, circuit	M	29.7	7.1
	F	24.3	5.8
Nautilus, circuit	M	22.6	5.4
Universal, circuit	M	33.1	7.9
	F	28.5	6.8
Isokinetic, slow	M	40.2	9.6
Isokinetic, fast	M	41.4	9.9
Isometric and free-weight	M	25.1	6.0
Hydra-Fitness, circuit	M	37.7	9.0
Walking on level	M	22.6	5.4

Data from Katch, F.I., et al.: Evaluation of acute cardiorespiratory responses to hydraulic resistance exercise. *Med. Sci. Sports Exerc.*, 17:168, 1985.
[a]Based on a body weight of 68 kg.

produced a significant increase in muscular strength, a decrease in blood pressure, and a modest improvement in body composition.

ENERGY COST OF DIFFERENT METHODS OF RESISTANCE EXERCISE

A number of studies have evaluated the caloric cost of different forms of resistance exercise. Table 22.3 displays the resulting caloric expenditures, expressed per minute, for exercise performed using free weights, Nautilus® (eccentric), Universal Gym® (concentric/eccentric), Cybex® (isokinetic), and Hydra-Fitness® (hydraulic-concentric).

The results show that caloric expenditure for the hydraulic exercises averaged 9.0 kcal · min⁻¹ (37.7 kJ); this was approximately 35% higher than exercise with free weights, 29.4% greater than the average caloric cost based on exercise using Nautilus®, and 11.5% higher than circuit resistance exercise with Universal® equipment. The energy expenditure values for hydraulic exercise averaged about 6.4% less than slow- and fast-speed isokinetic circuit exercise. As a frame of comparison, the caloric cost is also presented for walking at a normal pace on a level surface.

MUSCLE SORENESS AND STIFFNESS

Following an extended layoff from exercise, most of us have experienced soreness and stiffness in the exercised joints and muscles. A temporary soreness may persist for several hours immediately after unaccustomed exercise,

whereas a residual soreness, or **delayed onset muscle soreness (DOMS),** may appear later and last for 3 or 4 days.[39] Any one of at least five factors may be the causative agent:

• Minute tears in the muscle tissue itself or damage to its contractile components,
• Osmotic pressure changes that cause retention of fluids in the surrounding tissues,
• Muscle spasms,
• Overstretching and perhaps tearing of portions of the muscle's connective tissue harness,
• Acute inflammation,
• Alteration in the cell's mechanism for calcium regulation, or
• A combination of the above factors.

Soreness Occurs Predominantly with Eccentric Actions

Although the precise cause of muscle soreness is unknown, the degree of discomfort depends to a large extent on the intensity and duration of effort and the type of exercise performed.[123, 159] It is not the absolute muscle force per se but rather the magnitude of active strain imposed on a muscle fiber that precipitates muscle damage and resulting soreness.[96] *Eccentric, and to some extent isometric, muscle actions generally cause the greatest postexercise discomfort, which is more apparent among older individuals.*[39, 103, 142, 148, 151a, 161] It does not appear that existing muscle damage or soreness from previous exercise exacerbates subsequent muscle damage or the repair process.[116a]

During one study, for which muscle soreness was rated by subjects both immediately after exercise and 24, 48, and 72 hours after exercise, soreness was greater when the exercise involved repeated high strain during active lengthening in eccentric actions than when it involved concentric and isometric actions. This effect did not relate to lactate buildup because high-intensity, level running (concentric actions) produced no residual soreness despite significant elevations in blood lactate. Downhill running (eccentric actions), on the other hand, caused moderate-to-severe DOMS with no elevation in lactate during exercise.

Actual Cell Damage

Running downhill at a −10° slope for 30 minutes produced significant DOMS 42 hours after exercise.[17] There also were corresponding increases in serum levels of the muscle-specific enzyme creatine kinase (CK) and myoglobin (Mb), both commonly used markers of muscle injury. (There is also a greater mobilization of leukocytes and neutrophils that are associated with the process of acute inflammation.[123]) The subjects then were retested on the same exercise after 3, 6, and 9 weeks. Figure 22.25 shows the perceived soreness rating for the leg muscles as a function of elapsed postexercise time for the three study durations. For the 3- and 6-week comparisons, the differences between bouts were significant, with diminished DOMS noted in the second trial (red squares). The patterns of results for CK and Mb were similar to the perception of muscle soreness. Interestingly, peak soreness ratings achieved at 48 hours did not relate to the absolute or relative changes in CK or Mb. This means that individuals reporting the greatest soreness did not necessarily have the highest CK and Mb values. These data agree with the findings of others that the first bout of repetitive, high-force

exercise may disrupt the integrity of the sarcolemma and produce temporary ultrastructural muscle damage in a pool of stress-susceptible or degenerating muscle fibers.[44, 64, 98] Particularly vulnerable are the fast-twitch fibers with low oxidative capacities.[43] Damage to these becomes more extensive several days after exercise than in the immediate postexercise period.[44, 119]

Cellular damage and accompanying soreness from eccentric exercise is associated with mitochondrial swelling as well as increases in the serum levels of cytosolic muscle enzymes and myoglobin. *Importantly, a single bout of exercise has a significant prophylactic effect on the development of muscle soreness in subsequent exercise, and this effect appears to last for as long as 6 weeks.*[17, 114] Such results support the wisdom of initiating a training program with light exercise to protect against the muscle soreness that is almost sure to follow an initial heavy-exercise bout containing an eccentric component. However, even prior lower-intensity exercise of specific muscles does not provide complete protection from subsequent soreness with more intense exercise.[24]

Table 22.4 displays the results for muscle soreness and CK activity following an exercise circuit of either concentric-only or concentric and eccentric muscle actions.[16] Group 1 performed three sets of 8 exercises (concentric-eccentric) at 60% of 1-RM on Universal Gym® equipment: one set was equal to 20 seconds of exercise followed by 40 seconds of rest; total exercise time was 24 minutes. Group 2 followed the same exercise protocol, but they exercised maximally for each repetition on hydraulic resistance devices (Hydra-Fitness®) that utilized concentric only actions. Blood samples and ratings of perceived muscle soreness were obtained before exercise and 5, 10, and 25 hours after exercise. The major difference in soreness ratings between exercise groups occurred 25 hours after exercise; the concentric-eccentric workout produced significantly higher perceived ratings of soreness for the major muscle groups exercised. For serum CK, the magnitude of the increase was the same between groups from 5 to 25 hours postexercise. Whereas both modes of exercise resulted in elevations in serum CK, the concentric-only muscle actions did not produce significant DOMS. This finding of no DOMS with concentric-only exercise has been reported by others.[28]

An Altered Sarcoplasmic Reticulum. Changes in pH, high-energy phosphate levels, ionic balance, or temperature with unaccustomed exercise can produce major alterations in the structure and function of the sarcoplasmic reticulum. This results in a depression in the rate of Ca^{2+} uptake and its rate of release, and an increase in the concentration of free Ca^{2+} as it rapidly moves into the cytosol of the damaged fibers. This overload in intra-cellular Ca^{2+} may contribute to the autolytic process that degrades both contractile and noncontractile structures within damaged muscle.[15, 98] This leads

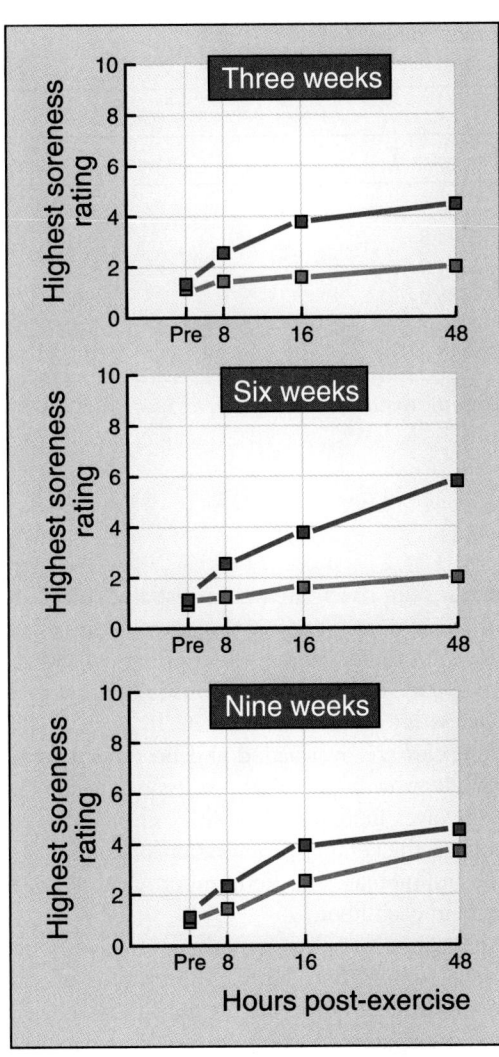

FIGURE 22.25

Highest soreness rating before and 6, 18, and 48 hours after exercise bout 1 *(blue square)* and exercise bout 2 *(red square)*, which is performed either 3, 6, or 9 weeks later. Similar results were obtained for creatine kinase and myoglobin. (From Byrnes, W.C., et al.: Delayed onset muscle soreness following repeated bouts of downhill running. *J. Appl. Physiol.*, 59:710, 1985.)

TABLE 22.4
ACUTE EFFECTS OF CONCENTRIC-ONLY AND CONCENTRIC-ECCENTRIC EXERCISE ON DELAYED ONSET MUSCLE SORENESS 25 HOURS AFTER EXERCISE[a]

	Soreness Ratings			Soreness Ratings	
Site	Concentric $\overline{X}$	Concentric-Eccentric $\overline{X}$	Site	Concentric $\overline{X}$	Concentric-Eccentric $\overline{X}$
Chest	2.3	5.1	Forearm (front)	1.7	3.4
Back (upper)	2.6	2.8	Forearm (back)	1.7	2.9
Shoulders (front)	2.2	3.6	Back (lower)	1.7	2.9
Shoulders (back)	1.9	3.6	Buttocks	1.8	2.5
Biceps (mid)	1.9	4.3	Quads (mid)	2.0	4.1
Biceps (lower)	1.8	3.5	Quads (lower)	2.1	3.8
Triceps (mid)	1.9	3.4	Hamstrings (mid)	2.1	3.5
Triceps (lower)	1.9	3.0	Hamstrings (lower)	2.1	3.0

		CK Activity ($mU \cdot mL^{-1}$)	
Sample time		Concentric $\overline{X}$	Concentric-Eccentric $\overline{X}$
Pre		86.7	126.9
5 h post		344.8	232.0
10 h post		394.3	368.5
25 h post		288.0	482.2
	Absolute increase	319.3	399.9
	Relative increase	435.6	355.4

From Byrnes, W.C.: Muscle soreness following resistance exercise with and without eccentric contractions. *Res. Q. Exerc. Sport*, 56:283, 1985.
[a]All differences between groups were statistically significant.

to a reduction in force-producing capability and eventual muscle soreness.

Current Model for DOMS. Figure 22.26 is a flow diagram that lists the probable steps in the development of DOMS and subsequent recuperation. An area of current controversy is whether the liberal use of nonsteroidal anti-inflammatory agents (e.g., flurbiprofen) as treatment for soft tissue injury or acute pain from DOMS is of any benefit (or harm) in the acute and long-term recuperative process.[110a]

■ SUMMARY ■

1. Muscle strength is largely determined by physiologic factors such as size and type of muscle fibers and by the anatomic-lever arrangement of bone and muscle. This strength capacity also is greatly affected by influences from the central nervous system that activate the prime movers in a specific action.
2. Genetic, exercise, nutritional, hormonal, environmental, and neural factors interact to regulate skeletal muscle mass and corresponding strength development.

3. Increases in strength with resistance training result from an improved capacity for motor unit recruitment, changes in the efficiency of the firing pattern of motor nerves, and significant alterations in the contractile elements within the muscle fiber itself.
4. As muscles are overloaded and become stronger, they normally grow larger. This process of muscle hypertrophy involves increased protein synthesis with resulting myofibril thickening, proliferation of connective tissue cells, and increases in the number of satellite cells that surround each fiber.
5. Muscle hypertrophy generally involves structural changes within the contractile apparatus of individual fibers, particularly the fast-twitch fibers, as well as increases in anaerobic energy stores. If new muscle fibers actually develop, their relative contribution to muscle enlargement is as yet undetermined.
6. Heavy resistance training does not induce adaptations in cellular components that would contribute to an enhanced aerobic energy transfer.
7. With short-term resistance training, strength improvements for women on a percentage basis are similar to

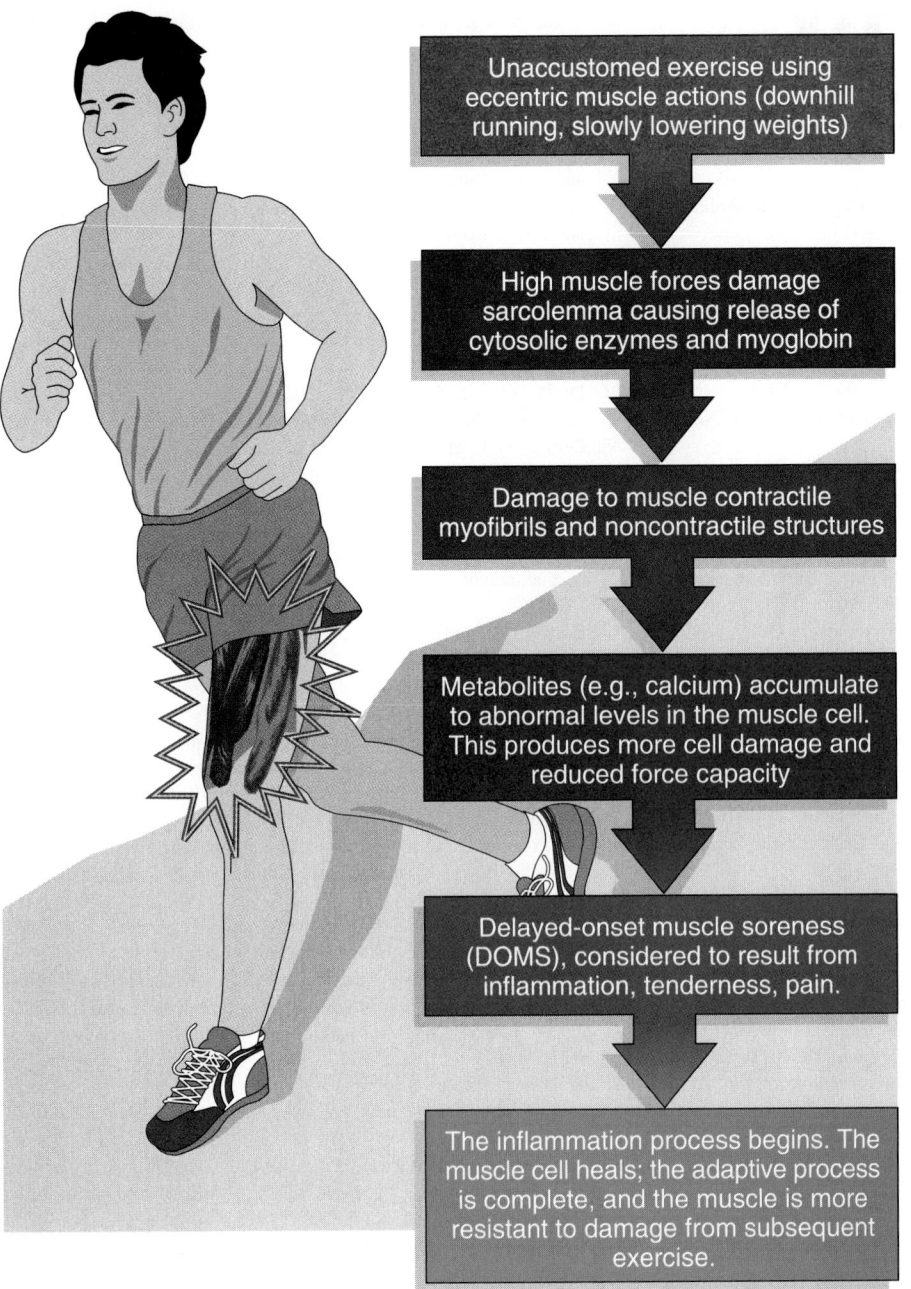

Unaccustomed exercise using eccentric muscle actions (downhill running, slowly lowering weights)

High muscle forces damage sarcolemma causing release of cytosolic enzymes and myoglobin

Damage to muscle contractile myofibrils and noncontractile structures

Metabolites (e.g., calcium) accumulate to abnormal levels in the muscle cell. This produces more cell damage and reduced force capacity

Delayed-onset muscle soreness (DOMS), considered to result from inflammation, tenderness, pain.

The inflammation process begins. The muscle cell heals; the adaptive process is complete, and the muscle is more resistant to damage from subsequent exercise.

FIGURE 22.26
Proposed sequence for the development of delayed-onset muscle soreness following unaccustomed exercise. Cellular adaptation to short-term exercise provides enhanced resistance to subsequent damage and pain.

those of men. Women also are capable of significant increases in muscle mass with resistance training.

8. Conventional resistance training exercises contribute little to the development of aerobic fitness. Because of the relatively low caloric cost of such exercises, they would not be effective, major activities in weight-reducing programs.

9. By employing lower resistance and higher repetitions, circuit resistance training offers an effective alternative for combining the muscle-training benefits of resistance exercise with the cardiovascular benefits of more continuous dynamic exercise.

10. Significantly greater delayed onset muscle soreness (DOMS) occurs with eccentric muscle actions compared to concentric-only or isometric actions, even though serum markers of muscle damage (such as creatine kinase and myoglobin) are elevated following all three modes of exercise.

11. A single bout of exercise has a significant protective effect on the development of muscle soreness and damage from subsequent exercise. This factor supports the wisdom of gradual progression when beginning an exercise program.

■ REFERENCES ■

1. Adams, G.R., et al.: Skeletal muscle myosin heavy chain composition and resistance training. *J. Appl. Physiol.*, 74:911, 1993.

2. Allerheiligen, W.B.: Speed development and plyometric training. In *Essentials of Strength Training and Conditioning.* T.R. Baechle (Ed.), Champaign, IL, Human Kinetics, 1994.

3. Alway, S.E., et al.: Functional and structural adaptations in skeletal muscle of trained athletes. *J. Appl. Physiol.*, 64:1114, 1988.

4. Alway, S.E., et al.: Contrasts in muscle and myofibers of elite male and female body builders. *J. Appl. Physiol.*, 67:24, 1989.

5. Antonio, J., and Gonyea, W.J.: Skeletal muscle fiber hyperplasia. *Med. Sci. Sports Exerc.*, 25:1333, 1993.

6. Antoino, J., and Gonyea, W.J.: Muscle fiber splitting in stretch-enlarged avian muscle. *Med. Sci. Sports Exerc.*, 26:973, 1994.

7. Åstrand, P.O., and Rodahl. K.: *Textbook of Work Physiology.* New York, McGraw-Hill, 1986.

8. Baker, D., et al.: Periodization: the effect on strength of manipulating volume and intensity. *J. Strength Cond. Res.*, 8:235, 1994.

9. Ballor, D.L., et al.: Metabolic response during hydraulic resistance exercise. *Med. Sci. Sports Exerc.*, 19:363, 1987.

10. Ballor, D.L., et al.: Physiological response to nine different exercise: rest protocols. *Med. Sci. Sports Exerc.*, 21:90, 1989.

11. Bergh, U.: The influence of body mass in cross-country skiing. *Med. Sci. Sports Exerc.*, 19:324, 1987.

12. Bergh, U., et al.: The relationship between body mass and oxygen uptake during running in humans. *Med. Sci. Sports Exerc.*, 23:205, 1991.

13. Boocock, M.G., et al.: Changes in stature following drop jumping and post-exercise gravity inversion. *Med. Sci. Sports Exerc.*, 22:385, 1990.

14. Braith, R.W., et al.: Effect of training on the relationship between maximal and submaximal strength. *Med. Sci. Sports Exerc.*, 25:132, 1993.

15. Byrd, S.K.: Alterations in the sarcoplasmic reticulum: a possible link to exercise-induced muscle damage. *Med. Sci. Sports Exerc.*, 24:531, 1992.

16. Byrnes, W.C.: Muscle soreness following resistance exercise with and without eccentric contractions. *Res. Q. Exer. Sport*, 56:283, 1985.

17. Byrnes, W.C., et al.: Delayed onset muscle soreness following repeated bouts of downhill running. *J. Appl. Physiol.*, 59:710, 1985.

18. Campbell, K.: Biomechanics of pitching. In *Proceedings of the 11th Symposium of the International Society of Sport Biomechanics: Biomechanics XI.* University of Massachusetts, Amherst, 1993.

19. Castro, M.J., et al.: Peak torque per unit cross-sectional area differs between strength-trained and untrained young adults. *Med. Sci. Sports Exerc.*, 27:397, 1995.

20. Charette, S.L., et al.: Muscle hypertrophy response to resistance training in older women. *J. Appl. Physiol.*, 70:912, 1991.

21. Cho, D.A.: Plyometric exercise. *NSCA Journal*, 5:56, 1984.

22. Clarke, D.H.: Adaptations in strength and muscular endurance resulting from exercise. In *Exercise and Sport Science Reviews.* Vol. 1, J.H. Wilmore (Ed.). New York, Academic Press, 1973.

23. Clarke, D.H., and Clarke, H.H.: *Research Processes in Physical Education, Recreation, and Health.* Englewood Cliffs, N.J., Prentice-Hall, 1984.

24. Clarkson, P.M., and Tremblay, I.: Exercise induced muscle damage, repair, and adaptation in humans. *J. Appl. Physiol.*, 65:1, 1988.

25. Coggan, A.R., et al.: Skeletal muscle adaptations to endurance training in 60- to 70-yr old men and women. *J. Appl. Physiol.*, 72:1780, 1992.

26. Colliander, E.B., and Tesch, P.A.: Effects of detraining following short term resistance training on eccentric and concentric muscle strength. *Acta Physiol. Scand.*, 144:23, 1992.

27. Cooney, M.M., and Walker, J.B.: Hydraulic resistance exercise benefits cardiovascular fitness in spinal cord injured. *Med. Sci. Sports Exerc.*, 18:522, 1986.

28. Cote, C., et al.: Isokinetic strength training protocols: do they induce skeletal muscle fiber hypertrophy? *Arch. Phys. Med. Rehab.*, 69:281, 1988.

29. Coyle, E.F., et al.: Leg extension power and muscle fiber composition. *Med. Sci. Sports*, 11:12, 1979.

30. Coyle, E.F., et al.: Specificity of power improvements through slow and fast isokinetic training. *J. Appl. Physiol.*, 51:1437, 1981.

31. Cureton, K.J., et al.: Muscle hypertrophy in men and women. *Med. Sci. Sports Exerc.* 20:338, 1988.

32. DeLorme, T.L., and Watkins, A.L.: *Progressive Resistance Exercise.* New York, Appleton-Century-Crofts, 1951.

33. Duchateau, J., and Hainaut, K.: Isometric or dynamic training: differentiated effects on mechanical properties of human muscle. *J. Appl. Physiol.*, 56:296, 1984.

34. Dudley, G., and Djamil, R.: Incompatibility of endurance and strength training modes of exercise. *J. Appl. Physiol.*, 59:1446, 1985.

35. Dudley, G.A., et al.: Importance of eccentric actions in performance adaptations to resistance training. *Aviat. Space Environ. Med.* 62:543, 1991.

36. Edström, L., and Ekblom, B.: Differences in sizes of red and white muscle fibers in vastus lateralis of musculus quadriceps femoris of normal individuals and athletes. *Scand. J. Clin. Lab. Invest.*, 30:175, 1972.

37. Edström L., and Grimby, L.: Effects of exercise on the motor unit. *Muscle Nerve*, 9:104, 1986.

38. Enoka, R.: *Neuromechanical Basis of Kinesiology.* Champaign, IL, Human Kinetics, 1988.

39. Evans, W.J., and Cannon, J.G.: The metabolic effects of exercise-induced muscle damage. *Exerc. Sport Sci. Rev.*, 19:99, 1991.

40. Fiatarone, A., et al.: High-intensity strength training in nonagenarians. *JAMA*, 263:3029, 1990.

41. Fiatarone, M.A., et al.: Exercise training and nutritional supplementation for physical frailty in very elderly people. *N. Engl. J. Med.*, 330:1769, 1994.

42. Foster, D.N., et al.: Effect of training frequency on lumbar extension strength. *Med. Sci. Sports Exerc.*, 21:S88, 1989.

43. Frieden, J., and Lieber, R.L.: Structural and mechanical basis of exercise-induced muscle injury. *Med. Sci. Sports Exerc.*, 24:521, 1992.

44. Friden, J., et al.: Myofibrillar damage following eccentric exercise in man. *Int. J. Sports Med.*, 4:170, 1983.

45. Frontera, W.R., et al.: Strength conditioning in older men: skeletal muscle hypertrophy and improved function. *J. Appl. Physiol.*, 64:1038, 1988.

46. Garhammer, J., and Takano, B.: Training for weightlifting. In *Strength And Power In Sport.* P.V. Komi, (Ed.), Oxford, Blackwell Scientific Publications. 1993.

47. Gettman, L.R.: Physiologic effects on adult men of circuit strength training and jogging. *Arch. Phys. Med. Rehab.*, 60:115, 1979.

48. Goldberg, A.L., et al.: Mechanism of work-induced hypertrophy of skeletal muscle. *Med. Sci. Sports*, 7:185, 1975.

49. Gollnick, P.D., et al.: Effect of training on enzyme activity and fiber composition of human skeletal muscle. *J. Appl. Physiol.*, 34:107, 1973.

50. Gonyea, W.J., et al.: Exercise induced increases in muscle fiber number. *Eur. J. Appl. Physiol.*, 55:137, 1986.

51. Graves, J.E., et al.: Effect of reduced training frequency on muscular strength. *Int. J. Sports Med.*, 9:316, 1988.

52. Graves, J.E., et al.: Specificity of limited range of motion variable resistance training. *Med. Sci. Sports Exerc.*, 21:84, 1989.

53. Gunther, B.: Dimensional analysis and theory of biological similarity. *Phys. Rev.*, 55:659, 1975.

54. Haennel, R., et al.: Effects of hydraulic circuit training on cardiovascular function. *Med. Sci. Sports Exerc.*, 21:605, 1989.

55. Harmon, E.A.: Resistive torque analysis of 5 Nautilus exercise machines. *Med. Sci. Sports Exerc.*, 15:113, 1983.

56. Harmon, E.A., et al.: Effect of a belt on intra-abdominal pressure during weight lifting. *Med. Sci. Sports Exerc.*, 21:186, 1989.

57. Harris, K.A., and Holly, R.G.: Physiological response to circuit weight training in borderline hypertensive subjects. *Med. Sci. Sports Exerc.*, 19:246, 1987.

58. Hather, B.M., et al.: Influence of eccentric actions on skeletal muscle adaptations to resistance training. *Acta Physiol. Scand.*, 143:177, 1991.

59. Hay, J.G., et al.: Effects of lifting rate on elbow torques exerted during arm curl exercise. *Med. Sci. Sports Exerc.*, 15:63, 1983.

60. Hennessy, L.C., and Watson, A.W.S.: The interference effects of training for strength and endurance simultaneously. *J. Strength Cond. Res.*, 8:12, 1994.

61. Hettinger, T.L., and Muller, E.A.: Muskelleistung und muskeltraining. *Int. Z. Angew. Physiol.*, 15:111, 1953.

62. Heyward, V.H., et al.: Gender differences in strength. *Res. Q. Exerc. Sport*, 57:154, 1986.

63. Hickson, R.C., et al.: Strength training effects on aerobic power and short-term endurance. *Med. Sci. Sports Exerc.*, 12:336, 1980.

64. Hikida, R.S., et al.: Muscle fiber necrosis associated with marathon running. *J. Neurol. Sci.*, 59:185, 1983.

65. Ho, K.W., et al.: Skeletal muscle fiber splitting with weight-lifting exercises in rats. *Am. J. Anat.*, 157:433, 1980.

66. Hochschuler, S.: *Back In Shape*. Boston, Houghton Mifflin Co., 1991.

67. Hortobágyi, T., and Katch, F.I.: Role of concentric force in limiting improvement in muscular strength. *J. Appl. Physiol.*, 68:650, 1990.

68. Hortobágyi, T., et al.: Day-to-day reliability for measures of force, velocity, power, peak time and rise time during isokinetic and isotonic squat and bench press exercise. *J. Appl. Sport Sci. Res.*, 2:56, 1988.

69. Hortobágyi, T., et al.: Interrelationships among various measures of upper body strength assessed by different contraction modes. *Eur. J. Appl. Physiol.*, 58:749, 1989.

70. Hortobágyi, T., et al.: Effects of simultaneous training for strength and endurance on upper and lower body strength and running performance. *J. Sports Med. Phys. Fitness*, 31:20, 1991.

71. Hortobágyi, T., et al.: The effects of detraining on power athletes. *Med. Sci. Sports Exerc.*, 25:929, 1993.

72. Housh, T., et al.: Anthropometric estimation of muscle group cross-sectional area. *J. Strength Cond. Res.*, 7:250, 1993.

73. Hurley, B.F., et al.: Effects of high intensity strength training on cardiovascular function. *Med. Sci. Sports Exerc.*, 16:483, 1984.

74. Häkkinen, K., and Komi, P.V.: Electromyographic changes during strength training and detraining. *Med. Sci. Sports Exerc.*, 15:455, 1983.

75. Häkkinen, K., et al.: Effect of explosive type strength training on isometric force- and relaxation-time, electromyographic and muscle fiber characteristics of leg extensor muscles. *Acta Physiol. Scand.*, 125:587, 1985.

76. Häkkinen, K., et al.: Neuromuscular and hormonal adaptations in athletes to strength training in two years. *J. Appl. Physiol.*, 65:2406, 1988.

77. Ikai, M., and Fukunaga, T.: Calculation of muscle strength per unit cross-sectional area of a human muscle by means of ultrasonic measurements. *Int. Z. Angew. Physiol.*, 26:26, 1968.

78. Ikai, M., and Steinhaus, A.H.: Some factors modifying the expression of human strength. *J. Appl. Physiol.*, 16:157, 1961.

79. Jackson, A.S.: Preemployment physical evaluation. *Exerc. Sport Sci. Rev.*, 22:55, 1994.

80. Janney, C., et al.: Maximum muscular strength differs in postmenopausal women with and without osteoporosis. *Med. Sci. Sports Exerc.* (abstract), 19:561, 1987.

81. Johnson, B.L., et al.: A comparison of concentric and eccentric muscle training. *Med. Sci. Sports*, 8:35, 1976.

82. Jones, D.A., and Rutherford, O.M.: Human muscle strength training: the effects of three different regimes and the nature of the resultant changes. *J. Physiol.*, 391:1, 1987.

83. Kanehisa, H., and Miyashita, M.: Specificity of velocity in strength training. *Eur. J. Appl. Physiol.*, 52:104, 1983.

84. Katch, F.I., et al.: Evaluation of acute cardiorespiratory responses to hydraulic resistance exercise. *Med. Sci. Sports Exerc.*, 17:168, 1985.

85. Katch, V.L.: Use of the oxygen/body weight ratio in correlational analyses: spurious correlations and statistical considerations. *Med. Sci. Sports Exerc.*, 5:253, 1973.

86. Katch, V.L., and Katch, F.I.: Use of weight-adjusted oxygen uptake scores that avoid spurious correlations. *Res. Q.*, 45:447, 1974.

87. Kelemen, M.H.: Resistance training safety and assessment guidelines for cardiac and coronary prone patients. *Med. Sci. Sports Exerc.*, 21:675, 1989.

88. Keller, B.: The influence of body size variables on gender differences in strength and maximum aerobic capacity. Unpublished doctoral dissertation, University of Massachusetts, Amherst, 1989.

89. Kitai, T.A., et al.: Specificity of joint angle in isometric training. *Eur. J. Appl. Physiol.*, 58:744, 1989.

90. Knapik, J.J., et al.: Angular specificity and test mode specificity of isometric and isokinetic strength training. *J. Orthop. Sports Phys. Ther.*, 5:58, 1983.

91. Kokkinos, P.F., et al.: Strength training does not improve lipoprotein-lipid profiles in men at risk for CHD. *Med. Sci. Sports Exerc.*, 23:1134, 1991.

92. Kraemer, W.J., et al.: Changes in hormonal concentrations after different heavy-resistance exercise protocols in women. *J. Appl. Physiol.*, 75:594, 1993.

92a. Kraemer, W.J., et al.: Compatibility of high-intensity strength and endurance training on hormonal and skeletal muscle adaptations. *J. Appl. Physiol.*, 78:976, 1995.

93. LaChance, P.F., et al.: Day-to-day reliability during high and low resistance bi-directional hydraulic exercise. *J. Appl. Sport Sci. Res.*, 2:57, 1988.

94. LaGasse, P., et al.: Neuromuscular facilitation of muscle tension output by reciprocal muscle work. *Ann. French-Canadian Assoc. Adv. Sciences*, 50:222, 1983.

95. Lees, A.: Methods of impact force absorption when landing from a jump. *Engineering Med.*, 10:207, 1981.

96. Lieber, R.L., and Fridén, J.: Muscle damage is not a function of muscle force but active muscle strain. *J. Appl. Physiol.*, 74:520, 1993.

97. Lindh, M.: Increase of muscle strength from isometric quadriceps exercises at different knee angles. *Scand. J. Rehabil. Med.*, 11:36, 1979.

98. Lowe, D.A., et al.: Eccentric contraction-induced injury of mouse soleus muscle: effect of varying $[Ca^{++}]$. *J. Appl. Physiol.*, 76:1445, 1994.

99. MacDougall, J.D.: Morphological changes in human skeletal muscle following strength training and immobilization. In *Human Muscle Power*. N.L. Jones et al. (Eds.), Champaign, IL, Human Kinetics, 1986.

100. MacDougall, J.D., et al.: Muscle ultrastructural characteristics of the elite powerlifters and bodybuilders. *Med. Sci. Sports*, 2:131, 1980.

101. MacDougall, J.D., et al.: Muscle fiber number in biceps brachii in bodybuilders and control subjects. *J. Appl. Physiol.*, 57:1399, 1984.

101a. Mayhew, T.P., et al.: Muscular adaptation to concentric and eccentric exercise at equal power levels. *Med. Sci. Sports Exerc.*, 27:868, 1995.

102. Malmivaara, A., et al.: The treatment of acute low back pain—bed rest, exercises, or ordinary activity. *N. Eng. J. Med.*, 332:351, 1995.

103. Manfredi, T.G., et al.: Serum creatine kinase activity and exercise-induced muscle damage in older men. *Med. Sci. Sports Exerc.*, 23:1028, 1991.

104. Manning, J.M., et al.: Effects of a resistive training program on lipoprotein-lipid levels in obese women. *Med. Sci. Sports Exerc.*, 23:1222, 1991.

105. Manning, R.M., et al: Constant vs variable resistance knee extension training. *Med. Sci. Sports Exerc.*, 22:397, 1990.

106. Marcinik, E.J., et al.: Aerobic/calisthenic and aerobic/circuit weight training for Navy men: a comparative study. *Med. Sci. Sports Exerc.*, 17:482, 1985.

107. Masterson, G., and Brown, S.P.: Effects of weighted rope jump training on power performance tests in collegians. *J. Strength Cond. Res.,* 7:108, 1993.

108. Mateyev, L.: *aPeriodisierang des Sportlichen Training.* Berlin, Berles & Wernitz, 1972.

109. McArdle, W.D., and Foglia, G.F.: Energy cost and cardiorespiratory stress of isometric and weight training exercises. *J. Sports Med. Phys. Fitness,* 9:23, 1969.

110. Miller, A.E.J., et al.: Gender differences in strength and muscle fiber characteristics. *Eur. J. Appl. Physiol.,* 66:254, 1993.

110a. Mishra, D.K., et al.: Anti-inflammatory medication after muscle injury. *J. Bone Joint Surg.,* 77-A:1510, 1995.

111. Moritani, T., and DeVries, H.: Neural factors versus hypertrophy in the time course of muscle strength gain. *Am. J. Phys. Med.,* 58:115, 1979.

111a. Morrissey, M.C., et al.: Resistance training modes: specificity and effectiveness. *Med. Sci. Sports Exerc.,* 27:648, 1995.

112. Morrow, J.R., Jr., and Hosler, W.W.: Strength comparisons in untrained men and trained women. *Med. Sci. Sports Exerc.,* 13:194, 1981.

113. Nevill, A.M., et al.: Scaling physiological measurements for individuals of different body size. *Eur. J. Appl. Physiol.,* 65:110, 1992.

114. Newham, D.J., et al.: Repeated high force eccentric exercise; effects on muscle pain and damage. *J. Appl. Physiol.,* 63:1381, 1987.

115. Nichols, D.L., et al.: Relationship of regional body composition to bone mineral density in college females. *Med. Sci. Sports Exerc.,* 27:178, 1995.

116. Nindl, B.C., et al.: The validity of using strength scores divided by fat-free body mass to compare lifting capacities of men and women. *J. Strength Cond. Res.,* 7:183, 1993.

116a. Nosaka, K., and Clarkson, P.M.: Muscle damage following repeated bouts of high force eccentric exercise. *Med. Sci. Sports Exerc.,* 27:1263, 1995.

117. O'Bryant, H.S., et al.: Cycle ergometer performance and maximum leg and hip strength adaptations to two different methods of weight training. *J. Appl. Sport Sci. Res.,* 2:27, 1988.

117a. O'Hagan, F.T., et al.: Comparative effectiveness of accommodating and weight resistance training modes. *Med. Sci. Sports Exerc.,* 27:1210, 1995.

118. Ozmun, J.C., et al.: Neuromuscular adaptations following prepubescent strength training. *Med. Sci. Sports Exerc.,* 26:510, 1994.

119. Paul, G.L.: Serum and urinary markers of skeletal muscle tissue damage after weight lifting exercise. *Eur. J. Appl. Physiol.,* 58:786, 1989.

120. Pavone, E., and Moffat, M.: Isometric torque of the quadriceps femoris after concentric, eccentric and isometric training. *Arch. Phys. Med. Rehabil.,* 66:168, 1985.

121. Petersen, S.R., et al.: The influence of isokinetic concentric resistance training on concentric and eccentric torque outputs and cross-sectional area of the quadriceps femoris. *Can. J. Sport Sci.,* 13:76, 1988.

122. Pipes, T.V., and Wilmore, J.H.: Isokinetic vs. isotonic strength training in adult men. *Med. Sci. Sports,* 7:262, 1975.

123. Pizza, F.X., et al.: Exercise-induced muscle damage: effect on circulating leukocyte and lymphocyte subsets. *Med. Sci. Sports Exerc.,* 27:363, 1995.

124. Ploutz, L.L., et al.: Effect of resistance training on muscle use during exercise. *J. Appl. Physiol.,* 76:1675, 1994.

125. Pollock, M.L., et al.: Effect of resistance training on lumbar extension strength. *Am. J. Sports Med.,* 17:624, 1989.

126. Rians, C.B., et al.: Strength training for prepubescent males: is it safe? *Am. J. Sports Med.,* 15:483, 1987.

127. Roman, W.J., et al.: Adaptations in the elbow flexors of elderly males after heavy-resistance training. *J. Appl. Physiol.,* 74:750, 1993.

128. Ross, W.D., and Marfell-Jones, M.J.: Kinanthropometry. In *Physiological Testing of the Elite Athlete.* J.D. MacDougall, et al. (Eds.), Canadian Association of Sport Sciences, Sport Medicine Council of Canada, 1982.

129. Roy, M.A., et al.: Changes in alpha motoneuron excitability following isokinetic training in sedentary males and females. *Can. J. Appl. Sport Sci.,* 9:20P, 1984.

130. Roy, R.R., et al.: The plasticity of skeletal muscle: effects of neuromuscular activity. In *Exercise and Sport Sciences Reviews.* Vol. 19, J.O. Holloszy (Ed.), Baltimore, Williams & Wilkins, 1991.

131. Sale, D.G.: Influence of exercise and training on motor unit activation. In *Exercise and Sport Sciences Reviews.* Vol. 15, K.B. Pandolf (Ed.), New York, Macmillan, 1987.

132. Sale, D.G.: Neural adaptations to resistance training. *Med. Sci. Sports Exerc.,* 20:S135, 1988.

133. Sale, D.G., et al.: Effect of strength training upon motoneuron excitability in man. *Med. Sci. Sports Exerc.,* 15:57, 1983.

134. Salleo, A., et al.: New muscle fiber production during compensatory hypertrophy. *Med. Sci. Sports,* 12:268, 1980.

135. Schantz, P.G., and Källman, M.: NADH shuttle enzymes and cytochrome b_5 reductase in human skeletal muscle: effect of strength training. *J. Appl. Physiol.,* 67:123, 1989.

136. Schmidtbleicher, D.: Training for power events. In *Strength and Power in Sport.* P.V. Komi, (Ed.), Oxford, Blackwell Scientific Publications, 1993.

137. Sergo, C., and Boatwright, D.: Training methods using various weighted bats on the effects on bat velocity. *J. Strength Cond. Res.,* 7:115, 1993.

138. Sewall, L., and Michelli, L.J.: Strength training for children. *J. Pediatr. Orthop.,* 6:143, 1986.

139. Sipalä, S., and Suominen, H.: Effects of strength and endurance training on thigh and leg muscle mass and composition in elderly women. *J. Appl. Physiol.,* 78:334, 1995.

140. Sjöström, M., et al.: Evidence of fiber hyperplasia in human skeletal muscles from healthy young men. *Eur. J. Appl. Physiol.,* 62:301, 1992.

141. Smith, J.L., et al.: Rapid ankle extension during paw shakes. Selective recruitment of fast ankle extensors. *J. Neurophysiol.,* 43:612, 1980.

142. Smith, L.L.: Acute inflammation: the underlying mechanism in delayed onset muscle soreness. *Med. Sci. Sports Exerc.,* 23:542, 1991.

143. Sparling, P.S., and Cantwell, J.A.: Strength training guidelines for cardiac patients. *Phys. Sportsmed.,* 17:191, 1989.

144. Staff, P.H.: The effects of physical activity on joints, cartilage, tendons, and ligaments. *Scand. J. Soc. Med.,* 29(Suppl.):59, 1982.

145. Starron, R.S., et al.: Muscle hypertrophy and fast fiber type conversions in heavy resistance-trained women. *Eur. J. Appl. Physiol.,* 60:71, 1990.

146. Staron, R.S., et al.: Strength and skeletal muscle adaptations in heavy-resistance-trained women after detraining and retraining. *J. Appl. Physiol.,* 70:631, 1991.

147. Staron, R.S., et al.: Skeletal muscle adaptations during the early phase of heavy-resistance training in men and women. *J. Appl. Physiol.,* 76:1247, 1994.

148. Stauber, W.T.: Eccentric action of muscles: physiology, injury, and adaptation. In *Exercise and Sport Sciences Reviews.* Vol. 17, K.B. Pandolf (Ed.), New York, Macmillan, 1989.

149. Stock, J.L., et al.: Dynamic muscle strength is decreased in postmenopausal women with low bone density. *J. Bone Min. Res.,* 2:338, 1987.

150. Stone, M.H.: Implications for connective tissue and bone alterations resulting from resistance exercise training. *Med. Sci. Sports Exerc.,* 20:S162, 1988.

151. Taylor, C.R., et al.: Scaling and energetic cost of running to body size in mammals. *Am J. Physiol.,* 219:1104, 1970.

151a. Teague, B.N., and Schwane, J.A.: Effect of intermittent eccentric contractions on symptoms of muscle microinjury. *Med. Sci. Sports Exerc.,* 27:1378, 1995.

152. Ter Haar Romeny, B.M., et al.: Relation between location of a motor unit in the human biceps brachii and its critical firing levels for different tasks. *Exp. Neurol.,* 85:631, 1984.

153. Tesch, P.A.: Enzyme activities of FT and ST muscle fibers in heavy-resistance trained athletes. *J. Appl. Physiol.,* 83:67, 1989.

154. Tesch, P.A., and Karlsson, J.: Muscle fiber types and size in trained and untrained muscles of elite athletes. *J. Appl. Physiol.*, 59:1716, 1985.

155. Tesch, P.A., and Larsson, L.: Muscle hypertrophy in body builders. *Eur. J. Appl. Physiol.*, 49:301, 1982.

156. Tesch, P.A., et al.: Muscle capillary supply and fiber type characteristics in weight and power lifters. *J. Appl. Physiol.*, 56:35, 1984.

157. Thorstensson, A.: Muscle strength, fiber types and enzyme activities in man. *Acta Physiol. Scand.*, Suppl. 443, 1976.

158. Thorstensson, A., et al.: Force-velocity relations and fiber composition in human knee extensor muscles. *J. Appl. Physiol.*, 40:12, 1976.

159. Tiidus, P.M., and Ianuzzo, C.D.: Effects of intensity and duration of muscular exercise on delayed soreness and serum enzyme activities. *Med. Sci. Sports Exerc.*, 15:461, 1983.

160. Tittel, K., And Wutscherk, H.: Anthropometric Factors. In *Strength And Power In Sport*. P.V. Komi (Ed.), Oxford, Blackwell Scientific Publications, 1993.

161. Triffletti, P., et al.: Creatine kinase and muscle soreness after repeated isometric exercise. *Med. Sci. Sports Exerc.*, 20:242, 1988.

162. Vailas, A.C., and Vailas, J.C.: Physical activity and connective tissue. In *Physical Activity, Fitness, and Health*. C. Bouchard et al. (Eds.), Champaign, IL, Human Kinetics, 1994.

163. Van Etten, L.M.L.A., et al.: Effect of body build on weight-training-induced adaptations in body composition and muscular strength. *Med. Sci. Sports Exerc.*, 26:515, 1994.

164. Vanderburgh, P.M., and Katch, F.I.: Ratio scaling of VO₂max penalizes women with larger percent body fat but not lean body mass. *Med. Sci. Sports Exerc.* (In press, 1996).

165. Vanderburgh, P.M., and Mahar, M.T.: Scaling of two-mile run times by body weight and fat-free weight in college-age men. *J. Strength Cond. Res.*, 92:67, 1995.

166. Vanderburgh, P.M., et al.: Allometric scaling of grip strength by body mass in college-age men and women. *Res. Q. Exerc. Sport*, 85:80, 1995.

167. Wathan, D.: Periodization: concepts and applications. In *Essentials of Strength Training and Conditioning*. T.R. Baechle (Ed.), Champaign, IL, Human Kinetics, 1994.

168. Weir, J.P., et al.: Electromyographic evaluation of joint angle specificity and cross-training after isometric training. *J. Appl. Physiol.*, 77:1927, 1994.

169. Weir, J.P., et al.: The effect of rest interval length on repeated maximal bench press. *J. Strength Cond. Res.*, 8:58, 1994.

170. Weltman, A., et al.: The effects of hydraulic resistance strength training in pre-pubertal males. *Med. Sci. Sports Exerc.*, 18:629, 1986.

171. Willoughby, D.: The effects of mesocycle-length weight training programs involving periodization and partially equated volumes on upper and lower body strength. *J. Strength. Cond. Res.*, 7:2, 1993.

172. Wilmore, J.H., et al.: Energy cost of circuit weight training. *Med. Sci. Sports*, 10:75, 1978.

173. Wilmore, J.H., et al.: Physiological alterations consequent to circuit weight training. *Med. Sci. Sports*, 10:79, 1978.

174. Winter, E.M.: Scaling: partitioning out differences in size. *Ped. Exerc. Sci.*, 4:296, 1992.

175. Winter, E.M., and Maughan, R.J.: Strength and cross-sectional area of the quadriceps in men and women. *J. Physiol (London)*, 438:175, 1991.

176. Wolpaw, J.R.: Acquisition and maintenance of the simplest motor skill: investigation of CNS mechanisms. *Med. Sci. Sports Exerc.*, 26:1475, 1994.

177. Wong, T.S., and Booth, F.W.: Protein metabolism in rat tibialis anterior muscle after stimulated chronic eccentric exercise. *J. Appl. Physiol.*, 69:1718, 1990.

178. Yarasheski, K.E., et al.: Acute effects of resistance exercise on muscle protein synthesis in young and elderly adults. *Am. J. Physiol.*, 265:E210, 1993.

Costill, D.L., et. al.: Effects of caffeine ingestion on metabolism and exercise performance. *Med. Sci. Sports.* 10:155, 1978.

The potential ergogenic benefits of various substances and procedures have always interested sports competitors and exercise physiologists. Costill and coworkers tested the hypothesis that in-

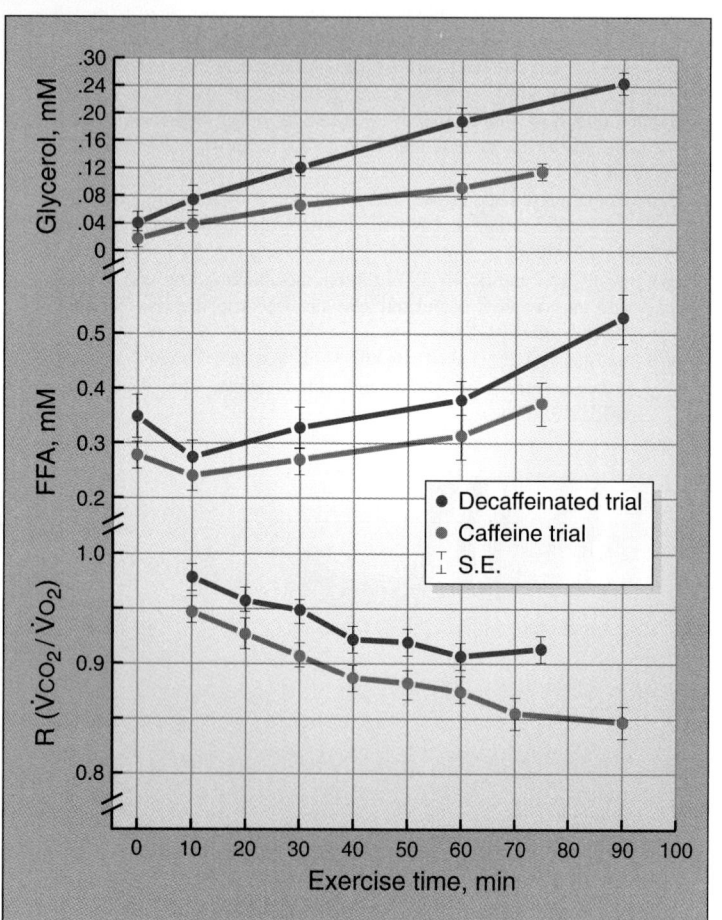

Average values for plasma glycerol, free fatty acids (FFA) and the respiratory exchange ratio (R) during endurance exercise trials after ingestion of caffeine and decaffeinated liquid.

gesting caffeine stimulated free fatty acid (FFA) mobilization, retarded the depletion of muscle glycogen, and consequently enhanced endurance exercise performance. Previous research with animals and humans demonstrated that elevating plasma FFA spared muscle glycogen and extended the exercise capacity. FFA typically became elevated when injecting heparin, a substance that

stimulated increases in FFA mobilization and subsequent oxidation. Because caffeine mobilizes FFA, its effects were tested on muscle glycogen sparing and endurance performance in humans.

Subjects were two female and seven male competitive cyclists (average $\dot{V}O_2$max of 60 mL · kg^{-1} · min^{-1}) who performed a cycle ergometer $\dot{V}O_2$max test and two additional exercise trials separated by 3 days while consuming the same diet. In one trial, subjects consumed 200 mL of hot water containing 5 g decaffeinated (D) coffee 60 minutes before the exercise trial. The cycling test continued as long as possible at a work rate of 80% $\dot{V}O_2$max. In the other trial, subjects consumed a hot drink containing 5 g decaffeinated coffee and 330 mg of caffeine (C) 60 minutes before the cycle ergometer test. The amount of C equaled that contained in 2.5 cups of percolated coffee. The subjects were unaware of the experiment's purpose, and test order was randomized for the D and C trials. Blood samples were taken before and during each trial; blood analysis included lactate, FFA, glycerol, glucose, and triglyceride. In addition, respiratory gas exchange was determined throughout testing, and the respiratory quotient (RQ) was computed to evaluate the non-protein metabolic mixture.

The figure displays the major findings of the study. Total exercise time to exhaustion increased 19.5% during trial C compared to trial D. In C, subjects performed an average of 90.2 minutes compared to a significantly shorter 75.5 minutes without caffeine. Although FFA did not differ significantly between conditions, the caffeinated drink produced significantly higher plasma glycerol levels and significantly lower RQ values (indicated as R in the researchers' figure) at all time comparisons. Using the RQ values enabled the researchers to calculate carbohydrate oxidation during the exercise (about 240 g of carbohydrate in both exercise trials). In contrast, lipid oxidation in C (118 g) exceeded that in D (57 g). Subjects also perceived the exercise as easier in the C condition.

This research demonstrated that caffeine ingestion increased the rate of lipolysis during sustained exercise. An increased rate of lipolysis could spare liver and skeletal muscle glycogen depletion during exercise and subsequently enhance performance. Subsequent research has clarified the role of caffeine in endurance performance (see pages 461 to 463).

Special Aids to Performance and Conditioning

Considerable literature exists on the topic of ergogenic aids and athletic performance. (*Ergogenic* refers to the application of a nutritional, physical, mechanical, psychologic, or pharmacologic procedure or aid to improve physical work capacity or athletic performance.) This literature includes studies of the potential performance benefits of alcohol, amphetamines, hormones, carbohydrates, proteins, additional red blood cells, caffeine, phosphates, oxygen-rich breathing mixtures, massage, wheat-germ oil, vitamins, minerals, ionized air, music, hypnosis, and even marijuana and cocaine! Only a few of these alleged aids, however, are used routinely by athletes, and only a few cause real controversy. Of specific interest are the use of anabolic steroids and other exogenous hormones and amphetamines and the unique procedure of "blood doping." Because warm-up and oxygen inhalation are commonly used to enhance performance, we also include these in our discussion of the effectiveness and practicality of ergogenic aids for human physiology and exercise performance. Nutritional requirements of the macro and micronutrients for active individuals were presented in the specific chapters dealing with these nutrients.

PHARMACOLOGIC AGENTS

Many male and female athletes use a variety of pharmacologic agents in the belief that a specific drug will have a positive influence on skill, strength, power, or endurance. In our drug-oriented, competitive culture, it is not surprising to find drug use for ergogenic purposes on the upswing among high school and even junior high school athletes. When winning becomes all important, one can do little to prevent the use **and** abuse of drugs by athletes, even if little "hard" scientific evidence exists to indicate a performance-enhancing effect. It is ironic that athletes who go to great lengths to promote all aspects of their health—by training hard, eating well-balanced meals, receiving medical care even for minor injuries—will ingest synthetic agents, many of which can precipitate side effects ranging from nausea, hair loss, itching, and nervous irritability to severe consequences such as sterility, liver disease, drug addiction, and even death caused by liver and blood cancer.

ANABOLIC STEROIDS

Anabolic steroids came into prominence for medical use in the early 1950s to treat patients who were deficient in natural androgens or had muscle-wasting diseases.[30] Other legitimate uses are for the treatment of osteoporosis in women and to counter an excessive decline in lean body mass and increase in body fat often observed in elderly men. Anabolic steroids now, however, have also become an integral part of the high-technology scene of competitive sports with an estimated 90% of male and 80% of female professional body builders using them in the belief that they improve performance.[22, 35]

Structure and Action

An anabolic steroid is a drug that functions in a manner similar to the chief male hormone testosterone. By binding with special receptor sites on muscle and various other tissues, this hormone greatly contributes to the male secondary sex characteristics and to the sex differences in muscle mass and strength that begin to develop at the onset of puberty. The hormone's androgenic or masculinizing effects can be minimized by synthetically manipulating the chemical structure of the steroid so that the cell's anabolic tissue-building, nitrogen-retaining process is emphasized for purposes of promoting increased muscle growth. Nevertheless, the masculinizing effect is still noticeable, especially when the drug is used by females. Athletes who take these drugs do so usually during the active years of their athletic careers, often taking a progressively increasing combined steroid dose in both oral and injectable form—a practice called "stacking"—far in excess of the recommended medical dose.[16, 17, 91] The dosage is then progressively reduced in the months prior to competition to reduce the chance of detection.

Anabolic steroids frequently are taken in conjunction with a resistance training program and an augmented protein intake. The aim is to improve performance in sports that require strength, speed, and power. In fact, a recent survey of U.S. Powerlifting Team members indicated that two-thirds of the respondents (60% response rate) had used androgenic-anabolic steroids.[121a] In the United States, more than 300,000 men and women used anabolic steroids over the 1-year period from 1992 to 1993.[142] Federal authorities conservatively estimate that the emerging business of illegally trafficking steroids exceeds 100 million dollars yearly—a figure that is growing rapidly. That many athletes get their steroids on the "black market" raises the fear that misinformed individuals may take a massive and prolonged dose of the drug without any medical monitoring for possible harmful alterations in physiologic function. Particularly worrisome is steroid use among young boys and girls and its accompanying effects, including extreme virilization and premature cessation of bone growth.[134] Approximately 1 of 15 high school students, or about a half-million adolescents (250,000 high school seniors), have used steroids.[16] These are the same young people who are likely to abuse a variety of other drugs, as well as share needles in the process.[38, 74] Improved athletic performance was the most common reason cited for steroid use among teenagers, although 25% said the main reason was enhanced appearance.[19]

Are They Effective?

Many athletes and trainers give testimony to the increased muscle size and performance benefits derived from steroid use. The widespread use of steroids is further illustrated by the disqualification and suspension of numerous elite amateur and professional athletes for taking them. Aside from the moral and ethical issues, this common use of steroids is unfortunate because of the conflicting scientific data on the degree to which they exert a positive influence on muscle growth and performance in normal, healthy athletes.

Much of the confusion regarding the ergogenic effectiveness of anabolic steroids has resulted from variations in experimental design: poor selection of controls; differences in drug selection, dosage, treatment duration, nutritional supplementation, training intensity, measurement technique, and previous experience of subjects; and individual variations in response. There is also speculation that the relatively small residual androgenic effect of the steroid acts through the central nervous system to facilitate improvements by making the athlete more aggressive, competitive, and fatigue resistant. This enables the person to train harder for a longer time when the drug is being taken, or begin to believe that augmented training effects are taking place.[31, 75, 114]

Research with animals has suggested that treatment with anabolic steroids, when combined with exercise and adequate protein intake, stimulates the process of protein synthesis and increases the muscle's protein content (myosin, myofibrillar, and sarcoplasmic factors).[98] Other research, however, has shown no benefit from steroid treatment on the leg muscle weight of rats subjected to functional overload by surgical removal of the synergistic muscle.[80] The researchers concluded that treatment with anabolic steroids does not complement functional over-

load to stimulate muscle development. The situation with humans is also conflicting because some studies have shown augmented body mass gains and reduced fat with steroid use in men who train. In contrast, other studies have shown no effects on strength and power or body composition, even when caloric and protein intake were sufficient to support an anabolic effect.[47, 58, 69, 132] When body mass gain does occur with steroid use, it often is unclear whether the compositional nature of this gain is primarily muscle tissue or water.

Are There Risks?

In our opinion, the infrequent but distinct possibility of harmful side effects from anabolic steroid treatment greatly outweighs any potential ergogenic effect. In addition, prolonged high dosages of these steroids can lead to a long-lasting impairment of normal testosterone endocrine function. A study of five male power athletes showed that the cessation of steroid use after 26 weeks reduced serum testosterone levels to less than half the level measured at the beginning of the study. This effect lasted throughout the 12- to 16-week follow-up period.[47] Other accompanying hormonal alterations during steroid use in males include a sevenfold increase in the concentration of the major female hormone estradiol.[2] This level was representative of the average value for normal females and possibly explains the **gynecomastia** (palpable breast tissue) often reported among male users of anabolic steroids.[48] Additional data from both animals and humans suggests that steroid use with exercise training may lead to connective tissue damage that decreases the tensile strength and elastic compliance of tendons.[22, 71, 115, 118] Furthermore, aside from negative effects on lipoprotein concentrations (see below), steroid use has caused injury to and functional alterations in myocardial cell cultures and an increased tendency for blood platelet aggregation that easily could compromise the health and function of the cardiovascular system and possibly increase the risk of stroke and acute myocardial infarction.[1a, 45, 60, 84, 100]

Steroid Use and Life-Threatening Disease. Table 23.1 presents the negative side effects and medical risks of anabolic steroid use. Of special concern is the evidence of a possible link between steroid use and alterations in normal liver function.[19, 65] We present these data not as a scare tactic, but to emphasize the potentially serious side effects even when a physician prescribes the drug in the recommended dosage. Although the duration of drug treatment for patients is often greater than that usually used by athletes, some athletes take steroids on and off for years, with the dosage greatly exceeding that typically prescribed for therapeutic purposes (50 to 200 mg per day versus the usual dosage of 5 to 20 mg per day). Preliminary data also suggest that anabolic steroid use as practiced by many athletes may interfere with the responsiveness of the body's immune system.[20] The precise clinical significance of these findings awaits further research. We believe that any potential ergogenic effect from anabolic steroid use is simply outweighed by the risk of undesirable and harmful side effects.

Steroid Use and Plasma Lipoproteins. In healthy men and women, anabolic steroid use produces a rapid and profound reduction in high-density lipoprotein cholesterol and elevations in both low-density lipoprotein cholesterol and total cholesterol.[28, 61, 122] In one study, weight lifters who used anabolic steroids had an average HDL cholesterol value of 26 mg · dL^{-1}, compared to 50 mg · dL^{-1} for weight lifters not on this drug.[66] A reduction of HDL to this level significantly increases the risk of heart disease to steroid users.

American College of Sports Medicine Position Statement on Anabolic Steroids

As part of their long-range educational program, the **American College of Sports Medicine (ACSM)** has taken a stand on the use and abuse of anabolic-androgenic steroids.[3] We endorse their position paper, which follows.

- Anabolic-androgenic steroids in the presence of an adequate diet and training can contribute to increases in body weight, often in the lean mass compartment.
- The gains in muscular strength achieved through high-intensity exercise and proper diet can occur by the increased use of anabolic-androgenic steroids in some individuals.
- Anabolic-androgenic steroids do not increase aerobic power or capacity for muscular exercise.

- Anabolic-androgenic steroids have been associated with adverse effects on the liver, cardiovascular system, reproductive system, and psychologic status in therapeutic trials and in limited research on athletes. Until further research is completed, the potential hazards of the use of the anabolic-androgenic steroids in athletes must include those found in therapeutic trials.
- The use of anabolic-androgenic steroids by athletes is contrary to the rules and ethical principles of athletic competition as set forth by many of the sports governing bodies. The American College of Sports Medicine supports these ethical principles and deplores the use of anabolic-androgenic steroids by athletes.

Steroid Use by Females

Besides the broad range of side effects discussed previously, females are susceptible to additional specific dangers from anabolic steroid use. These include masculinization, disruption of normal growth pattern by premature closure of the plates for bone growth (also for boys), deepened voice, increased facial hair, altered menstrual function, dramatic increase in sebaceous gland size, acne, hirsutism, decreased breast size, and enlargement of the clitoris. The long-term effects of steroid use on reproductive function are unknown.

GROWTH HORMONE: THE NEXT MAGIC PILL?

Human growth hormone (GH), also known as somatotropin, is now competing with anabolic steroids in the illicit market

TABLE 23.1
SIDE EFFECTS AND MEDICAL RISKS OF ANABOLIC STEROID USE

Males		Females	
Increase	*Decrease*	*Increase*	*Decrease*
Testicular atrophy	Sperm count	Voice change	Breast tissue
Gynecomastia	Testosterone levels	Facial hair	
		Menstrual irregularities	
		Clitoral enlargement	

Males and Females		
Increase	*Decrease*	*Possible*
LDL	HDL	Hypertension
LDL/HDL		Connective tissue damage
Potential for neoplastic disease of the liver		Myocardial damage
Aggressiveness, hyperactivity, irritability		Myocardial infarction
Withdrawal and depression upon stopping steroid use		Impaired thyroid function
Acne		Altered myocardial structure
Peliosis hepatitis		

TABLE 23.2
MAXIMAL FORCE PRODUCTION OF KNEE EXTENSOR AND FLEXOR MUSCLE GROUPS PRIOR TO AND FOLLOWING TRAINING WITH OR WITHOUT GH SUPPLEMENTS[a]

	Exercise plus Placebo			Exercise plus GH		
	Initial	Final	% Change	Initial	Final	% Change
Concentric						
Knee extensors	212 ± 13	248 ± 10	17	191 ± 11	214 ± 9	12
Knee flexors	137 ± 11	158 ± 7	15	122 ± 12	143 ± 6	17
Isometric						
Knee extensors	220 ± 13	252 ± 13	14	198 ± 15	207 ± 7	4
Knee flexors	131 ± 8	158 ± 8	20	127 ± 13	140 ± 16	10

From Yarasheski, K.F., et al.: Effect of growth hormone and resistance exercise on muscle growth in young men. *Am. J. Physiol.*, 262: E261, 1992.
[a]Values are mean ± SE. Maximum force (N · m) determined using a Cybex dynamometer. Concentric force measured at $60° \cdot s^{-1}$ angular velocity. Isometric force measured at 135° of knee extension. The maximum concentric force production of the knee flexor and extensor muscles increased in both groups ($P<0.05$), but these increments and the increments in maximum isometric force production were not greater in the exercise plus GH group.

of alleged tissue-building, performance-enhancing drugs. This hormone is produced endogenously by the adenohypophysis of the pituitary gland and is intimately involved in tissue-building processes and human growth. More specifically, GH stimulates bone and cartilage growth and enhances fatty acid oxidation while reducing glucose and amino acid breakdown.[138] Some of the decrease in fat-free body mass and increase in fat mass that occurs with aging is caused by a reduction in growth hormone secretion.[99] If excessive GH production occurs while the skeleton is still developing, the result is the endocrine and metabolic disorder of gigantism. If growth is completed before the onset of excessive GH production, the result is acromegaly, characterized by enlarged hands, feet, and facial features. Medically, GH is given to children who are deficient in GH to help them achieve near-normal size.

On the surface, the use of GH is attractive to the strength and power athlete because at physiologic levels, this hormone stimulates amino acid uptake and protein synthesis by muscle while enhancing lipid breakdown and conserving glycogen stores.[76] However, few well-controlled studies have evaluated the effectiveness of GH supplements on healthy subjects undergoing exercise training. In one study, six well-trained men, while maintaining a high-protein diet, were administered either biosynthetic GH or a placebo.[32] During 6 weeks of standard resistance training with GH, percent body fat decreased and fat-free mass increased significantly. No changes in body composition were noted for the group who trained with the placebo. These findings have not been supported by more recent investigations.[36, 139, 140] For example, 16 previously sedentary young men participated in a 12-week resistance training program.[139] They received either recombinant human GH supplements (40 $\mu g \cdot kg^{-1} \cdot d^{-1}$) or a placebo. Although fat-free body mass, total body water, and whole body protein synthesis increased more in the GH recipients, there were no significant differences between groups in their fractional rate of protein synthesis in skeletal muscle and no differences in torso and limb circumference or muscle function, as reflected in dynamic and static measures of muscle strength (Table 23.2). The authors attributed the greater increase in whole body protein synthesis in the group receiving GH to a possible increase in nitrogen retention in lean tissue other than skeletal muscle—for example, connective tissue, fluid, and noncontractile protein.

Because GH occurs naturally in the body, there is as yet no foolproof way to detect its use as an ergogenic aid. At present, the hormone is usually only available on the black market and often in a highly adulterated form. With the techniques of genetic engineering, it now is possible to produce a synthetic form of GH (such as Protoropin or Humantrope). Its use is approved for the treatment (cost of $20,000 to $40,000 per year) of children whose bodies produce inadequate quantities of GH. Undoubtedly, as more athletes use GH in the hope of attaining a competitive edge, there will be an increased incidence of diabetes and, in severe cases, gigantism in children and acromegalic syndrome—coarsening of the skin, thickening of bones, and overgrowth of soft tissue—in adults, as well as less overt side effects of insulin resistance, water retention, and carpal tunnel compression.[97]

NUTRITIONAL SUPPLEMENTS FOR AN ANABOLIC EFFECT

Although anabolic-androgenic steroids continue to be abused by an alarmingly high number of resistance-trained athletes, an emerging trend is to use nutrition as a legal alternative for "activating" the body's normal anabolic mechanisms. Specifically, many weight lifters and body builders use commercial nutritional supplements, particularly amino acids either singularly or in combination, in the belief that these products will boost the body's natural production of the anabolic hormones testosterone, GH, or insulin to improve muscle size and strength and facilitate body fat loss.[55] The rationale for this practice is based on the clinical use of amino acid infusion or ingestion to regulate various anabolic hormones in deficient patients.

In general, research on healthy subjects does not offer evidence of an ergogenic effect of oral amino acid supplements on hormone secretion or exercise performance. For example, in studies having appropriate design and statistical analyses, no effect occurred from supplements of arginine, lysine, ornithine, tyrosine, and other amino acids, either singularly or in combination, on levels of GH,[46, 70, 110] insulin secretion,[15, 46] diverse measures of anaerobic power,[45a] or all-out running performance at $\dot{V}O_2$max.[109] Furthermore, when supplements of all 20 amino acids were given to elite junior weight lifters, no effect was shown on physical performance or the resting or exercise-induced responses of testosterone, cortisol, or GH.[49] Such findings support the position that the ingestion of amino acids in the quantities recommended in commercial supplements is of **no benefit** to the body's hormonal milieu or to body composition and muscle size and subsequent exercise performance.

AMPHETAMINES

Amphetamines, or "pep pills," are pharmacologic compounds that exert a powerful stimulating effect on central nervous system function. Amphetamine (Benzedrine) and dextroamphetamine sulfate (Dexedrine) are the compounds used most frequently by athletes. Amphetamines are sympathomimetic in that their actions mimic those of the sympathetic hormones epinephrine and norepinephrine. These hormones cause a rise in blood pressure, pulse rate, cardiac output, breathing rate, metabolism, and blood sugar. Ingesting 5 to 20 mg of amphetamine usually produces an effect for 30 to 90 minutes, although the influence of the drug can persist for much longer. Aside from causing an aroused level of sympathetic function, amphetamines are supposed to increase alertness and wakefulness and to provide the capacity to perform increased amounts of work by depressing the sensation of muscle fatigue.[23] It should come as little surprise that athletes frequently use amphetamines with the hope of gaining an ergogenic edge when, in reality, there is little or no advantage.

Dangers of Amphetamines

The use of amphetamines in athletics is ill-advised for the following reasons:

• Continual use can lead to either physiological or emotional drug dependency. This often causes a cyclical dependency on "uppers" (amphetamines) or "downers" (barbiturates)—the barbiturates are taken to reduce or tranquilize the "hyper" state brought on by amphetamines.
• General side effects are headaches, tremulousness, agitation, fever, dizziness, and confusion, all of which negatively affect performance in sports requiring rapid reaction and judgment and a high level of steadiness and mental concentration.
• Larger doses are eventually required to achieve the same effect because tolerance to the drug increases with prolonged use; these larger doses may aggravate and even precipitate certain cardiovascular disorders.
• Agents like amphetamines that inhibit or suppress the body's normal mechanisms for perceiving and responding to pain, fatigue, or heat stress can severely jeopardize the athlete's health and safety.
• The effects of prolonged intake of high doses of amphetamines are unknown.

Amphetamine Use and Athletic Performance

Table 23.3 summarizes the results of seven experiments that evaluated the effects of amphetamines on physical performance. In almost all instances, amphetamines had little or no effect on exercise capacity or on performance of simple psychomotor skills.

The major reason athletes take amphetamines is to get and stay "up" for the event and be psychologically ready to compete. On the day or evening before a contest, however, competitors are often nervous and irritable and have difficulty relaxing. Under these circumstances, a barbiturate is used to induce sleep. The athlete then regains the "hyper" condition by popping an "upper." Not only is this cycle of depressant-to-stimulant undesirable and potentially dangerous, but the stimulant does not act in its normal manner when it follows the intake of a barbiturate. Knowledgeable and prudent people urge that amphetamines be banned from sports competitions. The International Olympic Committee, the American Medical Association, and most athletic governing groups have rules to disqualify athletes who use amphetamines. Ironically, most research has indicated that amphetamines do **not** enhance physical performance. Perhaps their greatest influence is in the psychologic realm, whereby athletes are easily convinced that any supplement will bring on a superior performance. A placebo containing an inert substance often produces identical results!

CAFFEINE

Caffeine is a possible exception to the rule against taking stimulants.[6, 10, 24, 53a, 75a, 82] Caffeine is one of a group of lipid-soluble compounds called methylxanthines found naturally in coffee beans, tea leaves, chocolate, cocoa beans, and cola nuts and is often added to carbonated beverages and nonprescription medicines. Depending on prepara-

TABLE 23.3
SUMMARY OF RESULTS ON THE EFFECTS OF AMPHETAMINES ON ATHLETIC PERFORMANCE

Study	Dose (mg)	Type of Experiment	Effect of Amphetamines
(1[a])	10–20	Two all-out treadmill runs with 10-min rest between runs	None
		Consecutive 100-yd swims with 10-min rest intervals	None
		220–440-yd swims for time	None
		220-yd track runs for time	None
		100-yd to 2-mile track runs for time	None
(2[b])	10	Bench stepping to fatigue carrying weights equal to $\frac{1}{3}$ body mass, 3 times with 3-min rest intervals	None
(3[c])	5	100-yd swim for speed	None
(4[d])	15	All-out treadmill runs	None
(5[e])	10	Stationary cycling at work rates of 275–2215 kgm · min^{-1} for 25–35 min followed by treadmill run to exhaustion	None on submaximal or maximal oxygen uptake, heart rate, ventilation volume, or blood lactic acid; work time on the bicycle and treadmill increased significantly
(6[f])	20	Reaction and movement time to a visual stimulus	None; subjective feelings of alertness or lethargy unrelated to reaction or movement time
(7[g])	5	Psychomotor performance during a simulated airplane flight	Enhanced performance and lessened fatigue, but if preceded by secobarbital (barbiturate), decreased performance

[a]Karpovich, P.V.: Effect of amphetamine sulfate on athletic performance. *JAMA*, 170:558, 1959.
[b]Foltz, E.E., et al.: The influence of amphetamine (Benzedrine) sulfate and caffeine on the performance of rapidly exhausting work by untrained subjects. *J. Lab. Clin. Med.*, 28:601, 1943.
[c]Haldi, J., and Wynn, W.: Action of drugs on efficiency of swimmers. *Res. Q.*, 17:96, 1959.
[d]Golding, L.A., and Barnard, R.J.: The effects of d-amphetamine sulfate on physical performance. *J. Sports, Med. Phys. Fitness*, 3:221, 1963.
[e]Wyndham, C.H., et al.: Physiological effects of the amphetamines during exercise. *S. Afr. Med. J.*, 45:247, 1971.
[f]Pierson, W.R., et al.: Some psychological effects of the administration of amphetamine sulfate and meprobamate on speed of movement and reaction time. *Med. Sci. Sports*, 12:61, 1961.
[g]McKenzie, R.E., and Elliot, L.L.: Effects of secobarbital and D-amphetamine on performance during a simulated air mission. *Aerospace Med.*, 36:774, 1965.

tion, one cup of brewed coffee contains between 150 and 250 mg of caffeine, instant coffee about 120 mg, brewed tea between 70 and 130 mg, and caffeinated soft drinks about 50 mg. Caffeine is absorbed rapidly from the intestinal tract and reaches peak plasma concentrations approximately 1 hour after ingestion, exerting an influence on the nervous, cardiovascular, and muscular systems.

Although all research does not support the ergogenic benefits of caffeine, consuming the amount of caffeine commonly found in 2.5 cups of percolated coffee (350 mg) 60 minutes before exercising has significantly extended endurance in moderately strenuous exercise.[25] With caffeine, subjects were able to perform an average of 90.2 minutes of exercise compared to 75.5 minutes of exercise without caffeine. Even though values for heart rate and oxygen uptake during the two trials were similar, the caffeine also made the work feel easier. Consumption of caffeine before exercise led to a high level of lipid catabolism and a corresponding reduced rate of carbohydrate oxidation, based on measurements of plasma glycerol and free fatty acid levels and the respiratory quotient. (See Focus on Research, p. 456).

Proposed Mechanism For Ergogenic Action

The ergogenic effect of caffeine in high-intensity endurance exercise likely results from the facilitated use of lipid as a fuel for exercise, perhaps mediated by catecholamine release from the adrenal medulla, thus sparing the body's limited carbohydrate reserves.[5, 53, 72, 116a] Caffeine acts either directly or through the action of epinephrine as an antagonist of the adenosine receptors on adipocyte cells. These are the receptors that normally inhibit lipolysis. The inhibition of adenosine receptors by caffeine causes cellular levels of cyclic AMP to increase; this reaction, in turn, activates hormone-sensitive lipases to promote lipolysis, which increases the release of free fatty acids into the plasma.[37]

The conservation of muscle and liver glycogen would be of benefit during prolonged exercise, when glycogen depletion is intimately related to a diminished endurance capacity. A lessening of the subjective rating of physical effort during exercise possibly results from a central analgesic effect of caffeine or its effect on neuronal excitability, possibly through a lowering of the threshold for motor unit recruitment and nerve transmission.[25] It also is possible that caffeine favorably affects maximal aerobic exercise because a small increase in $\dot{V}O_2$max follows ingestion of a beverage containing 350 mg of caffeine 1 hour prior to exercise.[116]

Endurance Effects Are Often Inconsistent

The effect of caffeine ingestion on the mobilization of free fatty acids is significantly blunted, and the metabolic mixture is unaltered during prolonged submaximal exercise in individuals who maintain a high carbohydrate intake.[124] The influence of prior nutrition may partly account for the wide and often inconsistent variations in individual response to exercise following caffeine ingestion. Individual differences in caffeine sensitivity, tolerance, and hormonal response resulting from short- and long-term patterns of caffeine consumption are probably important factors affecting the ergogenic nature of this drug.[21, 117, 133] Ergogenic effects are not consistently found among habitual caffeine users.[113, 117]

Effects on Muscle

Caffeine may act directly on muscle to enhance its capacity for exercise.[73, 111] By means of a double-blind research design, both voluntary and electrically stimulated muscle actions were evaluated under normal conditions and following the oral administration of 500 mg of caffeine.[73] Electrical stimulation of the motor nerve enabled the researchers to remove central nervous system control and look at the direct effects of caffeine on skeletal muscle. The results showed no effect of caffeine on maximal muscle force during either voluntary or electrically stimulated muscle actions. During submaximal effort, however, caffeine ingestion produced an increase in force for a given low frequency of electrical stimulation before and after muscle fatigue. These findings suggest a specific ergogenic effect of caffeine on skeletal muscle during repetitive low-frequency stimulation. The effect appears to be mediated by caffeine's direct action on muscle. One hypothesis is that caffeine acts on the sarcoplasmic reticulum to increase its permeability to Ca^{2+}, thus making this mineral readily available for the contraction process. It also is likely that caffeine influences the myofibril's sensitivity to Ca^{2+}.

Warning: the use of caffeine is not without its hazards for certain individuals, particularly those who normally avoid this drug. Caffeine is a stimulant to the central nervous system: it can cause headaches, insomnia, and nervous irritability and trigger premature left ventricular contractions. From the standpoint of temperature regulation, caffeine is a potent diuretic. This causes an unnecessary pre-exercise loss of fluid that could have a negative effect on thermal balance and exercise performance in a hot environment. Although small amounts of caffeine ingestion are permitted by the International Olympic Committee, consuming about 600 to 800 mg (four to seven cups of coffee) over a 30-minute period will significantly raise urine levels and lead to disqualification from competition.[129]

PANGAMIC ACID

Pangamic acid, commonly known as "vitamin" B_{15}, has been widely touted among athletes for its alleged ergogenic benefits in aerobic exercise. The proponents of pangamic acid use argue that studies conducted in Russia indicated that this compound increased the cell's ability to use oxygen, reduced lactic acid buildup, and enhanced endurance. As with many proposed ergogenic aids, testimonials from athletes abound as to its effectiveness as a training aid and performance enhancer. On careful scrutiny of the early studies of pangamic acid, it is difficult to interpret the validity of the findings in light of the significant limitations in research design. Research conducted in this country has been unable to show any benefit of this compound to aerobic capacity, endurance performance, or circulating levels of blood glucose and lactate.[50, 54] From a nutritional perspective, pangamic acid has no vitamin or provitamin properties and appears to serve no particular need in the body. Concern has been expressed that synthetic mixtures sold as B_{15} may be harmful to humans.[56] The Food and Drug Administration guidelines make it illegal to sell this compound as a dietary supplement or drug.

BUFFERING SOLUTIONS

All-out exercise of between 30 and 120 seconds is accompanied by dramatic alterations in the chemical balance between the intracellular and extracellular fluids because the muscle fibers rely predominantly on anaerobic means of energy transfer. As a result, significant quantities of lactic acid accumulate, accompanied by a concurrent fall in intracellular pH.[26, 112] The increase in acidity ultimately may inhibit the energy-transfer and contractile capabilities of the active muscle fibers.[57, 90] In the blood, the condition of acidosis reflects increases in the concentrations of both H^+ and lactate.

A major line of defense against an increase in intracellular H^+ concentration is the bicarbonate aspect of the body's buffering system (refer to Chapter 14). Maintaining extracellular bicarbonate at a high level causes H^+ to leave the cell more rapidly and reduce intracellular acidosis.[77] This fact has led to speculation that an increase in the body's bicarbonate reserve before short-term anaerobic exercise might enhance performance by delaying the fall in intracellular pH associated with this type of effort. The research in

TABLE 23.4

PERFORMANCE TIME AND ACID-BASE PROFILES FOR SUBJECTS UNDER CONTROL (PLACEBO) AND INDUCED PRE-EXERCISE ALKALOSIS CONDITIONS IMMEDIATELY PRIOR TO AND FOLLOWING AN 800-M RACE

Variable	Condition	Pre-treatment	Pre-exercise	Post-exercise
	Control	7.40	7.39	7.07
pH	Placebo	7.39	7.40	7.09
	Alkalosis	7.40	7.49[a]	7.18[b]
Lactate	Control	1.21	1.15	12.62
$(mmol \cdot L^{-1})$	Placebo	1.38	1.23	13.62
	Alkalosis	1.29	1.31	14.29[b]
Standard	Control	25.8	24.5	9.90
HCO_3^{-1}	Placebo	25.6	26.2	11.00
$(mEq \cdot L^{-1})$	Alkalosis	25.2	33.5[a]	14.30[b]

	Control	Placebo	Alkalosis
Performance time (min:s)	2:05.8	2:05.1	2:02.9[c]

From Wilkes, D., et al.: Effects of induced metabolic alkalosis on 800-m racing time. *Med. Sci. Sports Exerc.*, 15:277, 1983.
[a]Pre-exercise values significantly higher than pre-treatment values.
[b]Alkalosis values significantly higher than placebo and control values after exercise.
[c]Alkalosis time significantly faster than control and placebo times.

this area, however, has produced conflicting results, perhaps owing to variations in the pre-exercise doses of sodium bicarbonate and the types of exercise used to evaluate the ergogenic effects of alkalosis.[27, 59, 67, 78, 123] In an attempt to negate some of these previous limitations, one study investigated the effects of acute metabolic alkalosis on maximal short-term exercise during which fatigue was associated with a significant increase in anaerobic metabolites.[128] Six trained middle-distance runners were evaluated during an 880-m race under control conditions and following induced alkalosis via ingestion of a sodium bicarbonate solution (300 mg per kilogram body mass) or a calcium carbonate placebo of similar concentration. As shown in Table 23.4, ingestion of an alkaline drink raised the subjects' pH and standard bicarbonate levels before exercise. In addition, subjects ran an average of 2.9 seconds faster under alkalosis and achieved higher postexercise blood lactate, pH, and extracellular H^+ concentrations than under the placebo condition.

These results suggest that the ergogenic effect of pre-exercise alkalosis is the result of an augmented level of anaerobic energy transfer during exercise. It is possible that the increased extracellular buffering provided by ingesting pre-exercise sodium bicarbonate facilitates H^+ efflux from the working muscle fibers. This would delay the fall in intracellular pH and its subsequent negative effects on muscle function. The improvement of 2.9 seconds in an 800-m race time noted above represents rather dramatic performance results. This time period transposes to a distance of 19 m at

race pace, which, in most 800-m races, would bring a last-place finisher to first place!

Effect Related to Dosage and Degree of Anaerobiosis. Bicarbonate dosage and the cumulative anaerobic nature of the exercise interact to influence the potential ergogenic effect of pre-exercise "bicarbonate loading."[27, 59] Dosages of at least 0.3 g per kilogram body mass appear to facilitate H^+ efflux from the cell, significantly enhancing a single 1- to 2-minute bout of maximal effort[12, 52, 79] or longer-term arm or leg exercise that leads to exhaustion within 6 to 8 minutes.[96] No ergogenic effect occurs for the type of performance typically used in heavy resistance training.[123] An all-out effort lasting less than 1 minute may be improved only when the exercise is repetitive in nature.[27] Such intermittent anaerobic exercise produces a high intracellular H^+ concentration, the buffering of which would benefit from a higher level of bicarbonate in the extracellular fluid.

More research is needed concerning the ergogenic benefits and possible dangers of acute induced metabolic alkalosis. Many individuals who bicarbonate-load often experience urgent gastrointestinal distress in the form of abdominal cramps and diarrhea about 1 hour after ingestion. Such a side effect in the susceptible athlete could negate any potential ergogenic benefit. Adverse gastrointestinal effects can be reduced or eliminated by substituting the buffering agent sodium citrate (0.5 g per kilogram body mass) for sodium bicarbonate.[83]

TEMPOROMANDIBULAR JOINT (TMJ) REPOSITIONING

During the past 20 years, a number of reports in the popular and dental literature have claimed either real or potential benefits to exercise performance from temporomandibular joint (TMJ) repositioning by means of a specially designed, custom-fitted bite splint that optimizes the alignment of the upper and lower jaw.[49a, 62, 130] At the same time, the sports performance benefits of such jaw appliances have been extolled by elite athletes in a variety of sports including football, tennis, baseball, boxing, luge, field events, and sprint and distance running.[86] The proponents of this form of "sports dentistry" argue that improper TMJ alignment negatively affects the skeletal frame in general and the relatively large neural and vascular component in the jaw region in particular. Consequently, correct positioning and proper stability of the mandible will align the cervical vertebrae and alleviate negative neural and vascular input from the orofacial area to the brain. This adjustment, it is argued, will ultimately translate into optimal exercise performance.

Well-controlled research concerning the ergogenic effects of TMJ repositioning is sparse. Most claims of improved exercise performance are based on case studies, anecdotal "success stories," and subjective evaluation. Even under objective measurement, the research design often has been flawed and poorly controlled. In one of our laboratories, we evaluated the effects of a mandibular orthopedic repositioning appliance (MORA) on maximal and submaximal physiologic and performance measures in young adult men and women with documented TMJ malalignment.[81] The subjects were randomly assigned to each of four conditions: (*a*) normal, without a MORA, (*b*) with a placebo MORA having no bite surface to maintain normal jaw position, (*c*) with a MORA that optimized jaw position, and (*d*) with a MORA that magnified the subject's normal degree of malocclusion. To ensure a double-blind nature to the study, each of the three bite splints was coded for a particular subject and the code maintained by the dentists. Because the dentists did not take part in the laboratory measurements, neither the subjects nor the staff had knowledge of what particular bite splint was being used during testing. Data analysis revealed that the use of a MORA device had **no effect** on measures of visual reaction and movement time; muscular strength of the grip, elbow flexors, and leg extensors; submaximal and maximal oxygen uptake; perception of effort; running economy; or all-out anaerobic working capacity of the arms and legs. Placing the jaw in a less-than-optimal position (greater than the subject's normal degree of malocclusion) had no deleterious effect on any performance measures. Clearly, these findings were contrary to that predicted by advocates of mandibular repositioning appliances and in agreement with several studies showing no effect of TMJ repositioning on isometric and isokinetic measures of muscular strength and power.[87, 105, 141] Such findings support the contention that the beneficial effects of short-term TMJ repositioning on exercise performance noted in previous articles are the results of inadequacies in research design rather than real ergogenic effects of MORA devices.

RED BLOOD CELL REINFUSION—BLOOD DOPING

Red blood cell reinfusion, often called induced erythrocythemia, blood boosting, or "blood doping," came into public prominence as a possible ergogenic technique during the 1972 Munich Olympics, when a champion endurance athlete was alleged to have used this procedure in preparation for his eventual double gold-medal-winning endurance runs.

How It Works

In this procedure, a certain amount—usually between 1 and 4 units (1 unit = 450 mL of blood)—of a person's blood is withdrawn, the plasma is removed and immediately reinfused, and the packed red cells are placed in frozen storage. To prevent a dramatic reduction in blood cell concentration, each unit of blood is withdrawn over a 3- to 8-week period because it generally takes this long for the person to reestablish normal red blood cell levels. The stored blood cells are then infused (**autologous transfusion**) 1 to 7 days before an endurance event. In **homologous transfusion,** a type-matched donor's blood is infused. This causes the red blood cell count and hemoglobin level of the blood to rise, often by as much as 8 to 20%. In men, this hemoconcentration translates to an average increase in hemoglobin from a normal of 15 g per 100 mL of blood to 19 g per 100 mL (or from a hematocrit of 40% to one of 60%). These hematological characteristics remain elevated for at least 14 days.[51] It is theorized that the added blood volume contributes to a greater maximal cardiac output and that the red blood cell packing increases the blood's oxygen-carrying capacity and, thus, the quantity of oxygen available to the working muscles. Enhanced oxygen availability is particularly beneficial to the endurance athlete for whom oxygen transport and delivery often are limiting factors in exercise.[13, 121]

Usually, 900 to 1800 mL of freeze-preserved autologous blood is the amount infused to bring about an ergogenic effect. For each infusion of 500 mL of whole blood or its equivalent of 275 mL of packed red cells, about 100 mL of oxygen is theoretically added to the total oxygen-carrying capacity of the blood (each 100 mL of whole blood carries about 20 mL of oxygen). Because an endurance athlete's total blood volume circulates five or six times each minute during heavy exercise, the potential "extra" oxygen available to the tissues from red cell reinfusion is about 0.5 L. It also is possible that blood doping could have effects opposite to those intended. A large infusion of red blood cells (and resulting increase in blood cell concentration) could increase blood viscosity, or "thickness," causing a **decrease** in cardiac output, a **decrease** in blood flow velocity, and a **reduction** in peripheral oxygen content—all of which would **reduce** aerobic capacity. Certainly, any increase in blood viscosity could also compromise blood flow through the narrowed, atherosclerotic vessels of people with significant coronary artery disease.

Does Blood Doping Work?

A theoretical basis for blood doping exists, and there is experimental evidence to justify the procedure.[102] Much of the early conflict regarding the ergogenic benefits was the result of poor experimental design, inconsistent criteria for exercise performance, variations in techniques for storing blood, and in timing and quantity of blood withdrawn and replaced. The early research in this area noted a significant and rapid increase in $\dot{V}O_2$max following the infusion of whole blood.[41] One study even reported a 23% overnight increase in performance and a 9% increase in maximal oxygen uptake after blood doping.[43] Although many of these early studies were flawed in terms of research design, subsequent investigations, including a study by one of the past critics of this technique, support the previous findings and indicate physiologic and performance improvements from red blood cell reinfusion.[14, 94, 95, 108]

The differences in results among the various research studies of exercise performance following red blood cell reinfusion are based largely on blood storage methods. Frozen red blood cells can be stored in excess of 6 weeks without a

significant loss of cells compared to conventional storage at 4°C (used in some earlier studies): at 4°C, substantial hemolysis occurs after only 3 weeks. This limitation is important because, as shown in Figure 23.1, it usually takes a person 5 to 6 weeks to re-establish the blood cells lost after the withdrawal of 2 units of whole blood.[51]

When the appropriate method of blood storage is used, the procedure of red blood cell reinfusion significantly elevates hematological characteristics in both men and women. This, in turn, translates to a 5 to 13% increase in aerobic capacity, reduced submaximal heart rate and blood lactate for a standard exercise task, and augmented endurance both at altitude and sea level. In addition, significant thermoregulatory benefits (reduced body-heat storage and improved sweating responses) during exercise in the heat are noted following pre-exercise red blood cell reinfusion.[103, 104] The increased oxygen content of arterial blood in the infused state likely "frees" more blood for delivery to the skin for purposes of heat dissipation during exercise heat stress. Table 23.5 illustrates hematologic, physiologic, and performance responses in five adult men during submaximal and maximal exercise before and 24 hours after the comparatively large infusion of 750 mL of packed red blood cells. These response patterns are generally representative of the more recent research in this area.

A NEW TWIST—HORMONAL BLOOD BOOSTING

To eliminate the somewhat cumbersome and lengthy process of blood doping, endurance athletes are now experimenting with **erythropoietin,** a hormone normally produced by the kidneys. This hormone stimulates the bone

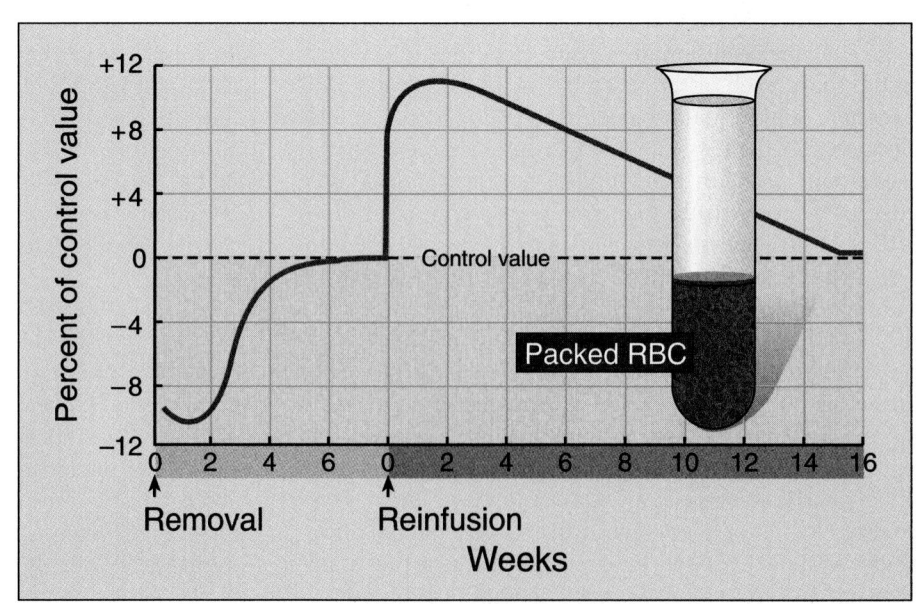

FIGURE 23.1
Time course of hematological changes after removal and reinfusion of 900 mL of freeze-preserved blood. (From Gledhill, N.: Blood doping and related issues: a brief review. *Med. Sci. Sports Exerc.*, 14:183, 1982.)

TABLE 23.5

PHYSIOLOGIC, PERFORMANCE, AND HEMATOLOGIC CHARACTERISTICS PRIOR TO AND 24 HOURS AFTER THE REINFUSION OF 750 ML OF PACKED RED BLOOD CELLS[a]

Variable	Pre-Infusion	Post-Infusion	Difference	Difference, %
Hemoglobin, g · 100 mL blood^{-1}	13.8	17.6	3.8[b]	+27.5[b]
Hematocrit[a], %	43.3	54.8	11.5[b]	+26.5[b]
Submaximal $\dot{V}o_2$, L · min^{-1}	1.60	1.59	−0.01	−0.6
Submaximal HR, beats · min^{-1}	127.4	109.2	18.2	−14.3[b]
$\dot{V}o_2$max, L · min^{-1}	3.28	3.70	0.42[b]	+12.8[b]
Max HR, beats · min^{-1}	181.6	180.0	−1.6	−0.9
Treadmill run time, s	793	918	125[b]	+15.8

From Roberston, R.J., et al.: Effect of induced erythrocythemia on hypoxia tolerance during exercise. *J. Appl. Physiol.*, 53:490, 1982.
[a]Hematocrit is presented as the percent (%) of 100 mL of whole blood occupied by the red blood cells.
[b]Difference is statistically significant.

marrow to produce red blood cells. From a medical standpoint, exogenous erythropoietin has proven quite useful in combating the anemia often observed in patients with severe renal disease.[44] Normally, when the blood count is low or the pressure of oxygen in arterial blood decreases—as in severe pulmonary disease or during an ascent to high altitude—this hormone is released, stimulating red blood cell production. Unfortunately, if self-administered in an unregulated and unmonitored manner (simply injecting the hormone requires much less sophistication than the procedures for blood doping), the hematocrit can increase in excess of 60%. Such a dangerously high hemoconcentration (and thus blood viscosity) greatly increases the likelihood of a stroke or heart attack, heart failure, and pulmonary edema.

WARM-UP (PRELIMINARY EXERCISE)

Engaging in some type of physical activity or warm-up before vigorous exercise is a procedure generally accepted by coaches, trainers, and athletes at all levels of competition. The underlying belief is that this preliminary exercise aids the performer in preparing either physiologically or psychologically for an event and may reduce the chances of joint and muscle injury. In a study of animals, greater forces and increases in muscle length were required to injure a "warmed-up" muscle compared to a muscle in the "cold" condition.[101] The warming-up process stretches the muscle-tendon unit and, thereby, possibly allows for greater length and less tension when a given external load is placed on the unit.

Warm-ups generally are classified under one of two categories, though overlap often exists.

• **General warm-up**—Examples of this type of warm-up include calisthenics, stretching, and general body movements or "loosening-up" exercises that are unrelated to the specific neuromuscular actions of the anticipated performance.

• **Specific warm-up**—This type of preliminary exercise provides a skill rehearsal for the actual activity in which the participant is preparing. Swinging a golf club, throwing a baseball or football, practicing tennis, and performing preliminary lead-up in the high jump or pole vault are examples of specific warm-up.

PSYCHOLOGICAL CONSIDERATIONS

Competitors at all levels often feel that performing some prior skill-related activity prepares them mentally for their events, allowing their concentration and "psyche" to become clearly focused on the upcoming performance. Some evidence supports the contention that a specific warm-up related to the activity itself improves the necessary skill and coordination. Consequently, sports that require accuracy, timing, and precise movements generally benefit from some type of specific, or "formal," preliminary practice.

There is also a notion that prior exercise before strenuous effort gradually prepares a person to go "all out" without fear of injury. A good example is the ritual warm-up of baseball pitchers. Is it conceivable that a pitcher would ever enter a game, throwing at competitive speeds, without previously warming up? Would any athlete begin competition without first engaging in a particular form, intensity, or duration of warm-up? Although in most instances the answer is a definite "no," it would be nearly impossible to design a proper experiment with top-flight athletes to resolve whether warm-up is really necessary and whether it facilitates improved subsequent performance with a reduced risk of injury.

In certain situations, peak performance is expected as soon as play begins, and little time is available for warming up. For example, a reserve player who enters a game during the last few minutes has no time for stretching, vigorous calisthenics, or practice shots. The player is expected to go all out and achieve optimal performance with no warm-up other than that done before the game or during intermission. Are more injuries recorded in such cases? Are physical performances such as shooting, rebounding, or playing defense in basketball, for example, poorer during the first few minutes of this "unwarmed" condition than they are during a performance preceded by a warm-up? Hopefully, future research will address such questions.

Psychological factors such as an athlete's ingrained belief in the importance of warming up establish a definite bias in comparing performances with and without warm-up. It is difficult (if not impossible) for a subject to perform at maximum effort with no warm-up if he or she believes that it is important. In this regard, some researchers have used hypnosis on their subjects to neutralize preconceived notions about warm-up.

PHYSIOLOGICAL CONSIDERATIONS

In one study, the effect of warm-up was evaluated during a 2-minute sprint ride on a bicycle ergometer at 120% of the power output and at $\dot{V}O_2$max.[93] During the first minute of exercise in the warmed-up condition, muscle temperatures were higher, muscle and blood lactate levels lower, and oxygen uptake higher compared to the same exercise with no warm-up. This outcome suggests that the warm-up exercise augmented local blood flow, which remained higher at the onset of exercise, increasing the aerobic contribution to muscle energy metabolism early during the exercise.

On purely physiologic grounds, there are five possible mechanisms through which warm-up should improve physical performance and exercise capacity as a result of subsequent increases in blood flow and muscle and core temperatures:[9]

- Increased speed of muscle action and relaxation.
- Greater economy of movement because of lowered viscous resistance within active muscles.
- Facilitated oxygen delivery by the muscles because hemoglobin releases oxygen more readily at higher temperatures.
- Facilitated nerve transmission and muscle metabolism resulting from the direct effect temperature has on accelerating the rate of bodily processes; a specific warm-up may also facilitate the recruitment of motor units required for physical activity.
- Increased blood flow through active tissues as the local vascular bed dilates with higher levels of metabolism and muscle temperature.

EFFECTS ON PERFORMANCE

Although there is little research on the ergogenic effect of warming up, it likely is beneficial. Because of the strong psychological and possibly physiological benefits of warming up, be it passive (massage, heat applications, and diathermy), general (calisthenics, jogging), or specific (practice of the actual movements), we recommend continuation of such procedures. Until there is substantial evidence justifying its elimination, a brief warm-up is certainly a comfortable way to lead up to more vigorous exercise. *The warm-up should be gradual and sufficient to increase muscle and core temperature without causing fatigue or reducing energy stores.* This consideration is highly individualized: adequate warm-up for an Olympic swimmer would totally exhaust the recreational swimmer. To reap the possible benefits of increased body temperature, the subject should begin the actual event or activity within several minutes of the end of the warm-up. In warming up, the specific muscles should be used in a way that mimics the anticipated activity and brings about a full range of joint motion.

SUDDEN STRENUOUS EXERCISE

Sudden exertion can trigger the onset of myocardial infarction, particularly in sedentary people.[85] With this in mind, the consideration of possible benefits from warming up takes on added significance. Several studies have evaluated the effects of preliminary exercise on the cardiovascular response to sudden, strenuous exercise. The findings provide a different physiologic framework for justifying warm-up. This framework is particularly important to those involved in programs of adult fitness and cardiac rehabilitation and to those in occupations and sports requiring a sudden burst of high-intensity exercise.

In one study, 44 men free of overt symptoms of coronary artery disease ran on a treadmill at high intensity for 10 to 15 seconds without prior warm-up.[7] An evaluation of the postexercise electrocardiogram (ECG) revealed that 70% of the subjects displayed abnormal electrocardiographic changes that could be attributed to an inadequate oxygen supply to the myocardium. These changes were not related to age or fitness level. To evaluate the effect of warm-up, 22 of the men with abnormal ECGs during the treadmill run jogged in place at a moderate intensity (heart rate about 145 beats per min) for 2 minutes before treadmill running. With warm-up, 10 of the men then had normal tracings during sudden exertion, while another 10 men had improved electrocardiographic responses; only two subjects still showed significant abnormalities. In a subsequent study, blood pressure response also improved with prior warm-up.[8] For seven men not engaging in prior warm-up, systolic blood pressure averaged 168 mm Hg immediately following the 15-second treadmill run. This was reduced to 140 mm Hg when exercise was preceded by a 2-minute jog-in-place warm-up.

These observations indicate that the adaptation of coronary blood flow to a sudden increase in myocardial work is not instantaneous and that transient myocardial ischemia (poor oxygen supply) can occur in apparently healthy and fit individuals. *The effect of prior warm-up (at least 2 minutes of easy jogging) on the subsequent electrocardiogram and blood pressure response to vigorous exercise indicates a benefit of warming up in establishing a favorable relationship between myocardial oxygen supply and demand.* Although warm-up preceding strenuous exercise is probably a prudent practice for all people, it is most important to those having limitations in myocardial blood flow, such as those suffering from coronary artery disease. A brief warm-up probably facilitates more optimal blood pressure and hormonal adjustment at the onset of strenuous exercise. Prior exercise would serve either one or both of two beneficial purposes at the onset of sudden exercise: *(a)* reduce the myocardial work load and, thus, the myocardial oxygen requirement, and/or *(b)* augment the flow of blood through the coronary arteries.

OXYGEN INHALATION (HYPEROXIA)

It is common to observe athletes breathing oxygen-enriched gas mixtures, or **hyperoxic** gas mixtures, during time-outs or half-times of football games or immediately after strenuous exercise. The assumption is that this procedure significantly enhances the blood's oxygen-carrying capacity and, thus, facilitates oxygen transport to the exercising or recovering muscles. The fact is, however, that when healthy people breathe ambient air at sea level, the hemoglobin in the blood leaving the lungs is normally 95 to 98% saturated with oxygen. In physiological terms:

• Breathing high concentrations of oxygen could increase oxygen transport by hemoglobin to only a small extent, or about 1 mL of extra oxygen for every 100 mL (10 mL per liter) of blood.
• The oxygen dissolved in plasma during the breathing of a hyperoxic mixture also increases about 0.4 mL per 100 mL of blood (4.0 mL per liter), from its normal quantity of 0.3 mL to about 0.7 mL per 100 mL (7.0 mL per liter) of blood.

Consequently, the blood's oxygen-carrying capacity under hyperoxic conditions would potentially be increased by about 14 mL of oxygen for every 1000 mL of blood—10 mL "extra" attached to hemoglobin and 4 mL "extra" dissolved in plasma.

PRE-EXERCISE OXYGEN BREATHING

A 70-kg person has about 5000 mL (5.0 L) of blood. Breathing a hyperoxic mixture could potentially add or "store" about 70 mL of oxygen in the total blood volume (5.0 L blood × 14 mL "extra" O_2 per liter of blood). Thus,

despite any potential psychological benefit from the athlete believing that pre-exercise oxygen breathing helps subsequent performance, this procedure confers only a trivial physiologic advantage owing to the added oxygen per se. Furthermore, this small advantage could be attained only if the subsequent exercise took place almost immediately following oxygen inhalation and ambient air was not breathed in the interval between hyperoxic breathing and exercise. The football player who breathes oxygen on the sideline before returning to the game or the swimmer who takes a few breaths of oxygen before moving to the blocks for the starting instructions really does not gain a competitive edge resulting from physiologic benefits. This is particularly ironic in football, because the energy to power each play is generated almost totally by metabolic reactions that do **not** utilize oxygen! The positive psychological influence of oxygen breathing should not be discounted, however, for it may provide a useful rationale for continuing this practice (if the player believes it is beneficial).

OXYGEN BREATHING DURING EXERCISE

There is considerable evidence that breathing hyperoxic gas during submaximal and maximal aerobic exercise enhances physical performance.[125, 131] Oxygen breathing during exercise has resulted in reduced blood lactate, heart rate, and pulmonary ventilation volume and a significant increase in maximal oxygen uptake.[1, 18, 42] In one study, subjects performed a 6.5-minute endurance ride on a bicycle ergometer, at an exercise level equivalent to 115% of $\dot{V}O_2$max, while breathing either room air or 100% oxygen.[127] To mask a subject's knowledge of the breathing mixture, both air and oxygen were supplied from tanks of compressed gas. Figure 23.2*A* illustrates that endurance was superior (with less drop-off in pedal revolutions) while the subject breathed pure oxygen. Figure 23.2*B* presents the oxygen uptake curves during the endurance ride while the subject breathed oxygen and room air. Oxygen uptake was higher in the 100% oxygen condition, which produced a higher level of oxygen uptake early in exercise.

Because breathing hyperoxic gas does not increase maximal cardiac output, the increase in $\dot{V}O_2$max must be the result of an expanded a-$\bar{v}$ O_2 difference.[125] During strenuous exercise, even a small increase in arterial hemoglobin saturation and dissolved oxygen in plasma with hyperoxic breathing increases total oxygen availability because the total blood volume is circulated 4 to 7 times each minute. More specifically, the additional 14 mL of oxygen in each liter of blood that results from breathing a hyperoxic mixture is a considerable amount of extra oxygen during exercise at a 20- to 30-L cardiac output. If this added oxygen were utilized by the active muscles during exercise, it would produce a 5 to 10% increase in $\dot{V}O_2$max. The increase in the partial pressure of oxygen in solution when hyperoxic gas is breathed also facilitates the diffusion of oxygen across the

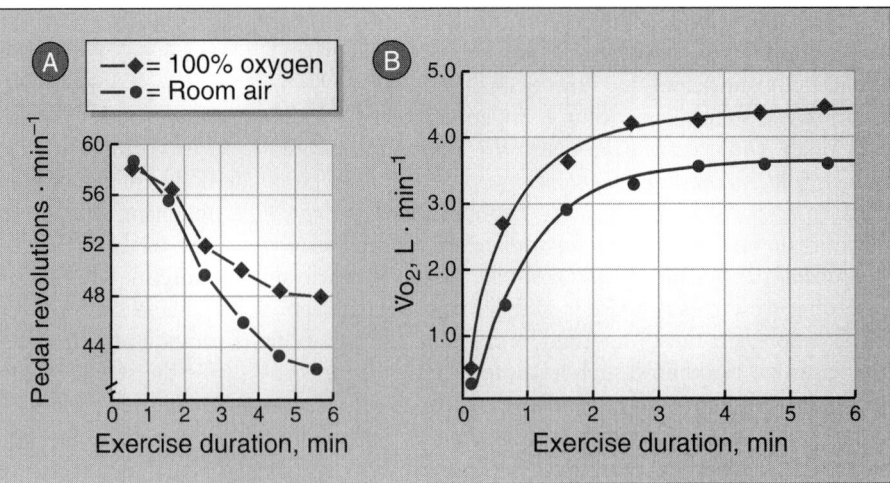

FIGURE 23.2

A, Superiority of endurance (measured by pedal revolutions each minute) that results from breathing 100% oxygen versus breathing ambient air. **B,** Oxygen uptake curves during the endurance rides demonstrate an enhanced level of oxygen uptake from breathing oxygen. (Data from Weltman, A., et al.: Effects of increasing oxygen availability on bicycle ergometer endurance performance. *Ergonomics*, 21:427, 1978.)

tissue-capillary membrane to the mitochondria. This diffusion may account for the higher rate of oxygen uptake at the beginning of exercise. A reduction in pulmonary ventilation that results from breathing hyperoxic gas reduces the oxygen cost of breathing. Theoretically, this liberates oxygen for use by the active muscles. Hyperoxia also may increase sustained local muscle performance in intense static and dynamic movements unaffected by central circulatory factors. The proposed mechanism for this ergogenic effect is high oxygen pressure within the local muscle environment enhancing sustained energy release.[39, 40]

Although breathing hyperoxic mixtures appears to offer positive ergogenic benefits **during** endurance performance, its practical application seems limited in sports. Even if an appropriate breathing system were devised, its "legality" would be unlikely during actual competition.

OXYGEN BREATHING DURING RECOVERY

Figure 23.3 illustrates the effects of breathing hyperoxic gas during recovery from strenuous exercise on subsequent exercise performance.[126] Following 1 minute of all-out exercise on a bicycle ergometer, subjects recovered passively (sat quietly) or actively (pedaled lightly) while breathing either room air or 100% oxygen for 10 or 20 minutes. They then repeated the all-out bicycle ride. There were no significant differences in the numbers of 6-second revolutions or cumulative revolutions (top graph) during the 1-minute ride after breathing room air or 100% oxygen while recovering from previous all-out exercise. During the 10- or 20-minute recovery periods, there also were no significant differences in blood lactate measurements resulting from breathing room air or oxygen. This indicated that breathing oxygen during recovery did not facilitate lactate removal. More recent research by others supports these findings and

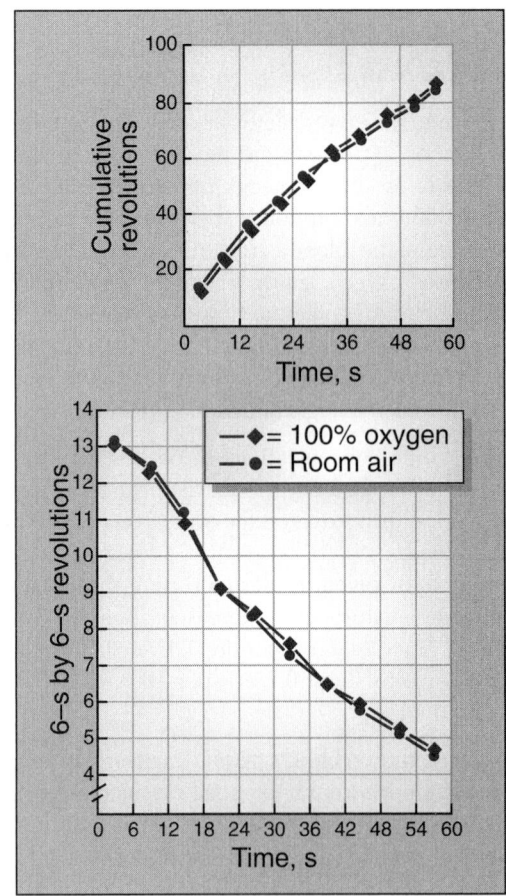

FIGURE 23.3

Cumulative *(Top)* and absolute *(Bottom)* pedal revolutions on a bicycle ergometer during 1 minute of maximal exercise after breathing either 100% oxygen or ambient air while recovering from a previous maximal exercise bout. (From Weltman, A., et al.: Exercise recovery, lactate removal, and subsequent high intensity exercise performance. *Res. Q.*, 48:786, 1977.)

has shown that oxygen breathing following short intervals of submaximal and maximal exercise had no effect on the recovery kinetics of minute ventilation, heart rate, or serum lactate levels, or on the level of subsequent exercise performance.[92, 135] In summary, research does not support the use of hyperoxic breathing mixtures as ergogenic aids in recovering from exercise or as adjuvants to improve subsequent performance following recovery from previous exercise.

MODIFICATION OF CARBOHYDRATE INTAKE

Carbohydrate loading is one of the more popular methods of nutritional modification used by endurance athletes to improve performance. Although the judicious adherence to this dietary technique can significantly improve specific exercise performance, some negative aspects of carbohydrate loading could prove detrimental.

NUTRIENT-RELATED FATIGUE DURING PROLONGED EXERCISE

The energy requirement during intense aerobic exercise is supplied largely by glycogen stored in the liver and active muscles.[88] If intense steady-rate exercise continues and the body's glycogen reserves are reduced, a progressively greater percentage of the energy for exercise is supplied through the catabolism of lipid. This energy nutrient is mobilized from storage sites in the adipose tissue and liver and delivered to the muscles via the circulation. If exercise is performed to a point at which muscle glycogen becomes severely lowered, fatigue occurs even though sufficient oxygen is available to the muscles and the potential energy from stored lipid remains almost unlimited. If a solution of glucose and water is ingested at the point of fatigue, exercise can sometimes be prolonged for an additional period of time, but for all practical purposes, the muscles' "fuel tank" reads empty, and a high level of energy transfer can no longer take place. This occurrence, accompanied by sensations of fatigue and muscle pain, has been termed "hitting the wall" by marathon runners.

In the late 1930s, scientists observed that endurance performance could be markedly improved by consuming a carbohydrate-rich diet. Conversely, endurance capacity was drastically reduced if the diet consisted predominantly of lipid. Because of this important relationship between diet and physical performance, researchers have evaluated possible ways to increase the body's glycogen reserves. As discussed in Chapter 1, simply modifying the diet's macronutrient composition greatly alters carbohydrate stores and profoundly affects subsequent performance in prolonged submaximal exercise.[91a] In one series of experiments, the endurance capacities of subjects who were fed a high-carbohydrate diet was more than three times greater

than when the same subjects consumed a high-fat diet of similar caloric content.[11] The recognition of carbohydrate as an important energy substrate during prolonged exercise has led researchers to focus on additional means to elevate the body's glycogen reserves.

GLYCOGEN SUPERCOMPENSATION

Research has shown that a particular combination of diet and exercise results in a significant "packing" of muscle glycogen. The procedure to achieve this is termed **carbohydrate loading,** or **glycogen supercompensation,** and often is used by endurance athletes preparing for competition. The result is an even greater increase in muscle glycogen than occurs with the high-carbohydrate diet discussed previously. Glycogen loading packs as much as 4 to 5 g of glycogen into each 100 g of muscle (in contrast to its normal value of about 1.7 g). (It is noteworthy that recent data suggest a sex-specific response to carbohydrate loading, with women showing no increased glycogen storage when dietary carbohydrate was increased from 60 to 75% of total caloric intake.[113a])

Classic Carbohydrate Loading Procedure

The classic procedure for achieving the supercompensation effect outlined in Table 23.6 is to first reduce the muscle's glycogen content with prolonged steady-rate exercise about 6 days before competition. Because glycogen supercompensation occurs **only** in the specific muscles depleted by exercise, athletes should be sure to engage the muscles involved in their sports. In preparation for a marathon, a 15- or 20-mile run is usually necessary, whereas for swimming and bicycling, approximately 90 minutes of moderately intense submaximal exercise in these activities is required. The athlete then maintains a low-carbohydrate diet (about 60 to 100 g per day) for several days to further deplete glycogen stores. (Note: Although the precise mechanism is poorly understood, glycogen depletion causes the formation of intermediate forms of the glycogen-storing enzyme **glycogen synthetase** in the muscle fiber.) Moderate training is continued during this time. Then, at least 3 days before competition, the athlete switches to a high-carbohydrate diet (400 to 600 g per day) and maintains it up to, and as part of, the precompetition meal. Of course, adequate daily protein, minerals and vitamins, and abundant water also must be part of the supercompensation diet.

It is noteworthy that the potential benefits of carbohydrate loading apply **only** to intense and prolonged aerobic activities. In most instances of sports competition and intense training, a daily diet containing about 60 to 70% of calories as carbohydrate provides for adequate muscle and liver glycogen reserves. Athletes who normally maintain this or a higher carbohydrate intake will have a level of

---

TABLE 23.6
TWO-STAGE DIETARY PLAN FOR INCREASING MUSCLE GLYCOGEN STORAGE

Stage 1—Depletion
  Day 1: Exhausting exercise performed to deplete muscle glycogen in specific muscles
  Days 2, 3, 4: Low-carbohydrate food intake (high percentage of protein and lipid in the daily diet)

Stage 2—Carbohydrate Loading
  Days 5, 6, 7: High-carbohydrate food intake (normal percentage of protein in the daily diet)

Competition Day
  Follow high-carbohydrate pre-competition meal

---

muscle glycogen that is usually about twice that of untrained individuals. To these athletes, the supercompensation effect would be relatively small. During periods of intense training, however, athletes who do not upgrade their daily caloric and carbohydrate intakes to meet energy demands may experience chronic muscle fatigue and staleness.[29]

Carbohydrate Loading Not Necessary for All Competition. It is not necessary to supercompensate fully for all competitions. Normal carbohydrate intake and glycogen reserves are adequate for exercise that lasts less than 60 minutes. Carbohydrate loading and the associated high levels of muscle and liver glycogen, for example, were of no benefit to performance of trained runners in a 20.9-km (13-mile) run compared to a run following a low-carbohydrate diet.[107] For most sport competitions, it only is necessary to increase the carbohydrate percentage of the diet to 60 to 70% for a day or two before the event. This will ensure that glycogen stores are adequate to meet the demands of the performance.

Athletes should be well informed about carbohydrate loading before trying to manipulate their diets and exercise habits to achieve a supercompensation effect. If, after weighing all of the pros and cons (see next section), an athlete decides to supercompensate, it should be tried in stages during training, not for the first time before competition. For example, the athlete should start with a long run followed by a high-carbohydrate diet. A detailed log should be kept of what is done and what happens. Subjective feelings should be noted during both exercise depletion and replenishment phases. If the results are positive, then the entire series of depletion, low-carbohydrate diet, and high-carbohydrate diet should be tried—but the low-carbohydrate diet should be tried for only 1 day. If no adverse effects appear, the low-carbohydrate diet should gradually be extended to a maximum of 3 or 4 days.

SAMPLE DIETS FOR ACHIEVING THE SUPERCOMPENSATION EFFECT

Table 23.7 provides an example of meal plans for carbohydrate depletion (Stage 1) and carbohydrate loading (Stage 2) preceding an endurance event.

NEGATIVE ASPECTS

The addition of 2.7 g of water stored with each gram of muscle glycogen makes it a heavy fuel compared to equivalent calories stored as lipid. This added body mass may make the athlete feel "too heavy" and uncomfortable; any extra load also directly adds to the energy cost of weight-bearing activities such as running, skiing, or hiking. The extra weight may actually negate the potential benefits derived from the increased glycogen storage. On the positive side, the water liberated during glycogen breakdown is available for temperature regulation that would be beneficial during exercise in the heat.

The classic model for supercompensation is potentially hazardous for individuals with specific health problems. A severe and chronic carbohydrate overload, interspersed with periods of high lipid or protein intake, can increase blood cholesterol and urea nitrogen levels. This could pose problems for individuals susceptible to adult-onset diabetes and heart disease or for those who have certain muscle enzyme deficiencies or renal disease.[4, 64] During the low-carbohydrate phase of the loading procedure, the potential exists for a marked ketosis often observed among individuals who exercise in carbohydrate-depleted states. Failure to eat a balanced diet may eventually lead to deficiencies of some minerals and vitamins, particularly the water-soluble vitamins; these deficiencies may require dietary supplementation. The glycogen-depleted state certainly reduces one's capability to engage in hard training, possibly resulting in an actual detraining effect during the loading period. Adverse alterations in mood state also have been reported in individuals who train while intaking low-carbohydrate diets.[68] It also is possible that dramatically reducing dietary carbohydrate for 3 or 4 days could set the stage for a loss of lean tissue because muscle protein is used as gluconeogenic substrate for maintaining blood-glucose levels.

MODIFIED LOADING PROCEDURE

Many of the negative aspects of the classic glycogen-loading sequence can be eliminated by following the less-stringent modified dietary protocol outlined in Figure 23.4.[91a,107] This 6-day protocol is achieved without prior exercise to exhaustion. The athlete trains at about 75% of $\dot{V}O_2$max (85% HRmax) for 1.5 hours and gradually reduces (tapers) the duration of exercise on successive days. Carbohydrates represent about 50% of total caloric intake during the first 3 days. The carbohydrate content of the diet is then increased to about 70% of total caloric intake for the 3 days before competition. This results in an accumulation of glycogen reserves to about the **same** point as that achieved with the classic loading protocol.[106] One reason for the effectiveness of the modified approach to carbohydrate loading is that increases in the glycogen-storing enzyme glycogen synthetase do not require dramatic glycogen depletion with exercise.[137]

L-CARNITINE

L-Carnitine is a vitamin-like compound that facilitates the influx of long-chain fatty acids into the mitochondria during energy metabolism. With prolonged exercise, the level of free fatty acids in the plasma is frequently elevated above the actual energy requirement. This elevation in plasma lipids might be the result of inadequate mitochondrial fatty acid uptake caused by an insufficient concentration of L-carnitine. If this were true, increasing the intracellular L-carnitine level through dietary supplementation would promote lipid oxidation, thereby conserving the body's limited glycogen reserves during exercise. The benefits of supplementation would be most apparent under conditions of glycogen depletion, when the demands are greatest for fatty acid oxidation.

The evidence does not indicate any ergogenic effect from L-carnitine supplementation.[119, 120] For one thing, it does not appear that an L-carnitine deficit will result from long-term exercise or heavy training.[33, 63, 89] When

---

TABLE 23.7
SAMPLE MEAL PLAN FOR CARBOHYDRATE DEPLETION AND CARBOHYDRATE LOADING DIETS PRECEDING AN ENDURANCE EVENT[a]

Meal	Stage 1 Depletion	Stage 2 Carbohydrate Loading
Breakfast	½ cup fruit juice 2 eggs 1 slice whole-wheat toast 1 glass whole milk	1 cup fruit juice 1 bowl hot or cold cereal 1 to 2 muffins 1 tbsp butter coffee (cream/sugar)
Lunch	6-oz hamburger 2 slices bread salad 1 tbsp mayonnaise and salad dressing 1 glass whole milk	2–3 oz hamburger with bun 1 cup juice 1 orange 1 tbsp mayonnaise pie or cake
Snack	1 cup yogurt	1 cup yogurt, fruit, or cookies
Dinner	2 to 3 pieces chicken, fried 1 baked potato with sour cream ½ cup vegetables iced tea (no sugar) 2 tbsp butter	1–1½ pieces chicken, baked 1 baked potato with sour cream 1 cup vegetables ½ cup sweetened pineapple iced tea (sugar) 1 tbsp butter
Snack	1 glass whole milk	1 glass chocolate milk with 4 cookies

[a]During Stage 1, the intake of carbohydrate is approximately 100 g, or 400 kcal; in Stage 2, the carbohydrate intake is increased to 400 to 625 g, or about 1600 to 2500 kcal.

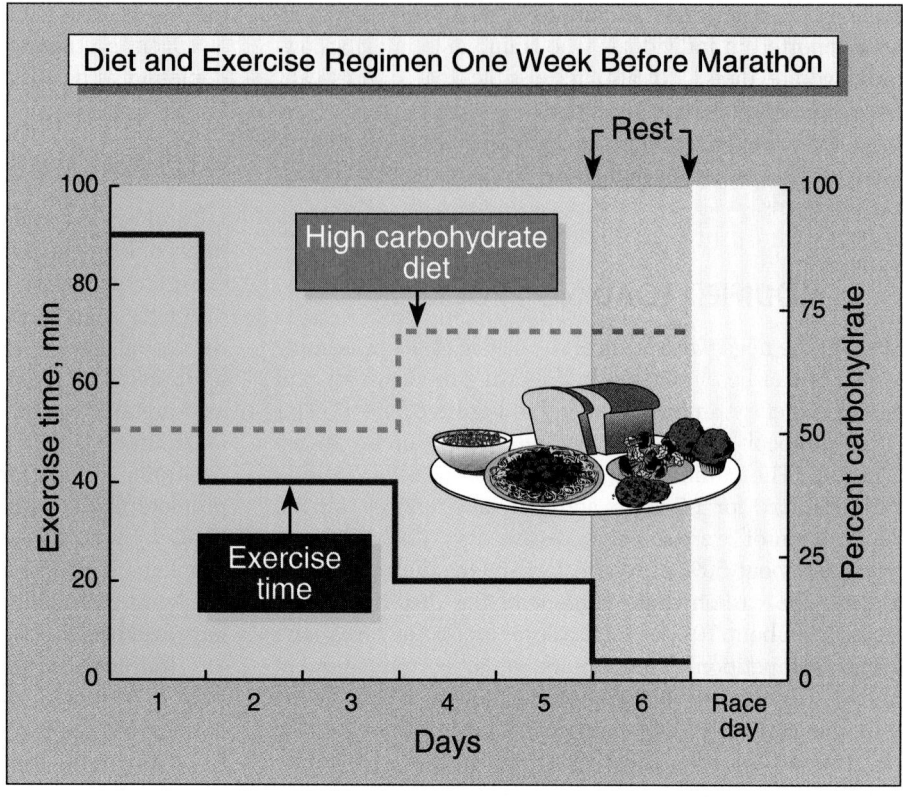

FIGURE 23.4
The modified approach. Recommended combination of diet and exercise for overloading muscle glycogen stores in the week before an important endurance contest. Exercise is gradually reduced during the week, and the carbohydrate content of the diet is increased for the last three days. (From Sherman, W.M., et al.: Effect of exercise-diet manipulation on muscle glycogen and its subsequent utilization during performance. *Int. J. Sports Med.*, 2:114, 1981.)

L-carnitine supplements of up to 2000 mg per day were ingested in one study, no effect was noted on the fuel mixture metabolized during aerobic exercise or on the levels of OBLA, endurance performance, or aerobic capacity.[136] Even under exercise conditions during which glycogen became depleted, individuals receiving L-carnitine supplements showed no alteration in substrate metabolism.[34]

■ SUMMARY ■

1. Ergogenic aids are substances or procedures believed to improve physical work capacity, physiologic function, or athletic performance.

2. Anabolic steroids are common pharmacologic agents used as ergogenic aids. These drugs function in a manner similar to the hormone testosterone. Although research findings often are inconsistent and the precise mechanism unclear, steroids may help to increase muscle size, strength, and power in some individuals.

3. Conflict exists as to whether administration of exogenous GH to normal, healthy people augments increases in muscle mass when combined with resistance training. As with anabolic steroids, significant potential health risks will probably affect those who abuse this chemical.

4. There is little evidence that amphetamines, or "pep pills," aid exercise performance or psychomotor skills in any way other than what can be derived from a simple placebo effect. The side effects of amphetamines include drug dependency, headache, dizziness, confusion, and upset stomach.

5. In some individuals, caffeine ingestion exerts an ergogenic effect by extending endurance in prolonged aerobic exercise. This is achieved by increasing the utilization of lipid for energy and conserving the body's glycogen reserves. These effects are less apparent in individuals who maintain a high-carbohydrate diet or who are habitual users of caffeine.

6. Relatively concentrated buffering solutions consumed before exercise significantly improve all-out anaerobic performance. There is no apparent ergogenic effect of TMJ repositioning or pangamic acid ingestion.

7. Red blood cell reinfusion, or "blood doping," involves the drawing, storage, and reinfusion several weeks later of concentrated (packed) red blood cells. The added blood volume contributes to a larger maximum cardiac output and an increase in the blood's oxygen-carrying capacity and, hence, $\dot{V}O_2$max. Studies applying appropriate methods of blood storage and research design support the ergogenic benefits of this process to both aerobic exercise and thermoregulation.

8. There is a physiologic rationale to why warm-up should enhance exercise performance. This rationale includes the possible ergogenic effects of warm-up on muscle-shortening velocity and efficiency, enhanced oxygen delivery and utilization, and facilitated transmission of nerve impulses. Research that supports the benefits of warm-up beyond a strong psychological component, however, is limited. Likewise, there is little evidence justifying its elimination if the performer feels that warm-up is important.

9. Moderate warm-up is useful before sudden strenuous exercise. It reduces myocardial work, and it may augment coronary blood flow when subsequent strenuous exercise begins. This may prevent transient myocardial ischemia and its potentially dangerous side effects.

10. Breathing hyperoxic gas during exercise extends endurance by increasing oxygen uptake, reducing blood lactate levels, and lowering pulmonary ventilation. Using this procedure before or following exercise is of no ergogenic effect.

11. Techniques for carbohydrate loading are generally effective in augmenting endurance in prolonged submaximal exercise. Because of potential negative effects, athletes should become well informed about this procedure. A modification of the classic loading procedure provides for the same high-level of glycogen storage without dramatic alterations in one's diet and exercise routine.

12. It does not appear that cellular levels of L-carnitine are adversely affected by long-term exercise or heavy training. This explains why most research has failed to demonstrate an ergogenic effect from supplements of this compound.

■ REFERENCES ■

1. Adams, R.P., and Welch, H.G.: Oxygen uptake, acid-base status, and performance with varied inspired oxygen fractions. *J. Appl. Physiol.*, 49:863, 1980.

1a. Ajayi, A.A.L., et al.: Testosterone increases human platelet thromboxane A_2 receptor density and aggregation responses. *Circulation*, 91:2742, 1995.

2. Alén, M., et al.: Response of serum hormones to androgen administration in power athletes. *Med. Sci. Sports Exerc.*, 17:354, 1985.

3. American College of Sports Medicine: The use of anabolic-androgenic steroids in sports. *Sports Med. Bull.*, 19:13, 1984.

4. American Medical Association Council on Food and Nutrition: *JAMA*, 224:1418, 1973.

5. Anderson, D.E., and Hickey, M.S.: Effects of caffeine on the metabolic and catecholamine response to exercise in 5 and 28°C. *Med. Sci. Sports Exerc.*, 26:453, 1994.

6. Anselme, F., et al.: Caffeine increases maximal anaerobic power and blood lactate concentration. *Eur. J. Appl. Physiol.*, 65:188, 1992.

7. Barnard, R.J., et al.: Cardiovascular responses to sudden strenuous exercise: heart rate, blood pressure, and ECG. *J. Appl. Physiol.*, 34:883, 1973.

8. Barnard, R.J., et al.: Ischemic response to sudden strenuous exercise in healthy men. *Circulation*, 48:936, 1973.

9. Bergh, U., and Ekblom, B.: Physical performance and peak aerobic power at different body temperatures. *J. Appl. Physiol.*, 46:885, 1979.

10. Berglund, B., and Hemmingsson, P.: Effects of caffeine ingestion on exercise performance at low and high altitudes in cross-country skiers. *Int. J. Sports Med.*, 3:234, 1982.

11. Bergstrom, J., et al.: Diet, muscle glycogen and physical performance. *Acta Physiol. Scand.*, 71:140, 1967.

12. Bouissou, P., et al.: Metabolic and blood catecholamine responses to exercise during alkalosis. *Med. Sci. Sports Exerc.*, 20:228, 1988.

13. Brechue, W.F., et al.: Blood flow and pressure relationships which determine VO_{2max}. *Med. Sci. Sports Exerc.*, 27:37, 1995.

14. Brien, A.J., and Simon, T.L.: The effects of red blood cell infusion on 10-km race time. *JAMA*, 257:2761, 1987.

15. Bucci, L., et al.: Ornithine supplementation and insulin release in bodybuilders. *Int. J. Sports Nutr.*, 2:287, 1992.

16. Buckley, W.E., et al.: Estimated prevalence of anabolic steroid use among male high school seniors. *JAMA*, 260:3441, 1988.

17. Burkett, L.N., and Falduto, M.T.: Steroid use by athletes in a metropolitan area. *Phys. Sportsmed.*, 12:69, 1984.

18. Byrnes, W.C., et al.: Submaximal exercise quantified as percent of normoxic and hyperoxic maximum oxygen uptakes. *Med. Sci. Sports Exerc.*, 16:572, 1984.

19. Cabasso, A.: Peliosis hepatitis in a young adult bodybuilder. *Med. Sci. Sports Exerc.*, 26:2, 1994.

20. Calabrese, L.H., et al.: The effects of anabolic steroids and strength training on the human immune response. *Med. Sci. Sports Exerc.*, 21:386, 1989.

21. Casal, D.C., and Leon, A.S.: Failure of caffeine to affect substrate utilization during prolonged exercise. *Med. Sci. Sports Exerc.*, 17:174, 1985.

22. Catlin, P., et al.: Assessing the threat of anabolic steroids. *Phys. Sportsmed.*, 21(8):37, 1993.

23. Chandler, J.V., and Blair, S.N.: The effect of amphetamines on selected physiological components related to athletic success. *Med. Sci. Sports*, 12:65, 1980.

24. Clarkson, P.: Nutritional ergogenic aids: Caffeine. *Int. J. Sports Nutr.*, 3:103, 1993.

25. Costill, D.L., et al.: Effects of caffeine ingestion on metabolism and exercise performance. *Med. Sci. Sports*, 10:155, 1978.

26. Costill, D.L., et al.: Leg muscle pH following sprint running. *Med. Sci. Sports Exerc.*, 15:325, 1983.

27. Costill, D.L., et al.: Acid-base balance during repeated bouts of exercise: influence of HCO_3. *Int. J. Sports Med.*, 5:228, 1984.

28. Costill, D.L., et al.: Anabolic steroid use among athletes: changes in HDL-C levels. *Phys. Sportsmed.*, 12:112, 1984.

29. Costill, D.L., et al.: Effects of repeated days of intensified training on muscle glycogen and swimming performance. *Med. Sci. Sports Exerc.*, 20:249, 1988.

30. Cowart, V.: Steroids in sports: After four decades, time to return to the genie's bottle? *JAMA*, 257:421, 1987.

31. Crist, D.M., et al.: Effects of androgenic anabolic steroids on neuromuscular power and body composition. *J. Appl. Physiol.*, 54:366, 1983.

32. Crist, D.M., et al.: Body composition response to exogenous GH during training in highly conditioned adults. *J. Appl. Physiol.*, 65:579, 1988.

33. Décombaz, J., et al.: Muscle carnitine after strenuous endurance exercise. *J. Appl. Physiol.*, 72:423, 1992.

34. Décombaz, J., et al.: Effect of L-carnitine on submaximal exercise metabolism after depletion of muscle glycogen. *Med. Sci. Sports Exerc.*, 25:773, 1993.

35. Delbeke, F.T., et al.: The abuse of doping agents in competing body builders in Flanders (1988 - 1993). *Int. J. Sports Med.*, 16:60, 1995.

36. Deyssig, R., et al.: Effect of growth hormone treatment on hormonal parameters, body composition and strength in athletes. *Acta Endocrinol.*, 128:313, 1993.

37. Dodd, S., et al.: Caffeine and exercise performance. *Sports Med.*, 15:14, 1993.

38. Durant, R.H., et al.: Use of multiple drugs among adolescents who use anabolic steroids. *N. Engl. J. Med.*, 328:922, 1993.

39. Eiken, O., and Tesch, P.A.: Effects of hyperoxia and hypoxia on dynamic and sustained static performance of the human quadriceps muscle. *Acta Physiol. Scand.*, 122:629, 1984.

40. Eiken, O., et al.: Human skeletal muscle function and metabolism during intense exercise at high O_2 and N_2 pressures. *J. Appl. Physiol.*, 63:571, 1987.

41. Ekblom, B.: Response to exercise after blood loss and reinfusion. *J. Appl. Physiol.*, 33:175, 1972.

42. Ekblom, B., et al.: Effect of changes in arterial oxygen content on circulation and physical performance. *J. Appl. Physiol.*, 39:71, 1975.

43. Ekblom, B., et al.: Central circulation during exercise after venesection and reinfusion of red blood cells. *J. Appl. Physiol.*, 40:379, 1976.

44. Eschbach, J.W., et al.: Correction of the anemia of end-stage renal disease with recombinant human erythropoietin. Results of a combined Phase I and II clinical trials. *N. Engl. J. Med.*, 316:73, 1987.

45. Ferenclick, G.S., and Adelman, S.: Myocardial infarction associated with anabolic steroid use in a previously healthy 37-year-old weightlifter. *Am. Heart J.*, 124:507, 1992.

45a. Fleck, S.J., et al.: Anaerobic power effects of an amino acid supplement containing no branched amino acids in elite competitive athletes. *J. Strength Cond. Res.*, 9:132, 1995.

46. Fogelholm, G.M., et al.: Low-dose amino acid supplementation: no effects on serum human growth hormone and insulin in male weight lifters. *Int. J. Sports Nutr.*, 3:290, 1993.

47. Forbes, G.B., et al.: Sequence of changes in body composition induced by testosterone and reversal of changes after drug is stopped. *JAMA*, 267:397, 1992.

48. Friedl, K.E., and Yesalis, C.E.: Self-treatment of gynecomastia in body builders who use anabolic steroids. *Phys. Sportsmed.*, 17:67, 1989.

49. Fry, A., et al.: Endocrine and performance responses to high volume training and amino acid supplementation in elite junior weightlifters. *Int. J. Sports Nutr.*, 3:306, 1993.

49a. Gelb, H., et al.: Relationship of muscular strength to jaw posture in sports dentistry. *NYSDJ*, Nov:58, 1995.

50. Girondola, R.N., et al.: Effects of pangamic acid (B_{15}) ingestion on metabolic response to exercise. *Biochem. Med.*, 24:218, 1980.

51. Gledhill, N.: Blood doping and related issues: a brief review. *Med. Sci. Sports Exerc.*, 14:183, 1982.

52. Goldfinch, J., et al.: Induced metabolic alkalosis and its effects on 400-m racing time. *Eur. J. Appl. Physiol.*, 57:45, 1988.

53. Grahm, T.E., and Spriet, L.L.: Performance and metabolic responses to a high caffeine dose during exercise. *J. Appl. Physiol.*, 71:2292, 1991.

53a. Graja, T.E., and Spirit, L.L.: Metabolic, catecholamine, and exercise performance responses to various doses of caffeine. *J. Appl. Physiol.*, 78:867, 1995.

54. Gray, M.E., and Titlow, L.W.: B_{15}: myth or miracle? *Phys. Sportsmed.*, 10(1):107, 1982.

55. Grunewald, K., and Bailey, R.: Commercially marketed supplements for bodybuilding athletes. *Sports Med.*, 15:90, 1993.

56. Herbert, V.: Pangamic acid ("vitamin B_{15}"). *Am. J. Clin. Nutr.*, 32:1534, 1979.

57. Hermansen, L.: Effect of metabolic changes on force generation in skeletal muscle during maximal exercise. In *Human Muscle Fatigue: Physiological Mechanisms.* R. Porter and J. Whelan (Eds.), CIBA Foundation, London, Pitman Medical, 1981.

58. Hervey, G.R., et al.: Effects of methandienone on the performance and body composition of men undergoing athletic training. *Clin. Sci.*, 60:457, 1981.

59. Horswill, C.A., et al.: Influence of sodium bicarbonate on sprint performance: relationship to dosage. *Med. Sci. Sports Exerc.*, 20:566, 1988.

60. Huie, M.J.: An acute myocardial infarction occurring in an anabolic steroid user. *Med. Sci. Sport Exerc.*, 26:408, 1994.

61. Hurley, B.F., et al.: High density lipoprotein cholesterol in body builders vs. power-lifters. Negative effects of androgen use. *JAMA*, 252:4, 1984.

62. Jakush, J.: Divergent views: can dental therapy enhance athletic performance? *J. Am. Dent. Assoc.*, 104:292, 1982.

63. Janssen, G., et al.: Muscle carnitine level in endurance training and running a marathon. *Int. J. Sports Med.*, 10:S153, 1989.

64. Jetté, M., et al.: The nutritional and metabolic effects of a carbohydrate-rich diet in a glycogen supercompensation training regimen. *Am J. Clin. Nutr.*, 31:2140, 1978.

65. Johnson, F.L.: The association of oral androgenic steroids and life-threatening disease. *Med. Sci. Sports,* 7:284, 1975.

66. Kantor, M.A., et al.: Androgens reduce HDL_2-cholesterol and increase hepatic triglyceride lipase activity. *Med. Sci. Sports Exerc.*, 17:462, 1985.

67. Katz, A., et al.: Maximal exercise tolerance after induced alkalosis. *J. Sports Med.*, 5:107, 1984.

68. Keith, R.E., et al.: Alterations in dietary carbohydrate, protein, and fat intake and mood state in trained female cyclists. *Med. Sci. Sports Exerc.*, 23:212, 1991.

69. Lamb, D.R.: Anabolic steroids and athletic performance. In *Hormones and Sport.* Z. Laron and A. Rogol (Eds.), Rome, Serono, 1989.

70. Lambert, M.I., et al.: Failure of commercial oral amino acid supplements to increase serum growth hormone concentrations in male body-builders. *Int. J. Sports Nutr.*, 3:298, 1993.

71. Laseter, J.T., and Russell, J.A.: Anabolic steroid-induced tendon pathology: a review of the literature. *Med. Sci. Sports Exerc.*, 23:1, 1991.

72. LeBlanc, J., et al.: Enhanced metabolic response to caffeine in exercise-trained human subjects. *J. Appl. Physiol.*, 59:832, 1985.

73. Lopes, J.M., et al.: Effect of caffeine on skeletal muscle function before and after fatigue. *J. Appl. Physiol.*, 54:1303, 1983.

74. Lutekemeier, M.J., et al.: Anabolic-androgenic steroids: prevalence, knowledge, and attitudes in junior and senior high school students. *J. Health Educ.*, 26:4, 1995.

75. MacDougall, D.: Anabolic steroids. *Phys. Sportsmed.*, 11:95, 1983.

75a. MacIntosh, B.R., and Wright, B.M.: Caffeine ingestion and performance of a 1,500-metre swim. *Canad. J. Appl. Physiol.*, 20:168, 1995.

76. MacIntyre, J.G.: Growth hormone and athletes. *Sports Med.*, 4:129, 1987.

77. Mainwood, G.W., and Worsley-Brown, P.: The effects of extracellular pH and buffer concentration on the efflux of lactate from frog sartorious muscle. *J. Physiol. (London)*, 250:1, 1975.

78. Margaria, R.: Effect of alkalosis on performance in supramaximal exercise. *Int. Z. Agnew. Physiol.*, 29:215, 1971.

79. Matson, L.G., and Tran, Z.V.: Effects of sodium bicarbonate ingestion on anaerobic performance: a meta-analytic review. *Int. J. Sports Nutr.*, 3:2, 1993.

80. Max, S.R., and Rance, N.E.: No effect of sex steroids on compensatory muscle hypertrophy. *J. Appl. Physiol.*, 56:1589, 1984.

81. McArdle, W.D., et al.: Temporomandibular joint repositioning and exercise performance: a double-blind study. *Med. Sci. Sports Exerc.*, 16:228, 1984.

82. McNaughton, L.: Two levels of caffeine ingestion on blood lactate and free fatty acid responses during incremental exercise. *Res. Q. Exerc. Sport.*, 58:255, 1987.

83. McNaughton, L.R.: Sodium citrate and anaerobic performance: implications of dosage. *Eur. J. Appl. Physiol.*, 61:392, 1990.

84. Melchert, R.B., and Lelder, A.A.: Cardiovascular effects of androgenic-anabolic steroids. *Med. Sci. Sports Exerc.*, 27:1252, 1995.

85. Mittleman, M.A., et al.: Triggering of acute myocardial infarction by heavy physical exertion. *N. Engl. J. Med.*, 329:922, 1993.

86. Moore, M.: Corrective mouth guards: performance aids or expensive placebos? *Phys. Sportsmed.*, 9:127, 1981.

87. Moore, T.J., et al.: Temporomandibular orthopedic repositioning appliance and its effect on power production in conditioned athletes. *Phys. Sportsmed.*, 14:137, 1986.

88. O'Brien, M.J., et al.: Carbohydrate dependence during marathon running. *Med. Sci. Sports Exerc.*, 25:1009, 1993.

89. Oyono-Enguelle, S., et al.: Prolonged submaximal exercise and L-carnitine in humans. *Eur. J. Appl. Physiol.*, 58:53, 1988.

90. Parkhouse, W.S., and McKenzie, D.C.: Possible contribution of skeletal muscle buffers to enhanced anaerobic performance: a brief review. *Med. Sci. Sports Exerc.*, 16:328, 1984.

91. Pope, H.G., Jr., and Katz, D.L.: Affective and psychotic symptoms associated with anabolic steroid use. *Am. J. Psychiatry*, 145:487, 1988.

91a. Rauch, L.H.G., et al.: The effects of carbohydrate loading on muscle glycogen content and cycling performance. *Int. J. Sports Nutr.*, 5:25, 1995.

92. Robbins, M.K., et al.: Effect of oxygen breathing following submaximal and maximal exercise on recovery and performance. *Med. Sci. Sports Exerc.*, 24:270, 1992.

93. Robergs, R.A., et al.: Effects of warm-up on muscle glycogenolysis during intense exercise. *Med. Sci. Sports Exerc.*, 23: 7, 1991.

94. Robertson, R.J., et al.: Effect of induced erythrocythemia on hypoxia tolerance during physical exercise. *J. Appl. Physiol.*, 53:490, 1982.

95. Robertson, R.J., et al.: Hemoglobin concentration and aerobic work capacity in women following induced erythrocythemia. *J. Appl. Physiol.*, 57:568, 1984.

96. Robertson, R.J., et al.: Effect of induced alkalosis on physical work capacity during arm and leg exercise. *Ergonomics*, 30:19, 1987.

97. Rogol, A.D.: Growth hormone: physiology, therapeutic use, and potential for abuse. In *Exercise and Sport Sciences Reviews*. Vol. 17, K.B. Pandolf (Ed.), New York, Macmillan, 1989.

98. Rogozkin, V.: Metabolic effects of anabolic steroids on skeletal muscle. *Med. Sci. Sports*, 11:160, 1979.

99. Rudman, D., et al.: Effects of human growth hormone in men over 60 years old. *N. Engl. J. Med.*, 323:1, 1990.

100. Sachtleben, T.R., et al.: The effects of anabolic steroids on myocardial structure and cardiovascular fitness. *Med. Sci. Sports Exerc.*, 25:1240, 1993.

101. Safran, M.R., et al.: The role of warm up in muscular injury prevention. *Am. J. Sports Med.*, 16:123, 1988.

102. Sawka, M.N., and Young, A.J.: Acute polycythemia and human performance during exercise and exposure to extreme environments. *Exercise and Sport Sciences Reviews*. Vol. 17, K.B. Pandolf (Ed.), New York, Macmillan, 1989.

103. Sawka, M.N., et al.: Influence of polycythemia on blood volume and thermoregulation during exercise heat stress. *J. Appl. Physiol.*, 62:912, 1987.

104. Sawka, M.N., et al.: Polycythemia and hydration: effects on thermoregulation on blood volume during exercise-heat stress. *Am. J. Physiol.*, 255:R456, 1988.

105. Schubert, M.M., et al.: Changes in shoulder and leg strength in athletes wearing mandibular orthopedic repositioning appliances. *J. Am. Dent. Assoc.*, 108:334, 1984.

106. Sherman, W.M.: Carbohydrates, muscle glycogen, and muscle glycogen super-compensation. In *Ergogenic Aids in Sports*. M.H. Williams (Ed.), Champaign, IL, Human Kinetics, 1983.

107. Sherman, W.M., et al.: Effect of exercise-diet manipulation on muscle glycogen and its subsequent utilization during performance. *Int. J. Sports Med.*, 2:114, 1981.

108. Spiret, L.L., et al.: Effect of graded erythrocythemia on cardiovascular and metabolic responses to exercise. *J. Appl. Physiol.*, 61:1942, 1986.

109. Stensrud, T., et al.: L-Tryptophan supplementation does not improve running performance. *Int. J. Sports Med.*, 13:481, 1992.

110. Suminski, R., et al.: The effect of amino acid ingestion and resistance exercise on growth hormone responses in young males. *Med. Sci. Sports Exerc.*, 25:S77(Abstract), 1993.

111. Supinski, G.S., et al.: Caffeine effect on respiratory muscle endurance and sense of effort during loaded breathing. *J. Appl. Physiol.*, 60:2040, 1986.

112. Sutton, J.R., et al.: Effect of pH on muscle glycolysis during exercise. *Clin. Sci.*, 61:331, 1981.

113. Tarnopolsky, M.A., et al.: Physiological responses to caffeine during endurance running in habitual caffeine users. *Med. Sci. Sports Exerc.*, 21:418, 1989.

113a. Tarnopolsky, M.A., et al.: Carbohydrate loading and metabolism during exercise in men and women. *J. Appl. Physiol.*, 78:1360, 1995.

114. Taylor, W.N.: Synthetic anabolic–androgenic steroids: a plea for controlled substance status. *Phys. Sportsmed.*, 15:140, 1987.

115. Tingus, S.J., and Carlsen, R.C.: Effect of continuous infusion of an anabolic steroid on murine skeletal muscle. *Med. Sci. Sports Exerc.*, 25:485, 1993.

116. Toner, M.M., et al.: Metabolic and cardiovascular responses to exercise with caffeine. *Ergonomics*, 25:1175, 1982.

116a. Trice, I., and Haymes, E.M.: Efects of caffeine ingestion on exercise-induced changes during high-intensity, intermittent exercise. *Int. J. Sports Nutr.*, 5:37, 1995.

117. Van Socren, M.H., et al.: Caffeine metabolism and epinephrine responses during exercise in users and nonusers. *J. Appl. Physiol.*, 75:805, 1994.

118. Visuri, T., and Lindholm, H.: Bilateral distal biceps tendon avulsions with use of anabolic steroids. *Med. Sci. Sports Exerc.*, 26:941, 1994.

119. Vukovich, M.D., et al.: Carnitine supplementation: effect on muscle carnitine and glycogen content during exercise. *Med. Sci. Sports Exerc.*, 26:1122, 1994.

120. Wagenmarkers, A.J.M.: L-Carnitine supplementation and performance in man. In *Advances in Nutrition and Top Sport*. Vol. 32, F. Brouns (Ed.), Basel, Karger, 1991.

121. Wanger, P.D.: Muscle O_2 transport and O_2 dependent control of metabolism. *Med. Sci. Sports Exerc.*, 27:47, 1995.

121a. Wagman, D.F., et al.: An investigation into anabolic androgenic steroid use by elite U.S. powerlifters. *J. Strength Cond. Res.*, 9:149, 1995.

122. Webb, O.L., et al.: Severe depression of high density lipoprotein cholesterol levels in weight lifters and body builders by self-administered exogenous testosterone and anabolic-androgenic steroids. *Metabolism*, 33:11, 1984.

123. Webster, M.J., et al.: Effect of sodium bicarbonate ingestion on exhaustive resistance exercise performance. *Med. Sci. Sports Exerc.*, 25:960, 1993.

124. Weir, J., et al.: A high carbohydrate diet negates the metabolic effects of caffeine during exercise. *Med. Sci. Sports Exerc.*, 19:100, 1987.

125. Welch, H.G.: Hyperoxia and human performance: a brief review. *Med. Sci. Sports Exerc.*, 14:253, 1982.

126. Weltman, A.L., et al.: Exercise recovery, lactate removal, and subsequent high intensity exercise performance. *Res. Q.*, 48:786, 1977.

127. Weltman, A.L., et al.: Effects of increasing oxygen availability on bicycle ergometer endurance performance. *Ergonomics*, 21:427, 1978.

128. Wilkes, D., et al.: Effect of acute induced metabolic alkalosis on 800-m racing time. *Med. Sci. Sports Exerc.*, 15:277, 1983.

129. Williams, M.H.: Ergogenic and ergolytic substances. *Med. Sci. Sports Exerc.*, 24:S344, 1992.

130. Williams, M.O., et al.: The effect of mandibular position on appendage muscle strength. *J. Prosthet. Dent.*, 49:560, 1983.

131. Wilson, B.A., et al.: Effects of hyperoxic gas mixtures on energy metabolism during prolonged work. *J. Appl. Physiol.*, 30:267, 1975.

132. Wilson, J.D.: Androgen abuse by athletes. *Endocrine Rev.*, 9:181, 1988.

133. Winder, W.W.: Effect of intravenous caffeine on liver glycogenolysis during prolonged exercise. *Med. Sci. Sports Exerc.*, 18:192, 1986.

134. Windsor, R., and Dumitrv, D.: Prevalence of anabolic steroid use by male and female adolescents. *Med. Sci. Sports Exerc.*, 21:494, 1989.

135. Winter, F.D., et al.: Effects of 100% oxygen on performance of professional soccer players. *JAMA*, 262:227, 1989.

136. Wyss, V., et al.: Effects of ʟ-carnitine administration on V̇o₂max and the aerobic-anaerobic threshold in normoxia and acute hypoxia. *Eur. J. Appl. Physiol.*, 60:1, 1990.

137. Yan, Z., et al.: Effect of low glycogen on glycogen synthase in human muscle during and after exercise. *Acta Physiol. Scand.*, 145:345, 1992.

138. Yarasheski, K.E.: Growth hormone effects on metabolism, body composition, muscle mass, and strength. *Exerc. Sport Sci. Rev.*, 22:285, 1994.

139. Yarasheski, K.E., et al.: Effect of growth hormone and resistance exercise on muscle growth in young men. *Am. J. Physiol.*, 262:E261, 1992.

140. Yarasheski, K.E., et al.: Short-term growth hormone treatment does not increase muscle protein synthesis in experienced weight lifters. *J. Appl. Physiol.*, 74:3073, 1993.

141. Yates, J.W., et al.: Effect of a mandibular orthopedic repositioning appliance on muscular strength. *J. Am. Dent. Assoc.*, 108:331, 1984.

142. Yesalis, C.E., et al.: Anabolic-androgenic steroid use in the United States. *JAMA*, 270:1217, 1993.

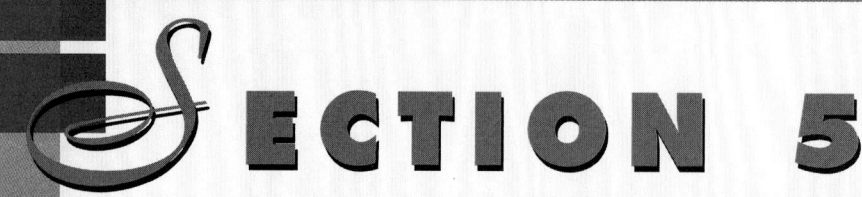

SECTION 5

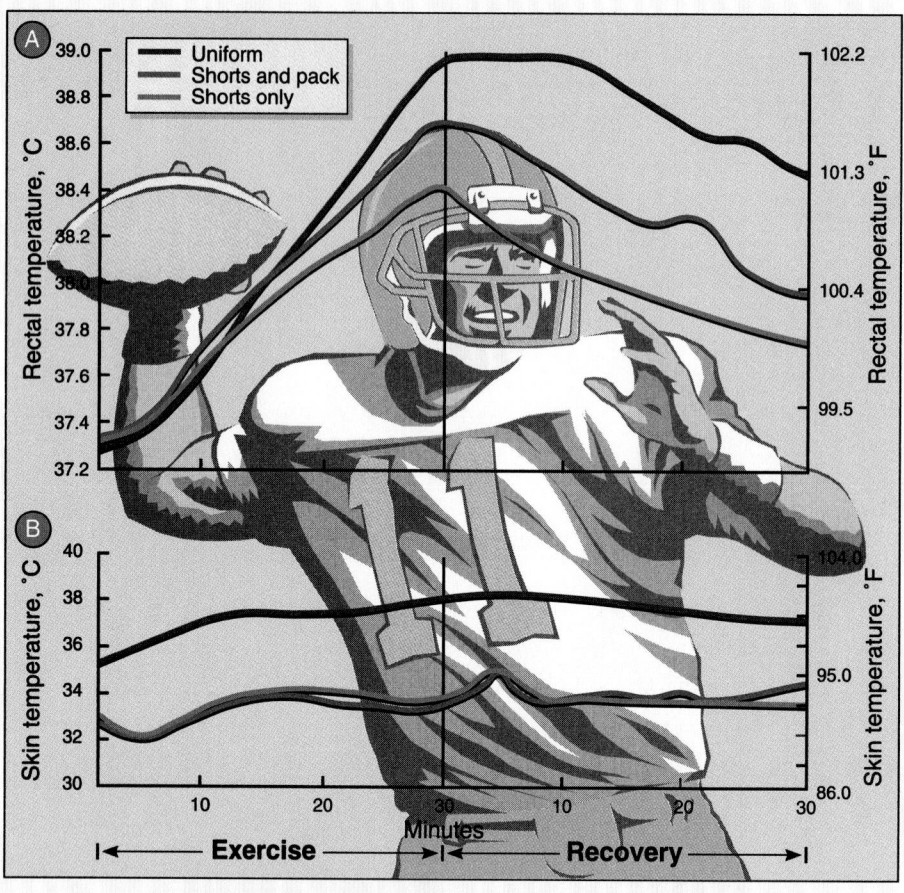

"THE TOTAL EFFECT OF

EACH ENVIRONMENTAL STRESSOR

IS DETERMINED BY THE DEGREE

TO WHICH IT DEVIATES FROM

NEUTRAL CONDITIONS, AND BY

THE DURATION OF EXPOSURE"

Exercise Performance and Environmental Stress

Previous chapters focused on the physiologic and metabolic adjustments that enable humans to generate energy for exercise in "normal" environments. In this context, the stress on the organism is largely that imposed by the specific form of work, such as walking or running, bicycling, or swimming in relatively warm water. In many instances, however, environmental conditions compound the stress of exercise.

Sport activities often are held at altitudes that impair the oxygenation of blood flowing through the lungs. Above a certain elevation, capacity is severely limited to generate aerobic energy for exercise. At the other extreme, to explore beneath the water's surface poses a different challenge. Beneath the water, divers must bring their sea level environment with them in the form of air compressed into scuba tanks carried on their backs. For some enthusiasts, however, there is no external assistance, and the length of an underwater excursion generally is limited by the quantity of air inhaled into the lungs just before diving and the buildup of arterial carbon dioxide during the dive. In both breath-hold diving and diving with scuba, the environment provides unique challenge and dangers for the participant. These risks often are independent of the stress of exercise. Consideration also must focus on the thermal quality of the environment. Exercising in a hot, humid environment or under conditions of extreme cold can impose severe thermal stress. These environmental demands not only impair one's capacity for exercise but, in the extreme, pose a threat to health and safety.

The total effect of each environmental stressor is determined by how much it deviates from neutral conditions, as well as by the duration of the exposure. In addition, several environmental stressors operating at the same time (e.g., extreme cold exposure at high altitude) may exceed and override the simple additive effects of each stressor if imposed separately. We recommend three textbooks for the student interested in the specifics of human adaptation to diverse forms of environmental stress.[1,2,3]

In the three chapters that follow, the specific problems encountered at altitude and during exercise in hot and cold environments are explored. We also discuss the immediate physiological adjustments and long-term adaptations as the body strives to maintain internal consistency despite an environmental challenge. The chapter on sport diving considers the unique problems associated with this popular form of sport and recreation.

■ REFERENCES ■

1. Dill, D.B.: *Handbook of Physiology. Section 4. Adaptation to the Environment.* Washington, DC, American Physiological Society, 1964.
2. Frisancho, A.R.: *Human Adaptation and Accommodation.* Ann Arbor, MI, University of Michigan Press, 1993.
3. Pandolf, K., et al. (eds.): *Human Performance Physiology and Environmental Medicine at Terrestrial Extremes.* Carmel, IN, Cooper Publishing Group, 1988.

Henry, F.M.: The role of exercise in altitude pain. *Am. J. Physiol.* 145:279, 1945.

Traveling to high altitude induces a variety of adaptive physiological responses and potentially debilitating physical symptoms. Being at extremely high altitudes (beyond terrestrial elevations) often results in intense pain, usually localized in or near the joints. This condition is termed "aviator bends" and is experienced by pilots in nonpressurized aircraft. The pain associated with bends increases in frequency and magnitude in relation to the increase in altitude and the accompanying decrease in barometric pressure.

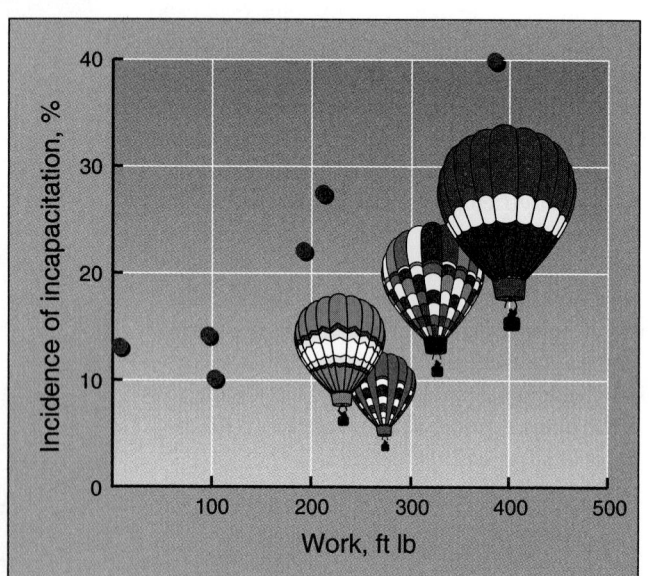

Incidence of incapacitating pain symptoms in relation to work performance at a simulated altitude of 38,000 ft.

The pain experienced at extreme altitude is unrelated to the adequacy of oxygen loading of blood, because the aviator normally breathes hyperoxic mixtures at the ambient-altitude barometric pressure to increase the inspired PO_2. Rather, symptoms of aviator bends generally result from the same process that occurs in rapid ascent from the underwater environment. Rapid ascent causes the expansion of dissolved nitrogen, which forms extravascular bubbles or embolic ischemia in the body tissues from bubbles within the vascular circuit. Joint pain can sometimes be prevented by removal of the body's dissolved gaseous nitrogen by breathing pure oxygen before travel to extreme altitude. The occurrence and severity of aviator bends vary in individuals who exercise on reaching high altitude. Some individuals experience symptoms during heavy exercise but not moderate exercise, while others experience severe symptoms when performing only moderate work.

Henry studied aviator bends by systematically varying the severity of exercise and observing the effect of such variation on bends pain. Three-hundred ninety subject-exposures took place in a decompression chamber at a barometric pressure of 155 mm Hg (38,000 ft; 11,582 m). Pure oxygen, administered by mask, supplied oxygen except during the first 10,000-ft ascent to simulated altitude. The ascent to 38,000 ft required 12 minutes, and subjects remained at that "altitude" for 90 minutes unless they required recompression and return to sea-level pressure because of incapacitating symptoms. On reaching high altitude, subjects performed one of six standard arm exercises designed to isolate such factors as continuous versus intermittent strain, total work, and the nature of joint movement. The exercises included holding a metal bar (1.5-in. diameter, 16 in. long) with added weights (16 and 36 lb). The cadence for moving the bar plus weights equaled $80 \text{ beats} \cdot \text{min}^{-1}$. The tasks included raising and lowering the bar to different heights. Exercise consisted of 2.5-minute on-off cycles, with the presence and severity of pain evaluated during each work cycle.

Sixty-three percent of total exposures resulted in pain to the hand, wrist, elbow, or shoulder, while only 16% resulted in pain in the foot, ankle, knee, and hip. Moderate or severe pain occurred in the arms 42% of the time, while incapacitating arm pain occurred in 22% of the exposures. In total, 80% of all pain, 86% of moderate to severe pain, and 90% of incapacitating pain occurred in the arms. The evidence clearly indicated that although altitude pain occurred in unexercised limbs, it was more prevalent and severe in exercised limbs. The figure plots the incidence of incapacitating pain symptoms with work performance. A direct, linear relationship existed between total work performed and the appearance of incapacitating pain in joints and muscles.

The Henry study, a simple but elegant experiment, first showed that exercise increased the incidence and severity of high-altitude pain symptoms. Paradoxically, exercise also hastened the rate that symptoms disappeared after their maximum effect. Exercise presumably caused a nitrogen-flushing function from the increased circulation. Henry's research showed that muscle strain, the number of intermittent movements, severity of strain, and joint angle were not related to the onset or severity of altitude pain. The only variable consistently related to pain was total work or "some factor directly related to it." The implications for the military included a better understanding of how exercise affects altitude pain at extremely low barometric pressures.

Exercise at Medium and High Altitude

More than 40 million people live, work, and recreate at terrestrial elevations between 3,048 m (10,000 ft) and 5,486 m (18,000 ft) above sea level. In the earth's topography, these elevations encompass the range of what is generally considered **high altitude**. Although high-altitude natives living in permanent settlements as high as 5486 m in the Andes and Himalayan mountains are self sustaining, prolonged exposure of an unacclimatized person to such altitude may cause death from hypoxia even if the person remains inactive. The physiologic challenge of even a medium altitude becomes readily apparent during physical activity.[64] In the United States, close to 1 million people per year ascend to Pikes Peak, Colorado (4300 m) within an hour by train, car, or railroad, and thousands of others do so by climbing, cycling, and even running. Many millions more throughout the world ascend to high altitudes for purposes of mountaineering, trekking, tourism, business, and scientific and military excursions. Whatever the purpose, many newcomers to altitude have not had time to acclimatize to the physiologic challenge caused by reduced partial pressure of oxygen (PO_2) at altitude.

THE STRESS OF ALTITUDE

The challenge of altitude is directly from the decreased ambient PO_2 and not the reduced total barometric pressure per se or from any change in the relative concentrations of the gases in the inspired air. The barometric pressure, the pressures of the respired gases, and the percent saturation of hemoglobin at various terrestrial elevations are illustrated in Figure 24.1. The data in Figure 24.2 show the changes that occur to oxygen availability (for PO_2) in ambient air, alveolar air, and arterial and mixed-venous blood as one ascends from sea level to the top of Pikes Peak. This progressive change in the pressure of oxygen in the environment (and in various components of the body) is known as the **oxygen transport cascade**.

The density of air decreases progressively as one ascends above sea level. For example, the barometric pressure at sea level averages 760 mm Hg, whereas at 3048 m the barometer reads 510 mm Hg; at an elevation of 5486 m, the pressure of a column of air at the earth's surface is about one-half its pressure at sea level. Although dry, ambient air at both sea level and altitude contains 20.93% oxygen, the PO_2 or density of the oxygen molecules in air is reduced in direct proportion to the fall in barometric pressure upon ascending to higher elevations ($PO_2 = 0.2093 \times$ barometric pressure). Thus, ambient PO_2 averages approximately 150 mm Hg at sea level but only 107 mm Hg at 3048 m. At the summit of Mt. Everest (8,848 m; 29,028 ft) the pressure of ambient air is approximately 250 mm Hg; the concomitant alveolar PO_2 is 25 mm Hg. This represents only approximately 30% of the oxygen available in air at sea level.[76] It is this reduction in PO_2 (and accompanying arterial hypoxia) that precipitates the immediate physiologic adjustments to altitude as well as the longer-term process of acclimatization.[a]

OXYGEN LOADING AT ALTITUDE

Because of the S-shaped nature of the oxyhemoglobin dissociation curve (see Chapter 13, Fig. 13.4), there only is a small change in the percent saturation of hemoglobin, with decreasing PO_2 until one reaches an altitude of approximately 3048 m. At 1981 m (6500 ft), for example, the alveolar PO_2 is reduced from its sea level value of 100 mm Hg to 78 mm Hg, although hemoglobin is still approximately 90% saturated with oxygen. Although this relatively small decrease in the amount of oxygen carried by the blood has little effect on a person at rest or even during mild exercise, vigorous aerobic activities are altitude sensitive. The relatively poor performances of men and women in middle-distance and distance running and swimming during the 1968 Olympics in Mexico City (altitude 2300 m; 7546 ft) have been attributed to the small reduction in oxygen transport at this altitude.[11, 17] No world records were established in events lasting longer than 2.5 minutes. The short-term anaerobic power activities such as sprint running, jumping, shot-put, and discus are not negatively affected at altitude. Enhanced performance often oc-

---

[a] "Acclimatization" refers to adaptations produced by a change in the natural environment, whether by a change in season or place or residence. In contrast, "acclimation" refers to adaptation produced in a controlled laboratory environment as occurs in special chambers that can simulate high-altitude and hypoxic environments, as well as extremes of thermal stress.

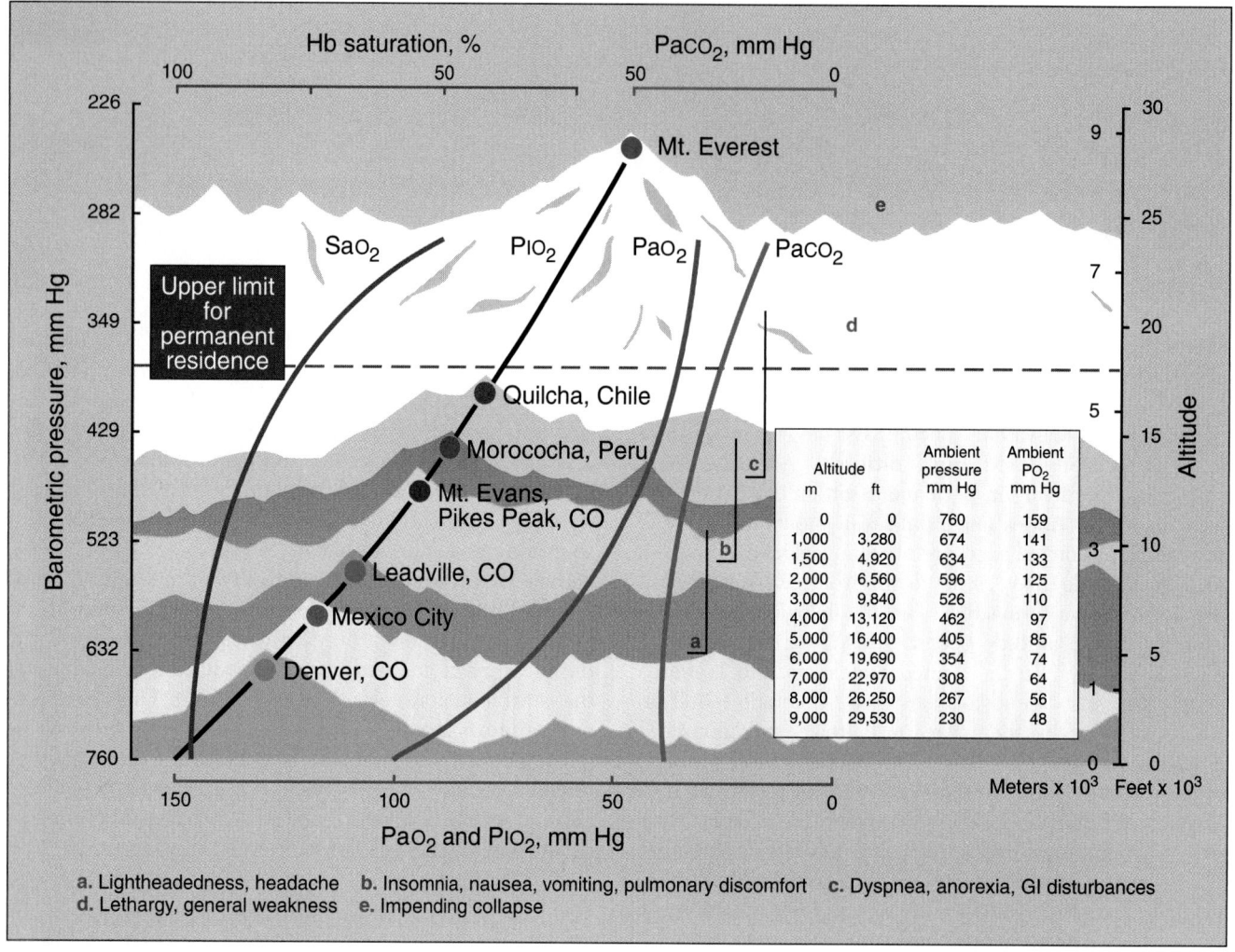

a. Lightheadedness, headache   b. Insomnia, nausea, vomiting, pulmonary discomfort   c. Dyspnea, anorexia, GI disturbances
d. Lethargy, general weakness   e. Impending collapse

FIGURE 24.1

Changes in environmental and physiologic variables with progressive elevations in altitude (PaO_2, partial pressure of arterial oxygen; $PaCO_2$, partial pressure of arterial carbon dioxide; PIO_2, partial pressure of oxygen in inspired air; SaO_2, oxygen saturation of hemoglobin). (From Kollias, J., and Buskirk, E.: Exercise and altitude. In *Science and Medicine of Exercise and Sports.* Edited by W. Johnson and E. Buskirk. New York, Harper and Row, 1974.)

curs because of the reduced air density (air resistance) at altitude compared to sea level.

At high elevations such as in the Andes and Himalayas, the reduced loading of hemoglobin with oxygen is readily apparent, and it is difficult to sustain physical activity. Acute exposure to 4,300 m, for example, causes a 32% reduction in aerobic capacity compared to sea level values.[5, 79] At altitudes above 5,182 m (17,000 ft), permanent living is nearly impossible, and mountain climbing above this elevation is usually done with the aid of oxygen equipment.[51] At 5,486 m (18,000 ft), arterial PO_2 is 38 mm Hg and hemoglobin is 73% saturated. Because this PO_2 is on the steep part of the oxyhemoglobin dissociation curve, any further increase in altitude (decrease in PO_2) brings about a relatively large decrease in hemoglobin saturation and oxygen transport capacity. Amazingly, however, there are reports of acclimatized mountaineers who lived for weeks at 6,706 m (22,000

ft) breathing only ambient air.[31] Members of two Swiss expeditions to Mt. Everest remained at the summit for 2 hours without using oxygen equipment![50] This is an impressive feat considering that arterial PO_2 is only approximately 25 mm Hg with a corresponding arterial blood oxygen saturation of 58%; under these conditions, an unacclimatized person would become unconscious within 30 seconds.[76] For acclimatized men at simulated extreme altitudes that approach the summit of Mt. Everest, $\dot{V}O_2max$ was reduced by approximately 70% from 4.13 L · min^{-1} to 1.17 L · min^{-1}, or from 49.1 mL · kg^{-1} · min^{-1} to 15.3 mL · kg^{-1} · min^{-1}.[25] These lower values represent the sea level aerobic capacity of a 70- to 80-year-old man! Although exceptional performances at high altitude are clearly the exception and not the rule, they do demonstrate the enormous adaptive capability of humans to survive and even work without external support at extreme terrestrial elevations.

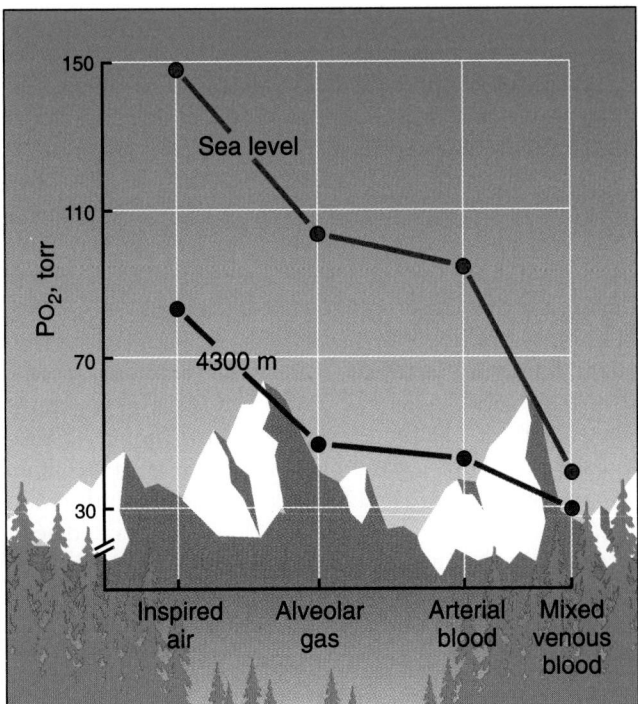

FIGURE 24.2
Oxygen transport cascade at sea level and at 4300 m (14,108 ft).

ACCLIMATIZATION

During the many years that mountaineers have attempted to climb the world's highest peaks, it was known that weeks were required for sea-level residents to adjust to successively higher elevations. *The adaptive responses in physiology and metabolism that improve one's tolerance to altitude hypoxia are broadly termed* **acclimatization.** Each adjustment to a higher altitude is progressive, and full acclimatization requires time. Successful adjustment to medium altitude represents only partial adjustment to a higher elevation. Residents of moderate altitudes, however, do show less decrement in physiological capacity and exercise performance compared to lowlanders when both groups travel to a high altitude.[46]

As summarized in Table 24.1, certain compensatory responses to altitude occur almost immediately, whereas other adaptations take weeks or even months. Although the rapidity of the body's response is largely altitude-dependent, considerable individual variability exists for both the rate and success of acclimatization.[53]

IMMEDIATE RESPONSES TO ALTITUDE

Upon arrival at elevations of 2300 m and higher, rapid physiological adjustments occur to compensate for the thinner

TABLE 24.1
IMMEDIATE AND LONGER-TERM ADJUSTMENTS TO ALTITUDE HYPOXIA

System	Immediate	Longer-Term
Pulmonary acid-base	Hyperventilation Body fluids become more alkaline due to reduction in CO_2 with hyperventilation	Hyperventilation Excretion of base via the kidneys and concomitant reduction in alkaline reserve
Cardiovascular	Increase in submaximal heart rate Increase in submaximal cardiac output Stroke volume remains the same or is slightly lowered Maximum cardiac output remains the same or is slightly lowered	Submaximal heart rate remains elevated Submaximal cardiac output falls to or below sea-level values Stroke volume is lowered Maximum cardiac output is lowered
Hematologic		Decreased plasma volume Increased hematocrit Increased hemoglobin concentration Increased total number of red blood cells
Local		Possible increased capillarization of skeletal muscle Increased red-blood-cell 2,3-DPG Increased mitochondrial density Increased aerobic enzymes in muscle Loss of body weight and lean body mass

air and accompanying reduced alveolar P_{O_2}. The most important of these responses are:

- An increase in the respiratory drive that results in a relative hyperventilation.
- An increase in blood flow both at rest and during submaximal exercise.

Hyperventilation. *The most important and clear-cut immediate response of the native lowlander to altitude exposure is hyperventilation brought on by the reduced arterial P_{O_2}.*[14, 62] Once initiated, this "hypoxic drive" increases during the first few weeks and may remain elevated for a year or longer during prolonged altitude residence.[38]

Special receptors sensitive to reduced oxygen pressure are located in the aortic arch and at the branching of the carotid arteries in the neck. Any significant reduction in arterial P_{O_2}, which occurs at an altitude above approximately 2000 m, progressively stimulates these peripheral chemoreceptors. This, in turn, modifies inspiratory activity to increase alveolar ventilation and cause alveolar P_{O_2} to increase toward the level in ambient air—the greater the hyperventilation, the more closely alveolar air resembles inspired air. The increase in alveolar P_{O_2} with hyperventilation facilitates oxygen loading in the lungs and provides the rapid first line of defense against the reduced ambient P_{O_2} at altitude.[71] Mountaineers who respond with a strong, hypoxic ventilatory drive perform exercise tasks better at extreme altitudes and can reach a higher altitude compared to other climbers who have a blunted ventilatory response when exposed to a reduced ambient P_{O_2}.[62]

Increased Cardiovascular Response. In the early stages of altitude adaptation, submaximal exercise heart rate and cardiac output may increase by 50% above sea-level values, whereas the heart's stroke volume remains unchanged.[35, 73] Because the oxygen cost of exercising at altitude is no different than at sea level, the increase in blood flow at altitude partially compensates for the reduced oxygen in arterial blood. For example, a 10% increase in cardiac output at rest or in moderate exercise offsets a 10% reduction in arterial oxygen saturation, at least for the total oxygen circulated through the body. As illustrated in Figure 24.3, although the oxygen cost of submaximal exercise at 100 watts on a bicycle ergometer remains unchanged at approximately 2.0 L · min^{-1} at both sea level and high altitude, the relative strenuousness of the effort can be considerable at altitude. In this example, submaximal exercise that represents 50% of a subject's $\dot{V}_{O_2}$max at sea level is equivalent to 70% of aerobic capacity at an altitude of 4,300 m (14,108 ft).

The increase in systemic arterial blood pressure noted during high-altitude exposure is related to an increase in the level of norepinephrine from an augmented sympathetic activity.[77] The 24-hour urinary excretion of norepinephrine and epinephrine during control (sea level) and following altitude exposure at 4300 m for seven days is displayed in

Figure 24.4. There were no changes in epinephrine, but norepinephrine increased significantly by the fourth day. Although not shown in the figure, the levels of urinary norepinephrine remain elevated for approximately 1 week following return to sea level.[67]

The effects of acute altitude exposure on the metabolic and cardiorespiratory response to moderate and maximal bicycle exercise in young men are presented in Table 24.2. Physiologic measures were obtained at sea level and during a brief exposure to a simulated altitude of 4,000 m (13,124 ft).[65] Even with the increase in pulmonary ventilation during submaximal exercise at "altitude," arterial oxygen saturation reduced from 96% at sea level to approximately 70% at all altitude exercise levels. During submaximal exercise, however, the blood's reduced oxygen content was entirely compensated for by an increased cardiac output. The increase in blood flow was due to an elevated heart rate because the heart's stroke volume remained unchanged during short-term altitude exposure. With this circulatory adjustment, oxygen uptake was nearly identical during submaximal exercise at sea level and altitude. The greatest effect of altitude on aerobic metabolism was observed during maximal exercise, when the $\dot{V}_{O_2}$max was reduced to 72% of the sea-level value. With maximal exercise, the ventilatory and circulatory adjustments to acute altitude exposure cannot compensate for the lower arterial oxygen content. The compensatory effects of pulmonary ventilation and oxygen uptake at a given exercise level on the bicycle ergometer from sea level to simulated altitudes from 1,000 to 4,000 m are illustrated in Figure 24.5. For each 1,000-m increase

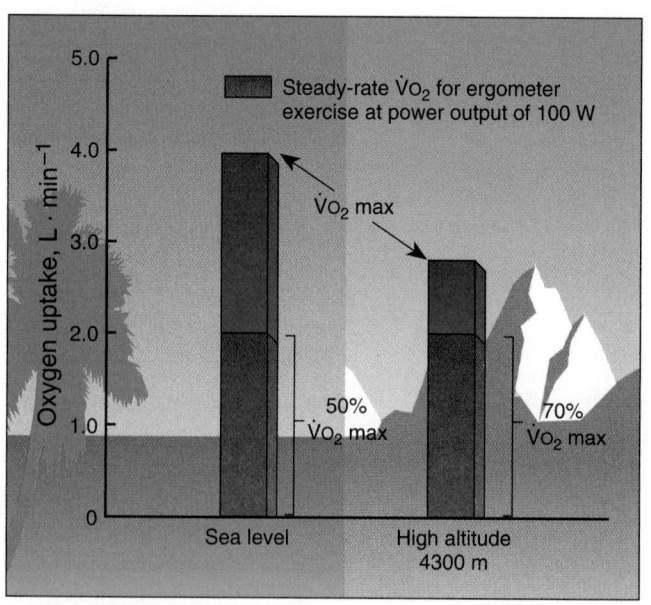

FIGURE 24.3

Comparison of oxygen cost and relative strenuousness of submaximal exercise at sea level and high altitude.

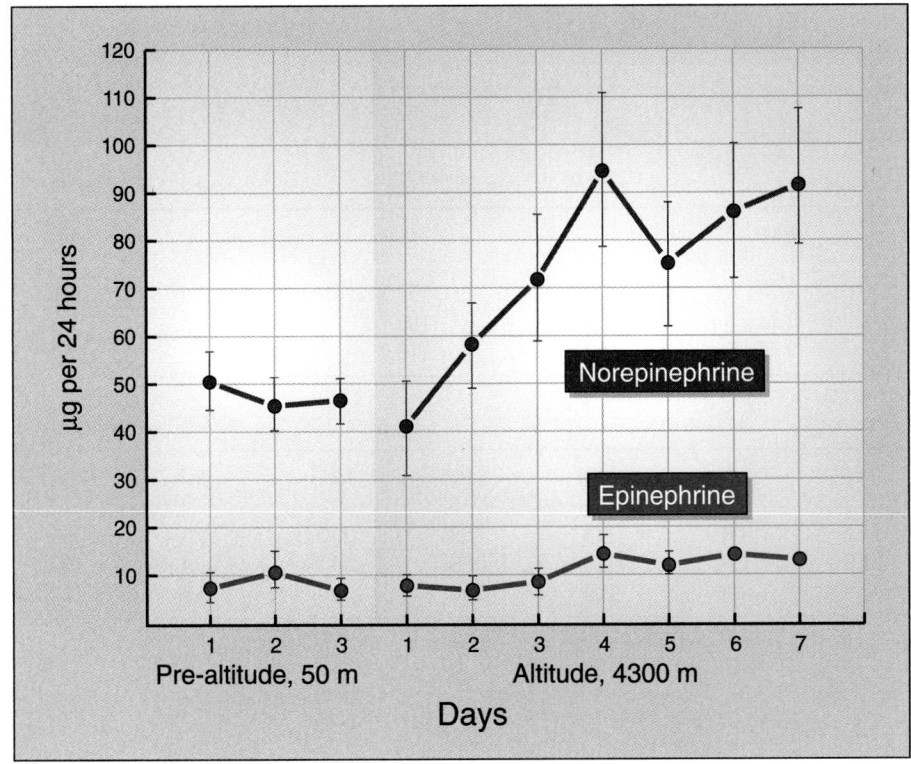

FIGURE 24.4

Effects of a 7-day stay at 4,300-m (14,108 ft) altitude in eight male sea-level residents on urinary norepinephrine and epinephrine. (Modified from Surks, M.J., et al.: Changes in plasma thyroxine concentration and metabolism, catecholamine excretion and basal oxygen uptake during acute exposure to high altitude (14,100 ft). *J. Clin. Invest.*, 45:1442, 1966.)

in altitude, there is a proportionate increase in ventilation volume up to about 2.0 L · min⁻¹ oxygen uptake; thereafter, the increase in ventilation increases disproportionately as ascent continues.

ALTITUDE-RELATED MEDICAL PROBLEMS

Natives who live and work at high altitudes, as well as newcomers to altitude, often encounter a variety of medical problems associated with the reduced PO_2 at higher elevations. Some of these problems are transient and mild and dissipate within hours or several days, depending on the rapidity of the ascent and degree of exposure; other medical complications can be severe and can significantly compromise the person's overall health and safety. Three medical conditions pose potential problems to those who ascend to high altitude: (*a*) acute mountain sickness (AMS), the most common of the maladies; (*b*) high-altitude pulmonary edema (HAPE), which can be reversed if the person is returned quickly to a lower altitude; and (*c*) high-altitude cerebral edema (HACE), a potentially fatal condition if not diagnosed and treated immediately.

The changes in a variety of sensory and mental functions in relation to the changes in arterial oxygen saturation with increasing altitude are shown in Figure 24.6. These neurological alterations range from a 5% decrease in sensitivity to light at 1,524 m (5,000 ft), to a further decrease of 25% in light sensitivity and a 30% decrease in visual acuity when altitude doubles to 3,048 m (10,000 ft), to a 25% deterioration in coding tasks and simple reaction time at 6,096 m (20,000 ft).

Acute Mountain Sickness. Despite the body's rapid defense against the stress of altitude, many people experience the acute discomfort of **mountain sickness** during the first few days at altitudes of 3,000 m and higher. This relatively benign condition is most frequently seen in people who ascend rapidly to a high altitude without benefiting from a gradual and progressive acclimatization to lower altitudes. These symptoms, which are usually resolved within several days, include headache (most frequent symptom, probably due to dilation of cerebral blood vessels), dizziness, nausea, constipation, vomiting, depressed urine output (even with adequate hydration), dimness of vision, insomnia, and generalized weakness.[29, 40] The onset of symptoms usually begins within 4 to 12 hours after reaching high altitude, and symptoms usually are resolved within the first week. Some people will experience symptoms at only 2,500 m (8,000 ft), but most symptoms become prevalent at altitudes above 3,000 m (10,000 ft). Rapid ascent to 4,200 m (14,000 ft) will almost guarantee some form of AMS.[44]

Appetite suppression can be severe during the early stages of a high-altitude stay, resulting in an average reduction in energy intake of approximately 40% and an accompanying loss of body mass. Diets low in salt and high in carbohydrates are well tolerated early during the stay

TABLE 24.2
CARDIORESPIRATORY AND METABOLIC RESPONSE DURING SUBMAXIMAL AND MAXIMAL EXERCISE AT SEA LEVEL AND SIMULATED ALTITUDE OF 4,000 M (13,115 FT)

Exercise Level	$\dot{V}O_2 (L \cdot min^{-1})$		$\dot{V}E (L \cdot min^{-1} BTPS)$		Arterial Saturation (%)	
Altitude, m	0	4000	0	4000	0	4000
600 kg · m · min⁻¹	1.50	1.56	39.6	53.7	96	71
900 kg · m · min⁻¹	2.17	2.23	59.0	93.7	95	69
Maximum	3.46	2.50	123.5	118.0	94	70

Exercise Level	$\dot{Q} (L \cdot min^{-1})$		H R (beats · min⁻¹)		S V (mL)		a-$\overline{v}$ O_2 Diff (mL O_2 · 100 mL⁻¹)	
Altitude, m	0	4000	0	4000	0	4000	0	4000
600 kg · m · min⁻¹	13.0	16.7	115	148	122	113	10.8	9.4
900 kg · m · min⁻¹	19.2	21.6	154	176	125	123	11.4	10.4
Maximum	23.7	23.2	186	184	127	126	14.6	10.8

From Sternberg, J., et al.: Hemodynamic response to work at simulated altitude 4000 m. *J. Appl. Physiol.*, 21:1589, 1966.

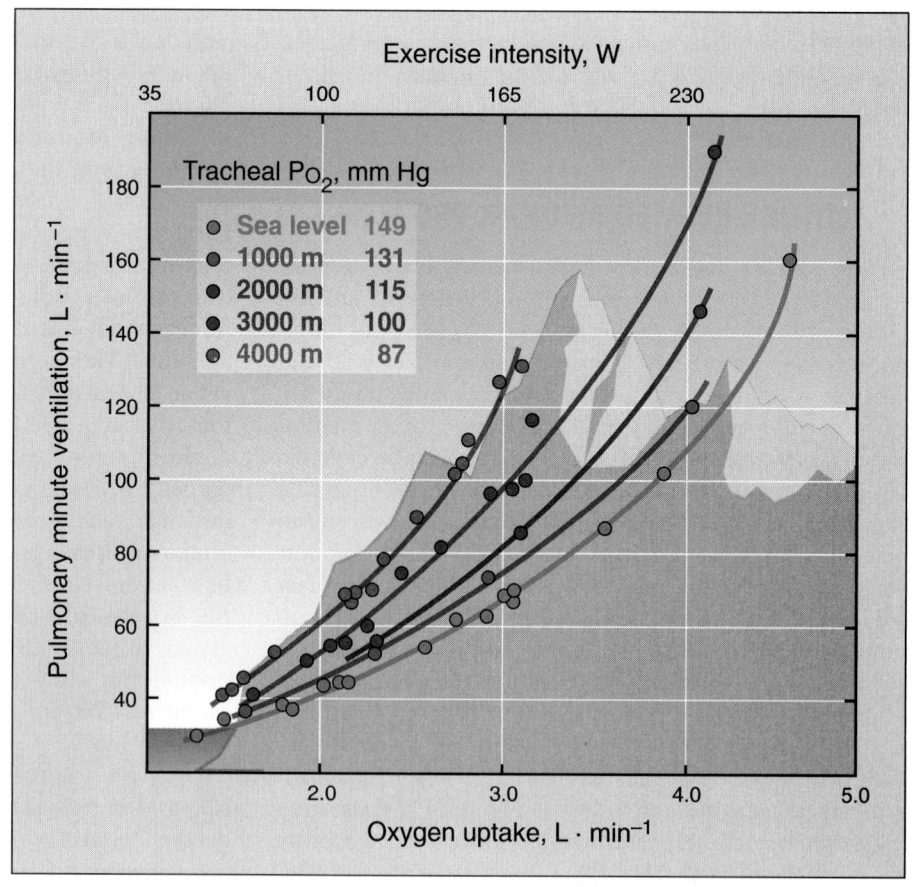

FIGURE 24.5
Effects on pulmonary ventilation and oxygen uptake of increasing simulated altitude exposure from sea level to 4,000 m (13,124 ft) during cycle ergometry. (Modified from Åstrand, P.O.: The respiratory activity in man exposed to prolonged hypoxia. *Acta Physiol. Scand.*, 30:343, 1954.)

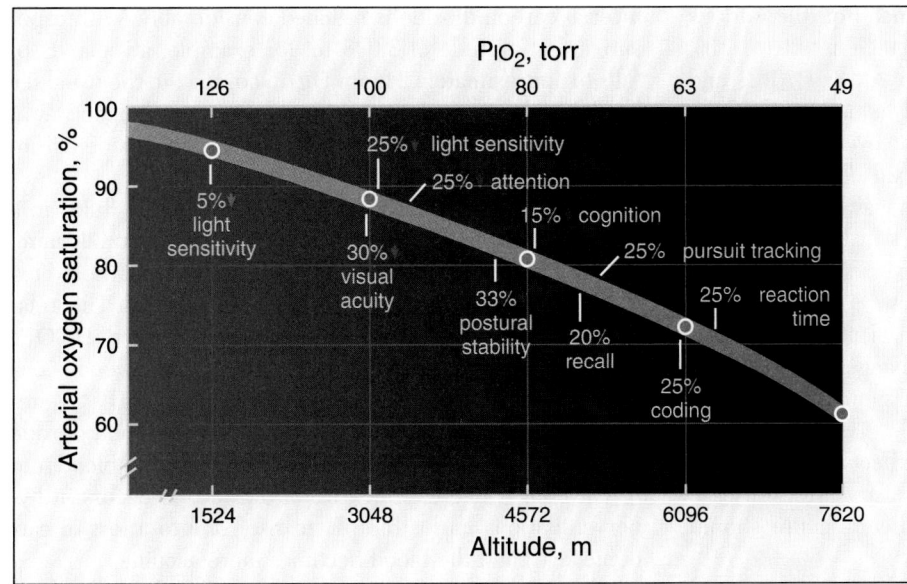

FIGURE 24.6
Arterial saturation as a function of increasing altitude and the corresponding changes in a variety of sensory and mental functions. (Modified from Fulco, C.S., and Cymerman, A.: Human performance and acute hypoxia. In *Human Performance Physiology and Environmental Medicine at Terrestrial Extremes*. Edited by Pandolf, K.B., et al. Carmel, IN, Cooper Publishing Group, 1994.)

at high altitude. A potential benefit of this diet is that the energy liberated per unit of oxygen consumed is greater in carbohydrate than in lipid breakdown (5.0 kcal versus 4.7 kcal per liter O_2). Also, high levels of circulating lipids after a high-fat meal may reduce arterial oxygen saturation. In general, a high-carbohydrate diet tends to (*a*) enhance altitude tolerance, (*b*) reduce the severity of mountain sickness, and (*c*) lessen the physical performance decrements during the early stages of altitude exposure.

Even moderate exercise can be intolerable for people suffering the effects of mountain sickness. With acclimatization, symptoms subside and many disappear. Concurrently, a person's ability to exercise improves and considerably more work can be accomplished. Mountain sickness usually can be prevented by acclimatizing slowly to moderate altitudes below 3,048 m, followed by a slow progression to higher elevations. Physical activity also should be minimized during the first days of altitude exposure.

High-Altitude Pulmonary Edema (HAPE). For unknown reasons, approximately 2% of sojourners to altitudes above 3,048 m experience a severe complication from acute mountain sickness termed **high-altitude pulmonary edema** or **HAPE**. Symptoms of HAPE usually manifest within 12 to 96 hours after a rapid ascent to high altitudes. In this life-threatening condition, fluid accumulates in the brain and lungs.[40, 61] At first, the symptoms do not seem too severe (general fatigue, dyspnea upon exertion, persistent dry, irritating cough without phlegm and without preexisting pulmonary infection, pain or pressure in the substernal area, headache, and nausea). This leads to pulmonary edema and fluid retention by the kidneys.[29] Chest examination reveals wheezy and raspy sounds known as rales. Even in well-acclimatized individuals, HAPE can develop upon severe exertion at elevations above 5,486 m (18,000 ft) and probably is related to increases in pulmonary artery pressure. The best treatment to prevent severe disability or even death from HAPE is immediate descent to lower altitude on a stretcher (or flown to safety) because an increase in physical activity from walking can potentiate complications. For a 10-year period before the 1968 Mexico City Olympics (2,300 m), there were no cases of HAPE in approximately 10,000 athletes who competed in various world championships at that altitude. Therefore, HAPE should be of little concern in apparently healthy individuals who journey to and recreate without acclimatization at relatively low altitudes not exceeding approximately 1,676 m (5,500 ft).

High-Altitude Cerebral Edema (HACE). If left untreated, this condition of increased intracranial pressure can lead to coma and ultimately death. The early symptoms are similar to AMS and HAPE, but the symptoms eventually become more severe. HACE occurs in approximately 1% of people exposed to altitudes usually above 2700 m (9000 ft). In addition to debilitating headache and severe fatigue, there is disruption of vision, bladder and bowl dysfunction, loss of coordination involving the trunk muscles, paralysis on one side of the body, generally poor reflexes, and mental confusion. Cerebral edema is probably due to cerebral vasodilation and an elevated capillary hydrostatic pressure. The additional cerebral fluid then distorts brain structures, which exacerbates symptoms of mountain sickness and increases the activity of the sympathetic nervous system. Because diagnosis at high altitude is often difficult, immediate descent to a lower elevation is mandatory for treating this condition.

Other High-Altitude Conditions. For the serious mountaineer that ventures beyond 6,069 m (20,000 ft), there are medical dangers other than AMS, HAPE, and HACE, including high-altitude retinal hemorrhage. If the hemorrhage occurs in the macula of the eye (the oval "yellow spot" region in the back of the eyeball close to the optic disc), then visual defects can persist and may be irreversible. The hemorrhages are due to increases in blood pressure surges from exercise that cause blood vessels in the eye to dilate from increased cerebral blood flow.[48, 68]

Generally, individuals with normal electrocardiograms (ECGs) at sea level show no adverse changes in these tracings to indicate myocardial ischemia at simulated high altitudes, even during maximal exercise.[58, 66] One researcher cautions that little is known about the effects of altitude exposure on individuals with known coronary artery disease and that individuals with congestive heart failure should avoid altitude exposure.[44]

Fluid Loss. Because the air in mountainous regions is usually cool and dry, considerable body water can be lost through evaporation as inspired air is warmed and moistened in the respiratory passages. This fluid loss often leads to a moderate dehydration and accompanying symptoms of dryness of the lips, mouth, and throat. This is particularly true for active people who have a large daily total sweat loss and pulmonary ventilation volume (and, hence, water loss). For these individuals, body weight should be checked frequently and water should be readily available at all times.

LONGER-TERM ADJUSTMENTS TO ALTITUDE

Hyperventilation and increased submaximal exercise cardiac output provide a rapid and relatively effective counter to the acute challenge of altitude exposure. Concurrently, other slower-acting adjustments occur during a prolonged high-altitude stay.[80] The most important of these involve:

- Regulation of the acid-base balance of body fluids that become altered by hyperventilation.
- Increased production of hemoglobin and red blood cells and accompanying changes in local circulation and cellular function.

Both of these adaptations generally reduce distress and improve tolerance to the relative hypoxia of medium and high altitudes.

Acid-Base Readjustment. Although hyperventilation at altitude favorably increases alveolar P_{O_2}, it has the opposite effect on carbon dioxide. Because ambient air contains essentially no carbon dioxide, the increased breathing volumes at altitude tends to "wash out" or dilute this gas in the alveoli. This creates a larger-than-normal gradient for the diffusion of carbon dioxide from the blood to the lungs, and

arterial carbon dioxide is reduced considerably. With exposure to an altitude of 3,048 m, for example, alveolar P_{CO_2} falls to approximately 24 mm Hg, in contrast to the usual sea level alveolar P_{CO_2} of 40 mm Hg. During a prolonged stay at high altitude, the pressure of alveolar carbon dioxide falls to as low as 10 mm Hg.

The loss of carbon dioxide from the body's fluids in a hypoxic environment causes a physiologic disequilibrium. As noted in Chapter 13, the largest quantity of carbon dioxide is normally carried as carbonic acid (H_2CO_3). This relatively weak acid readily dissociates into H^+ and HCO_3^-, which are then transported to the lungs by the venous circulation. In the pulmonary capillaries, H^+ and HCO_3^- recombine to form H_2CO_3, which then forms carbon dioxide and water; carbon dioxide then diffuses from the blood into the alveoli. A decrease in carbon dioxide, as occurs in hyperventilation, causes the pH to rise (due to a loss of carbonic acid) and the blood becomes more alkaline.

Because hyperventilation is a normal and sustained response to altitude exposure, adjustments must be made during acclimatization to minimize the accompanying "side effects" that disrupt the acid-base balance. This control of respiratory alkalosis is accomplished slowly as the kidneys excrete base (HCO_3^-) through the renal tubules. In turn, the restoration of a normal pH increases the responsiveness of the respiratory center, thus enabling ventilation to increase to even higher levels to adjust to altitude hypoxia.

Reduced Buffering Capacity and the "Lactate Paradox." The establishment of acid-base equilibrium with acclimatization occurs at the expense of a loss of absolute alkaline reserve. Thus, although the pathways of anaerobic metabolism are unaffected at high altitude, the blood's buffering capacity for acids is gradually decreased, and the critical level for the accumulation of acid metabolites is lowered. A general depression in maximum lactate concentration is particularly apparent during maximal exercise at altitudes above 4000 m.[54]

The phenomenon of a reduced maximal lactate concentration during exercise with large muscle groups after altitude acclimatization has been termed the "lactate paradox." This term is used to identify an apparent physiological contradiction in that the hypoxemia associated with high altitude should promote lactate accumulation. Furthermore, this reduction in exercise blood lactate levels during chronic high-altitude hypoxia is not accompanied by an increase in $\dot{V}_{O_2}$max or an increase in oxygen delivery to active tissues after acclimatization. The lower blood lactate has been attributed partly to a reduced output of the glucose-mobilizing catecholamines (glucose being the only anaerobic macronutrient) during exercise at high altitude. The reduction in maximum lactate levels during chronic hypoxia has also been attributed to a reduced drive from the central nervous system, which blunts one's capacity for all-out effort.[34, 47] Reduced blood lactate accumulations at high altitude do not appear to be due to the decrease in buffering capacity that accompanies high-altitude acclimatization.[33]

Hematological Changes. *An increase in the blood's oxygen-carrying capacity is the most important longer-term adaptation to altitude.* Two factors are responsible for this adaptation: (*a*) an initial decrease in plasma volume, which is followed by (*b*) an increased synthesis of erythrocytes and hemoglobin.

Decrease in Plasma Volume. During the first several days of altitude exposure, the body's fluid balance is altered in a direction that causes fluid to shift from the intravascular space into the interstitial and intracellular spaces. This decrease in plasma volume causes the red blood cells to become more concentrated in the plasma.[3, 26] After 1 week at 2,300 m, for example, the plasma volume decreased by approximately 8%, whereas the concentrations of red blood cells (hematocrit) increased by 4% and hemoglobin increased by 10%. A 1-week stay at 4,300 m (14,108 ft) caused a 16 to 25% decrease in plasma volume, whereas the hematocrit rose 6% and hemoglobin increased 20%.[8, 26] This rapid reduction in plasma volume and accompanying hemoconcentration causes the oxygen content of arterial blood to increase significantly above values observed upon arrival at altitude. During the normal acclimatization process, the shift in fluid volume is accompanied by diuresis (increased urine output) so that fluid balance is maintained at a lower total body water content.

Increase in Red Blood Cell Mass. The reduced arterial PO_2 at high altitude also stimulates an increase in the total number of red blood cells, a condition termed **polycythemia**. This response is mediated by an erythrocyte-stimulating hormone, **erythropoietin**, which is released from the kidneys and other tissues within 15 hours after altitude ascent.[1] In the weeks that follow, the production of erythrocytes in the marrow of the long bones increases considerably and remains elevated during the stay at altitude.[25, 57] A typical miner in the Andes, for example, has 38% more circulating red blood cells than his low-altitude counterpart. In some apparently healthy high-altitude natives, the red cell count may be more than 50% above normal—8 million cells per cubic millimeter compared to 5.3 million for the native lowlander![45] During a 1973 Mt. Everest Expedition, a 40% increase in hemoglobin concentration and a 66% increase in hematocrit were noted for climbers acclimatized at 6500 m.[10] This probably approaches the upper limit of a beneficial concentration of red blood cells. Any further erythrocyte packing would increase the blood's viscosity and probably restrict blood flow and oxygen diffusion to the tissues.

Polycythemia directly translates into an increase in the blood's capacity to transport oxygen. For example, the oxygen-carrying capacity of blood for high-altitude residents of Peru is 28% above sea-level averages.[32] For well-acclimatized mountaineers, the blood's oxygen-carrying capacity is 25 to 31 mL of oxygen per 100 mL of blood compared to 19.7 mL for lowland residents.[51, 75] Therefore, even with the reduced saturation of hemoglobin at high altitude, the actual quantity of oxygen in arterial blood approaches or even equals sea-level values.

The general trend for the increase in hemoglobin and hematocrit during altitude acclimatization is illustrated in Figure 24.7A. These data were obtained for eight young women at the University of Missouri (altitude 213 m) who lived and worked for 10 weeks at the 4267-m summit of Pikes Peak.[26] Because the researchers' previous work showed markedly fewer hematological changes during acclimatization in women than in men (possibly due to inadequate iron intake), each woman received iron supplementation before, during, and upon return from altitude. Upon reaching Pikes Peak, red blood cell concentration increased rapidly. This hemoconcentration was caused by a reduction in plasma volume that occurred during the first 24 hours at high altitude. In the month that followed, hemoglobin concentration and hematocrit continued to increase and then stabilized for the remainder of the stay. Pre-altitude values were reestablished 2 weeks after the women returned to Missouri.

As shown in Figure 24.7B, iron supplementation increased the pre-altitude values for hematocrit and hemoglobin. This finding is not surprising. As noted in Chapter 2, young women frequently suffer from a mild dietary iron insufficiency with depressed iron reserves. When the acclimatization curves for the iron-supplemented women were compared with those of another group of women not given additional iron, there was a greater hematocrit increase in the group given supplements. Therefore, at least for these women, iron supplementation enhanced the rate of hematocrit increase at altitude to a level similar to men at the same location. These findings indicate that athletes who have borderline iron stores may not respond to the acclimatization process as well as individuals who arrive at altitude with iron reserves adequate to sustain an increase in red blood cell production.

Cellular Adaptations. A topic of considerable debate is whether vascular and cellular adaptations to extremes of hypoxia take place that could improve local oxygen extraction and maximize oxidative function in humans.[22, 30, 70] Capillaries are more concentrated in the skeletal muscle of animals born and raised at high altitude compared to sea level.[72] This modification in local circulation reduces the distance for oxygen diffusion between the blood and tissues. Also, muscle biopsies from humans living at high altitude indicate an increase in myoglobin by as much as 16% after acclimatization. This was complemented by an increase in the number of mitochondria and the concentration of enzymes required for aerobic energy transfer.[43, 56] Such adaptations increase the "storage" of oxygen in specific muscles and facilitate intracellular oxygen release and utilization at low tissue PO_2.

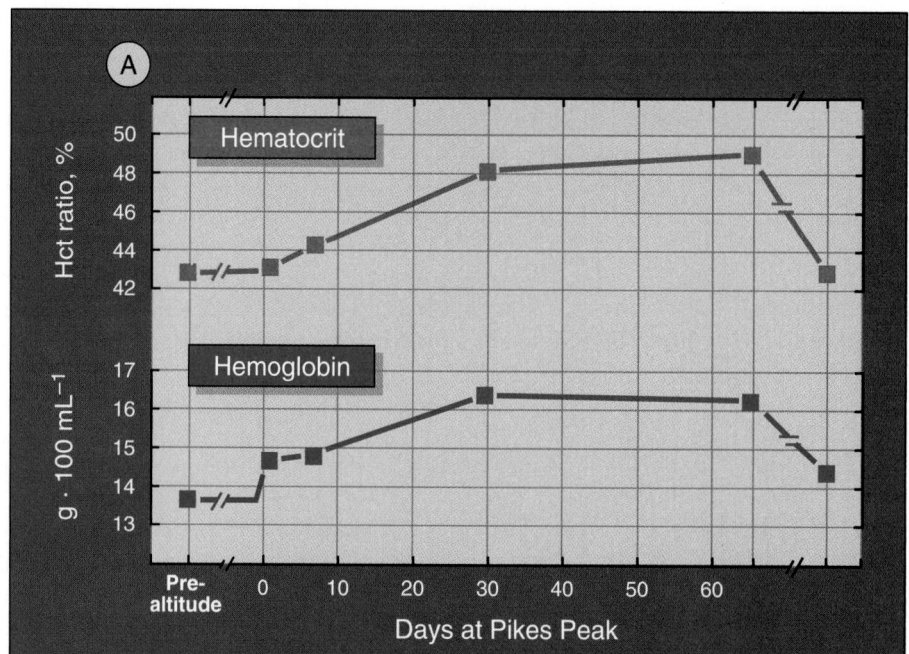

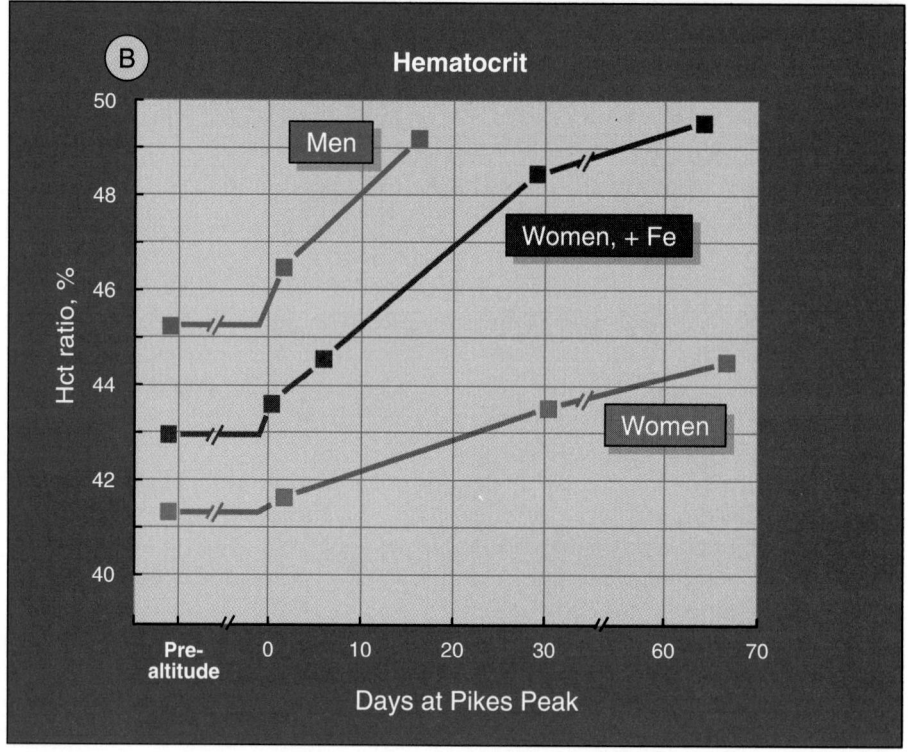

FIGURE 24.7

A, Effects of altitude on hemoglobin and hematocrit levels of eight young women before, during, and 2 weeks after exposure to altitude of 4267 m. (From Hannon, J. P., et al.: Effects of altitude acclimatization on blood composition of women. *J. Appl. Physiol.,* 26:540, 1968.) **B,** Hematocrit response of young women receiving supplemental iron (+ Fe) before and during altitude exposure compared to groups of male and female subjects receiving no supplemental iron. (Courtesy of Dr. J.P. Hannon.)

High-altitude natives benefit from a slight shift to the right of the oxyhemoglobin dissociation curve. This decreases the oxygen affinity of hemoglobin and favors the release of available oxygen to the tissues for a given drop in cellular P_{O_2}. This adaptation occurs because of an increase in the concentration of 2,3-diphosphoglycerate (2,3-DPG) in red blood cells (see Chapter 13) during long-term high-altitude residency.[16, 41] An increase in 2,3-DPG coupled with an increased quantity of circulating hemoglobin (and red blood cells) places the long-term high-altitude resident in a favorable physiologic position for supplying oxygen to active tissue during physical activity.

Changes in Body Mass and Composition. *Long-term exposure to high altitude produces a significant loss in lean body mass and body fat; the magnitude of weight loss is directly related to the terrestrial elevation.* Six men participated in progressive decompression in a hyperbaric chamber over 40 days to an ambient pressure of 249 mm Hg to simulate ascent to the top of Mt. Everest. Daily caloric intake decreased by 43% during the exposure period. This represented a loss of 7.4 kg of body mass, predominantly derived from the muscle component of the fat-free body mass.[59] In addition to a reduced energy intake during high-altitude exposure, the efficiency of intestinal absorption may be reduced, which further compounds the difficulty in maintaining body weight.[15] There is also a marked increase in the basal metabolic rate upon arrival at high altitude, which facilitates weight loss. To some extent, this accelerated metabolic rate can be overridden, and weight loss can be minimized by consciously increasing the energy intake during the high-altitude stay.[9]

TIME REQUIRED FOR ACCLIMATIZATION

The length of the acclimatization period depends on the altitude. Acclimation at one altitude ensures only partial adjustment to a higher elevation.[46] As a broad guideline, approximately 2 weeks are required to adapt to altitudes up to 2300 m. Thereafter, for each 610-m increase in altitude, an additional week is necessary to fully adapt up to an altitude of approximately 4600 m. For athletes desiring to compete at altitude, intense training should commence as soon as possible during the acclimatization period. This will minimize any detraining effects because it is difficult to engage in hard training during the early days of one's altitude stay.[39] The benefits of acclimatization are lost within 2 or 3 weeks after returning to sea level.

METABOLIC, PHYSIOLOGIC, AND EXERCISE CAPACITIES AT ALTITUDE

The stress of high altitude imposes significant restrictions on work capacity and physiologic function. Even at lower altitudes, the body's adjustments do not fully compensate for the reduced oxygen pressure and performance is compromised. Certain circulatory parameters, particularly stroke volume and maximum heart rate, are altered in a direction that contributes to a reduced capacity for oxygen transport.[19, 60]

MAXIMAL OXYGEN UPTAKE

The relationship between the reduction in $\dot{V}O_2$max as a percentage of the sea level value in relation to altitude exposure is depicted in Figure 24.8. Aerobic capacity is not

measurably altered until the altitude exceeds 1,500 m. Thereafter, $\dot{V}O_2$max decreases linearly at a rate of approximately 10% per 1,000-m increase in altitude.[8, 12, 52, 64] Thus, the aerobic capacity at 4,000 m is approximately 70% of the value at sea level. At 6,248 m (20,500 ft), the $\dot{V}O_2$max is approximately one-half the sea level value, whereas the aerobic capacity of a relatively fit man atop Mt. Everest is approximately 1,000 mL of oxygen per minute.[50, 80] This value corresponds to an exercise power output of only about 50 watts on a bicycle ergometer.

The degree of physical conditioning before high-altitude exposure offers little protection because the percentage reduction in $\dot{V}O_2$max is equal in both trained and untrained individuals. In well-conditioned individuals, a standard exercise task at altitude still provides relatively

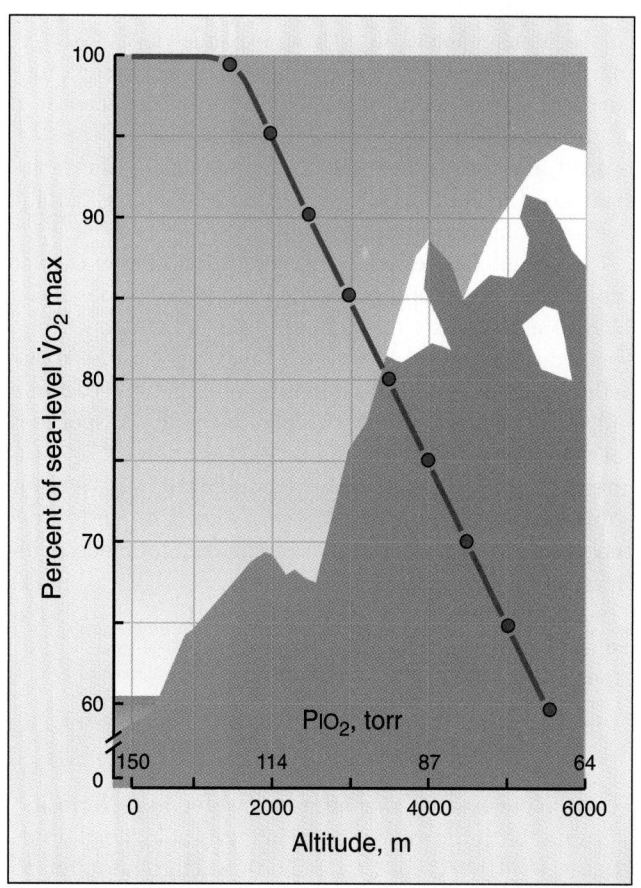

FIGURE 24.8
Reduction in $\dot{V}O_2$max as a percentage of the sea-level value in relation to altitude exposure. Aerobic capacity is not measurably altered until the altitude exceeds 1500 m (or inspired PO_2 less than 120 torr). Thereafter, a linear decrease in $\dot{V}O_2$max at the rate of 10% per 1000 m occurs. (Modified from Fulco, C.S., and Cymerman, A.: Human performance and acute hypoxia. In *Human Performance Physiology and Environmental Medicine at Terrestrial Extremes.* Edited by Pandolf, K.B., et al. Carmel, IN, Cooper Publishing Group, 1994.)

less stress because it can be performed at a lower percentage of the trained person's $\dot{V}O_2$max.

CIRCULATORY FACTORS

Even after several months of acclimatization, the $\dot{V}O_2$max remains significantly below sea-level values.[18, 38] This occurs because the benefits of acclimatization are offset by a reduction in circulatory efficiency in both submaximal and maximal exercise.[3, 24, 36]

Submaximal Exercise. Although the immediate altitude response to exercise involves an increase in submaximal cardiac output (Table 24.2), this response becomes reduced in the days and weeks of acclimatization that follow and does not improve with longer altitude exposure.[3, 35] This reduction in exercise cardiac output is due mainly to a decrease in the heart's stroke volume as the altitude stay progresses. With a reduced cardiac output, submaximal oxygen uptake is maintained through an expanded a-$\bar{v}$ O_2 difference. To some extent, the decrease in stroke volume observed during a stay at altitude is offset by an increase in submaximal heart rate. Even at altitudes as high as Mt. Everest, the rate and contractile function of the heart are maintained in reasonable fashion despite the considerable level of chronic hypoxia.[55]

Maximal Exercise. A reduction in maximum cardiac output occurs after approximately 1 week at altitudes above 3048 m and persists throughout one's altitude stay.[23, 52, 73] This reduction in blood flow during maximal exercise is due to the combined effect of a decrease in maximum heart rate and stroke volume.[24, 35-38, 60] This blunted cardiac response is not due to myocardial hypoxia, at least as reflected by measurement of ECG and coronary blood flow during vigorous exercise at high altitudes.[27, 60] The reduced stroke volume may result from a decrease in plasma volume and an increase in total peripheral vascular resistance. The reduction in maximum heart rate at altitude may be influenced by enhanced parasympathetic tone induced by prolonged altitude exposure.[28]

PERFORMANCE MEASURES

The absolute exercise load must be lowered to perform aerobic exercise at the same relative intensity at higher altitude as at sea level. If it is not, a larger portion of the energy for exercise will be provided by anaerobic metabolism and fatigue develops.[78] For example, a 2 to 13% decrement in exercise performance is observed for fit subjects in the 1-mile and 3-mile runs at the medium altitude of 2300 m.[18] This agrees with the 7.2% increase in 2-mile run times reported for highly trained middle-distance runners at the same altitude.[2] Even after 29 days of acclimatization, significant decrements in 3-mile running performance at high altitude occur compared to run times over the same distance near sea level.[54]

ALTITUDE TRAINING AND SEA-LEVEL PERFORMANCE

It is clear that altitude acclimatization improves one's capacity for aerobic exercise at altitude, especially high altitude. What is not clear, however, is the effect of previous altitude exposure and altitude training on aerobic capacity and endurance performance immediately upon return to sea level. Certainly, altitude adaptations in local circulation and cellular metabolism, as well as the compensatory increase in the blood's oxygen-carrying capacity, should facilitate subsequent sea-level performance. Also, the pulmonary adaptations and responses during prolonged hypoxic exposure are not lost immediately upon descent from altitude.[63] Furthermore, if tissue hypoxia is an important training stimulus, altitude and training should act synergistically so that the total effect exceeds that of similar training at sea level. Unfortunately, much of the previous exercise-altitude research has not been designed to adequately evaluate this possibility. Often, the activity level of the subjects was poorly controlled, making it difficult to determine whether an improved $\dot{V}O_2$max or performance score on return from altitude represents a training effect, an altitude effect, or a synergism between altitude and training.[8, 18]

AEROBIC CAPACITY UPON RETURN TO SEA LEVEL

When $\dot{V}O_2$max is used as the criterion, sea-level performance is not significantly improved after living at altitude.[4, 7, 18, 42, 49] For example, there was no significant change in the original 25% reduction in aerobic capacity in young runners during an 18-day stay at 3,100 m.[23] Upon return to sea level, the $\dot{V}O_2$max was about the same as the pre-altitude measures. These observations have been duplicated at even higher altitudes.[7] More specifically, highly trained male varsity track members were flown to Nunoa, Peru (altitude 4,000 m; 13,124 ft), where they continued to train and acclimatize for 40 to 57 days. After the initial 3 days at high altitude, $\dot{V}O_2$max was reduced 29% below sea-level values; after 48 days, it was still 26% lower. Running performance after acclimatization was measured in the 440-yard, 880-yard, 1-mile, and 2-mile runs during a "track meet" with the altitude natives. Run times were still considerably slower than pre-altitude times, particularly in the longer runs. Furthermore, when the athletes returned to sea level, $\dot{V}O_2$max and running performance were generally **no different** than in the pre-altitude measures. On no occasion did a runner improve his previous pre-altitude run time! Running times in the longer events remained approximately 5% below pre-altitude trials. In other studies, training in chambers designed to simulate high altitude provided no additional benefit to sea level performance compared to similar training at sea level. Of course, the "altitude"-trained group showed significantly better exercise performance at the simulated altitude compared to sea-level counterparts.[69] Even in those studies in which there was a small improvement in either $\dot{V}O_2$max or exercise performance at altitude and upon return to sea level, the change often was attributed to an increase in physical activity (i.e., the effects of training and/or repeated testing) during the altitude exposure.[13, 17, 21, 37]

Possible Negative Effects. Some of the physiological changes that occur during prolonged altitude exposure may actually negate adaptations that possibly could improve exercise performance upon return to sea level. For example, the residual effects of a loss in muscle mass and a reduced maximum heart rate and stroke volume frequently observed during a stay at altitude certainly would not enhance sea-level performance. Any reduction in maximum cardiac output at altitude would offset the benefits derived from an increase in the blood's oxygen-carrying capacity. Although circulatory function does return to normal after a few weeks at sea level, so also do the potentially positive hematological adaptations.[26] Within a physiological context, the controversial use of blood doping (see Chapter 23) mimics the hematological benefits of a stay at altitude without the potential negative effects on cardiovascular dynamics and body composition.[20]

CAN TRAINING BE MAINTAINED AT HIGH ALTITUDE?

Exposure to altitudes of 2300 m and higher makes it nearly impossible for athletes to train at the same intensity as at sea level. This reduction in training intensity in relation to sea-level standards for six competitive college athletes is shown in Table 24.3.[39]

At successively higher elevations, the absolute training intensity was progressively below what was possible at a lower altitude. At 4000 m, for example, the runners were only able to train at 39% of the sea-level $\dot{V}O_2$max compared to an intensity of 78% when training at sea level. This reduction in the absolute exercise training level is possibly of such magnitude that at high altitude, an athlete may be unable to maintain peak condition for sea-level competition. In this regard, elite athletes might benefit by periodically returning from high altitude to sea level for intensive training to help offset any "detraining" that takes place during a prolonged high-altitude stay. Such a procedure would not interfere with acclimatization and might even be beneficial to altitude performance.[13] If this approach is impractical, athletes should be sure to include high-intensity speed work in their altitude training programs to maintain muscle mass and power.[5]

IS ALTITUDE TRAINING MORE EFFECTIVE THAN TRAINING AT SEA LEVEL?

Equivalent groups were used to determine whether altitude training was more effective than similar sea-level training.[2] Six highly trained middle-distance runners trained at sea level for 3 weeks at 75% of the sea-level $\dot{V}O_2$max, whereas another group of six runners trained an equivalent distance at the same percentage of their $\dot{V}O_2$max at 2300 m. The groups then exchanged training sites and continued training for 3 weeks at an intensity similar to that of the preceding group. Initially, 2-mile run times were 7.2% slower at altitude than at sea level. This improved approximately 2.0% for both groups after altitude training, but post-altitude performance at sea level was unchanged when compared to pre-altitude sea-level runs. As shown in Figure 24.9, $\dot{V}O_2$max for both groups at altitude was reduced initially by approximately 17.4%. This improved only slightly after 20 days of altitude training. When the runners were then measured at sea level, aerobic capacity was 2.8% **below** pre-altitude sea-level values! Clearly, for these well-conditioned middle-distance runners, there was no synergistic effect of hard aerobic training at medium altitude over an equivalent program of severe training pursued at sea level.

TABLE 24.3
EFFECT OF ALTITUDE ON TRAINING INTENSITY OF SIX COLLEGIATE ATHLETES

	Altitude (m)			
	300	2300	3100	4000
Intensity of workout (% of $\dot{V}O_2$max at 200 m)	78	60	56	39

From Kollias, J., and Buskirk, E.R.: Exercise and altitude. In *Science and Medicine of Exercise and Sports*, 2nd ed. W.R. Johnson and E.R. Buskirk (Eds.). New York, Harper and Row, 1974.

FIGURE 24.9

Maximal oxygen uptakes of two equivalent groups during training for 3 weeks at altitude and 3 weeks at sea level. Group 1 trained first at sea level and then continued training for 3 weeks at altitude. For Group 2, the procedure was reversed as they trained first at altitude and then at sea level. (From Adams, W.C., et al.: Effects of equivalent sea-level and altitude training on $\dot{V}O_2$max and running performance. *J. Appl. Physiol.*, 39:262, 1975.)

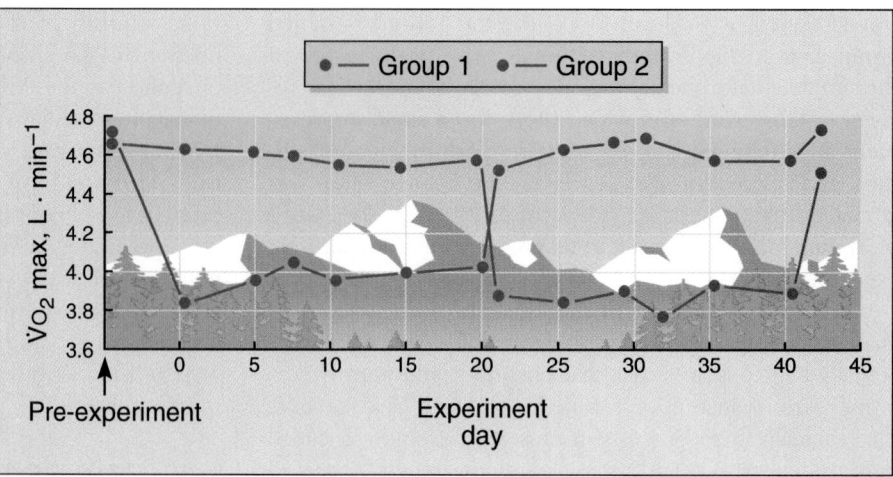

■ SUMMARY ■

1. The progressive reduction in ambient PO_2 as one ascends in altitude eventually leads to inadequate oxygenation of hemoglobin. This produces noticeable performance decrements in aerobic activities at altitudes of 2000 m and higher. Short-term sprint and power performances that depend on energy from the stored intramuscular high-energy phosphates are not adversely affected at altitude.

2. The reduced PO_2 and accompanying hypoxia at altitude stimulate physiologic responses and adjustments that improve one's altitude tolerance at rest and during exercise. The primary immediate responses are a relative hyperventilation and an increase in submaximal cardiac output via an elevated heart rate.

3. Medical problems ranging from mild to life-threatening are often observed upon ascent to altitude. The most prominent of these are acute mountain sickness (AMS), high-altitude pulmonary edema (HAPE), and high-altitude cerebral edema (HACE). Both HAPE and HACE are potentially lethal. They require the patient's immediate removal to a lower altitude.

4. The longer-term acclimatization process involves physiologic and metabolic adjustments that greatly improve tolerance to altitude hypoxia. The main adjustments involve (*a*) reestablishing the acid-base balance of the body fluids, (*b*) increased formation of hemoglobin and red blood cells, and (*c*) possible changes in local circulation and cellular metabolism. The latter two adjustments would significantly facilitate oxygen transport and utilization.

5. The rate of altitude acclimatization depends on the altitude. Noticeable improvements are generally observed within several days, and the major adjustments require approximately 2 weeks, although 4 to 6 weeks may be required to acclimatize to relatively high altitudes.

6. The alveolar PO_2 is approximately 25 mm Hg at a simulated altitude that approaches the summit of Mt. Everest. In acclimatized men, this results in a 70% reduction in $\dot{V}O_2$max to approximately 15 mL $O_2 \cdot kg^{-1} \cdot min^{-1}$. Unacclimatized individuals at this altitude would become unconscious within 30 seconds.

7. Acclimatization does not fully compensate for the stress of altitude. Even after acclimatization, the $\dot{V}O_2$max is lowered by approximately 2% for every 300 m above 1500 m. This is paralleled by a significant decrement in performance in endurance-related activities.

8. The inability to achieve sea-level $\dot{V}O_2$max values at altitude is partially explained by the fact that the beneficial effects of acclimatization are somewhat offset by altitude-related decrements in physiologic function. The latter involve mainly a reduction in maximum heart rate and stroke volume.

9. Although some adaptations during acclimatization to altitude should enhance aerobic capacity and endurance performance upon return to sea level, research results do not support this effect. This is probably the result of the altitude-related decrease in both maximum heart rate and stroke volume.

10. Training at altitude provides no additional benefit to sea-level performance compared to equivalent training at sea level.

■ REFERENCES ■

1. Abbrecht, P.H., and Littell, J.K.: Plasma erythropoietin in men and mice during acclimatization to different altitudes. *J. Appl. Physiol.*, 32:54, 1972.

2. Adams, W.C., et al.: Effects of equivalent sea-level and altitude training on $\dot{V}O_2$max and running performance. *J. Appl. Physiol.*, 39:262, 1975.

3. Alexander, J.K., et al.: Reduction of stroke volume during exercise in man following ascent to 3,100 m altitude. *J. Appl. Physiol.*, 23:849, 1967.

4. Balke, B., et al.: Effects of altitude acclimatization on work capacity. *Fed. Proc.,* 15:7, 1966.

5. Balke, B., et al.: Variation in altitude and its effects on exercise performance. In *Exercise Physiology.* Edited by H.B. Falls. New York, Academic Press, 1968.

6. Burse, R.L., et al.: Respiratory functions and muscle function during isometric handgrip exercise at high altitude. *Aviat. Space Environ. Med.,* 58:39, 1987.

7. Buskirk, E.R., et al.: Maximal performance at altitude and on return from altitude in conditioned runners. *J. Appl. Physiol.,* 23:259, 1967.

8. Buskirk, E.R., et al.: Physiology and performance of track athletes at various altitudes in the United States and Peru. In *The International Symposium on the Effects of Altitude on Physical Performance.* Edited by R.F. Goddard. Chicago, The Athletic Institute, 1967.

9. Butterfield, G.E., et al.: Increased energy intake minimizes weight loss in men at altitude. *J. Appl. Physiol.,* 72:1741, 1992.

10. Cerretelli, P.: Limiting factors to oxygen transport on Mount Everest. *J. Appl. Physiol.,* 40:658, 1976.

11. Craig, A.B., Jr.: Olympics 1968: a post-mortem. *Med. Sci. Sports,* 1:177, 1969.

12. Cymerman, A., et al.: Operation Everest II: maximal oxygen uptake at extreme altitude. *J. Appl. Physiol.,* 66:2446, 1989.

13. Daniels, J., and Oldridge N.: The effects of alternate exposure to altitude and sea level on world-class middle-distance runners. *Med. Sci. Sports,* 2:107, 1970.

14. Dempsey, J.A.: Effects of acute through life-long hypoxic exposure on exercise pulmonary gas exchange. *Respir. Physiol.,* 13:62, 1971.

15. Dinmore, A.J., et al.: Intestinal carbohydrate absorption and permeability at high altitude (5,730 m). *J. Appl. Physiol.,* 76:1903, 1994.

16. Eaton, J.W., et al.: Role of red cell 2,3-diphosphoglycerate (DPG) in adaptation of men to altitude. *J. Lab. Clin. Med.,* 73:603, 1969.

17. Faulkner, J.A., et al.: Effects of training at moderate altitude on physical performance capacity. *J. Appl. Physiol.,* 23:85, 1967.

18. Faulkner, J.A., et al.: Maximum aerobic capacity and running performance at altitude. *J. Appl. Physiol.,* 24:685, 1968.

19. Ferretti, G., et al.: Oxygen transport system before and after exposure to chronic hypoxia. *Int. J. Sports Med.,* 11:S15, 1990.

20. Gledhill, N.: Blood doping and related issues: a brief review. *Med. Sci. Sports Exerc.,* 14:183, 1982.

21. Gold, A.J., et al.: Effects of altitude stress on mitochondrial function. *Am. J. Physiol.,* 224:946, 1973.

22. Green, H.J., et al.: Operation Everest II: adaptations in human skeletal muscle. *J. Appl. Physiol.,* 66:2454, 1989.

23. Grover, R.F., and Reeves, J.T.: Exercise performance of athletes at sea level and 3,100 meters altitude. In *The Effects of Altitude on Physical Performance.* Edited by R.F. Goddard. Chicago, IL, Athletic Institute, 1967.

24. Grover, R.F., et al.: Alterations in coronary circulation of man following ascent to 3,100 m altitude. *J. Appl. Physiol.,* 4:832, 1976.

25. Groves, B.M., et al.: Operation Everest II: elevated high-altitude pulmonary resistance unresponsive to oxygen. *J. Appl. Physiol.,* 63:521, 1987.

26. Hannon, J.P., et al.: Effects of altitude acclimatization on blood composition of women. *J. Appl. Physiol.,* 26:540, 1969.

27. Harris, C.W., and Hansen, J.E.: Electrocardiographic changes during exposure to high altitude. *Am. J. Cardiol.,* 18:183, 1966.

28. Hartley, L.H., et al.: Reduction of maximal exercise heart rate at altitude and its reversal with atropine. *J. Appl. Physiol.,* 36:362, 1976.

29. Honigman, B., et al.: Acute mountain sickness in a general tourist population at moderate altitude. *Ann. Intern. Med.,* 118:587, 1993.

30. Hoppeler, H., and Desplanches, D.: Muscle structural modifications in hypoxia. *Int. J. Sports Med.,* 13:S166, 1992.

31. Hunt, J., and Hillary, E.: *The Conquest of Everest.* New York, E.P. Dutton Co., 1954.

32. Hurtado, A.: Animals in high altitudes: resident man. In *Handbook of Physiology.* Edited by D.B. Dill, et al. Baltimore, Williams & Wilkins, 1964.

33. Kayser, B., et al.: Maximal lactate capacity at altitude: effect of bicarbonate loading. *J. Appl. Physiol.,* 75:1070, 1993.

34. Kayser, B., et al.: Fatigue and exhaustion in chronic hypobaric hypoxia: influence of exercising muscle mass. *J. Appl. Physiol.,* 76:634, 1994.

35. Klausen, K.: Cardiac output in man in rest and work during and after acclimatization to 3800 m. *J. Appl. Physiol.,* 21:609, 1969.

36. Klausen, K.: Exercise under hypoxic conditions. *Med. Sci. Sports,* 1:43, 1969.

37. Klausen, K., et al.: Effect of high altitude on maximal working capacity. *J. Appl. Physiol.,* 21:1191, 1966.

38. Klausen, K., et al.: Exercise at ambient and high oxygen pressure at high altitude and at sea level. *J. Appl. Physiol.,* 29:456, 1970.

39. Kollias, J., and Buskirk, E.R.: Exercise at altitude. In *Science and Medicine of Exercise and Sports.* Edited by W.R. Johnson and E.R. Buskirk. New York, Harper and Row, 1974.

40. Krasney, J.A.: Brief review: a neurogenic basis for acute altitude sickness. *Med. Sci. Sports Exerc.,* 26:195, 1994.

41. Lenfant, C.P., et al.: Effect of chronic hypoxic hypoxia on the O_2-Hb dissociation curve and respiratory gas transport in man. *Respir. Physiol.,* 7:7, 1969.

42. Levine, B.D., et al.: Altitude training does not improve running performance more than equivalent training near sea level in trained runners. *Med. Sci. Sports Exerc.,* 24:769, 1992.

43. MacDougall, J.D., et al.: Operation Everest II: Structural adaptations in skeletal muscle in response to extreme simulated altitude. *Acta Physiol. Scand.,* 142:421, 1991.

44. Malconian, M.K., and Rock, P.B.: Medical problems related to altitude. In *Human Performance Physiology and Environmental Medicine at Terrestrial Extremes.* Edited by K. Pandolf, et al. Carmel, IN, Cooper Publishing Group, 1994.

45. Manier, G., et al.: Pulmonary gas exchange in Andean natives with excessive polycythemia—effect of hemodilution. *J. Appl. Physiol.,* 65:2107, 1988.

46. Maresh, C.M., et al.: Maximal exercise during hypobaric hypoxia (447 Torr) in moderate-altitude natives. *Med. Sci. Sports Exerc.,* 15:360, 1983.

47. Mazzeo, R., et al.: β-Adrenergic blockade does not prevent the lactate response to exercise after acclimatization to high altitude. *J. Appl. Physiol.,* 76:610, 1994.

48. McFaddan, D.M., et al.: High altitude retinopathy. *JAMA,* 245:581, 1981.

49. Mizuno, M., et al.: Limb skeletal muscle adaptation in athletes after training at altitude. *J. Appl. Physiol.,* 68:496, 1990.

50. Pugh, L.C.G.E.: Muscular exercise on Mount Everest. *J. Physiol. (Lond.),* 141:233, 1958.

51. Pugh, L.C.G.E.: Physiological and medical aspects of the Himalayan Scientific and Mountaineering Expedition, 1960-61. *BMJ,* 2:621, 1962.

52. Pugh, L.C.G.E.: Animals in high altitudes: an above 5000 meters-mountain exploration. In *Handbook of Physiology.* Edited by D.B. Dill, et al. Baltimore, Williams & Wilkins, 1964.

53. Pugh, L.C.G.E.: Muscular exercise at great altitudes. *J. Appl. Physiol.,* 19:431, 1964.

54. Pugh, L.C.G.E.: Athletes at altitude. *J. Physiol. (Lond.),* 192:619, 1967.

55. Reeves, J.T.: Operation Everest II; preservation of cardiac function at extreme altitude. *J. Appl. Physiol.,* 63:531, 1987.

56. Reynafarje, C.: Myoglobin content and enzymatic activity of muscle and altitude adaptation. *J. Appl. Physiol.,* 17:301, 1962.

57. Reynafarje, C.: Hematologic changes during rest and physical activity in man at high altitude. In *The Physiological Effects of High Altitude.* Edited by W.H. Weihe. New York, Macmillan, 1964.

58. Rock, P.B., et al.: Operation Everest II. Electrocardiography during maximal exercise at extreme altitude. *Med. Sci. Sports Exerc.,* 18:S74, 1986.

59. Rose, M.S., et al.: Operation Everest II: nutrition and body composition. *J. Appl. Physiol.,* 65:2545, 1988.

60. Saltin, B., et al.: Maximal oxygen uptake and cardiac output after 2 weeks at 4300 m. *J. Appl. Physiol.,* 25:400, 1968.

61. Schoene, R.B.: High-altitude pulmonary edema: the disguised killer. *Phys. Sportsmed.,* 16:103, 1988.

62. Schoene, R.B., et al.: Relationship of hypoxic ventilatory response to exercise performance on Mount Everest. *J. Appl. Physiol.,* 56:1478, 1984.

63. Schoene, R.B., et al.: Operation Everest II: ventilatory adaptations during gradual decompression to extreme altitude. *Med. Sci. Sports Exerc.,* 22:804, 1990.

64. Squires, R.W., and Buskirk, E.R.: Aerobic capacity during acute exposure to simulated altitude, 914 to 2,286 meters. *Med. Sci. Sports Exerc.,* 14:36, 1982.

65. Stenberg, J., et al.: Hemodynamic response to work at simulated altitude, 4,000 m. *J. Appl. Physiol.,* 21:1589, 1966.

66. Suarez, J.M., et al.: Operation Everest II. Left ventricular systolic function in man at high altitude assessed by two dimensional echocardiography. *Am. J. Cardiol.,* 60:137, 1987.

67. Surks, M.J., et al.: Changes in plasma thyroxine concentration and metabolism, catecholamine excretion and basal oxygen uptake during acute exposure to high altitude (14,100 ft). *J. Clin. Invest.,* 45:1442, 1966.

68. Sutton, J.R.: High altitude retinal hemorrhage. *Sem. Resp. Med.,* 5:159, 1983.

69. Terrados, N., et al.: Effects of training at simulated altitude on performance and muscle metabolic capacity in competitive road cyclists. *Eur. J. Appl. Physiol.,* 57:203, 1988.

70. Terrados, N., et al.: Is hypoxia a stimulus for synthesis of oxidative enzymes and myoglobin? *J. Appl. Physiol.,* 68:2369, 1990.

71. Torre-Bueno, J.R., et al.: Diffusion limitation in normal humans during exercise at sea-level and simulated altitude. *J. Appl. Physiol.,* 58:989, 1985.

72. Valdivia, E.: Total capillary bed in striated muscle of guinea pigs native to Peruvian mountains. *Am. J. Physiol.,* 194:585, 1958.

73. Vogel, J.A., et al.: Cardiovascular responses in man during exhaustive work at sea level and high altitude. *J. Appl. Physiol.,* 23:531, 1967.

74. West, J.B.: Do climbs to extreme altitudes cause brain damage? *Lancet,* 2:387, 1986.

75. West, J.B., et al.: Arterial oxygen saturation during exercise at high altitude. *J. Appl. Physiol.,* 17:617, 1962.

76. West, J.B., et al.: Pulmonary gas exchange on the summit of Mount Everest. *J. Appl. Physiol.,* 55:678, 1983.

77. Wolfel, E.E., et al.: Systemic hypertension at 4,300 m is related to sympathoadrenal activity. *J. Appl. Physiol.,* 76:1643, 1994.

78. Young, A.J.: Energy substrate utilization during exercise in extreme environments. In *Exercise and Sport Sciences Reviews.* Vol. 18. Edited by K.B. Pandolf. Baltimore, Williams & Wilkins, 1990.

79. Young, A.J., and Young, P.M.: Human acclimatization to high terrestrial altitude. In *Human Performance Physiology and Environmental Medicine at Terrestrial Extremes.* Edited by K.B. Pandolf, et al. Indianapolis, Benchmark Press, 1988.

80. Young, P.M., et al. Altitude acclimatization attenuates plasma ammonia accumulation during submaximal exercise. *J. Appl. Physiol.,* 63:758, 1987.

Asmussen, E. and Bøje, O.: Body temperature and capacity for work. *Acta. Physiol. Scand.,* 10:1, 1945.

Research on the relationship between the rise in body temperature and exercise capacity has produced conflicting results. Some researchers have suggested that increased core and muscle temperature signals a failing thermoregulatory mechanism that reduces exercise performance. Others have hypothesized that temperature increases might accelerate neuromuscular processes and thus augment exercise capacity. Increases in blood and muscle temperature could also hasten the dissociation of oxyhemoglobin, thereby facilitating aerobic processes in exercise. Asmussen and Bøje reasoned

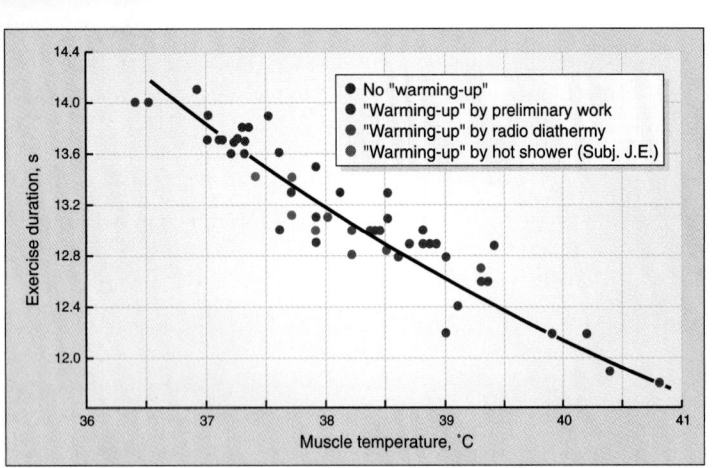

Performance time for sprint-type exercise in relation to the temperature of vastus lateralis muscle.

that if increased body temperature facilitated physiologic function and exercise capacity per se, then passive "warm-up" prior to exercise would enhance subsequent exercise performance.

To test the passive warm-up hypothesis, subjects performed bicycle exercise at predetermined rates for specified durations under different conditions. Measurements included muscle and rectal

(core) temperatures and respiratory gas exchange. In addition to studying the effects of prior warm-up, the researchers determined the independent effects of increased muscle and core temperature on exercise capacity. In each experimental protocol, subjects performed more work in a given time when the exercise was preceded by warming up. The warm-up benefit occurred predominantly for exercise lasting 12 to 15 seconds and in longer performances of 4 to 5 minutes. The researchers speculated that the beneficial effect of active warm-up resulted from increased temperature per se and other cardiorespiratory and hormonal changes accompanying the prior muscular activity. Also, using more intense active warm-up progressively increased core and muscle temperatures and improved subsequent short-duration (less than 20 seconds) work output. Further experiments confirmed the body temperature increased with passive warm-up that included such procedures as radio diathermy or hot (47°C for 10 minutes) showers. And, as occurred with active warm-up, passive warm-up increased exercise capacity.

The figure illustrates the relationship between vastus lateralis temperature and sprint cycling performance. The time required to perform the assigned exercise task decreased steadily with increasing muscle temperature in the range from 36.5 to 40.8°C. To determine if the ergogenic effects of increased temperature were related to increased muscle or rectal temperature, other experiments manipulated each thermal variable independently. The results showed that enhanced work output was related more to muscle temperature than to core temperature. The authors suggest that a "local" temperature effect decreased local blood viscosity and increased elastic properties (mechanical factors) and/or chemical factors within the active muscles that favored energy release.

Contemporary research concerning the efficacy of prior exercise on muscle performance remains controversial. Nevertheless, the Asmussen and Bøje study demonstrated that active or passive prior warm-up enhanced exercise performance.

Exercise and Thermal Stress

The requirements for thermoregulation can be considerable; the price of failure is death. A drop in deep body temperature[a] of 10°C and an increase of only 5°C can be tolerated. This has been vividly illustrated during the past 20 years in more than 100 football players who died as a direct result of excessive heat stress during practice or actual competition. Heat injury is also an unfortunate common occurrence in a variety of longer-duration athletic events. Such tragedies are avoidable with proper understanding of thermoregulation and the best ways to support these mechanisms. A major part of this responsibility rests with the people who organize and guide athletic and physical activity programs.

PART 1

MECHANISMS OF THERMOREGULATION

THERMAL BALANCE

As shown in Figure 25.1, body temperature, or more specifically the temperature of the deeper tissues (core), is in dy-

namic equilibrium between factors that add and subtract body heat. This balance is maintained by the integration of mechanisms that alter heat transfer to the periphery (shell), regulate evaporative cooling, and vary the body's rate of heat production. If heat gain exceeds heat loss, as can occur readily during vigorous exercise in a warm environment, core temperature rises; in a cold environment, on the other hand, heat loss often exceeds heat production and core temperature falls.

Thermal data for heat production and heat loss by sweating at rest and during maximal exercise are presented in Table 25.1. Body heat is gained directly from the reactions of energy metabolism. The heat contribution from muscular activity can be considerable. From shivering alone, the total metabolic rate can increase threefold to fivefold.[59, 118] During sustained vigorous exercise, the metabolic rate can increase 20 to 25 times above the resting level or to about 20 kcal · min^{-1}; this theoretically can increase core temperature by about 1°C (1.8°F) every 5 to 7 minutes! Heat also is absorbed from the environment by solar radiation and from objects that are warmer than the body. Heat is lost by the physical mechanisms of radiation, conduction, and convection, and, most importantly, by the vaporization of water from the skin and respiratory passages. Under op-

---

[a]"Temperature" is technically defined as the mean kinetic energy of the molecules of a substance. A functional definition of temperature is the potential for heat exchange between substances (e.g., blood to capillary walls) or objects (e.g., playing surface to participant's body).

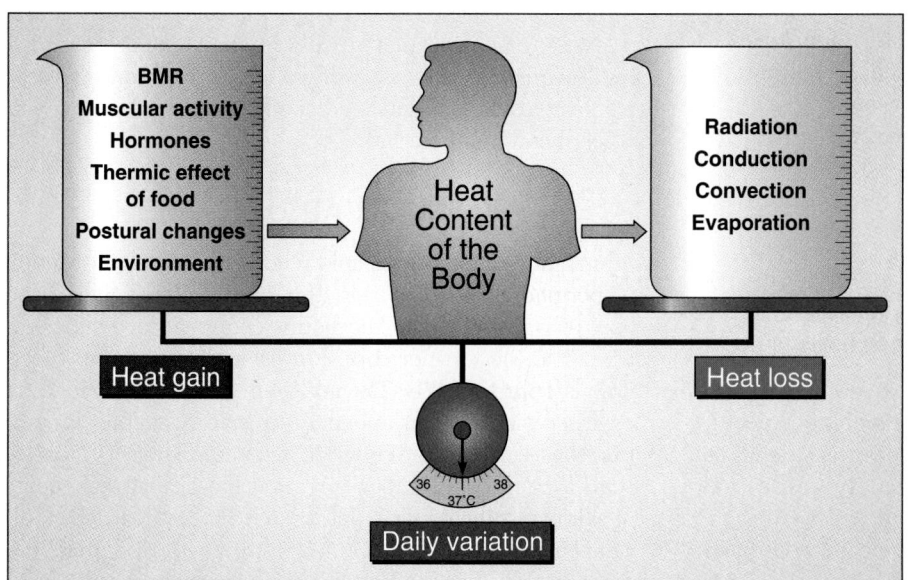

FIGURE 25.1
Factors that contribute to heat gain and heat loss to regulate core temperature at about 37°C.

TABLE 25.1
THERMODYNAMICS AT REST AND DURING EXERCISE

Condition	Rest	Maximal Exercise
Body's heat production	~0.25 L O_2 · min^{-1}	~4.0 L O_2 · min^{-1}
(1 L O_2 uptake = ~4.82 kcal)	~1.2 kcal · min^{-1}	~20.0 kcal · min^{-1}
Body's capacity for evaporative cooling		*Maximal Sweating*
(Each 1 mL sweat evaporation		30 mL · min^{-1} = ~18 kcal · min^{-1}
= ~0.6 kcal body heat loss)		
Core temperature increase	No increase	~1°C every 5 to 7 minutes

timal conditions, evaporative cooling can account for a heat loss of about 18 kcal · min^{-1}.

Circulatory adjustments provide the "fine tuning" for temperature regulation. Heat is conserved by rapidly shunting blood deep to the cranial, thoracic, and abdominal cavities and portions of the muscle mass. This optimizes the insulation from subcutaneous fat and other portions of the body's shell. Conversely, when internal heat becomes excessive, peripheral vessels dilate and warm blood is channeled to the cooler periphery. The drive for thermal balance is so strong that it may elicit a sweat rate of 3.5 L per hour during exercise in the heat or an oxygen uptake of 1000 mL per minute brought on by shivering in severe cold.

HYPOTHALAMIC REGULATION OF TEMPERATURE

The **hypothalamus** *contains the central coordinating center for the various processes of temperature regulation.* This group of specialized neurons at the floor of the brain acts as a "thermostat" (usually set and carefully regulated at 37°C ± 1°C) that makes thermoregulatory adjustments to deviations from a temperature norm. Unlike a thermostat in a building, however, the hypothalamus cannot "turn off" the heat; it can only initiate responses to protect the body from a buildup or loss of heat.

Heat-regulating mechanisms are activated in two ways:

• By thermal receptors in the skin that provide input to the central control center.
• By direct stimulation of the hypothalamus through changes in blood temperature perfusing this area.

Peripheral thermal receptors, or sensors responsive to rapid changes in heat and cold, are distributed predominantly as free nerve endings in the skin. The cutaneous cold receptors are generally toward the skin surface and are more abundant than the deeper heat receptors. Cold receptors play an important role in initiating the regulatory response to a cold environment. The cutaneous thermal receptors act as an "early warning system" that relays sensory information to the hypothalamus and cortex to cause appropriate heat-conserving or heat-dissipating adjustments and to cause the individual to consciously seek relief from a thermal challenge.

The central regulatory center plays the most important role in maintaining thermal balance. In addition to receiving peripheral input, cells in the anterior portion of the hypothalamus are capable of detecting changes in blood temperature. These cells then activate other hypothalamic regions to initiate coordinated responses for heat conservation (posterior hypothalamus) or heat loss (anterior hypothalamus). In contrast to the importance of peripheral receptors in detecting cold, body warmth is monitored mainly by the temperature of the blood perfusing the hypothalamus.

THERMOREGULATION IN COLD STRESS: HEAT CONSERVATION AND HEAT PRODUCTION

The normal heat transfer gradient is from the body to the environment, and core temperature generally is maintained without physiologic strain. In extreme cold, however, excessive heat loss can occur, particularly when the person is resting. In this situation, the body's heat production increases and heat loss is retarded as adjustments are made to prevent a fall in core temperature.

VASCULAR ADJUSTMENTS

Stimulation of cutaneous cold receptors causes constriction of peripheral blood vessels; this immediately reduces the flow of warm blood to the body's cooler surface and redirects it to the warmer core. For example, cutaneous blood flow is approximately 250 mL · min^{-1} in a thermoneutral environment, whereas under severe cold stress this flow approaches zero.[60] Consequently, skin temperature falls toward the ambient temperature, and the insulatory benefits of skin and subcutaneous fat are used to their maximal advantage. An overfat person, therefore, can derive great benefits from this heat-conserving mechanism when exposed to cold stress.[75, 83] For a thinly clad person who is not overfat, the regulation of cutaneous blood flow generally provides effective thermoregulation at ambient temperatures between 25 and 29°C (77 and 84°F).

MUSCULAR ACTIVITY

Although significant metabolic heat is generated through shivering, the greatest contribution of muscle to defend against cold occurs during physical activity. Exercise energy metabolism can sustain a constant core temperature in air temperature as low as −30°C (−22°F) without the need for heavy, restrictive clothing. It should be noted that the thermoregulatory defense against cold is mediated by internal temperature, not by the body's heat production per se.[85] Therefore, shivering occurs even during exercise if the core temperature is low. As a result, exercise oxygen uptake is proportionally higher (due directly to shivering) in cold stress than it is during the same exercise in a warmer environment.[25, 75]

HORMONAL OUTPUT

During acute cold exposure, increased heat production is due partially to the action of two "calorigenic" hormones of the adrenal medulla, epinephrine and norepinephrine. It is also possible that prolonged cold stress increases the release of the thyroid hormone, thyroxine, which leads to sustained elevation in resting metabolism.

THERMOREGULATION IN HEAT STRESS: HEAT LOSS

The body's thermoregulatory mechanisms are primarily geared to protect against overheating.[107] This is important during exercise in hot weather, when an inherent competition exists between mechanisms that maintain a large muscle blood flow and those that provide adequate thermoregulation. The potential avenues for heat exchange in an exercising human are illustrated in Figure 25.2. Body heat is lost by radiation, conduction, convection, and evaporation.

HEAT LOSS BY RADIATION

Objects are continually emitting electromagnetic heat waves. Because our bodies are usually warmer than the environment, the net exchange of radiant heat energy is through the air to the solid, cooler objects in the environment. This form of heat transfer does not require molecular contact between objects and is the means for the sun's rays to warm the earth. A person can remain warm by absorbing radiant heat energy from direct sunlight (or reflected from the snow, sand, or water), even in subfreezing temperatures. When the temperature of objects in the environment exceeds skin temperature, radiant heat energy is absorbed from the surroundings. Under these conditions, the only avenue for heat loss is evaporative cooling.

HEAT LOSS BY CONDUCTION

Heat loss by conduction involves the direct transfer of heat through a liquid, solid, or gas from one molecule to another. Although most of the body heat is transported to the shell by the circulation, a small amount continually moves by conduction directly through the deep tissues to the cooler surface. Heat loss by conduction then involves

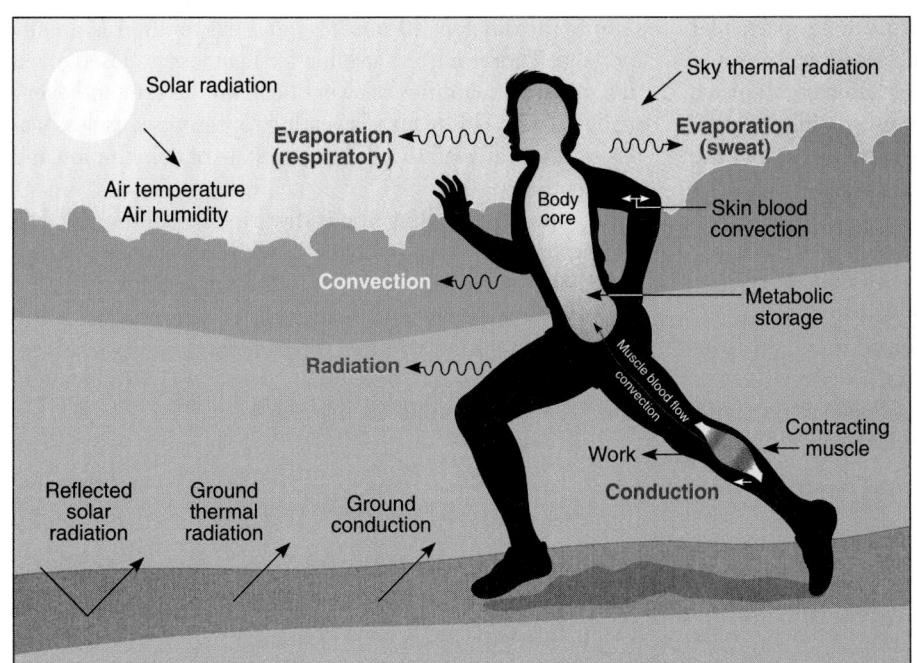

FIGURE 25.2

Heat production within active muscle and its subsequent transfer from the core to the skin. Under appropriate environmental conditions, excess body heat is dissipated to the environment and core temperature is regulated within a narrow range. (From Gisolfi, C.V., and Wenger, C.B.: Temperature regulation during exercise: old concepts, new ideas. *Exerc. Sport Sci. Rev.*, 12:339, 1984.)

the warming of air molecules and cooler surfaces in contact with the skin.

The rate of conductive heat loss depends on the temperature gradient between the skin and surrounding surfaces and their thermal qualities. For example, heat loss in water can be considerable. This is clearly illustrated by placing one hand in water at room temperature. The hand feels much colder than the hand in air—even though the water and air are the same temperature. This occurs because water can absorb several thousand times more heat than air and can conduct it away from the warmer body. For this reason, sitting immersed in an indoor swimming pool is uncomfortable compared to sitting out of water on the pool deck, even when the air and water are at the same temperature. Warm-weather hikers can gain considerable body heat from both exercise and the environment. Some relief can be obtained by lying on a cool rock that has been shielded from the sun. This conductance between the rock's cold surface and the warmer surface of the hiker can facilitate a favorable loss of body heat.

HEAT LOSS BY CONVECTION

The effectiveness of heat loss by conduction depends on how rapidly the air (or water) near the body is exchanged once it becomes warmed. If air movement or convection is slow, the air next to the skin is warmed and acts as a zone of insulation. This minimizes further conductive heat loss. Conversely, if the warmer air surrounding the body is continually replaced by cooler air (as occurs on a breezy day, in a room with a fan, or during running), heat loss increases as convective currents carry the heat away. For example, air currents at 4 miles per hour are about twice as effective for cooling as air moving at 1 mile per hour. This is the basis of the Wind Chill Index (see p. 521), which shows the equivalent still-air temperature for a particular ambient temperature at different wind velocities. In water, convection is also an important factor affecting thermal balance because the body loses heat more rapidly by convection while swimming than while lying motionless in the water.

HEAT LOSS BY EVAPORATION

Evaporation provides the major physiologic defense against overheating. Heat is continually transferred to the environment as water is vaporized from the respiratory passages and skin surface. For each liter of water that vaporizes, 580 kcal are extracted from the body and transferred to the environment.

Approximately 2 to 4 million sweat glands are distributed over the body's surface. In response to heat stress, these eccrine glands, which are controlled by cholinergic sympathetic nerve fibers, secrete large quantities of hypotonic saline solution (0.2 to 0.4% NaCl). When sweat reaches the skin, a cooling effect occurs as the fluid evaporates. The cooled skin then serves to cool the blood that has been shunted from the interior to the surface. Along with heat loss through sweating, approximately 350 mL of water seeps through the skin each day and evaporates to the environment as insensible perspiration. Also, approximately 300 mL of water vaporizes daily from the moist mucous membranes of the respiratory passages. This is seen as "foggy breath" in cold weather.

Evaporative Heat Loss at High Ambient Temperatures. As ambient temperature increases, the effectiveness of heat loss decreases by conduction, convection, and radiation. When ambient temperature exceeds body temperature, heat is actually gained by these mechanisms of thermal transfer. In such environments (or when conduction, convection, and radiation are inadequate to dissipate a large metabolic heat load), sweat evaporation and the small contribution to cooling provided by the vaporization of water from the respiratory tract is the only means of heat dissipation. In fact, the rate of sweating increases directly with the ambient temperature.[89]

Heat Loss in High Humidity. The total sweat vaporized from the skin depends on three factors: (*a*) the surface exposed to the environment, (*b*) the temperature and relative humidity of the ambient air, and (*c*) the convective air currents around the body. *By far, relative humidity is the most important factor that determines the effectiveness of evaporative heat loss.*

Relative humidity is defined as the ratio of the water in ambient air at a particular temperature to the total quantity of moisture that could be carried in that air, expressed as a percentage. For example, 40% relative humidity means that ambient air contains only 40% of the air's moisture-carrying capacity at the specific temperature. When humidity is high, the ambient vapor pressure approaches that of the moist skin (approximately 40 mm Hg) and evaporation is greatly reduced. Therefore, this avenue for heat loss is closed, even though large quantities of sweat bead on the skin and eventually roll off. This form of sweating represents a useless water loss that can lead to a dangerous state of dehydration and overheating.

Evaporative cooling also is thwarted by continually drying the skin with a towel before sweat has a chance to evaporate. *Sweat does not cool the skin; evaporation of sweat cools the skin.* As long as the humidity is low, relatively high environmental temperatures can be tolerated. For this reason, hot, dry desert climates are more comfortable than cooler but more humid tropical climates.

INTEGRATION OF HEAT-DISSIPATING MECHANISMS

Mechanisms for heat loss remain the same whether heat load is imposed internally (metabolic heat) or externally (environmental heat).

Circulation. The circulatory system is the "work-horse" in maintaining thermal balance. At rest in hot weather, heart rate and cardiac output increase while superficial arterial and venous blood vessels dilate to divert warm blood to the body shell. This is seen as a flushed or reddened face on a hot day or during vigorous exercise. With extreme heat stress, 15 to 25% of the cardiac output will pass through the skin. This greatly increases the thermal conductance of peripheral tissues and favors radiative heat loss to the environment, especially from the hands, forehead, forearms, ears, and tibial areas.

Evaporation. Sweating begins within several seconds of the start of vigorous exercise, and, after about 30 minutes, reaches an equilibrium that is in direct relation to the exercise load.[11, 46] An effective thermal defense is established when evaporative cooling is combined with a large cutaneous blood flow. The cooled peripheral blood then returns to the deeper tissues to pick up additional heat as it returns to the heart.

Hormonal Adjustments. Because both water and electrolytes are lost through sweating, hormonal adjustments are initiated in heat stress as the body attempts to conserve salts and fluid.[29, 43] The pituitary gland releases vasopressin or antidiuretic hormone (ADH), which increases water reabsorption from the kidney tubules. This causes the urine to become more concentrated during heat stress. Concurrently, during repeated days of exercise in hot weather, or with just a single bout of exercise, the sodium-conserving hormone aldosterone is released from the adrenal cortex.[22] This hormone acts on the renal tubules to increase the reabsorption of sodium. Aldosterone also acts to reduce the osmolality of sweat. Thus, sodium concentration in sweat is decreased during repeated heat exposure, which further aids in conserving electrolytes.

EFFECTS OF CLOTHING ON THERMOREGULATION

Clothing insulates the body from its surroundings. It can reduce radiant heat gain in a hot environment or retard conductive and convective heat loss in the cold.

COLD-WEATHER CLOTHING

In providing insulation from the cold, the mesh of cloth fibers traps air, which then becomes warm. Because cloth and air are poor heat conductors, a barrier to heat loss is established; the thicker the zone of trapped air next to the skin, the more effective the insulation. For this reason, several layers of light clothing or garments lined with animal fur, feathers, or synthetic fabrics (with numerous layers of trapped air) provide much greater insulation than a single bulky layer of winter clothing. The clothing layer against the skin must also be effective in transporting moisture (wicking action) away from the body's surface to the next insulating clothing layer for subsequent evaporation. Wool or synthetics such as polypropylene, which insulates well and dries quickly, can serve this purpose. Furthermore, a wool cap contributes considerably to heat conservation because nearly 30 to 40% of body heat can be lost through the highly vascularized head region, which represents only about 8% of the body's total surface area. Conversely, cooling the head during exercise in hot weather is beneficial in reducing symptoms of thermal discomfort. When clothing becomes wet, through either external moisture or condensation from sweating, it loses almost 90% of its insulating properties. This actually facilitates heat loss from the body because water conducts heat much faster than air.

When exercising in cold air, the thermoregulatory problem is usually not adequate insulation but the dissipation of metabolic heat through a thick air-clothing barrier. Cross-country skiers alleviate this problem by removing layers of clothing as the body becomes warm. In this way, core temperature is maintained without reliance on evaporative cooling. *The ideal winter garment in cold, dry weather is impermeable to air movement but permits the escape of water vapor from the skin if sweating occurs.*

WARM-WEATHER CLOTHING

Dry clothing, no matter how lightweight, retards heat exchange more than the same clothing soaking wet. The practice of switching to a dry tennis, basketball, or football uniform in hot weather makes little sense from the standpoint of temperature regulation. Evaporative heat loss occurs only when the clothing becomes wet throughout. A dry uniform simply prolongs the time between sweating and cooling.

Different materials absorb water at different rates. Cottons and linens readily absorb moisture. On the other hand, heavy "sweat shirts" and clothing made of rubber or plastic produce high relative humidity close to the skin and retard the vaporization of moisture from the skin surface; this significantly inhibits or even prevents evaporative cooling. Warm-weather clothing should be loose fitting to permit the free circulation of air between the skin and environment to promote evaporation from the skin. Color is also important because dark colors absorb light rays and add to the radiant heat gain, whereas clothing of lighter color reflects heat rays.

FOOTBALL UNIFORMS

Of all athletic uniforms and equipment, those used in football present the most significant barrier to heat dissipation. Even with loose-fitting porous jerseys, the wrappings, the padding (with its plastic covering), the helmet, and other objects of "armor" effectively seal off 50% of the body's surface from the benefits of evaporative cooling. To this is added the metabolic cost of carrying the 6 or 7 kg of equipment, often on a relatively hot artificial playing surface. This situation is further magnified by the large size of these athletes, particularly the offensive and defensive linemen, who possess a relatively small surface area-to-mass ratio and a higher percentage of body fat than players at other positions.[120]

The metabolic and thermal stress provided by the football uniform is shown in Figure 25.3. In this experiment,[73] nine men were tested at 25.6°C (78°F) and 35% relative humidity while running for 30 minutes. In one test, the men wore only shorts; in another, they wore the complete football uniform, including helmet and plastic-covered padding. In a third series of measurements, they wore shorts and carried a backpack containing 6.2 kg, exactly the weight of the uniform and equipment.

When exercising wearing football gear, rectal temperature and skin temperature were significantly higher during both exercise and recovery than with either of the other exercise conditions. The temperature directly beneath the padding averaged only 1°C less than rectal temperature. This meant that subcutaneous blood in these areas was cooled only about one-fifth as much as at the skin surface directly exposed to the environment. Because rectal temperature remained elevated during recovery with uniforms, it appears that a "rest" period is of limited value in normalizing thermal status unless the uniform is removed. As shown

by the blue line in Figure 25.3, a large portion of the heat load was provided simply by the weight of the uniform. Skin temperatures, however, were much cooler and sweat rates were less when the uniform was not worn. Without the uniform, evaporation from the skin was relatively free, whereas the uniform insulated the athlete and reduced the evaporative surface.

■ SUMMARY ■

1. Humans can tolerate only relatively small variations in internal temperature. Consequently, exposure to heat or cold stress initiates thermoregulatory mechanisms that generate and conserve heat at low ambient temperatures and dissipate heat at high temperatures.

2. The "thermostat" for temperature regulation is located in the hypothalamus. This coordinating center initiates adjustments in response to input from thermal receptors in the skin as well as changes in the temperature of blood perfusing the hypothalamic regions.

3. Heat conservation in cold stress is achieved by vascular adjustments that shunt blood from the cooler periphery to the warmer deep tissues of the body's core. If this is ineffective, shivering provides a significant input of

FIGURE 25.3

Effects of full football uniform and its equivalent weight on rectal temperature (**A**) and skin temperature (**B**) during exercise. Subjects ran at 9.6 km · hr[-1] for 30 minutes at 25.6°C and 35% relative humidity. Owing to its effect in retarding evaporative cooling, the uniform caused the largest heat stress as indicated by significant elevations in rectal and skin temperatures. (From Mathews, D.K., et al.: Physiological responses during exercise and recovery in a football uniform. *J. Appl. Physiol.*, 26:611, 1969.)

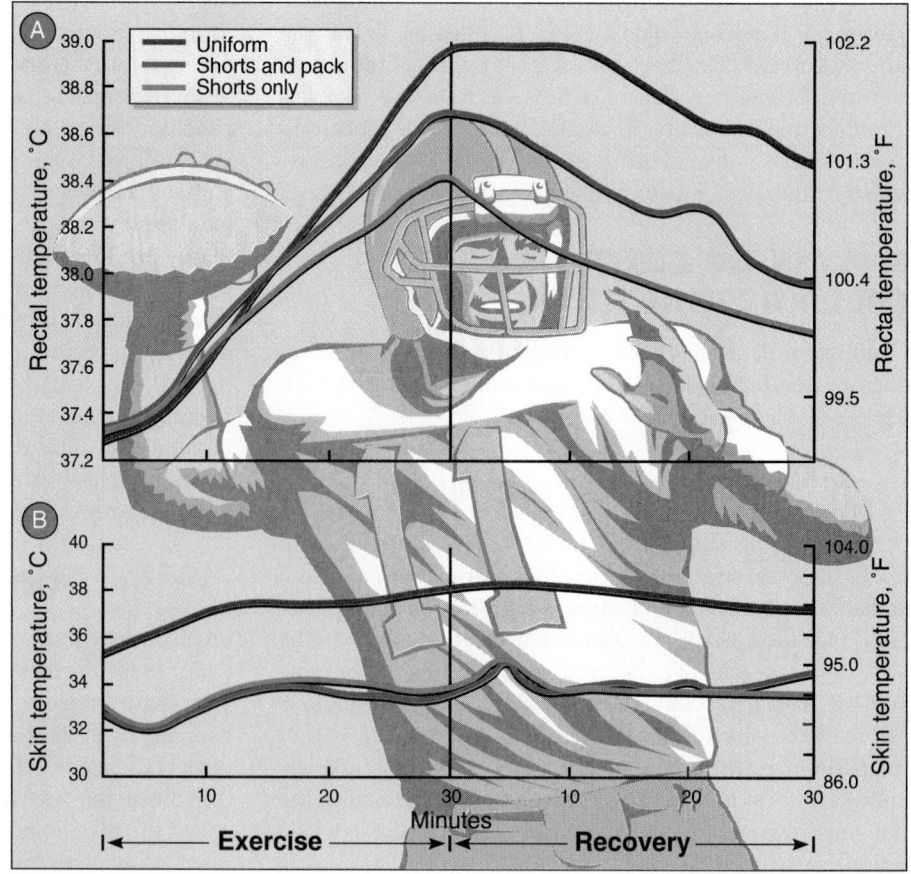

metabolic heat. Hormones that cause a sustained elevation in resting metabolism are also released.

4. In response to heat stress, warm blood is diverted from the body's core to the shell. Body heat is lost by radiation, conduction, convection, and evaporation. At high ambient temperatures and during exercise, evaporation provides the major physiologic defense against overheating.

5. In warm, humid environments, the effectiveness of evaporative heat loss is dramatically reduced. This makes a person particularly vulnerable to a dangerous state of dehydration and spiraling core temperature.

6. Several layers of light clothing provide a relatively thick zone of trapped air against the skin. This gives a more effective insulation from the cold than a single thick layer of winter clothing. When clothing becomes wet, insulation is lost and heat flow from the body is greatly facilitated.

7. The metabolic heat generated during vigorous exercise generally maintains core temperature in cold-air environments, even if the person wears relatively little clothing.

8. The ideal warm-weather clothing is lightweight, loose-fitting, and light in color. Even wearing this clothing, heat loss is retarded until the clothing becomes wet and evaporative cooling can proceed.

9. Football uniforms impose a significant barrier to heat dissipation because they effectively seal off about 50% of the body's surface from the benefits of evaporative cooling.

PART 2

THERMOREGULATION AND ENVIRONMENTAL STRESS DURING EXERCISE

EXERCISE IN THE HEAT

In addition to cardiovascular adjustments, the dissipation of metabolic heat during exercise (particularly in hot weather) depends on the refrigeration mechanism of evaporative cooling. A price is paid, however, as demands are placed on the body's fluid reserves and a relative state of dehydration frequently occurs. Excessive sweating leads to more serious fluid loss and an accompanying reduction in plasma volume. This can cause circulatory failure, and core temperature may rise to lethal levels.

CIRCULATORY ADJUSTMENTS

When exercising in hot weather, the body is faced with two competitive cardiovascular demands:

- The muscles require oxygen to sustain energy metabolism.
- The metabolic heat generated during exercise must be transported via the blood from the deep tissues to the periphery. Therefore, this blood cannot deliver its oxygen to the active muscles.

Cardiac output during submaximal exercise is similar in both hot and cold environments.[102, 104] However, the heart's stroke volume is usually lower in the heat, in proportion to the fluid deficit created during exercise, which causes the heart rate to be higher at all levels of submaximal exercise.[82] Maximal cardiac output and $\dot{V}O_2$max are reduced during exercise in the heat because the reflex compensatory increase in heart rate is insufficient to offset the stroke volume decrease.

Vascular Constriction and Dilation. In the heat, adequate cutaneous and muscle blood flow is achieved at the expense of other tissues, which can temporarily compromise their blood supply. For example, vasodilation of the subcutaneous vessels is rapidly countered by compensatory constriction of the splanchnic vascular bed and renal tissues. Such a significant and often prolonged reduction in blood flow to these tissues may contribute to the large number of liver and renal complications noted with exertional heat stress.

Maintenance of Blood Pressure. In addition to redirecting blood to areas in great need, vasoconstriction in the viscera increases total vascular resistance. As a result, arterial blood pressure is usually maintained during exercise in the heat. During heavy exercise, with its accompanying dehydration, relatively less blood is shunted to peripheral areas for heat dissipation.[42] This probably reflects the body's attempt to maintain cardiac output in the face of a diminishing plasma volume caused by sweating. Under these conditions, circulatory regulation and muscle blood flow take precedence over temperature regulation.[84]

Even when submaximal exercise in the heat is well tolerated, work is generally accomplished with a greater dependence on anaerobic metabolism than in cooler conditions.[127] This results in the early accumulation of lactic acid and encroachment on glycogen reserves.[18, 40] An increased lactic acid level is probably due to (*a*) a decreased lactate uptake by the liver because of a reduction in hepatic blood flow during exercise in the heat and (*b*) a reduced muscle circulation as a large portion of the cardiac output is shunted to the periphery for heat dissipation. Both of these factors contribute to the early fatigue noted during only moderate exercise in the heat.

CORE TEMPERATURE DURING EXERCISE

The heat generated by active muscles can raise core temperature to fever levels that would incapacitate a person if caused by external heat stress alone.[5] Champion distance runners show no ill effects from rectal temperatures as high as 41°C (105.8°F) recorded at the end of a 3-mile race.[56]

Higher Core Temperatures are Regulated. Within limits, the increase in core temperature during exercise does not reflect a failure of the heat-dissipating mechanisms. To the contrary, a well-regulated response occurs even during exercise in the cold. The relationship between esophageal (core) temperature and oxygen uptake for five men and two women of varying fitness levels during exercise of increasing severity is illustrated in Figure 25.4A. Core temperature increases to a higher level in all subjects as exercise becomes more intense. However, there was wide variability in temperature response among subjects. When core temperature is plotted in relation to exercise oxygen uptake, expressed as a percentage of each person's $\dot{V}O_2$max (Fig. 25.4B), the lines move closer together. This indicates that it is the relative workload (i.e., the percentage of one's capacity) that determines the change in core temperature with exercise. *More than likely, a modest rise in core temperature reflects a favorable internal adjustment that creates an optimal thermal environment for physiologic and metabolic function* (refer to Focus on Research, p. 500).

Generally, exercise in a comfortable environment at 50% of $\dot{V}O_2$max increases temperature to a new steady level of approximately 37.3°C (99°F), whereas work at 75% of maximum elevates core temperature to 38.5°C (101°F), regardless of the absolute level of oxygen uptake. Therefore, at the same percentage of $\dot{V}O_2$max, a fit person generates more total energy during exercise but still has about the same core temperature as a less fit counterpart.[105] This extra metabolic heat is dissipated via a larger sweat output by the person working at the higher absolute level of exercise. Of course, at the same workload, the trained person exercises with a lower core temperature.

WATER LOSS IN THE HEAT—DEHYDRATION

A few hours of heavy exercise in a hot environment can cause water loss to reach a significant level. This fluid deficit or dehydration occurs from both the intracellular and extracellular compartments and can rapidly reach levels that impede heat dissipation, reduce heat tolerance, and severely compromise cardiovascular function and exercise capacity. Because sweat is hypotonic with other body fluids, the hypovolemia caused by sweating is associated with a corresponding increase in the osmolality of the blood plasma.

Magnitude of Fluid Loss. In an acclimatized person, water loss by sweating may reach a peak of approximately 3 L per hour during intense exercise in the heat and may average nearly 12 L (26 lb) on a daily basis. Furthermore, several hours of intense sweating can cause sweat-gland fatigue, which ultimately leads to an inability to regulate core temperature. Elite marathon runners frequently experience fluid losses in excess of 5 L during competition.[96] In these athletes, this fluid loss represents between 6 and 10% of body mass. For a slower-paced marathon or ultramarathon, the average fluid loss probably rarely exceeds 500 mL per hour.[91] *The exceptional potential for evaporative cooling of acclimatized humans can only be sustained with adequate fluid replacement.*

Distance running is not the only sport in which a large sweat output and subsequent fluid loss occur. Football, basketball, and hockey players may lose similar large quantities of fluid during a contest. High school wrestlers often lose 9 to 13% of their preseason body mass before certification; the greatest portion of this weight loss comes from voluntarily reducing water intake and excessive sweating before weigh-in. Collegiate wrestlers, excluding heavyweights, regained an average of 3.7 kg (8.1 lb) during the 20-hour pe-

FIGURE 25.4

Relationship between esophageal temperature and oxygen uptake (absolute exercise intensity expressed as power output) **(A)** and oxygen uptake as a percent of $\dot{V}O_2$max **(B)**. (From Saltin, B., and Hermansen, L.: Esophageal, rectal, and muscle temperature during exercise. *J. Appl. Physiol.*, 21:1757, 1966.)

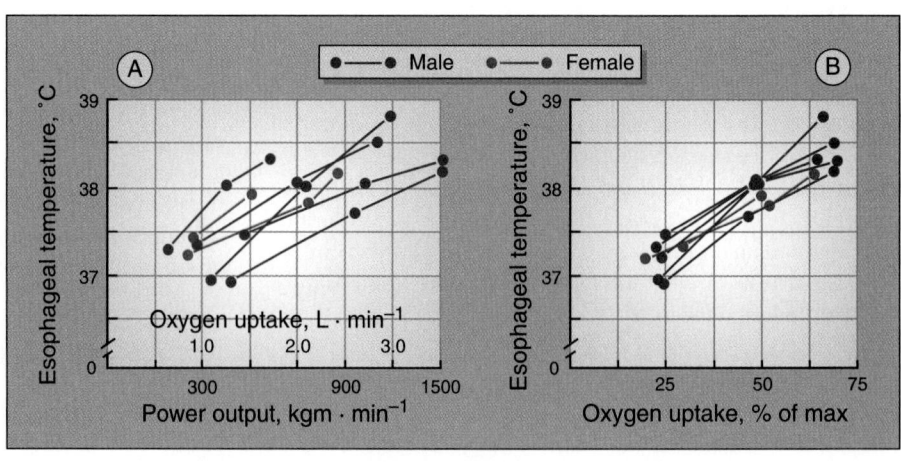

riod between weigh-in and the start of competition.[110] In their desire to "make weight," high school and collegiate wrestlers usually compete in a dehydrated state.[128]

Significant Consequences. As dehydration progresses and plasma volume decreases, peripheral blood flow and sweating rate are reduced and thermoregulation becomes progressively more difficult. For men and women, a pre-exercise dehydration equivalent to 5% of body mass significantly increases rectal temperature and heart rate and decreases sweating rate, $\dot{V}O_2$max, and exercise capacity compared to conditions of normal hydration.[108] The elevated heart rate in the dehydrated state is attributed to a reduced central blood volume, which leads to a lower ventricular filling pressure and a 25 to 30% reduction in the heart's stroke volume. This reduced stroke volume often is not offset by a proportional increase in heart rate; consequently, the cardiac output and arterial blood pressure decline.[24, 45] The elevation in core temperature is related to a reduction in both sweating rate and blood flow to the skin.[41, 86]

Fluid loss is particularly apparent during exercise in hot, humid environments. In this situation, the effectiveness of evaporative cooling is thwarted by the high vapor pressure of ambient air. As illustrated in Figure 25.5, a linear relationship exists between sweating rate, both at rest and during exercise, and the air's moisture content. Ironically, the excessive output of sweat in high humidity contributes little to cooling because evaporation is at a minimum.

Physiologic and Performance Decrements. The reduction in peripheral blood flow and increase in core temperature during exercise are proportionate to the level of dehydration. A fluid loss equivalent to as little as 1% of body mass is associated with a significant increase in rectal temperature compared to the same exercise with normal hydration.[18, 32] For each liter of sweat-loss dehydration, the exercise heart rate becomes elevated by about 8 beats per minute with a corresponding 1.0 L · min⁻¹ decrease in cardiac output.[24] When water loss reaches 4 to 5% of body mass (a value commonly seen among high school wrestlers), a definite impairment is noted in physical work capacity and physiologic function.[14, 19, 104] Although wrestlers weigh in about 5 hours before their matches, this may not be enough time to ensure complete rehydration and electrolyte balance at the time of competition.[125]

Because a large portion of water loss through sweating comes from the blood plasma, circulatory capacity is adversely affected as sweat loss progresses (if water is not continually replenished). This is manifested by a decrease in plasma volume, a reduced skin blood flow for a given core temperature, a fall in stroke volume and a compensatory increase in heart rate, and a general deterioration in circulatory and thermoregulatory efficiency during exercise.[106] For exercise capacity, a 48% reduction in walking endurance occurred when subjects dehydrated to 4.3% of body mass; at the same time, $\dot{V}O_2$max decreased by 22%.[26] In these same

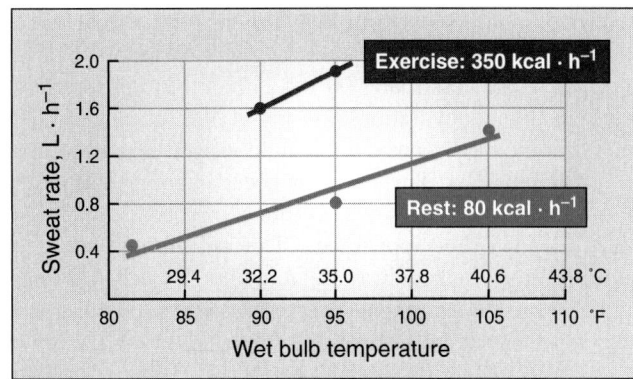

FIGURE 25.5
The effect of humidity (wet-bulb temperature) on sweat rate at rest and during exercise in the heat. Ambient temperature (dry-bulb) was 43.4°C (110°F). (From Iampietro, P.F.: Exercise in hot environments. In *Frontiers of Fitness*. Edited by R.J. Shephard. Springfield, IL, Charles C. Thomas, 1971.)

experiments, endurance performance was reduced by 22% and $\dot{V}O_2$max was reduced by 10% when dehydration averaged only 1.9% of body mass. Clearly, dehydration reduces the capability of the thermoregulatory system to meet the metabolic and thermal stress of exercise.

Use of Diuretics. A greater percentage of water is drawn from the plasma if body water is lost as a result of diuretic-induced dehydration.[19] Therefore, wrestlers who use diuretics to lose body water rapidly to "make weight" are at a distinct disadvantage because of a disproportionate reduction in plasma volume and the negative effect of this reduction on thermoregulation and cardiovascular function. In addition, drugs that induce a diuretic effect may also cause a marked impairment in neuromuscular function that is not noted when comparable fluid loss is brought on by exercise.[15] Chemicals that induce vomiting and diarrhea are also used by athletes for acute weight loss. Not only does this abuse lead to dehydration, but it may also cause excessive mineral loss with accompanying muscle weakness and impaired neuromuscular function; this would clearly give the competitive "edge" to the opponent.

WATER REPLACEMENT: REHYDRATION

The primary aim of fluid replacement is to maintain plasma volume so that circulation and sweating can progress at optimal levels. Ingesting fluid during exercise increases blood flow to the skin for more effective cooling, independent of any change in plasma volume.[81] Prevention of dehydration and its consequences, particularly hyperthermia, can only be achieved with an adequate water replacement schedule that is strictly followed.[16, 74, 87] This may be "easier said than done," because some coaches and athletes feel that ingesting water hinders performance. When left on their own, most athletes will voluntarily replace only about one-half of the water lost (less than 500 mL · hr^{-1}) during exercise.[90] For wrestlers, dehydration is a "way of life," because young boys and men lose considerable fluid weight to wrestle in a lower-weight class. This also may occur in young and older ballet dancers who have a continual preoccupation with maintaining a thin appearance. The enlightened exercise specialist must be keenly aware of the importance of proper hydration for thermoregulation, exercise performance, and safety.

"Cold treatments" such as periodic application of cold towels to the forehead and abdomen during exercise or a cold shower before exercise in a hot environment is of only small benefit in facilitating heat transfer at the body's surface compared to the same exercise without skin wetting.[10, 38] *The most effective defense against heat stress is adequate hydration.* This is achieved by balancing water loss with water intake, not by pouring water over the head or body. There is simply no evidence to indicate that restricting fluid intake during training in some way makes an athlete better able to adjust to subsequent work in the heat. *A well-hydrated athlete always functions at a higher level than one who exercises in a dehydrated state.* Specific factors that influence gastric emptying and subsequent intestinal absorption of ingested fluids, as well as practical recommendations for oral rehydration beverages and possible complications from excessive water intake with prolonged exercise (hyponatremia), have been discussed in Chapters 2 and 3.

Ingestion of "extra" water, or **hyperhydration** before exercising in a hot environment, provides some protection because it delays the development of dehydration, increases sweating during exercise, and brings about a smaller rise in core temperature.[46, 86] In this regard, it is wise to consume 400 to 600 mL (13 to 20 oz) of cold water about 20 minutes before exercising in the heat. This not only provides pre-exercise fluid uptake, but increasing the stomach's volume is a major factor to optimize gastric emptying (see Chapter 3). This procedure, however, does not replace the need for continual fluid replacement during exercise. In activities such as distance running, matching fluid loss with fluid intake may be virtually impossible, because only about 1000 mL of fluid can be emptied from the stomach each hour during such vigorous exercise. This is insufficient to match a water loss that may average nearly 2000 mL per hour. Consequently, athletes must be carefully monitored during exercise, even if they are permitted free access to water.

Adequacy of Rehydration. *Changes in body weight can be used to indicate water loss during exercise and the adequacy of rehydration during and after exercise or athletic competition.* Recommendations for fluid intake with weight loss during exercise are presented in Table 25.2. Although these standards were developed for a 90-minute football practice, they are easily adapted to most exercise situations.

TABLE 25.2
RECOMMENDED FLUID AVAILABILITY AND INTAKE FOR A STRENUOUS 90-MINUTE ATHLETIC PRACTICE^a

Weight Loss		Minutes Between Water Breaks	Fluid per Break		Fluid Availability for an 11-Member Squad	
lb	kg		oz	mL	Gallons	Liters
8	3.6	No practice	—		—	
7½	3.4	recommended	—		—	
7	3.2	10	8–10	266	6½–8	27.4
6½	3.0	10	8–9	251	6½–7	25.5
6	2.7	10	8–9	251	6½–7	25.5
5½	2.5	15	10–12	325	5½–6½	22.7
5	2.3	15	10–11	311	5½–6	21.8
4½	2.1	15	9–10	281	5–5½	19.9
4	1.8	15	8–9	251	4½–5	18.0
3½	1.6	20	10–11	311	4–4½	16.1
3	1.4	20	9–10	281	3½–4	14.2
2½	1.1	20	7–8	222	3	11.4
2	0.9	30	8	237	2½	9.5
1½	0.7	30	6	177	1½	5.7
1	0.5	45	6	177	1	3.8
½	0.2	60	6	177	½	1.9

^{a}Based on an 80% replacement of weight loss.

Coaches may have their athletes weigh in before and after practice and insist that weight loss be minimized by periodic water breaks during activity. (Each 1-lb weight loss represents 450 mL, or 15 fluid oz, of dehydration.) Water must be available and consumed during practice and competition. Because the thirst mechanism is generally an imprecise guide to water needs, athletes must be urged to rehydrate themselves. If rehydration were left entirely to a person's thirst, it might take several days to reestablish fluid balance after severe dehydration.[100]

ELECTROLYTE REPLACEMENT

Because sweat is hypotonic to the body fluids, replacing water is much more of an immediate concern than replacing minerals. For a fluid loss of less than 2.7 kg (6 lb) in adults, electrolytes are readily replenished by adding a slight amount of salt to food when the need exists. For example, the addition of the electrolytes sodium and potassium chloride to the drinking water was of minimum value in men and women who were dehydrated because of sweating by about 3% of body mass on 5 successive days but were permitted food and water ad libitum during each daily recovery period.[21] Furthermore, sodium losses during prolonged exercise are balanced by the sodium-conservation mechanisms of the kidney, which are activated during such exercise.[58]

A Small Amount of Salt May Be Beneficial. As discussed in Chapter 3, a small amount of electrolytes (and glucose) added to a rehydration beverage may bring about a more complete rehydration than plain water.[17, 74, 86, 92, 93] It is postulated that pure water absorbed from the gut rapidly dilutes the plasma concentration of sodium. This, in turn, stimulates urine production and blunts the sodium-dependent stimulation of the thirst mechanism. Maintaining a relatively high plasma concentration of sodium by adding a small amount of this electrolyte to the ingested fluid may sustain the thirst drive and more rapidly restore lost plasma volume.

With prolonged exercise in the heat, sweat loss may deplete the body of 13 to 17 g of salt (2.3 to 3.4 g per L of sweat) per day. This amount is approximately 8 g more than that normally provided in the daily diet. In this case, some extra sodium may be necessary, which can be provided by adding about one-third teaspoon of table salt to a liter of water. It is doubtful if potassium supplements are needed, because the potassium loss through sweating is negligible except under the most extreme conditions.[23, 31] In this case, potassium loss can be replaced by increasing the intake of potassium-rich foods such as citrus fruits and bananas. A glass of orange juice or tomato juice replaces almost all the potassium, calcium, and magnesium excreted in about 3 L of sweat. For all but unusual cases, dietary modifications and electrolyte conservation by the kidneys adequately compensate for mineral loss through sweating.

FACTORS THAT MODIFY HEAT TOLERANCE

Acclimatization. Tasks that are relatively easy when performed in cool weather become taxing if attempted on the first hot day of spring. The early stages of spring training are often the most hazardous for heat injury, because thermoregulatory mechanisms have not adjusted to the dual challenge of exercise and environmental heat. Repeated exposure of men and women to hot environments, particularly when combined with exercise, results in an improved capacity for exercise and less discomfort upon heat exposure.[27, 108, 113, 121]

The physiologic adaptive changes that improve heat tolerance are collectively termed **heat acclimatization.** As depicted in Figure 25.6, the major acclimatization occurs during the first week of heat exposure and essentially is complete after 10 days.[69, 116] Only 2 to 4 hours of daily heat exposure are required. In practical terms, the first several exercise sessions in a hot environment should be light and should last about 15 to 20 minutes. Thereafter, exercise sessions can increase systematically in duration and intensity.

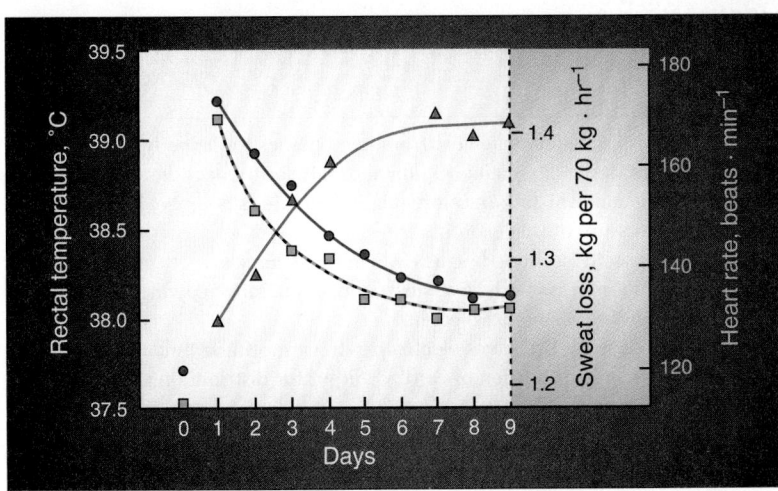

FIGURE 25.6

Average rectal temperature (●), heart rate (■), and sweat loss (▲) during 100 minutes of daily heat-exercise exposure for 9 consecutive days. On day 0, the men walked on a treadmill at an exercise intensity of $300 \cdot kcal \cdot h^{-1}$ in a cool climate. Thereafter, the same daily exercise was performed in the heat at 48.9°C (26.7°F wet bulb). (From Lind, A.R., and Bass, D.E.: Optimal exposure time for development of acclimatization to heat. *Fed. Proc.*, 22:704, 1963.)

The main physiologic adjustments during heat acclimatization are summarized in Table 25.3. In this process, larger quantities of blood are shunted to cutaneous vessels during exercise to facilitate heat transfer from the core to the periphery. A more effective distribution of cardiac output also is achieved to maintain blood pressure during exercise. This "circulatory acclimatization" is complemented by a lowered threshold for sweating. Consequently, the cooling process is initiated before temperature increases too markedly. After 10 days of heat exposure, the capacity for sweating is nearly doubled, and the sweat becomes more diluted (less salt is lost) and more evenly distributed on the skin surface. These adjustments in circulation and evaporative cooling enable a heat-acclimatized person to exercise with a lower skin and core temperature and heart rate than an unacclimatized individual.[1, 9] This lower core temperature results in less need to divert blood to the skin, thus freeing a greater portion of the cardiac output for distribution to the working muscles. For substrate metabolism, acclimatization reduces the level of carbohydrate use during exercise; this is associated with reductions in plasma epinephrine concentrations.[39] It is noteworthy that the acclimatization process is less than optimal unless adequate hydration is maintained. Also, the major benefits of acclimatization are lost within 2 to 3 weeks after returning to a more temperate environment.

Training. The regular exercise-induced "internal" heat stress of training in a cool environment causes adjustments in peripheral circulation and evaporative cooling that are qualitatively similar to those observed at hot ambient temperatures. These responses generally occur within an 8- to 12-week training period at an exercise intensity that exceeds 50% of the person's aerobic capacity. As a result, well-conditioned men and women respond more effectively to severe heat stress than their sedentary counterparts.[4, 32] Exercise training increases the sensitivity and capacity of the sweating response so that sweating begins at a lower core temperature, producing larger volumes of more diluted sweat. This is partly the result of a training-induced intrinsic adaptation in the sweat glands.[13] A significant increase in plasma volume is also noted early with aerobic training.[20, 70] This added fluid supports the needs of sweat glands during heat stress while maintaining an adequate plasma volume for the cardiovascular (skin and muscle blood flow) demands of exercise.[70, 72] Therefore, a trained person stores less heat early during exercise and arrives at a thermal steady state sooner and at a lower core temperature than an untrained person. This training advantage for thermoregulation occurs only if the individual is fully hydrated during exercise.[109]

As might be expected, exercise "heat conditioning" in cool weather is considerably less effective than acclimatization derived from similar exercise training in the heat. *Full heat acclimatization cannot be achieved without actual exposure to environmental heat stress.* Athletes who train and compete in hot weather have a distinct advantage over athletes who train in cool climates but only periodically compete in hot weather.

Age. Debate exists regarding whether the ability to tolerate and acclimatize to moderate heat stress appreciably deteriorates with age.[3, 49, 62, 94, 99, 102] In an early study, men and women aged 60 to 93 years were exposed to 70 minutes of heat stress as they progressively exercised at intensities ranging from 2 to 5 times the resting metabolic rate (MET).[51] The relationship between heart rate and exercise intensity during work in the heat for these subjects and for young men and women is displayed in Figure 25.7.

As expected, heart rates were higher for the generally less fit elderly subjects than for the young adults of the same sex. The heat imposed no greater physiologic strain on the older subjects because their body temperature increased an average of only 0.3°C compared to 0.2°C in the younger

TABLE 25.3
PHYSIOLOGIC ADJUSTMENTS DURING HEAT ACCLIMATIZATION

Acclimatization Response	Effect
Improved cutaneous blood flow	Transports metabolic heat from deep tissues to the body's shell
Effective distribution of cardiac output	Appropriate circulation to skin and muscles to meet demands of metabolism and thermoregulation; greater stability of blood pressure during exercise
Lowered threshold for start of sweating	Evaporative cooling begins early during exercise
More effective distribution of sweat over skin surface	Optimum use of effective surface for evaporative cooling
Increased sweat output	Maximizes evaporative cooling
Lowered salt concentration of sweat	Dilute sweat preserves electrolytes in extracellular fluid
Lower skin and core temperature and heart rate for standard exercise	Frees greater portion of cardiac output for distribution to active muscles
Less reliance on carbohydrate catabolism during exercise	Carbohydrate-sparing effect

group. The elderly subjects were also tested in the spring and fall to evaluate the extent of natural heat acclimatization during the summer months. After the summer, heart rates during the standard thermal-exercise stress were significantly lower for all subjects.

Comparisons between young and middle-aged competitive runners indicate no age-related decrements in thermoregulatory ability during marathon running.[98] Likewise, for physically trained 50-year-old men, little impairment in thermoregulatory function was noted in comparison to young men.[94] Supporting these findings is a report that the capacity for sweating is fully adequate to regulate body temperature during desert walks for men aged 58 to 84 years.[30] *Studies that control such factors as body size and composition, aerobic fitness level, level of hydration, degree of acclimatization, and chronological age generally show little or no age-related effects on thermoregulatory capacity or the ability to acclimatize to heat stress.*[63, 115]

Despite an equivalence in the capacity for thermoregulation during heat stress, age-related factors that could affect thermoregulation do exist. If an age effect on thermoregulation does occur, it could be attributed to an apparent delayed onset in sweating with advancing age, as well as a blunted sweating response due to either a limitation in sweat gland output or to a dehydration-limited sweat output if fluid replacement is insufficient.[62] Peripheral vascular responsiveness that impairs local vasodilation also occurs with aging. Older athletes show a 25 to 40% reduction in skin blood flow compared to younger athletes.[64] Such age-related changes are intrinsic to the structure and function of the skin and its vasculature and probably are not the result of an autonomic nervous system dysfunction.[61, 64, 101] Furthermore, older adults do not recover from dehydration as effectively as younger individuals, which seems to be related to a blunted thirst drive.[63, 115] This could make elderly individuals prone to a chronic state of hypohydration with a less than optimal plasma volume that would affect thermoregulatory capacity. An altered thirst mechanism, as well as a shift in the operating point for the control of body fluid volume and composition, also may contribute to the observed decrease in total blood volume with aging.[28, 71]

Children. Children show a lower rate of perspiration and a higher core temperature during heat stress compared to adolescents and adults. This occurs even though children have a larger number of heat-activated sweat glands per unit skin area.[7, 36] This difference probably lasts through puberty and generally does not limit exercise capacity except during extreme environmental heat stress.[35] Sweat composition also differs between children and adults; in children, the concentrations of sweat sodium and chlorine are higher, and lactate, H^+, and potassium concentrations are lower.[36, 80] Also, children may require a longer time to acclimatize to heat compared to adolescents and young adults.[57] *From a practical standpoint, exercise levels should be reduced for children exposed to heat and additional time should be allowed for acclimatization compared to the mature competitor.*

Sex. Early comparisons of thermoregulation between men and women indicated that men showed a greater tolerance to environmental heat stress during exercise. A major flaw in this research, however, was that the women studied were consistently exercising at higher intensities in relation to their aerobic capacity. When this factor was controlled and men and women of equal fitness were compared, the thermoregulatory differences between the sexes were much less pronounced.[44, 48, 54] *The general consensus is that women can tolerate the physiologic and thermal stress of exercise at least as well as men of comparable fitness and level of acclimatization; both sexes can acclimatize to a similar degree.*[2, 113, 123]

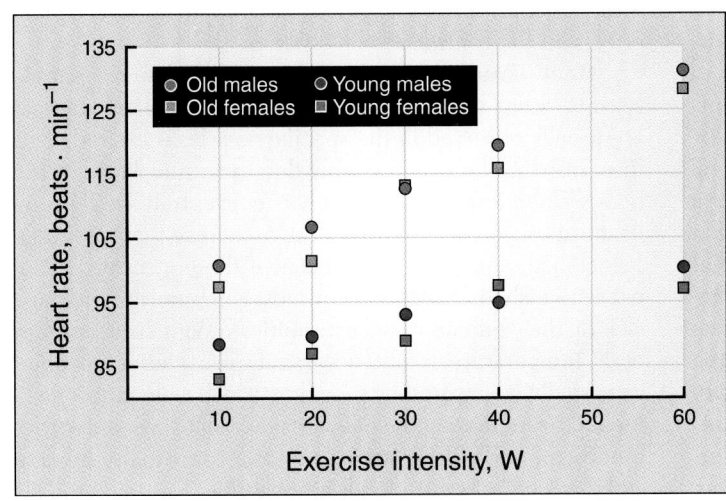

FIGURE 25.7

Heart rate during moderate exercise in the heat for young and old men and women. Dry-bulb ambient temperature was 33.5°C and wet-bulb was 28.5°C. (Adapted from Henshel, A.: The environment and performance. In *Physiology of Work Capacity and Fatigue.* Edited by E. Simonsen. Springfield, IL, Charles C. Thomas, 1971.)

Sweating. *Sweating is the distinct sex difference in thermoregulation.* Although women possess more heat-activated sweat glands per unit skin area than men, they are less prolific in sweating.[13] Women start to sweat at higher skin and core temperatures; they also produce less sweat than men for a comparable heat-exercise load, even after acclimatization comparable to that achieved by men.[31, 122]

Evaporative versus Circulatory Cooling. Despite a lower sweat output, women show heat tolerance similar to men of equal aerobic fitness at the same exercise level.[6, 8, 44] Women probably rely more on circulatory mechanisms for heat dissipation, whereas men make greater use of evaporative cooling. Clearly, less sweat production to maintain thermal balance would provide significant protection from dehydration for women during exercise at high ambient temperatures.

Ratio of Body Surface Area to Body Mass. A favorable dimensional characteristic for heat dissipation generally possessed by women compared to men is a relatively large surface area-to-mass ratio; that is, the smaller female has a larger external surface per unit of body mass exposed to the environment. Consequently, under identical conditions of heat exposure, women tend to cool at a faster rate than men through a smaller body mass across a relatively large surface area. In this regard, children would also possess a "geometric" advantage during heat stress, in that both boys and girls have a larger surface area per unit body mass compared to adults.

Effect of Menstruation. The sweating response at the forearm in relation to esophageal temperature during cycle ergometer exercise at 60% of $\dot{V}o_2$max at 35°C during the follicular and luteal phases of the menstrual cycle is illustrated in Figure 25.8 (*top*).[114] The rightward shift of the curve during the luteal phase indicates that a significantly higher core temperature threshold is required to initiate the sweating response with exercise during this phase of menstruation. This response has also been observed during heavier exercise at 80% of aerobic capacity.[65] Such data and corroborating experiments indicate that a unique feature of the hormonally sensitive menstrual cycle is an alteration in the control of core temperature, which is shifted upward to reflect a resetting of the thermoregulatory "set-point" during the luteal phase.[47, 52, 114] Figure 25.8 (*bottom*) is a schematic diagram of the normal hormonal responses during the follicular and luteal phases of the menstrual cycle, including an upward shift of approximately 0.4°C in oral temperature (an amount equal to the increase in central core temperature shown in the top part of the figure) that persists for about 6 days during the luteal phase. Note that estradiol exhibits a biphasic upward shift (once in the follicular and luteal phases), but that the surge in progesterone coincides with the increase in oral temperature during the luteal phase. *The change in thermoregulatory sensitivity during the luteal phase of the menstrual cycle does not appear to affect a woman's ability to exercise or perform hard physical work during the menstrual cycle.*[33, 124] It is clear,

however, that the changing phases of the monthly cycle must be considered when evaluating the thermoregulatory response of women to exercise and thermal stress.

Level of Body Fat. Excess body fat is a liability when working in a hot environment. Because the specific heat of fat is greater than that of muscle tissue, fat increases the insulatory quality of the body shell and retards conduction of heat to the periphery. The large, overfat person also has a small body surface area-to-body mass ratio for the evaporation of sweat compared to a leaner, smaller person.

In addition to thwarting effective heat exchange, excess body fat directly adds to the metabolic cost of weight-bearing activities. When this effect is compounded by the additional demands of the weight of equipment such as football gear, intense competition, and a hot, humid environment, the overfat person is at a distinct disadvantage in terms of temperature regulation and exercise performance. Fatal heat stroke occurs 3.5 times more frequently in young adults who are obese than in individuals whose body mass is within reasonable limits.[50]

COMPLICATIONS FROM EXCESSIVE HEAT STRESS

If the normal signs of heat stress—thirst, tiredness, grogginess, and visual disturbances—are not heeded, cardiovascular compensation begins to fail and a series of disabling complications, termed **heat illness,** can result. The major forms of heat illness, in order of increasing severity, are heat cramps, heat exhaustion, and heat stroke. There is often no clear-cut demarcation between these maladies because symptoms often overlap.[55] When heat illness does occur, however, immediate action must be taken to reduce the heat stress and rehydrate the person until medical help is available. The salient features of the cardiovascular response patterns during three distinct stages of exercise hyperthermia are listed in Table 25.4. These states—compensation, crises, and failure—apply to the conditions of heat exhaustion and heat stroke. The response patterns are characterized in terms of central circulatory effects, peripheral effects, and effects on the central nervous system.

Heat Cramps. Heat cramps, or involuntary muscle spasms, occur during or after intense physical activity and are usually observed in the specific muscles exercised. This form of heat illness is probably due to an imbalance in the body's fluid level and electrolyte concentrations. During heat exposure, salts can be lost as a result of sweating. Muscle pain and spasm may occur if these electrolytes are not replenished. (Spasms occur most commonly in the muscles of the abdomen and extremities.) With heat cramps, body temperature is not necessarily elevated. Prevention can usually be ensured by providing copious amounts of water and by increasing the daily intake of salt several days before the period of heat stress; the easiest way to do this is to add a "pinch" of salt to foods at mealtime.

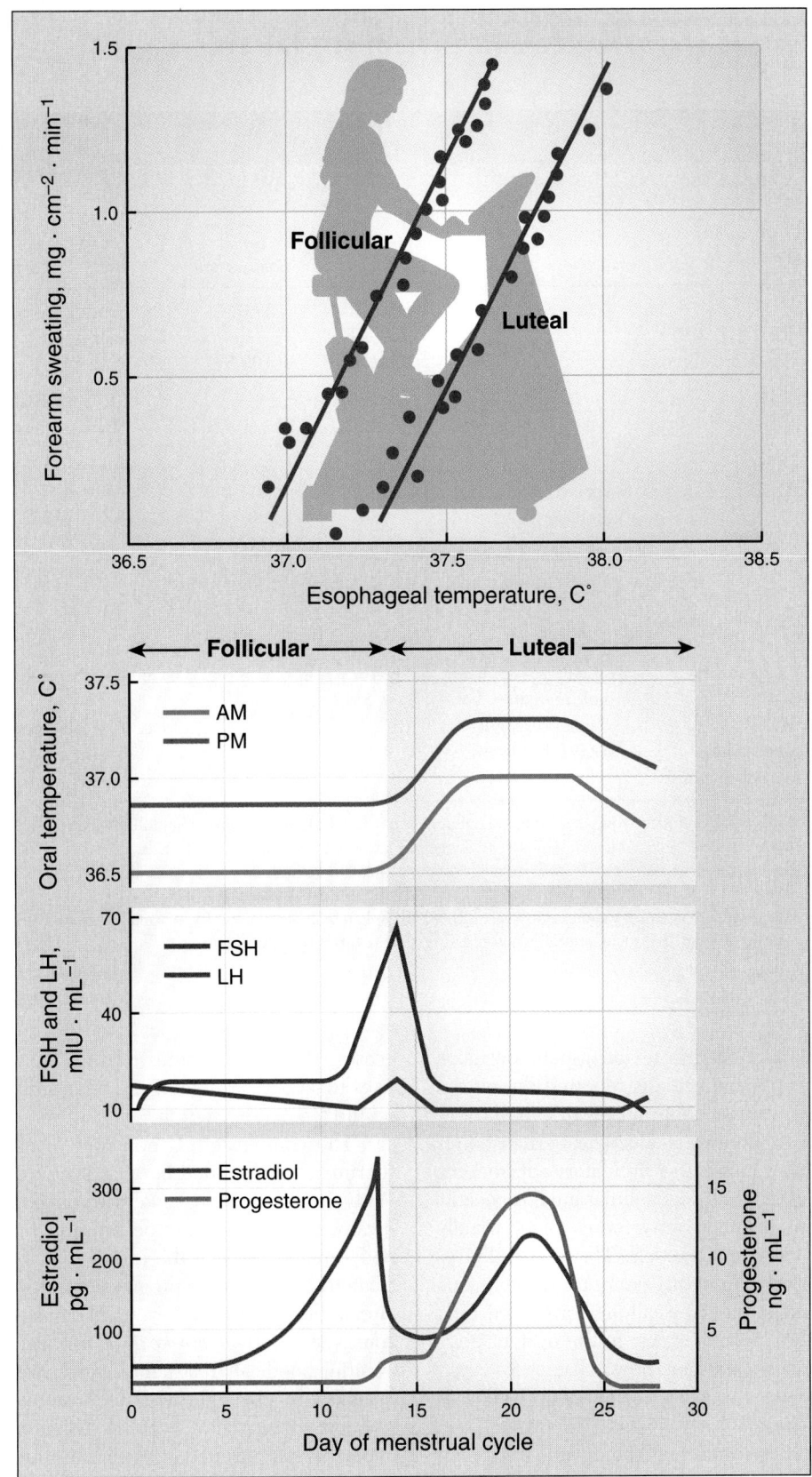

FIGURE 25.8

Top, Sweating response at the forearm in relation to esophageal temperature during cycle ergometer exercise performed at 60% of V̇o₂max at 35°C during the follicular and luteal phases of the menstrual cycle. (Modified from Stephenson, L.A., and Kolka, M.A.: Menstrual cycle phase and time of day alter reference signal controlling arm blood flow and sweating. *Am. J. Physiol.,* 249:R186, 1985.) *Bottom,* Oral temperature and hormonal changes during the follicular and luteal phases of the menstrual cycle. Menses typically occurs during days 1 to 5. (Modified from Stephenson, L.A., and Kolka, M.A.: Effect of gender, circadian period and sleep loss on thermal responses during exercise. In *Human Performance Physiology and Environmental Medicine at Terrestrial Extremes.* Edited by K.B. Pandolf, et al. Carmel, IN, Cooper Publishing Group, 1994.)

TABLE 25.4
CARDIOVASCULAR RESPONSES DURING THREE STAGES OF EXERCISE HYPERTHERMIA

	Central Circulation		Peripheral	Rectal Temperature	Central Nervous System Status
Compensation	↑ CO ↑ SV, ↑ HR ↓ PV Respiratory alkalosis	↓ Low SPBF	↓ Low TPVR ↑ Skin BF ↑ Muscle BF	37.0° C to 39.5	Premonitory signs Dizziness Headache Euphoria Psychoses
Crises	↑↓ CO, ↑ MABP, ↓ SV ↑↑ HR Tachycardia (180 bpm) Metabolic acidosis	↑↓ SPBF ↓ PI Volume Moderate CVP	↓ TPVR ↑↓ Skin BF	39.5° C 41.5° C	Cerebral congestion ↓ Cerebral edema ↓ Intracranial hypertension
Failure	↓↓ CO ↓↓ MABP ↑ HR Tachycardia Metabolic acidosis	↑↑ SPBF (autoregulatory escape); High CVP but low if hypovolemic	↓ TPVR ↓ Low Skin BF	41.5° C	Coma, decreased cerebral perfusion ↓ Cerebral ischemia ↓ Neurologic damage, seizures

Data reported by Hubbard, R.W., and Armstrong, L.E.: The heat illnesses: biochemical, ultrastructural, and fluid-electrolyte considerations. In: *Human Performance Physiology and Environmental Medicine at Terrestrial Extremes.* Pandolf, K., et al. (Eds.). Carmel, IN, Cooper Publishing Group, 1994. Original data of Kielblock, A.J., et al.: Cardiovascular origins of heatstroke pathophysiology: An anesthetized rat model. *Aviat. Space Environ. Med.* 53:171, 1982.

Abbreviations: CO, cardiac output; SV stroke volume; HR, heart rate; SPBF, splanchnic blood flow; PV, plasma volume; TPVR, total peripheral vascular resistance; BF, blood flow; MABP, mean arterial blood pressure; CVP, central venous pressure.

Heat Exhaustion. Heat exhaustion usually develops in unacclimatized people and often is reported during the first heat wave of the summer or during the first hard training session on a hot day. Exercise-induced heat exhaustion is believed to be caused by ineffective circulatory adjustments compounded by a depletion of extracellular fluid, especially plasma volume, owing to excessive sweating. Blood usually pools in the dilated peripheral vessels. This drastically reduces the central blood volume necessary to maintain cardiac output. Heat exhaustion is usually characterized by a weak, rapid pulse, low blood pressure in the upright position, headache, dizziness, and general weakness. Sweating may be reduced somewhat, but body temperature is not elevated to dangerous levels (i.e., above 104°F or 40°C). A person experiencing these symptoms should stop exercising and move to a cooler environment; fluids should be administered, usually via intravenous therapy.

Heat Stroke. *Heat stroke is the most serious and complex heat-stress malady and requires immediate medical attention.* Heat stroke reflects a failure of the heat-regulating mechanisms brought on by an excessively high body temperature. When thermoregulation fails, sweating usually ceases, the skin becomes dry and hot, body temperature rises to 41.5°C or higher, and an inordinate strain is placed on the circulatory system.

The complexity of the problem of emergency hyperthermia is confounded because symptoms are often subtle. With intense exercise, usually in young, highly motivated individuals, sweating may be present, but heat gain by the body greatly exceeds the avenues for heat loss. If left untreated, the disability progresses and death ensues due to circulatory collapse and eventual damage to the central nervous system. *Heat stroke is a medical emergency!* While awaiting medical treatment, aggressive steps must rapidly be taken to lower the elevated core temperature because mortality is related to both the magnitude and duration of hyperthermia. Immediate treatment includes alcohol rubs, application of ice packs, and whole-body immersion in cold or even ice water.

Don't Rely on Oral Temperature. Oral temperature is often a highly inaccurate measure of core temperature after strenuous exercise. In one report, large and consistent differences were noted between oral and rectal temperatures—the average rectal temperature following a 14-mile race in a tropical climate was 103.5°F, whereas oral temperature was a normal 98°F![103] Part of the reason for this discrepancy is that oral temperature is influenced by evaporative cooling of the mouth and airways during pulmonary ventilation. This cooling effect can be considerable with the relatively high ventilatory volumes during and immediately after heavy exercise.

HOW HOT IS "TOO HOT"?

Factors other than air temperature determine the physiologic strain imposed by heat. These factors include individual variations in body size and fatness, state of training and acclimatization, and external factors such as convective air currents, radiant heat gain, intensity of exercise, amount, type, and color of clothing, and, most importantly, the relative humidity. Several football deaths have been reported when the air temperature was below 75°F (23.9°C) but the relative humidity exceeded 95%.

The most effective way to control heat-stress injuries is to prevent them. Acclimatization greatly reduces the chance for heat injury. Another consideration is to evaluate the environment for its potential thermal challenge. This can be done with the use of the **wet bulb-globe temperature (WB-GT).** This index of environmental heat stress was developed by the United States military and is derived from measures of ambient temperature, relative humidity, and radiant heat. It is calculated as follows:

$$\text{WB-GT} = 0.1 \times \text{DBT} + 0.7 \times \text{WBT} + 0.2 \times \text{GT}$$

where DBT is the dry-bulb or air temperature recorded by an ordinary mercury thermometer that records air temperature. WBT is the wet-bulb temperature recorded by a similar thermometer, except that a wet wick surrounds the mercury bulb that is exposed to rapid air movement. When the relative humidity is high, little evaporative cooling occurs from the wetted bulb, so the temperature of this thermometer is similar to that of the dry-bulb. On a dry day, however, significant evaporation occurs from the wetted bulb and the difference is maximized between the two thermometer readings. A small difference between readings indicates a high relative humidity, whereas a large difference indicates little air moisture and a high rate of evaporation. GT is the globe temperature recorded by a thermometer in which the bulb is enclosed in a metal sphere that has been painted black. The black globe absorbs radiant energy from the surroundings to provide a measure of this important source of heat gain.

WB-GT guidelines that can be applied to athletic activities to reduce the chance of heat injury are presented in Figure 25.9 (*top*). These standards apply to lightly clothed humans but do not take into account the specific heat load imposed by uniforms or equipment such as that used in football. For this sport, the lower end of each temperature range serves as a more prudent guide. An indication of the ambient heat load also can be obtained from the wet-bulb thermometer, because this reading reflects both air temperature and relative humidity. The thermometer is fairly inexpensive and can be purchased at most industrial supply companies. Heat stress recommendations based on the wet-bulb temperature are presented in Figure 25.9 (*bottom*). If WBT is not available but the relative humidity is known, the **Heat Stress Index** illustrated in Figure 25.10 can be consulted to determine the relative degree of heat stress.

WB-GT Range °F	WB-GT Range °C	Recommendations
80–84	26.5–28.8	• Use discretion, especially if unconditioned or unacclimatized
85–87	29.5–30.5	• Avoid strenuous activity in the sun
88	31.2	• Avoid exercise training

WBT Range °F	WBT Range °C	Recommendations
60	15.5	• No prevention necessary
61–65	16.2–18.4	• Alert all participants to problems of heat stress and importance of adequate hydration
66–70	18.8–21.1	• Insist that appropriate quantity of fluid be ingested
71–75	21.6–23.8	• Rest periods and water breaks every 20 to 30 minutes; limits placed on intense activity
76–79	24.5–26.1	• Practice curtailed and modified considerably
80	26.5	• Practice cancelled

FIGURE 25.9
Wet Bulb-Globe Temperature (WB-GT) for outdoor activities and Wet-Bulb Temperature (WBT) guide. (Modified from Murphy, R.J., and Ashe, W.F.: Prevention of heat illness in football players. *JAMA,* 194:650, 1965.)

FIGURE 25.10
How hot is too hot? The Heat-Stress Index.

Air temperature, °F

Relative humidity	70°	75°	80°	85°	90°	95°	100°	105°	110°	115°	120°
					Heat Sensation						
0%	64°	69°	73°	78°	83°	87°	91°	95°	99°	103°	107°
10%	65°	70°	75°	80°	85°	90°	95°	100°	105°	111°	116°
20%	66°	72°	77°	82°	87°	93°	99°	105°	112°	120°	130°
30%	67°	73°	78°	84°	90°	96°	104°	113°	123°	135°	148°
40%	68°	74°	79°	86°	93°	101°	110°	123°	137°	151°	
50%	69°	75°	81°	88°	96°	107°	120°	135°	150°		
60%	70°	76°	82°	90°	100°	114°	132°	149°			
70%	70°	77°	85°	93°	106°	124°	144°				
80%	71°	78°	86°	97°	113°	136°					
90%	71°	79°	88°	102°	122°						
100%	72°	80°	91°	108°							

Heat sensation	Risk of heat injury
90°–105°	Possibility of heat cramps
105°–130°	Heat cramps or heat exhaustion likely Heat stroke possible
130°+	Heat stroke a definite risk

■ S U M M A R Y ■

1. Core temperature normally increases during exercise; the magnitude of the rise is determined by the relative stress of a particular exercise. This well-regulated temperature adjustment probably creates a more favorable environment for physiologic and metabolic function.

2. Sweating places demands on the body's fluid reserves and creates a relative state of dehydration. If sweating is excessive and fluids are not continually replaced, plasma volume falls and core temperature may rise to lethal levels.

3. Exercise in hot, humid environments poses a great thermoregulatory challenge because the large sweat loss in high humidity contributes little to evaporative cooling.

4. Fluid loss in excess of 4 to 5% body mass significantly impedes heat dissipation and compromises cardiovascular function and exercise capacity.

5. The primary aim of fluid replacement is to maintain plasma volume so that circulation and sweating progress at optimal levels. The ideal replacement schedule during exercise matches fluid intake to fluid loss. This can be monitored effectively by changes in body mass.

6. About 1000 mL of water can be absorbed each hour from the intestine. Factors that affect this rate of absorption include the volume contained in the stomach and the temperature and the osmolality of the oral rehydration beverage.

7. A small amount of electrolytes added to a rehydration beverage will facilitate fluid replacement more than drinking plain water.

8. Minerals lost through sweating generally can be replaced through the diet. With prolonged exercise in a hot environment, sodium replacement can be augmented by adding a small amount of salt (1 tsp per liter) to the replacement fluid.

9. Repeated heat stress initiates thermoregulatory adjustments that result in improved exercise capacity and less discomfort on subsequent heat exposure. This heat acclimatization triggers a favorable distribution of cardiac output and a greatly increased capacity for sweating. Full acclimatization generally occurs in about 10 days of heat exposure.

10. Although changes in thermoregulatory function have been noted with aging, the ability to tolerate and acclimatize to moderate heat stress probably does not appreciably deteriorate with age.

11. When factors such as level of fitness and acclimatization are accounted for, women are at least as efficient as men in thermoregulation during exercise. However, women tend to produce less sweat than men while maintaining the same core temperature.

12. The major forms of heat illness are heat cramps, heat exhaustion, and heat stroke. Heat stroke is by far the most serious and complex of these maladies.

13. Various practical heat-stress indices (e.g., wet bulb-globe temperature, Heat Stress Index) make use of ambient temperature, radiant heat, and relative humidity to evaluate the environment's potential heat challenge of an environment to an exercising person.

EXERCISE IN THE COLD

Human exposure to extremes of cold produces significant physiological and psychological strain and ranks high among different terrestrial environments for potentially lethal consequences.[118] Water is an excellent medium through which to study physiologic adjustment to cold because heat conduction in water is about 25 times that of air at the same temperature. Consequently, immersion in cool water of only 28 to 30°C can impose a thermal stress that causes considerable thermoregulatory adjustments in a relatively short time. Shivering is frequently observed if people remain inactive in a pool or ocean environment because of a large conductive heat loss. Even with moderate exercise in cold water, the metabolic heat generated is often insufficient to counter the large thermal drain. An example occurs during swimming because heat transfer by convection markedly increases with the rapid movement of water past the skin surface.

During light and moderate exercise in cold water, oxygen uptake is higher and body temperature is lower compared to identical exercise in warmer water.[25, 76] For example, swimming at a submaximal pace in a flume at 18°C (64°F) requires about 500 mL of oxygen more per minute than swimming at the same speed in 26°C (79°F) water.[83] This additional oxygen uptake is directly related to the added energy cost of shivering as the body attempts to combat heat loss in colder water.

BODY FATNESS, EXERCISE, AND COLD STRESS

Differences in body fat content between individuals have a significant effect on physiologic function in a cold environment both at rest and during exercise.[77, 78, 111] Successful ocean swimmers, for example, usually possess a relatively large amount of subcutaneous fat compared to highly trained non-ocean swimmers.[95] This additional fat greatly increases the effective insulation when peripheral blood is redirected from the body's shell to the core in cold water. With this advantage, athletes with greater thermal insulation from fat accretion can swim in cool ocean water with almost no fall in core temperature. In leaner swimmers, however, the heat generated during exercise is insufficient to counter the heat drain to the water and the body core cools.

To a large extent, stress from cold is highly relative. The physiologic strain imposed by the cold depends not only on the environmental temperature but also on one's level of metabolism and the resistance to heat flow provided by body fat, particularly in water colder than 25°C.[78, 97, 117, 119] An overfat person who is comfortable resting immersed to the neck in 26°C water may sweat about the forehead during vigorous exercise. For this person, 18°C may be a more favorable water temperature for heavy exercise. In a lean person, on the other hand, water at 18°C is debilitating at rest and during exercise. Therefore, there is an optimum water temperature for each person and for each activity. For most people, water temperatures between 26°C (78.8°F) and 30°C (86.0°F) provide effective heat dissipation during exercise but are not excessively cold to compromise exercise capacity. For short-term intense exercise, even cooler water may be optimal, especially for fatter people. For an unexplained reason, older adults do not withstand the challenge of cold at rest and during low-intensity exercise as effectively as younger individuals with similar aerobic capacity.[37] Variations in body composition or hormone-related functions may provide part of the explanation.

Children. Cold water can be an exceptionally stressful thermoregulatory environment for children. Children have distinctly larger body surface area-to-body mass ratios than adults; while facilitating heat loss in a warm environment, this becomes a liability during cold stress and body heat is lost more rapidly. In the less "stressful" environment of air, children compensate for their relatively large body surface during cold stress because they show a greater increase in oxygen uptake and a more effective peripheral vasoconstriction of the limbs compared to adults.[112]

ACCLIMATIZATION TO THE COLD

Humans possess much less capacity for adaptation to prolonged cold exposure than to long-term exposure to heat.[126] Indeed, the basic response of Eskimos and Lapps is to avoid the cold or minimize its effect. For example, the clothing of these cold-weather inhabitants provides a near-tropical microclimate, and the temperature inside an igloo is generally maintained at about 21°C (70°F).

Some indication of cold adaptation has been provided from studies of the Ama, the women professional breathhold divers of Korea and southern Japan.[53] These women can tolerate daily prolonged exposure to diving for food in cold water that is about 10°C (50°F) in winter. During the summer, when water temperature is 25°C, the Ama perform three bouts of diving, each about 45 minutes in duration. In the winter, only one bout of diving is performed for 15 minutes each day. In both summer and winter, the women generally remain in the water until oral temperature declines to about 34°C (93.2°F). The temperature responses of the Ama with time spent in the water are shown in Figure 25.11 (*top*). During the summer, the women could stay in the water for 15 minutes longer than in winter. The winter versus summer dives also preserved the differences between mean skin temperature and mean body temperature, which were always lower during the winter dives. Results for shivering response to different immersion temperatures for a group of Ama divers compared to groups of nondiving Korean women and men are shown in Figure 25.11 (*bottom*). The response curve for the Ama was shifted to the right, indicating a blunted thermogenic response (higher shivering threshold) until water temperature reached 28.2°C

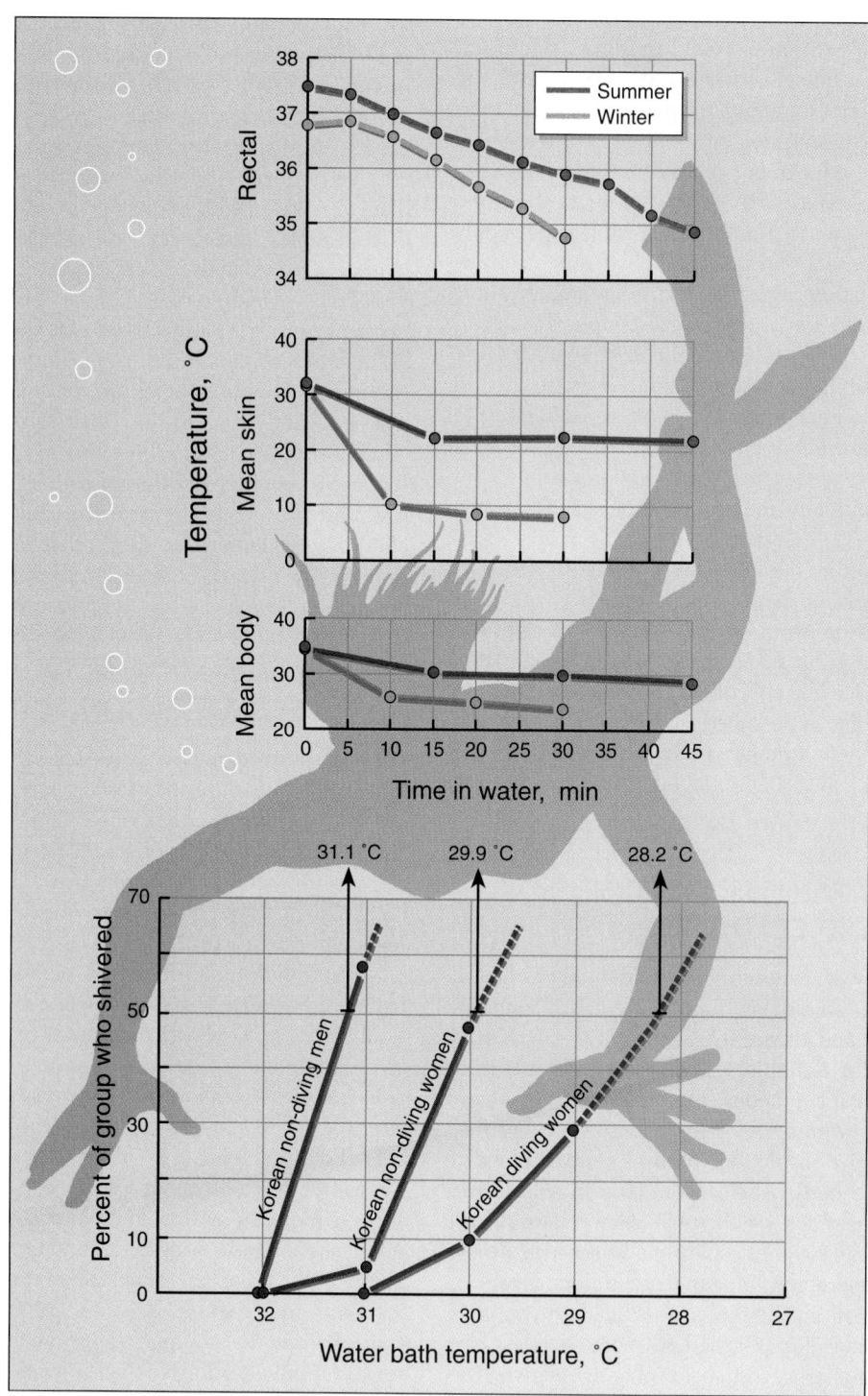

FIGURE 25.11

Top, Differences in rectal temperature, mean skin temperature, and mean body temperature in relation to dive duration during the summer and winter for a group of Ama professional breath-hold divers immediately upon surfacing from a dive. (Modified from Kang, D.H., et al.: Energy metabolism and body temperature of the Ama. *J. Appl. Physiol.,* 18:483, 1965.) *Bottom,* Shivering response in Ama professional breath-hold divers compared to groups of nondiving Korean men and women in response to different immersion temperatures. The temperatures indicated at the top of the figure represent the temperature at which 50% of a group started shivering (Modified from Hong, S.K.: Comparison of diving and nondiving women of Korea. *Fed. Proc.,* 22:831, 1963.)

(82.8°F), the coldest water temperature at which at least 50% of the group started shivering. Clearly, the Ama divers show a higher shivering threshold to cold-water immersion than the other nondiving groups.

In addition to an apparent psychological toughness, the capability of the Ama to tolerate extreme cold has been attributed to an elevated resting metabolism. In winter, this is increased by about 25% compared to nondiving women living in the same community. Interestingly, the body fat content of the Ama is no greater than their nondiving female counterparts. It is possible, therefore, that circulatory adaptations aid these divers by retarding heat transfer from the core to the skin.

A type of general cold adaptation appears to occur following regular and prolonged cold-air exposure. As a result, heat loss is not compensated for by increased heat production; the body "regulates" at a lower core temperature in response to cold.[66] Some peripheral adaptations also reflect a form of acclimation with severe local cold exposure.[67, 68, 88] Repeated cold exposure of the hands or feet causes an increased blood flow through these areas. This is readily apparent in fishermen, who handle nets and fish in extreme cold. Although this local adaptation actually results in a loss of body heat from the periphery, it does represent a form of "self-defense," because a vigorous circulation of warm blood in the exposed areas aids in preventing tissue damage due to hypothermia. Although not specifically a form of cold acclimatization, improved physical fitness, as reflected by a high aerobic capacity and relatively large muscle mass, enhances a person's thermoregulatory defense against cold stress. This manifests in a larger shivering response as well as an earlier (more sensitive) onset of this response with cold exposure.[12]

HOW COLD IS "TOO COLD"?

Cold injuries from overexposure are occurring more frequently because of the increasing popularity of outdoor winter activities such as ice skating, ice fishing, cross-country skiing, snowmobiling, and all-season walking, jogging, and cycling. Owing to the pronounced peripheral vasoconstriction during severe cold exposure, the temperature of the skin and the extremities may fall to dangerous levels. Early warning signs of possible cold injury include a tingling and numbness in the fingers and toes or a burning sensation of the nose and ears. If these signs are not heeded, overexposure can lead to tissue damage in the form of frostbite; in extreme cases, the damage is irreversible and the tissue must be surgically removed.

The Wind Chill Index. One dilemma in evaluating the thermal quality of an environment is that ambient temperature alone is not always a valid indication of "coldness." For instance, the winds of a spring day can be very chilling, even though the temperature is well above freezing. On the other hand, a calm subfreezing day may feel quite comfortable. *The important factor is the wind—on a windy day, air currents magnify heat loss as the warmer insulating air layer surrounding the body is continually replaced by cooler, ambient air.*

The cooling effect of wind is clearly shown by the Wind Chill Index presented in Figure 25.12. This figure illustrates the effects of wind velocity on bare skin for different temperatures and wind velocities. For example, a 30°F reading is equivalent to 0°F when the wind speed is 25 mph, whereas a 10°F reading is equivalent to 29°F at the same wind velocity. In addition, if a person runs, skis, or skates into the wind, the effective cooling from the wind is in-

Wind speed, mph	Ambient temperature, °F*															
	40	35	30	25	20	15	10	5	0	−5	−10	−15	−20	−25	−30	
	Equivalent temperature, °F															
Calm	40	35	30	25	20	15	10	5	0	−5	−10	−15	−20	−25	−30	Calm
5	37	33	27	21	16	12	6	1	−5	−11	−15	−20	−26	−31	−35	5
10	28	21	16	9	4	−2	−9	−15	−21	−27	−33	−38	−46	−52	−58	10
15	22	16	11	1	−5	−11	−18	−25	−36	−40	−45	−51	−58	−65	−70	15
20	18	12	3	−4	−10	−17	−25	−32	−39	−46	−53	−60	−67	−76	−81	20
25	16	7	0	−7	−15	−22	−29	−37	−44	−52	−59	−67	−74	−83	−89	25
30	13	5	−2	−11	−18	−26	−33	−41	−48	−56	−63	−70	−79	−87	−94	30
35	11	3	−4	−13	−20	−27	−35	−43	−49	−60	−67	−72	−82	−90	−98	35
*40	10	1	−6	−15	−21	−29	−37	−45	−53	−62	−69	−76	−85	−94	−101	40**

■ Little danger ■ Danger ■ Great danger

* °C= 0.556 (°F −32)
** Convective heat loss at wind speeds above 40 mph has little additional effect on body cooling

FIGURE 25.12

How cold is too cold? The Wind Chill Index.

creased in direct relation to the exerciser's velocity. Therefore, running at 8 mph into a 12-mph headwind is the equivalent of a 20-mph wind speed. Conversely, running at 8 mph with a 12-mph wind at one's back creates a relative wind speed of only 4 mph. In the lightly shaded zone at the left of Figure 25.12, there is relatively little danger from cold injury for a properly clothed person. In contrast, in the medium-shaded zone that generally begins at about 22°F, there is increasing danger to exposed flesh, particularly the ears, nose, and fingers. In the heavily shaded zone on the right, the equivalent "wind-chill" temperatures pose a serious danger to the freezing of exposed flesh within a matter of minutes.

THE RESPIRATORY TRACT DURING COLD-WEATHER EXERCISE

Cold ambient air generally does not pose a special danger of damage to the respiratory passages. Even in extreme cold, the incoming air generally is warmed to between 26.5 and 32.2°C by the time it reaches the bronchi, although values as low as 20°C have been observed while breathing large volumes of cold, dry air.[79] When the incoming breath of air is warmed, its capacity to hold moisture increases greatly and humidification occurs at the expense of water from the respiratory passages. Therefore, significant amounts of water and heat can be lost from the respiratory tract in cold weather, particularly during exercise, when ventilatory volumes are quite large. This often contributes to frequent respiratory complaints during cold-weather exercise. General dehydration can also accompany exercise, as well as dryness of the mouth, burning sensation in the throat, and irritation of the respiratory passages. These symptoms can be greatly reduced by wearing a scarf or mask-type "balaclava" that covers the nose and mouth and traps the water in the exhaled air. This action subsequently warms and moistens the next breath of incoming air.

■ SUMMARY ■

1. Because water conducts heat about 25 times more than air, immersion in water of only 28 to 30°C can provide considerable thermal stress and bring about thermoregulatory adjustments in a relatively short period of time.
2. Heat flux to a cold environment is somewhat offset by heat production from shivering and physical activity. In the average man, shivering can increase the metabolic rate by between 3 to 6 METs.
3. Subcutaneous fat provides excellent insulation against cold stress. It greatly enhances the effectiveness of vasomotor adjustments, which enable fat individuals to retain a large percentage of metabolic heat. This enhanced insulation is apparent in cold water, in which relatively overfat individuals show proportionally

smaller thermal and cardiovascular stress and greater exercise tolerance than their leaner counterparts.
4. The body is much less capable of adapting physiologically to prolonged cold stress than to prolonged heat exposure. In most instances, appropriate clothing enables humans to tolerate some of the coldest climates on earth.
5. The "coldness" of an air environment is influenced by the ambient temperature and the wind. The cooling effect of the wind can be determined by the Wind Chill Index.
6. Although considerable water can be lost from the respiratory passages when exercising on a cold day, the temperature of the inspired ambient air generally does not pose a danger to the respiratory tract.

■ REFERENCES ■

1. Adams, W.C., et al.: Thermoregulation during marathon running in cool, moderate, and hot environments. *J. Appl. Physiol.*, 38:1030, 1975.
2. American College of Sports Medicine: American College of Sports Medicine position stand on prevention of thermal injuries during distance running. *Sports Med. Bull.*, 19:8, 1984.
3. Anderson, R.K., and Kenney, W.L.: Effect of age on heat-activated sweat gland density and flow during exercise in dry heat. *J. Appl. Physiol.*, 63:1089, 1987.
4. Armstrong, L.E., and Pandolf, K.B.: Physical training, cardiorespiratory physical fitness and exercise-heat tolerance. In *Human Performance Physiology and Environmental Medicine at Terrestrial Extremes*. Edited by K.B. Pandolf, et al. Indianapolis, Benchmark Press, 1988.
5. Asmussen, E., and Bøje, O.: Body temperature in muscular work. *Acta Physiol. Scand.*, 10:1, 1945.
6. Avellini, B.A., et al.: Physiological responses of physically fit men and women to acclimation to humid heat. *J. Appl. Physiol.*, 49:254, 1980.
7. Bar-Or, O.: Temperature regulation during exercise in children and adolescents. In *Perspectives in Exercise Science and Sports Medicine*. Vol. 2. Edited by C.V. Gisolfi and D.R. Lamb. Indiana, Benchmark Press, 1989.
8. Bar-Or, O., et al.: Heat tolerance of exercising obese and lean women. *J. Appl. Physiol.*, 26:403, 1969.
9. Bass, D.E., et al.: Mechanisms of acclimatization to heat in man. *Medicine*, 34:323, 1955.
10. Bassett, D.R. Jr., et al.: Thermoregulatory responses to skin wetting during prolonged treadmill running. *Med. Sci. Sports Exerc.*, 19:28, 1987.
11. van Beaumont, W., and Bullard, R.W.: Sweating: its rapid response to muscular work. *Science*, 141:643, 1963.
12. Bittel, J.H.M., et al.: Physical fitness and thermoregulatory reactions in a cold environment. *J. Appl. Physiol.*, 65:1984, 1988.
13. Buono, M.J., and Sjoholm, N.T.: Effect of physical training on peripheral sweat production. *J. Appl. Physiol.*, 65:811, 1988.
14. Burge, C.M., et al.: Rowing performance, fluid balance, and metabolic function following dehydration and rehydration. *Med. Sci. Sports Exerc.*, 25:1358, 1993.
15. Caldwell, J.E., et al.: Diuretic therapy, physical performance, and neuromuscular function. *Phys. Sportsmed.*, 12:73, 1984.
16. Candas, V., et al.: Hydration during exercise: effects on thermal and cardiovascular adjustments. *Eur. J. Appl. Physiol.*, 55:113, 1986.
17. Carter, J.E., and Gisolfi, C.V.: Fluid replacement during and after exercise in the heat. *Med. Sci. Sports Exerc.*, 21:532, 1989.

18. Claremont, A.D., et al.: Comparison of metabolic, temperature, heart rate and ventilatory responses to exercise at extreme ambient temperature (0° and 35°C). *Med. Sci. Sports*, 7:150, 1975.

19. Claremont, A.D., et al.: Heat tolerance following diuretic induced dehydration. *Med. Sci. Sports*, 8:239, 1976.

20. Convertino, V.A.: Blood volume: its adaptation to endurance training. *Med. Sci. Sports Exerc.*, 23:1338, 1991.

21. Costill, D.L., et al.: Water and electrolyte replacement during repeated days of work in the heat. *Aviat. Space Environ. Med.*, 46:795, 1975.

22. Costill, D.L., et al.: Exercise induced sodium conservation: changes in plasma renin and aldosterone. *Med. Sci. Sports*, 8:209, 1976.

23. Costill, D.L., et al.: Muscle water and electrolytes following varied levels of dehydration in man. *J. Appl. Physiol.*, 40:6, 1976.

24. Coyle, E.F., and Montain, S.J.: Benefits of fluid replacement with carbohydrate during exercise. *Med. Sci. Sports Exerc.*, 24:S324, 1992.

25. Craig, A.B., Jr., and Dvorak, M.: Thermal regulation of man exercising during water immersion. *J. Appl. Physiol.*, 25:28, 1968.

26. Craig, F.N., and Cummings, E.G.: Dehydration and muscular work. *J. Appl. Physiol.*, 21:670, 1966.

27. Davies, C.T.M.: Effect of acclimatization to heat on the regulation of sweating during moderate and severe exercise. *J. Appl. Physiol.*, 50:741, 1981.

28. Davy, K.P., and Seals, D.R.: Total blood volume in healthy young and older men. *J. Appl. Physiol.*, 76:2059, 1994.

29. DeSouza, M.J., et al.: Menstrual status and plasma vasopressin, renin and aldosterone exercise responses. *J. Appl. Physiol.*, 67:736, 1989.

30. Dill, D.B., et al.: Cardiovascular responses and temperature in relation to age. *Aust. J. Sports Med.*, 7:99, 1975.

31. Dill, D.B., et al.: Capacity of young males and females for running in desert heat. *Med. Sci. Sports*, 9:137, 1977.

32. Drinkwater, B.L.: Thermoregulatory response of women to intermittent work in the heat. *J. Appl. Physiol.*, 41:57, 1976.

33. Drinkwater, B.L.: Women and exercise: physiological aspects. In *Exercise and Sport Sciences Reviews.* Lexington, MA, Collomore Press, 1984.

34. Drinkwater, B.L., et al.: Aerobic power as a factor in women's response to work in hot environments. *J. Appl. Physiol.*, 41:815, 1976.

35. Falk, B., et al.: Longitudinal analysis of the sweating response of pre-, mid-, and late-pubertal boys during exercise in the heat. *Am. J. Human Biol.*, 4:527, 1992.

36. Falk, B., et al.,: Thermoregulatory responses of pre-, mid-, and late pubertal boys to exercise in dry heat. *Med. Sci. Sports Exerc.*, 24:688, 1992.

37. Falk, B., et al.: Response to rest and exercise in the cold: effects of age and aerobic fitness. *J. Appl. Physiol.*, 76:72,1994.

38. Falls, H.B., and Humphrey, L.D.: Cold water application effects on responses to heat stress during exercise. *Res. Q.*, 42:21, 1971.

39. Feblruio, M.A., et al.: Muscle metabolism during exercise and heat stress in trained men: effect of acclimatization. *J. Appl. Physiol.*, 76:589, 1994.

40. Fink, W.J., et al.: Leg muscle metabolism during exercise in the heat and cold. *Eur. J. Appl. Physiol.*, 34:183, 1975.

41. Fortney, S.M., et al.: Effect of blood pressure on sweating rate and blood lipids in exercising humans. *J. Appl. Physiol.*, 51:1594, 1981.

42. Fortney, S.M., et al.: Effect of hyperosmolarity on control of blood flow and sweating. *J. Appl. Physiol.*, 57:1668, 1984.

43. Francesconi, R.P.: Endocrinological responses to exercise in stressful environments. In *Exercise and Sport Sciences Reviews.* Vol. 16. Edited by K.B. Pandolf. New York. Macmillan, 1988.

44. Frye, A.J., and Kamon, E.: Responses to dry heat of men and women with similar capacities. *J. Appl. Physiol.*, 50:65, 1981.

45. Gonzalez-Alonso, J.R., et al.: Reductions in cardiac output, mean blood pressure and skin vascular conductance with dehydration are reversed when venous return is increased. *Med. Sci. Sports Exerc.*, 26:S163, 1994.

46. Greenleaf, J.E.: Hyperthermia in exercise. In *International Review of Physiology: Environmental Physiology III.* Vol. 20. Edited by D. Robertshaw. Baltimore, University Park Press, 1979.

47. Haslag, S.W.M., and Hertzman, A. B.: Temperature regulation in young women. *J. Appl. Physiol.*, 20:1283, 1965.

48. Haymes, E.M.: Physiological responses of female athletes to heat stress: a review. *Phys. Sportsmed.*, 12:45, 1984.

49. Hellon, R.F., et al.: The physiological reactions of men of two age groups to a hot environment. *J. Physiol. (Lond.)*, 133:118, 1956.

50. Henshel, A.: Obesity as an occupational hazard. *Can. J. Public Health*, 58:491, 1967.

51. Henshel, A.: The environment and performance. In *Physiology of Work Capacity and Fatigue.* Edited by E. Simonsen. Springfield, IL, Charles C Thomas, 1971.

52. Hessemer, V., and Bruck, K.: Influence of menstrual cycle on thermoregulatory, metabolic, and heart rate responses to exercise at night. *J. Appl. Physiol.*, 59:1902, 1985.

53. Hong, S. K., and Rahn, H.: The diving women of Korea and Japan. *Sci. Am.*, 216:34, 1967.

54. Horstman, D.H., and Christensen, E.: Acclimatization to dry heat: active men vs. active women. *J. Appl. Physiol.*. 52:825, 1982.

55. Hubbard, R.W., et al.: The heat illnesses: biochemical, ultrastructural and fluid-electrolyte considerations. In *Human Performance, Physiology and Environmental Medicine at Terrestrial Extremes.* Edited by K.B. Pandolf, et al. Indianapolis, IN, Benchmark Press, 1988.

56. Iampietro, P.F.: Exercise in hot environments. In *Frontiers of Fitness.* Edited by R.J. Shephard. Springfield, IL, Charles C Thomas, 1971.

57. Inbar, O., et al.: Conditioning vs. work-in-the-heat as methods for acclimatizing 8-10 year old boys to dry heat. *J. Appl. Physiol.: Environ. Exer. Physiol.*, 50:406, 1981.

58. Irving, R.A., et al.: The immediate and delayed effects of marathon running on renal function. *J. Urol.*, 136:1176, 1986.

59. Jacobs, I., et al.: Thermoregulatory thermogenesis in humans during cold stress. *Exerc. Sport Sci. Rev.*, 22:221, 1994.

60. Johnson, J.M., et al.: Regulation of the cutaneous circulation. *Fed. Proc.*, 45:2841, 1986.

61. Kastello, G.M., et al.: Young and old subjects matched for aerobic capacity have similar noradrenergic responses to exercise. *J. Appl. Physiol.*, 74:49, 1993.

62. Kenney, W.L., and Anderson, R.K.: Response of older and younger women in dry and humid heat without fluid replacement. *Med. Sci. Sports Exerc.*, 20:155, 1988.

63. Kenney, W.L., and Johnson, J.M.: Control of skin blood flow during exercise. *Med. Sci. Sports Exerc.*, 24:303, 1992.

64. Kenney, W.L., et al.: Alpha 1-adrenergic blockage does not alter control of skin blood flow during exercise. *Am. J. Physiol.*, 260:H855, 1991.

65. Kolka, M.A., and Stephenson, L.A.: Thermoregulation during active and passive heating during the menstrual cycle (Abstract). *Physiologist*, 28:368, 1985.

66. LeBlanc, J.: Factors affecting cold acclimation and thermogenesis in man. *Med. Sci. Sports Exerc.*, 20:S193, 1988.

67. LeBlanc, J.: Local adaptation to cold of Gaspé fisherman. *J. Appl. Physiol.*, 17:950, 1962.

68. Leftheriotis, G., et al.: Finger and forearm vasodilatory changes after local acclimation. *Eur. J. Appl. Physiol.*, 60:49, 1990.

69. Lind, A.R., and Bass, D.E.: Optimal exposure time for development of acclimatization to heat. *Fed. Proc.*, 22:704, 1963.

70. Luetkemeier, M.J., and Thomas, E.L.: Hypervolemia and cycling time trial performance. *Med. Sci. Sports Exerc.*, 26:503, 1994.

71. Mack, G.W., et al.: Body fluid balance in dehydrated healthy older men: thirst and renal osmoregulation. *J. Appl. Physiol.*, 76:1615, 1994.

72. Mack, G.W., et al.: Influence of exercise intensity and plasma volume on active cutaneous vasodilatation in humans. *Med. Sci. Sports Exerc.*, 26:209, 1994.

73. Mathews, D.K., et al.: Physiological responses during exercise and recovery in a football uniform. *J. Appl. Physiol.*, 26:611, 1969.

74. Maugham, R.F.: Fluid and electrolyte loss and replacement in exercise. In *Foods, Nutrition and Sports Performance.* Edited by C. Williams and J.T. Devlin. London, E. & F. Spoon, 1992.

75. McArdle, W.D., et al.: Metabolic and cardiovascular adjustment to work in air and water at 18, 25, 33°C. *J. Appl. Physiol.*, 40:85, 1976.

76. McArdle, W.D., et al.: Thermal adjustment to cold-water exposure in exercising men and women. *J. Appl. Physiol.*, 56:1572, 1984.

77. McArdle, W.D., et al.: Thermal adjustment to cold-water exposure in resting men and women. *J. Appl. Physiol.*, 56:1565, 1984.

78. McArdle, W.D., et al.: Thermal responses of men and women during cold-water immersion: influences of exercise intensity. *Eur. J. Appl. Physiol.*, 65:265, 1992.

79. McFadden, E.R., Jr.: Respiratory heat and water exchange: physiological and clinical implications. *J. Appl. Physiol.*, 54:331, 1984.

80. Meyer, F., et al.: Sweat electrolyte loss during exercise in the heat: effects of gender and maturation. *Med. Sci. Sports Exerc.*, 24:776, 1992.

81. Montain, S.J., and Coyle, E.F.: Fluid ingestion during exercise increases skin blood flow independent of increases in blood volume. *J. Appl. Physiol.*, 73:903, 1992.

82. Montain, S.J., and Coyle, E.F.: The influence of graded dehydration on hyperthermia and cardiovascular drift during exercise. *J. Appl. Physiol.*, 73:1340, 1992.

83. Nadel, E.R.: Thermal and energetic exchanges during swimming. In *Problems With Temperature Regulation During Exercise.* New York, Academic Press, 1977.

84. Nadel, E.R.: Circulatory regulation during exercise in different ambient temperatures, *J. Appl. Physiol.*, 46:430, 1979.

85. Nadel, E.R., et al.: Thermoregulatory shivering during exercise. *Life Sci.*, 13:983, 1973.

86. Nadel, E.R., et al.: Effect of hydration state on circulatory and thermal regulation. *J. Appl. Physiol.*, 49:751, 1980.

87. Nadel, E.R., et al.: Influence of fluid replacement beverages on body fluid homeostasis during exercise and recovery. In *Perspectives in Exercise Science and Sports Medicine.* Vol. 3. Edited by C.V. Gisolfi and D.R. Lamb. Carmel, Benchmark, Press, 1990.

88. Nelms, J.D., and Soper, J.G.: Cold vasodilatation and cold acclimatization in the hands of British fish filleters. *J. Appl. Physiol.*, 17:444, 1962.

89. Nielsen, B., and Nielsen, M.: On the regulation of sweat secretion in exercise. *Acta Physiol. Scand.*, 64:314, 1965.

90. Noakes, T.D.: Fluid replacement during exercise. *Exerc. Sports Sci. Rev.*, 21:297, 1993.

91. Noakes, T.D., et al.: The danger of an inadequate water intake during prolonged exercise. A novel concept re-visited. *Eur. J. Appl. Physiol.*, 57:210, 1988.

92. Nose, H., et al.: Role of osmolality and plasma volume during rehydration in humans. *J. Appl. Physiol.*, 65:325, 1988.

93. Nose, H., et al.: Recovery of blood volume and osmolality after thermal dehydration in rats. *Am. J. Physiol.*, 251:R492, 1986.

94. Pandolf, K.B., et al.: Thermoregulatory responses of middle-aged and young men during dry-heat acclimatization. *J. Appl. Physiol.*, 65:65, 1988.

95. Pugh, L.C.G.E.: A physiological study of channel swimming. *J. Clin. Invest.*, 37:538, 1960.

96. Pugh, L.C.G.E., et al.: Rectal temperatures, weight losses and sweat rates in marathon running. *J. Appl. Physiol.*, 21:1251, 1966.

97. Rennie, D.W.: Tissue heat transfer in water: lessons from the Korean divers. *Med. Sci. Sports Exerc.*, 20:S177, 1988.

98. Robinson, S.: Training, acclimatization and heat tolerance. *Can. Med. Assoc. J.*, 96:795, 1967.

99. Robinson, S., et al.: Acclimatization of older men to work in the heat. *J. Appl. Physiol.*, 20:583, 1965.

100. Rolls, B.J., et al.: Thirst following water deprivation in humans. *Am. J. Physiol.*, 239(Regulatory Integrative Comp. Physiol. 8):476, 1980.

101. Rooke, G.A., et al.: Maximal skin blood flow is decreased in elderly men. *J. Appl. Physiol.*, 77:11, 1994.

102. Rowell, L.B.: *Human Cardiovascular Control.* Cary, NC, Oxford University Press, 1994.

103. Rozycki, T.J.: Oral and rectal temperatures in runners. *Phys. Sportsmed.*, 12:105, 1984.

104. Saltin, B.: Circulatory response to submaximal and maximal exercise after thermal dehydration. *J. Appl. Physiol.*, 19:1125, 1964.

105. Saltin, B., and Hermansen, L.: Esophageal, rectal and muscle temperature during exercise. *J. Appl. Physiol.*, 21:1757, 1966.

106. Sawka, M.N.: Physiological consequences of hypohydration: exercise performance and thermoregulation. *Med. Sci. Sports Exerc.*, 24:657, 1992.

107. Sawka, M.N., and Wegner, C.B.: Physiological responses to acute-exercise heat stress. In *Human Performance Physiology and Environmental Medicine at Terrestrial Extremes.* Edited by K.B. Pandolf, et al. Indianapolis, IN, Benchmark Press, 1988.

108. Sawka, M.N., et al.: Hypohydration and exercise: effects of heat acclimatization, gender, and environment. *J. Appl. Physiol.*, 55:1147, 1983.

109. Sawka, M.N., et al.: Influence of hydration level and body fluids on exercise performance in the heat. *JAMA*, 252:1165, 1984.

110. Scott, J.R., et al.: Acute weight gain in collegiate wrestlers following a tournament weigh-in. *Med. Sci. Sports Exerc.*, 26:1181, 1994.

111. Shiraki, K., and Claybaugh, J.R.: Effects of diving and hyperbaria on responses to exercise. *Exerc. Sport Sci. Rev.*, 23:459, 1995.

112. Smolander, J., et al.: Thermoregulation during rest and exercise in the cold in pre- and early-pubescent boys and young men. *J. Appl. Physiol.*, 72:1589, 1992.

113. Stephenson, L.A., and Kolka, M.A.: Thermoregulation in women. *Exerc. Sport Sci. Rev.*, 21:231, 1993.

114. Stephenson, L.A., and Kolka, M.A.: Effect of gender, circadian period and sleep loss on thermal responses during exercise. In *Human Performance Physiology and Environmental Medicine at Terrestrial Extremes.* Edited by K.B. Pandolf, et al. Carmel, IN, Cooper Publishing Group, 1994.

115. Tankersley, G.G., et al.: Sweating and skin blood flow during exercise: effects of age and maximal oxygen uptake. *J. Appl. Physiol.*, 71:230, 1991.

116. Taylor, H.L., et al.: Cardiovascular adjustments of man at rest and work during exposure to dry heat. *Am. J. Physiol.*, 139:583, 1955.

117. Toner, M.M., and McArdle, W.D.: Physiological adjustments of a man to cold. In *Human Performance Physiology and Environmental Medicine at Terrestrial Extremes.* Edited by K.B. Pandolf, et al. Indianapolis, IN, Benchmark Press, 1988.

118. Toner, M.M., and McArdle, W.D.: Human thermoregulatory responses to acute cold stress with special reference to water immersion. *Handbook of Physiology. Section 4: Environmental Physiology,* vol. 1 Fregly, M.J., and Blatteis, C.M. (Eds.). New York, Oxford University Press, 1996.

119. Toner, M.M., et al.: Thermal responses during arm and leg and combined arm-leg exercise in water. *J. Appl. Physiol.*, 56:1355, 1984.

120. Wailgum, T.D., and Paolone, A.M.: Heat tolerance of college football lineman and backs. *Phys. Sportsmed.*, 12:81, 1984.

121. Wegner, C.B.: Human heat acclimatization. In *Human Performance Physiology and Environmental Medicine at Terrestrial Extremes.* Edited by K.B. Pandolf, et al. Indianapolis, IN, Benchmark Press, 1988.

122. Wells, C.L.: Sexual differences in heat stress response. *Phys. Sportsmed.*, 5:79, 1977.

123. Wells, C.L.: Responses of physically active and acclimatized men and women to exercise in a desert environment. *Med. Sci. Sports*, 12:9, 1980.

124. Wells, C.L., and Horvath, S.M.: Responses to exercise in a hot environment as related to the menstrual cycle. *J. Appl. Physiol.,* 36:299, 1974.

125. Widerman, P.M., and Hagen, R.D.: Body weight loss in a wrestler preparing for competition: a case study. *Med. Sci. Sports Exerc.,* 14:413, 1982.

126. Young, A.J.: Human adaptation to cold. In *Human Performance Physiology and Environmental Medicine at Terrestrial Extremes.*

Edited by K.B. Pandolf, et al. Indianapolis, IN, Benchmark Press, 1988.

127. Young, A.J.: Energy substrate utilization during exercise in extreme environments. In *Exercise and Sport Sciences Reviews.* Vol. 18. Edited by K.B. Pandolf and J.O. Holloszy. Baltimore, Williams & Wilkins, 1990.

128. Zambraski, E.J., et al.: Iowa wrestling study: weight loss and urinary profiles of collegiate wrestlers. *Med. Sci Sports,* 8:105, 1976.

Craig, A.B., Jr.: Summary of 58 cases of loss of consciousness during underwater swimming and diving. *Med. Sci. Sports* **8:171, 1976.**

Death in the water can occur even among those with considerable experience. Craig describes the specifics of 58 cases of losing consciousness during underwater swimming, his objective being to uncover commonalities among diving incidences and prevent further tragedies. The review by Craig showed that most diving accident victims were males, typically between the ages of 16 and 20 years. All swimmers or divers exhibited good or excellent swimming skills. In most instances, the person competed with himself or others for distance swum underwater or length of underwater breath-hold while at rest. For every person that survived and could recount the experience, hyperventilation occurred prior to the subsequent breath-hold and dive. In 80% of the cases, the accident occurred in a pool with a lifeguard.

Among the 34 survivors, most reported an urge to breathe but lost consciousness without other recognizable warning signs. In several cases, victims passed out without remembering any feelings associated with reaching the "breaking point" for breath-holding. Of the 23 drownings, most divers attempted to determine how long they could remain underwater. In most fatalities, the person used hyperventilation to prolong breath-hold time. Craig speculated that the combination of prolonged breath-hold augmented by prior hyperventilation caused total relaxation of respiratory muscles. If lung volume exceeded the expiratory reserve volume, then exhaling air would occur passively. The effect of the previous severe hypoxia during breath-holding could prevent an inspiratory effort following expiration, and death would occur shortly thereafter.

There is poor documentation on the pathophysiology of those who survive diving accidents. In some instances, victims surface and begin breathing spontaneously. Craig hypothesized that these swimmers or divers are breath-holding during ascent just before (or during) loss of consciousness but spontaneously continue patterned respiratory motor activity. If lucky, the diver arrives at the surface just before final collapse and requires minimal resuscitative effort to re-establish arterial oxygen partial pressure (PaO_2) and regain consciousness. In these cases, medical attention is not necessary.

Static and dynamic measures of pulmonary function using simulated breath-hold provide insight about the mechanism responsible for loss of consciousness during underwater swimming and diving. In a series of experiments, Craig investigated the time course of decreases in alveolar partial pressure of oxygen (PAO_2) at different oxygen uptake levels using a rebreathing technique that simulated breath-holding during an underwater breath-hold dive. This technique permitted calculation of time to death at a critical PAO_2 value. Craig calculated that if the PAO_2 decreased from 109 to 44 mm Hg in 1 minute (resting $\dot{V}O_2 = 0.30$ L $\cdot$ min^{-1}), death would occur in about 8 minutes if breathing did not resume. If the $\dot{V}O_2$ increased to about 1.0 L $\cdot$ min^{-1} (as occurs during recreational swimming underwater), the initial decline in PAO_2 would take about 30 seconds, and death would follow in about 4 minutes. At $\dot{V}O_2$ values above 1.0 L $\cdot$ min^{-1}, the estimated time before death would be shorter.

"Hyperventilation done in preparation for the breath hold decreases the body stores and partial pressure of carbon dioxide (PCO_2). During the breath hold and exercise of swimming or diving, the signal which warns a person to come to the surface and which is related to the increase in PCO_2 is delayed. In the meantime the partial pressure of oxygen (PO_2) in the arterial blood reaches a low value below which the brain no longer functions."

All divers and those responsible for swimming-pool safety must learn the dangers of hyperventilation and prolonged breath-hold before diving or swimming underwater.

Sport Diving

In the United States, there are an estimated 4 to 5 million scuba divers, and an additional 200,000 divers are trained each year. With this interest in diving, pool directors and physical educators are being called upon to initiate, teach, and supervise instructional programs in diving. The following sections outline general principles of diving, as well as potential dangers as a person descends and ascends in the water. Unquestionably, safe diving requires thorough knowledge of diving physics and physiology. Within this framework, emphasis is on the relationship between diving depth, pressure, and gas volume, as well as the potentially toxic effects of various gases respired in diving.[1, 3, 7, 16, 20]

PRESSURE-VOLUME RELATIONSHIPS AND DIVING DEPTH

DIVING DEPTH AND PRESSURE

Because water is essentially noncompressible, water pressure against a diver's body increases directly with the depth of the dive. This pressure is the result of two forces: (*a*) the weight of the column of water directly above the diver and (*b*) the weight of the atmosphere at the water's surface. As shown in Table 26.1, a column of fresh water exerts a force of one sea level atmosphere (atm), or 760 mm Hg (14.7 lb

per square inch), for each 33 ft (10 m) one descends below the water's surface. (Because salt water is more dense than fresh water, a depth of about 32 ft corresponds to the pressure equivalent of 1 atm in ocean diving.) Consequently, a person diving to a depth of 33 ft is exposed to a pressure of 2 atm—1 atm due to the weight of the ambient air at the surface and the other due to the weight of the column of water itself. Diving from sea level to a depth of 66 ft (20 m) exposes the diver to an absolute external pressure of 3 atm; at 99 ft (30 m), the pressure is 4 atm, and so on. Clearly, considerable pressure is exerted when diving relatively short distances below the surface.

Because the tissues of the body are largely water, they too are incompressible and not particularly susceptible to the increased external pressure in diving. The body, however, also contains air-filled cavities—notably the lungs, respiratory passages, and sinus and middle-ear spaces. Volume and pressure in these spaces are greatly modified by any increase or decrease in diving depth.[3, 20] *Pain, injury, and even death can occur unless adjustments are made to equalize the rapid and significant changes in pressure that occur during diving.*

DIVING DEPTH AND GAS VOLUME

According to **Boyle's law,** the volume of any gas varies inversely with the pressure on it. When the pressure is dou-

TABLE 26.1
RELATIONSHIP OF DEPTH IN WATER TO PRESSURE AND VOLUME

Depth		Pressure		Hypothetical Lung Volume (mL)	Inspired Air (mm Hg)	
ft	*m*	*atm*	*mm Hg*		P_{O_2}	P_{N_2}
	Sea level	1	760	6,000	159	600
33	10	2	1,520	3,000	318	1,201
66	20	3	2,280	2,000	477	1,802
99	30	4	3,040	1,500	636	2,402
133	40	5	3,800	1,200	795	3,003
166	50	6	4,560	1,000	954	3,604
200	60	7	5,320	857	1,113	4,204
300	90	10	7,600	600	1,590	6,006
400	120	13	9,880	461	2,068	7,808
500	150	16	12,160	375	2,545	9,610
600	180	19	14,440	316	3,022	11,412

bled, the volume is halved; conversely, reducing the pressure by one-half causes the volume of any gas to expand to twice its previous size.

As shown in Table 26.1 and illustrated in Figure 26.1, if a diver fills his or her lungs with 6 L of air at sea level and then descends to a depth of 10 m, the lung volume is compressed to 3 L; diving an additional 10 m to a depth of 20 m (where the external pressure is now 3 atm), the original 6-L lung volume is reduced one-third to 2 L. At a depth of 91 m (300 ft), the lung volume is compressed to approximately 0.6 L simply due to the compressive force of water acting against the air-filled chest cavity. For most of us, any further increase in diving depth would cause the air volume in the respiratory tract to become small enough to produce serious damage to the chest wall and lung tissue. When the diver returns to the surface, the air volume reexpands to its original 6-L volume. Of great significance to the scuba diver who breathes pressurized air is that 6 L of air in the lungs at a depth of 10 m will expand to 12 L at the water's surface; this 6-L volume at 50 m will occupy 36 L at sea-level pressure. If this "extra" air volume is not permitted to escape through the nose or mouth during ascent, the lung tissue will rupture under the force of expanding gases.

SNORKELING AND BREATH-HOLD DIVING

Swimming at the surface of the water with fins, mask, and snorkel is a common form of recreation and sport. This "skin diving" is popular for spear-fishing and exploring shallow areas of clear water. The snorkel is a J-shaped tube that allows the swimmer to breathe continually with the face immersed in water. The swimmer periodically takes a full breath of air and dives beneath the water for a closer look. After about 30 seconds, the carbon dioxide level in the blood increases, the diver senses the need to breathe and surfaces quickly. This activity basically is an extension of swimming and is limited entirely by the swimmer's breath-hold ability.

LIMITS TO SNORKEL SIZE

Novice skin divers often speculate that if only the snorkel were longer, it would be possible to swim deeper in the water and still breathe ambient air through the top of the snorkel. Some novices even believe that they could sit at the pool bottom and breathe through a garden hose extending up to the pool deck! Although the idea of a longer snorkel is

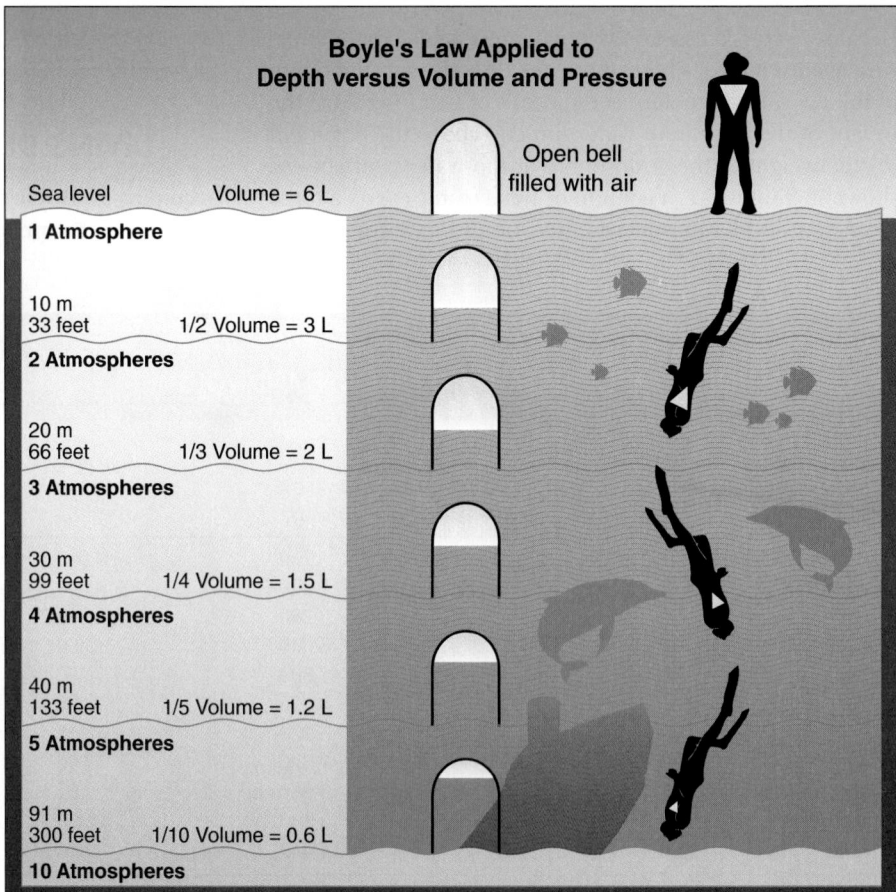

FIGURE 26.1
Any gas volume varies inversely with the pressure to which it is exposed. A 6-L volume, whether in an open bell or in the flexible thoracic cavity, is compressed to 3 L in 33 ft (10 m) of water. This occurs because the external water pressure has been doubled. At 99 ft or 4 atm, the gas is reduced to 25% of its original volume or 1.5 L.

intriguing, two factors must be considered: (*a*) the increased water pressure on the chest cavity as one descends beneath the water and (*b*) the increase in pulmonary dead space brought about by enlarging the snorkel.

Inspiratory Capacity with Diving Depth. When breathing through a snorkel, the diver must inspire air at atmospheric pressure. At a depth of about 3 ft (1 m), the compressive force of water against the chest cavity becomes so large that the inspiratory muscles are usually unable to overcome external pressure and expand thoracic dimensions. Consequently, inspiration is impossible unless air is supplied at a pressure sufficient to counter the compressive force of water at the particular depth. This is the basic principle of scuba, which is discussed fully later in this chapter.

Snorkel Size with Pulmonary Dead Space. As stated in the discussion of pulmonary ventilation in Chapter 12, not all inspired air enters the alveoli. Approximately 150 mL of each breath fills the nose, mouth, and other nondiffusible portions of the respiratory tract. The use of a snorkel adds to the volume of this anatomic dead space. Consequently, the ideal snorkel should be about 15 inches (38 cm) long with an inside diameter of five-eighths to three-quarters of an inch.[18] Any further increase in snorkel size significantly increases the dead space, thus encroaching on one's capacity for alveolar ventilation.

BREATH-HOLD DIVING

If a person takes a full inspiration of ambient air, approximately 1 L of oxygen is brought into the lungs. If the breath is then held, approximately 650 mL of this oxygen can be used to sustain metabolism before the partial pressures of arterial oxygen and carbon dioxide (the most important chemical factor controlling breath-holding) signal the need for renewed breathing.[4] With some training, most people can breath-hold for up to 1 minute. During this time, arterial P_{O_2} drops to approximately 60 mm Hg, whereas P_{CO_2} rises to 50 mm Hg, thus signaling an urgency to breathe. During exercise, breath-hold time is greatly reduced because oxygen uptake and carbon dioxide production increase directly with the severity of the activity. *Breath-hold diving, when preceded by hyperventilation, will significantly extend the breath-hold period; at the same time, the risks to the diver are greatly increased.*

Hyperventilation and Breath-Hold Diving: Blackout. The problem of sudden loss of consciousness or **blackout** is unique to skin diving and usually occurs in divers who attempt to extend the duration of a dive beyond reasonable limits. The cause is probably either a critical reduction in arterial P_{O_2}, an increase in arterial P_{CO_2}, or the combined effects of both (see Focus on Research, p. 526).

The breakpoint for breath-hold usually corresponds to an increase in arterial P_{CO_2} to approximately 50 mm Hg. *For some people, it is possible to "ignore" this stimulus and continue the breath-hold until arterial carbon dioxide reaches levels that cause severe disorientation and even blackout.*[5] With hyperventilation before breath-hold, arterial P_{CO_2} may decrease from its normal value of 40 mm Hg to 15 mm Hg. This lowering of the body's carbon dioxide content significantly extends the duration of breath-hold until the arterial P_{CO_2} increases to a level to stimulate ventilation. For example, the longest breath-hold recorded while breathing air without prior hyperventilation is 270 seconds. Breath-holds of 15 to 20 minutes have been reported with hyperventilation followed by several breaths of pure oxygen.[13]

The attempt to extend breath-hold time in diving is not without serious risks.[5, 6, 13] Consider the following scenario. A skin diver hyperventilates at the surface before a dive. This reduces arterial P_{CO_2} and the potential for the length of the breath-hold is extended. The diver now takes a full inhalation and descends beneath the water. Alveolar oxygen continually moves into the blood and is delivered to the working muscles. Owing to the previous hyperventilation, the arterial carbon dioxide level remains low and the diver is essentially "free" from the urge to breathe. Concurrently, as the diver goes deeper, the external water pressure compresses the thorax. This increased pressure maintains a relatively high P_{O_2} within the alveoli. Therefore, even though the absolute quantity of alveolar oxygen is lowered (as oxygen moves into the blood during the dive), an adequate P_{O_2} is maintained to load hemoglobin as the dive progresses. Now, as the diver senses the need to breathe and begins the ascent, significant reversals occur in pressure. As water pressure on the thorax decreases, and lung volume expands and the partial pressure of alveolar oxygen becomes reduced. As the diver nears the surface, the alveolar P_{O_2} may be so low that dissolved oxygen actually leaves the venous blood and flows into the alveoli. In this situation, the diver may suddenly lose consciousness before reaching the surface.

Additional Considerations. Two other physiologic effects must be considered in assessing the risks of hyperventilation preceding a breath-hold dive.

- A normal quantity of arterial carbon dioxide is necessary to maintain the acid-base balance of the blood. This is mediated by the release of H^+ as carbonic acid is formed from the union of carbon dioxide and water. By reducing the blood's carbon dioxide content through hyperventilation, the H^+ concentration is lowered, causing the pH of the blood to shift in the direction of increased alkalinity.
- Maintaining a normal level of arterial P_{CO_2} provides a continuous stimulus for the dilation of the small arteries in the brain. The significant reduction of arterial carbon dioxide during hyperventilation can reduce cerebral blood flow and cause dizziness or even loss of consciousness. This would obviously create a dangerous situation in the water.

Depth Limits with Breath-Hold Diving: Thoracic Squeeze. The body's air cavities are subjected to tremendous compressive forces as the skin diver progresses deeper beneath the water. Generally, if the lung volume is compressed below 1.0 to 1.5 L (to the residual lung volume), internal and external pressures are unable to equalize and **lung squeeze** occurs. This effect of excessive hydrostatic pressure can cause extensive damage to respiratory tissue.

There is considerable variability among individuals in the safe depth for breath-hold diving without danger of lung squeeze.[a] This critical depth is generally determined by the ratio of the diver's total lung volume to residual lung volume; this ratio usually averages about 4:1 at the surface. *There is no danger from lung squeeze if the lung volume remains greater than the residual volume.* This is because sufficient air remains in the lungs and rigid respiratory passages to equalize pressure and prevent damage due to compression. For most people, this critical depth is usually about 30 m. If the lung volume during a dive is reduced below residual volume—that is, if the ratio of total lung volume to residual lung volume is less than 1.00—the pulmonary air pressure becomes less than the external water pressure. This unequalized pressure creates a relative vacuum within the lungs, which can cause serious damage to alveolar tissue. In severe cases of lung squeeze, blood is literally sucked from the pulmonary capillaries through the alveoli into the lungs. In this situation, the diver actually drowns in his own blood. Further increases in depth cause compression fracture of the ribs as the chest cavity begins to cave in from the excessive external pressure.

Other Problems. If gas pressure in the internal cavities does not equalize with the external hydrostatic pressures during a dive, problems other than lung squeeze will limit the depth of the dive. For example, if air at ambient pressure remains trapped in the middle ear (owing to inflamed tissue or a mucus plug) and cannot equilibrate with air in the lungs, the hydrostatic pressure will cause the eardrum to move inward and eventually rupture.[7] This can occur at relatively shallow depths.

The sinuses are also a source of difficulty for skin divers. Air that is compressed in the lungs by the external force of water will attempt to move into the paranasal sinuses. However, inflamed and irritated sinuses (due to infection) have extremely narrow openings and often are unable to equilibrate with small pressure changes within the respiratory tract. This creates a relative vacuum in the sinus cavities and distorts the shape of these tissues, causing intense sinus pain. In severe cases, fluid and blood move into the sinuses to fill the vacuum.

SCUBA DIVING

In the discussion of snorkeling, it was noted that at depths below 1 m, the inspiratory muscles are unable to overcome the compressive force of the column of water against the chest cavity. To counteract this external force, air under pressure must be supplied from an external source to promote inspiratory action. The **self-contained underwater breathing apparatus** or **scuba** is the most common apparatus used for this purpose. The scuba system, strapped to the diver's chest or back, consists of a tank of compressed air and a regulator with a hose and mouthpiece or full face mask. Two basic scuba designs are used: (*a*) the popular **open-circuit system** and (*b*) the **closed-circuit system,** which is useful for military operations and special applications that require mixed gases.

OPEN-CIRCUIT SCUBA

The typical open-circuit scuba system is illustrated in Figure 26.2. This is the only form of scuba that should be used in sport diving. For most diving purposes, the tanks are constructed of aluminum and contain 1000 to 2000 L of air compressed to a pressure of about 3000 pounds per square inch (p.s.i.). One tank supplies enough air for 0.5 to 1 hour at moderate depths. The compressed air flows through a regulator valve that reduces the tank pressure to the "ambient" pressure at a particular depth. A slight negative pressure is created as the diver begins inspiration. This causes

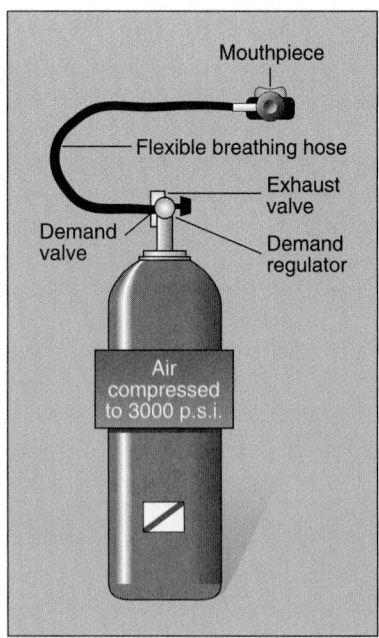

FIGURE 26.2
Open-circuit scuba system.

---

[a]The world record for apnea or breath-hold diving depth following a single breath of air is an amazing 417 feet, which is about 20 yards above the cruising depth of nuclear submarines. This remarkable physiological feat was achieved by Francisco Ferreras (height, 6 ft 3 in.; weight, 220 lb). While wearing fins and a hooded wet suit, he was lowered aboard a slide down a cable anchored to the ocean floor. At the desired depth, a balloon-like bag was inflated that facilitated ascent to the surface. The total round trip took about 2.5 minutes!

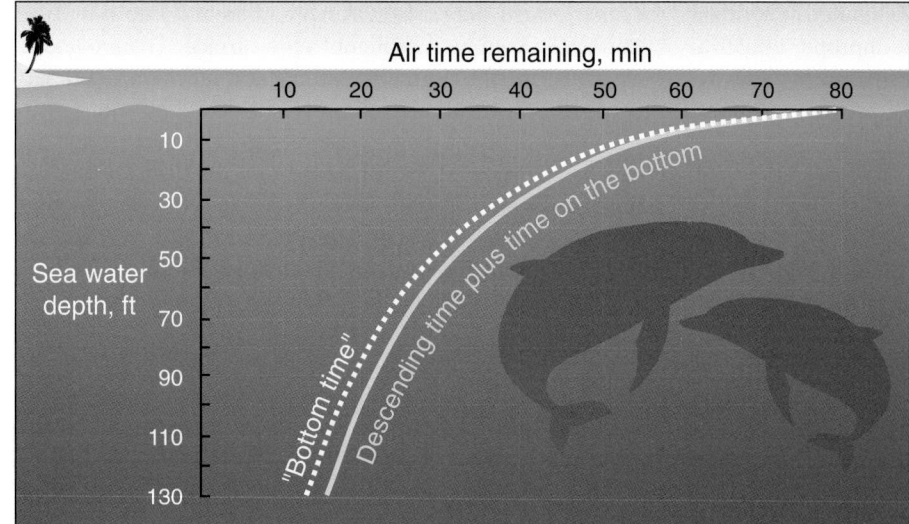

FIGURE 26.3
Theoretical air time for a single tank containing 80 cubic ft of air. The solid line includes the time spent while descending (at a rate of 60 ft · min⁻¹) plus the time on the bottom; the dashed line represents only "bottom time."

the demand valve to open and release air to the diver at a pressure about equal to the external pressure of the water. Upon exhalation, the inspiratory valves close and the exhaled air is discharged into the water.

Open-circuit scuba is not without its drawbacks. Because expired air generally contains about 16 to 17% oxygen, the open-circuit system is wasteful because about 75% of the total oxygen in the tank is ultimately exhaled into the water. In addition, a significant mass of air must be supplied to the diver at increased depths to provide the appropriate tidal volume for adequate pulmonary ventilation. As an extreme example, the equivalent of 50 L of air at sea level must be pumped to a diver at 300 ft (90 m) to provide a 5-L volume. This effect of pressure on air volume greatly limits the time one can remain at a great depth before the air is depleted in the scuba tank.

The theoretical air time limits for a diver doing similar work at various depths are shown in Figure 26.3. These times are based on a completely filled standard compressed air tank and a 60-ft-per-minute rate of ascent and descent. For example, a single aluminum tank with 80 cubic ft of air compressed to 3000 p.s.i. normally supplies an 80-minute dive near the surface. At a depth of 10 m, however, this tank supplies enough air for about 40 minutes, whereas at 3 atm or 20 m, the diving time is reduced by one-third to about 27 minutes. Of course, these time limits will vary due to the diver's body size, type and intensity of activity, level of fitness, and experience, all of which have an impact on the ventilatory volumes during exercise.

CLOSED-CIRCUIT SCUBA

The closed-circuit underwater breathing apparatus operates in the same manner as the closed-circuit spirometer described in Chapter 8. A small cylinder of pure oxygen feeds into a bellows or bag from which the diver breathes. This breathing bag acts as a pressure regulator. Appropriate valves in the breathing mask direct the exhaled gas through a canister containing soda lime, which absorbs carbon dioxide; the carbon dioxide–free gas is then passed back to the diver. The cylinder of oxygen replenishes the oxygen used in metabolism. Consequently, oxygen is continually rebreathed, and the only gas eliminated from the tank is the oxygen used to supply the metabolic requirements of the dive. With only a small cylinder of oxygen, the diver can remain submerged for several hours. Because no expired air is released into the water, the system also provides for an almost completely silent and "bubble-free" operation in contrast to open-circuit diving systems.

Two main problems exist with closed-circuit scuba. First, serious injury can occur if the carbon dioxide output exceeds its rate of absorption, or if the absorption fails altogether. With a faulty rebreathing system, the diver may not receive warning symptoms and can drown as a result of being anesthetized by a buildup in arterial carbon dioxide. Second, high concentrations of inspired oxygen, especially when breathed under pressure, have a variety of adverse effects on physiologic functions. At more than 2 atm pressure, inspired oxygen becomes a deadly poison. This phenomenon is discussed more fully in the section on oxygen poisoning later in this chapter.

SPECIAL PROBLEMS BREATHING GASES AT HIGH PRESSURES

Underwater breathing systems must supply air, oxygen, or other gas mixtures at sufficient pressure to overcome the force of water against the diver's chest. At 20 m or 3 atm of pressure, for example, the respired gas must be delivered at approximately 2280 mm Hg (3 × 760 mm Hg), whereas at 60 m, the gas is delivered at a pressure of 5320 mm Hg. In the following sections, the specific dynamics of breathing gases at high pressures are considered and their effects on physiologic function, as well as on the physical responses of gas to abrupt changes in pressure, are examined. The main hazards of scuba diving that result from improper equalization of pressure within the body's air spaces (and diving mask) in response to changes in external pressure are summarized in Figure 26.4.

AIR EMBOLISM

An air volume breathed underwater expands in direct proportion to the reduction in external pressure as the diver ascends toward the surface. Air breathed at a depth of 10 m doubles in volume if brought to the surface. This expanding air vents freely if normal breathing continues during the ascent. If a diver takes a full breath at this depth but fails to exhale while ascending to the surface, the progressive and rapid expansion of gas on ascent eventually ruptures the lungs before the surface is reached. The potential for **lung burst** is quite real. Many inexperienced divers react to a perceived underwater danger by filling their lungs and then holding their breath while rapidly swimming to the surface.

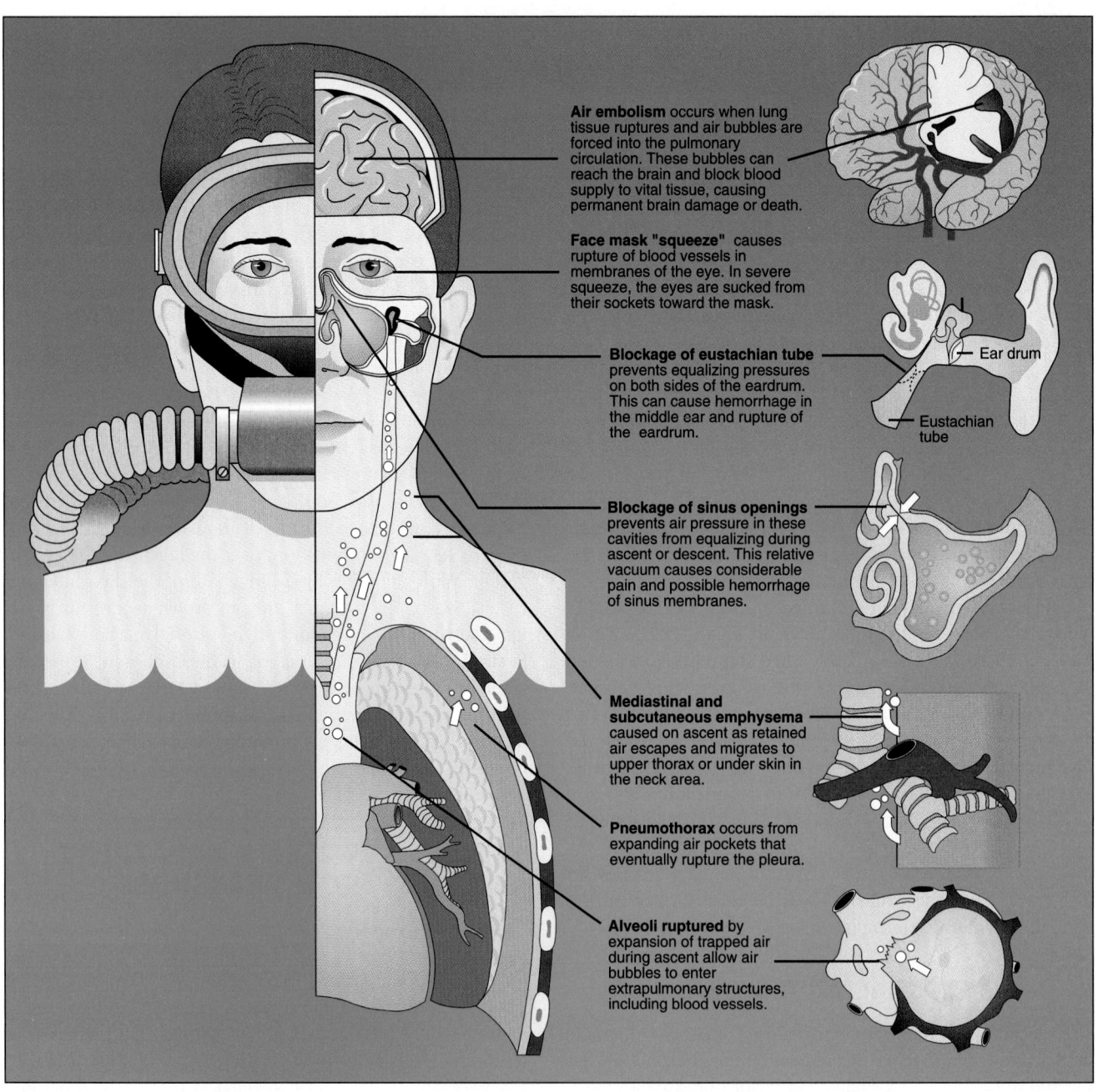

Air embolism occurs when lung tissue ruptures and air bubbles are forced into the pulmonary circulation. These bubbles can reach the brain and block blood supply to vital tissue, causing permanent brain damage or death.

Face mask "squeeze" causes rupture of blood vessels in membranes of the eye. In severe squeeze, the eyes are sucked from their sockets toward the mask.

Blockage of eustachian tube prevents equalizing pressures on both sides of the eardrum. This can cause hemorrhage in the middle ear and rupture of the eardrum.

Ear drum

Eustachian tube

Blockage of sinus openings prevents air pressure in these cavities from equalizing during ascent or descent. This relative vacuum causes considerable pain and possible hemorrhage of sinus membranes.

Mediastinal and subcutaneous emphysema caused on ascent as retained air escapes and migrates to upper thorax or under skin in the neck area.

Pneumothorax occurs from expanding air pockets that eventually rupture the pleura.

Alveoli ruptured by expansion of trapped air during ascent allow air bubbles to enter extrapulmonary structures, including blood vessels.

FIGURE 26.4
Hazards of scuba diving due to the inability to equalize internal and external pressure.

This particular diving hazard is not necessarily related to deep dives. Accidents caused by breath-hold ascent with scuba frequently occur in shallow dives; changes in pressure have the greatest effect on the expanding lung volume near the water's surface. *A full inhalation of compressed air in 6 ft of water can cause serious overdistension of lung tissue during ascent if the diver does not exhale on the way up.* Fatal **air embolism** can occur in swimming pools as shallow as 8 ft for an inexperienced diver using scuba.[10]

During ascent, if expansion of air in the respiratory tract causes lung tissue to rupture, air bubbles may be forced into the pulmonary venous system. These bubbles or **emboli** are then carried to the heart and passed into the systemic circulation. Because the diver is usually in the head-up, vertical position on ascent, the bubbles move upward in the body. Eventually, they become lodged in the small arterioles or capillaries and can restrict the blood supply to vital tissue. General symptoms of air embolism include confusion, weakness, dizziness, and blurred vision. Severe blockage of pulmonary, coronary, and cerebral circulation causes collapse, unconsciousness, and frequently death. The only effective treatment for air embolism is rapid decompression to reduce the size of the bubbles and to force them into solution to open the plugged vessels. Even with rapid, expert treatment, death occurs in approximately 16% of air embolism victims.

PNEUMOTHORAX: LUNG COLLAPSE

Often, when lung tissue ruptures and air is forced through the alveoli, it migrates laterally to burst through the pleural sac covering the lungs. This causes an air pocket to form in the chest cavity, outside the lungs between the chest wall and lung tissue. Continued expansion of this trapped air during ascent causes the ruptured lung to collapse and the heart and other organs to be pushed out of their normal positions. Treatment for this condition of **pneumothorax** often requires surgical intervention using a syringe to "extract" the air bubble.

To eliminate the danger of air embolism and pneumothorax, all divers must be instructed to ascend slowly and breathe normally when using scuba gear. It is imperative that the diver's lungs be free of any disease that could lead to the trapping of air (e.g., chronic obstructive pulmonary disease) and could make it difficult for alveolar pressure to equalize to external pressure during ascent.

MASK SQUEEZE

Before a dive, air in the face mask or goggles is at the same pressure as ambient air at the surface. However, a considerable pressure differential develops between the inside and outside of the mask as the diver progresses beneath the water. This creates a relative vacuum within the mask. For example, wearing swimming goggles to protect the eyes from chemical irritants and to improve vision beneath the water

can cause the eyes to bulge or "squeeze" from their sockets, leading to capillary rupture and hemorrhage of the eyes and surrounding soft tissue. This will occur at depths as shallow as 8 ft—a depth that represents the deep end of many pools.[8] The squeeze effect occurs because most goggles are made of rigid materials. Consequently, the only means to equalize air pressure between the goggle space and external pressure during breath-hold diving is through the movement of the eye and surrounding soft tissue into the air space between the eye and the goggles. As many newer pools with separate diving wells reach depths of 14 ft (4.3 m), the use of goggles could pose a unique problem to swimmers who frequently dive to the bottom to explore or retrieve a lost object.

Breath-hold diving with a face mask that covers both the eyes and nose represents a somewhat different situation than that with only swim goggles. Because the eyes and nose are covered by the mask, the air pressure within the mask can equalize to the external water pressure because the nasal passages are connected to the other air compartments, most notably to the relatively large volume of air in the lungs. In breath-hold diving, the air in the lungs becomes compressed and is passed through the nose to equalize the mask pressure. With scuba, the inspired air is automatically adjusted to the outside water pressure. Therefore, periodically exhaling through the nose into the mask balances the pressures on both sides of the face mask.

AEROTITIS: MIDDLE-EAR SQUEEZE

Another significant problem often encountered by the diver is equalizing the air space within the **eustachian tubes,** the passages that connect the middle ear with the back of the throat.[1] These mucus-lined channels are relatively narrow and generally resist the flow of air. In healthy individuals, the tubes are clear so that changes in external pressure against the eardrum can be equalized by the same pressure changes transmitted from the air within the lungs through the eustachian tubes. In both skin and scuba diving (as well as in air travel in nonpressurized aircraft), middle-ear pressure can usually be equalized to external pressure by blowing gently against closed nostrils. Swallowing, yawning, or moving the jaws from side to side is also helpful in "popping" the ears.

If upper respiratory tract infection is present, the eustachian tube membranes swell and produce mucus, which may plug these air passages. The greatest difficulty is usually experienced in equalizing middle-ear pressure during descent, because a change in pressure against the outer surface of the eardrum is not readily met by an equal force from the interior. In diving, the magnitude of pressure changes are considerable compared to those experienced in air travel. The diver can suffer severe pain with only a few feet of descent under water because the eardrum becomes stretched and moves inward toward the plugged canal. With further pressure disequilibrium, the relative vacuum in the middle ear causes tissue to hemorrhage. When the eustachian tubes are totally blocked, the eardrums rupture and water rushes into the middle ear, which is at a considerably lower pressure.

Never Dive with Earplugs. *Earplugs should never be worn while diving.* The external water pressure pushes the earplug deep into the external ear canal. If a pocket of ambient air is trapped between the plug and eardrum, the eardrum may rupture outward during descent. People who have the following conditions should not dive: respiratory disease, perforated eardrums, or temporary blockage of the eustachian tubes due to infection. In the latter case, diving can be resumed again when the infection subsides and the ear canals clear.

Aerosinusitis. Inflamed and congested sinuses prevent the air pressure in these cavities from equalizing during diving. If sinus air pressure does not equalize during descent, the air in these spaces remains at atmospheric pressure while external pressure increases. This relative vacuum creates "sinus squeeze," causing bleeding in the sinus membranes as blood moves in to equalize the pressure differential.

NITROGEN NARCOSIS: RAPTURE OF THE DEEP

During diving, the total pressure of the respired gas increases in direct proportion to the depth of the dive. Likewise, the partial pressure of each gas in the breathing mixture increases, so that at 10 m, the partial pressure of nitrogen is double the sea-level value or 1200 mm Hg. With each additional 10 m, the partial pressure of nitrogen increases by 600 mm Hg—at a depth of 60 m, the inspired P_{N_2} is approximately 4200 mm Hg. Therefore, at each successive depth, a gradient exists for the net flow of nitrogen across the alveolar membrane into the blood and eventually into the tissue fluids for equilibration. At 20 m, for example, all tissues will eventually contain about three times as much nitrogen as they did before the dive. Factors such as tissue perfusion, solubility coefficients of tissue, body composition, and temperature all influence the uptake of nitrogen at the tissue level.

An increase in the pressure and quantity of dissolved nitrogen causes physical and mental reactions characterized by a general state of euphoria similar to alcohol intoxication; this has been termed **rapture of the deep.** This effect at a depth of 30 m is similar to the feelings one often experiences after consuming alcohol on an empty stomach; at 60 m, the feelings are similar to the effects of two or three martinis. Eventually, high nitrogen levels produce a numbing or anesthetic effect on the central nervous system. These symptoms are collectively termed **nitrogen narcosis.** At the extreme, mental processes are affected to the extent that a diver may feel that the scuba gear is unnecessary and may actually remove it and swim deeper instead of toward the surface.

Because nitrogen diffuses slowly into the body tissues, the narcosis effect depends not only on depth but also on the duration of the dive.[19] Although great individual variation in sensitivity exists, a mild narcosis usually appears after an hour or more at a depth of 30 to 40 m. *This is usually the maximum recommended depth range for recreational scuba divers.* The treatment for nitrogen narcosis simply requires

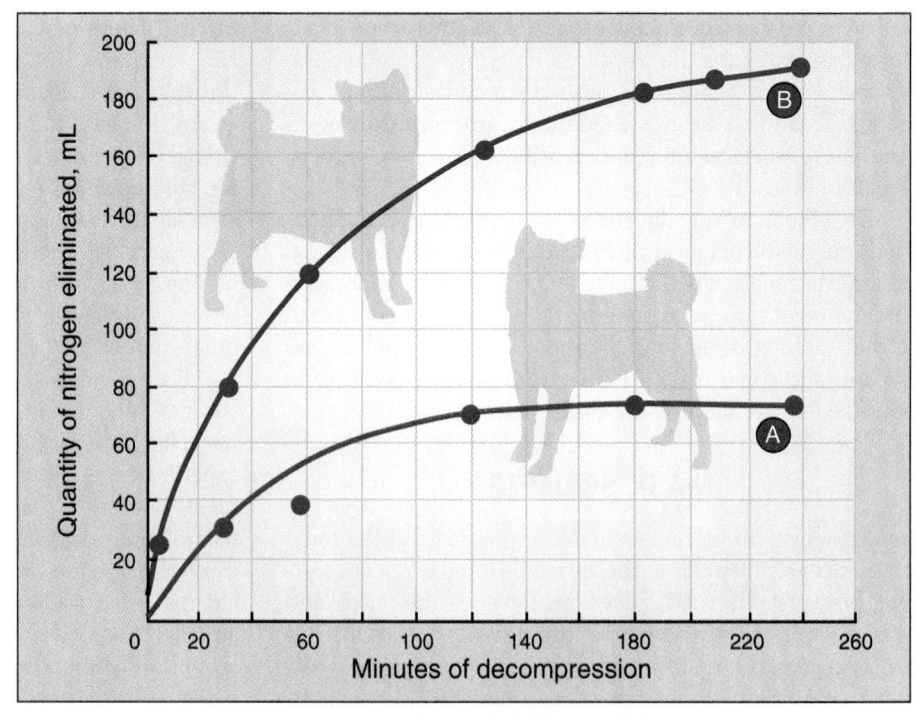

FIGURE 26.5

Elimination of nitrogen from the body tissues during decompression in a chamber of a relatively lean dog (*A*) and one that was high in body fat (*B*). (Courtesy of Dr. A.R. Behnke.)

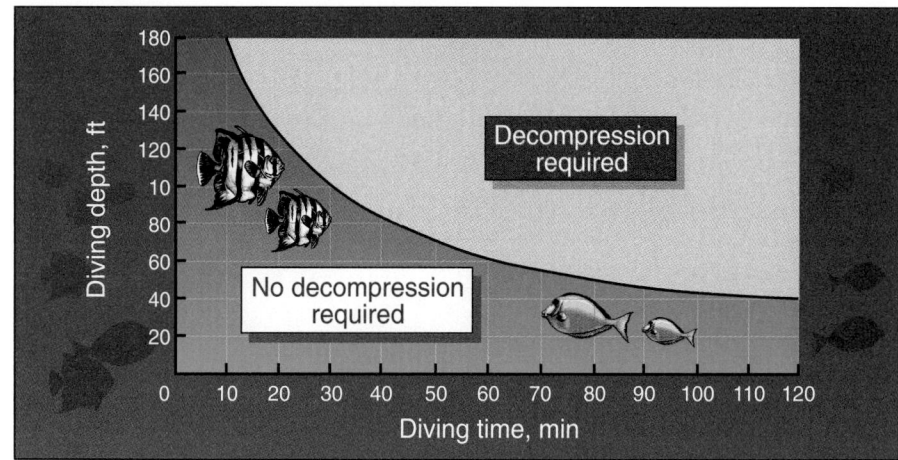

FIGURE 26.6

Zero decompression limits. Any single dive falling on the left side of the curve requires no decompression as long as the rate of ascent does not exceed 60 ft per minute (m = ft × 0.34048). Dives on the right side of the line require a decompression period, the specifics of which can be obtained from Navy Standard Decompression Tables.[18]

that the diver ascend to a shallower depth—recovery is usually immediate and complete.[18]

DECOMPRESSION SICKNESS: THE BENDS

Decompression sickness or *"the bends" occurs when dissolved nitrogen moves out of solution and forms bubbles in body tissues and fluids.* It is caused by ascending to the surface too rapidly after a deep, prolonged dive that often is made possible with the use of double and triple air tanks. Because nitrogen reaches equilibrium slowly in many tissues, especially fatty tissues, it leaves the body slowly.[19] This means that women, who generally possess a greater percentage of body fat than men, and men who are obese may be at a greater risk for decompression sickness.[11] The relationship of body fat to nitrogen elimination from the body is illustrated for two dogs in Figure 26.5. Dog B was relatively fat and dog A was lean, which is reflected by the large difference in nitrogen content in proportion to body mass between animals.

Nitrogen Elimination. If a diver ascends at a prescribed, relatively slow rate, all of the body's excess dissolved nitrogen has sufficient time to diffuse from the tissues into the blood and is eliminated through the lungs. If the ascent is too rapid and the external pressure against the diver's body is reduced dramatically, the excess nitrogen begins to separate from the dissolved state and eventually forms bubbles in the tissues. This effect is not unlike the formation of carbon dioxide bubbles when removing the cap from a carbonated beverage. As long as the cap is in place, the gas is under pressure and remains dissolved. When the cap is removed, bubbles form and pressure is reduced suddenly.

Zero Decompression Limits. Diving at 30 m for up to 30 minutes is the upper limit before sufficient nitrogen becomes dissolved to pose danger from the bends. About 18 minutes is the limit at 40 m, whereas almost an hour can be spent at 20 m without danger from decompression sickness.

If a diver exceeds the depth-duration recommendations for compressed-air diving shown in Figure 26.6, the ascent to the surface must be accomplished in stages at a specified rate to specific depths in a stepwise fashion. Such pauses or decompression stops give sufficient time for excess nitrogen to diffuse from the tissues by way of the blood to exit through the lungs without the formation of bubbles.[18, 19] For example, a dive to 30 m for 50 minutes requires one, 2-minute decompression stop at 6 m (20 ft) and another 24-minute stop at 3 m (10 ft).

For the sport diver, a conservative approach is recommended and the diver should not exceed a 20- to 25-m depth (maximum 30 m). Furthermore, the diver should never approach the time limits indicated by the decompression tables during single or repetitive dives.[9] The recommendations in Figure 26.6 assume a single dive with a minimum of 12 hours between dives. For repeated dives performed within 12 hours of each other, the diver must consult the appropriate repetitive dive decompression schedules, which account for the residual nitrogen remaining in the body at the start of the next dive if it occurs within the 12-hour period.

Consequences of Inadequate Decompression. The evidence that bubbles within the vascular circuit initiate the complications responsible for decompression injury is overwhelming. With the exception of bubbles forming in central nervous tissue, the primary bubbles occur in the venous and arterial vascular bed.[2] Symptoms of decompression sickness usually appear within 4 to 6 hours after the dive. If decompression procedures have been severely violated, when a diver runs out of air and ascends rapidly, symptoms may appear immediately and progress to paralysis within minutes.[17] The most common symptoms of inadequate decompression are dizziness, itchy skin, and pain in the legs and arms, especially in the "tight" tissues such as ligaments and tendons. The degree of injury depends on the size of the bubbles and where they are formed. Bubbles in the lungs can cause choking and asphyxia, whereas bubbles in the brain and coronary arteries block the flow of blood. The bubbles deprive these vital tissues of oxygen and nutrients, which leads to subsequent cellular damage and death. Central nervous system "bends" are relatively common and serious, because permanent neural damage can result if treatment is delayed.

Treatment for the bends involves the lengthy process of recompression in a specialized chamber (hyperbaric) to force the nitrogen gas back into solution. This is followed by slow decompression so the expanding gas has sufficient time to leave the body as the diver is brought back to the "surface." For the sport diver, the chances of having a recompression chamber nearby are slim. This makes it imperative that the recommendations not be exceeded for diving depth and duration.

OXYGEN POISONING

In general, when inspired P_{O_2} exceeds 2 atm, or 1520 mm Hg, the diver becomes highly susceptible to **oxygen poisoning**.[12] For this reason, the use of closed-circuit scuba systems that use pure oxygen places severe restrictions on both the depth and duration of a dive. At depths of more than 25 ft (7.6 m), rebreathing pure oxygen is not recommended, except in extraordinary circumstances (Table 26.2).

High oxygen pressures affect bodily functions in several ways: (*a*) a high P_{O_2} directly irritates respiratory passages and eventually induces bronchopneumonia if exposure is continued; (*b*) at pressures of about 2 atm, oxygen tends to constrict cerebral blood vessels and has a profound negative effect on central nervous system function; and (*c*) high pressures of inspired oxygen also may cause dysfunction by blunting carbon dioxide elimination. Specifically, a high inspired P_{O_2} may force sufficient oxygen into solution in the plasma to supply the metabolic needs of the diver. Oxygen is therefore returned to the lungs still in combination with hemoglobin. This causes carbon dioxide buildup because a normal route is no longer available for elimination of this gas combined with deoxygenated hemoglobin. The treatment for oxygen poisoning consists of breathing air at sea-level pressure.

CARBON MONOXIDE POISONING

Carbon monoxide is a lethal gas that combines with hemoglobin 200 times more readily than oxygen. Therefore, tissue hypoxia can occur easily, with only a small quantity of carbon monoxide in the inspired mixture. This becomes a problem during deep dives, because the partial pressures of all gases in the breathing mixture (including the impurities) increase greatly.

Contaminants from automotive and industrial exhausts, including carbon monoxide and oxides of sulfur, may be high in urban areas. For this reason, it is not advisable to fill scuba tanks when an air pollution alert is in effect. Aside

TABLE 26.2
U.S. NAVY RECOMMENDED DEPTH/TIME LIMITS BREATHING PURE OXYGEN DURING WORKING DIVES[a]

Normal Operations		
Depth		
(ft)	(m)	Time (min)
10	3.0	240
15	4.6	150
20	6.1	150
25	7.6	75

Exceptional Operations		
Depth		
(ft)	(m)	Time (min)
30	9.2	45
35	10.7	20
40	12.2	10

[a]No symptoms of oxygen poisoning were noted at these depths and durations.

from the contaminants present in free air, carbon monoxide and oil impurities also can be added during the operation of the gasoline or diesel engine compressor. This potential source of contamination can be eliminated by placing the engine's exhaust downstream from the air intake that provides the compressed air.

■ SUMMARY ■

1. Underwater divers are exposed to high pressures and to the possibility of rapid changes in pressures. Divers can suffer severe injury and even death unless adjustments are made to equalize pressures in the body's air-filled cavities.

2. Snorkel size is limited by two factors: (*a*) the underwater depth at which the skin diver can generate sufficient inspiratory force to breathe, and (*b*) the additional pulmonary dead space created by the snorkel's volume.

3. Hyperventilation increases breath-hold time but also can contribute to underwater blackout. This extremely dangerous consequence of hyperventilation probably is brought on by a critical reduction in oxygen, an abnormal increase in carbon dioxide, an acid-base imbalance, or the combined effects of these factors.

4. The maximum depth for breath-hold diving is generally determined by the point at which the diver's lung volume is compressed to residual volume. Below this criti-

cal depth, internal and external pressures are unable to equalize and lung squeeze results.

5. Because scuba systems supply breathing mixtures at great depths and pressures, specific hazards result from improper equalization of pressure in the lungs, sinus, and middle-ear spaces with the external water pressure. The most significant dangers are from air embolism, pneumothorax, mask and middle-ear squeeze, and aerosinusitis.

6. Gases breathed at high pressures move across the alveolar membrane and eventually dissolve and equilibrate in the fluids of all tissues of the body. High tissue pressures of oxygen and nitrogen have profound effects on physiologic function. Because of these problems, the maximum recommended depth for breathing compressed air is generally about 30 m.

7. As a scuba diver ascends toward the surface, a gradient is created for the net flow of nitrogen from the body fluids into the lungs. If the ascent is too rapid, the excess nitrogen that cannot exit through the lungs escapes from the dissolved state and forms bubbles in the tissues. This extremely painful condition is termed decompression sickness or the "bends."

■ REFERENCES ■

1. Becker, G.D.: Barotrauma resulting from scuba diving: an otolaryngological perspective. *Phys. Sportsmed.*, 13:113, 1985.
2. Behnke, A.R.: Decompression sickness: advances and interpretations. *Aerosp. Med.*, 42:255, 1971.
3. Bove, A., and Davis, J.: *Diving Medicine.* Philadelphia, W.B. Saunders, 1990.
4. Corteix, C., et al.: Chemical and nonchemical stimuli during breath holding in divers are not independent. *J. Appl. Physiol.*, 75:2022, 1993.
5. Craig, A.B., Jr.: Causes of loss of consciousness during underwater swimming. *J. Appl. Physiol.*, 16:583, 1961.
6. Craig, A.B., Jr.: Summary of 58 cases of loss of consciousness during underwater swimming and diving. *Med. Sci. Sports*, 8:171, 1976.
7. Craig, A.B., Jr.: Principles and problems of underwater diving. *Phys. Sportsmed.*, 8:72, 1980.
8. Craig, A.B., Jr.: Physics and physiology of swimming goggles. *Phys. Sportsmed.*, 12:107, 1984.
9. Davis, J.C.: Decompression sickness in sport scuba diving. *Phys. Sportsmed.*, 16(2):108, 1988.
10. Kindwall, E.P.: Medical aspects of sport scuba diving. *Aqua Notes*, 3:1, 1976.
11. Kizer, K.W.: Women and diving. *Phys. Sportmed.*, 9:84, 1981.
12. Lambertsen, C.J.: Effects of oxygen at high partial pressure. In *Handbook of Physiology.* Edited by W.O. Fenn and H. Rahn. Washington, DC, American Physiological Society, 1965.
13. Lanphier, E.H., and Rahn, H.: Alveolar gas exchange during breath-hold diving. *J. Appl. Physiol.*, 18:471, 1963.
14. Lin, Y. -C.: Breath-hold diving in terrestrial mammals. In *Exercise and Sport Sciences Reviews.* Vol. 10. Edited by R.L. Terjung. Philadelphia, Franklin Institute, 1982.
15. Miller, J.W.: *NOAA Diving Manual.* Washington, DC, U.S. Department of Commerce, U.S. Government Printing Office, 1979.
16. Strauss, R.H.: Diving medicine. *Am. Rev. Respir. Dis.*, 119:1001, 1979.
17. Strauss, R.H., and Yount, D.E.: Decompression sickness. *Am. Sci.*, 65:598, 1977.
18. *The NOAA Diving Manual.* Washington, DC, US Government Printing Office, 1991.
19. Wienke, B.R.: *Basic Decompression Theory and Applications.* Flagstaff AZ, Best Publishing Co., 1991.
20. Wienke, B.R.: *Basic Diving Physics and Applications.* Flagstaff, AZ, Best Publishing Co., 1994.

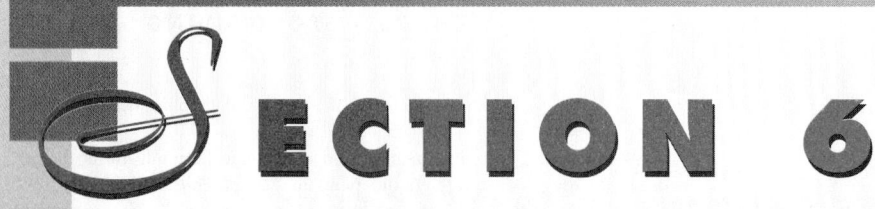

SECTION 6

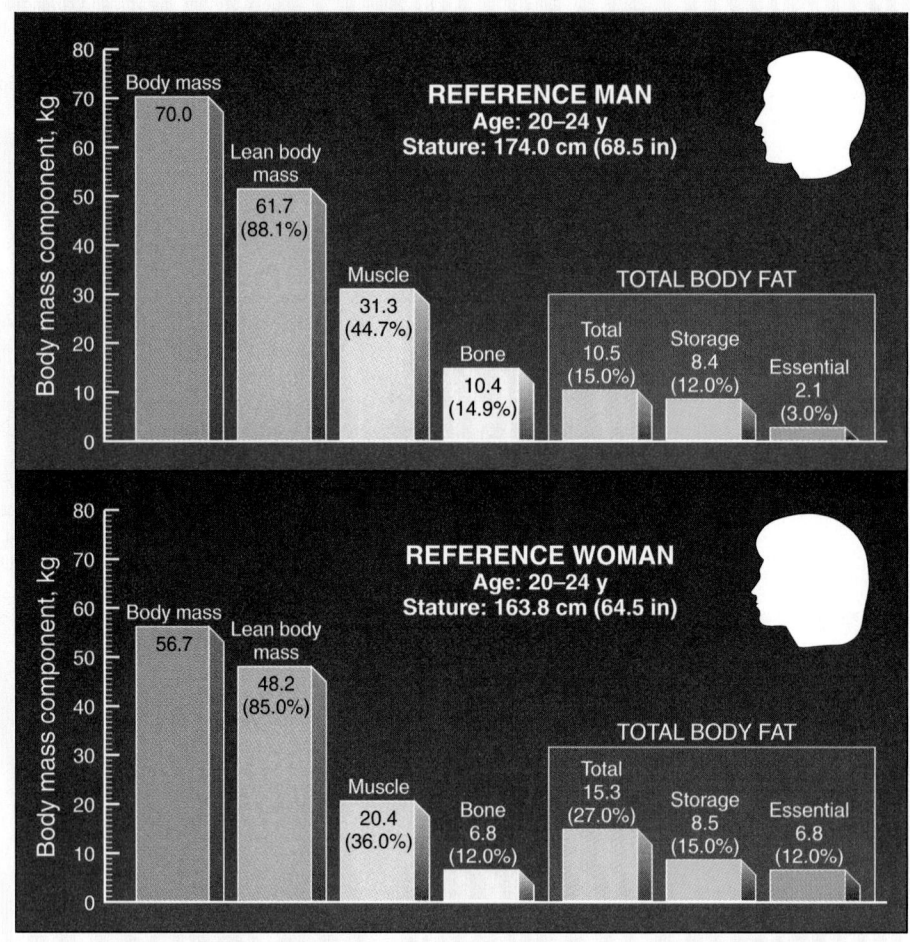

"**COMBINATIONS OF REGULAR**

AEROBIC EXERCISE AND DIET OFFER

MORE FLEXIBILITY IN ACHIEVING

BODY FAT LOSS THAN EITHER

EXERCISE ALONE OR DIET ALONE."

Body Composition, Energy Balance, and the Health-Related Aspects of Exercise

The accurate appraisal of body composition is an important component in a comprehensive program of total physical fitness. In this regard, the height-weight tables—a frequently used standard—are of limited value in evaluating physique because "overweight" and "overfat" are not necessarily synonymous. This point is clearly illustrated in athletes, many of whom are muscular and exceed some average weight for their sex and height but are otherwise quite lean in body composition. For such individuals, a weight-loss program is unnecessary and may even be detrimental to sports performance. In contrast, comprehensive dietary management programs are surely needed by the 60 million overfat dieters in the United States. This group of people spends more than $40 billion per year, purchasing 54 million diet books and services and products at 1500 weight-control clinics in the hope of permanently reducing excess fat! In 1995, spending inflated to approximately 51 billion dollars as dieters intensified their weight-loss efforts. Also of importance is the need for effective programs of weight control among those adults who suffer the insidious consequences of physical inactivity and consuming high-fat foods. For many of these men, women, and children, body fat exceeds even the most liberal limits for normalcy. In this regard, exercise can play a crucial role and is, in our opinion, the key ingredient to long-term success in maintaining a healthful body composition.

With regard to aging effects, there is no question that the physiological and exercise capacities of older people are generally below those of their younger counterparts. What is uncertain is whether these differences are caused by true biologic aging or are simply the results of a lack of use brought on by alterations in lifestyle and activity opportunities as people age. No longer can older men and women be stereotyped as sedentary with little or no initiative for active pursuits. There is currently a tremendous upswing in the participation of "senior citizens" in a broad range of physical activities and exercise programs. Research clearly demonstrates that if an active lifestyle is continued into later years, a relatively high level of function is retained, and vigorous activities can be engaged in safely and successfully. In addition, regular exercise throughout life offers significant protection against a variety of diseases and risk factors, particularly those related to the cardiovascular system.

In this section, we discuss body composition—its components and assessment and the differences that exist between men and women and trained and untrained. We also deal with topics relevant to obesity and weight-control programs that use diet and exercise. The final chapter explores several aspects of the aging process with special emphasis on exercise and its relation to cardiovascular disease.

Welham, W.C., and Behnke, A.R.: The specific gravity of healthy men; Body weight/volume and other physical characteristics of exceptional athletes and of naval personnel. *JAMA* 118:498, 1942.

The Welham and Behnke research is one of the most frequently cited papers in the body composition and exercise physiology literature. These researchers tested the hypothesis that differences in body fat among men are chiefly related to the

gravity values were known for the body's fat and nonfat (fat-free) tissue components. This research was the first to show that body density is mainly related to adipose tissue and that differences in body density among individuals are primarily related to relative differences in the body's fat content. Consequently, the standard height-weight tables were inadequate to determine a person's "desirable body weight." The researchers postulated that body density could serve as a useful indicator of whether a person has attained a desirable body mass.

Twenty-five professional football players, the majority of whom had been designated as All-Americans, were classified as being unfit for military service because they were overweight according to standard height-weight tables. Welham and Behnke's measurements for the basic analysis included stature, body mass, and body density determined by hydrostatic weighing. A unique aspect of the measurement process was the correction of body volume using estimates of residual lung volume.

The figure shows the relationship between body density and "weight by height" for the 25 athletes. The vertical line at a weight-to-height ratio of 2.65 represents the upper limit of the ratio for classification as "fit" for military duty. For this age group, men whose data fell to the right of the vertical line were not qualified for life insurance because of their overweight condition. Adopting this criterion of overweight, 17 of the All-American players were classified as obese. In eleven of these athletes, their high body density values indicated a low percentage of body fat. The average body mass for the football players equaled 90.9 kg (200 lb), and average body density was 1.080 g · cm^{-3}. For the six heaviest men, body mass averaged 230 lb and body density 1.059 g · cm^{-3}. These observations supported the hypothesis that adipose tissue, not body mass per se, largely determined an individual's body density and thus quantity of body fat.

Welham and Behnke suggested that a density value of 1.060 g · cm^{-3} should serve as the dividing line for classifying excessive body fatness. Using this criterion, 23 of the 25 lean but heavy football players would have qualified as "fit" (and not overfat) for military induction.

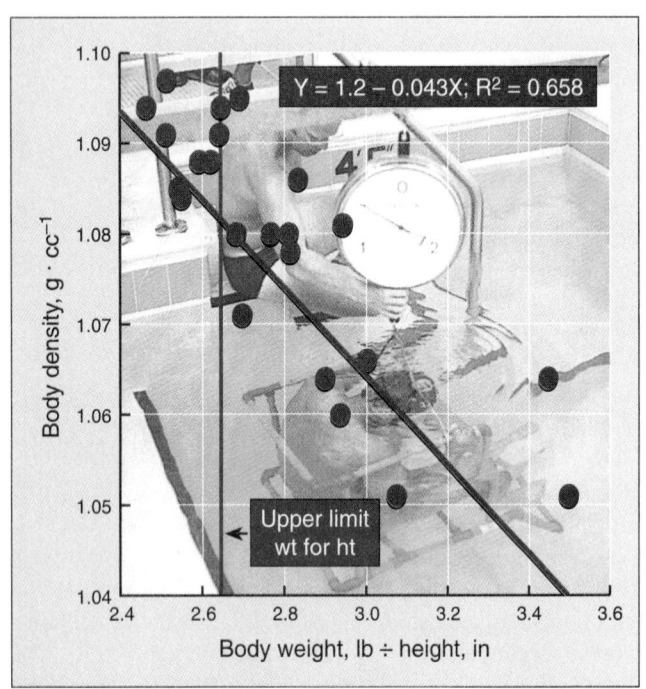

$$Y = 1.2 - 0.043X; R^2 = 0.658$$

Upper limit wt for ht

Relationship between body density and weight to height ratio for 25 All-American football players. The *vertical line* represents the upper limit of the weight-to-height ratio to permit classification as fit for military duty.

body's specific gravity and not body mass. The hypothesis predicted that men who are heavy but lean would have higher values for specific gravity, thus confirming that body mass per se should not substitute as an appropriate measure of excessive fatness.

In 1942, the relation between body specific gravity (or body density) and estimates of body fatness were not yet determined, although specific

Body Composition Assessment

The evaluation of body composition permits quantification of the major structural components of the body—muscle, bone, and fat. Although the actuarial-based height-weight tables often are used to assess the extent of "overweightness" based on sex and bony frame size, such tables do not provide reliable information on the relative composition, or quality, of an individual's body. (Note: The proper scientific term for height is stature [SI unit, cm] and for weight, mass [kg]. We acknowledge the distinction and have changed weight to mass and height to stature as long as it preserves readability.) These tables are statistical landmarks, based on the average ranges of body mass in relation to stature, where the mortality rate is lowest, for people aged 25 to 59 years. They do not consider specific causes of death or quality of health (morbidity) before death. A person may weigh much more than the average weight-for-height standards of life insurance company statistics, yet still be "underfat" in his or her body's total fat quantity. The "extra" weight could simply be additional muscle mass. According to the tables, assuming a "large" frame size, the desirable body mass range for a professional football player who is 188 cm tall and weighs 116 kg is between 78 and 88 kg. Similarly, the average weight, regardless of frame size, for young adult males who are 188 cm tall is 85 kg. Using either criterion, the player is clearly "overweight" and, based on conventional standards, should reduce his body mass at least 28 kg just to achieve the upper limit of the desirable weight range! He must reduce an additional 3 kg to match his "average" American male counterpart.

If the player followed these guidelines, it is a good bet he would no longer be playing football and might even jeopardize his overall health by undertaking a crash or bizarre diet regimen that prohibits the proper intake of essential nutrients. Although some larger-sized persons are indeed "overweight," they are not necessarily too fat and may not need to lose weight. The total fat content of the football player was only 12.7% of body mass compared with 15.0% body fat typically reported for untrained young men, even though he weighed 31 kg more than the average!

Such observations among trained men were first noted in 25 football players by Navy physician Dr. Albert Behnke in the early 1940s. Seventeen of these men were deemed unfit for military service because they were overweight and presumably too fat.[8] A careful evaluation of each player's body composition, however, revealed that their excess weight was due primarily to extreme muscular development. These observations clearly point out that the term **overweight** generally refers only to a body mass greater than some standard, usually the average body mass for a given stature. Being above some "average," "ideal," or "desirable" body mass based on height-weight tables should not necessarily dictate whether or not someone starts a weight-reducing regimen. A more desirable alternative is to determine body composition using one of the laboratory or field techniques reviewed in this chapter.

The Body Mass Index: A Somewhat Better Alternative

The **body mass index (BMI),** derived from body mass and stature, is used frequently by clinicians and researchers to evaluate the "normalcy" of one's body weight. The BMI has a somewhat higher association with body fat than do estimates based simply on stature and mass. BMI is computed as follows:

$$BMI = Body\ mass,\ kg \div Stature,\ m^2$$

The importance of this easy-to-obtain index, illustrated in Figure 27.1, lies in its curvilinear relationship to the all-cause mortality ratio: as the BMI becomes larger, so also does the risk of a variety of diseases, such as cardiovascular complications (including hypertension), diabetes, and renal disease. The classification schema at the bottom of the figure represents the degree of risk with each 5-unit increase in BMI. Thus, the lowest health-risk category is that of individuals whose BMIs range from 20 to 25, and the highest risk category is that of individuals whose BMIs exceed 40. Within this context, the suggested desirable BMI range for women is 21.3 to 22.1; for men, it is 21.9 to 22.4. BMI values above 27.8 for men and 27.3 for women are associated with an increased incidence of high blood pressure, diabetes, and coronary heart disease.[34] The Surgeon General has defined being overweight as having a BMI between 25 and 30, with obesity defined as a BMI in excess of 30; this value corresponds to a moderate category of risk. The National Center for Health Statistics[112] conducts the National Health and Nutrition Examination Survey (NHANES[111]) through surveying and direct physical examination of a representative civilian, noninstitutionalized U.S. population. This organization defines being overweight as having a BMI greater than or equal to the 85th percentile values for the BMI distributions in 20- to 29-year-old

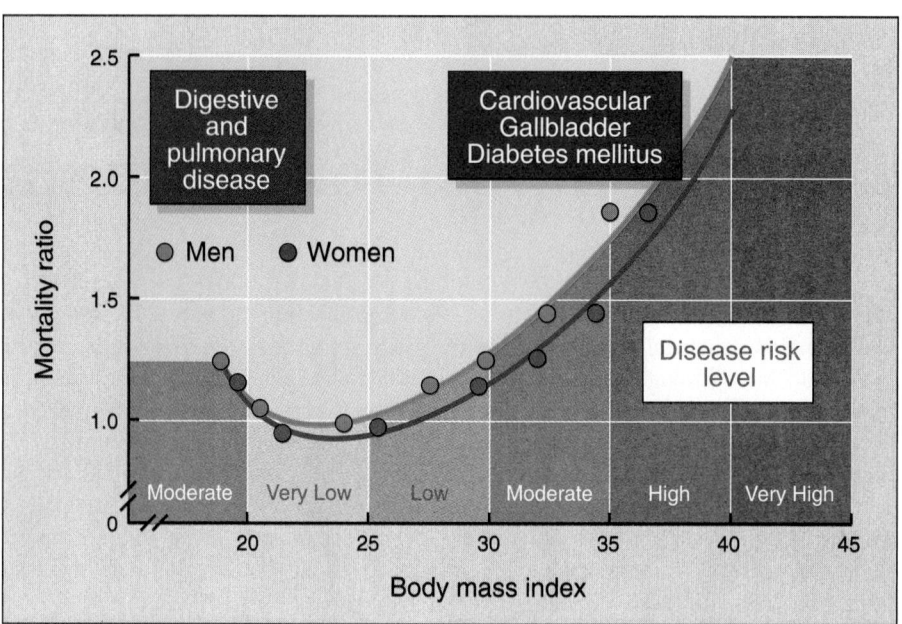

FIGURE 27.1
Curvilinear relationship based on American Cancer Society data between all-cause mortality and body mass index. The classification schema proposed for very low to very high risk includes a classification relating risk to one of a number of treatments (reduced food intake, exercise, drug therapy, and surgery). (Modified from Bray, G.A.: Pathophysiology of obesity. *Am. J. Clin. Nutr.*, 55:488S, 1992.)

men and women. This corresponds to a BMI exceeding 27.3 for females and 27.8 for males. The definition of severely overweight corresponds to a BMI equal to or greater than the 95th percentile (BMI for men, 31.1; BMI for women, 32.3).

Sample Computation of BMI

> *Male:* Stature = 175.3 cm, 1.753 m (69 in.);
> mass = 97.1 kg (214.1 lb)
>
> BMI = 97.1 ÷ (1.753)²
>
> BMI = 31.6 kg · m⁻²

In this example, the person clearly is overweight and outside the range deemed to be the cutoff of the desirable upper range of BMI values for men. This example is not atypical: the prevalence of overweight in the United States using the BMI index from NHANES II[111] included 34 million adults (15.4 million males, 18.6 million females) and represented about 26% of the adult population.[84] When the NHANES II data were analyzed by ethnicity and sex, significantly more black, Mexican, Cuban, and Puerto Rican males and females were overweight compared to white males and females. Mexican males exhibited the greatest degree of BMI determined overweight (31.2%), while 45.1% of black females were designated as overweight using the BMI standards.

Limitations of BMI. As with the height-weight tables, the BMI fails to consider the proportional composition of the body.[132] Specifically, the numerator of the BMI equation is affected by factors other than excess body fat, such as bone and muscle mass and even the quantity of plasma volume that increases with exercise training. In relatively lean individuals with excessive muscle mass in relation to stature because of genetic makeup or exercise training, a high BMI could lead to an incorrect interpretation of overfatness.

The possibility of misclassifying someone as overweight using BMI standards applies particularly to large-size athletes such as professional football players. For example, the average BMI for defensive linemen of a former NFL Super Bowl team was 31.9, and the team average BMI was 28.7. Clearly, these professional athletes were overweight and would be classified, by BMI standards, in the moderate category for mortality risk. However, evaluation of the body fat content for these players was 18.0% for the linemen and 12.1% for the team. Obviously, the large-size players were misclassified for fatness using BMI as the standard of overweight. In comparison to the pro football players, the average BMI was 24.5 for average players in the National Basketball Association in the 1993 to 1994 season. The relatively low BMIs for these athletes would place them in the very-low-risk category and also keep them from being categorized as overweight, although by the height-weight standards, they would be.

COMPOSITION OF THE HUMAN BODY

The current evaluation of body composition is based on partitioning the total body mass into different compartments, the sum of which is equal to body mass. In 1921, a Czech anthropologist, Matiegka,[100] described a four-component system, or model, consisting of the weights of the skeleton (S), skin plus subcutaneous tissue ([SK + ST]), skeletal muscles

(M), and a remainder (R), such that the four components would equal the body mass as follows:

$$\text{Total body mass} = S + [SK + ST] + M + R$$

In this early attempt to analytically describe human physique, Matiegka used anthropometric measurements to approximate the first three anatomic entities in his proposed four-component model. The weight of S was estimated from the thickness of four bony structures (wrists, ankles, and humeral and femoral condyles) plus stature. The weight of SK + ST was determined from six fatfolds (upper arm, forearm, thigh, calf, thorax, and abdomen) plus body surface area. The weight of M was based on girth measurements of the upper arm, thigh, and calf (subtracting a fatfold and determining the radius of the area to compute cross-sectional area). In essence, the three major structural components of the human body include the masses of muscle, fat, and bone.

Over the past 65 years, thousands of research articles have been published on the topic of body composition and how best to measure its various components. Most of the methodologies have attempted to further partition the body into two distinct compartments, fat-free body mass and body mass composed of fat. The composition of homogenized samples of fat-free body tissue has a density of approximately $1.100 \text{ g} \cdot \text{cm}^{-3}$ at 37°C in small mammals,[119] a water content of about 73.2%,[108] and a potassium content of 60 to 70 $\text{mmol} \cdot \text{kg}^{-1}$ in men and 50 to 60 $\text{mmol} \cdot \text{kg}^{-1}$ in women.[10, 11] Fat stored in the adipose tissue has a density of $0.900 \text{ g} \cdot \text{cm}^3$ at 37°C.[106] In subsequent studies of body composition, the two-component model was enhanced to a model consisting of four distinct components—water, protein, bone mineral, and fat.[80] Because there are marked sex differences in the relative quantities of these components, reference standards have been devised in an attempt to quantify the constituents of the different components. Among the most useful of the reference standards are the concepts proposed by Behnke of a reference man and reference woman.[7]

BEHNKE REFERENCE MAN AND WOMAN

Figure 27.2 depicts the different body composition compartments for Behnke's reference man and reference

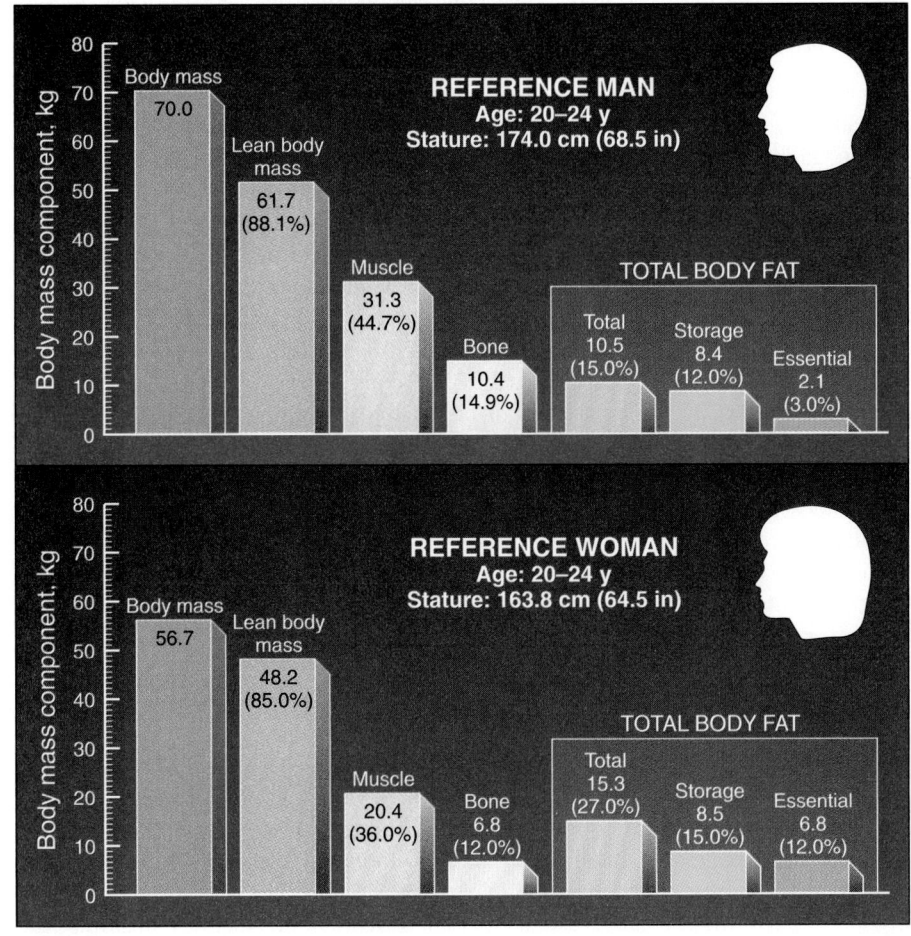

FIGURE 27.2
Behnke's theoretical model for the reference man and reference woman.

woman. This classification schema partitions the body mass into lean body mass, muscle, and bone, with total body fat further subdivided into storage and essential fat components. This theoretical model is based on the average physical dimensions obtained from detailed measurements of thousands of individuals in large-scale anthropometric surveys, and on a synthesis of information about the body's biological composition and structure.[7]

The reference man is taller and heavier, his skeleton weighs more, and he has a larger muscle mass and lower body fat content than the reference woman. These differences exist even when the quantity of fat, muscle, and bone are expressed as percentages of body mass. It is not known how much of the sex difference in body fat is biological and how much is related to behavioral factors, owing perhaps to the more sedentary lifestyle of the average female. More than likely, hormonal differences play an important role. The concept of reference standards does not mean that men and women should strive to achieve the body composition of the reference models or that the reference man and woman are in fact "average." The model, however, is useful as a frame of reference for statistical comparison and interpretation of data from other studies of diverse groups such as athletes, individuals involved in physical training programs, and the underweight and obese.

ESSENTIAL AND STORAGE FAT

Body fat exists in two storage sites, or depots. The first depot, termed **essential fat,** is the fat stored in the marrow of bones and in the heart, lungs, liver, spleen, kidneys, intestines, muscles, and lipid-rich tissues of the nervous system. This fat is required for normal physiologic functioning. In the heart, for example, the quantity of dissectable fat determined from cadaver studies represents about 18.4 g, or 5.3%, for an average heart weight of 349 g in males, and 22.7 g, or 8.6%, for an average heart weight of 256 g in females.[150] Essential fat in females also includes **sex-specific,** or sex-characteristic, fat. It is not at all clear whether this fat depot is expendable or serves as reserve storage for metabolic fuel.

The other major fat depot, **storage fat,** consists of fat that accumulates in adipose tissue. This nutritional reserve includes the visceral fatty tissues that protect the various internal organs from trauma and the larger subcutaneous fat volume deposited beneath the skin's surface. Although the proportional distribution of storage fat in men and women is similar (12% in men, 15% in women), the total percentage of essential fat in women, including the sex-specific fat, is four times higher than in men. More than likely, the additional essential fat is biologically important for child-bearing and other hormone-related functions. Considering the reference body's total quantity of storage fat (about 8.25 kg), this depot, at least theoretically, represents approximately 74,250 kcal of stored energy, or the

energy equivalent of running nonstop at a 9-minute per mile pace for 133 hours!

Figure 27.3 illustrates the theoretical model for body fat distribution in Behnke's reference woman. Note that as part of the 5 to 9% sex-specific reserve fat, the contribution of breast fat is probably no more than about 4% of body mass for women, whose total fat content varied from 14 to 35%.[78] We interpret this to mean that other substantial sex-specific fat depots must be present in the female, such as in the pelvic, buttock, and thigh regions, that contribute quantitatively to the female's body fat stores.[122]

Fat-Free Body Mass and Lean Body Mass

The terms fat-free body mass and lean body mass are often considered interchangeable when they should not be. The lean body mass contains a small percentage of essential fat stores (perhaps as much as 3%), chiefly within the central nervous system, marrow of bones, and internal organs. In contrast, use of the term "fat-free" mass refers to the body mass devoid of **all** extractable fat. Behnke points out that fat-free mass is an in vitro entity and is the appropriate term for carcass analysis.[6] Behnke views lean body mass, on the other hand, as an in vivo entity that remains relatively constant throughout the active adult life span with regard to compositional components such as water, organic matter, and minerals. *In normally hydrated, healthy adults, the only difference between fat-free body mass and lean body mass is the "essential" lipid-rich stores in bone marrow, brain, spinal cord, and internal organs.* Thus, in calculating lean body mass (LBM), the small quantity of essential fat is still present, whereas in computing fat-free body mass "total" body fat is subtracted (FFM = Body mass − Fat mass).

As displayed in Figure 27.2, lean body mass in men and minimal body mass in women are composed chiefly of essential fat (plus sex-specific fat for females), muscle, water, and bone. The density of the reference man having 12% storage fat is $1.070 \text{ g} \cdot \text{cm}^{-3}$, including the 3% essential fat. The density of his fat-free body mass is $1.094 \text{ g} \cdot \text{cm}^{-3}$. If the total body fat of the reference man is 15.0% (storage plus essential fat), the density of the hypothetical "fat-free" body attains the upper limit of $1.100 \text{ g} \cdot \text{cm}^{-3}$.

In the reference woman, the average body density is $1.040 \text{ g} \cdot \text{cm}^{-3}$ at a body fat percentage of 27%; of this, about 12% is considered to be essential body fat. The density of the minimal body mass of 48.5 kg is $1.072 \text{ g} \cdot \text{cm}^{-3}$. In actual practice, densities of 1.075 to $1.080 \text{ g} \cdot \text{cm}^{-3}$ are rarely exceeded except in lean male and female athletes.

MINIMAL STANDARDS FOR LEANNESS

There seems to be a biologic lower limit beyond which a person's body mass cannot be reduced without impairing health status. This lower limit in men is the lean body mass and is calculated as body mass minus the mass of storage fat.

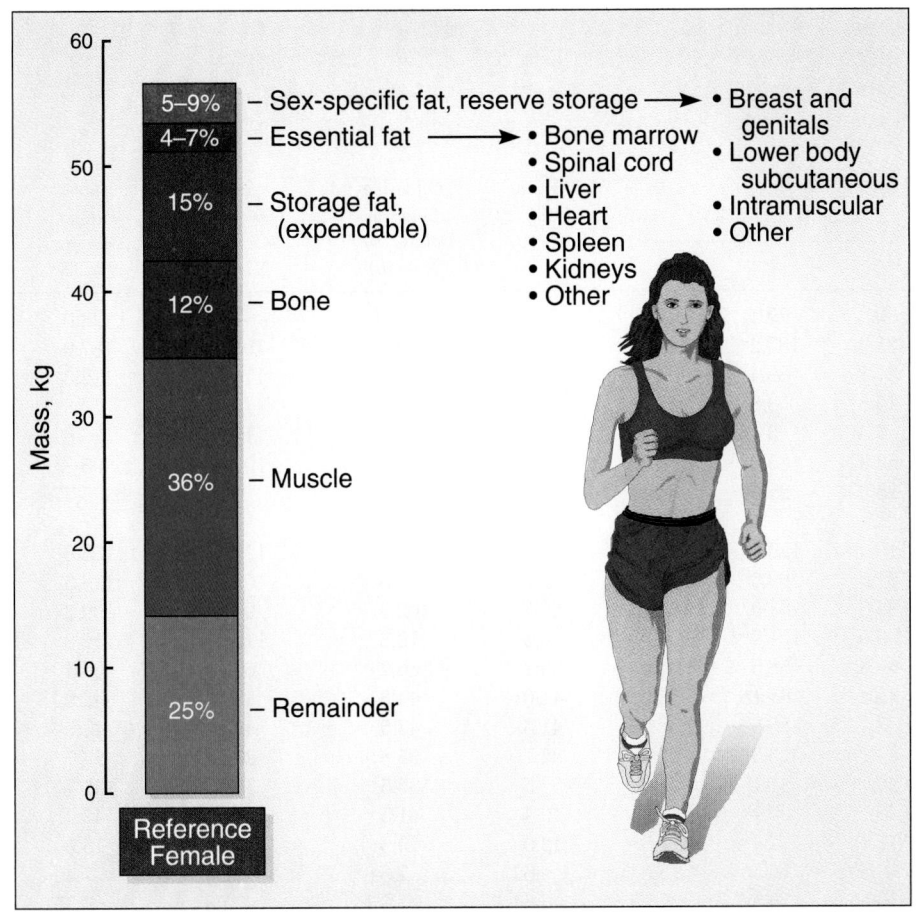

FIGURE 27.3
Theoretical model for body fat distribution for a reference woman whose body mass is 56.7 kg (stature = 163.8 cm) and percent body fat is 23.6. (From Katch, V.L., et al.: Contribution of breast volume and weight to body fat distribution in females. *Am. J. Phys. Anthropol.*, 53:93, 1980.)

For the reference man, the lean mass is equivalent to 61.7 kg; this includes approximately 3%, or 2.1 kg, of essential body fat. According to Behnke, this amount of body fat is a lower limit, and any encroachment into this reserve may impair one's normal physiologic function and capacity for vigorous exercise.[6]

Low body fat values have been reported for champion male athletes such as world-class marathon runners and some conscientious objectors who voluntarily reduced their body fat stores during a prolonged experiment with semi-starvation.[81] The low fat levels of marathon runners, ranging from 1 to 8% of body mass, probably reflect an adaptation to the severe training for distance running. This minimal fat level reduces the energy cost of weight-bearing exercise and provides an effective gradient for the transfer of metabolic heat produced during high-intensity endurance running.

Considerable variation is found in the fat-free body mass of different athletes, with values ranging from a low of 48.1 kg in some jockeys to over 100 kg in football offensive linemen and shot-putters.[7] Seven elite Sumo wrestlers (seki-tori) had fat-free body masses averaging 109 kg.[83] Table 27.1 presents data on the physique statuses and body compositions of selected professional athletes who could be classified as "underfat" and "overweight." There are striking differences in body size between these groups, as well as in relative body fat, fat-free body mass, lean-to-fat ratio, and various girth measures. The defensive and offensive backs in football were "underfat" compared to the reference man (or any other nonathletic standard), whereas the linemen and shot-putters were clearly "overweight" for their statures: their body masses relative to stature (mass per unit size) represented the 90th percentile for nonathletic males.

Minimal Body Mass

In contrast to the lower limit of body mass for the reference man, which includes about 3% essential fat, the lower limit of body mass for the reference woman includes about 12% essential fat. This theoretical limit, termed **minimal body mass,** is equivalent to 48.5 kg for the reference woman. Generally, the leanest women in the population do not have body fat levels below about 10 to 12% of body mass: this probably represents the lower limit of fatness for most women in good health.[68] *This concept of minimal body mass in women, incorporating about 12% essential fat, corresponds to the lean body mass in men, including 3% essential fat.* It should be emphasized that Behnke's concept of min-

TABLE 27.1
PHYSIQUE AND BODY COMPOSITION OF "UNDERFAT" PROFESSIONAL FOOTBALL PLAYERS AND "OVERWEIGHT" OFFENSIVE AND DEFENSIVE PROFESSIONAL FOOTBALL LINEMEN AND SHOT-PUTTERS

Variable	Defensive Backs (All-Pro) 1	2	3	4	Offensive Back (All-Pro, N = 1)	Offensive Linemen (Dallas, 1977, N = 10)	Defensive Linemen (Dallas, 1977, N = 5)	Shot-Putters (Olympic, N = 13)
Age	27.1	30.2	29.4	24.0	32	—	—	24.0
Stature, cm	184.7	181.9	187.2	181.5	184.7	193.8	197.6	187.0
Mass, kg	87.9	87.1	88.4	88.9	90.6	116.0	116.5	112.3
Relative fat, %	3.9	3.8	3.8	2.5	1.4	18.6	13.2	14.8
Absolute fat, kg	3.4	3.3	3.4	2.2	1.3	21.6	15.4	16.6
Fat-free body mass, kg	84.5	83.8	85.0	86.7	89.3	94.4	101.1	95.7
Lean/fat ratio	24.85	25.39	25.00	39.41	68.69	4.37	6.57	5.77
Girths, cm								
Shoulders	122.1	119.0	120.5	117.2	121.8	129.5	122.5	133.3
Chest	101.6	101.0	99.5	107.5	102.0	116.5	109.9	118.5
Abdomen, average	81.8	85.5	81.0	82.6	81.7	102.0	97.0	100.3
Buttocks	98.0	99.0	101.9	102.0	96.5	112.8	111.5	112.3
Thigh	61.0	61.0	58.5	64.0	63.2	66.2	69.3	69.4
Knee	39.5	41.3	41.1	38.0	41.0	44.8	45.8	42.9
Calf	37.6	38.8	38.8	37.8	41.3	43.5	42.4	43.6
Ankle	21.8	23.1	23.5	22.4	22.7	25.8	25.7	24.7
Forearm	31.8	29.1	31.1	31.8	33.5	33.5	34.8	33.7
Biceps	38.0	35.8	37.1	37.7	40.4	41.5	41.7	42.2
Wrist	18.5	17.2	17.4	17.5	18.0	19.3	19.3	18.9
D[a]	6.51	6.50	6.50	6.64	6.62	7.34	7.20	7.40
3F[b]	6.54	6.56	6.52	6.58	6.64	7.35	7.28	7.35
us-W[c]	113.5	115.4	111.5	118.2	117.0	138.0	134.1	141.9

From Katch, F.I., and Katch, V.L.: The body composition profile: techniques of measurement and applications. *Clin. Sports Med.*, 3:30, 1984.
[a]D = sum of 11 girths/100.
[b]$3F = 3 \times \sqrt{(mass, kg/stature, dm)}$.
[c]us-W = unit size-Weight (mean body mass relative to mean stature). For men, us-W = $183.6 \, W/h^{1.7}$, where W = mass, kg, and h = stature, dm. For women, us-W = $204.4 \, W/h^{1.7}$. The 90th percentile for us-W is 126 for men and 123 for women. For the reference man and woman, us-W = 100.

imal body mass in women is a theoretical construct based on this researcher's observations.

Calculation of Minimal Mass. Behnke has proposed a relatively simple method for estimating a woman's minimal body mass based on bone diameter measurements.[7] If body mass is lower than the computed minimal body mass, the woman is clearly underweight and should not reduce further without medical supervision. The following equation is used to calculate minimal body mass, where D is the sum of eight bone diameters (cm), h is stature in decimeters (dm), and 33.5 and 0.111 are constants:

$$\text{Minimal body mass} = (D/33.5)^2 \times h \times 0.111$$

The example shown in Table 27.2 illustrates the computation of minimal body mass in a young, thin-appearing woman weighing 38.7 kg (85.3 lb) and standing 166.7 cm, or

16.67 dm (65.6 in.) tall. The eight bone diameter measurements were taken according to standard procedures.[7] Clearly, by Behnke's standards, this woman would be classified as underweight because her body mass of 38.7 kg is about 8% below her recommended minimal body mass.

FIVE-LEVEL MODEL OF BODY COMPOSITION

Figure 27.4 displays a newly proposed five-level component model for quantifying body composition.[144] Each level of the model becomes more complex (atoms → molecules → cells → tissue systems → whole body) with increases in the body's levels of biological organization. Note that there are subdivisions within each of the five levels. One of the aims in developing the model was to identify and then attempt to quantify the various components of each of the levels. An es-

TABLE 27.2
PROCEDURE FOR COMPUTING A WOMAN'S MINIMAL BODY MASS (STATURE, 16.67 DM)

Diameter	Measurement, cm
Biacromial	34.4
Chest	23.8
Bi-iliac	22.7
Bitrochanteric	29.8
Knees[a]	16.1
Ankles[a]	11.5
Elbows[a]	11.1
Wrists[a]	10.0
	Sum = 159.4

[a]Sum of right and left sides.

Step 1. Compute D, which is the sum of the eight diameters. Note that the last four measurements represent the sum of the right and left sides.

Step 2. Substitute in the equation for minimal body mass:

Minimal body mass

$= (D/33.5)^2 \times h \times 0.111$

$= (159.4/33.5)^2 \times 16.67 \times 0.111$

$= 41.9 \text{ kg}$

sential feature of the model is that each level is separate and distinct, and that either direct or indirect methods of measurements can quantify a particular characteristic within a level. Examples of measurement procedures in relation to each classification level include the following:

- **Atomic level.** The body mass is the sum of all of the elements in the body (Body mass = O + C + H + N + Ca + remainder). Elemental composition can be determined from cadaver or tissue biopsy samples. Total body potassium can be determined by whole-body ^{40}K counting;[110] total body sodium, chlorine, phosphorus, and calcium can be determined by delayed-g neutron activation;[27] total body nitrogen can be determined by prompt-g neutron activation;[27] and total body carbon can be determined by inelastic neutron scattering.[79]

- **Molecular level.** The elements of body mass form molecules that constitute more than 100,000 different chemical compounds. The major components are water, lipids (essential and storage), glycogen, protein (nitrogen-containing compounds), and minerals (metallic and nonmetallic elements). The elements are sampled from body fluids and directly estimated using isotopic dilution,[36] and osseous (bone containing more than 99% Ca and 86% P) and nonosseous mineral is quantified by single-photon[101, 117] and dual-photon absorptiometry.[116]

- **Cellular level.** There are three main compartments to the body mass: cells (cell mass = cells from muscles + connective [includes fat cells], epithelial, and nervous tissues); extracellular fluids (plasma + interstitial fluid); and extracellular solids (organic and inorganic extracellular solids). Isotopic dilution procedures directly measure extracellular fluid and plasma volumes.[114]

- **Tissue level.** The body is composed of eleven subsystems (circulatory, respiratory, nervous, integumentary, muscular, endocrine, respiratory, lymphatic, digestive, skeletal, and reproductive), but for body composition evaluation, the following four tissue-systems can be more easily grouped to represent total body mass (adipose tissue + skeletal muscle + bone + blood). CT, MRI, and ultrasound procedures can be used to estimate the volumes of subcutaneous fat, visceral adipose tissue, and segmental muscle mass.

- **Whole body level.** The common anthropometric procedures include fatfolds, girths, bone diameters, body mass, stature, BMI, surface area, segment lengths, segmental and total body volume, and body density.

UNDERWEIGHT AND THIN

The terms *underweight* and *thin* are not necessarily synonymous. In some cases they describe physical conditions that differ considerably. Measurements in our laboratories have focused on the structural characteristics of apparently "thin" females.[75] Subjects were initially screened subjectively as appearing thin or "skinny." Each of the 26 women then underwent a thorough anthropometric evaluation, including measurements of fatfolds, circumferences, and bone diameters, and determination of percent body fat and fat-free body mass by hydrostatic weighing. (These techniques are discussed in detail beginning on page 550.)

The results were unexpected because the women's percent body fat measurements averaged 18.2%, about 7 percentage points below the average value of 25% body fat typically reported for young adult women. The other striking finding was the lack of significant differences in four trunk and four extremity bone-diameter measurements between the thin-appearing women, 174 women who averaged 25.6% fat, and 31 women who averaged 31.4% body fat. These findings indicated that appearing thin or skinny does not necessarily mean that skeletal frame size is diminutive or that the body's total fat content is excessively low, as would be the case for the lower limits of minimal body mass and essential body fat proposed by Behnke.

We believe that three criteria can be used to designate an adult female as underweight: (*a*) body mass less than minimal body mass, calculated from skeletal measurements as outlined in Table 27.2; (*b*) body mass lower than the 20th percentile by stature, and (*c*) body fat less than 17%.

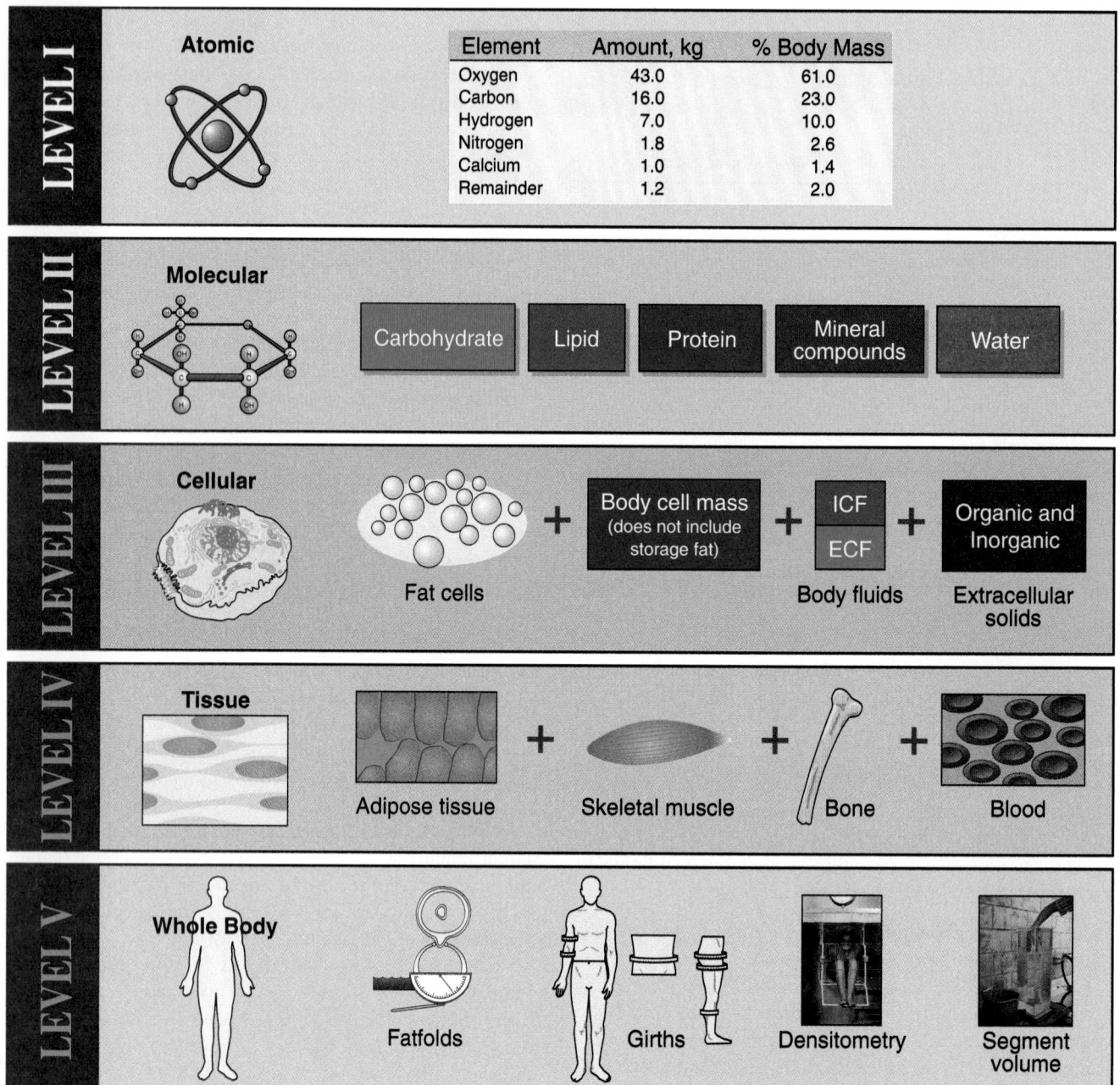

Element	Amount, kg	% Body Mass
Oxygen	43.0	61.0
Carbon	16.0	23.0
Hydrogen	7.0	10.0
Nitrogen	1.8	2.6
Calcium	1.0	1.4
Remainder	1.2	2.0

FIGURE 27.4

Five-level, multicomponent model for assessment and interpretation of body composition. Each component within a level becomes more complex with an increase in the body's level of biological organization. A key feature of the five-level model is the use of appropriate measurement techniques within each level. This allows the researcher to focus on a particular aspect of body composition, particularly in relation to specific or general biological effects. These could include changes in tissue composition resulting from body weight gain or loss or more theoretical aspects related to cellular and tissue function. (Modified from Wang, Z.M., et al.: The five-level model: a new approach to organizing body composition research. *Am. J. Clin. Nutr.*, 56:19, 1992.)

LEANNESS, REGULAR EXERCISE, AND MENSTRUAL IRREGULARITY

Physically active women in general, and particularly athletes in sports that require a low percentage of body fat for success, increase their chances of either a delayed onset of menstruation, an irregular menstrual cycle (**oligomenorrhea**), or a complete cessation of the menses (**amenorrhea**).[46, 91, 93, 143] In support of this position are studies of female ballet dancers who, as a group, are quite lean and report greater incidences of menstrual dysfunction, eating disorders, and higher mean ages at menarche compared to age-matched, non-dance females.[39, 145] One-third to one-half of female athletes in endurance-type sports are believed to have some menstrual irregularity.[142] When menstrual function is irregular or absent in premenopausal women, these women face an increased risk of bone loss and musculoskeletal injury when they participate in vigorous exercise.[46, 88] The speculation is that, in some way, the body "senses" when physical stress is high and energy reserves are inadequate to sustain a pregnancy and, thus, ceases ovulation to prevent conception. Often cited is the maintenance of at least 17% body fat as the "critical level" for the onset of menstruation and 22% fat as the level required to maintain a normal cycle.[39, 41] It is argued that hormonal and metabolic disturbances that affect the menses are triggered if body fat falls below these levels. A critical lower level of body fat, however, may be an inadequate explanation.

Leanness is Not the Only Factor

Although the lean-to-fat ratio is important for normal menstrual function (perhaps through the role of peripheral fat in the conversion of androgens to estrogens), other factors are probably also operating. *This is because there are many physically active females who are significantly below the supposed critical level of 17% body fat but have normal menstrual cycles and maintain high levels of physiologic and performance capacity.*[15, 38, 124] Conversely, some amenorrheic athletes have average levels of body fat. In a study from one of our laboratories, for example, 30 female athletes and 30 nonathletes, all having less than 20% body fat, were compared for menstrual cycle regularity.[72] Four of the athletes and three nonathletes ranging from 11 to 15% body fat had regular cycles, whereas seven athletes and two nonathletes had irregular cycles or were amenorrheic. For the total sample, 14 athletes and 21 nonathletes had regular menstrual cycles. These data corroborate other findings and support the contention that the hypothesis that a critical body fat level of 17 to 22% is required for normal menstrual function is simply not valid.

The complex interplay of physical, nutritional, genetic, hormonal, regional fat distribution, psychological, and environmental factors must be considered when evaluating potential causes of menstrual dysfunction.[12, 14, 99, 127, 128, 151] Within the realm of strenuous physical activity, research indicates that an intense bout of exercise triggers the release of an array of hormones, some of which have anti-reproductive properties.[17] For example, the release of cortisol and other stress-related hormones during intense and/or prolonged exercise suggests that the stimulation of the hypothalamic-pituitary-adrenal axis in exercise may disrupt normal ovarian function.[28, 93] It remains to be determined, however, whether regular bouts of heavy exercise have a cumulative hormonal effect sufficient to alter a normal menses. In this regard, it is noteworthy that when young amenorrheic ballet dancers had injuries that prevented them from exercising regularly, normal menstruation resumed even though body weight remained unchanged.[145] In addition, nutritional inadequacy and an exercise-induced energy deficit with heavy training among athletes having reproductive endocrine dysfunction have been identified as possible predisposing factors.[15, 58, 124] Proper nutrition may prevent or reverse athletic amenorrhea without requiring a reduction in exercise training volume or intensity.[92]

Based on current knowledge, approximately 13 to 17% body fat should be regarded as an estimate of the as-yet undetermined minimal level of body fat associated with regular menstrual function. The effects and risks of sustained amenorrhea on the reproductive system are also undetermined. However, failure to menstruate or cessation of the normal cycle should be evaluated by a gynecologist/endocrinologist because it may reflect a significant medical condition such as pituitary or thyroid gland malfunction or premature menopause.[129] Furthermore, as discussed in Chapter 2, prolonged menstrual dysfunction can have a profound negative effect on the density of the body's bone mass.

DELAYED ONSET OF MENSTRUATION AND CANCER RISK

The delayed onset of menarche generally observed in chronically active young females may provide a positive health benefit.[41, 42, 44, 133] Female athletes who start training in high school or earlier show lower lifetime occurrences of cancer of the breast and reproductive organs, as well as nonreproductive-system cancers, compared to their less active counterparts. Women who exercise an average of 4 hours per week after menarche reduce their risk of breast cancer 50% compared to that of age-matched inactive women.[9] It is speculated that one mechanism for the lower cancer risk is linked to the production of less total estrogen, or a less potent form of estrogen, over the athlete's lifetime, with a lower number of ovulatory cycles accompanying the delayed onset of menstruation.[9, 40, 137] Lower body fat levels in athletes may also be contributing factors because peripheral fatty tissues convert androgens to estrogen.

COMMON TECHNIQUES FOR ASSESSING BODY COMPOSITION

Two general procedures are used to evaluate body composition:

- Direct evaluation by chemical analysis of the animal carcass or human cadaver, and
- Indirect evaluation by hydrostatic weighing or with simple fatfold and girth measurements or other procedures.

DIRECT ASSESSMENT

Two approaches have been used in the direct assessment of body composition. In one technique, the body is literally dissolved in a chemical solution and a determination made of the fat and fat-free components of the mixture. The other technique involves the physical dissection of a variety of body components such as fat, fat-free adipose tissue, muscle, and bone. Although considerable research has been done on the direct chemical assessment of body composition in various animal species, few studies have chemically determined human fat content.[23, 37, 107] Such analyses are time consuming and tedious, require specialized laboratory equipment, and involve many ethical and legal problems in obtaining cadavers and human tissues for research purposes.

Direst assessment of body composition has indicated that while considerable variation exists in total body fatness, the compositions of the skeletal mass and lean and fat tissues remain relatively stable. The assumed chemical constancy of these tissues has enabled researchers to develop mathematical equations to determine the body's fat percentage. This is indeed fortunate, as the direct method for assessing the fat content of cadavers, while of considerable theoretical importance, obviously cannot be used with live subjects.

INDIRECT ASSESSMENT

A variety of indirect procedures are commonly used to assess body composition. The first involves Archimedes' principle as applied to **hydrostatic weighing** (also referred to as densitometry or underwater weighing). With this method, percent body fat is computed from body density (the ratio of body mass to body volume). Other procedures include the prediction of body fat from fatfold and girth measurements, x-ray, total body electrical conductivity or impedance, near-infrared interactance, ultrasound, computed tomography, and magnetic resonance imaging.

HYDROSTATIC WEIGHING: ARCHIMEDES' PRINCIPLE

The Greek mathematician Archimedes discovered the physical principle that serves as the basis for indirect body composition evaluation. When King Hieron asked Archimedes to determine the gold content of his crown, he was in fact asking for an analysis of a two-compartment system of gold and some other metal that was supposedly diluting the crown's gold content. In solving this problem, Archimedes reasoned that the volume of water that overflowed when he entered his bath was equal to the volume of his submerged body. He also reasoned that an object either submerged or floating in water is buoyed up by a counterforce that equals the weight of the volume of water displaced. This buoyant force helps support the submerged object against the downward pull of gravity. Thus, an object is said to lose weight in water. *Because the object's loss of weight in water equals the weight of the volume of water it displaces, its specific gravity can be defined as the ratio of its weight in air divided by its loss of weight in water.*[a]

Archimedes used quantities of silver and gold, each having the same weight as the crown. When the silver and gold were submerged in a container filled with water, each caused a different volume to overflow. When the crown was submerged, it displaced more water than the gold but less than the silver. Thus, Archimedes deduced that the King's gold crown had been adulterated and was indeed composed of **both** gold and silver. Figure 27.5 illustrates the application of Archimedes' principle of buoyant force in determining the volume and specific gravity of the king's crown.

Validity of Hydrostatic Weighing for Estimating Body Fat

There is experimental evidence that establishes the validity of hydrostatic weighing for estimating body fat content. In Behnke's early studies of Navy divers, 64 subjects were placed into two groups based on body density. The mean difference between the groups in body mass was 12.4 kg, and in body volume, 13.29 liters. The ratio of these average differences (Δ weight ÷ Δ volume), was 0.933 g · cm^{-3}, a value within the densitometric range of 0.92 to 0.96 g · cm^{-3} for human adipose tissue. Thus, the difference in body mass between the high- and low-density groups was equivalent to the density of adipose tissue. When the density of a group of heavy but lean professional football players was determined by hydrostatic weighing, the players had an average body density of 1.080 g · cm^{-3} and an average lean body mass that was 20 kg higher than that of the Navy divers. As Behnke has stated, "Here indeed was a presumptive demonstration that fat could be separated from bone and muscle in vivo or 'the silver from the gold' by application of a principle renowned in antiquity."[7]

The lower and upper limits of body density among humans are approximately 0.93 g · cm^{-3} in the very obese and 1.10 g · cm^{-3} in the leanest males. These values coincide nicely with the 1.10 density of fat-free and 0.90 density of samples of homogenized whole body fatty tissue in small mammals at 37°C.[82]

Possible Limitations

The validity of body density in estimating total body fat is based on several assumptions, some not yet verified in hu-

---

[a]Specific gravity can be thought of as an object's degree of "heaviness" in relation to its volume. Objects of the same volume may vary considerably in density, density being defined as mass per unit volume (density = mass ÷ volume). The volume of 1 g of water is exactly 1 cm^{-3} at a temperature of 39.2°F (4°C). Its density would be 1 g per cubic centimeter. Because the density of water is greatest at 4°C, increasing the temperature would increase the volume of 1 g of water and decrease its density. It is necessary, therefore, to correct the volume of an object weighed in water to the water's density at the weighing temperature. This temperature effect distinguishes density from specific gravity.

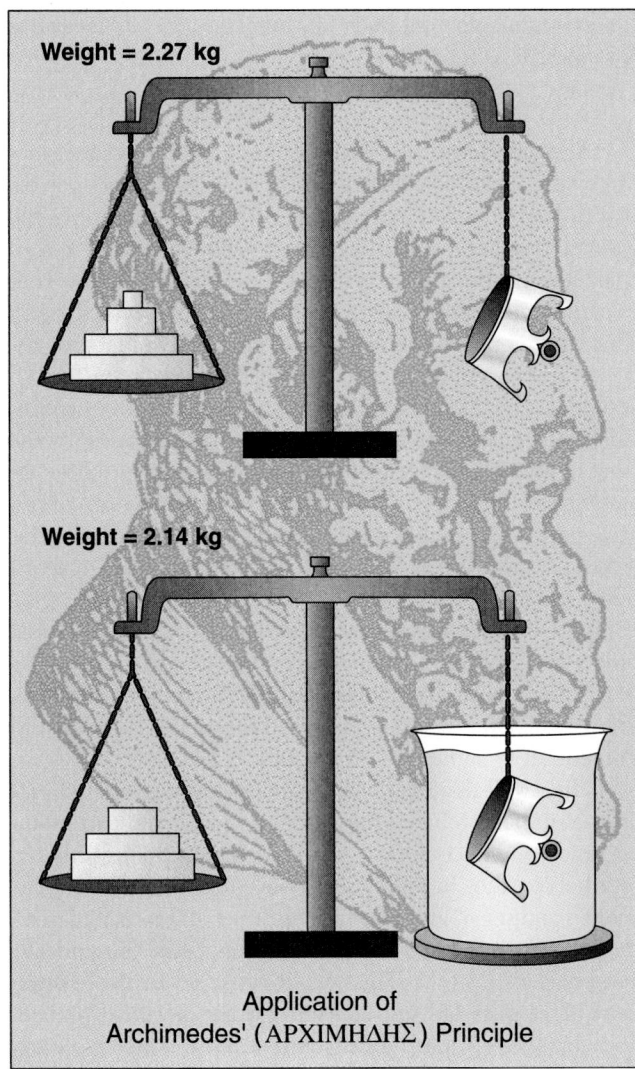

Weight = 2.27 kg

Weight = 2.14 kg

Application of
Archimedes' (ΑΡΧΙΜΗΔΗΣ) Principle

FIGURE 27.5
Use of Archimedes' principle of buoyant force for determining the volume and, subsequently, the specific gravity of the king's crown. (The solution: The crown weighs 2.27 kg in air and 0.13 kg less, or 2.14 kg, when immersed under water. Specific gravity of the crown, computed by dividing the weight of the crown [2.27 kg] by its loss of weight in water [0.13 kg], is 17.5. Because this ratio is considerably different than the specific gravity of pure gold, which has a value of 19.3, Archimedes can conclude: "Eureka, the crown is a fraud!")

mans. Although 19th-century German anatomists had conducted experiments on the gross composition of various body tissues, only six adult human bodies had been analyzed for skin, muscle, adipose tissue, bone, and organ components until more recent cadaver analysis studies. In 1984, anatomic data were presented from analyses of 12 embalmed (six male, six female) and 13 nonembalmed (six male, seven female) cadavers ranging in age from 55 to 94 years.[23]

The time-consuming and meticulous nature of the cadaver experiments revealed that several of the basic assumptions were not consistent with the two-compartment model (fat and fat-free compartments) for body composition assessment. The basic assumption that the densities of the fat-free components (bone, mineral, muscle, and water) are constant among individuals could not be confirmed. For example, the range for muscle as a percent of fat-free mass was 41.9% (female) to 59.4% (male); similarly, the range for bone was 17.4% (male) to 25.7% (female). Also, other experiments have demonstrated large individual variations in bone density in living humans.[3] Such possible variations in the densities and percentage contributions of the fat-free tissue components indicate that the application of whole-body density computed by hydrostatic weighing to estimating one's percent body fat and fat-free body mass may have limitations as far as being the "gold standard." Hopefully, more cadaver studies over a broad age range in "healthy" men and women will improve the precision of the theoretical model for predicting body composition.

Computing Body Density

According to Archimedes' principle, if a person weighs 75 kg in air and 3 kg when submerged in water, the loss of weight in water of 72 kg is equal to the weight of the displaced water. Because the density of water at any temperature is known, the volume of water displaced can easily be computed. In the example, 72 kg of water is equal to 72 L, or 72,000 cm³ (1 g of water = 1 cm³ in volume). If the water temperature is 4°C, there is no correction factor. (Refer to Appendix G for the correction factors at higher water temperatures.) The density of this person, computed as mass divided by volume, would be 75,000 g ÷ 72,000 cm³, or 1.0416 g · cm⁻³. The laboratory procedures for measuring body density are discussed on pages 553 to 555. Once the body density is known, the next step is to convert the density value to an estimate of percent body fat.

Computing Percent Body Fat

The percentage of fat in the body can be determined using an equation that incorporates whole body density. (Note: An algebraic expression that incorporates the assumed densities of the fat and fat-free tissues can be represented by D, the density of the whole system; F, having a density of f, and L, having a density of l, are the fat and fat-free tissue components. The object is to solve for F.) The simplified equation derived by Berkeley scientist William Siri is obtained by substituting 0.90 g · cm⁻³ for the density of fat (F) tissues and 1.10 g · cm⁻³ for the density of fat-free (L) tissues.[130]

$$D = F + L \div (F/f) + (L/l)$$

Because the density of the whole system equals the sum of its parts, F + L = 1.00. Substituting in the above formula,

$$D = 1.00 \div (F/f) + (L/l)$$

By rearranging terms, the proportional contribution of F becomes:

$$F = 1.00 \div D \times f \times 1 \div (1 - f) - f \div (1 - f)$$

Its final derivation, referred to as the "Siri equation," is:

$$\text{Percent body fat} = 495 \div \text{Body density} - 450$$

This equation was derived from a two-compartment model of the body consisting of fat and fat-free tissues. Fat extracted from adipose tissue has a density of 0.90 g · cm^{-3} at 36°C, whereas fat-free tissue has a density of about 1.10 g · cm^{-3}. The assumption of early research in this area was that each of these densities remains relatively constant among individuals, even among those having large individual variations in total fat and fat-free body mass. In addition, it is assumed that the density of the fat-free tissue components of bone and muscle are the same among different individuals.

In the previous example, where body mass = 75 kg and body volume = 72 L, the density of 1.0416 g · cm^{-3} when converted to percent fat by the Siri equation = 25.2%.

$$\text{Percent body fat} = (495 \div 1.0416) - 450 = 25.2\%$$

Several formulas other than Siri's equation have also been devised to estimate percent body fat from body density.[16] The basic difference in calculations of body fat between the formulas is generally less than about 1% body fat units for levels of body fat that range between 4 and 30%.

Limitations of Density Assumptions

The generalized density values for fat-free (1.10 g · cm^{-3}) and fat (0.90 g · cm^{-3}) tissues of the body are average values for young and middle-aged adults. The assumed densities of the components of fat-free body mass at 37°C are: water, 0.993 g · cm^{-3}; mineral, 3.042 g · cm^{-3}; and protein, 1.340 g · cm^{-3}. Although it is assumed that these values are constants, this may not be the case.[32, 97, 98] Any variation from these assumed constants would therefore create inaccuracies in the partitioning of the body mass into fat and fat-free components by hydrostatic weighing. For example, the densities of fat-free body mass in adult blacks were estimated to be significantly greater than those of a corresponding group of whites (1.113 g · cm^{-3} versus 1.100 g · cm^{-3}).[123] This racial difference apparently also exists among adolescents.[136] Consequently, the existing equations used to calculate body composition from body density in whites would tend to **overestimate** fat-free body mass (**underestimate** percent body fat) when applied to blacks.[25] A proposed modification

for computing percent body fat from body density measures for blacks is as follows:

$$\text{Percent body fat} = 437.4 \div \text{Body density} - 392.8$$

Applying constant density values to the various tissues of growing children or aging adults could also introduce errors in predicting body composition.[89, 90, 149] For example, the water and mineral contents of fat-free body mass are in continual change during the growth period and during the well-documented demineralization of osteoporosis with aging.[146] This condition would make the actual density of fat-free tissue in young children and the elderly lower than the assumed constant of 1.10 g · cm^{-3}. This lower value would invalidate the assumptions of the two-compartment model (that is, assumed constant composition, or density, of the fat and fat-free masses) and result in an **overestimation** of relative body fat by densitometry for these individuals. For this reason, many researchers have not attempted to convert body density to percent body fat in children and aging adults. Others, however, have used a multicompartmental model in an attempt to adjust for such factors in computing percent body fat from body density in prepubertal children.[131, 148] (One equation proposed for use with children is: Percent fat = 530 ÷ Density − 489.[89])

The well-documented, exercise-training-related increases in bone mineral mass, muscle mass, and extracellular fluid volume could also affect the assumptions underlying the densities in the two-compartment model. In highly trained and select groups of athletes such as football players, the densities of the fat-free components could theoretically exceed 1.10 g · cm^{-3}. This would cause an **underestimation** of relative fat and account for the negative percent body fat values reported for some of these athletes.[1] A significantly large residual volume may have also caused the discrepancy in these results. In our experiences measuring several thousand elite white and black performers (Olympic athletes, professional football, baseball, basketball, and soccer players, as well as champion body builders and gymnasts), we have never recorded a whole-body density value greater than 1.10 g · cm^{-3} (which would produce a negative value for percent body fat) when residual volume has been measured directly and found to be in the range appropriate for body size and age.

Recent studies of the fractional contributions of water, protein, and minerals to fat-free body masses (as well as the ratios of total body potassium and total body water to fat-free mass) in white, male long-distance runners have indicated no differences in these measurements compared to untrained counterparts,[115] even though fat-free body mass constituted a larger proportion of the total body mass in the runners. Such data support the use of the classic two-compartment model for evaluating body composition in athletes, at least among trained groups of white, male runners.

Computing the Mass of Fat

The total quantity of body fat using data from the prior example is computed by multiplying percent fat by body mass.

$$\text{Fat mass} = (\text{Percent fat}/100) \times \text{Body mass}$$
$$= 0.252 \times 75 \text{ kg}$$
$$= 18.9 \text{ kg}$$

Further calculations could be done to subdivide the total fat mass for this person into essential and storage fat. A female of 25.2% body fat has about 12% essential fat, or 9.0 kg (0.12 × 75 kg); the remaining 13.2%, or 9.9 kg, would be in the form of storage fat (0.132 × 75 kg). A male with 3% essential fat and 22.2% storage fat (based on a percent body fat of 25.2) would have corresponding values of 2.3 kg for essential fat and 16.65 kg for storage fat. Clearly, if a man and woman have the same percent body fat, the man could be considered "fatter" because a larger percentage of his total fat is in the form of storage fat. Because each gram of lipid contains about 9 kcal (9,000 kcal per kilogram), a rough approximation can also be made of the potential energy stored in each fat depot. For storage fat, the values would be 89,100 kcal for the woman and 149,850 kcal for the man; for essential fat, including the female sex-specific fat, the values would be 81,000 kcal for the woman and 20,250 kcal for the man. The kcal values for storage fat are considerably larger in obese men and women, whose percentage of body fat can equal 50% or more of total body mass.[60, 147]

Computing Fat-Free Body Mass

Fat-free body mass is calculated by subtracting the mass of fat from body mass.

$$\text{Fat-free body mass} = \text{Body mass} - \text{Fat mass}$$
$$= 75 \text{ kg} - 18.9 \text{ kg}$$
$$= 56.1 \text{ kg}$$

MEASUREMENT OF BODY VOLUME

The principle discovered by Archimedes is applied to the measurement of body volume in one of two ways: (*a*) water displacement or (*b*) hydrostatic weighing. Body volume must be measured accurately because small variations in volume can have a substantial effect on the density calculation and, hence, on the computed values of percent fat and fat-free body mass.

Water Displacement

The volume of an object submerged in water can be measured based on the corresponding rise in the level of water within a container. Using this technique, the rise of water is measured in a thin tube secured to the side of a tank. This finely calibrated tube permits accurate volume measurements. When the volume of the body is measured in this manner, the volume of air that remains in the subject's lungs during submersion must be considered. This lung volume is usually determined before the subject enters the tank and subtracted from the total body volume determined by water displacement.

Hydrostatic Weighing

This is the most common application of Archimedes' principle for determining body volume. In this procedure, body volume is computed as the difference between body mass measured in air (M_a) and body weight measured during water submersion (W_w; the term weight is appropriate here, because the body's mass remains unchanged under water). *Body volume is equal to the loss of weight in water, with the appropriate temperature correction for the density of water.*

Figure 27.6 illustrates the procedure for measuring body volume through hydrostatic weighing. The subject's body mass is first determined in air on a balance scale accurate to ±50 g. When fatter-appearing subjects are weighed, a diver's belt is secured around the waist to ensure they do not float upward during submersion. The underwater weight of this belt and chair is determined beforehand and subtracted from the subject's total weight under water. The subject, who wears a thin nylon swim suit, sits in a lightweight, plastic tubular chair suspended from the scale and submerged beneath the surface of the water. A swimming pool can serve the same purpose as the tank, and the scale and chair assembly can be suspended from a support at the side of the pool. In the tank, water temperature is maintained at about 95°F, a value close to the person's skin temperature. Water temperature is recorded to correct for the density of water at the weighing temperature.

The subject makes a forced maximal exhalation as the head is lowered under water. After all possible air is exhaled, the breath is then held for about 5 to 10 seconds while underwater weight is recorded on a sensitive scale accurate to ±10 g, or on a force transducer system with digital readout. The underwater weighing procedure is repeated 8 to 12 times because unaccustomed subjects "learn" to expel progressively more air from their lungs with each additional underwater trial. An average of the last two or three weighings is used because these trials represent the subject's "true" weight under water with minimal intraindividual variation.[61] As occurs with the water-displacement method, residual volume (preferably measured, not predicted to eliminate a potential source of significant error) must be subtracted from total body volume determination.[109] Reproducibility of body volume scores measured several times on the same day or on consecutive days is always high, with the test-retest reliability coefficient usually above r = 0.94.[73] In subjects that

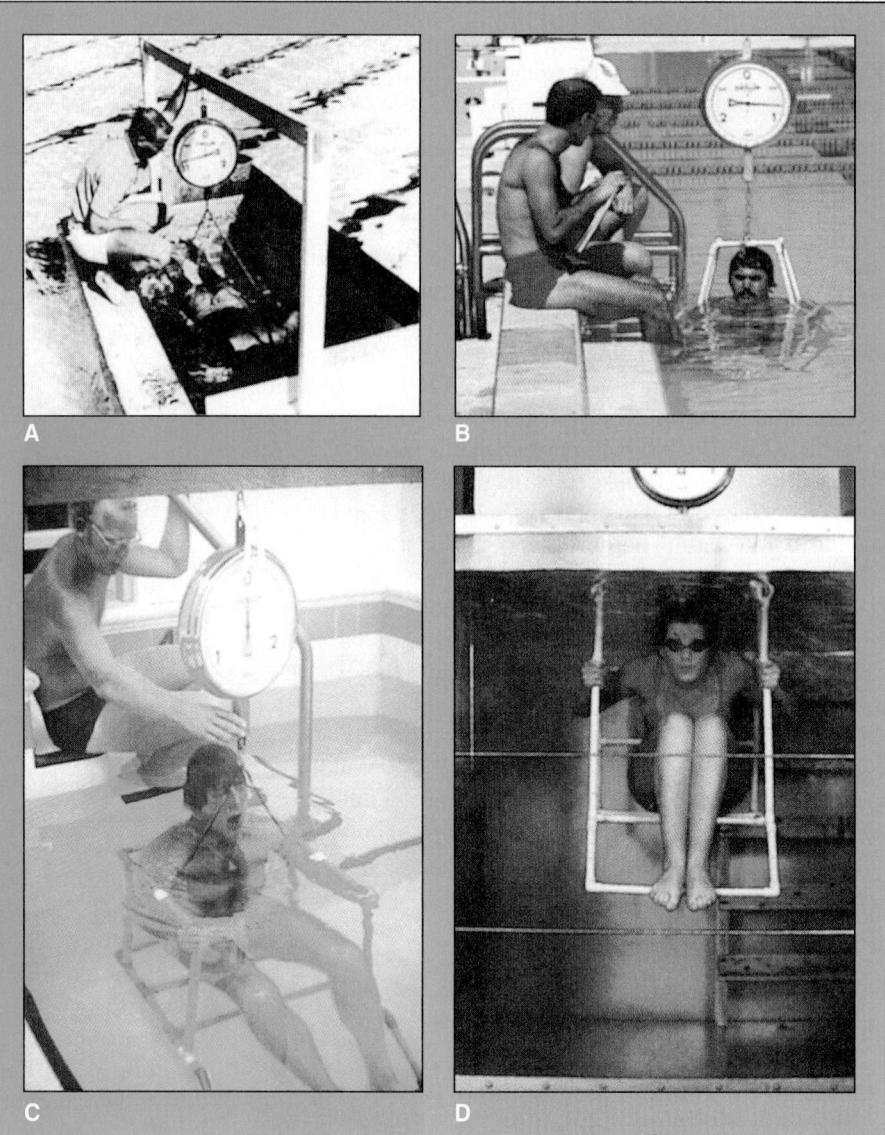

FIGURE 27.6

Measuring body volume by the procedure of underwater weighing. Prone and supine methods can be used for underwater weighing with no difference in results, and residual lung volume can be measured either before, during, or after the underwater weighing.[51] Measurements are taken (**A**) prone, (**B**) seated in a swimming pool, (**C**) seated in a therapy pool, and (**D**) upright in a stainless steel tank with Plexiglas® front in the laboratory. For any of the methods, a snorkel with nose clip can be used by subjects who are apprehensive about submersion. The underwater weight of these objects must then be accounted for in the final calculation of the subject's underwater weight.

exhibit anxiety while making forced maximal exhalations during submersion (or in younger or older subjects, the infirm or handicapped, or other special populations), a modified underwater weighing procedure can be substituted that does not require full-head submersion (subject seated with water level just below the chin) but yields values for body density almost identical to the standard, full-head-submersion procedure.[31]

Variations with Menstruation. Normal fluctuations in body mass (chiefly body water) related to the menstrual cycle are not large enough to affect body density and body fat assessed by hydrostatic weighing.[19, 135] In the small number of females who do experience perceptible changes in body mass (less than 1.0 kg) during menstruation, this alteration in total body water will affect body density and introduce some error in computing percent body fat.[18]

Calculating Body Composition from Body Mass, Body Volume, and Residual Lung Volume

Data from measurements on two professional football players who were "All-Pro" and played on Super Bowl teams are shown in Table 27.3.

The conventional formula for density is mass divided by volume, where density is expressed in $g \cdot cm^{-3}$, mass is in kilograms, and volume is in liters. The difference between M_a and W_w is equal to the body volume when the appropriate water temperature correction (D_w) is applied. Because air remaining in the lungs and any other gas remaining in the "spaces" of the body (abdominal viscera, sinuses) contribute to buoyancy at the time of underwater weighing, these volumes must be considered. In most subjects, abdominal gas and sinus air volumes are small (less than 100 mL) and can be ignored. *This is in contrast to the residual*

TABLE 27.3
BODY COMPOSITION MEASUREMENTS OF TWO PROFESSIONAL FOOTBALL PLAYERS USING THE UNDERWATER WEIGHING METHOD

Variable	Symbol	Defensive Lineman	Running Back
Body mass, kg	M_a	121.73	97.37
Net underwater weight, kg	M_w	7.30	6.52
Water temperature correction	D_w	0.99336	0.99336
Residual lung volume, L	RLV	1.213	1.374
Total body volume, L	TBV	113.89	90.08
Body density, g · cm⁻³	D_b	1.0688	1.0809

Body Composition			
Relative percent body fat, %[a]	% Fat	13.1	8.0
Absolute body fat, kg	FM	15.9	7.2
Fat-free body mass, kg	FFM	105.8	90.2

[a]Siri equation; % fat = [495/density] − 450.

lung volume, which is large and variable; it must be measured and subtracted from the total body volume.

Whereas the residual lung volume tends to be slightly less when measured while the subject is in water rather than air, probably a result of the compressing force of water against the thoracic cavity, the effect on computed body fat is small.[113, 120] Residual lung volume (RLV) can therefore be measured in air before underwater weighing without a loss in accuracy compared to the simultaneous measurement of residual volume with underwater weighing.[51]

The formula for calculating the density of the body (D_b) is as follows:

$$D_b = Mass_b \div Volume_b$$

$$= \frac{M_a}{\dfrac{M_a - W_w}{D_w} - RLV}$$

The lower part of Table 27.3 presents the body composition results based on the computation of body density.

FATFOLD AND GIRTH MEASUREMENTS

Hydrostatic weighing is the most widely used indirect laboratory method for assessing body volume. When laboratory facilities are unavailable, alternative and simpler procedures can be used to predict body fatness. Two of these procedures, measuring subcutaneous **fatfolds** and

girths (circumferences), require relatively inexpensive equipment.

Measurement of Subcutaneous Fatfolds

The rationale for fatfold measurements to estimate total body fat is based on a relationship between the fat located in the depots directly beneath the skin and both internal fat and body density.

The Caliper. By 1930, a special pincer-type caliper was being used to accurately measure subcutaneous fat at selected sites on the body. The caliper works on the same principle as the micrometer used to measure the distance between two points. The procedure for measuring fatfold thickness requires grasping firmly with the thumb and forefingers a fold of skin and subcutaneous fat and pulling it away from the underlying muscle tissue, following the natural contour of the fatfold. A constant tension of 10 g · mm⁻² is exerted by the pincer jaws of the calipers, regardless of jaw opening at the point of contact with the skin. The thickness of the double layer of skin and subcutaneous tissue is then read directly from the caliper dial and recorded in millimeters within two seconds after applying the full force of the caliper. This time limitation is imposed to avoid fatfold compression when taking the measurements.[5]

The Sites. The most common areas for taking fatfold measurements are at the triceps, subscapular, suprailiac, abdominal, and upper thigh sites. All measurements are taken on the right side of the body while the subject stands. A minimum of two or three measurements are made at each site, and the average value is used as the fatfold score. When fatfolds are measured for research purposes, the investigator generally has had considerable experience and should be consistent in duplicating values for the same subject made on the same day, consecutive days, or even weeks apart. Figure 27.7 illustrates the anatomic location of the five most frequently measured fatfold sites:

- Triceps—vertical fold measured at the midline of the upper arm halfway between the tip of the shoulder and the tip of the elbow.
- Subscapular—oblique fold measured just below the bottom tip of the scapula.
- Suprailiac—slightly oblique fold measured just above the hip bone; the fold is lifted to follow the natural diagonal line at this point.
- Abdominal—vertical fold measured 1 in. to the right of the umbilicus.
- Thigh—vertical fold measured at the midline of the thigh, two-thirds the distance from the middle of the patella (knee cap) to the hip.

Fatfolds also are sometimes taken on the medial, lateral, and posterior calf and on the anterior chest wall (men) at the level of the armpit. However, these measurements are

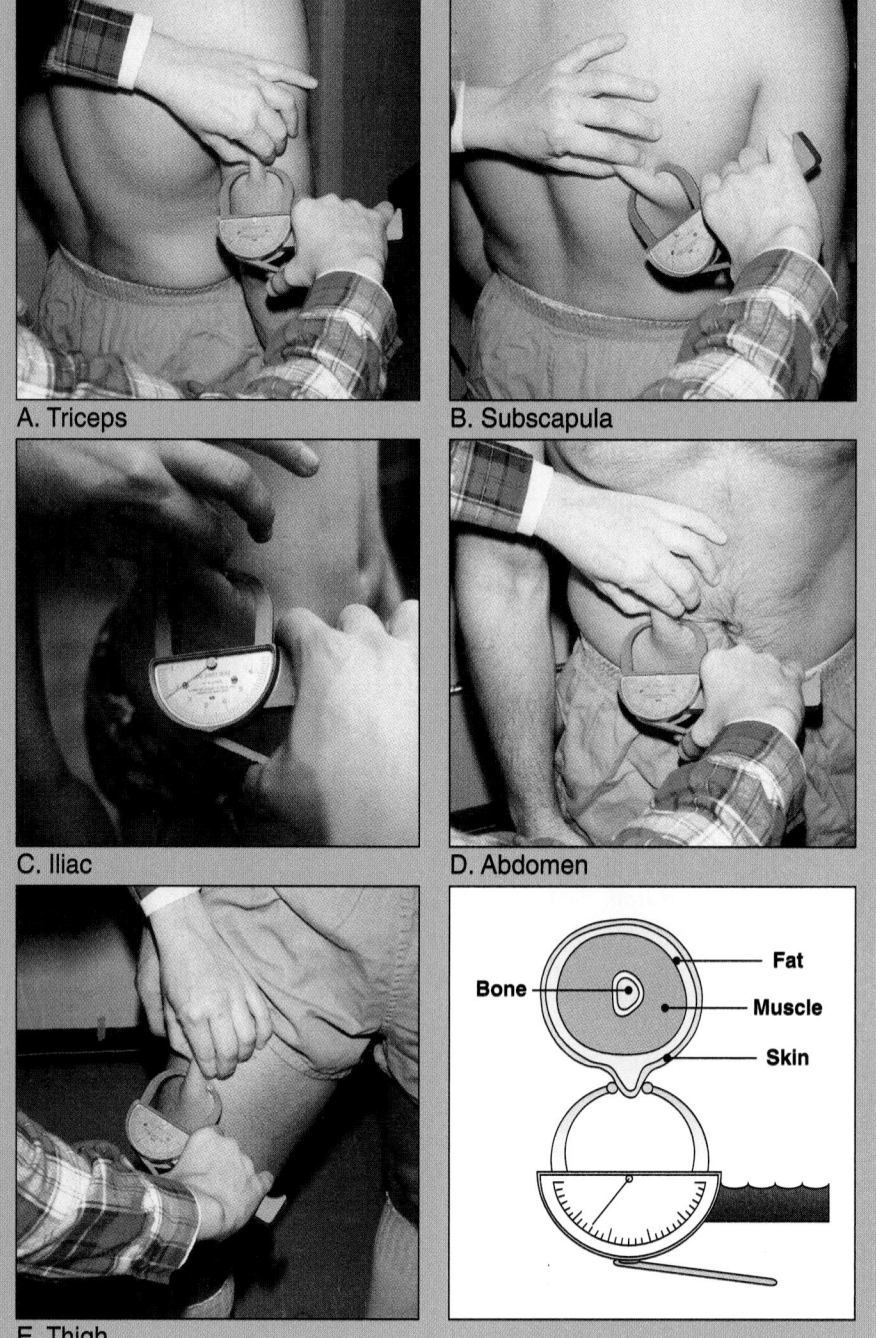

FIGURE 27.7

Anatomic location of five common fatfold sites: (**A**) triceps, (**B**) subscapula, (**C**) iliac (suprailiac), (**D**) abdomen, and (**E**) thigh. A schematic diagram of a fatfold caliper is shown at the lower right. Note that a double layer of skin and underlying tissue is compressed during the measurement. The measurements are taken in the vertical plane except at the subscapular and suprailiac, sites where they are taken diagonally.

often difficult to take depending on the degree of fatness of the individual.

Usefulness of Fatfold Scores

Fatfold measurements provide fairly consistent and meaningful information concerning body fat and its distribution.[45] There are basically two ways to use fatfolds. The first is to sum the scores as an indication of the relative degree of fatness among individuals. This "sum of fatfolds" can then also be used to reflect body fat changes "before" and "after" an intervention program. Changes in individual fatfold values and total scores can then be evaluated on either an absolute or percentage basis. From the fatfold data given in Table 27.4, obtained from a 22-year-old female college student before and after a 16-week exercise program, the following observations can be made:

- The largest changes in fatfold thickness occurred at the suprailiac and abdominal sites.
- The triceps showed the largest decrease and the subscapular the smallest decrease when changes were expressed as percentages.
- The total reduction in subcutaneous fatfolds at the five sites was 16.6 mm, or 12.6% of the "before" condition.

A second way to use fatfolds is in conjunction with mathematical equations designed to predict body density or percent body fat. These equations are "population specific" in that they predict fatness fairly accurately for subjects similar in age, sex, state of training, fatness, and probably race, when used with a similar group of individuals on which the equations were derived.[55, 66, 118] *When these criteria are met, the predicted value of fatness for an individual is usually within 3 to 5% of the body fat based on body density measurements using hydrostatic weighing.*

As a result of several experiments conducted in our laboratories, equations have been developed to predict body fat from triceps and subscapular fatfolds.[69–71] The equations most useful for predicting total body fat in young women and men are the following:

Young women, ages 17 to 26 years

Percent body fat = 0.55(A) + 0.31(B) + 6.13

Where A = triceps fatfold, mm
B = subscapular fatfold, mm

Young men, ages 17 to 26 years

Percent body fat = 0.43(A) + 0.58(B) + 1.47

Where A = triceps fatfold, mm
B = subscapular fatfold, mm

Using the fatfold data of the young woman who participated in the 16-week physical conditioning program, we can compute her percent body fat before and after the condition-

ing program using the equation for young women. Substituting the pretraining values for triceps (22.5 mm) and subscapular (19.0 mm) fatfolds, percent body fat equals 24.4%.

$$\text{Percent body fat} = 0.55(A) + 0.31(B) + 6.13$$
$$= 0.55(22.5) + 0.31(19.0) + 6.13$$
$$= 12.38 + 5.89 + 6.13$$
$$= 24.4\%$$

Substituting the values for triceps (19.4 mm) and subscapular (17.0 mm) fatfolds, the post-training value for percent body fat of 22.1% is computed in a similar fashion.

$$\text{Percent body fat} = 0.55(19.4) + 0.31(17.0) + 6.13$$
$$= 10.67 + 5.27 + 6.13$$
$$= 22.1\%$$

The determination of percent body fat before and after a physical conditioning and weight-control program provides a convenient means to evaluate alterations in body composition that often are independent of changes in body mass.

Fatfolds and Age

In young adults, approximately one-half of the body's total fat is subcutaneous fat, and the remainder is internal or organ fat. With advancing age, a proportionately greater quantity of total fat is deposited internally compared to subcutaneous fat.[43] Thus, the same fatfold score reflects a greater total percent body fat as one gets older. *For this reason, age-adjusted equations, or* **generalized equations,** *must be used when predicting body fat from fatfolds or girths in older adult men and women.*[55, 90, 118, 139]

User Beware

Although the use of fatfolds to predict percent body fat has been widespread in the allied health professions, a major drawback is that to obtain consistent values, the person taking the measurements must have considerable experience in the proper techniques. With extremely obese people, the thickness of the fatfold often exceeds the width of the caliper's jaws. The particular caliper used may also contribute to the measurement error.[90] It is difficult to determine which sets of fatfold data are the best to use because there are no standards to compare the results between different investigators in diverse geographic regions. Thus, prediction equations developed by a particular researcher (which may be highly valid for the sample measured) may result in large predictive errors when applied by another person to fatfolds taken from a dissimilar group. The error in predicting body fat could be ±200% or higher![66]

The surface area formula method described below may provide a more valid estimate of body fat for use with diverse populations, although limitations are still present.[74]

**TABLE 27.4
CHANGES IN SELECTED FATFOLDS FOR A
YOUNG WOMAN DURING A 16-WEEK
EXERCISE PROGRAM**

Fatfolds, mm	Before	After	Absolute Change	Percent Change
Triceps	22.5	19.4	−3.1	−13.8
Subscapular	19.0	17.0	−2.0	−10.5
Suprailiac	34.5	30.2	−4.3	−12.8
Abdomen	33.7	29.4	−4.3	−12.8
Thigh	21.6	18.7	−2.9	−13.4
Sum	131.3	114.7	−16.6	−12.6

The basic equation is as follows:

$$\% \text{ Fat} = \frac{\Sigma \text{ fatfolds}}{3F \times k(sf)}$$

Where Σ fatfolds is the sum of two or more fatfold sites, depending on availability; $3F = 3\sqrt{\text{mass/stature}}$ (where mass is in kilograms and stature is in decimeters); and k(sf) = fatfolds/3F × % fat. Percent fat is based on a criterion method such as underwater weighing and on the observed average of the group or population (of a particular age, sex, state of training, or sport) to which the equation is being applied. Thus, different k(sf) constants are required for diverse populations. For example, consider the mean values for a population that represents relatively sedentary young men: stature = 18.42 dm, mass = 72.16 kg, fatfolds = 67.3 mm, and % fat = 15.3. The k(sf) constant is calculated as follows:

$$k(sf) = \frac{67.3}{3\sqrt{3.9175 \times 15.3}} = 0.741$$

By first calculating a k(sf) constant based on group data, the percent body fat for any similar individual can be computed with the basic equation. If mass = 74.0 kg, stature = 17.52 dm, and the sum of 5 fatfolds = 57.5 mm, percent fat for this particular young man is computed as follows:

$$\% \text{ fat} = \frac{\Sigma \text{ fatfolds}}{3F \times k(sf)}$$

$$\% \text{ fat} = \frac{57.5}{6.166 \times 0.741}$$

$$\% \text{ fat} = 12.6\%$$

This was the method used to estimate the body fat content of the two champion body builders whose data are displayed in Chapter 28, Figure 28.10. For the reference group of body builders, 3F was 6.666, percent fat was 6.4, the sum of five fatfolds was 30.4 mm, and k(sf) was 0.71818.

Measurement of Girths

A linen or plastic measuring tape is applied lightly to the skin surface so that the tape is taut but not tight. This procedure avoids the skin compression that produces lower than normal scores. Duplicate measurements are taken at each site, and the average is used. Figure 27.8 displays the anatomic landmarks for the various girths commonly used to assess fatness.

- **Abdomen**—1 in. above the umbilicus.
- **Hips**—maximum protrusion with the heels together.
- **Right thigh**—upper thigh just below the buttocks.
- **Right upper arm (biceps)**—palm up, arm straight and extended in front of the body, measurement taken at midpoint between the shoulder and elbow.
- **Right forearm**—maximum girth with the arm extended in front of the body and palm up.
- **Right calf**—widest girth midway between the ankle and knee.

Different prediction equations have been developed for each sex and various age groups.[69, 138, 139] The equations developed for these subgroups, although cross-validated on different samples with good results, are nevertheless population specific and should not be used to predict fatness in individuals who (a) appear very thin or very fat or (b) have been involved for a number of years in strenuous endurance sports or activities with substantial resistance training components.[70]

Usefulness of Girth Measurements

The girth-based prediction equations are most useful in ranking or ordering individuals within a group according to relative fatness. As with fatfold measures, girths can also be used to predict body density and/or percent body fat. *If one uses the equations and constants presented in Appendix E for young and older men and women, the error in predicting an individual's body fat is generally ±2.5 to 4.0%.* These relatively small prediction errors make the equations particularly useful to those without access to laboratory facilities: a tape measure is inexpensive and the measurements are easy to take. Specific equations based on girth have been developed to estimate the body compositions of obese adult men and women.[146] Along with predicting percent body fat, girth measurements are also well suited, in obese people, to determining patterns of fat distribution in the body as well as changes in body fat during weight loss.[56, 141]

Target Body Fat from Changes in Abdominal Girth

A method has been devised to calculate a desired percent body fat based on a target change in abdominal girth.[77] The individual attempts to achieve a target percent body fat through a fat loss as reflected by a reduced waist girth. In this different approach, the question is asked, "How much does the abdominal girth need to be reduced to achieve a desired percent body fat?"

In the following example, excess abdominal girth (measured at the level of the umbilicus) is calculated based on a "desired" level of fatness representing the 50th percentile for the population:

Step 1. A target abdominal girth expressed in centimeters is computed as the product of (body mass, kg ÷ stature, m) and a constant (Q) (at the 50th percentile for percent body fat: Q is 12.36 for males and 14.25 for females). For example, in a male with an abdominal girth of 89.7 cm, body mass of 85.5 kg, and stature of 1.876 m, 85.5 ÷ 1.876 = 6.751. This value is then multiplied by Q (12.36) to yield the target abdominal girth of 83.4 cm.

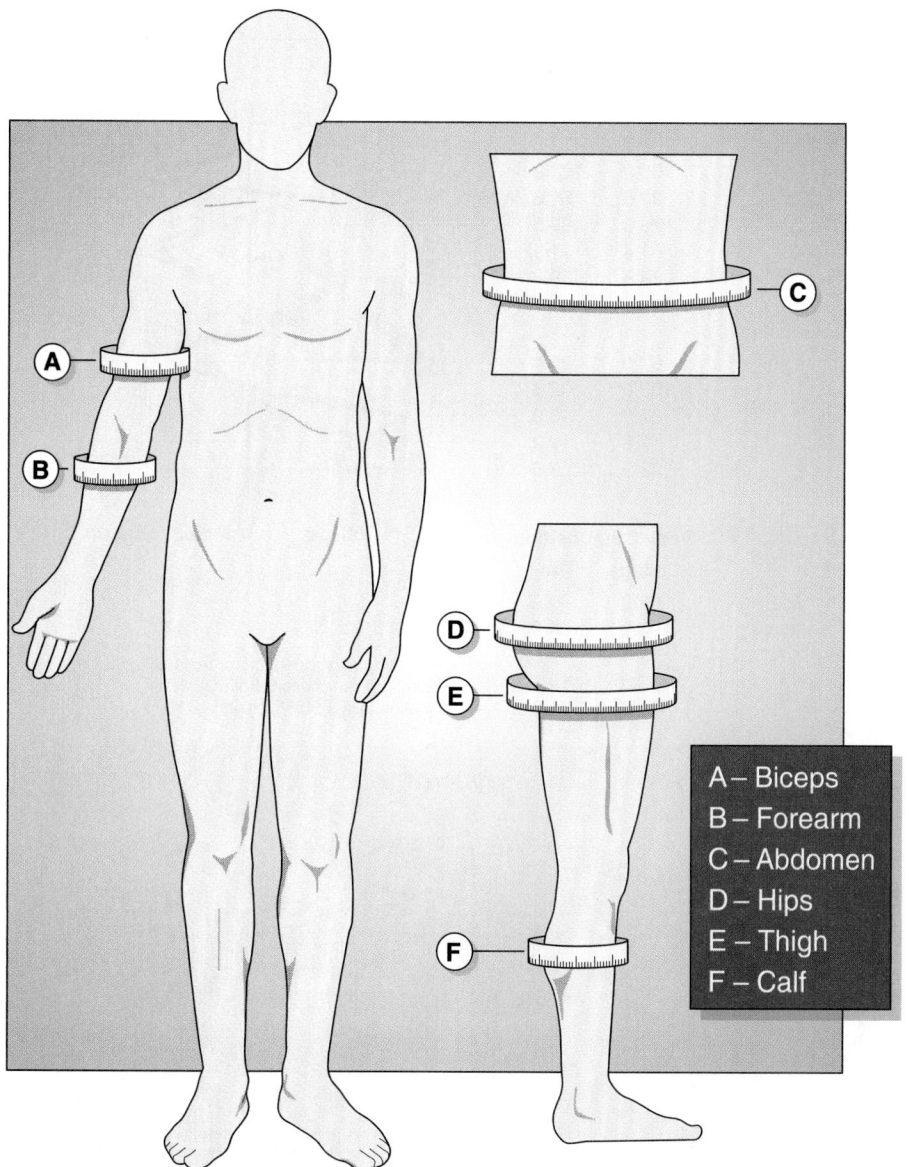

FIGURE 27.8
Anatomic landmarks for measuring various body girths.

A – Biceps
B – Forearm
C – Abdomen
D – Hips
E – Thigh
F – Calf

Step 2. Excess abdominal girth is computed as the measured abdominal girth, 89.7 cm in the above example, minus the target abdominal girth of 83.4 cm from Step 1. This difference of 6.3 cm (89.7 cm − 83.4 cm) is the excess girth. This person would then attempt to reduce abdominal girth by 6.3 cm. When this goal is reached, percent body fat will correspond to approximately the 50th percentile.

An important consideration with this approach is to decide the target or desired level of percent body fat. If different percentile values for body fat are desired, then different Q values must be used in Step 1. (See reference 77 for specific Q values.) Because this is a new approach to the quantification of determining excess body fat based on abdominal girth, future research is needed to refine and extend the applicability of the different Q constants used in Step 1.

APPLICATION OF SURFACE ANTHROPOMETRY: THE BODY PROFILE

A matrix of 11 girths can be integrated into a muscular and nonmuscular "body profile," illustrated in Figure 27.9, to provide a quantitative assessment of body shape.[6, 68, 76] If the anthropometric proportions of the individual conformed to group symmetry, all of the deviation values on the body profile would fall within ±2% units of the vertical, or zero-deviation, reference line.

The practical application of the body profile method of analysis allows one to quantify the relative proportions of the body's girth dimensions and chart any **changes** in these physical dimensions resulting from such factors as acute and chronic training, dietary intervention, or the influence of aging.[67] The body profile method also permits quantification of

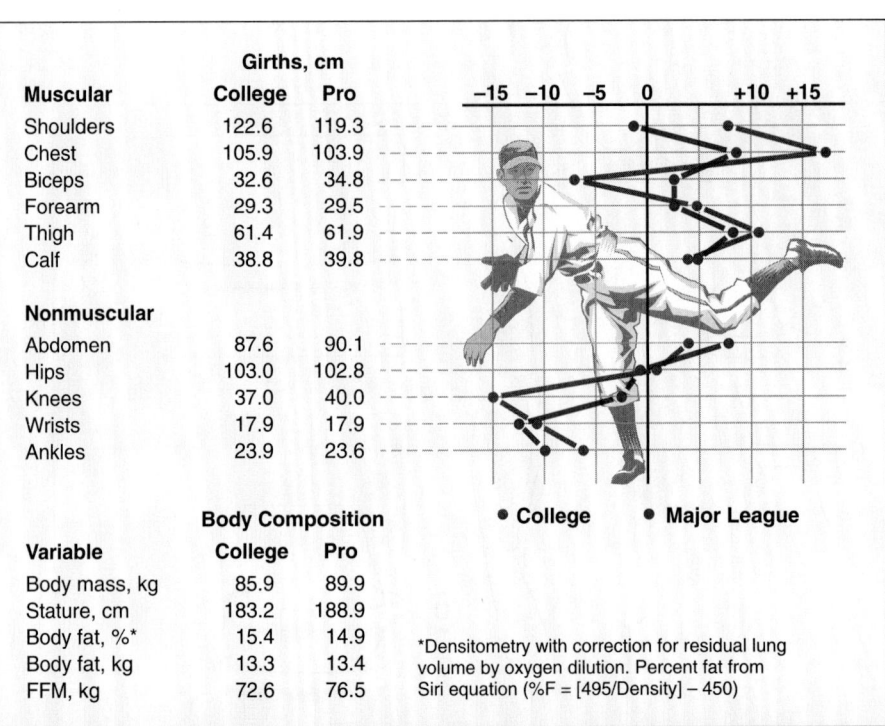

Girths, cm		
Muscular	**College**	**Pro**
Shoulders	122.6	119.3
Chest	105.9	103.9
Biceps	32.6	34.8
Forearm	29.3	29.5
Thigh	61.4	61.9
Calf	38.8	39.8
Nonmuscular		
Abdomen	87.6	90.1
Hips	103.0	102.8
Knees	37.0	40.0
Wrists	17.9	17.9
Ankles	23.9	23.6

● College   ● Major League

Body Composition		
Variable	**College**	**Pro**
Body mass, kg	85.9	89.9
Stature, cm	183.2	188.9
Body fat, %*	15.4	14.9
Body fat, kg	13.3	13.4
FFM, kg	72.6	76.5

*Densitometry with correction for residual lung volume by oxygen dilution. Percent fat from Siri equation (%F = [495/Density] − 450)

FIGURE 27.9

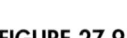

Top, Body profile analysis using the girth technique to display the muscular and nonmuscular areas of the body in relation to standards established for the reference man and reference woman as indicated by the vertical line. The examples are Division I university baseball pitchers (N = 9; University of Massachusetts, Amherst) and major league baseball pitchers (N = 23; Boston Red Sox). *Bottom,* Age trends in girth patterns for females ages 4 to 64 years. Note that the waist (designated a nonmuscular region) increases progressively in girth from age 30 to age 64. If all of the girths were to remain in relative proportion as individuals aged, there would be no positive deviations in the body profile, and all of the measurements would plot as a vertical line, as they do for the reference woman at ages 20 to 24. Refer to references 68 and 76 for details about constructing the body profile.

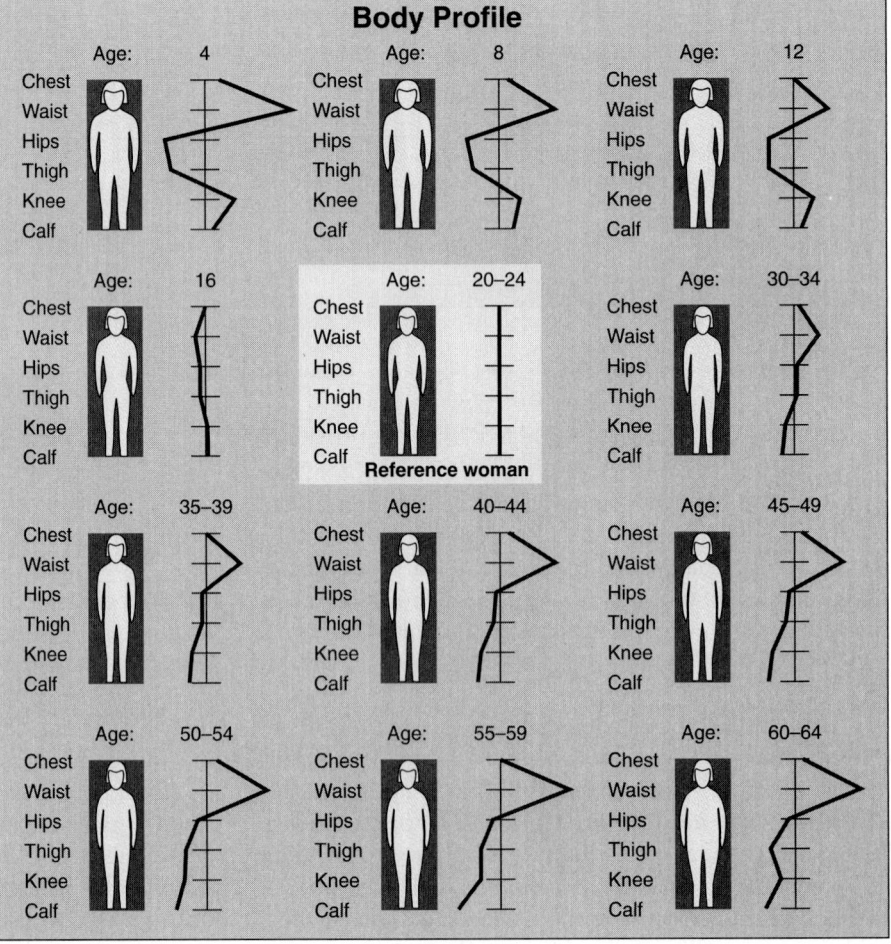

differences in physique between athletes in different sports (for example, gymnasts versus long distance swimmers) or within the same sport (football defensive linemen versus quarterbacks, or small versus large body builders).

BIOELECTRICAL IMPEDANCE ANALYSIS

Bioelectrical impedance analysis (BIA) is based on the concept that electrical flow is facilitated through hydrated fat-free body tissues and extracellular water compared to fat tissue because of the greater electrolyte content (and, thus, lower electrical resistance) of the fat-free component. Consequently, impedance to the flow of electric current will be directly related to the quantity of body fat. In the BIA technique, injector electrodes are placed on the dorsal surfaces of the foot and wrist, and detector electrodes are placed between the radius and ulna (styloid process) and at the ankle (between the medial and lateral malleoli). A painless, localized electrical signal is introduced, and the impedance or resistance to current flow is determined. The impedance value is then converted to body density (adding body mass and stature and sometimes several girths to the equation), which in turn is converted to percent body fat by use of the Siri or other similar equation (see p. 551).

One factor affecting the accuracy of BIA is the subject's hydration level, as either hypohydration or hyperhydration will alter the normal electrolyte concentrations in the body, which affects current flow independent of real changes in body composition.[4, 57, 63, 96] More specifically, a loss of body water will decrease the impedance measure and yield a lower percent fat, whereas hyperhydration produces the opposite effect. Skin temperature (influenced by ambient conditions) also affects whole-body resistance and, thus, the prediction of body fat using BIA. Predicted body fat is significantly lower in a warm environment (less impedance to electrical flow) than in a cold environment.[4, 21] Even under conditions of normal hydration and environmental temperature, the resulting prediction of body fat may be questionable compared to values obtained from hydrostatic weighing, with the tendency being to overpredict body fat in lean and athletic subjects and underpredict fat in the obese.[49, 94, 125] The technique may be less accurate than the various anthropometric methods that use girths and fatfolds to predict body fat.[57, 134] There also is the complicating statistical consideration of including body size variables (stature, body mass, girths) in the regression equation to predict body fat because the factors all are highly intercorrelated. This practice can generate spurious relationships and essentially invalidate the very criterion variables of interest. There is also conflicting evidence as to whether the technique can detect small changes in body composition during weight loss.[35, 121] *At best, BIA is another noninvasive, indirect, relatively easy means for a general assessment of body composition, provided measurements are made under conditions strictly standardized in terms of ambient temper-* *ature and level of hydration, and with the understanding that the validity of the "software" used to generate the resulting criterion values may be subject to statistical uncertainty.*

NEAR-INFRARED INTERACTANCE

Near-infrared interactance, or **NIR,** is based on technology developed by the U.S. Department of Agriculture to assess the body composition of livestock. The commercial version used with humans (Futrex-5000) employs principles of light absorption and reflection to assess the composition of the body. A fiber optic probe, or light "wand," emits a low-energy beam of near-infrared light into the single measuring site at the anterior midline surface of the biceps of the dominant arm. A detector within the same probe measures the intensity of the re-emitted light, expressed as optical density. Shifts in the wavelength of the reflected beam as it interacts with organic material in the arm are entered into the manufacturer's prediction equation (along with the subject's stature and mass, estimated frame size, sex, and physical activity level) to provide a rapid determination of percent body fat and fat-free body mass. The equipment is safe, portable and lightweight, and requires minimal training to use. In addition, there is relatively little physical contact with the subject during measurement. These aspects of test administration help to explain the popularity of this technique for body composition assessment in health clubs, hospitals, and weight-loss centers. However, many concerns have been expressed about this technology.

Questionable Validity of NIR

Early research with this technology indicated a significant relationship between spectrophotometric measures of light interactance at various sites on the body and body composition assessed by total body water.[29] Subsequent research with humans, however, was less than supportive in documenting the validity of NIR when compared to a variety of techniques such as hydrostatic weighing and fatfold measurements. From the objective data available, it appears that NIR is of limited value in accurately predicting body fat across a broad range of body fat levels. Several investigations indicate that NIR is less accurate than fatfold measures in assessing percent body fat.[22, 54, 134] In one study, NIR overestimated body fat in lean men and women and underestimated fat in fatter subjects.[104] As shown in Figure 27.10, fatfold measurements more accurately predicted body fat than NIR, especially at extremes of the body fat continuum when hydrostatic weighing was used as the criterion for percent body fat. An error of greater than 4% body fat units was noted in more than 47% of the subjects, with the greatest errors noted at the extremes of body fatness. Furthermore, NIR produced large errors (both standard error of estimate and total prediction error) when estimating percent body fat in both children and adolescents[20] and underestimated body fat in college football players.[50] *Currently, available objective data do not support the use of NIR as an important measurement technique for validly assessing the composition of the human body.*

ULTRASOUND ASSESSMENT OF FAT

Ultrasound is used for body composition assessment in a variety of disciplines to determine either the thicknesses of different tissues (fat and muscle) or obtain an image of deeper tissues, such as a limb's muscle cross-sectional area. The basic idea of ultrasound is to convert electrical energy through a probe and receiver into high-frequency (pulsed) sound waves that penetrate the skin surface and enter the tissues, then reflect back to the probe. After the sound waves pass through adipose tissue, they then pass through the muscle layer and are reflected from the fat-muscle interface (after reflection from a bony surface), producing an echo, which returns to the probe. In the simplest type of ultrasound, for which there is no image of the underlying tissues (known as A-mode), the time required for sound wave

transmission through the tissues and back to the transducer is converted to a distance score and displayed on a light-emitting diode scale that represents fat or muscle thickness. It is then simply a matter of comparing fatfolds or cross-sectional area of a muscle with the corresponding data from ultrasound.[62] In the more expensive and technically demanding B-mode ultrasound, a two-dimensional image provides considerable detail and differentiation of tissues.[53]

The reliability of repeat measurements of subcutaneous fat thickness at multiple sites and with the subject in the lying and standing positions is high ($r > 0.85$), as is the association between measures made on different days.[52, 62] The ultrasound technique may be especially useful with the obese, for whom variation in compression of subcutaneous body fat with fatfold measures is greatest.[85] The uses of ultrasound for "mapping" muscle and fat thicknesses at different body regions and quantifying changes in topographical fat patterns are valuable adjuncts in the assessment of body composition.[53] In hospitalized patients, ultrasonic determination of fat and muscle thickness can help in evaluation of nutritional status during periods of weight loss and gain. Ultrasonic imaging techniques also are available as medical

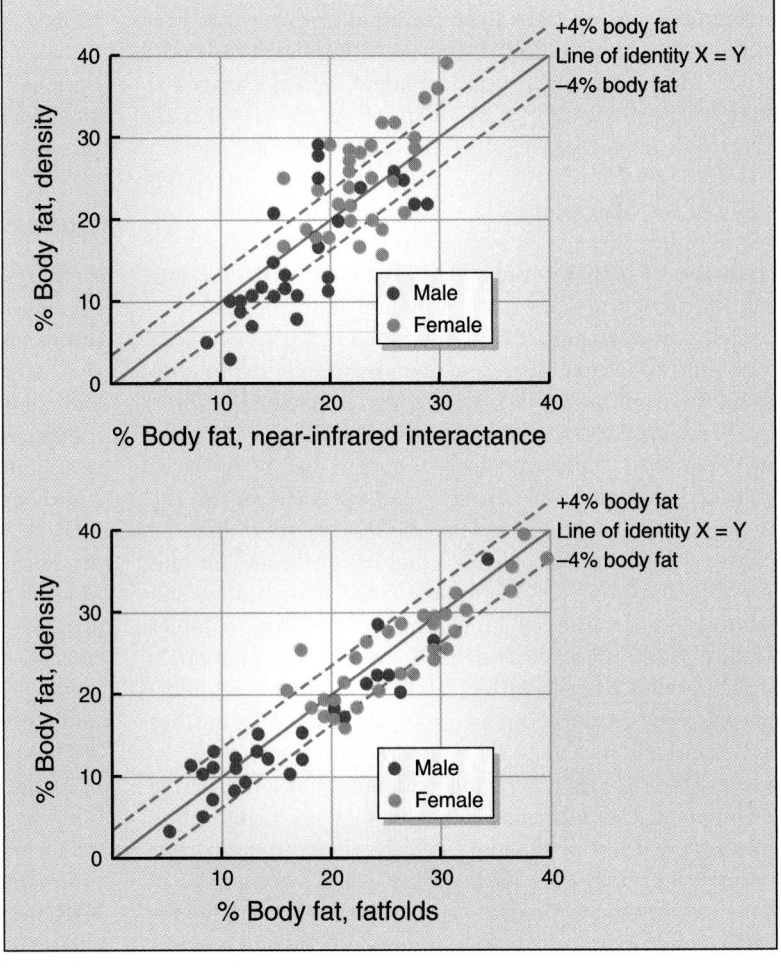

FIGURE 27.10

Comparison of near-infrared interactance (Futrex-5000) (*top*) and fatfolds (*bottom*) for assessing percent body fat. (From McLean, K., and Skinner, J.S.: Validity of Futrex-5000 for body composition determination. *Med. Sci. Sports Exerc.*, 24:253, 1992.)

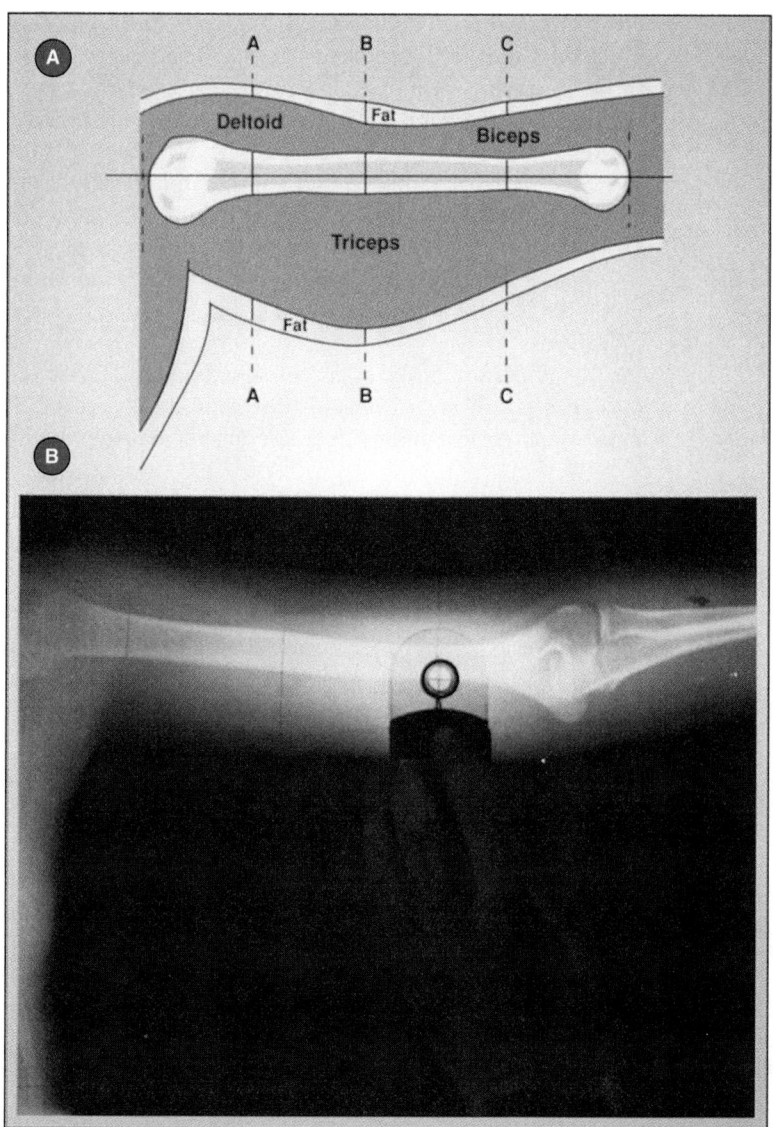

FIGURE 27.11

A, Schematic drawing of a radiograph of the arm of a 24-year-old female. The six fat widths are represented by the vertical lines drawn perpendicular to the long axis of the humerus at points *A, B,* and *C.* There is a demarcation on the radiograph between fat, muscle, and bone that permits an accurate assessment of radiographic widths. Total body fat determined from this radiograph was 23.6%; by underwater weighing, body fat was 23.3%. **B,** The technician is using a digitizer to calculate fat width on the radiograph. The information from the digitizer is processed by a computer to a printer and graphics plotter. (Line art and photo from Drs. A.R. Behnke and F.I. Katch.)

diagnostic devices to assess growth and development of various tissues, including fetal development, and assess structural function in the heart and other organs. In imaging devices, the reflected sound waves from the soft tissues are converted to a real-time image for convenient visualization or measurement via computer digitization (area, volume, diameter) directly from the image. With the introduction of color and multiple-frequency imaging, it now is possible to more easily trace the course of blood flow through organs and tissues or make use of miniaturized probes for much clearer identification of internal tissues, vessels, and organs.

ARM X-RAY ASSESSMENT OF FAT

The arm radiograph is a useful method for analyzing body composition; it permits reliable and valid quantification of body fat.[64, 65] The objective of x-ray assessment is to provide a direct and unambiguous estimate of fat deposition. The thicknesses of the fat layers at points A, B, and C shown in Figure 27.11 are transformed into a body fat value for the individual using the fatfold-surface area equation on page 557. The only difference in the equation is that the fat thickness from the roentgenogram is substituted for fatfolds. The k constant is derived in the same manner and differs among individuals depending on age, level of fitness, and race.[63, 64] The validity of the x-ray procedure was determined by comparing values of fatness based on the roentgenogram with body fat values determined by hydrostatic weighing. The relationship between the two methods was high (correlation of r = 0.90 in young and older, white and black men and women). For an individual, the conversion of the x-ray widths of fat to total body fat percentage was accurate to within ±3% units of body fat determined hydrostatically. This degree of accuracy is slightly higher than that for estimates of body fat derived from fatfolds or girths. Applications of the x-ray procedure also include the assessment of muscle size, which is useful in studying body composition with training and aging, as well as in clinical evaluations of nutritional status.[33]

COMPUTED TOMOGRAPHY (CT), MAGNETIC RESONANCE IMAGING (MRI), AND DUAL-ENERGY X-RAY ABSORPTIOMETRY (DEXA)

Computed Tomography (CT)

CT imaging procedures produce radiographic images of different segments of the body. In the CT method, detailed cross-sectional, two-dimensional images of the body are obtained when an x-ray beam (ionizing radiation) passes through tissues of different densities. Through the use of appropriate computer software, pictorial and quantitative information can be obtained from the CT scan for the areas of total tissue, total fat and muscle, and thickness and volume of tissues within an organ. Figure 27.12A to C illustrates CT scans of both upper legs and a cross section at the midthigh in a professional walker who completed an 11,200-mile walk through the 50 United States in 50 weeks.

A comparison of CT scans before and after the walk indicated a significant increase in the total cross section of muscle and corresponding decrease in subcutaneous fat in

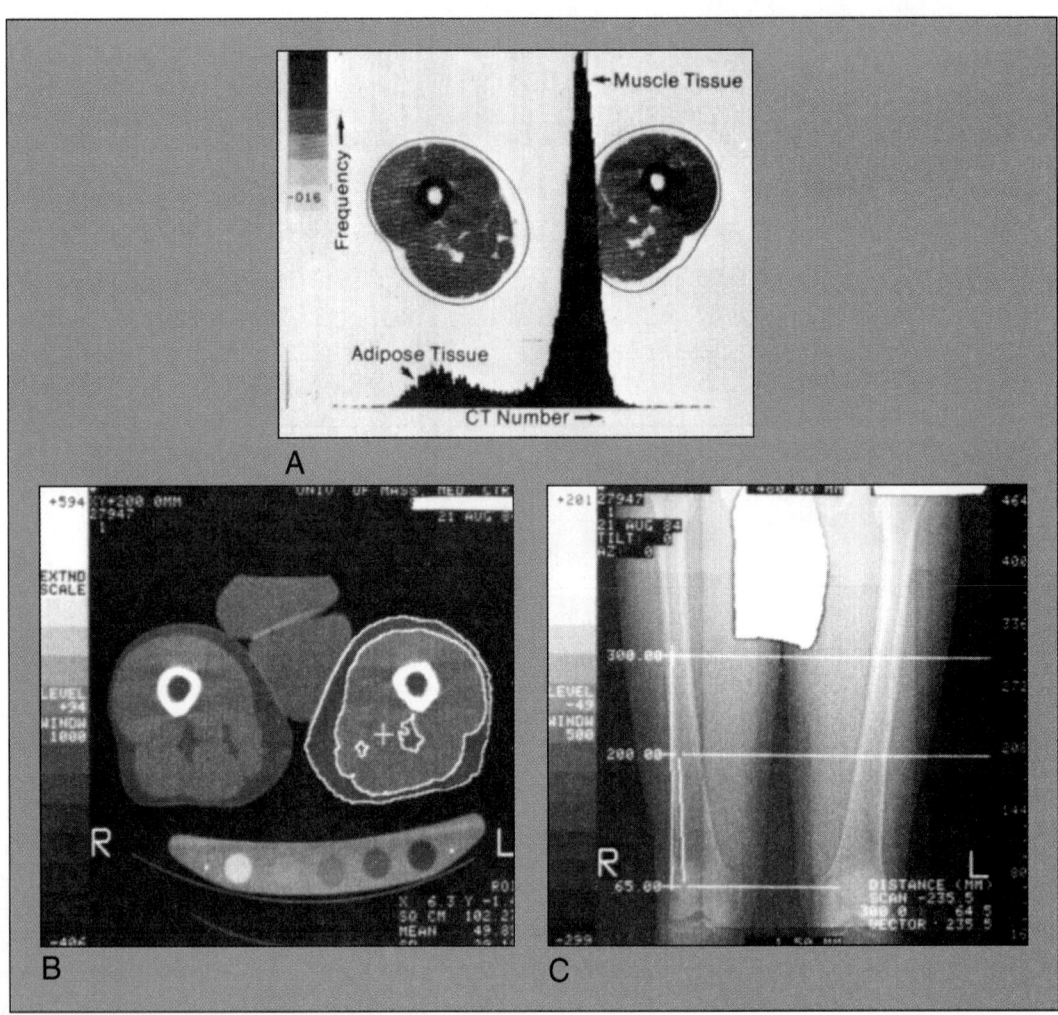

FIGURE 27.12
Computed tomography (CT) scans. **A,** Plot of pixel elements illustrates the extent of adipose and muscle tissue in a cross-section of the thigh. The two other views show a cross section of the midthigh (**B**) and an anterior view of the upper legs (**C**) before a 1-year walk across the United States by a champion walker. (CT scans are courtesy of Dr. Steven Heymsfeld, Obesity Research Center, St. Luke's-Roosevelt Hospital, Columbia University, College of Physicians and Surgeons, New York.)

the midthigh region. Many other studies have demonstrated the efficacy of using CT scans to evaluate the relationship between simple anthropometric measures at the abdominal region (fatfolds and girths) and total adipose tissue volume measured from single or multiple "slices" through the abdominal region.[2, 13, 86, 126] In a Canadian cohort of 110 men, deep and total abdominal adipose tissue accumulation was determined by CT scan at the L4-L5 region, including subcutaneous fat thickness and waist girth.[30] Figure 27.13 illustrates the significant correlation of r = 0.82 between waist girth and deep abdominal adipose tissue (AT) area, showing that men with larger waist girth had a greater amount of AT located deep within the abdominal region. This relationship using abdominal girth was stronger than that between subcutaneous fat thickness and deep AT. When the subjects were separated by BMI (less than 28 and greater than 28), the relationship between waist girth and AT was considerably stronger for the men with BMIs less than 28. In other words, a higher percent body fat was an important correlate of total AT in the visceral region in both subgroups. For men with BMIs greater than 28, it also was clear that a greater degree of total body fat was associated with a greater amount of abdominal AT evaluated by CT scan. For both groups, the amount of error in predicting abdominal AT from CT scan was approximately 30% of the mean amount of abdominal AT. Nevertheless, a higher abdominal AT was associated with a greater risk of diabetes, disorders of the blood lipid profile, hypertension, and cardiovascular disease. In Chapter 29, we discuss risk factors associated with abdominal obesity of the AT type.

Magnetic Resonance Imaging (MRI)

The newer technology of MRI provides valuable, noninvasive information about the body's tissue compartments. With MRI, electromagnetic radiation (not ionizing radiation as in CT scans) in the presence of a strong magnetic field is used to excite the hydrogen nuclei of the body's water and lipid molecules. This causes the nuclei to give off a detectable signal that can then be rearranged under computer control to visually represent the various body tissues. Figure 27.14 is a color-enhanced MRI transaxial image of the midthigh of a 30-year-old, male middle-distance runner. Using appropriate computer software, the muscle cross-sectional area of the thigh (blue area) is computed minus the fat and bony tissues (lighter color areas). MRI has been used effectively to quantify total and subcutaneous adipose tissue in individuals of varying degrees of body fatness. These values are used to evaluate changes in such parameters as a muscle's lean and fat components following resistance exercise training or during different stages of growth and aging. Because the MRI procedure is widely accepted for purposes of medical diagnosis, the question can be raised as to whether MRI imaging is valid for body compo-

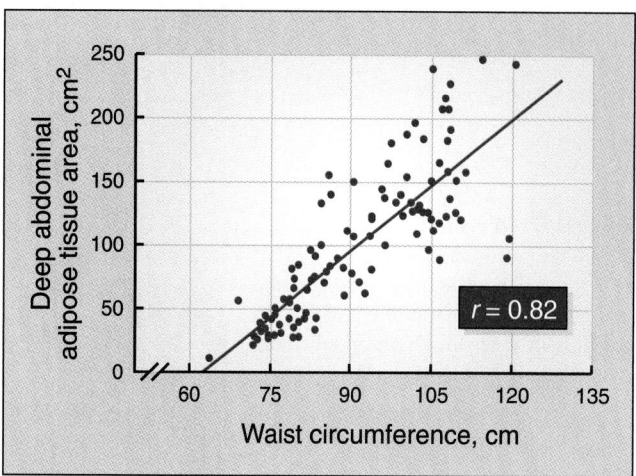

FIGURE 27.13

Relationship between deep abdominal adipose tissue determined by CT scan and waist girth in 110 men, ages 18 to 42 years, who varied widely in percent body fat determined by densitometry ($\bar{X}$ = 22.9%; range 2.2% to 39.9%). The best predictors of deep abdominal fat included (a) abdominal fatfold thickness in mm, (b) waist girth in cm, and (c) waist-hip ratio. Deep abdominal fat (cm²) = −363.12 + [−1.113 (a)] + [3.478 (b)] + [186.7 (c)]. For example, if abdominal fatfold = 23.0 mm, waist girth = 92.0 cm, and waist ÷ hip ratio = 0.929, then by substitution in the equation, deep abdominal fat = 104.7 cm². (Modified from Déspres, J.,-P., et al. Estimation of deep abdominal adipose-tissue accumulation from simple anthropometric measurements in men. *Am. J. Clin. Nutr.*, 54:471, 1991.)

sition evaluation in the exercise and sport sciences. In other words, how does MRI imaging for quantifying muscle mass or body fat compare to the standard criterion methods to evaluate body composition?

Figure 27.15 (*top*) is a plot of percent body fat determined by underwater weighing and MRI scanning in 20 Swedish women, ages 23 to 40. Underwater weighing was determined using the same procedures described on pages 553 to 554, and percent body fat based on MRI scanning was determined from 30 transaxial images taken along the length of the body. An area representing fat was determined within each image, and total body fat was computed as the sum of the fat determined from the calves, thighs, lower and upper trunk, and lower and upper arm components. Agreement between the two independent estimates of body fat (r = 0.84) was good, thus validating the MRI procedure for body fat quantification. The relationships were also of the same magnitude between total body fat determined by MRI, underwater weighing, and total body water, another valid procedure for estimating the body's fat content.[43, 105]

The bottom of Figure 27.15 displays the distributions of subcutaneous fat, nonsubcutaneous fat, and the sum of the

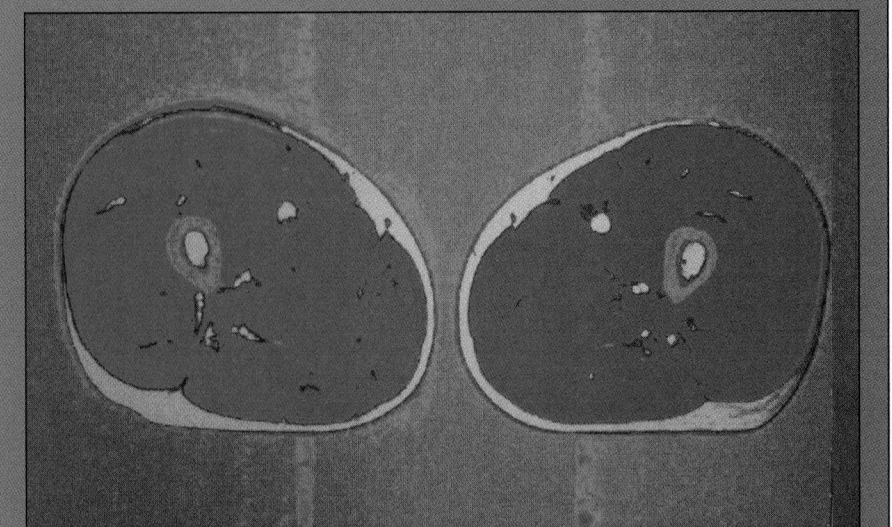

FIGURE 27.14
Magnetic resonance imaging (MRI) scan of the midthigh of a 30-year-old male middle-distance runner. (MRI scan courtesy of J. Staab, Department of the Army, USARIEM, Natick, MA.)

two in different body regions. The bar graphs are arranged left to right from the smallest to the largest depots of fat. There was more fat, both subcutaneous and nonsubcutaneous, compared to total body fat in the lower trunk region (38.5%) than in the other areas. The lower arm region contained the smallest amount of fat in the body (2.7%). The lower right graph displays the amount of body fat in each body compartment as a percentage of total MRI-determined fat. Of the total amount of fat determined by MRI (21,830 mL), subcutaneous fat accounted for 75.2%. Because nonsubcutaneous fat accounts for the remaining 24.8% of the total fat determined by MRI imaging, it seems fair to state that "excess" fat probably is deposited to a greater extent in the subcutaneous tissues than elsewhere.

Comparison of Lean and Obese

Seventeen tissue slices in a group of lean and obese females have been compared for total and subcutaneous AT volume at 4 anatomically defined sites measured between the top of the patella and the sternal notch. In the lean women, body fat determined by densitometry was 25.4% and BMI was 20.6; in contrast, the body fat of the obese women was 42.4% and BMI was 42.4. The family of graphs in Figure 27.16 displays the differences between the lean and obese females in total body fat (sum of fatty and nonfatty tissues), total AT, and subcutaneous AT at the 17 sites. The results show a fairly consistent pattern in the assessment of MRI-derived AT volumes. The obese subjects had 165% more subcutaneous AT and 155% greater total AT. The largest regions of fat accretion were in the abdominal and upper thigh areas. Interestingly, the lean women had greater nonfatty AT at some sites (upper thorax and lower thigh regions). The inset graph shows the strong relationship between percent

MRI-determined body adipose tissue (using 4 instead of 17 sites) and percent body fat determined by underwater weighing in the obese and lean subjects. The technique of MRI yields a wealth of information for accurately estimating aspects of body composition applied to total and regional areas of the body in diverse groups of subjects. Future acute and longer term studies should be conducted with different athletic groups and during separate and combined regimens of dietary manipulation and exercise training.

Dual-Energy X-Ray Absorptiometry

Dual-energy x-ray absorptiometry (DEXA) is another high-technology imaging procedure that permits quantification of fat and muscle, as well as bone mineral content (BMC) of the deeper bony structures of the body.[95, 101] DEXA is an accepted clinical tool for assessing spinal osteoporosis and other related bone disorders. The underlying principle of DEXA is that the bone and soft tissue areas can be penetrated to a depth of about 30 cm by two distinct energy peaks from a source of the high-activity isotope gadolinium-153 (^{153}Gd). The penetration is analyzed by a scintillation detector. With the subject lying supine on a table, the source and detector are passed across the body at a relatively slow speed of 1 cm · s^{-1}. A DEXA scan of the whole body takes about 12 minutes. Specialized computer software reconstructs an image of the underlying tissues, permitting the quantification of BMC, total fat mass, and fat-free body mass. Selected trunk and limb regions also can be pinpointed for a more in-depth analysis of tissue composition.

Previous studies have confirmed that DEXA provides excellent corroboration with other independent estimates of BMC, yielding estimates that are within approximately 1% of each other.[117] Strong relationships also were obtained be-

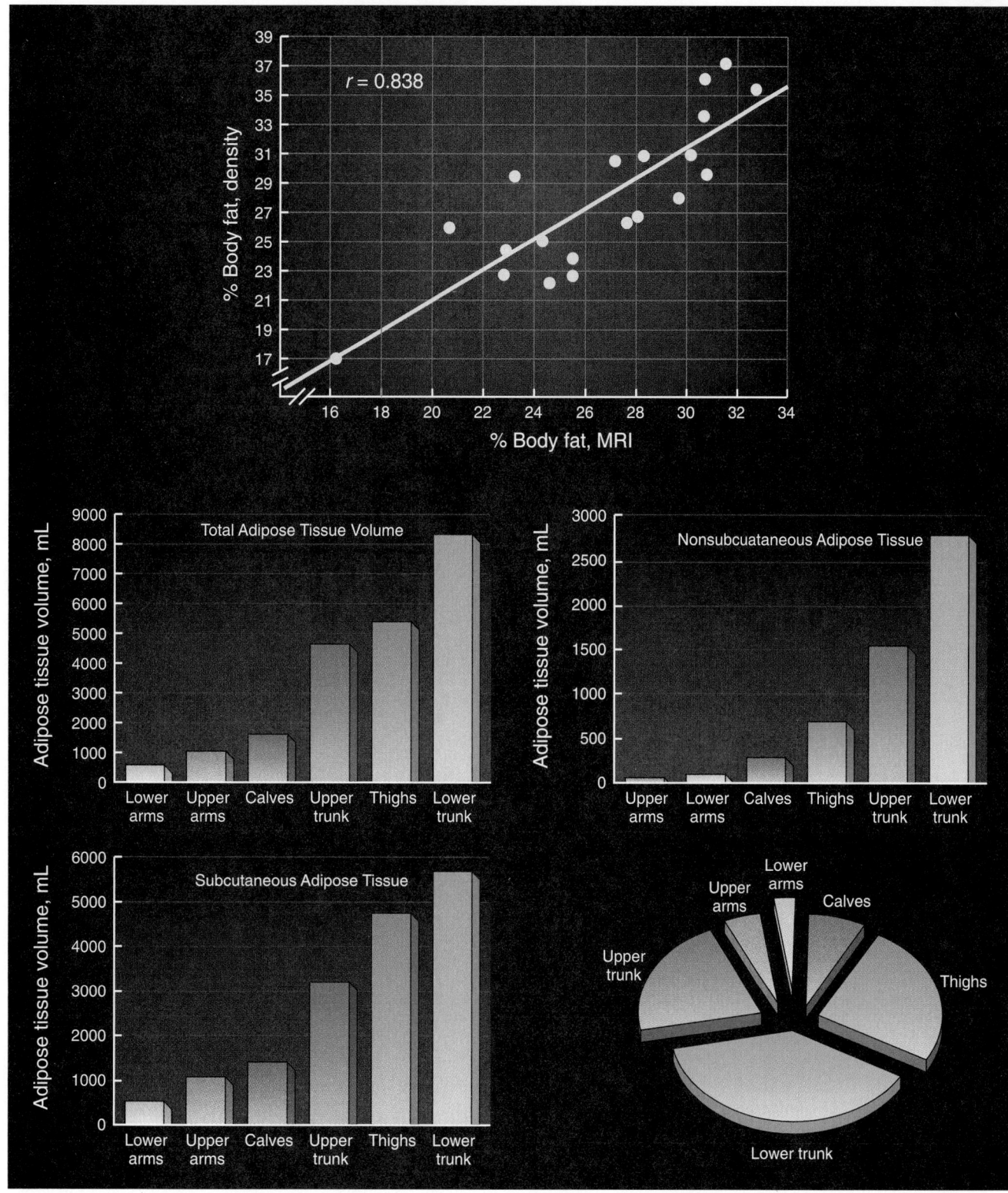

FIGURE 27.15

Top, Relationship between percent body fat determined by underwater weighing and MRI scanning (graph created from individual data points presented in the original article). The total amount of fat from the MRI scans was determined from each of 30 images taken along the length of the body. The area of fat was determined from each image by tracing the outline within the tissue slice. Adipose tissue was assumed to contain 80% lipid with a density of 0.9000 g · cm⁻³, 2% protein with a density of 1.34 g · cm⁻³, and 18% water with a density of 0.999 g · cm⁻³. This gave a density for adipose tissue of 0.9225 g · cm⁻³. The volume of adipose tissue was converted to fat weight as the product of 0.9225 × 0.8. Total fat was the sum of fat determined from the calves, thighs, lower and upper trunk, and lower and upper arms. *Bottom,* Distribution of adipose tissue (total, subcutaneous, nonsubcutaneous) within the various body compartments. Arrangement is from largest to smallest. The lower right graph displays the percentage distribution of adipose tissue in the different body regions. (Modified from Sohlstrom, A., et al.: Adipose tissue distribution as assessed by magnetic resonance imaging and total body fat by magnetic resonance imaging, underwater weighing, and body-water dilution in healthy women. *Am. J. Clin. Nutr.,* 58:830, 1993.)

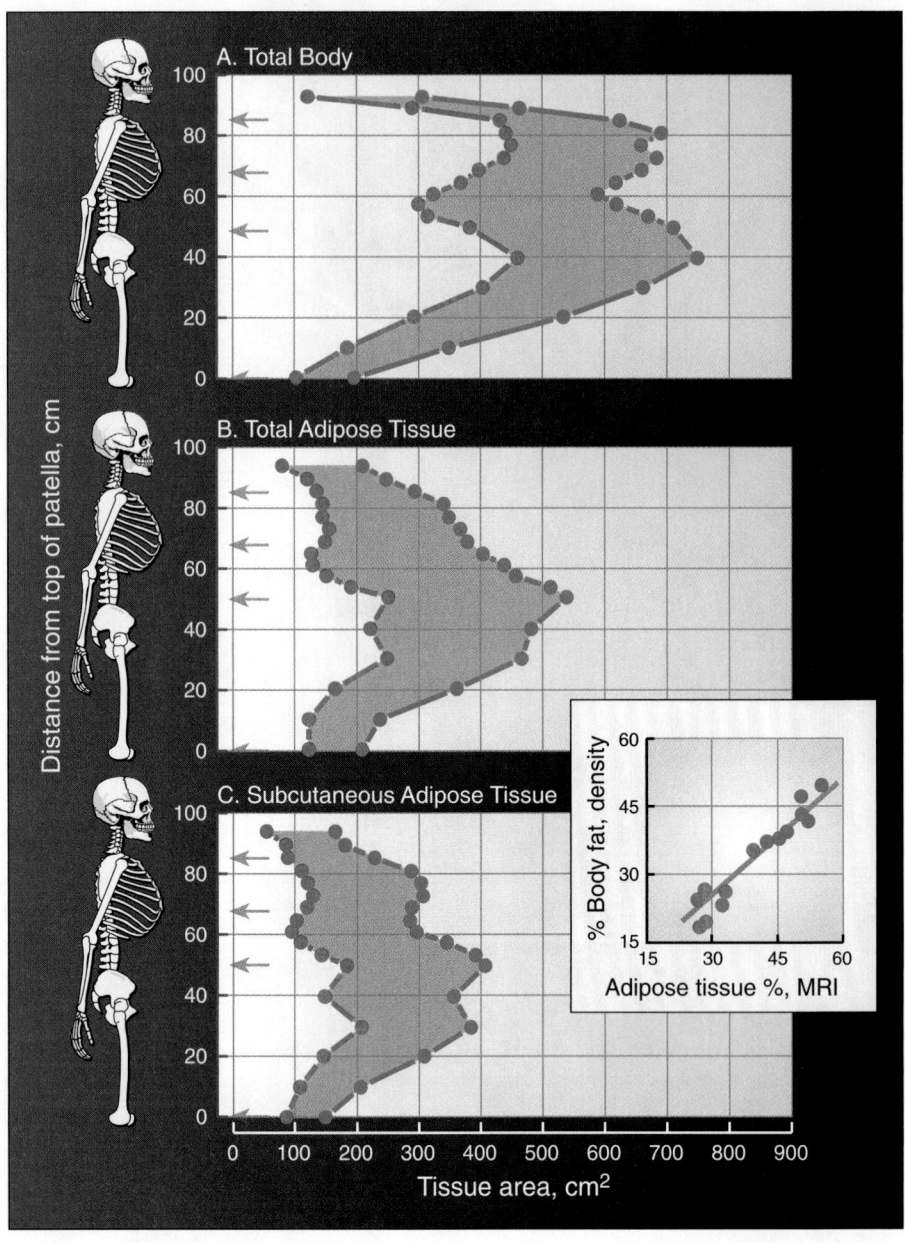

FIGURE 27.16

Distribution of total body tissues (sum of fatty and nonfatty tissues) (*top*), total adipose tissue (*middle*), and subcutaneous adipose tissue (*bottom*) in seven lean (red) and seven obese (blue) females. The four anatomical markers in relation to position on the skeleton are shown by arrows to the right of the y axis. The inset graph displays the relationship between percent body adipose tissue (using four instead of 17 sites) and percent total body fat determined by underwater weighing in the obese and lean subjects. (Modified from Fowler, P.A., et al.: Total and subcutaneous adipose tissue in women: the measurement of distribution and accurate prediction of quantity by using magnetic resonance imaging. *Am. J. Clin. Nutr.*, 54:18, 1991.)

tween total body fat determined by DEXA and percent body fat determined by densitometry,[47, 102] segmental body composition (upper and lower extremity mass), total body potassium (K^{40}), and total body nitrogen.[103] Figure 27.17 displays the nearly linear relationship obtained between DEXA and densitometric estimates of percent body fat in young, middle-aged, and older men and women. In this study, prediction of percent body fat (from densitometry) was not as strong for older and fatter subjects but within the range normally obtained between discrete methodologies. In contrast, using a more robust model of body composition assessment, the error was less than 2% between DEXA and densitometry in a heterogeneous age group of adults.[48]

DEXA and Body Composition in Anorexia Nervosa. DEXA is used to evaluate the skeletal and re-

gional body composition characteristics in anorexia nervosa. Figure 27.18 gives an example of an anorexic female and a typical female whose body fat percentage averages 25% of her total body mass of 56.7 kg (125 lb). The average body mass was 44.4 kg (97.9 lb) in the 10 anorexic women measured in this study; although their average fat-free mass was close to the normal value of 43.0 kg, body fat only was 7.5%, a value nearly three times lower than comparison groups of "normal" young females. All the women had been anorexic for at least 1 year, and the average length of amenorrhea was 3.1 years (range 1 to 8 years). The insert table compares the bone mineral density (BMD, g · cm^{-2}) in the anorexic females to a group of normal-fat females. The values in the right column represent the percentage values of BMD for different regional body areas in the anorexic group in rela-

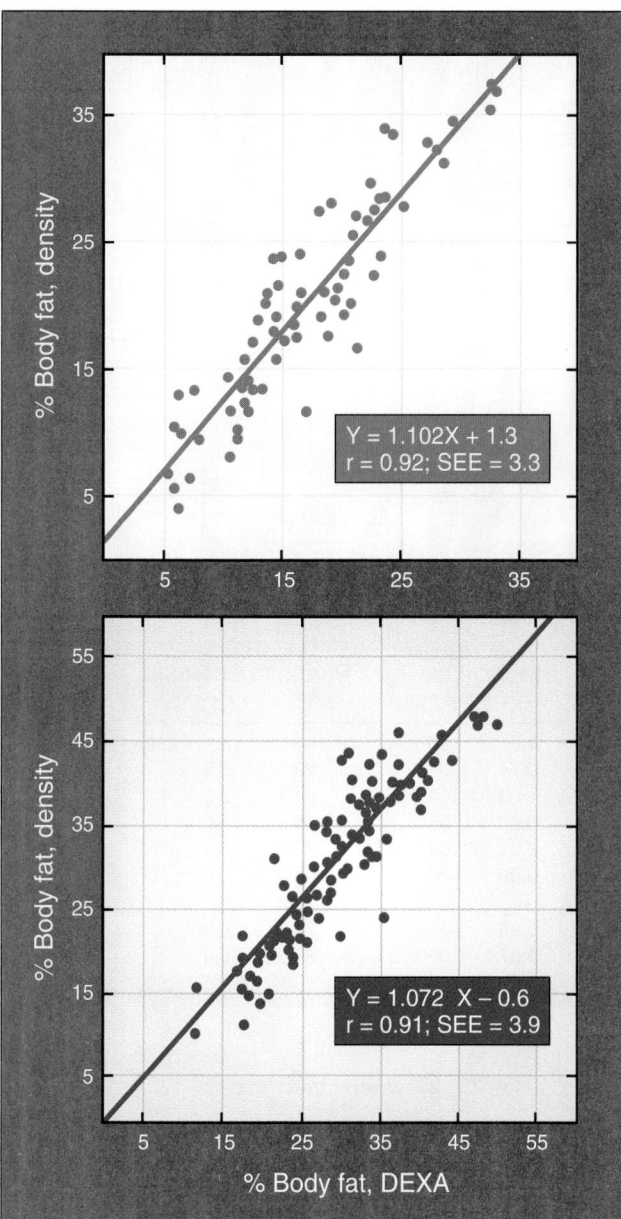

FIGURE 27.17

Comparison of total body fat determined by densitometry and DEXA in men (*top*) and women (*bottom*). The insert box includes the regression prediciton equation, correlation coefficient, and standard error of estimate. (Modified from Snead, D.B., et al.: Age-related differences in body composition by hydrodensitometry and dual-energy absorptiometry. *J. Appl. Physiol.,* 74:770, 1993.)

tion to a normal comparison group of 287 females age 20 to 40 years. Total body BMD was about 10% lower, the L2-L4 region of the spine was 27% less, and the femoral neck BMD was 13% below comparable values in the normal group. The spine BMD in the young anorexic group was identical to the average BMD in 70-year-old women. The researchers concluded that the diminished BMD in the anorexics, along with a small skeletal size, may render them

particularly susceptible to osteoporotic fractures at a younger age than expected for comparison groups.

WHAT IS AVERAGE FOR PERCENT BODY FAT?

Average values for body fat in samples of men and women throughout the United States are presented in Table 27.5. Also included are values representing ±1 standard deviation to give some indication of the amount of variation or spread from the average: the column headed "68% Variation Limits" indicates the range of values for percent body fat that fall within one standard deviation from the average, or about 68 of every 100 persons measured. As an example, the average percent body fat of young men from the New York sample is 15.0%, and the 68% variation limits are from 8.9 to 21.1% body fat. Interpreting this statistically, it could be expected that for 68 out of every 100 young men measured, values for percent fat would range between 8.9 and 21.1%. Of the remaining 32 young men, 16 would possess more than 21.1% body fat, while of the other 16 men, body fat would be less than 8.9%.

Representative Samples Are Lacking

Although considerable data are available concerning average body composition for many groups of men and women of different ages and fitness levels, there has been no systematic evaluation of the body composition of representative samples from the general population that would warrant setting up precise norms or recommended values for body composition. At this time, the best we can do is present the average values from various studies of different age groups.

A general conclusion based on the currently available data is that with increasing age, the percentage of body fat tends to rise in both men and women. This average change does not necessarily mean that the trend should be interpreted as desirable or "normal," because participation in vigorous physical activity throughout life can retard the "average" fat increase with age.[59, 87, 140] Changes in body composition with age could occur because the aging skeleton becomes demineralized and porous; such a process reduces body density because of the decrease in bone density. Another reason for the relative increase in body fat with age is a reduction in the level of daily physical activity. A more sedentary lifestyle could increase the deposition of storage fat and reduce the quantity of muscle mass. This would occur even if the daily caloric intake remained unchanged.

DESIRABLE BODY MASS

Although an excess of body fat is undesirable for good health and fitness, an optimal level of body fat or body mass for a particular individual cannot be precisely stated. More than likely, this optimum varies from person to

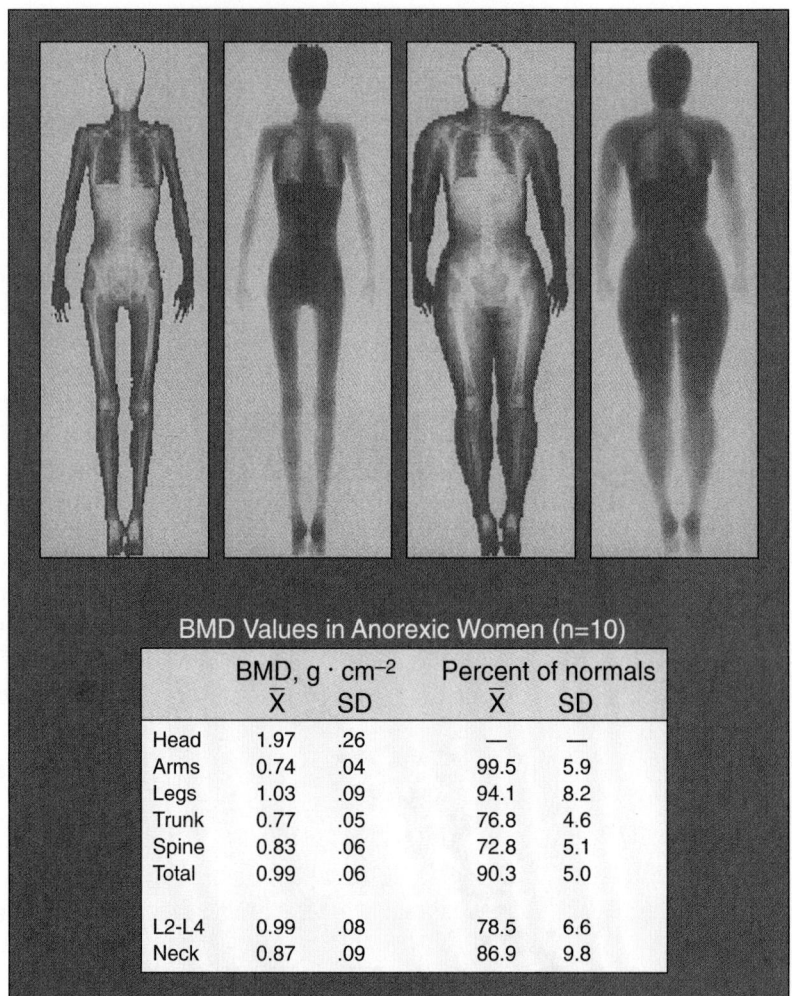

FIGURE 27.18

Example of an anorexic female *(two left images)* and a typical female *(two right images)* whose body fat percentage averages 25% of her total body mass of 56.7 kg (125 lb). The average anorexic subject weighed 44.4 kg (97.9 lb) and was 7.5% body fat estimated by DEXA from the fat percentages at the arms, legs, and trunk regions. The values in the right column of the insert table present the percentage values for bone mineral density (BMD) for different regional body areas in the anorexic group compared to a group of 287 normal females aged 20 to 40 years. (Photo courtesy of R.B. Mazess, Department of Medical Physics, University of Wisconsin, Madison, WI, and the Lunar Radiation Corporation, Madison, WI. Data from Mazess, R.B., et al.: Skeletal and body composition effects of anorexia nervosa. Paper presented at the International Symposium on In Vivo Body Composition Studies, June 20–23, Toronto, Ontario, Canada, 1989.)

BMD Values in Anorexic Women (n=10)

	BMD, g · cm^{-2}		Percent of normals	
	X̄	SD	X̄	SD
Head	1.97	.26	—	—
Arms	0.74	.04	99.5	5.9
Legs	1.03	.09	94.1	8.2
Trunk	0.77	.05	76.8	4.6
Spine	0.83	.06	72.8	5.1
Total	0.99	.06	90.3	5.0
L2-L4	0.99	.08	78.5	6.6
Neck	0.87	.09	86.9	9.8

person and is greatly influenced by genetic factors. *Based on data from physically active young adults, it would be desirable in our opinion to strive for a body fat content of 15% for men (certainly less than 20%) and about 25% for women (less than 30%).* An "optimal" or "desirable" body mass can be computed using a desired level of body fat as follows:

$$\text{Desirable body mass} = \frac{\text{Fat-free body mass}}{1.00 - \text{Desired \% fat}}$$

Suppose a 91-kg (200-lb) man with 20% body fat wishes to know how much weight to lose to attain a body fat composition of 10%. The computations would be as follows:

Fat mass

= 91 kg × .20

= 18.2 kg

Fat-free body mass

= 91 kg − 18.2 kg

= 72.8 kg

Desirable body mass

= 72.8 kg ÷ (1.00 − 0.10)

= 72.8 kg ÷ 0.90

= 80.9 kg (178 lb)

**Desirable fat loss =
Current body mass — Desirable body mass**

= 91 kg − 80.9 kg

= 10.1 kg (22.2 lb)

If this man lost 10.1 kg of body fat, his new body mass of 80.9 kg would have a fat content equal to 10% of body mass. These calculations assume no change in fat-free body mass with weight loss.

ON THE HORIZON

Recently, a procedure has been perfected for estimating body volume that holds considerable promise as an alternative to densitometry for assessing diverse groups of sub-

TABLE 27.5
AVERAGE VALUES OF PERCENT BODY FAT FOR YOUNGER AND OLDER WOMEN AND MEN FROM SELECTED STUDIES

Study	Age Range	Stature, cm	Mass, kg	% Fat	68% Variation Limits
Younger women					
North Carolina, 1962	17–25	165.0	55.5	22.9	17.5–28.5
New York, 1962	16–30	167.5	59.0	28.7	24.6–32.9
California, 1968	19–23	165.9	58.4	21.9	17.0–26.9
California, 1970	17–29	164.9	58.6	25.5	21.0–30.1
Air Force, 1972	17–22	164.1	55.8	28.7	22.3–35.3
New York, 1973	17–26	160.4	59.0	26.2	23.4–33.3
North Carolina, 1975		166.1	57.5	24.6	—
Army Recruits, 1986	17–25	162.0	58.6	28.4	23.9–32.9
Massachusetts, 1996	17–30	165.2	57.8	21.8	16.7–27.8
Older women					
Minnesota, 1953	31–45	163.3	60.7	28.9	25.1–32.8
	43–68	160.0	60.9	34.2	28.0–40.5
New York, 1963	30–40	164.9	59.6	28.6	22.1–35.3
	40–50	163.1	56.4	34.4	29.5–39.5
North Carolina, 1975	33–50	—	—	29.7	23.1–36.5
Massachusetts, 1993	31–50	165.2	58.9	25.2	19.2–31.2
Younger men					
Minnesota, 1951	17–26	177.8	69.1	11.8	5.9–11.8
Colorado, 1956	17–25	172.4	68.3	13.5	8.3–18.8
Indiana, 1966	18–23	180.1	75.5	12.6	8.7–16.5
California, 1968	16–31	175.7	74.1	15.2	6.3–24.2
New York, 1973	17–26	176.4	71.4	15.0	8.9–21.1
Texas, 1977	18–24	179.9	74.6	13.4	7.4–19.4
Army Recruits, 1986	17–25	174.7	70.5	15.6	10.0–21.2
Massachusetts, 1996	17–30	178.1	76.4	12.9	7.8–18.9
Older men					
Indiana, 1966	24–38	179.0	76.6	17.8	11.3–24.3
	40–48	177.0	80.5	22.3	16.3–28.3
North Carolina, 1976	27–50	—	—	23.7	17.9–30.1
Texas, 1977	27–59	180.0	85.3	27.1	23.7–30.5
Massachusetts, 1993	31–50	177.1	77.5	19.9	13.2–26.5

jects.[103a] The method is rapid (3–5 minutes), reproducibility of values is high, and validity is excellent compared to densitometry (r = 0.99; standard error of measurement less than 2% body fat). The method is an adaptation of air displacement plethysmography first reported in the late 1800s[87a] and in the 1950s using helium as the gas.[130a, 130b] With this new procedure, a subject sits inside a small chamber (marketed commercially as BOD POD.[29a] By means of electronics and computer software, body volume is measured accurately from the known physical relationships between the temperature, pressure, and volume of the ambient air surrounding the person in the chamber (taking into account air volume in the lungs and thorax). The ease of use, accuracy, and rapidity of measurement make this method potentially attractive for use in clinical and research settings.

■ SUMMARY ■

1. Standard "height-weight" tables reveal little about an individual's body composition and may vary considerably for any given body mass and stature. Studies of athletes clearly indicate that one can be overweight but not overfat.

2. Total body fat consists of essential fat and storage fat. Essential fat is the fat present in bone marrow, nerve tissue, and the various organs; it is not a labile energy reserve

but required for normal biologic function. Storage fat is the energy reserve that accumulates mainly as adipose tissue beneath the skin and in visceral depots.

3. Although storage fat values for men average 12% of body mass, and storage fat values for women average 15% of body mass, the essential fat differences are large between sexes and amount to 3% of body mass for men and 12% for women. This difference probably is related to child-bearing and hormonal functions.

4. It appears that a person cannot reduce fat below the essential fat level and still maintain good health.

5. Menstrual dysfunction occurs among certain groups of female athletes, particularly women who train hard and maintain low levels of body fat. The precise interaction between the physiological and psychological stress of intense, regular training, hormonal balance, energy and nutrient intake, and body fat requires further study.

6. The delayed onset of menarche observed in chronically active young females may confer health benefits because such individuals show a lower lifetime occurrence of reproductive organ and other cancers.

7. The two most popular indirect methods of body composition assessment are hydrostatic weighing and prediction methods from fatfolds and girths. Hydrostatic weighing involves the determination of body density and the subsequent estimation of percent body fat. This computation assumes a constant density for the body's compartments of fat and fat-free tissues. Fat-free body mass is calculated by subtracting fat mass from body mass.

8. Part of the error inherent in predicting body fat from whole-body density lies in the assumptions concerning the densities of the body's fat and fat-free components. These densities, especially that of the fat-free body mass, differ from assumed constants because of race, age, and athletic experience. Currently, firm data are lacking for improving the theoretically based constants.

9. Common methods to assess body composition employ equations developed from relationships between selected fatfolds and girths and body density and percent fat. These equations are "population specific": they are most accurate with subjects similar to those from whom the equations were derived. A surface-area formula based on body stature and body mass and fatfolds also can be used to estimate body composition in diverse groups of different ages.

10. Bioelectrical impedance analysis (BIA) is based on the concept that electrical flow is facilitated through hydrated fat-free body tissues and extracellular water compared to fat tissue because of the greater electrolyte content of the fat-free component. Consequently, impedance to the flow of electric current will be directly related to the quantity of body fat. BIA is a noninvasive, indirect means for general assessment of body composition, provided measurements are made under strictly standardized conditions.

11. Ultrasound, x-ray, computed tomography, magnetic resonance imaging, and dual-energy x-ray absortiometry are other indirect techniques for assessing body composition. Each has its unique application and special limitations for expanding our knowledge of the compositional components of the human body.

12. Based on data from physically active young adults, it is probably desirable to consider as average a body fat content of 15% for men and 25% for women. These averages serve as a frame of reference for evaluating deviations and excess accumulations of body fat.

■ REFERENCES ■

1. Adams, J., et al.: Total body fat content in a group of professional football players. *Can. J. Appl. Sport Sci.,* 7:36, 1982.
2. Ashwell, M., et al.: Obesity: new insight into the anthropometric classification of fat distribution shown by computed tomography. *Br. Med. J.* 290:1692, 1985.
3. Bakker, H.K., and Strvikenkamp, R.S.: Biological variability and lean body mass estimates. *Hum. Biol.,* 53:181, 1977.
4. Baumgartner, R.N., et al.: Bioelectric impedence for body composition. In *Exercise and Sport Sciences Reviews.* Vol. 18, K.B. Pandolf and J.O. Holloszy (Eds.), Baltimore, Williams & Wilkens, 1990.
5. Becque, M.D., et al.: Time course of skin-plus-fat compression in males and females. *Hum. Biol.,* 58:33, 1984.
6. Behnke, A.R.: New concepts in height-weight relationships. In *Obesity.* N. Wilson (Ed.), Philadelphia, F.A. Davis, 1969.
7. Behnke, A.R., and Wilmore, J.H.: *Evaluation and Regulation of Body Build and Composition.* Englewood Cliffs, N.J., Prentice- Hall, 1974.
8. Behnke, A.R., et al.: The specific gravity of healthy men. *JAMA,* 118:495, 1942.
9. Bernstein, L., et al.: Physical exercise and a reduced risk of breast cancer in young women. *J Natl. Cancer Inst.,* 86:1403, 1994.
10. Boddy, K., et al.: Body potassium and fat free mass. *Clin. Sci.,* 44:622, 1973.
11. Boling, E.A., et al.: Total exchangeable potassium and chloride, and total body water in healthy men of varying fat content. *J. Clin. Invest.,* 41:1840, 1962.
12. Bonen, A., et al.: Profiles of selected hormones during menstrual cycles of teenage athletes. *J. Appl. Physiol.,* 50:545, 1981.
13. Borkan, G.A., et al.: Relationships between computed tomography tissue areas, thicknesses and total body composition. *Ann. Hum. Biol.,* 10:537, 1983.
14. Boyden, T.: Prolactin responses, menstrual cycles and body composition of women runners. *J. Clin. Endocrinol. Metab.,* 54:712, 1982.
15. Brooks-Gunn, J., et al.: The relation of eating problems and amenorrhea in ballet dancers. *Med. Sci. Sports Exerc.,* 19:41, 1987.
16. Brožek, J., et al.: Densitometric analysis of body composition: revision of some quantitative assumptions. *Ann. N.Y. Acad. Sci.,* 110:113, 1963.
17. Bullen, B.A., et al.: Endurance training effects on plasma hormonal responsiveness and sex hormone excretion. *J. Appl. Physiol.,* 56:1453, 1984.
18. Bunt, J.C., et al.: Impact of total body water fluctuations on estimation of body fat from body density. *Med. Sci. Sports Exerc.,* 21:96, 1989.
19. Byrd, P.J., and Thomas, T.R.: Hydrostatic weighing during different stages of the menstrual cycle. *Res. Q. Exerc. Sport,* 54:296, 1983.

20. Cassady, S.L., et al.: Validity of near infrared body composition analysis in children and adolescents. *Med. Sci. Sports Exerc.*, 25:1185, 1993.

21. Caton, J.R., et al.: Body composition by bioelectrical impedence: effect of skin temperature. *Med. Sci. Sports Exerc.*, 20:489, 1988.

22. Clark, R.R., et al.: A comparison of methods to predict minimal weight in high school wrestlers. *Med. Sci. Sports Exerc.*, 25:1541, 1993.

23. Clarys, J.P., et al.: Gross tissue weights in the human body by cadaver dissection. *Hum. Biol.*, 56:459, 1984.

24. Clauser, C.E., et al.: Anthropometry of air force women. *AMRL-TR-70-5*, Ohio, Wright Patterson Air Force Base, 1972.

25. Côté and Adams, W.C.: Effect of bone density on body composition estimates in young adult black and white women. *Med. Sci. Sports Exerc.*, 25:290, 1993.

26. Cohn, S.H., and Dombrowski, C.S. Measurement of total body calcium, sodium, chlorine, nitrogen, and phosphorus in man by in-vivo neutron activation. *J. Nucl. Med.*, 12:499, 1971.

27. Cohn, S.N., et al.: Indexes of body cell mass: nitrogen versus potassium. *Am. J. Physiol.*, 244:E305, 1983.

28. Constantine, N.W., and Warren, M.P.: Physical activity, fitness, and reproductive health in women: Clinical observations. In *Physical Activity, Fitness, and Health*. C. Bouchard et al. (Eds.), Champaign, Ill., Human Kinetics 1994.

29. Conway, J.M., et al.: A new approach for the estimation of body composition: infrared interactance. *Am. J. Clin. Nutr.*, 40:1123, 1984.

29a. Dempster, P., and Aitkens, S.: A new air displacement method for the determination of human body composition. *Med. Sci. Sports Exerc.*, 27:1692, 1995.

30. Déspres, J-P., et al. Estimation of deep abdominal adipose-tissue accumulation from simple anthropometric measurements in men. *Am. J. Clin. Nutr.* 54:471, 1991.

31. Donnelly, J.E., et al.: Hydrostatic weighing without head submersion. Description of a method. *Med. Sci. Sports Exerc.*, 20:66, 1988.

32. Drinkwater, D.T., et al.: Validation by cadaver dissection of Matiegka's equations for the anthropometric estimation of anatomical body composition in adult humans. In *Perspectives in Kinathropometry*. J.A.P. Day (Ed.), Champaign, Ill., Human Kinetics, 1986.

33. Drumm, S., et al.: Changes in body composition, anthropometry, and arm radiography following 10 weeks of hydraulic resistive circuit exercise. *Med. Sci. Sports Exerc.*, 16:184, 1984.

34. Dulloo, A.G., et al.: Normal caffeine consumption: influences on thermogenesis and daily energy expenditure in lean and postobese human volunteers. *Am. J. Clin. Nutr.*, 49:44, 1989.

35. Durenberg, P., et al.: Changes in fat-free mass during weight loss measured by bioelectrical impedance and by densitometry. *Am. J. Clin. Nutr.*, 49:33, 1989.

36. Forbes, G.B.: *Human Body Composition*. New York, Springer-Verlag, 1987.

37. Forbes, R.M., et al.: The composition of the adult human body as determined by chemical analysis. *J. Biol. Chem.*, 203:349, 1953.

38. Freedson, P.S., et al.: Physique, body composition, and psychological characteristics of competitive female body builders. *Phys. Sportsmed.*, 11:85, 1983.

39. Frisch, R.E., et al.: Delayed menarche and amenorrhea in ballet dancers. *N. Engl. J. Med.*, 303:17, 1980.

40. Frisch, R.E., et al.: Lower prevalence of breast cancer and cancers of the reproductive system among former college athletes compared to non-athletes. *Br. J. Cancer*, 52:885, 1985.

41. Frisch, R.E., et al.: Lower lifetime occurence of breast cancer and cancers of the reproductive system among former college athletes. *Am. J. Clin. Nutr.*, 45:328, 1987.

42. Frisch, R.E., et al.: Lower prevalence of non-reproductive cancers among female former college athletes. *Med. Sci. Sports Exerc.*, 21:250, 1989.

43. Going, S., et al.: Aging and body composition: biological changes and methodological issues. *Exerc. Sport Sci. Revs.*, 23:459, 1995.

44. Hata, E., and Aoki, K.: Age at menarche and select menstrual characteristics in young Japanese athletes. *Res. Q. Exer. Sports*, 61:178, 1990.

45. Hayes, P.A., et al.: Subcutaneous fat thickness measured by magnetic resonance imaging, ultrasound, and calipers. *Med. Sci. Sports Exerc.*, 20:303, 1988.

46. Hetland, M.L., et al.: Running induces menstrual irregularities but bone mass is unaffected, except in amenorrheic women. *Am. J. Med.*, 95:53, 1993.

47. Heymsfield, S.B., et al.: Appendicular skeletal muscle mass: measurement by dual-photon absorptiometry. *Am. J. Clin. Nutr.* 52:214, 1990.

48. Heymsfield, S.B., et al.: Body composition of humans: comparison of two improved four-compartment models that differ in expense, technical complexity, and radiation exposure. *Am. J. Clin. Nutr.*, 52:52, 1991.

49. Hodgdon, J.A., and Fitzgerald, P.J.: Validity of impedance predictions at various levels of fatness. *Hum. Biol.*, 59:281, 1987.

50. Houmard, J.A., et al.: Validity of a near-infrared device for estimating body composition in a college football team. *J. Appl. Sport Sci. Res.*, 5:53, 1991.

51. Hsieh, S., et al.: Measurement of residual volume sitting and lying in air and water (and during underwater weighing) and its effects on computed body density. *Med. Sci. Sports Exerc.*, 17:204, 1985.

52. Ishida, Y., et al.: Reliability of B-mode ultrasound for the measurement of body fat and muscle thickness. *Am. J. Hum. Biol.*, 4:511, 1992.

53. Ishida, Y., et al.: Body fat and muscle thickness distributions in untrained young females. *Med. Sci. Sports Exerc.*, 27:270, 1995.

54. Israel, R.G., et al. Validity of near-infrared spectrophotometry devise for estimating human body composition. *Res. Q. Exerc. Sport.*, 60:379, 1989.

55. Jackson, A.S., et al.: Generalized equations for predicting body density of women. *Med. Sci. Sports*, 12:175, 1980.

56. Johnston, F.E.: Body fat deposition in adult obese women. I. Patterns of fat distribution. *Am. J. Clin. Nutr.*, 47:225, 1988.

57. Kahled, M.A., et al.: Electrical impedence in assessing human body composition: the BIA Method. *Am. J. Clin. Nutr.*, 47:789, 1988.

58. Kaiserauer, S., et al.: Nutritional, physiological, and menstrual status of distance runners. *Med. Sci. Sports Exerc.*, 21:120, 1989.

59. Kasch, F.W., and Wallace, J.P.: Physiological variables during 10 years of endurance exercise. *Med. Sci. Sports*, 8:5, 1976.

60. Katch, F.I.: Cross validation of body composition prediction equations in obese, adult males. *Am. J. Hum. Biol.*, In Press, 1996.

61. Katch, F.I.: Practice curves and errors of measurement in estimating underwater weight by hydrostatic weighing. *Med. Sci. Sports*, 1:212, 1969.

62. Katch, F.I.: Reliability and individual differences in ultrasound assessment of subcutaneous fat: effects of body position. *Hum. Biol.*, 55:789, 1983.

63. Katch, F.I.: Assessment of lean body tissues by radiography and bioelectrical impedance. In *Body Composition in Youth and Adults*. Columbus, Ohio, Ross Laboratories, 1985.

64. Katch, F.I., and Behnke, A.R.: Arm x-ray assessment of body fat in men and women. *Med. Sci. Sports Exerc.*, 16:316, 1984.

65. Katch, F.I., and Hortobágyi, T.: Validity of surface anthropometry to estimate upper-arm muscularity, including changes with body mass loss. *Am. J. Clin. Nutr.*, 52:591, 1990.

66. Katch, F.I., and Katch, V.L.: Measurement and prediction errors in body composition assessment and the search for the perfect prediction equation. *Res. Q. Exerc. Sport*, 51:249, 1980.

67. Katch, F.I., and Katch, V.L.: Computer technology to evaluate body composition, nutrition, and exercise. *Prev. Med.*, 12:619, 1983.

68. Katch, F.I., and Katch, V.L.: The body composition profile: techniques of measurement and applications. *Clin. Sports Med.*, 3:31, 1984.

69. Katch, F.I., and McArdle, W.D.: Prediction of body density from simple anthropometric measurements in college-age men and women. *Hum. Biol.*, 45:445, 1973.

70. Katch, F.I., and McArdle, W.D.: Validity of body composition prediction equations for college men and women. *Am. J. Clin. Nutr.*, 28:105, 1975.

71. Katch, F.I., and Michael, E.D.: Prediction of body density from skinfold and girth measurements of college females. *J. Appl. Physiol.*, 25:92, 1968.

72. Katch, F.I., and Spiak, D.L.: Validity of the Mellits and Cheek method for body-fat estimation in relation to menstrual cycle status in athletes and non-athletes below 22 percent fat. *Ann. Hum. Biol.*, 11:389, 1984.

73. Katch, F.I., et al.: Estimation of body volume by underwater weighing: description of a simple method. *J. Appl. Physiol.*, 23:811, 1967.

74. Katch, F.I., et al.: Estimation of body fat from skinfolds and surface area. *Hum. Biol.*, 51:411, 1979.

75. Katch, F.I., et al.: The underweight female. *Phys. Sportsmed.*, 8:55, 1980.

76. Katch, F.I., et al.: The ponderal somatogram: evaluation of body size and shape from anthropometric girths and stature. *Hum. Biol.*, 59:439, 1987.

77. Katch, F.I., et al.: A new approach for estimating excess body fat from changes in abdominal girth. *Am. J. Hum. Biol.*, 2:125, 1990.

78. Katch, V.L., et al.: Contribution of breast volume and weight to body fat distribution in females. *Am. J. Phys. Anthropol.*, 53:93, 1980.

79. Kehayias, J.J., et al.: Measurement of body fat by neutron inelastic scattering: comments on installation, operation, and error analysis. In *In Vivo Body Composition Studies*. S. Yasumura et al. (Eds.), New York, Plenum Press, 1990.

80. Keys, A., and Brožek, J.: Body fat in adult men. *Physiol. Rev.*, 33:245, 1960.

81. Keys, A., et al.: *The Biology of Human Starvation*. Minneapolis, University of Minnesota Press, 1950.

82. Kodama, A.A.: In vivo and in vitro determinations of body fat and body water in the hamster. *J. Appl. Physiol.*, 31:218, 1971.

83. Kondo, M., et al.: Upper limit of fat-free mass in humans: A study of Japanese Sumo wrestlers. *Am. J. Hum. Biol.*, 6: 613, 1994.

84. Kuczmarski, R.J.: Prevalence of overweight and weight gain in the United States. *Am. J. Clin. Nutr.*, 55:495S, 1992.

85. Kuczmarski, R.J., et al.: Ultrasonic assessment of body composition in obese adults: overcoming the limitations of the skinfold caliper. *Am. J. Clin. Nutr.*, 45:717, 1987.

86. Kvist, H., et al.: Total and visceral adipose-tissue volumes derived from measurements with computed tomography in adult men and women: predictive equations. *Am. J. Clin. Nutr.*, 48:1351, 1988.

87. Lewis, S., et al.: Body composition of middle-aged female endurance athletes. In *Biomechanics of Sports and Kinanthropometry*. Vol. 6, F. Landry and W.A.R. Orban (Eds.), Miami, Fla., Symposia Specialists, 1978.

87a. Lim, T.P.K.: Critical evaluation of the pneumatic method for determining body volume: Its history and technique.

88. Lloyd, T., et al.: Women athletes with menstrual irregularities have increased musculoskeletal injuries. *Med. Sci. Sports Exerc.*, 18:374, 1986.

89. Lohman, T.G., and Going, S.B.: Multicomponent models in body composition research: opportunities and pitfalls. *Basic Life Sci.*, 60:53, 1993.

90. Lohman, T.G., et al.: Methodological factors and the prediction of body fat in female athletes. *Med. Sci. Sports Exerc.*, 16:92, 1984.

91. Loucks, A.B.: Effects of exercise training on the menstrual cycle: existence and mechanisms. *Med. Sci. Sports Exerc.*, 22:275, 1990.

92. Loucks. A.B., and Callister, R.: Induction and prevention of low-T_3 syndrome in exercising women. *Am. J. Physiol.*, 264:R924, 1993.

93. Loucks, A.B., et al.: Hypothalamic-pituitary-thyroidal function in eumenorrheic and amenorrheic athletes. *J. Clin. Endocrin. Metabol.*, 75:514, 1992.

94. Lukaski, H.C.: Methods for the assessment of human body composition: traditional and new. *Am. J. Clin. Nutr.*, 46:537, 1987.

95. Lukaski, H.C.: Soft tissue composition and bone mineral status: evaluation by dual-energy x-ray absorptiometry. *J. Nutr.*, 123:438, 1993.

96. Malina, R.M.: Bioelectric methods for estimating body composition: an overview and discussion. *Hum. Biol.*, 59:329, 1987.

97. Martin, A.D., and Drinkwater, D.T.: Variability in the measures of body fat: assumptions or techniques? *Sports Med.*, 11:277, 1991.

98. Martin, A.D., et al.: Prediction of body fat by skinfold caliper: assumptions and cadaver evidence. *Int. J. Obesity.*, 9(Suppl. 1):31, 1985.

99. Martin, B.J.: Is athletic amenorrhea specific to runners? *Am. J. Obst. Gynecol.*, 143:859, 1982.

100. Matiegka, J.: The testing of physical efficiency. *Am. J. Phys. Anthrop.*, 4:223, 1921.

101. Mazes, R.A.B.: Estimation of bone and skeletal weight by direct photon absorptiometry. *Invest. Radiol.*, 6:52, 1971.

102. Mazes, R.A.B., et al.: Total body composition by dual photon (^{153}Gd) absorptiometry. *Am. J. Clin. Nutr.*, 40:834, 1984.

103. Mazes, R.A.B., et al.: Dual energy x-ray absorptiometry for total-body regional bone-mineral and soft-tissue composition. *Am. J. Clin. Nutr.*, 51:1106, 1990.

103a. McCrory, M.A., et al.: Evaluation of a new air displacement plethysmograph for measuring human body composition. *Med. Sci. Sports Exerc.*, 27:1686, 1995.

104. McLean, K., and Skinner, J.S.: Validity of the Futrex-5000 for body composition determination. *Med. Sci. Sports Exerc.*, 24:253, 1992.

105. McNeill, G., et al.: Body fat in lean and overweight women estimated by six methods. *Br. J. Nutr.*, 65:95, 1991.

106. Mendez, J., et al.: Density of fat and bone mineral of mammalian body. *Metabolism*, 9:472, 1960.

107. Mitchell, H.H., et al.: The chemical composition of the adult human body and its bearing on the biochemistry of growth. *J. Biol. Chem.*, 158:625, 1945.

108. Morales, M.F., et al.: Studies on body composition. *J. Biol. Chem.*, 158:677, 1945.

109. Morrow, J.R., Jr.: Accuracy of measured and predicted residual lung volume on body density measurement. *Med. Sci. Sports Exerc.*, 18:647, 1986.

110. Myhre, L.G., and Kessler, W.V.: Body density and potassium 40 measurements of body composition as related to age. *J. Appl. Physiol.*, 21:1251, 1966.

111. National Center for Health Statistics: Plan and operation of the second National Health and Nutrition Examination Survey. *Vital Health Stat.*, 1:15, 1981.

112. National Center for Health Statistics: *Health, United States.* Hyattsville, Md., Public Health Service, 1990.

113. Ostrove, S.M., and Vaccaro, P.: Effect of immersion on RV in young women: implications for measurement of body density. *Int. J. Sports Med.*, 3:220, 1982.

114. Pace, N., and Rathbun, E.N.: Studies on body composition. III. The body water and chemically combined nitrogen in relation to fat content. *J. Biol. Chem.*, 158:685, 1945.

115. Penn, I-W., et al.: Body composition and two-compartment model assumptions in male long distance runners. *Med. Sci. Sports Exerc.*, 26:392, 1994.

116. Peppler, W.W., and Mazes, R.B.: Total body bone mineral and lean body mass by dual photon absorptiometry. Theory and measurement procedure. *Calcif. Tissue Int.*, 33:353, 1981.

117. Pierson, R.N., Jr., et al.: High precision in-vivo neutron activation analysis: a new era for compartmental analysis in body composition. In *In Vivo Body Composition Studies*. S. Yasumura et al. (Eds.), New York, Plenum Press, 1990.

118. Pollock, M.L., and Jackson, A.S.: Measurement of cardiorespiratory fitness and body composition in the clinical setting: *Compr. Ther.*, 6:12, 1980.

119. Rathbun, E.N., and Pace, N.: Studies on body composition. *J. Biol. Chem.*, 158:667, 1945.

120. Robertson, C.H., et al.: Lung volumes in men immersed to the neck: dilution and plethysmographic techniques. *J. Appl. Physiol.*, 44:679, 1978.

121. Ross, R., et al.: Sensitivity of bioelectrical impedence to detect changes in body composition. *J. Appl. Physiol.*, 67:1643, 1989.

122. Rubeffe-Scrive, M.L., et al.: Fat cell metabolism in different regions in women: effect on menstrual cycle, pregnancy, and lactation. *J. Clin. Invest.*, 75:1973, 1985.

123. Schutte, J.E., et al.: Density of lean body mass is greater in Blacks than Whites. *J. Appl. Physiol.*, 56:1647, 1984.

124. Schweiger, V., et al.: Caloric intake, stress, and menstrual function in athletes. *Fertil. Steril.*, 49:447, 1988.

125. Segal, K., et al.: Lean body mass estimation by bioelectrical impedance analysis: a four-site cross-validation study. *Am. J. Clin. Nutr.*, 47:7, 1988.

126. Seidell, J.C., et al.: Abdominal fat depots measured with computed tomography: effects of degree of obesity, sex, and age. *Eur. J. Clin. Nutr.*, 42:805, 1988.

127. Shangold, M.M.: Sports and menstrual function. *Phys. Sportsmed.*, 8:66, 1980.

128. Shangold, M.M.: Do women's sports lead to menstrual problems? *Contemp. Obst. Gynecol.*, 17:52, 1981.

129. Shangold, M.M., et al.: Evaluation and management of menstrual dysfunction in athletes. *JAMA*, 262:1665, 1990.

130. Siri, W.E.: Gross composition of the body. In *Advances in Biological and Medical Physics*. Vol. 4, J.H. Lawrence and C.A. Tobias (Eds.), New York, Academic Press, 1956.

130a. Siri, W.E.: Apparatus for measuring human body volume. *Rev. Sci. Inst.*, 27:729, 1956.

130b. Siri, W.E.: Body volume measurement by gas dilution. In *Techniques for Measuring Body Composition*. Brožek, J., and Henschel, A. (Eds). Washington, D.C., National Academy of Sciences–National Research Council, 1961.

131. Slaughter, M.H., et al.: Skinfold equations for estimation of body fatness in children and youths. *Hum. Biol.*, 60:709, 1988.

132. Smalley, K.J., et al.: Reassessment of body mass indices. *Am. J. Clin. Nutr.*, 52:405, 1990.

133. Stager, J.M., and Hatler, L.K.: Menarche in athletes: the influence of genetics and prepubertal training. *Med. Sci. Sports Exerc.*, 20:369, 1988.

133a. Stern, H: Investigations on corporeal specific gravity and on the value of this factor in physical diagnosis. *Med. Rec.*, 59:204, 1901.

134. Stout, J.R., et al.: Validity of percent body fat estimations in males. *Med. Sci. Sports Exerc.*, 26:632, 1994.

135. Svboda, M.D., and Query, L.M.: Hydrostatic weighing of women throughout the menstrual cycle. In *Perspectives in Kinanthropometry. The 1984 Olympic Scientific Congress Proceedings*. Vol. 1, J.A.P. Day (Ed.), Champaign, Ill., Human Kinetics, 1984.

136. Thorland, W.G., et al.: Estimation of body composition in black adolescent male athletes. *Pediatric Exer. Sci.*, 5:116, 1993.

137. Toniolo, P.G., et al.: A prospective study of endogenous estrogens and breast cancer in postmenopausal women. *J. Natl. Cancer Inst.*, 87:190, 1995.

138. Tran, Z.V., and Weltman, A.: Predicting body composition of men from girth measurements. *Hum. Biol.*, 60:167, 1988.

139. Tran, Z.V., and Weltman, A.: Generalized equation for predicting body density of women from girth measurements. *Med. Sci. Sports Exerc.*, 21:101, 1989.

140. Vaccaro, P., et al.: Body composition and physiological responses of Masters female swimmers 20 to 70 years of age. *Res. Q. Exerc. Sport*, 55:278, 1984.

141. Wadden, T. A., et al.: Body fat deposition in adult obese women. II. Changes in fat distribution accompanying weight reduction. *Am. J. Clin. Nutr.*, 47:229, 1988.

142. Wakat, D.K., et al.: Reproductive system function in women cross-country runners. *Med. Sci. Sports Exerc.*, 14:263, 1982.

143. Walberg, J.L., and Johnston, C.S.: Menstrual function and eating behavior in female recreational weight lifters and competitive body builders. *Med. Sci. Sports Exerc.*, 23:30, 1991.

144. Wang, Z.M., et al.: The five-level model: a new approach to organizing body composition research. *Am. J. Clin. Nutr.*, 56:19, 1992.

145. Warren, M.P.: The effects of exercise on pubertal progression and reproductive function. *J. Clin. Endocrinol. Metab.*, 51:1150, 1980.

146. Webster, B.L., and Barr, S.I.: Body composition analysis of female adolescent athletes. *Med. Sci. Sports Exerc.*, 25:648, 1993.

147. Weltman, A., et al.: Accurate assessment of body composition in obese females. *Am. J. Clin. Nutr.*, 48:1179, 1988.

148. Weststrate, J.A., and Duerenberg, P.: Body composition in children: proposal for a method for calculating body fat percentage from total body density or skinfold-thickness measurements. *Am. J. Clin. Nutr.*, 50:1104, 1989.

149. Wilmore, J.H.: Body composition in sport and exercise: directions for future research. *Med. Sci. Sports Exerc.*, 15:21, 1983.

150. Womack, H.C.: The relationship between human body weight, subcutaneous fat, heart weight, and epicardial fat. *Human. Biol.*, 55:667, 1983.

151. Yeager, K.K., et al.: The female athlete triad: disordered eating, amenorrhea, osteoporosis. *Med. Sci. Sports Exerc.*, 25:775, 1993.

Clarys, J.P., et al.: Gross tissue weights in the human body by cadaver dissection. *Hum. Biol.* 56:459, 1984.

Chemical and anatomical dissection procedures are two direct methods for studying human body composition. The chemical method quantifies the amount of water, lipid, protein, and various mineral elements in the different tissues and the whole body. Anatomical dissection partitions the body into components including skin, muscle, adipose tissue, bone, and whole organs. Since 1940, the body com-

position literature reveals only eight complete analyses of adults, with only three done by chemical methods. Thus, the anatomical method provides information about gross tissue weights in only five adult humans. Commonly employed indirect assessment procedures include fatfolds, girths, ultrasound, underwater weighing, and electrical impedance. Until the research of Clarys and colleagues, no direct comparisons existed between indirect (particularly the body density method) and direct assessment of body composition (by dissection).

The researchers used anthopometry, radiography, photogrammetry, densitometry, and complete anatomical dissection of 25 cadavers for determining the gross tissue mass of skin, adipose tissue, muscle, bone, and vital organs. For each cadaver, analysis included removing skeletal muscle and other major organs (brain, heart, lungs, liver, kidneys, and spleen). The bones were separated by their articulations and scraped to leave their surfaces free of muscle and adipose tissue. Ligaments were included with muscle, and the cartilage on any articular surface was retained with the bone. Airtight plastic buckets stored all dissected tissues, including scrapings. The tissues were weighed within 0.1 g and their densities determined. The complete dissection of a cadaver took approximately 15 hours and required a team of 10 to 12 anatomists and kinesiologists. The cadavers ranged in age from 55 to 94 years and included 12 embalmed (six male, six female) and 13 nonembalmed (six male, seven female) Caucasians.

The figure shows an average adipose tissue mass of 40.5% of total body mass in females and 28.1% in males. The researchers introduced the concept of adipose tissue-free weight (ATFW) consisting of the whole body mass less the mass of all dissectable adipose tissue. Muscle accounted for 52% of the ATFW in males and 48.1% in females, while bone accounted for 19.9% of ATFW in males and 21.3% in females. Combining the male and female data, the average proportion of the ATFW included 8.5% for skin, 50.0% for muscle, and 20.6% for bone.

Using densitometry to estimate the fat and fat-free weight (FFW) of the body requires the assumption of a constant density for the FFW. This in turn requires that the composition of the components making up the FFW remain constant. The important components—the proportions of fat-free muscle, fat-free adipose tissue, fat-free bone, and other tissues—must remain unchanged from one person to another, including the densities for each tissue. Although Clarys' research did not include measurements of whole-body fat, considerable variation existed in the ATFW. The extent of this variation challenges the assumption of a constant density for the FFW component of the body.

Various tissue weights in the adult human body expressed as percentage of total body mass.

Physique, Performance, and Physical Activity

The evaluation of body composition provides an excellent opportunity to partition the gross size of a person into two major structural components: body fat and fat-free body mass. As discussed in Chapter 27, physique differs considerably between adult men and woman. There are pronounced differences in physique when comparisons are made among sports participants of the same sex, such as Olympic competitors, track-and-field specialists, wrestlers, and football players. These differences also are apparent in comparisons between highly proficient adolescent competitors. Besides describing physique by sports category and level of competition, some experiments have determined the effects of different forms of sports training and exercise on body composition and physique status. In this chapter, we take a closer look at the physiques of champion athletes in various sports and evaluate the relative effects of diet and exercise on body composition.

PHYSIQUE OF CHAMPION ATHLETES

Considerable research has dealt with the anthropometric methodology of quantifying physique status. Visual appraisal often describes individuals as small, medium, or large, or thin (ectomorphic), muscular (mesomorphic), or fat (endomorphic). A shortcoming of this approach, termed **somatotyping,** is that visual inspection does little more than describe body shape for a particular category such as thin or muscular. Visual appraisal really does not quantify the various body dimensions of how large the chest or shoulders are or how much the biceps are developed (or underdeveloped) compared to the thighs or calves. While the use of the somatotype technique is a valuable adjunct in the analysis of physique status and has been used extensively in evaluation of world-class athletes,[11, 13, 14, 18] our focus is on two main components of body composition, body fat and fat-free body mass. In our analysis, we quantify aspects of physique using girth and fatfold anthropometry, and densitometry in Olympic competitors, endurance runners, collegiate and professional football players, triathletes, high school wrestlers, champion male and female body builders, and diverse subgroups. We use the body profile technique discussed in Chapter 27.

OLYMPIC AND ELITE ATHLETES

Early studies of Olympic competitors revealed that physique was related to a high level of achievement in certain sports.[17, 32] Tables 28.1 and 28.2 list the anthropometric characteristics of male and female competitors in the 1964 Tokyo and 1968 Mexico City Olympics.[18, 23] Lean body mass and percent body fat were estimated from bone diameter measures and stature to show relative differences in body composition among the different specialists. Table 28.3 lists anthropometric data (body mass, stature, eight fatfolds) for male and female swimmers, divers, and water polo athletes at the Sixth World Championships held in Perth, Australia, in 1992. Also of interest are the body size differences among different groups of athletes within a particular sport. The top of Figure 28.1 compares 12 male swimmers rated as "best" in the 200 + 400 m freestyle with the rest of the competitors for body mass, stature, chest girth, and upper and lower limb lengths. Also compared at the bottom of the figure are the body size variables between the best 50 + 100 + 200 m breaststroke female swimmers (for rank in performance) and the rest of the competitors. There is little doubt that the best male swimmers are heavier and taller and have larger chest, upper arm, and thigh girths and upper and lower limb lengths than their counterparts who did not place among the top 12 finishers. Not only were the best female breaststroke swimmers taller and heavier, but they also had larger arm spans, foot and arm lengths, and hand and wrist breadth than their less successful counterparts.

Sex Differences

Table 28.1 indicates that for the men, basketball players, rowers, and weight throwers were the tallest and heaviest competitors; they also possessed the largest amount of lean body mass and percent body fat. For example, weight throwers in both Olympiads averaged 30% body fat, whereas 94 marathon and 133 long-distance runners averaged an exceptionally low 1.6% body fat. The biggest discrepancy in body composition within a particular sports category was between the Tokyo wrestlers, who averaged 12.7% body fat, and the wrestlers in Mexico City, who averaged only 1.2% body fat. This difference is even more re-

TABLE 28.1

AGE, BODY SIZE, AND BODY COMPOSITION OF MALE ATHLETES IN SELECTED EVENTS WHO COMPETED IN THE TOKYO AND MEXICO CITY OLYMPICS

Specialty	Event	Olympics	N	Age (y)	Stature (cm)	Mass (kg)	LBM[a] (kg)	Body Fat[b] (%)
Sprint	100–200 m; 4 × 100 m;	Tokyo	172	24.9	178.4	72.2	64.9	10.1
	110-m hurdles	Mexico City	79	23.9	175.4	68.4	62.8	8.2
Long-distance	3000, 5000,	Tokyo	99	27.3	173.6	62.4	61.5	1.4
running	10,000 m	Mexico City	34	25.3	171.9	59.8	60.1	−0.5
Marathon	42.2 km	Tokyo	74	28.3	170.3	60.8	59.2	2.7
		Mexico City	20	26.4	168.7	56.6	58.1	2.7
Decathlon		Tokyo	26	26.3	183.2	83.5	68.5	18.0
		Mexico City	8	25.1	181.3	77.5	67.1	13.4
Jump	High, long,	Tokyo	89	25.3	181.5	73.2	67.2	8.2
	triple jump	Mexico City	14	23.5	182.8	73.2	68.2	6.8
Weight	Shot, discus,	Tokyo	79	27.6	187.3	101.4	71.6	29.4
throwing	hammer	Mexico City	9	27.3	186.1	102.3	70.7	30.9
Swimming	Free, breast, back,	Tokyo	450	20.4	178.7	74.1	65.1	12.1
	butterfly, medley	Mexico City	66	19.2	179.3	72.1	65.6	9.0
Basketball		Tokyo	186	25.3	189.4	84.3	73.2	13.2
		Mexico City	63	24.0	189.1	79.7	73.0	8.4
Gymnastics	All events	Tokyo	122	26.0	167.2	63.3	57.0	9.9
		Mexico City	28	23.6	167.4	61.5	57.2	7.0
Wrestling	Bantam and	Tokyo	29	27.3	163.3	62.3	54.4	12.7
	featherweight	Mexico City	32	22.5	166.1	57.0	56.3	1.2
Rowing	Single and double	Tokyo	357	25.0	186.0	82.2	70.6	14.1
	skulls; pairs, fours, eights	Mexico City	85	24.3	185.1	82.6	69.9	15.4

Adapted from De Garay, et al.: *Genetic and Anthropological Studies of Olympic Athletes*. New York, Academic Press, 1974, and from Hirata, K.: *Physique and age of Tokyo Olympic champions. J. Sports Med. Phys. Fitness*, 6: 207, 1966.
[a]Calculated by Behnke's method: LBM = h^2 × 0.204, where h = stature, dm (see reference 6).
[b]Body fat (%) = (Body mass − LBM)/Body mass × 100.

markable because age, stature, and lean body mass were similar in both groups of wrestlers.

For female Olympic athletes (Table 28.2), the most striking observation is their relatively low body fat values. Except for the weight throwers, who averaged about 31% body fat, competitors in the other sports groups were close to the average body fat of 13.1% for all 676 female participants in both Olympics. For the aquatic athletes, whose data for body mass, stature, and fatfolds are displayed in Table 28.3, it is evident that there are basic differences in fatfold anthropometry among sports, and females in the aquatic sports have larger fatfolds at most sites than their male counterparts.

Prior studies have established a relationship between certain aspects of body composition and swimming performance. As noted previously, the swimmers' morphology significantly influences the horizontal components of lift and drag during swimming.[15] Selected anthropometric variables play important roles in the propulsive and resistive forces

acting on the swimmer. The combined influence of stroke length and stroke frequency on swimming velocity also relates positively to a swimmer's overall body size and shape.[22] In well-trained freestyle swimmers, arm length, leg length, and hand and foot size (factors governed mainly by genetics) are significantly related to stroke length and stroke frequency. Table 28.4 presents additional anthropometric comparisons between male and female Olympians in five different sports at the Montreal Olympics.

World Records. Figure 28.2 compares world record times for males and females in various running events (100 m to 10,000 m) through 1991. The percentage differences in performance average about 10% between males and females for all running events from 100 m through the marathon, including the 400-m hurdles and 400-m to 3200-m relay races. In strength and power comparisons of male and female weight lifters of the same body mass category, women in the 52-kg weight class are within 89.2%

TABLE 28.2
AGE, BODY SIZE, AND BODY COMPOSITION OF FEMALE ATHLETES WHO COMPETED IN THE TOKYO AND MEXICO CITY OLYMPICS IN SELECTED EVENTS

Specialty	Event	Olympics	N	Age (y)	Stature (cm)	Mass (kg)	LBM[a] (kg)	Body Fat[b] (%)
Sprint	100–200 m;	Tokyo	85	22.7	166.0	56.6	49.6	12.4
	100-m hurdles	Mexico City	28	20.7	165.0	56.8	49.0	13.7
Jump	High, long,	Tokyo	56	23.6	169.5	60.2	51.7	14.1
	triple jump	Mexico City	12	21.5	169.4	56.4	51.7	8.4
Weight	Shot, discus,	Tokyo	37	26.2	170.4	79.0	52.3	33.8
throwing	hammer	Mexico City	9	19.9	170.9	73.5	52.6	28.5
Swimming	Free, breast, back,	Tokyo	272	18.6	166.3	59.7	49.8	16.6
	butterfly, medley	Mexico City	28	16.3	164.4	56.9	48.6	14.5
Diving	Spring, high	Tokyo	65	18.5	160.9	54.1	46.6	13.9
		Mexico City	7	21.1	160.4	52.3	46.3	11.5
Gymnastics	All events	Tokyo	102	22.7	157.0	52.0	44.4	14.7
		Mexico City	21	17.8	156.9	49.8	44.3	11.0

Adapted from De Garay, et al.: *Genetic and Anthropological Studies of Olympic Athletes.* New York, Academic Press, 1974, and from Hirata, K.: Physique and age of Tokyo Olympic champions. *J. Sports Med. Phys. Fitness,* 6:207, 1966.
[a]Calculated by Behnke's method: LBM (lean body mass) = $h^2 \times 0.18$, where h = stature, dm (see reference 6).
[b]Body fat (%) = (Body mass − LBM)/Body mass $\times$ 100.

TABLE 28.3
COMPARISON OF BODY MASS, STATURE, AND EIGHT FATFOLDS IN MALE AND FEMALE SWIMMERS, DIVERS, AND WATER POLO ATHLETES AT THE SIXTH WORLD CHAMPIONSHIPS HELD IN PERTH, AUSTRALIA, IN 1992

Males	Mass (kg)	Stature (cm)	Tri[a]	Scap	Supra	Abd	Thi	Calf	Bic	Iliac
Swimming	78.4	183.8	7.0	7.9	6.3	9.4	9.6	6.5	3.7	9.2
Diving	66.7	170.9	6.8	7.9	6.0	9.6	9.6	6.0	3.8	8.5
Water polo	86.1	186.5	9.2	9.9	8.2	14.9	12.6	7.9	4.3	13.4
Females										
Swimming	63.1	171.5	12.1	8.8	7.3	12.1	19.1	11.4	5.9	9.8
Diving	53.7	161.2	11.4	8.5	6.8	11.1	18.2	9.7	4.9	7.9
Water polo	64.8	171.3	15.3	10.5	9.6	17.6	23.4	13.5	7.1	12.1

[a]These abbreviations are for fatfolds, mm: Tri, triceps; Scap, subscapula; Supra, supraspinale; Abd, abdomen; Calf, mid-calf; Bic, biceps; Iliac, iliac crest. Modified from Mazza, J.C., et al.: Absolute body size. In *Kinanthropometry in Aquatic Sports. A Study of World Class Athletes.* J.E. Carter and T.R. Ackland (Eds.), Human Kinetics Sport Science Monograph Series, Vol. 5, Champaign, IL, Human Kinetics Publishers, 1994.

of the male best performance; the percentage difference between sexes increases at the higher weight categories. In field events (not listed), the percentages of best performance by females compared to males are as follows: high jump (83.3%), long jump (84.0%), javelin throw (82.5%), and triple jump (83.2%). The bottom insert of Figure 28.2 demonstrates that the sex differences in the world record times expressed as maximum running speed

$(m \cdot s^{-1})$ remain remarkably similar for events of 100 m through 10,000 m. Running speed for males is identical for 100 and 200 m. After that, running speed declines steadily for both sexes. The percentage decline to 800 m is 29% for males and 35% for females. Thereafter, the rate of decline in speed is less. From 800 m to 10,000 m, the cumulative decrement is about 28% in maximum speed for both men and women.

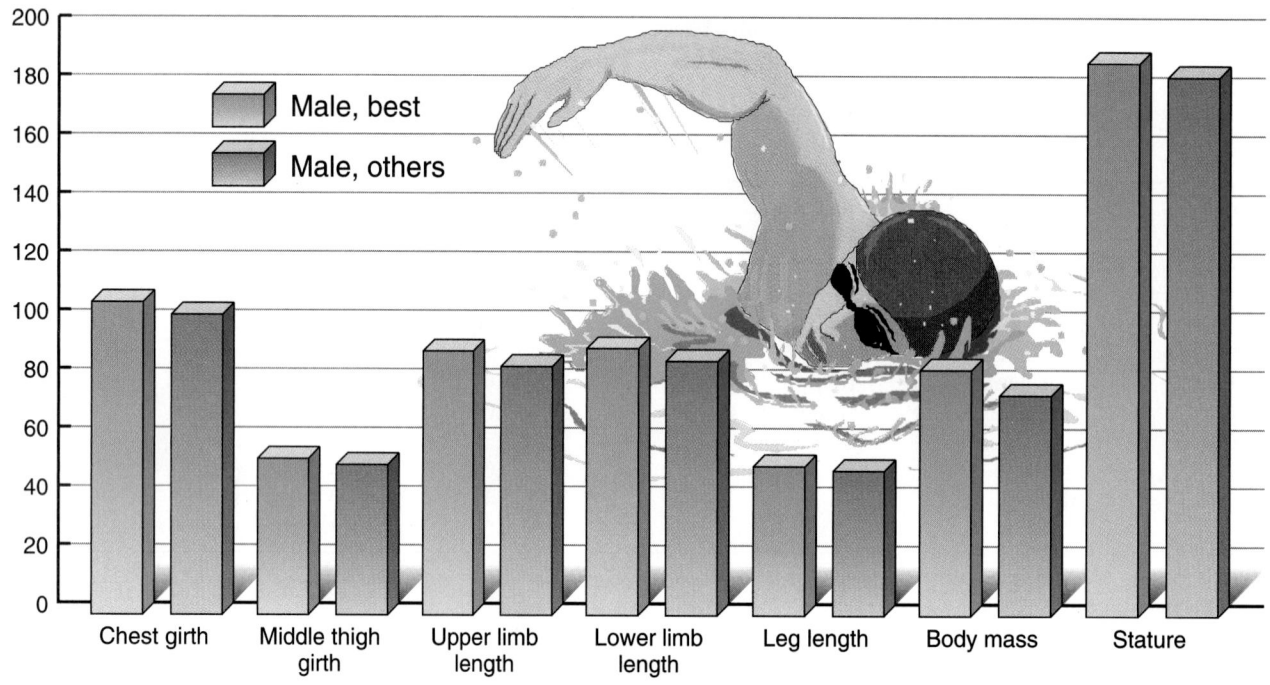

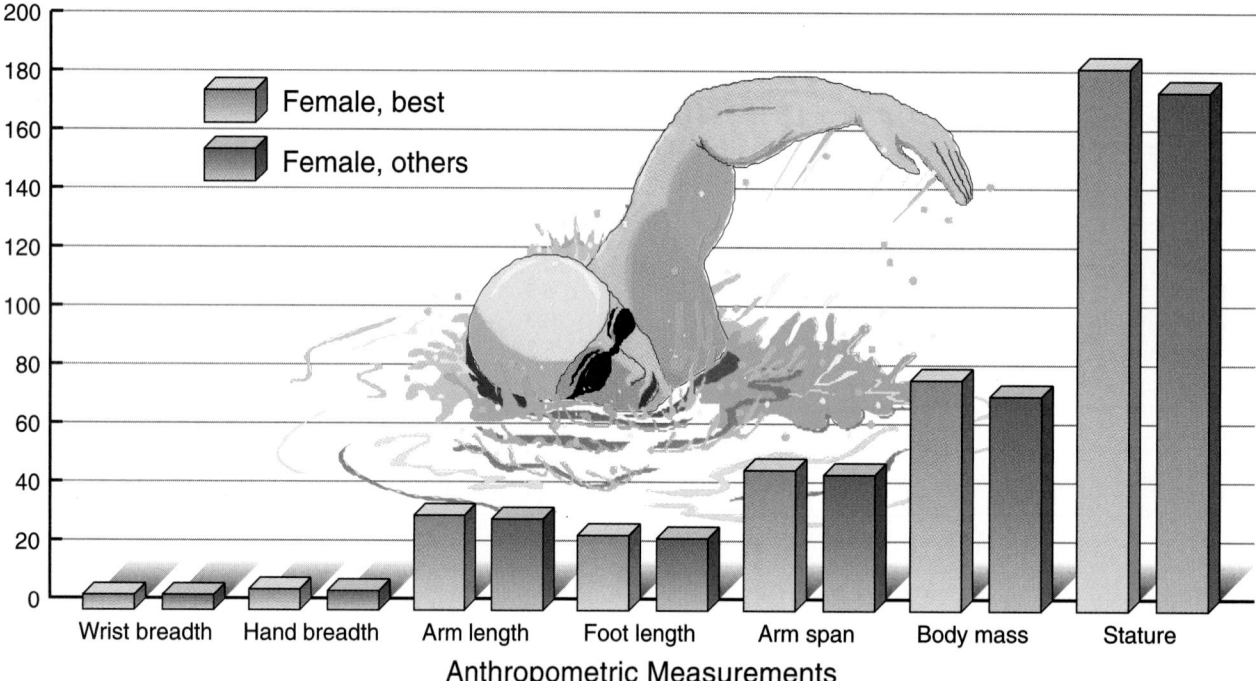

Anthropometric Measurements

FIGURE 28.1

Top, Comparison of 200 + 400 m freestyle male swimmers in body mass, stature, chest girth, arm span (actual values divided by 4), and upper and lower limb lengths, categorized as best performers (top 12 ranks) and the rest of the competitors. *Bottom,* Comparison of differences in body size variables between the best 50 + 100 + 200 m breaststroke female swimmers (top 12 ranks) versus the rest of the competitors. The *y*-axis is in centimeters for stature, girths, and lengths and in kilograms for body mass. (Modified from Mazza, J.C., et al.: Absolute body size. In *Kinanthropometry In Aquatic Sports. A Study of World Class Athletes.* J.E. Carter and T.R. Ackland (Eds.), Human Kinetics Sport Science Monograph Series, Vol. 5, Champaign, IL, Human Kinetics Publishers, 1994.)

TABLE 28.4

SELECTED ANTHROPOMETRIC MEASUREMENTS IN MALES AND FEMALES WHO COMPETED IN FIVE DIFFERENT SPORTS AT THE MONTREAL OLYMPIC GAMES[a]

Measurement	Canoe		Gymnastics		Rowing		Swimming		Track	
	M	F	M	F	M	F	M	F	M	F
Stature	185.4	170.7	169.3	161.5	191.3	174.3	178.6	166.9	179.1	168.5
Upper extremity L	82.4	76.0	76.0	72.2	85.2	76.0	80.2	74.7	80.9	74.8
Lower extremity L	88.0	81.8	78.9	76.5	91.7	82.3	84.1	78.1	86.9	80.3
Biacromial D	41.4	36.8	39.0	35.9	42.5	37.4	40.8	37.1	40.2	36.3
Bi-iliac D	28.1	27.3	25.8	25.0	30.2	28.2	27.9	26.7	27.1	27.2
Arm relaxed G	32.2	27.6	30.7	24.3	31.7	27.6	30.6	27.3	29.1	24.5
Arm flexed G	35.3	29.6	33.9	25.9	34.9	29.3	33.3	28.2	32.2	26.4
Forearm G	29.3	25.4	27.5	23.2	30.3	25.5	27.4	23.9	27.9	23.3
Chest G	102.6	88.9	95.1	83.5	103.7	89.6	98.6	88.0	94.3	83.8
Waist G	80.6	69.8	72.8	63.2	84.0	70.8	79.3	69.4	77.7	67.4
Thigh G	54.6	54.0	51.0	49.9	60.2	57.5	55.4	52.8	56.0	53.9
Calf G	37.5	34.9	34.7	33.3	39.3	37.0	36.9	34.0	37.6	34.9

Adapted from Carter, J.E., et al. Anthropometry of Montreal Olympic Athletes. In *Physical Structure of Olympic Athletes. Part 1: The Montreal Olympic Games Anthropological Project.* J.E. Carter (Ed.), Basel, Karger, 1982.
[a]L, length; D, diameter; G, girth; all values are centimeters.

Figure 28.3 shows further comparisons in world record performances between males and females for swimming, speed skating, and cycling. In the freestyle 400-, 800-, and 1500-m swims, the female times come closer to those of males (about 94% of best male times) compared to shorter running and swimming distances (90.7%). The percentage differences are approximately the same between sexes in speed skating and middle-distance swimming events (400 through 1500 m), but in 1-km to 100-km cycling events, females achieve only 87% of the best times for males. One can raise the question of whether continued improvement in training procedures and technique can overcome what appear to be sex-determined "genetic limits" to maximal performance, particularly in events that require extremes in muscular strength and power, or aerobic capacity. This question will persist until a female breaks through the apparent sex barrier in world record performance and achieves the superior performance. We may not witness such an occurrence in our lifetime, but when it does occur, it most likely will be in a middle-distance swimming event.

Fat-Free–to–Fat Ratio. Figure 28.4 compares the ratios of fat-free body mass to fat mass (FFM/FM) among male and female sport competitors. These FFM/FM values are from average body mass and percent body fat measurements from numerous studies in the world literature for the particular sport. The insert graphs present the data for average body mass, percent body fat, fat weight, and fat-free

body mass. Male marathon runners and gymnasts have the largest FFM/FM, while the values are smallest for football offensive and defensive lineman and shot-putters. The largest FFM/FM values for females are observed in body builders (same FFM/FM as in males), and the smallest FFM/FM occurs for field event participants. Surprisingly, female gymnasts and ballet dancers are about intermediate in the FFM/FM ratio compared to other female sport participants.

Percent Body Fat Grouped By Sport Category

Figure 28.5 categorizes sport activities into six classifications depending on the particular characteristics and requirements of the sport, and then ranks percent body fat within each category for male and female competitors. This method of organization provides a better overview of the distribution of percent body fat for broad sport categories.

Racial Differences. Racial differences in physique among Olympic competitors may significantly affect athletic performance.[46] Black sprinters and high jumpers, for example, have longer limbs and narrower hips than their white counterparts. From a mechanical perspective, a black sprinter with leg and arm sizes identical to those of a white sprinter would have a lighter, shorter, and slimmer body to propel. This might confer a more favorable power-to-body

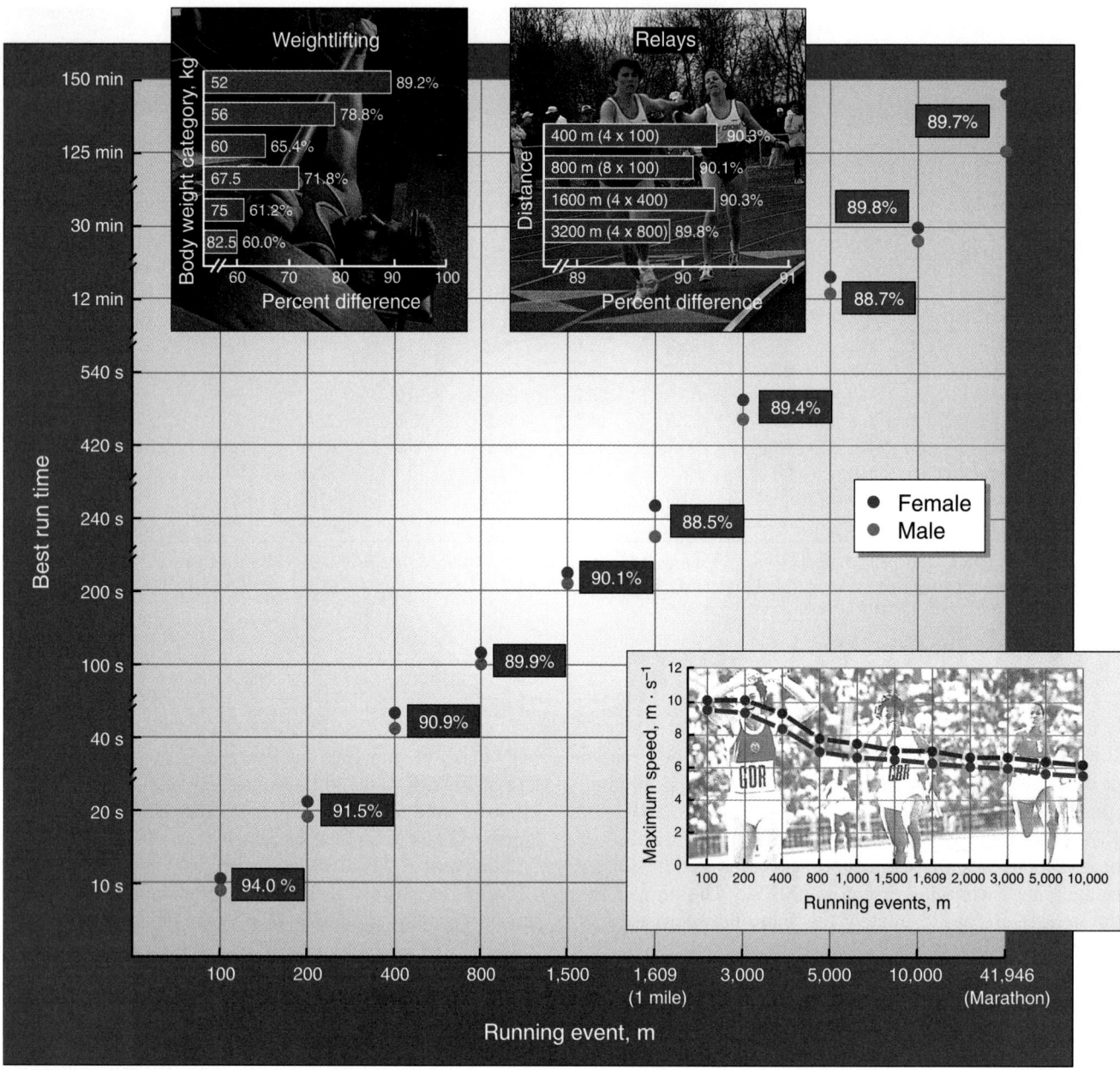

FIGURE 28.2

World records in various running events for men and women grouped by energy system requirement (100 m = anaerobic to marathon = aerobic). The *top left* inset displays the percentage differences between sexes for total weight lifted in the snatch and clean-and-jerk for six weight classifications. The *top right* inset displays the percentage differences in four popular relay events. The *bottom* insert expresses the differences in the world record times between sexes as maximum running speed for 100 m through 10,000 m. (Weightlifting data from U.S. Weightlifting Federation National Championships, Blaine, MN, April 26–28, 1991.)

mass ratio for black athletes at any given body size compared to white competitors. A greater power output would be advantageous in jumping events and in sprint running events, where the rapid generation of energy for short periods is crucial to successful performance. This advantage may be diminished somewhat in the various throwing events. Compared to whites and blacks, Asian athletes have short legs in relation to their upper torso components. This might confer some advantage in the short and longer distance races, as well as in weightlifting. Successful weight lifters of all races compared to other groups of athletes have relatively short arms and legs for their stature.

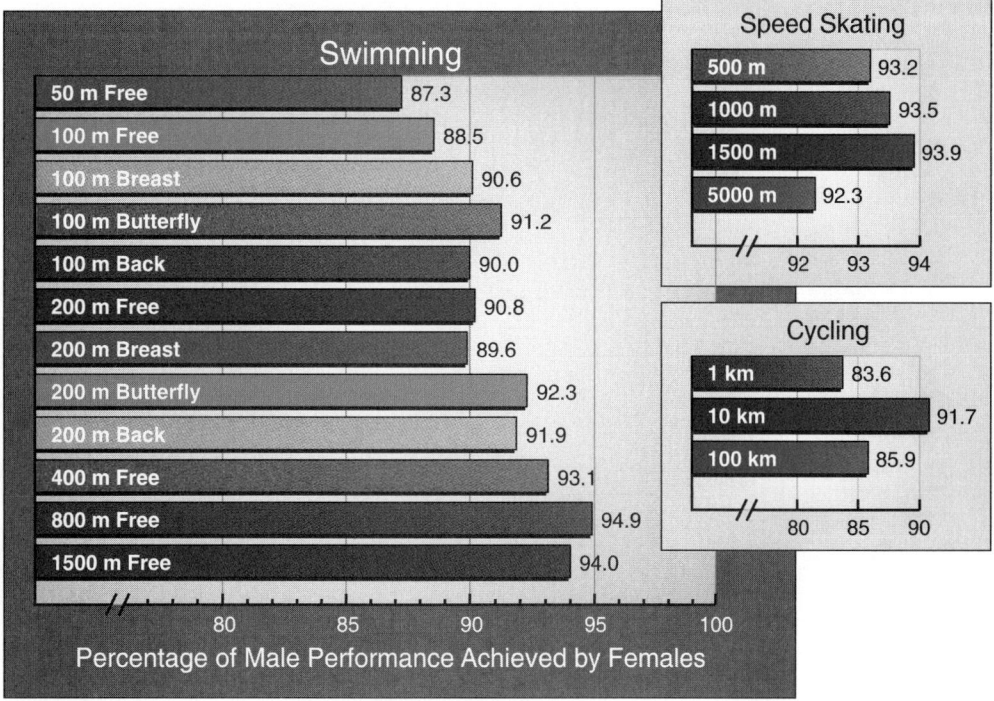

FIGURE 28.3

Sex differences in swimming, speed skating, and cycling world record performances through 1991.

FIELD EVENT ATHLETES

The body composition data for the ten top American athletes in the discus, shot put, javelin, and hammer throw were obtained by densitometry and anthropometry 2 years before the 1980 Moscow Olympics. Figure 28.6 displays the results for body composition (ranked from high to low in percent body fat, fat weight, fat-free body mass, and lean-to-fat ratio). Comparative data are presented for international elite middle- and long-distance runners (average treadmill $\dot{V}O_2$ max was 76.9 mL $\cdot$ kg^{-1} $\cdot$ min^{-1}) and the reference man (see Chapter 27). Table 28.5 lists the corresponding data for girth and fatfold anthropometry. Shot-putters clearly are the largest in overall size based on body mass and girths; they are followed in overall size by discus, hammer, and javelin athletes.

FEMALE LONG-DISTANCE RUNNERS

Table 28.6 presents data for body mass, stature, and body composition of 11 female long-distance runners of national and international caliber.[52] The runners averaged 15.2% body fat (determined by underwater weighing), similar to reports of high school cross-country runners[10] but considerably lower than the average value of about 26% reported for sedentary females of the same age, stature, and body mass.[28] Compared to other female athletes, the runners have a lower average fat value than collegiate basketball players (20.9%),[43] competitive gymnasts (15.5%),[44] younger distance runners (18%),[32] swimmers (20.1%),[29] or tennis players (22.8%).[29]

Interestingly, the average body fat for these runners is the same as the 15% average generally reported for males and is close to the quantity of essential fat proposed by Behnke in his model for the refzerence woman. The body fat values of several of the female distance runners listed in Table 28.6 were within the range of values reported for topflight male distance runners. The leanest women in the population, based on Behnke's reference woman, have essential fat equal to about 12 to 14% of body mass. This apparent discrepancy requires that further study be conducted between the estimated fat contents of distance runners and Behnke's theoretical lower limit for body fat in women. It is also difficult to explain the relatively high body fat content of one of the best runners, indicating that other factors often override the obvious limitations to distance running imposed by excess fat.

MALE LONG-DISTANCE RUNNERS

Table 28.7 presents body composition data for eleven male elite middle and long-distance runners and eight elite

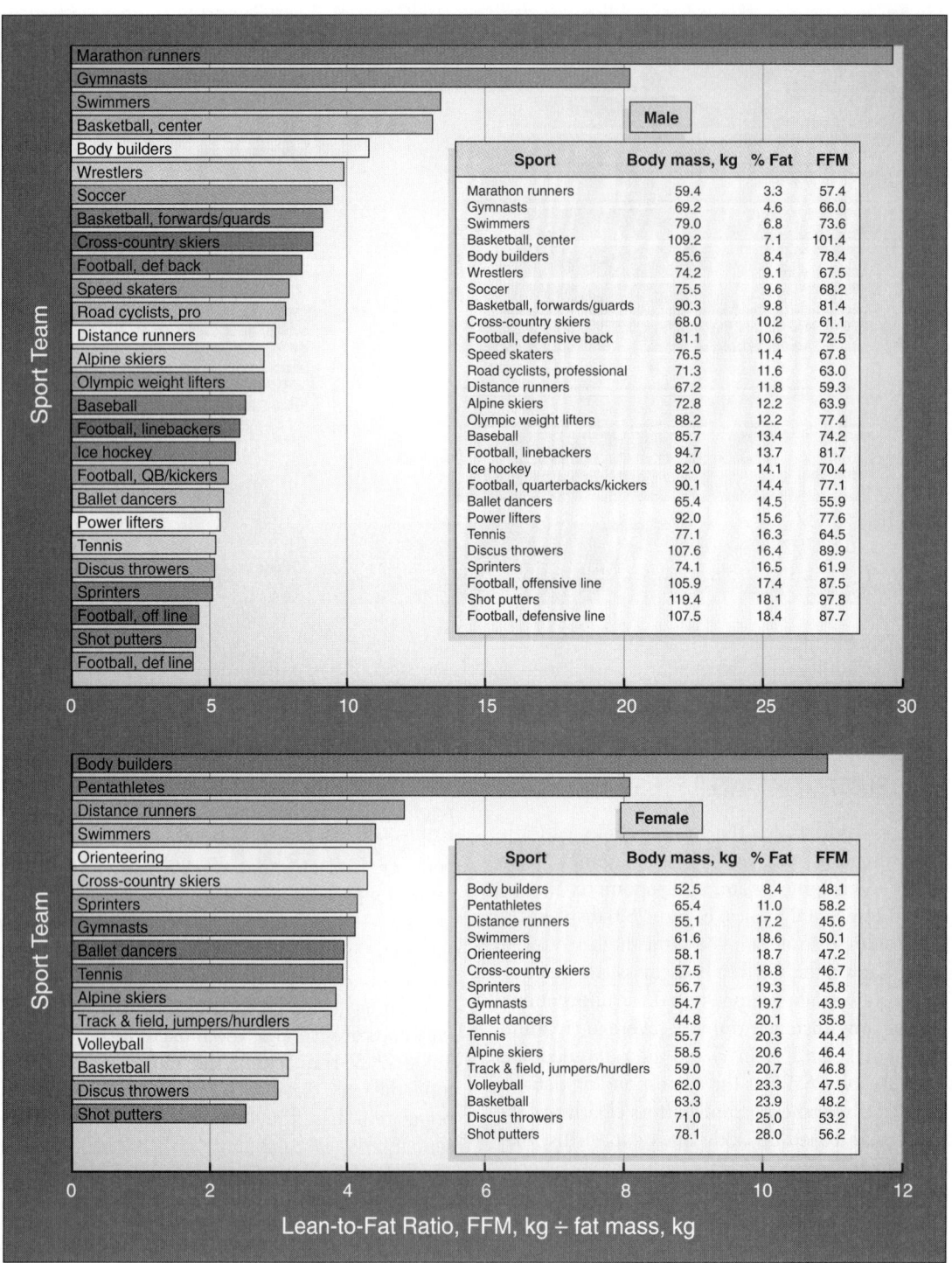

FIGURE 28.4

Comparison of the lean-to-fat ratios among male and female sports competitors. Values are based on the average body mass and percent body fat from various studies in the literature for each sport. The lean-to-fat ratio is computed as the fat-free body mass, kilograms ÷ fat mass, kilograms. The values in the insert tables represent averages for body composition when two or more literature citations were available on a specific sport. Body density was converted to percent body fat by the equation of Siri (refer to page 551, Chapter 27).

marathoners. Prefontaine was a former American record holder in the 800- and 1500-m runs, and Shorter was the 1976 Olympic Gold Medalist in the marathon. For comparative purposes, data are included for a typical sample of 95 untrained college-aged men.

Body fat values were extremely low for both groups of runners, considering that the quantity of essential fat for males is estimated at about 3% of body mass. Clearly, these endurance runners are at the lower end of the lean-to-fat continuum for topflight athletes. Apparently, this physique characteristic is a prerequisite for success in distance running. This makes sense for several reasons: first, the body's ability to dissipate heat during running is of primary importance in maintaining thermal balance during competition. Excess fat thwarts heat dissipation. Second, excess body fat is "dead weight" that adds directly to the energy cost of running.

With regard to body structure, elite male distance runners generally have smaller girths and bone diameters than untrained males.[17] One could consider that these structural differences, especially the bone diameters, are "genetic," as was the case for the anthropometric characteristics of the aquatic athletes (Fig. 28.1). The best long-distance runners inherit a physique that is slight of build, not only in stature but in skeletal dimensions. When this physique profile is combined with a lean body composition, highly developed aerobic system, and the proper psychological attitude for prolonged, intensive training, the ingredients are potentially there to create a champion.

TRIATHLETES

The triathlon combines endurance performance in three continuous activities—swimming, bicycling, and running. At the upper extreme of triathlon requirements is the ultra-endurance Ironman competition, for which performers are required to swim 3.9 km (2.4 miles), bicycle 180.2 km (112 miles), and run a standard marathon of 42.2 km (26.2 miles). Average training for the serious triathlete involves about 3 hours of training per day, covering 280 miles per week by swimming (7.2 mi; 30:00 pace), bicycling (227 mi; 18.6 mph), and running (45 mi; 7:42 pace).[24] Data for six males and three females who participated in the 1982 Ironman Triathlon indicated that body fat values ranged between 5.0 and 11.3% for males and between 7.4 and 17.2% for females. In the top 15 male finishers, body fat averaged 7.1%, with a corresponding $\dot{V}O_2$ max value of 72.0 mL $\cdot$ kg^{-1} $\cdot$ min^{-1}. From these data, it appears that the body fat and aerobic capacity of a triathlete are similar to values reported for athletes in single endurance sports.[38] A subsequent study of 14 triathletes training for the 1984 Ironman competition concluded that the physiques of both male and female triathletes are most similar to those of elite cyclists.[37] The aerobic capacity

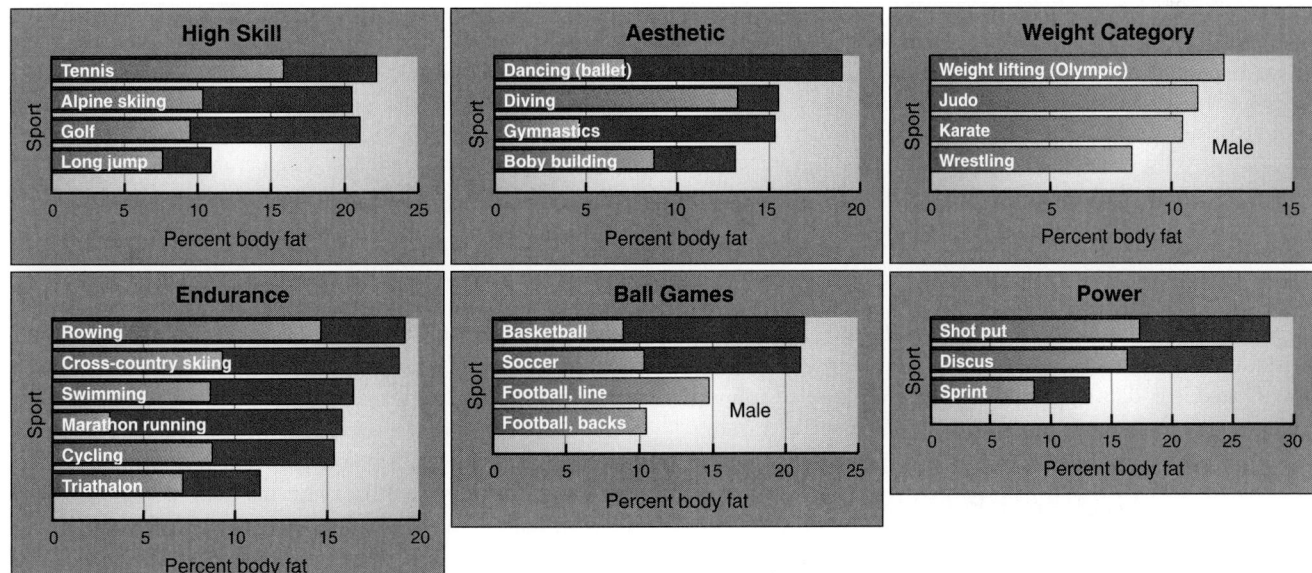

FIGURE 28.5

Percentage of body fat grouped by sports category. The value for males is displayed within the bar when there is a corresponding female value. A single bar represents data for males. The values for percent body fat represent averages from the literature.

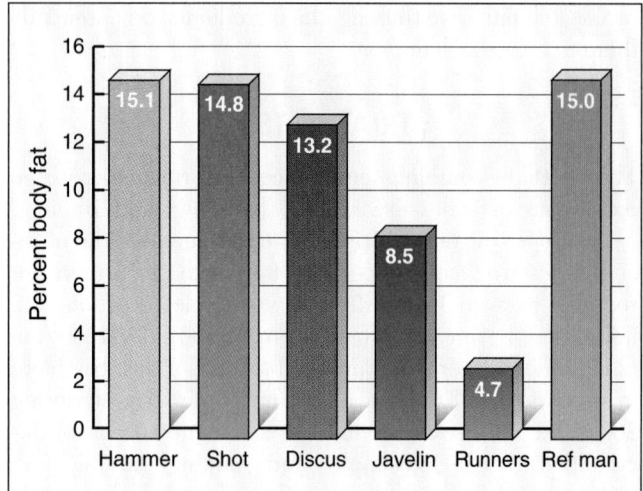
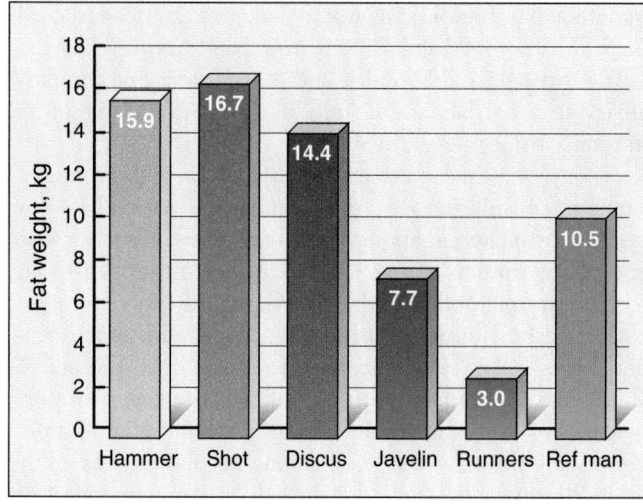
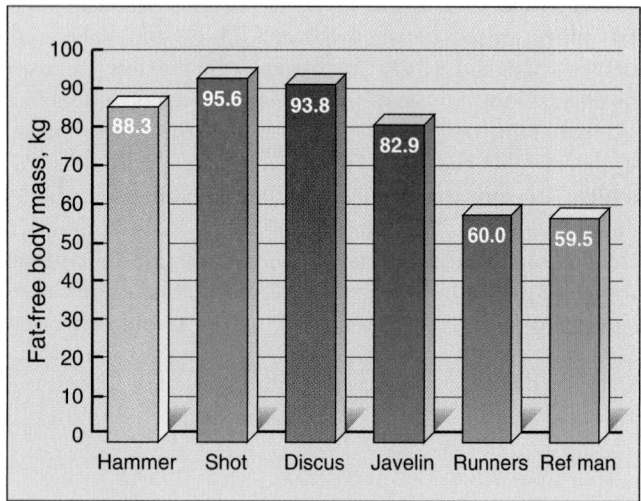
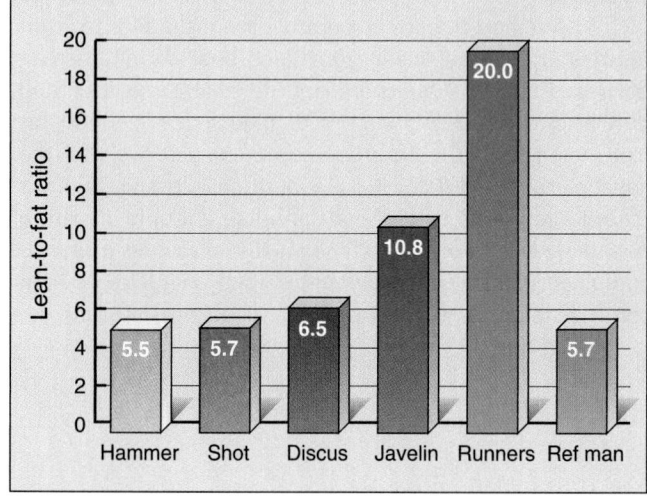

FIGURE 28.6

Body composition of the ten top American athletes in the discus, shot put, javelin, and hammer throw determined by densitometry using the procedures described in Chapter 27 for underwater weighing and residual lung volume (O_2 dilution). (Data collected by two of the authors (F.K. and V.K.) at a 1978 U.S. Olympic minicamp at the University of Houston, Houston, TX. Data include gold medalist Wilkins (discus) and world-record holder Powell (discus). Data for the international elite middle and long distance runners are from Pollock, M.L., et al.: Body composition of elite class distance runners. *Ann. NY Acad. Sci.*, 301:361, 1977. The reference man data are from Chapter 27.)

values for male triathletes were similar to those of trained swimmers, and the values for the females were at the upper range of data reported for elite endurance-trained runners.

FOOTBALL PLAYERS

The first detailed body composition analyses of football players vividly demonstrated the inadequacy of determining a person's "optimal" body mass from "height-weight" standards.[50] Football players as a group had a body fat content that averaged only 10.4% of body mass, while their fat-free body mass averaged 81.3 kg (179.3 lb). Certainly, these men were heavy, but they were not fat. The heaviest lineman weighed 118 kg (260 lb, 17.4% body fat, 215 lb of fat-free body mass), whereas the fattest lineman had 23.2% body fat and a body mass of 115.4 kg (252 lb). The player with the least fat was a defensive back; for his body mass of 82.3 kg (182 lb), body fat was 3.3% and fat-free body mass 79.6 kg (175 lb).

Table 28.8 presents a clearer picture of the average values for body mass, stature, percent body fat, and fat-free body mass of college and professional players grouped by position.[51, 53] The *Pro, older* group consists of 25 players from the 1942 Washington Redskins, the first professional players measured for body composition using densitometry to assess fat content. The *Pro, current* group consists of 164 players from 14 teams in the National Football League (NFL) (69% were veterans; 31% were rookies). The third group is 107 members of the 1976 to 1978 Dallas Cowboys and New York Jets football teams. For comparison, three groups of collegiate players are represented: (*a*) the St. Cloud State College, Minnesota, players who were candidates for spring practice; (*b*) players from the University of Massachusetts (UMass), also those who were

candidates for spring practice; and (*c*) members from the University of Southern California (USC) teams of 1973 to 1977, National Champions and participants in two Rose Bowls. For this data set, underwater weighing with correction for measured residual lung volume, as outlined in Chapter 27, was used to obtain the body composition measurements.

One would generally expect modern-day professional players to be larger in body size at each position than a representative collegiate group. Although this was generally true for the comparison with the St. Cloud and UMass play-

TABLE 28.5
FATFOLD AND GIRTH ANTHROPOMETRY OF THE TOP TEN AMERICAN ATHLETES IN THE DISCUS, SHOT PUT, JAVELIN, AND HAMMER THROW; DATA CORRESPOND TO THE ATHLETIC GROUPS PRESENTED IN FIGURE 28.1[a]

Measurement	Discus	Shotput	Javelin	Hammer	Runners	Ref. Man
Body mass, kg	108.2	112.3	90.6	104.2	63.1	70.0
Stature, cm	191.7	187.0	186.0	187.3	177.0	174.0
Fatfolds, mm						
Triceps	13.0	15.0	11.9	12.7	5.0	—
Scapula	18.0	23.8	12.5	21.5	6.4	—
Iliac	24.5	29.6	17.0	27.4	4.6	—
Abdomen	25.6	31.4	18.4	29.1	7.1	—
Thigh	16.4	15.7	13.3	17.3	6.1	—
Girths, cm						
Shoulders	129.8	133.3	121.5	127.4	106.1	110.8
Chest	113.5	118.5	104.6	111.3	91.1	91.8
Waist	94.1	99.1	86.6	94.8	74.6	77.0
Abdomen	97.5	101.5	87.8	98.0	74.2	79.8
Hips	110.4	112.3	102.0	108.7	87.8	93.4
Thighs	66.3	69.4	61.5	67.3	51.9	54.8
Knees	41.5	42.9	40.0	41.0	36.2[b]	36.6
Calves	42.6	43.6	39.5	41.5	35.4	35.8
Ankles	25.4	24.9	24.1	24.3	21.0	22.5
Biceps	41.8	42.2	37.7	39.9	28.2	31.7
Forearms	33.1	33.7	30.8	32.4	26.4	26.4
Wrists	18.7	18.9	18.2	18.4	16.0	17.3
Diameters, cm						
Biacromial	44.5	43.8	43.2	44.8	39.5	40.6
Chest	33.1	33.7	30.8	32.6	31.3	30.0
Bi-iliac	31.3	31.2	29.6	30.4	28.0	28.6
Bitrochanter	35.5	34.9	33.7	34.8	32.2	32.8
Knee	10.2	10.5	10.0	10.2	9.5	9.3
Wrist	6.3	6.2	6.0	6.2	5.6	5.6
Ankle	7.6	7.6	7.5	7.4	—	7.0
Elbow	7.6	7.6	7.6	7.2	—	7.0

[a]Details about measurement procedures from Katch, F.I., and Katch, V.L.: The body composition profile: techniques of measurement and applications. *Clin. Sports Med.*, 3:31, 1984.
[b]Not measured; value computed from the ratio for the reference man calf to knee.

TABLE 28.6
BODY COMPOSITION OF FEMALE LONG-DISTANCE RUNNERS

Subjects	Age (y)	Stature (cm)	Mass (kg)	FFM (kg)	Body Fat (kg)	Body Fat (%)
1[a]	24	172.7	52.6	49.5	3.1	5.9
2[b]	26	159.8	71.5	46.2	25.3	35.4
3[c]	28	162.6	50.7	47.6	3.1	6.1
4	31	171.5	52.0	47.3	4.7	9.0
5	33	176.5	61.2	50.8	10.4	17.0
6	34	166.4	52.9	44.8	8.1	15.2
7	35	168.4	55.0	48.7	6.3	11.6
8	36	164.5	53.1	44.3	8.8	16.6
9	36	182.9	61.5	50.4	11.1	18.1
10	36	182.9	65.4	55.7	9.7	14.8
11	37	154.9	53.6	44.0	9.6	18.0
Average	32.4	169.4	57.2	48.1	9.1	15.2

From Wilmore, J.H., and Brown, C.H.: Physiological profiles of women distance runners. *Med. Sci. Sports*, 6:178, 1974.
[a] World's best time in marathon (2:49:40) as of 1974.
[b] World's best time in 50-mile run (7:04:31); established 18 months after the body composition evaluation.
[c] Noted U.S. distance runner. Five consecutive national and international cross-country championships.

ers, the USC players were similar in physique to the professionals. With the exception of defensive linemen, the USC players at each position had almost the same body fat content, although they tended to weigh less than the current professional players at each position. In the all-important category of fat-free body mass, the USC players were no more than 4.4 kg lighter than the professionals at each position. The average defensive lineman in the NFL outweighed his USC counterpart in fat-free tissue by only 1.8 kg. The total body mass of the professional linemen, however, was significantly heavier than that of the USC counterparts. This difference existed because the professional linemen possessed 18.2% body fat, whereas the leaner collegians possessed 14.7%. It certainly seems that the body sizes and compositions of college and professional players are similar at the highest levels of collegiate competition.

It is of interest to note that as a group, the professional players of 50 years ago were lowest in total body fat (10.4%), and were shorter in stature and lighter in total body mass and fat-free body mass than modern players. The exceptions were the defensive and offensive backs and receivers; they were almost identical in body size and composition to current players. The biggest differences in physique status were in the defensive linemen: current players were taller by 6.7

cm, heavier by 20 kg, had 12.3 kg more fat-free body mass, and were 4.2 percentage points higher in percent body fat. Obviously, "bigness" was not yet an important factor in the line play of the 1940s. This is clearly demonstrated in Figure 28.7, which plots the average body mass of all roster players in the NFL for the 1994 season.

Maximal Running Performance and Body Composition

The maximal accelerations and velocities obtained during a 50-yd running performance (5-yd intervals for 50 yd) plotted in Figure 28.8 were obtained for a Super Bowl football team during the last week of spring practice before the season. Players started the sprint run from a crouched, bent-forward position with one hand touching the ground (similar to a football stance). Ten timing lights were placed at 5-yd intervals for 50 yd. Each player ran the distance twice, and the fastest time for the 50-yd sprint was used as the criterion performance. The offensive backs were the fastest players and the offensive linemen the slowest. There was no relationship between any time interval during the run and either body mass, fat mass, percent body fat, or fat-free body mass. Thus, a 50-yd maximal effort run was not related to individual differences in body composition.

HIGH SCHOOL WRESTLERS

Wrestlers represent a unique group of athletes who undergo both severe training and acute weight loss. Despite warnings from medical and professional groups of dangers related to rapid weight loss,[2, 3] most high school and college wrestlers (except heavyweights) attempt to reduce weight a few days before or on the day of competition. This weight loss is pursued with the hope of gaining a competitive advantage by wrestling at a lower weight category. The loss typically amounts to approximately 2 to 6 kg of body mass. This process of "making weight" usually is achieved by combining food restriction and dehydration, either through fluid and food deprivation or exercise in a hot environment while wearing plastic or rubber garments. Diuretics, laxatives, extended time in a sauna or steam room, and vomiting also are used to induce weight loss. In one study, approximately 2% of intercollegiate wrestlers exhibited bulimic behavior.[49] Unfortunately, it is other wrestlers, not the coach or parents, who are the source of information about how best to cut weight.[48] During a typical competitive season, an average wrestler can experience weight loss-gain 7 to 15 times, and this may be repeated more than 100 times during a career.[49] In a study of weight loss and gain during the NCAA Division I, II, and III wrestling championships, the pattern of weight gain and loss was consistent among wrestling weight categories but not levels of competition.[42] Following the official weigh-in, the wrestlers were weighed again 20 hours later before the first round of competition. The average wrestler gained 4.9% of body mass in 20 hours. The lightest weight wrestlers gained the most weight (4.5 kg, or 7.8% of body mass), while heavyweight wrestlers gained the least weight (0.7% of body mass). Wrestlers who advanced to the second round of the tournament all regained their lost weight, often as much as 7 kg (15.4 lb) in a 12-hour period! The American College of Sports Medicine (ACSM) recommends that weigh-ins be held immediately before competition to discourage rapid weight loss.[2] Thus, the NCAA rules currently are at odds with the recommended guidelines proposed by the ACSM.

To help reduce the possibility of injury and medical complications from acute weight loss and dehydration, the ACSM (and previously the American Medical Association[3]) recommends that each wrestler's body composition be as-

sessed several weeks before the competitive season to determine an acceptable minimal wrestling weight. A lower limit of 5% body fat (determined using hydrostatic weighing or population-specific regression equations based on anthropometry) is proposed as the lowest acceptable level for safe wrestling competition. The concern about rapid fluid loss relates to the potential for significant reductions in plasma volume, central blood volume, and blood flow to active tissues. With a 2% loss in body mass, significant alterations occur in the cardiovascular response to submaximal exercise. These alterations can increase central core temperature and produce undesirable shifts in the electrolyte concentration. The monitoring of relative leanness also may be appropriate for competitors below the high school level; research indicates that prepubescent wrestlers possess significantly less body fat than normally active boys.[41]

TABLE 28.7
BODY COMPOSITION CHARACTERISTICS OF ELITE MALE MIDDLE- AND LONG-DISTANCE RUNNERS AND ELITE MARATHONERS

Group	Stature (cm)	Mass (kg)	Density (g·mL⁻¹)	Body Fat (%)	FFM (kg)	Fat Mass (kg)	Sum 7 Fatfolds (mm)
Distance Runners							
Brown	187.3	72.10	1.07428	10.8	64.31	7.79	53.0
Castaneda	178.6	63.34	1.09102	3.7	61.00	2.34	32.5
Crawford	171.8	58.01	1.09702	1.2	57.31	0.70	32.5
Geis	179.1	66.28	1.07551	10.2	59.52	6.76	49.0
Johnson	174.6	61.79	1.08963	4.3	59.13	2.66	35.5
Manley	177.8	69.10	1.09642	1.5	68.06	1.04	32.0
Ndoo	169.3	53.97	1.08379	6.7	50.35	3.62	33.5
Prefontaine	174.2	68.00	1.08842	4.8	64.74	3.26	38.0
Rose	175.6	59.15	1.08248	7.3	54.83	4.32	31.5
Tuttle	176.8	61.44	1.09960	0.2	61.32	0.12	31.5
	170.5	60.92	1.08916	4.5	58.18	2.74	34.5
x̄	176.0	63.10	1.08794	5.0	59.89	3.21	36.7
(± SD)	(5.0)	(5.30)	(0.00832)	(3.5)	(4.90)	(2.38)	(7.4)
Marathon Runners							
Cusack	174.6	64.19	1.08096	7.9	59.12	5.07	45.5
Galloway	180.9	65.76	1.08419	6.6	61.42	4.34	43.0
Kennedy	167.0	56.52	1.09348	2.7	54.99	1.53	37.0
Moore	184.1	64.24	1.09193	3.3	62.12	2.12	37.0
Pate[a]	179.6	57.28	1.09676	1.3	56.54	0.74	32.5
Shorter	178.4	61.17	1.09475	2.2	59.82	1.35	45.0
Wayne	172.1	61.61	1.07859	8.9	56.13	5.48	42.5
Williams	177.2	66.07	1.09569	1.8	64.88	1.19	41.5
x̄	176.8	62.11	1.08954	4.3	59.38	2.73	40.5
(± SD)	(5.6)	(3.66)	(0.00718)	(3.0)	(3.38)	(1.92)	(4.6)

Data from Pollock, M.L., et al.: Body composition of elite class distance runners. *Ann. NY Acad. Sci.*, 301:361, 1977.
[a]Dr. Russel Pate is an exercise physiologist, Department of Exercise Science, University of South Carolina, Columbia, SC.

TABLE 28.8
COMPARISON OF BODY COMPOSITION BETWEEN COLLEGIATE AND PROFESSIONAL FOOTBALL PLAYERS GROUPED BY POSITION[a]

Position	Level	N	Stature (cm)	Mass (kg)	Body Fat (%)	FFM (kg)
Defensive backs	St. Cloud[b]	15	178.3	77.3	11.5	68.4
	U Mass[c]	12	179.9	83.1	8.8	76.8
	USC[d]	15	183.0	83.7	9.6	75.7
	Pro, current[e]	26	182.5	84.8	9.6	76.7
	Pro, older[f]	25	183.0	91.2	10.7	81.4
Offensive backs	St. Cloud	15	179.7	79.8	12.4	69.6
and receivers	U Mass	29	181.8	84.1	9.5	76.4
	USC	18	185.6	86.1	9.9	77.6
	Pro, current	40	183.8	90.7	9.4	81.9
	Pro, older	25	183.0	91.7	10.0	87.5
Linebackers	St. Cloud	7	180.1	87.2	13.4	75.4
	U Mass	17	186.1	97.1	13.1	84.2
	USC	17	185.6	98.8	13.2	85.8
	Pro, current	28	188.6	102.2	14.0	87.6
Offensive linemen	St. Cloud	13	186.0	99.2	19.1	79.8
and tight ends	U Mass	23	187.5	107.6	19.5	86.6
	USC	25	191.1	106.5	15.3	90.3
	Pro, current	38	193.0	112.6	15.6	94.7
Defensive linemen	St. Cloud	15	186.6	97.8	18.5	79.3
	U Mass	8	188.8	114.3	19.5	91.9
	USC	13	191.1	109.3	14.7	93.2
	Pro, current	32	192.4	117.1	18.2	95.8
	Pro, older	25	185.7	97.1	14.0	83.5
Total	St. Cloud	65	182.5	88.0	15.0	74.2
	U Mass	91	184.9	97.3	13.9	83.2
	USC	88	186.6	96.6	11.4	84.6
	Pro, current	164	188.1	101.5	13.4	87.3
	Pro, older	25	183.1	91.2	10.4	81.3
	Dallas-Jets[g]	107	188.2	100.4	12.6	87.7

[a]Grouping according to Wilmore, J.H., and Haskel, W.L.: Body composition and endurance capacity of professional football players. *J. Appl. Physiol.*, 33:564, 1972.

[b]Data from Wickkiser, J.D., and Kelly, J.M.: The body composition of a college football team. *Med. Sci. Sports*, 7:199, 1975.

[c]U Mass data from Coach Robert Stull and F. Katch, University of Massachusetts. Data collected during spring practice, 1985; % fat by densitometry.

[d]USC data from Dr. Robert Girandola, University of Southern California, Los Angeles, 1978, 1993.

[e]Data from Wilmore, J.H., et al.: Football pros' strengths–and CV weakness–charted. *Phys. Sportsmed.*, 4:45, 1976.

[f]Data from Dr. A.R. Behnke.

[g]Data from Katch, F.I., and Katch, V.L.: Body composition of the Dallas Cowboys and New York Jets football teams. Unpublished data, 1978.

Physical Characteristics of High School Wrestlers

The physical characteristics of three groups of high school wrestlers are presented in Table 28.9.[16, 25] The "certified" Iowa and Minnesota wrestlers were assigned to wrestle at one of 12 different weight categories; the "champion" wrestlers competed in the state or conference finals. Except for age and fatfolds, there was little difference in the physi-cal characteristics of the Iowa and Minnesota certified and champion wrestlers. As reflected by the fatfold measures, however, the champions were considerably leaner than their less successful teammates. Because differences in body mass were small among groups, the elite wrestlers actually competed at heavier fat-free body masses. This factor may have contributed greatly to their success in a particular

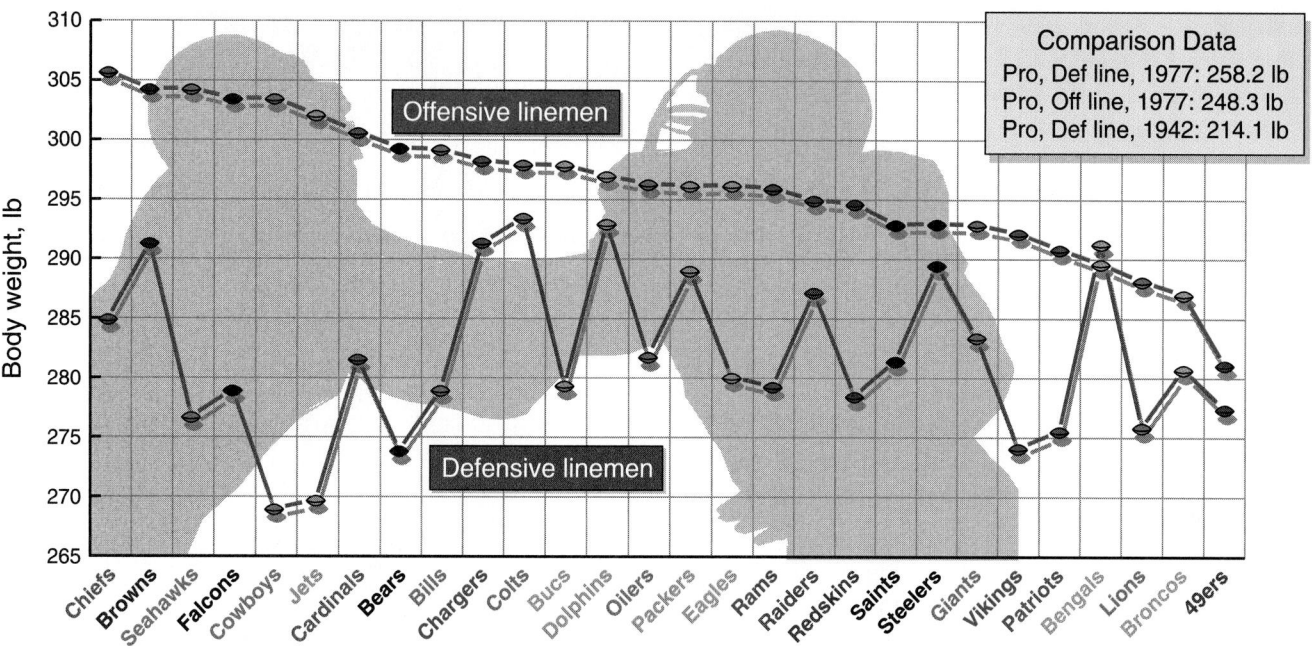

FIGURE 28.7

Average body weight of all roster offensive and defensive linemen in the National Football League for 1994. (From active team rosters for 28 NFL teams as of the first regular-season weekend, September 4–5, 1994. Data courtesy of the National Football League public relations department.)

Position	50-yd run time, s									
	5	10	15	20	25	30	35	40	45	50
Offensive line	1.30	2.03	2.68	3.26	3.84	4.40	4.95	5.51	6.05	6.61
Defensive line	1.31	1.98	2.62	3.19	3.72	4.28	4.81	5.34	5.87	6.41
Offensive backs	1.22	1.88	2.48	3.00	3.52	4.02	4.51	5.00	5.48	5.97
Wide receivers	1.25	1.91	2.50	3.03	3.54	4.02	4.50	4.98	5.45	5.94
Linebackers	1.24	1.93	2.54	3.10	3.60	4.15	4.66	5.18	5.70	6.19
Defensive backs	1.22	1.89	2.48	3.01	3.52	4.02	4.51	5.00	5.50	5.97

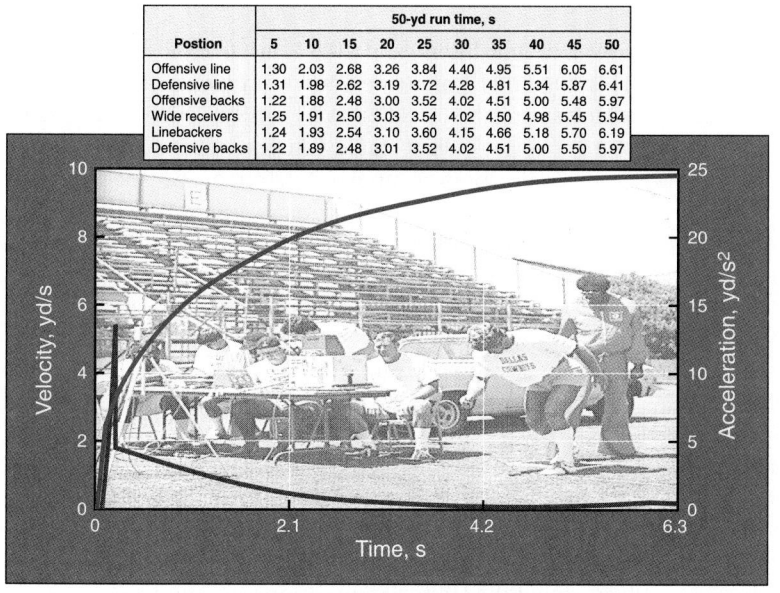

FIGURE 28.8

Maximal acceleration (red line) and velocity (blue line) during a 50-yd running performance (5-yd intervals for 50 yd) for 39 professional football players (Super Bowl Champions). Timing lights hooked in series were used to record sequential run times. The inset graph displays the results for raw run time (5-yd intervals) by player's position. (Data from Dr. Paul Ward.)

weight class. The last column in Table 28.9 presents additional data on 409 Nebraska high school wrestlers.[25] Their anthropometric characteristics are most similar to the Iowa and Minnesota certified wrestlers. The relative percent body fat of the Nebraska wrestlers, as determined by densitometry, was 11.0 ± 4.0% (range from 1.5 to 26.0%). Their minimal wrestling weights at 5% body fat averaged 59.1 kg.

Weight Loss Recommendations for Wrestlers

Prior to the season's start, suppose a high school wrestler who wishes to compete in the lowest possible weight category compatible with good health and performance weighs 70 kg and has 15% body fat. A prudent recommendation for weight loss would be to reduce body fat content to no lower than 5% of body mass.[47] The proposed weight loss would therefore be 10% of the

TABLE 28.9
ANTHROPOMETRIC COMPARISONS BETWEEN CERTIFIED AND CHAMPION IOWA AND MINNESOTA HIGH SCHOOL WRESTLERS[a] AND COMPARISON TO NEBRASKA WRESTLERS[b]

| Measurement | Certified Wrestlers | | Champion Wrestlers | | Nebraska Wrestlers |
	Iowa (N = 484)	Minn (N = 245)	Iowa (N = 382)	Minn (N = 164)	(N = 409)
Age, y	15.9	16.8	17.8	17.4	16.4
Stature, cm	169.9	172.0	171.7	172.5	171.0
Body mass, kg	64.3	65.3	64.6	64.7	63.2
Chest diameter, cm	26.8	26.5	27.7	26.6	27.9
Chest depth, cm	19.0	16.8	19.2	17.3	18.9
Bitrochanteric diameter, cm	31.0	31.4	31.1	31.5	31.0
Ankles diameter, cm	14.3	14.3	14.0	14.3	13.8
Fatfolds, mm					
Scapular	8.4	7.9	6.4	6.8	8.8
Triceps	8.6	9.1	6.0	5.6	8.9
Suprailiac	13.3	12.3	9.1	7.5	11.8
Abdominal	13.1	12.2	8.6	8.3	11.6
Thigh	10.8	13.6	7.7	8.3	9.4
Sum of 5 fatfolds	54.2	55.1	37.8	36.5	50.5

[a]From Clarke, K.S.: Predicting certified weight of young wrestlers; a field study of the Tcheng-Tipton method. *Med. Sci. Sports,* 6:52, 1974.
[b]From Housh, T.J., et al.: Validity of anthropometric estimations of body compositions in high school wrestlers. *Res. Q. Exerc. Sport,* 60:239, 1989.

wrestler's body mass, or about 7 kg, resulting in a final body mass of 63 kg. With increased training and moderate caloric restriction, a weight loss of 1 kg per week is a reasonable objective.[45] Thus, in about 7 weeks, the desired weight loss would be achieved and the wrestler could effectively compete in the 145-lb (65.8-kg) weight class. Interestingly, some coaches have used changes in hand grip strength in an attempt to evaluate lean body mass loss by its effects on maximal muscular force output. Unfortunately, maximum grip force does not decline correspondingly with body mass loss, even when the loss in body mass averages 15.6% and fat-free body mass declines by 6.9% in only 8.5 weeks.[27] Thus, when muscle mass declines, a change in grip strength would not be a good indicator of this negative alteration in body composition.

WEIGHT LIFTERS AND BODY BUILDERS

Men

Men who engage in resistance training often exhibit remarkable muscular development. Excess levels of muscle development and fat-free body mass have been quantified in competitive body builders, Olympic weight lifters, and power weight lifters.[31] For percent body fat, the values were quite similar, averaging 9.3% in the body builders, 9.1% in power weight lifters, and 10.8% in Olympic weight lifters. This degree of leanness existed even though each group of athletes could be classified as 14 to 19% "overweight" based on the "height-weight" tables! Also, no differences between groups were present in skeletal frame size, fat-free body mass, fatfolds, or bone diameter measurements. The only differences in anthropometry between the groups were in the shoulders, chest, biceps both relaxed and flexed, and forearm girths, with the body builders being larger at each site. Estimation of excess muscle revealed that the body builders possessed nearly 16 kg of excess muscle, while power weight lifters possessed 15 kg and Olympic weight lifters, 13 kg.

Women

Body building among females gained widespread popularity throughout the United States during the late 1970s. As more women undertook the vigorous demands of resistance training, competition became more intense, and the level of achievement increased markedly. Because success in body building is based on a "slim" and lean appearance, complemented by a well-defined yet enlarged musculature, interesting questions are raised with regard to body composition. How lean are such competitors, and is their presumably low level of body fat accompanied by a relatively large muscle mass?

A study of the body composition of 10 competitive female body builders revealed that these athletes were quite lean, averaging 13.2% body fat (range from 8.0 to 18.3%) and having an average fat-free body mass of 46.6 kg.[21] With the exception of champion gymnasts, who also average about 13% body fat, the body builders were 3 to 4% shorter in stature, 4 to 5% lower in body mass, and possessed 7 to 10% less total mass of body fat compared to other top female athletes. The most striking compositional characteristic of the female body builders was a dramatically large FFM/FM ratio of 7 : 1, compared to 4.3 : 1 for other female athletic groups. This difference occurred without the use of steroids, as reported by the women in a questionnaire. Interestingly, menstrual function was reported to be normal by eight of ten body builders despite their relatively low levels of body fat.

Men versus Women

Table 28.10 compares the body composition, girths, and excess muscle mass of male and female body builders. The latter was defined as the difference between scale mass and mass-for-stature taken from Metropolitan Life Insurance tables. The men are 14.8 kg (18%) overweight, and the women are 1.2 kg (12%) overweight. Obviously, in these athletes, excess mass is primarily fat-free body mass, primarily in the form of excess muscle.

The comparison of the girth data makes it possible to compare individuals (or groups) who differ in overall body size. The analysis indicates that sex differences in girths, when scaled to body size (referred to as "adjusted" in the table), are not as different as would be expected if only the raw girths were compared. Compared to their body sizes, the females are actually larger than the male body builders in 7 of the 12 body areas. *This suggests that women can probably alter muscle size to almost the same relative extent as males, at least when scaled to a body size factor.* The larger hips in the women are probably related to greater fat stores in this location.

COMPARATIVE DATA: ANALYSIS OF MUSCULAR AND NONMUSCULAR COMPONENTS

The body profile technique introduced in Chapter 27 provides a unique way to partition the anthropometric aspects

TABLE 28.10
BODY COMPOSITION AND ANTHROPOMETRIC GIRTHS OF MALE AND FEMALE BODY BUILDERS

Sex	Age (y)	Mass (kg)	Stature (cm)	Fat (%)	FFM (kg)	Excess Mass[a] (kg)
Male[b] (N = 18)	27.0	82.4	177.1	9.3	74.6	14.8
Female[c] (N = 10)	27.0	53.8	160.8	13.2	46.6	1.2

Body Part (cm)	Males		Females		% Difference (Males vs. Females)	
	Raw	Adjusted[d]	Raw	Adjusted[d]	Raw	Adjusted[d]
Shoulders	123.1	37.1	101.7	36.7	17.4	1.1
Chest	106.4	32.1	90.6	32.7	14.9	−1.9
Waist	82.0	24.7	64.5	23.3	21.3	5.7
Abdomen	82.3	24.8	67.7	25.1	15.3	−1.2
Hips	95.6	28.8	87.0	31.4	9.0	−9.0
Biceps relaxed	35.9	10.8	25.8	9.3	28.1	13.9
Biceps flexed	40.4	12.2	28.9	10.4	28.5	14.8
Forearm	30.7	9.2	24.0	8.7	21.8	5.4
Wrist	17.4	5.2	15.1	5.4	13.2	−3.8
Thigh	59.6	17.9	53.0	19.1	11.1	−6.7
Calf	37.3	11.2	32.4	11.7	13.1	−4.5
Ankle	22.8	6.9	26.3	7.3	11.0	−5.8

[a]Body mass minus body mass estimated from height-weight tables (Reference 1).
[b]Reference 31.
[c]Reference 21.
[d]Calculated as $G_i/\sqrt{mass}$, kg/stature, $dm^{0.7}$, where G_i equals any one of the girths. The term (mass/stature$^{0.7}$) is a frame structure estimate of perimetric (girth) size. The adjusted values are the perimetric equivalent adjusted girths due to sex differences because they are corrected for whatever differences may exist as a result of differences in body size.

of body size and shape into muscular and nonmuscular components. A major advantage of this approach is that diversity in overall body dimensions can readily be compared among individuals and groups. The technique also permits easy tracking of progress in the various body components that result from different modes of training, weight loss and gain, growth, and aging. Table 28.11 presents the percentage deviations in the muscular and nonmuscular components for ten different groups. The percentage deviation scores are directly comparable because the data analysis was based on the Behnke reference man and woman as standards of comparison, and adjustments were made among the groups to equalize their dimensions compared to stature.

Professional Ballet Dancers

The subjects of this study (Group 1) were ten prima ballerinas from the San Francisco Ballet Company. Not unexpectedly, six of the 11 percentage deviations were negative; the exceptions were the shoulders, chest, thigh, calf, and ankles.

Champion Male and Female Body Builders

The excessive muscular development in the champion group of 11 Mr. Universe body builders (Group 2) is evident for the six muscular sites, particularly the biceps, which exhibited the largest deviation (77.9%) of any body site among the groups. Expressed as the ponderal equivalent of the biceps, the 77.9% deviation is equivalent to 127.9 kg. This means that for a body builder weighing 84.2 kg, the mass of the biceps would be the projected size of biceps in an individual weighing 127.9 kg. The ratio of the muscular-to-nonmuscular girths was 1.396; this would verify the existence of excess muscle. In contrast, the muscular-to-nonmuscular ratios in the ten champion female body builders (Group 3) was considerably lower, at 1.097. Although visual appraisal of a female body builder gives the appearance that the muscular girths predominate, the body profile analysis suggests that the eye may be unable to detect excess muscle as well as it detects general refinement and muscular shaping in different body parts. Stated differently, female body builders as a group were more evenly

---

TABLE 28.11
PERCENTAGE DEVIATION FOR THE MUSCULAR AND NONMUSCULAR COMPONENTS AMONG INDIVIDUALS AND GROUPS THAT DIFFER MARKEDLY IN BODY SIZE AND SHAPE (GROUPS 1 TO 10 ARE IDENTIFIED IN THE FOOTNOTE[a])

Reference Data Group	Group									
	1	*2*	*3*	*4*	*5*	*6*	*7*	*8*	*9*	*10*
Age, y	21.8	32.1	27.1	18–22	17.2	17.2	17.0	17.4	17.2	21.2
Body mass, kg	51.4	84.2	53.4	78.5	69.3	58.2	43.4	141.8	59.1	64.6
Stature, cm	166.4	170.6	160.6	180.3	178.1	165.0	161.2	189.7	171.0	172.9
Muscular Girths					**Percentage Deviation**					
Shoulders	10.6	28.2	12.9	1.7	2.7	−1.0	0.7	−6.4	—	—
Chest	8.6	49.2	19.4	6.4	2.2	1.4	3.8	4.1	−1.2	2.0
Biceps	−9.2	77.9	14.9	2.3	−2.4	−2.9	5.4	3.1	−10.4	17.3
Forearm	−1.8	43.7	9.1	3.3	1.6	−0.8	2.0	−15.3	2.6	4.0
Thigh	0.0	17.9	−1.6	6.3	2.5	−2.2	−20.2	26.1	−4.1	−2.4
Calf	9.8	20.9	3.4	4.7	4.4	2.0	1.4	11.0	2.1	2.0
Nonmuscular Girths										
Abdomen	−1.2	−28.7	−7.0	−2.6	−4.5	0.2	−7.8	31.9	−5.9	−7.6
Hips	−3.7	−30.1	−11.0	−3.1	−0.4	−2.0	−1.4	3.2	2.4	−2.5
Wrist	−5.8	−26.4	−8.3	−7.8	−4.7	−3.9	16.4	−36.4	3.4	−7.0
Knee	−4.9	−29.0	−12.1	−3.8	−1.0	4.3	7.6	−12.2	8.7	−0.6
Ankle	0.6	−27.7	−6.1	−5.9	2.6	5.8	11.1	−4.7	—	—

[a]The numbers for the groups refer to the following: 1, professional ballet dancers; 2, champion male body builders; 3, champion female body builders; 4, male college students; 5, senior high school males; 6, senior high school females; 7, smallest boy in a 12th-grade class; 8, largest boy in a 12th-grade class; 9, entering class of Amherst College in 1882; 10, graduating class of Amherst College in 1886. More detailed anthropometric information about Groups 1 to 10, including original references, appears in: Katch, F.I., et al.: The ponderal somatogram: evaluation of body size and shape from anthropometric girths and stature. *Hum. Biol.*, 59:439, 1987.

proportional between their muscular and nonmuscular components.

College-Age Males

Group 4 was a representative sample of 100 males from Eastern Oregon College, all nonathletes.

Twelfth-Grade Caucasian Males and Females

Groups 5 and 6 were part of a large-scale multiracial nutrition and anthropometric survey of 9th- through 12th-grade students at Berkeley High School, Berkeley, California.[26] Despite substantial differences in body mass and stature at identical ages, the percentage deviations were surprisingly similar for the muscular and nonmuscular components. The absolute values for the various body parts, however, were larger for the males by approximately the same difference as those for the body masses.

Smallest and Largest Boy in the 12th Grade. Groups 7 and 8 represent the smallest and largest boy, respectively, of the same age in the 450-member 12th-grade class at Berkeley High School. The comparison is dramatic: the difference between the boys is 98.4 kg (217 lb) in body mass and 28.5 cm (almost 1 ft) in stature!

Table 28.12 compares the ponderal (mass) equivalents for the muscular and nonmuscular body components in these two boys. The listed ponderal values are the mass equivalents for a person possessing a specific girth. For example, the ponderal equivalent of 44.7 kg for the diminutive boy is the projected mass based on that particular girth. Note that the smallest boy weighed 43.4 kg, so his shoulder ponderal equivalent mass (44.7 kg) was certainly of "normal" development. This percentage deviation for the shoulder of 0.7, listed in Table 28.11 (Group 7), is much smaller than the −6.4% deviation for the largest boy (Group 8). His ponderal equivalent mass based on the shoulder measurement is 128.5 kg (Table 28.11), yet his body mass is 13.3 kg greater at 141.8 kg. Viewed somewhat differently, the largest boy in the class had a shoulder ponderal equivalent of someone who weighed 128.5 kg. It would certainly be fair to conclude that despite the boy's size, his shoulders were underdeveloped, as were the ponderal equivalent masses projected from his forearms (116.3 kg), wrists (90.6 kg), knees (125.1 kg), and ankles (135.8 kg).

In the nonmuscular abdominal component, the ponderal equivalent for the diminutive boy also was small (38.9 kg) for his scale mass of 43.4 kg. In the largest boy, the abdominal component was excessively large: it corresponded to a projected mass of 46.2 kg more, or 188.0 kg (415 lb)!

It may be that in relatively small children or large adolescents, the occurrence of a large positive deviation in the ponderal equivalent for the abdomen "signals" the onset of late-adolescent or even adult-onset obesity. If this is true, then determination of the abdominal ponderal

TABLE 28.12
PONDERAL EQUIVALENT (P-E) MUSCULAR AND NONMUSCULAR COMPONENTS FOR THE SMALLEST AND LARGEST BOYS IN A TWELFTH-GRADE CLASS[a]

	Smallest Boy Mass = 43.4 kg Stature = 161.2 cm		Largest Boy Mass = 141.8 kg Stature = 189.7 cm	
	Girth (cm)	P-E (kg)	Girth (cm)	P-E (kg)
Variable				
Muscular				
Shoulders	92.3	44.7	144.2	128.5
Chest	74.7	42.7	126.0	142.9
Biceps	25.6	42.0	43.3	141.6
Forearm	22.1	43.5	33.3	116.3
Thigh	40.6	35.4	82.8	173.2
Calf	29.9	45.0	50.7	152.4
Nonmuscular				
Abdomen	60.9	38.9	123.4	188.0
Hips	75.0	41.6	130.0	147.0
Wrist	15.1	49.1	18.9	90.6
Knee	30.7	45.4	47.0	125.1
Ankle	19.2	46.9	30.1	135.8

[a]Data are for Groups 7 and 8 in Table 28.11.

equivalent at an early age with subsequent follow-up could be useful as a clinical marker for preventive purposes.

Entering and Graduating Classes of Amherst College (1882–1886)

This remarkable data set for groups 9 and 10 in Table 28.11 was retrieved from the archival records of the pioneer exercise anthropometrist, Dr. Edward Hitchcock, Jr. Note the dramatic increase in biceps girth and decreases in the nonmuscular abdomen and hip regions. These changes coincided with the start of daily resistance training using weighted bowling pins (refer to Introduction Figure 4, p. 13).

EFFECTS OF EXERCISE TRAINING ON BODY COMPOSITION

In this section, we consider the effectiveness of walking, jogging, cycling, and resistance training in modifying the body composition of young and middle-aged adults. These findings have special meaning to health professionals and others involved in leading exercise programs because of the important role exercise can play in effective weight control as discussed more fully in Chapter 29.

TEN-WEEK JOGGING PROGRAM

Table 28.13 illustrates changes in physique for men aged 17 to 59 years who jogged 3 days per week for 10 weeks.[54] The average distance run by the end of 10 weeks was 84.4 km (51.8 miles), or about 2.8 km (1.7 miles) per day. Body composition changes did occur but were relatively small. Because fat-free body mass did not change, the decrease in body mass was attributed to a reduction in percent body fat from pretest (18.9%) to post-test (17.8%); this represented a fat loss of 1.07 kg. The reduction in individual fatfold values paralleled the decrease in body fat. It is possible that the small reduction in body fat was a result of the relatively short duration of the jogging program, or that the average body fat of the group before training was only slightly greater than the average for college-aged men. As such, these men were not overfat and did not need to greatly reduce body size.

WALKING-RUNNING FOR DIFFERENT DURATIONS

The duration of exercise has an effect on fat loss with training. Table 28.14 lists the changes in body fat (predicted from fatfolds) for three groups of men who trained walking and running for either 15, 30, or 45 minutes per workout.[36] Also

included are the distances run and total duration of the weekly workouts, training heart rate, body mass, sum of fatfolds (chest, axilla, triceps, abdomen, suprailiac, and anterior thigh), and waist girth.

Compared to the control group that remained unchanged over the 20-week training period, the three exercise groups significantly decreased their body fat, fatfolds, and waist girth. Body mass also was significantly lowered with exercise training except for the 15-minute group, whose mass remained stable. Comparisons made between the three groups indicated that the 45-minute training group lost a greater percentage of body fat than either the 30- or the 15-minute exercise group. This was attributed to the greater calorie-burning effect of the longer exercise period. Individuals desiring to use walking as their sole means of exercise training for weight loss can employ hand, wrist, and ankle weights to increase exercise intensity and caloric output as the program progresses.[9]

TWO-YEAR PROGRAM OF CALISTHENICS AND JOGGING

A 2-year calisthenics and jogging program was used to evaluate changes in body composition of seven middle-aged men.[12] Comparative data were also presented for six controls who were measured at the same 6-month intervals but did not take part in the exercise program. The exercisers participated in a supervised program 3 days per week. Initially, they walked and jogged for 10 minutes; thereafter, they jogged for 30 to 35 minutes. The average distance covered increased from 2.4 to 12.1 km per week, and the total distance run per subject after 2 years of training averaged 1188 km (738 miles).

Compared with control subjects whose body composition remained relatively constant during the 2-year period, the exercisers after the first year significantly reduced their body mass (5.7%), sum of fatfolds (27.4%), and girth measurements (3.1%). Thereafter, there was little further change in body mass and body composition. These results indicate that calisthenics and jogging can significantly alter the physiques of previously sedentary 40- to 60-year-old men. The changes paralleled a 25% improvement in aerobic capacity.

WALKING, RUNNING, AND BICYCLING

An evaluation of relative training effects on body composition of walking, running, or bicycling indicates that each mode of exercise significantly reduces body mass, body fat, fatfold thickness, and girths. *In addition, there generally is no selective effect of either running, walking, or bicycling, each training mode being equally effective in altering body composition.*

TABLE 28.13
BODY COMPOSITION CHANGES RESULTING FROM A 10-WEEK JOGGING PROGRAM

Variable	Pre-Training	Post-Training	Difference
Body mass, kg	79.59	78.58	−1.01[a]
Body fat, %	18.88	17.77	−1.11[a]
Body fat, kg	15.03	13.96	−1.07
FFM, kg	64.56	64.62	0.06
Fatfolds, mm			
Triceps	11.5	11.1	−0.4
Scapula	16.3	15.1	−1.2[a]
Suprailiac	24.9	24.4	−0.5
Mid axillary	17.3	14.3	−3.0[a]
Abdominal	24.4	23.5	−0.9
Thigh	16.9	16.0	−0.9[a]
Chest	12.7	11.5	−1.2[a]
Girths, cm			
Waist	84.8	84.4	−0.8[a]
Abdomen	88.2	87.7	−0.5

From Wilmore, J.H., et al.: Body composition changes with a 10-week program of jogging. *Med. Sci. Sports*, 2:113, 1970.
[a]Statistically significant.

TABLE 28.14
EFFECTS OF THREE TRAINING DURATIONS OF WALKING AND RUNNING ON BODY COMPOSITION CHANGES

| | | | | Training Group | | | | |
| | Control (N = 16) | | 15 Minute (N = 14) | | 30 Minute (N = 17) | | 45 Minute (N = 12) | |
Variable	Pre	Post	Pre	Post	Pre	Post	Pre	Post
Body mass, kg	72.1	73.2	76.9	76.3	80.6	78.9	70.9	69.9
Body fat, %	12.5	13.0	13.7	13.2	14.2	13.6	13.2	12.0
Sum fatfolds, mm	73.8	79.6	83.0	77.0	90.0	83.8	77.5	67.0
Waist girth, cm	82.7	84.9	84.3	82.8	88.2	86.1	83.6	81.8
Distance run per workout (miles)	week 4		1.56		2.89		4.13	
	8		1.54		2.95		4.46	
	13		1.79		3.19		4.82	
	17		1.75		3.24		5.06	
Total time of exercise (min:s)	week 4		14:58		30:25		41:18	
	8		14:11		28:40		42:48	
	13		15:51		29:43		43:19	
	17		14:53		30:12		42:27	
Training heart rate (beats · min^{-1})	week 4		179		175		174	
	8		179		174		169	
	13		182		175		177	
	17		180		175		175	
Intensity (% of max HR)	week 4		89.4		83.8		84.5	
	8		89.8		73.4		81.0	
	13		94.0		90.1		89.5	
	17		92.5		90.2		88.1	

From Milesis, C.A., et al.: Effects of different durations of physical training on cardiorespiratory function, body composition, and serum lipids. *Res. Q., 47:716, 1976.*

RESISTANCE TRAINING

Resistance training is a possible modality for inducing favorable changes in body composition.[8] Because the caloric expenditure of circuit resistance training averages about 9 kcal per minute, this form of exercise can potentially produce a substantial caloric output during a typical 30- to 60-minute workout.[5, 30] Table 28.15 presents the results of body composition changes of initially obese females who trained 3 days per week for 8 weeks without modifying daily caloric intake.[4] The exercise regimen consisted of an eight-station routine performed on a multistation hydraulic apparatus. Subjects performed 3 sets of 10 reps of the bench press, inverse leg press, lateral pull-down, biceps curl, triceps extension, calf raise, leg extension, and hamstring curl. Strength, evaluated by the 1-RM bench press (refer to Chapter 22), improved by 5.0 kg, from 35 kg to 40 kg.

Considering the relatively brief duration of training, there was an impressive 4.9% increase in biceps girth; this was more than likely a result of a 6.0% increase in muscle-plus-bone cross-sectional area, as measured by radiographic examination of the upper arm, and a corresponding decrease of 5.3% in the cross-sectional area in arm fat. Body composition changed favorably: percent fat decreased by 1.2% fat units (−3.4%), fat mass decreased by 0.6 kg (−2.3%), and fat-free body mass increased by 1.1 kg (2.3%).

FREQUENCY OF TRAINING

Research has investigated optimal training frequency.[40] Training consisted of either running or walking for 30 to 47 minutes a day for 20 weeks; exercise intensity was maintained always at 80 to 95% of maximum heart rate. Training 2 days per week did not significantly change body mass, fatfolds, or percent body fat, but training 3 and 4 days per week did alter these components. Subjects who trained 4 days per week reduced their body masses and fatfolds significantly more than the 3-day per week group. Reductions in percent body fat, however, were similar for both groups.

TABLE 28.15
BODY COMPOSITION AND ANTHROPOMETRIC AND X-RAY MEASUREMENTS IN 10 OBESE FEMALES BEFORE AND AFTER RESISTANCE TRAINING

| | Mean Value | | |
| | Before Training | After Training | Change (%) |
Variable			
Body Composition			
Body mass, kg	73.9	74.3	0.5
Body fat, %[a]	35.1	33.9	−3.4[d]
Fat mass, kg	26.2	25.6	−2.3
FFM, kg	47.7	48.8	2.3[d]
Anthropometry[b]			
Waist girth, cm	80.5	81.1	0.7
Thigh girth, cm	64.4	65.4	1.6
Calf girth, cm	38.5	38.8	0.8
Biceps girth, cm	32.8	34.4	4.9[d]
Forearm girth, cm	26.8	27.6	3.0
Sum 5 fatfolds, mm	170.1	170.6	0.3
Arm Radiography[c]			
Arm area, cm²	255.7	261.8	2.4
Muscle + bone area, cm²	173.8	184.3	6.0[d]
Fat area, cm²	81.8	77.5	−5.3[d]

From Ballor, D.L., et al.: Resistance weight training during caloric restriction enhances lean body weight maintenance. *Am. J. Clin. Nutr.*, 47:19, 1988.
[a]Densitometry.
[b]Measurement procedures discussed in Chapter 27 and Appendix E.
[c]Measurement procedures illustrated in Figure 27.11.
[d]Changes were statistically significant compared to control subjects matched for age, stature, fat-free body mass, and percent body fat.

Based on these findings, at least 3 days of training per week are required to change body composition through exercise; more frequent training may be even more effective. More than likely, such effects result from the added caloric stress provided by the extra training. In addition, the calorie-burning effect of each exercise session should reach a threshold of about 300 kcal.[39] Generally, this is achieved with 20 to 30 minutes of moderate to vigorous running, swimming, bicycling, or circuit resistance training, or walking programs of at least 60 minutes duration.

EFFECTS OF DIET AND EXERCISE ON BODY COMPOSITION DURING WEIGHT LOSS

The addition of exercise to a program of weight control can favorably modify the composition of the weight lost, resulting in more weight being lost in the form of fat.[4, 7, 34, 35] In one study, a daily caloric deficit of 500 kcal was maintained by each of three groups of adult women during a 16-week period of weight loss.[55] The diet group reduced daily food intake by 500 kcal, whereas women in the exercise group increased their energy outputs by 500 kcal through participation in a supervised walking and exercise program 5 days per week. The women using diet plus exercise achieved their daily 500 kcal deficit by reducing food intake by 250 kcal and increasing energy output by 250 kcal through exercise. In weight loss, there was no significant difference among the three groups: each group lost approximately 5 kg. This finding indicates that as long as a caloric deficit is created, body mass will be reduced, regardless of the method used to create the imbalance. *For reducing body fat, however, combining diet and exercise was the most effective approach to weight loss.* The most interesting observation concerned fat-free body mass. Although the exercise group increased its fat-free body mass by 0.9 kg, and the combination group increased its fat-free body mass by 0.5 kg, the dieters lost 1.1 kg of lean tissue!

Figure 28.9 displays the body composition changes that resulted when 40 obese women were placed in one of four groups: (*a*) control, with no exercise and no diet; (*b*) diet only, without exercise (DO); (*c*) diet plus resistance exercise (D + E); and (*d*) resistance exercise only, without diet (EO). The women trained 3 days per week for 8 weeks. They performed ten repetitions for each of three sets of eight strength exercises. Body mass decreased significantly for the DO (−4.5 kg) and D + E (−3.9 kg) groups, compared to EO (+0.5 kg) and controls (−0.4 kg). Interestingly, fat-free body mass increased significantly for EO (1.1 kg) compared to DO (−0.9 kg) and controls (−0.3 kg), and lean tissue was spared for D + E (+0.4 kg), compared to the loss in fat-free body mass for DO (−0.9 kg). The authors concluded that augmenting a caloric-restriction program with resistance exercise training preserves the fat-free body mass better than a diet program without such exercise.[4]

GAINING WEIGHT

For athletes, gaining weight poses a unique problem that is not easily resolved. Gaining weight per se is a relatively easy and often enjoyable task elicited by tilting the body's energy balance in favor of a greater caloric intake. In a sedentary person, an excess intake of 3,500 kcal results in a body mass gain of about 0.5 kg because the excess calories are stored as body fat. Weight gain for athletes, however, should be in the lean tissues, specifically muscle mass. Generally, this form of weight gain only is accomplished if an increased caloric intake accompanies an appropriate exercise program.[45] Although endurance exercise can increase fat-free body mass slightly,[40] the body composition

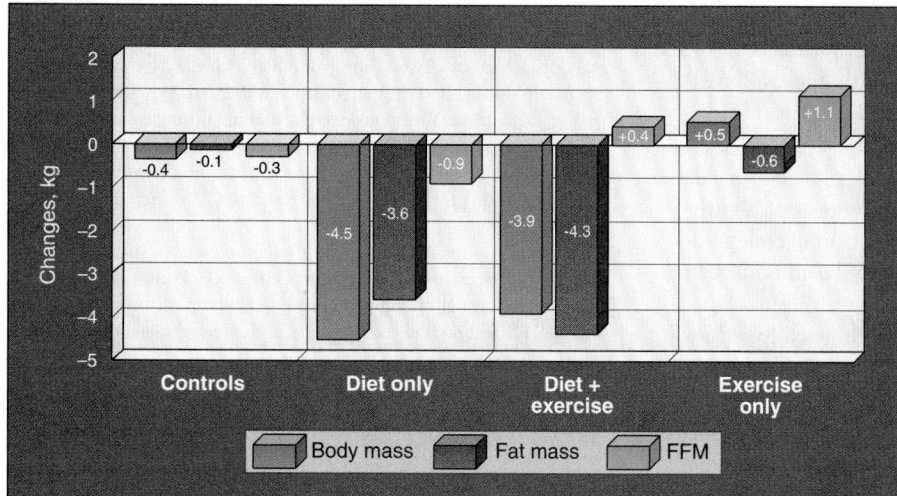

FIGURE 28.9
Changes in body composition with exercise and diet in obese females. (From Ballor, D.L., et al.: Resistance weight training during caloric restriction enhances lean body weight maintenance. *Am. J. Clin. Nutr.*, 47:19, 1988.)

change is frequently accompanied by a loss in body mass resulting from fat loss. This loss is probably the result of the calorie-burning and appetite-depressing effects of endurance exercise.

Heavy muscular overload (resistance training) supported by a prudent diet effectively increases muscle mass and strength. If all of the "extra" calories consumed during resistance training were used for muscle growth, then 2000 to 2500 extra kcal from a well-balanced diet would be required for each 0.5 kg increase in lean tissue. In a practical sense, 700 to 1000 kcal added to the daily diet supplies the nutrients needed to support a weekly 0.5- to 1.0-kg gain in lean tissue as well as the additional energy required for the training.[19] This ideal situation presupposes that all extra calories synthesize lean tissue. Variations from this ideal depend on many factors, such as the type, intensity, and frequency of training, including the hormonal characteristics and muscle fiber type of the athlete. Athletes who have relatively high androgen-to-estrogen ratios and greater percentages of fast-twitch muscle fiber probably increase lean tissue to the greatest extent. One way to verify whether the combination of training and increased food intake increases lean tissue (and not body fat) is to regularly monitor body mass and body fat. This is accomplished in the laboratory with appropriate body composition measurement procedures.

IS THERE AN UPPER LIMIT TO FAT-FREE BODY MASS?

In Chapter 27, data were presented on Japanese Sumo wrestlers (seki-tori) whose fat-free body masses averaged 109 kg. As a group, these athletes are possibly the largest in the world, with the exception of some individual participants in American professional football who have been reported to weigh 159 kg (350 lb). Because it is unlikely that such large athletes would have less than 15% body fat,

their fat-free masses at 15% body fat theoretically would be 135 kg. In reality, however, a football player whose body mass is 159 kg would more likely be in the range of 20 to 25% body fat. At 20% body fat, the fat-free mass would be about 127 kg, certainly the highest value ever using densitometry as the criterion method to evaluate body composition. But this is only hypothetical in the absence of reliable data. Even an extremely large professional basketball player (mass of 138.3 kg, or 305 lb, and stature of 210.8 cm, or 83 in.) is not likely to have a percent body fat of less than about 10% of body mass, or a fat weight of 13.8 kg and fat-free mass of 114.2 kg. This amount of fat-free body mass seems the more likely scenario for an upper limit value of 114 kg in an athlete of such body dimensions. To gain more insight into the question of an upper limit for fat-free body mass, over 20 years of densitometric data from the authors' laboratories were reviewed to determine the largest values for fat-free body mass. Sixteen athletes exceeded a fat-free body mass of 100 kg, the top five values being 114.3, 109. 5, 107.4, 105.4, and 105.2 kg. The two top values were larger than the two values of 106.5 kg reported for defensive football linemen from 1969–1971 data[6] and for other resistance trained athletes.[20] Until more data become available on the body composition of extremely large and relatively lean athletes, as determined by densitometry, the fat-free mass of 121.3 kg reported for one Sumo wrestler remains the largest ever reported.[33] In the absence of additional data, 121.3 kg represents the upper limit of fat-free body mass in humans.

■ SUMMARY ■

1. Body composition assessment reveals that athletes generally have physique characteristics unique to their specific sport. For example, field event athletes have relatively large quantities of lean tissue and high per-

centages of body fat, whereas long-distance runners have the least amount of lean tissue and fat mass.

2. Physique characteristics combined with highly developed physiologic support systems provide important ingredients for a champion performance.

3. Body composition analysis of football players reveals that they are among the heaviest and leanest of all athletes. At the highest levels of competition, collegiate and professional football players are similar in body size and composition.

4. Wrestlers should be discouraged from drastically reducing body fat, particularly if it brings them below 5% body fat.

5. The body profile technique provides a practical method to subdivide anthropometric dimensions into muscular and nonmuscular components and monitor the progress resulting from training, diet, growth, and aging.

6. Continuous moderate- to high-intensity exercise can be effective for weight reduction. The greater the caloric expenditure, the greater the potential will be for body fat loss. This effect is independent of mode of exercise as long as there is a sufficient caloric deficit caused by the exercise. Training at least 3 days per week is required, but seven days per week is preferred.

7. Thirty minutes of moderately strenuous running, bicycling, circuit-resistance exercise, or swimming, or at least 60 minutes of walking, will stimulate fat loss. This threshold level of exercise generally represents about a 300-kcal increase in daily energy expenditure.

8. A combination of diet and exercise offers the greatest flexibility for achieving a negative caloric balance and desirable body fat loss. The inclusion of exercise with diet in a weight-loss program provides protection against an excessive loss of lean tissue. This results in greater fat loss than would be achieved by diet alone.

9. For athletes, weight gain should be in the form of lean body tissue, that is, muscle mass. Increased caloric intake plus resistance training increases muscle mass and strength effectively. Ideally, 700 to 1000 extra kcal per day supports a weekly 0.5- to 1.0-kg gain in lean tissue and training energy requirements. Realistically, individual physiologic variations and training factors also affect weight gain. For this reason, changes in body mass and body fat should be monitored on a regular basis.

10. The largest fat-free mass reported in the literature is 121.3 kg for a Sumo wrestler; this probably represents the upper limit in this aspect of body composition.

■ REFERENCES ■

1. Abraham, S., et al.: Weight and height of adults 18 to 74 years of age. United States Vital and Health Statistics. Series H, No. 211, Washington, D.C., U.S. Government Printing Office, 1979.

2. American College of Sports Medicine: Weight loss in wrestlers. *Med. Sci. Sports,* 8:11, 1976.

3. American Medical Association Committee on the Medical Aspects of Sports: Wrestling and weight control. *JAMA,* 201:541, 1967.

4. Ballor, D.L., et al.: Resistance weight training during caloric restriction enhances lean body weight maintenance. *Am. J. Clin. Nutr.,* 47:19, 1988.

5. Ballor, D.L., et al.: Physiologic responses to nine different work:rest protocols during hydraulic resistive exercises. *Med. Sci. Sports Exerc.,* 21:90, 1989.

6. Behnke, A.R., and Wilmore, J.H.: *Evaluation and Regulation of Body Build and Composition.* Englewood Cliffs, N.J., Prentice Hall, 1974.

7. Bouchard, C., et al.: Long-term exercise training with constant energy intake. 1: Effect on body composition and selected metabolic variables. *Int. J. Obesity,* 14:57, 1990.

8. Brown, C.H., and Wilmore, J.H.: The effects of maximal resistance training on the strength and body composition of women athletes. *Med. Sci. Sports,* 6:174, 1974.

9. Buono, M.J., et al.: Effects of a diet and exercise program on blood lipids, cardiorespiratory function, and body composition in obese women. *Med. Sci. Sports Exerc.,* 17:189, 1985.

10. Butts, N.K.: Physiological profile of high school female cross-country runners. *Phys. Sportsmed.,* 10:103, 1983.

11. Carter, J.E.L., and Ackland, T.R.: *Kinanthropometry in Aquatic Sports. A Study of World Class Athletes.* J.E. Carter and T.R. Ackland (Eds.), Human Kinetics Sport Science Monograph Series, Vol. 5, Champaign, Ill., Human Kinetics, 1994.

12. Carter, J.E.L., and Phillips, W.H.: Structural changes in exercising middle-aged males during a 2-year period. *J. Appl. Physiol.,* 27:787, 1969.

13. Carter, L.E., and Lucio, F.D.: Body size, skinfolds, and somatotypes of high school and Olympic wrestlers. *Perspectives in Kinanthropometry.* J.A.P. Day (Ed.). The 1984 Olympic Scientific Congress Proceedings. Vol. 1, Champaign, Ill., Human Kinetics, 1986.

14. Carter, L.E., et al.: Advances in somatotype methodology and analysis. *Yearbook of Physical Anthropology,* 26:193, 1983.

15. Changalur, S.N., et al.: An analysis of male and female Olympic swimmers in the 200-meter events. *Can. J. Sport Sci.,* 17:104, 1992.

16. Clarke, K.C.: Predicting certified weight of young wrestlers: a field study of the Tcheng-Tipton Method. *Med. Sci. Sports,* 6:52, 1974.

17. Cureton, T.K.: *Physical Fitness of Champion Athletes.* Urbana, Ill., University of Illinois Press, 1951.

18. DeGaray, A.L., et al.: *Genetic and Anthropological Studies of Olympic Athletes.* New York, Academic Press, 1974.

19. Fahey, T., and Brown, C.: The effects of an anabolic steroid on the strength, body composition, and endurance of college males when accompanied by a weight training program. *Med. Sci. Sports,* 5:272, 1973.

20. Fahey, T., et al.: Body composition and $\dot{V}O_2$ max of exceptional weight-trained athletes. *J. Appl. Physiol.,* 39:559, 1975.

21. Freedson, P.S., et al.: Physique, body composition, and psychological characteristics of competitive female bodybuilders. *Phys. Sportsmed.,* 11:85, 1983.

22. Grimston, S.K., Hay, J.G.: Relationships among anthropometric and stroking characteristics of college swimmers. *Med. Sci. Sports Exerc.,* 18:60, 1986.

23. Hirata, K.: Physique and age of Tokyo Olympic champions. *J. Sports Med. Phys. Fitness,* 6:207, 1966.

24. Holly, R.G., et al.: Triathlete characterization and response to prolonged competition. *Med. Sci. Sports Exerc.,* 18:123, 1986.

25. Housh, T.J., et al.: Validity of anthropometric estimations of body composition in high school wrestlers. *Res. Q. Exerc. Sport.,* 60:239, 1989.

26. Huenemann, R.L., et al.: *Teenage Nutrition and Physique.* Springfield, Ill., Charles C. Thomas, 1974.

27. Johnson, M.J., et al.: Loss of muscle mass is poorly reflected in grip strength performance in healthy young men. *Med. Sci. Sports Exerc.,* 26:235, 1994.

28. Katch, F.I., and McArdle, W.D.: Prediction of body density from simple anthropometric measurements in college-age men and women. *Hum. Biol.,* 45:445, 1973.

29. Katch, F.I., et al.: Effects of physical training on the body composition and diet of females. *Res. Q.,* 40:99, 1969.

30. Katch, F.I., et al.: Evaluation of acute cardiorespiratory responses to hydraulic resistance exercise. *Med. Sci. Sports Exerc.,* 17:168, 1985.

31. Katch, V.L., et al.: Muscular development and lean body weight in body-builders and weight lifters. *Med. Sci. Sports,* 12:340, 1980.

32. Kohlraush, W.: Zusammenhang von Korperform und Leistung. Ergebnisse der anthropometrischen Messungen an der Athletern der Amsterdamer Olympiade. *Int. Z. Angrew. Physiol.,* 2:187, 1970.

33. Kondo, M., et al.: Upper limit of fat-free mass in humans: A study on Japanese Sumo wrestlers. *Amer. J. Hum. Biol.,* 6:613, 1994.

34. Konstantin, N.P., et al.: Effects of dieting and exercise on fat-free body mass, oxygen uptake, and strength. *Med. Sci. Sports Exerc.,* 17:446, 1985.

35. McMurray, R.G., et al.: Responses of endurance trained subjects to caloric deficits induced by diet or exercise. *Med. Sci. Sports Exerc.,* 17:574, 1985.

36. Milesis, C.A., et al.: Effects of different durations of physical training on cardiorespiratory function, body composition, and serum lipids. *Res. Q.,* 47:716, 1976.

37. O'Toole, M.L.: Training for ultraendurance triathletes. *Med. Sci. Sports Exerc.,* 21:209, 1989.

38. O'Toole, M.L., et al.: The ultraendurance triathlete: a physiological profile. *Med. Sci. Sports Exerc.,* 19:45, 1987.

39. Pollock, M.L., and Jackson, A.: Body composition: measurement and changes resulting from physical training. In *Toward an Understanding of Human Performance.* E.J. Burke (Ed.), Ithaca, N.Y., Mouvement Publications, 1977.

40. Pollock, M.L., et al.: Frequency of training as a determinant for improvement in cardiovascular function and body composition of middle-aged men. *Arch. Phys. Med. Rehabil.,* 56:141, 1975.

41. Sady, S.P., et al.: Physiological characteristics of high-ability prepubescent wrestlers. *Med. Sci. Sports Exerc.,* 16:72, 1984.

42. Scott, J.R., et al.: Acute weight gain in collegiate wrestlers following a tournament weigh-in. *Med. Sci. Sports Exerc.,* 26:1181, 1994.

43. Sinning, W.E.: Body composition, cardiorespiratory function, and rule changes in women's basketball. *Res. Q.,* 44:313, 1973.

44. Sinning, W.E., and Lindberg, G.D.: Physical characteristics of college age women gymnasts. *Res. Q.,* 43:226, 1972.

45. Smith, N.J.: Gaining and losing weight in athletics. *JAMA,* 236:149, 1976.

46. Tanner, J.M.: *The Physique of the Olympic Athlete.* London, Allen and Unwin, 1964.

47. Tcheng, T., and Tipton, C.M.: Iowa wrestling study: anthropometric measurements and the prediction of a "minimal" body weight for high school wrestlers. *Med. Sci. Sports,* 5:1, 1973.

48. Tipton, C.M.: Making and maintaining weight for interscholastic wrestling. Gatorade Sports Science Exchange, 2:1, 1990.

49. Tipton, C.M., and Oppliger, R.A.: Nutritional and fitness considerations for competitive wrestlers. In *Nutrition and Fitness for Athletes.* A.P. Simopoulos and K.N. Pavlou (Eds.), *World Rev. Nutr. Diet. Karger Basal.,* 71:84, 1993.

50. Welham, W.C., and Behnke, A.R.: The specific gravity of healthy men. *JAMA,* 118:498, 1942.

51. Wickkiser, J.D., and Kelly, J.M.: The body composition of a college football team. *Med. Sci. Sports,* 7:199, 1975.

52. Wilmore, J.H., and Brown, C.H.: Physiological profiles of women distance runners. *Med. Sci. Sports,* 6:178, 1974.

53. Wilmore, J.H., and Haskell, W.L.: Body composition and endurance capacity of professional football players. *J. Appl. Physiol.,* 33:564, 1972.

54. Wilmore, J.H., et al.: Body composition changes with a 10-week program of jogging. *Med. Sci. Sports,* 2:113, 1970.

55. Zuti, W.B., and Golding, L.A.: Comparing diet and exercise as weight reduction tools. *Phys. Sportsmed.,* 4:49, 1976.

Bouchard, C., et al.: The response to long-term overfeeding in identical twins. _N. Engl. J. Med._ 322:1477, 1990.

An area of current research in weight control and obesity is trying to explain individual differences in total and regional body fat content. Bouchard and colleagues studied differences in body fat acquisition by overfeeding 12 pairs of male monozygotic twins for 100 days to assess the role of inherited characteristics on body composition adaptations to long-term energy imbalance (consuming more calories than required for body mass maintenance).

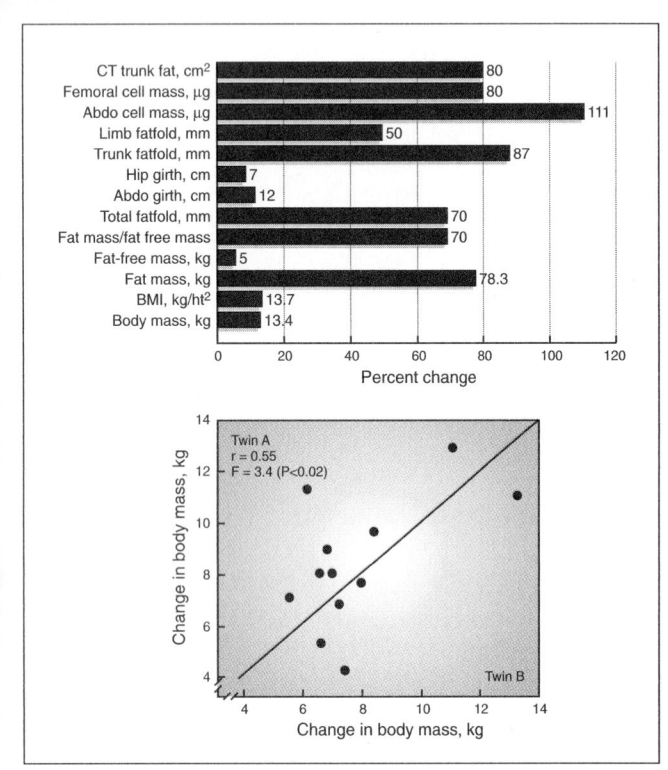

Top, Effects of 100 days of overfeeding in 12 pairs of male monozygotic twins. Values are percent changes from before to after overfeeding. _Bottom,_ Similarity within 12 pairs of male twins for changes in body mass in response to 100 days of overfeeding by 84,000 calories.

The twin pairs (mean age, 21 years; range, 19 to 27 years) lived in a dormitory under 24-hour supervision for 120 consecutive days. This included 14 days for baseline testing, 3 days for testing before overfeeding, 100 days for the period of overfeeding, and 3 days for post-testing. Subjects ate normally during baseline testing, and each meal was analyzed for nutrient composition and energy content. The subjects' body mass remained stable during baseline. For the pre- and post-overfeeding periods, subjects underwent testing for resting metabolic rate, body fat determination by underwater weighing, adipose tissue fat analysis by needle biopsy from the abdominal (umbilicus-level) and femoral (mid-thigh-level) areas, "trunk-fat"

mass by computed tomography (CT scans) of the abdominal and abdominal visceral areas, and anthropometric assessment that included 10 fatfolds (five trunk and five limb) and waist and hip circumference.

After baseline testing, subjects consumed a diet for 6 days a week containing 1000 kcal per day more than their established baseline energy requirement. Daily food consumption consisted of 50% carbohydrate, 35% lipid, and 15% protein. On day 7 of each week, subjects consumed their baseline number of calories. The total excess energy intake over the 100-day period was 84,000 kcal. Subjects ate three meals daily plus an evening snack, and daily activities included reading, playing video games, playing cards, watching television, and walking outdoors for 30 minutes. Measurements taken during overfeeding included body mass (daily), fatfolds (every 5 days), and waist and hip girth (every 25 days).

The _top_ figure displays the mean percentage changes from before to after overfeeding. Body mass increased significantly (average gain, 8.1 kg), as did fat mass and fat-free body mass, but the percentage gain in adipose cell mass (111%) exceeded the increase in fat-free body mass (5%). The sum of fatfold thickness (used to estimate change in subcutaneous fat) increased from 76 to 129 mm or 70%. Fatfold thickness also increased on the trunk and limbs, but more so on the trunk (87%) than the limbs (50%). Waist and hip girth increased significantly. The ratio of waist girth to hip girth also increased, indicating greater fat gain at the waist than the hip level. Overfeeding increased the adipose tissue fat mass in all subcutaneous and visceral anatomical sections estimated by CT scanning.

Considerable individual differences existed for changes in body mass and body composition, with greater variation between twin pairs compared to the variation within each pair of twins. The _bottom_ figure displays the within-pair differences for the changes in body mass with equivalent excess energy intake. Each point represents one pair of twins (A and B). The closer the points are to the diagonal line, the more similar the twins are to each other. The large differences between twin pairs for change in body mass exceed the differences within twin pairs.

A threefold difference occurred for the changes in body mass, body composition, trunk fat, and visceral fat between the high and low weight gainers. Thus, surplus energy intake (with other factors kept constant) did not produce similar responses in the outcome variables among twin pairs. Also, the increase in body mass or body fat did not predict the accumulation of visceral fat. The finding that some persons were more prone than others to store fat on the trunk, in the abdominal cavity, or at both anatomic areas is of considerable importance. The authors hypothesized that a person's genotype determines adaptation to sustained energy surplus, and that a yet-undetermined genetic characteristic produces large individual differences in the tendency toward obesity and distribution of body fat.

Obesity and Weight Control

PART 1
OBESITY

It is indeed unfortunate that in our modern era of technologic and scientific achievement, during which man has walked on the moon, developed miraculous surgical procedures to prolong and enhance the quality of life, and discovered many of the microscopic secrets of molecular interaction, there is no adequate explanation for a seemingly simple question: why do so many people become too fat, and what can be done to prevent it? The 22% of American men and 37% of women who are currently attempting to lose weight spend approximately $35 billion annually, often using harmful dietary practices.[12, 34] Despite these increasing attempts at weight loss, more Americans are overweight than a generation ago. Over the past 15 years, the average body weight of adult Americans has increased by about 8 lb. The recent data given in Figure 29.1 are from a national representative cross-sectional survey of the prevalence of overweight among adults in the U.S. population compared to the government's objective for the year 2000.[78] Between 1988 and 1991, one-third of adults aged 20 to 74 years were estimated to be overweight. This was a dramatic increase over previous surveys, with the incidence of obesity being particularly high among women and minority groups (insert table). These data are a considerable distance from the Healthy People 2000 goal of reducing the prevalence of overweight among U.S. adults to no more than 20% by the year 2000.[109] Particularly disturbing is that for about one in five American children and adolescents, obesity is the most common chronic disorder. Obesity in this age range has increased about 45% regardless of race and sex—and excessive fatness in one's youth may be even more of an adult health risk than obesity that begins in adulthood. Regardless of their final body weight as adults, people who are overweight in adolescence have a significantly greater risk of a broad range of illnesses as adults than adolescents of normal weight.[93]

Obesity Often Is a Long-Term Process. *Obesity is defined as an excess accumulation of body fat.* Obesity often begins early in childhood. When this is the case, the chances for adult obesity are three times greater than for children having a normal amount of body fat.[51, 115] Simply stated, a child generally does not "grow out of" an overfat condition. Children of obese parents are at two to three times increased risk of obesity as adults compared to children in families in which neither parent is morbidly obese. This is not only for genetic reasons, but also because of the family's poor dietary and exercise habits.[92] Excessive fatness also develops slowly during adulthood, ages 25 to 44 being the danger years. Middle-aged men and women invariably weigh more than their college-aged counterparts of the same stature. In the Western world, the average 35-year-old male gains between 0.2 and 0.8 kg of fat each year until the sixth decade of life, despite a progressive decrease in food intake. Women tend to be the biggest weight gainers, with about 14% putting on more than 30 pounds between the ages of 25 and 34. It is not known to what extent "creeping obesity" during adulthood reflects a normal biologic pattern.

Obesity Is Not Necessarily Related to Overeating. Overeating is often believed to be the major cause of obesity. If obesity were truly a unitary disorder, and gluttony and overindulgence were the only factors causing fat accumulation, then the easiest way to permanently reduce would surely be to cut back on food intake. Of course, if it were this simple, obesity would soon be eliminated as a major health problem. There obviously are other factors operative, such as genetic, environmental, social, and perhaps racial influences.[21, 134, 158] Differences in specific factors also may predispose humans to excessive weight gain. These factors include eating patterns and environment, food packaging, and body image. They also include differences in resting metabolic rate; dietary-induced thermogenesis; level of spontaneous activity ("fidgeting"); basal body temperature; levels of cellular adenosine triphosphatase, lipoprotein lipase, and other enzymes; and metabolically active brown adipose tissue.[6, 24a, 24b, 25, 75, 110] Individual differences in muscle fiber type distribution, however, do not appear to be determinants of body fat content or fat distribution in men and women.[123a] It is worth noting that glandular abnormalities are generally **not** the cause of obesity per se, except in certain instances of endocrinopathy. However, while the cause of obesity seldom is linked to hormonal aberrations, obesity can trigger a variety of abnormal hormonal responses.[104]

Genetics Plays a Role. Our genetic makeup does not necessarily cause obesity, but it does lower the thresh-

FIGURE 29.1
The fattening of America. Trends in age-adjusted prevalence of overweight in the U.S. population aged 20 through 74 years, compared with the year 2000 health objective. The inset table presents the age-adjusted percentages of overweight and severely overweight persons aged 20 to 74 years, from the National Health and Nutrition Examination Survey (NHANES) II and NHANES, categorized by ethnicity and sex. NHES is the National Health Examination Survey. (From Kuczmarski, R.J., et al.: Increasing prevalence of overweight among US adults. *JAMA*, 272:205, 1994. Insert from Kuczmarski, R.J., et al.: Prevalence of overweight and weight gain in the United States. *Am. J. Clin. Nutr.*, 55:495S, 1992.)

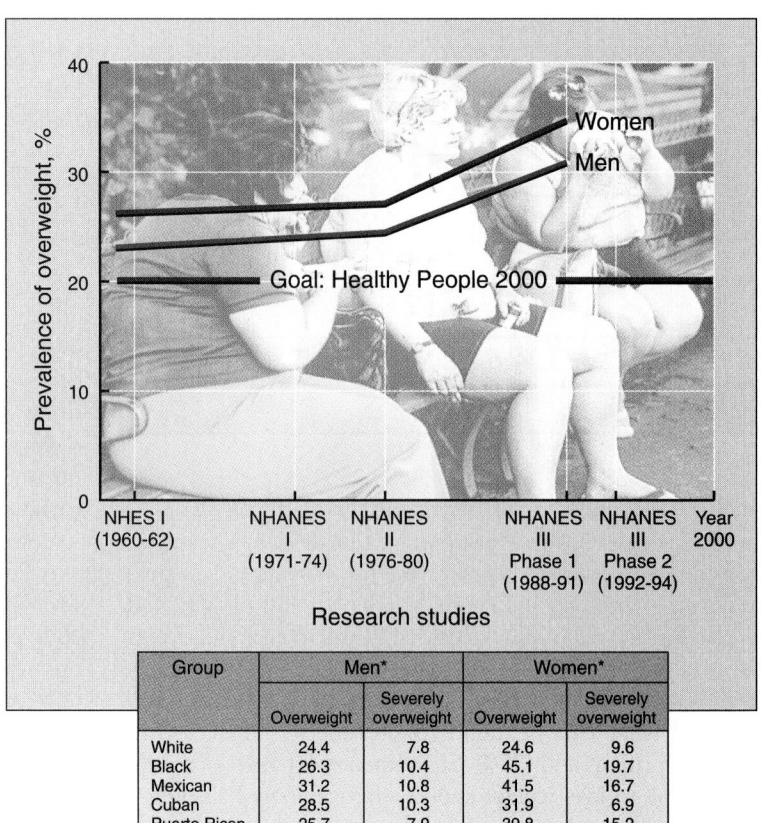

Group	Men*		Women*	
	Overweight	Severely overweight	Overweight	Severely overweight
White	24.4	7.8	24.6	9.6
Black	26.3	10.4	45.1	19.7
Mexican	31.2	10.8	41.5	16.7
Cuban	28.5	10.3	31.9	6.9
Puerto Rican	25.7	7.9	39.8	15.2

*Age-adjusted percentages of overweight and severely overweight persons aged 20-74 y living in the U.S.

FIGURE 29.2
Total transmissible variance for body fat. Total body fat and percent body fat were determined by hydrostatic weighing. (From Bouchard, C., et al.: Inheritance of the amount and distribution of human body fat. *Int. J. Obes.*, 12:205, 1988.)

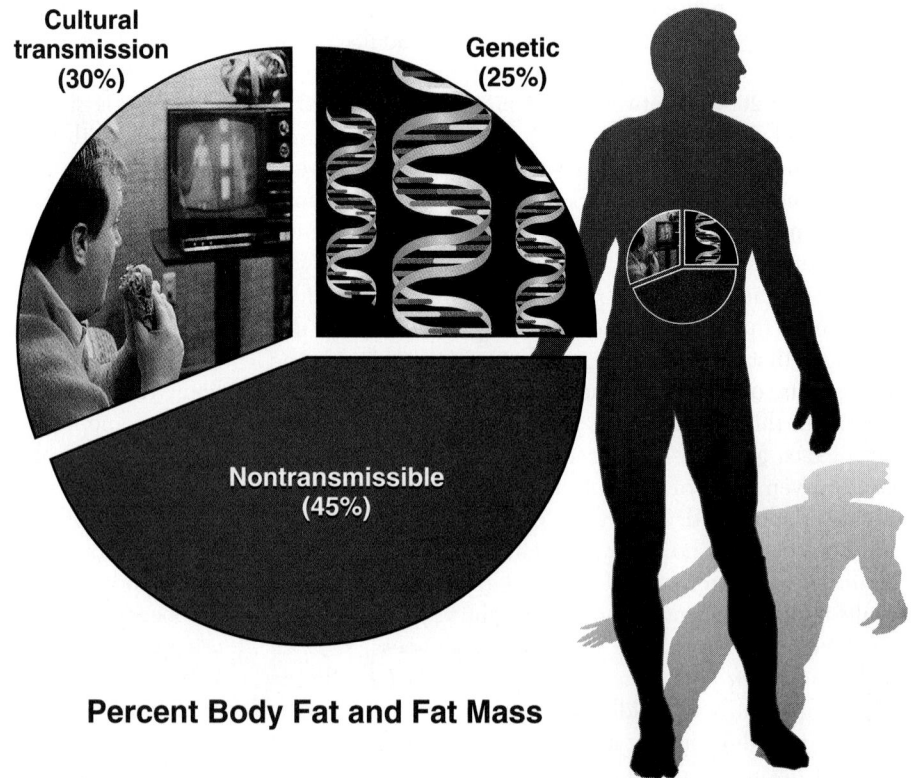

Percent Body Fat and Fat Mass

old for the development of the disease (susceptibility genes) and contributes significantly to the variability in weight gain observed among individuals fed identical daily caloric excesses.[24] The data in Figure 29.2 are based on a study of a relatively large number of individuals representing nine different types of relations. It appears that about 25% of the variation among people in percent body fat and total fat mass is biologically determined by genetic factors, while the larger percentage of variation is associated with a transmissible (cultural) effect.[20, 22] *In an obesity-producing environment (sedentary and stressful, with easy access to food), the genetically susceptible individual will gain weight, possibly lots of it.*

A Mutant Gene? Research with a strain of mice that balloon up to five times the girth of normal mice has pro-

vided evidence to support the contention that some people are genetically "destined" to become overfat.[6] The mutation of a gene called **obese,** or simply **ob,** is believed to disrupt hormonal signals that regulate the animal's metabolism, fat storage, and appetite, causing energy balance to tip in the direction of fat accumulation.[158]

As proposed in Figure 29.3, the ob gene normally is activated in adipose tissue, where it causes the production of a body-fat-signaling, hormone-like protein (a satiety protein called ob protein, or **leptin**) that is secreted into the bloodstream.[53a, 102a] This hormone is then transported to the ventromedial nucleus of the hypothalamus, the area of the brain considered the control center for appetite. Normally, the action of this hormone blunts the urge to eat when the caloric intake is sufficient to maintain ideal

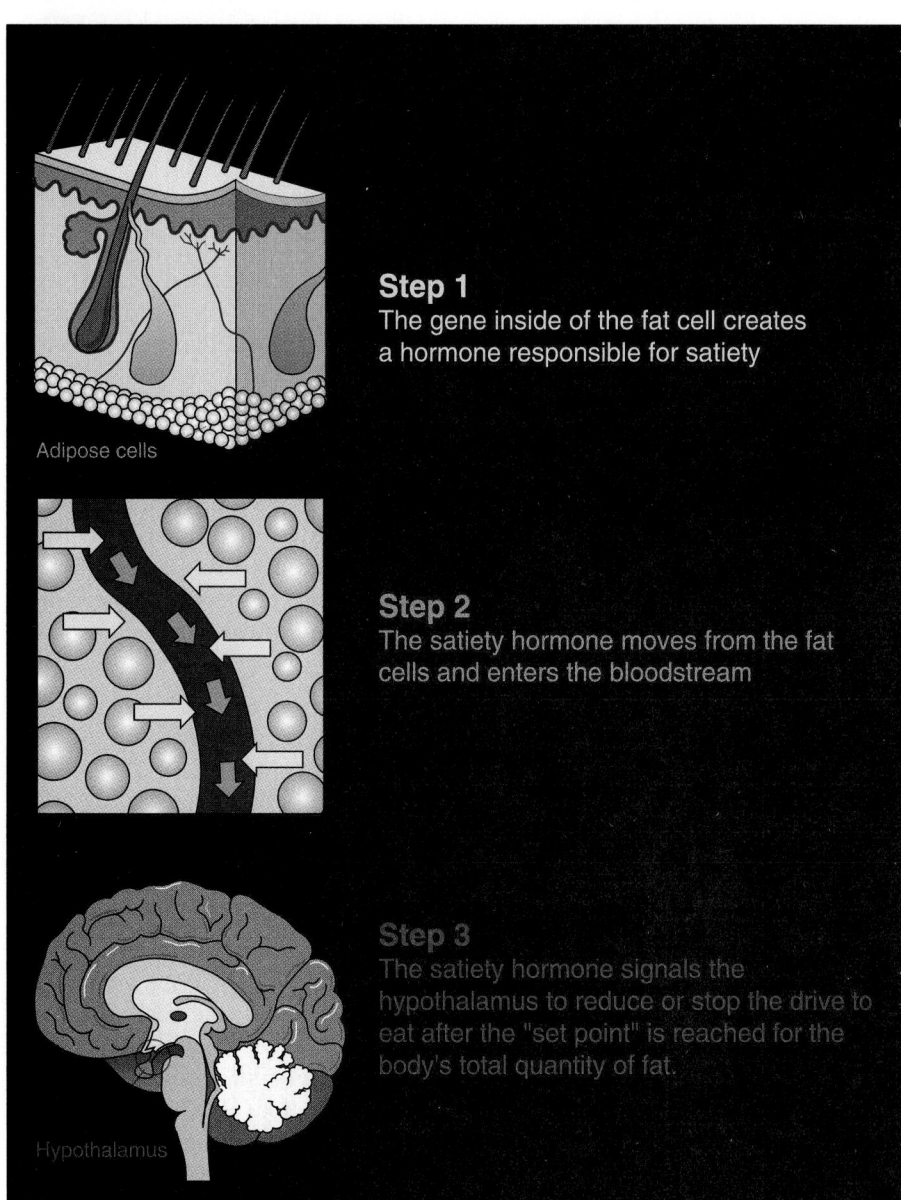

Step 1
The gene inside of the fat cell creates a hormone responsible for satiety

Adipose cells

Step 2
The satiety hormone moves from the fat cells and enters the bloodstream

Step 3
The satiety hormone signals the hypothalamus to reduce or stop the drive to eat after the "set point" is reached for the body's total quantity of fat.

Hypothalamus

FIGURE 29.3

A genetic model for obesity. A malfunction of the satiety gene can have a marked effect on production of the satiety hormone leptin (after the Greek word *leptos,* for thin). This would disrupt the events that occur in *Step 3* in the hypothalamus, the center responsible for adjusting the body's fat level. (This model is based on research conducted at Rockefeller University, New York.) The following are present and future fat-fighting drugs and hormone-like substances. *Present:* Dexfenfluramine—promotes release of serotonin and prevents its uptake by the brain thus decreasing appetite; sibutramine—decreases appetite by inhibiting brain uptake of both serotonin and norepinephrine; orlistat—facilitates weight loss by inhibiting intestinal digestion of lipids. *Three to five years:* Beta-3 adrenergic agonists—augment daily caloric output by elevating resting metabolism; CCK-A promoter—enhances the effect of CCK-A, an intestinal hormone that may inhibit appetite. *Five to ten years:* Ob-protein—natural body protein that may reduce appetite and accelerate lipid metabolism; ob-receptor stimulator—drugs that mimic the appetite-suppressing effect when the Ob protein binds to its receptor in the brain; neuropeptide-Y blockers—drugs that reduce appetite by blocking the effect of the brain chemical neuropeptide Y, which appears to stimulate appetite.

fat stores. In this way, the level of body fat is intimately "connected" to the brain by a physiological pathway that can then regulate caloric intake accordingly. This feedback loop between the brain and adipose tissue was first proposed by scientists about 40 years ago. With a defective gene, however, an inadequate amount of hormone is produced, or no hormone at all, and the brain is not given a proper assessment of the body's adipose status. Thus, the urge to eat is constant. This biological control mechanism (although no specific obesity gene has as yet been identified in humans) fits nicely with the setpoint theory (see page 618) to explain abnormal accumulations of body fat and the extreme difficulty encountered by obese people in sustaining a significant body fat loss.

The genetic connection to obesity provides a sound rationale for viewing the overfat condition as a disease rather than some psychological flaw or personality weakness that could be corrected if only the person had sufficient willpower. It is noteworthy that the discovery of the ob gene does not herald an instant "cure" for the obese condition that affects nearly 60 million Americans. Human obesity is the end result of a complex interaction of numerous factors and influences. In theory, however, it may eventually be possible to synthesize a drug that mimics the protein normally produced by the defective gene to produce a feeling of satiety. This would be achieved with a smaller caloric intake and less of the feelings of hunger and deprivation that often accompany conventional diet plans. It is also possible that identifying this genetic predisposition early in life would make it possible to begin diet and exercise intervention before the obese condition becomes firmly established. Once one becomes obese, it is exceedingly difficult to permanently reduce body fat.

Physical Activity: An Important Component. Observations of older men and women who maintain active lifestyles suggest that the "normal" pattern of fat gain in adulthood can be attenuated significantly.[72, 145] For both young and middle-aged men who exercised regularly, the time spent in physical activity was inversely related to body fat level.[55, 88] Surprisingly, no relationship emerged between body fat and caloric intake. This suggests that the greater levels of body fat observed among the active middle-aged men compared to their younger, more active counterparts were the consequences of less vigorous training, not greater food intake.

From age 3 months to 1 year, the total energy expenditure of infants who later became overweight was significantly lower, 21%, than that of infants who maintained normal weight gain.[113] In another study, 24-hour energy expenditure was measured in young-adult Native Americans and related to changes in body mass over a 2-year period.[110] The risk of gaining more than 7.5 kg was four times greater in people with low, rather than high, 24-hour energy expenditures.

This section deals with various aspects of obesity, including (a) health risks, (b) classification criteria, (c) fat cell characteristics in normal and obese persons before and after weight gain and loss, (d) development of adipose cellularity, and (e) possible modification of adipose cellularity through diet and exercise.

HEALTH RISKS OF OBESITY

Between 30 and 35% of adult American men and women weigh at least 20% more than their desirable body weights, and more than 15 million of these people are severely obese and at great risk of developing a variety of obesity-related diseases. This is truly remarkable considering that the boundaries of "desirable weight" have moved upward over the past decade. Figure 29.4 illustrates that the economic cost of obesity-related medical problems was 56.3 billion dollars in 1986—about 7.8% of the 715 billion dollar total cost of illness in the United States. This statistic in 1994 was almost 10% of the more than one trillion dollar cost of illness in the United States!

THE CULPRIT: BODY WEIGHT OR BODY FAT?

There is some debate as to whether being overweight without being overfat correlates to an excess risk for cardiovascular disease. Some studies have indicated that blood pressure, cholesterol, and risk for premature heart disease were greater in men who were significantly overweight but not obese compared to normal-weight, nonobese men.[147] When more rigorous standards are used for determining body fat levels, it is **excess fat,** rather than body weight per se, that is seen to drive the relationship between excess weight and an increased heart disease risk.[122] Such findings point up the importance of identifying the composition of "excess weight" when evaluating one's overall health profile.

Overweight in Adolescence Predicts Adverse Health Effects

A positive relationship exists between an overweight condition in adolescence (ages 13 to 18) and subsequent adverse health effects 55 years later.[93] Data were analyzed from the Harvard Growth Study, conducted from 1922 to 1935, in 3000 school children evaluated annually for a variety of health factors (including triplicate measures of body stature and mass at the same time each year) until they left or graduated from high school.[36] Of the initial group, 1857 subjects were studied for an additional 8 years. Subjects were designated as either lean (those who remained in the 25th to 50th percentile for BMI) or overweight (BMI cutoff exceeding 75th percentile). In the adult men, there was, overall, a greater relative risk of

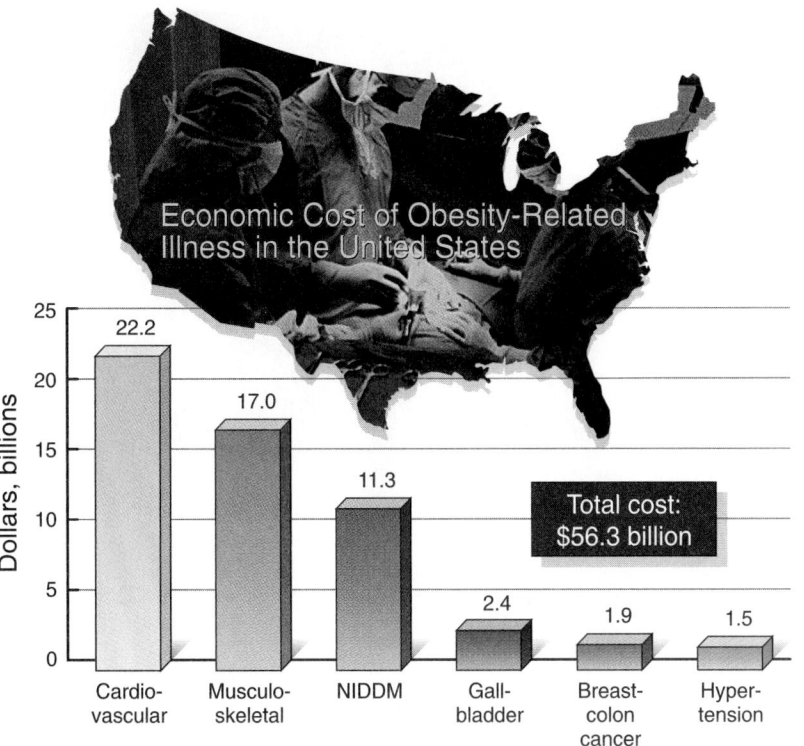

Economic Cost of Obesity-Related Illness in the United States

Total cost: $56.3 billion

FIGURE 29.4
Economic cost of obesity-related illnesses in the United States. Of the six major diseases, cardiovascular disease ranks first, followed by musculoskeletal complications and diabetes. (Modified from data of Colditz, G.A.: Economic costs of obesity. *Am. J. Clin. Nutr.*, 55:503S, 1992.)

mortality from all causes (including stroke and colorectal cancer), but coronary heart disease risk was about two times higher among the group that was overweight in adolescence than among the lean group. Overweight women in adolescence were eight times more likely to report problems with personal care concerns and routine living tasks (walking, stair climbing, lifting) than women who were lean during adolescence. This difference included a 1.6-fold increase in arthritis. The conclusion was straightforward: the prevention of overweight in youth may be the most effective means of decreasing adult morbidity and mortality.

SPECIFIC RISKS OF EXCESS FAT: BEING OVERWEIGHT SHORTENS ONE'S LIFE

There is considerable information regarding the association between obesity and a number of specific health risks in children, adolescents, and adults.[103, 132, 156] A report from the National Institutes of Health concludes that obesity should be viewed as a chronic, degenerative disease because there are multiple biologic hazards of premature illness and death at surprisingly low levels of excess fat, representing as little as 5 to 10 lb above desirable body weight.[94] Higher levels of body weight within the normal range significantly increase the risk of heart disease and cancer.[85a, 155] An 8-year study of nearly 116,000 female nurses suggested that all but the thinnest women were at increased risk of heart attack and chest pain.[85] Nurses of average weight had

30% more heart attacks than the thinnest women, while the risk to moderately overweight nurses was 80% higher. This means that a woman who gains 9 kg between her late teens and middle age doubles her heart attack risk. It is argued rather convincingly that obesity is an independent and powerful heart disease risk that may be equal to that of smoking, elevated blood lipids, and hypertension.[63] A major 16-year follow-up study of nurses (excluding people who were lean because of smoking or pre-existing disease) suggests that even a moderate weight gain (to a body mass index of 27 or greater) above a person's weight at age 18 can be deadly.[85a] The important findings were that more than one-half of cardiovascular deaths and one-third of cancer deaths (colon, endometrium, and breast) were linked to overweight. Women classified as obese (30% or more above desirable weight) were four times as likely to die of heart disease and two times as likely to die of cancer as age-matched women who were below average for body weight. Speculation is that before long, obesity will surpass cigarette smoking as a cause of death in this country. The specific health risks of obesity include (*a*) impaired cardiac function as a result of increased mechanical work and autonomic and left ventricular dysfunction;[116] (*b*) hypertension and stroke;[129] (*c*) adult-onset diabetes, as about 80% of these patients are overweight;[104, 133] (*d*) renal disease;[153] (*e*) pulmonary disease and impaired function resulting from the added effort needed to move the chest wall;[10] (*f*) problems in administering anesthetics during surgery;[152] (*g*) osteoarthritis, degenerative joint disease, and gout;[47] (*h*) several types of cancer;[124] (*i*) abnormal plasma lipid and lipoprotein levels;[117] (*j*) menstrual irregularities;[94] and (*k*) an enormous psychological burden.[25]

Weight loss in the obese often normalizes serum cholesterol and triglycerides and has a beneficial effect on blood pressure.[66a] The normally observed relationship between age and blood pressure is partially explained by the tendency to gain weight with age. Considering such factors as cigarette smoking and current disease status, a 27-year study of Harvard alumni showed that men whose body weights were 20% or more above their "desirable weights" had death rates 2.5 times greater that the leanest men. At all ages, the leanest men were the least likely to die.[79, 80]

CRITERIA FOR OBESITY: HOW FAT IS TOO FAT?

In Chapter 27, we discussed the limitations of the height-weight tables for assessing the body's composition. A more appropriate approach is to measure a person's fat content for the percent of body mass that is fat (percent body fat), the distribution or patterning of that fat on the body, or the size and number of individual fat cells.

PERCENT BODY FAT

Where is the line drawn between what is considered normal for body fat content and what is considered obese? In Chapter 27, we suggested "normal" ranges of body fat for adult men and women: an "average" value for body fat plus or minus one standard deviation unit of variation. For men and women aged 17 to 50, this variation unit is approximately 5% body fat. Using this statistical boundary, "over-fatness" would correspond to body fat that exceeds the average value plus 5% additional body fat units. For example, in young men whose body fat values average 15% of body mass, the borderline for obesity would be 20% body fat. In older men whose body fat values average about 25%, obesity could be defined as a body fat content in excess of 30%. In young women, obesity would correspond to a body fat content above 30%. In older women, the borderline for obesity would be about 37% body fat. We emphasize, however, that just because the "average" value for percent body fat tends to increase with age,[13] this does not necessarily mean that people should expect to get fatter as they grow older. In our opinion, one criterion for what is considered "too fat" should be based on the data for younger men and women—above 20% for men and above 30% for women. Using this criterion, average age-related population values do not become reference standards and, subsequently, accepted as "normal." We also recognize that this proposed classification standard based on an average for young adults is extremely rigorous when applied to all adults in the population. It would probably place

TABLE 29.1
PERCENTILE RANKINGS FOR TRICEPS FATFOLDS IN BOYS AND GIRLS

Age	Percentile			
	15th	50th	85th	95th
Boys				
6	6.2	8.4	11.1	14.1
8	6.1	8.8	13.7	17.2
10	6.0	9.1	16.0	20.7
12	5.8	9.4	17.3	23.3
14	5.6	8.9	16.4	23.5
16	5.5	8.5	15.8	21.5
18	5.6	8.5	16.6	21.8
Girls				
6	6.8	10.1	13.4	15.6
8	7.6	11.4	16.4	20.2
10	8.4	12.7	19.0	24.4
12	9.3	14.1	21.3	28.0
14	10.4	15.5	23.3	30.9
16	11.3	26.6	25.1	33.2
18	11.7	17.0	25.8	33.8

From Must, J., et al.: Reference data for obesity: 85th and 95th percentiles of body mass index (wt/ht²) and triceps skinfolds. *Am. J. Clin. Nutr.*, 53:89, 1991.

nearly 50% of U.S. adults in the obese category. Interestingly, however, this is not that divergent from the current data for overweight Americans presented in Figure 29.1.

Standards for Overfatness

Men—above 20%
Women—above 30%

It should be kept in mind that there is a gradation in obesity that progresses from the upper limit of normal—20% body fat for men and 30% for women—to as high as 50 to 70% of body mass in massively obese people. This group includes people who weigh in the range of 170 to 250 kg or more. In this weight range, body fat often exceeds fat-free body mass, and obesity becomes life-threatening.

Criterion for Children. The limitations of hydrostatic weighing in evaluating the body composition of growing children and adolescents were discussed in Chapter 27. It is still possible, however, to broadly assess a child's degree of excess fat by means of fatfold measures. Table 29.1 presents percentile rankings for boys and girls aged 6 to 18 years. Generally, a triceps fatfold at the 85th percentile or higher would raise concern for the child's nutritional status as related to excessive body fatness.

REGIONAL FAT DISTRIBUTION

The patterning of the body's adipose tissue distribution, independent of total body fat, alters the health risks of obesity.[45, 100, 119] *More specifically, ratios of waist-to-hip girth that exceed 0.80 for women and 0.95 for men are associated with an increased risk of death from coronary artery disease and other illnesses.*[14, 123, 138] In older women, this ratio is a better marker of the risk of death (in a dose-response manner) than the commonly used body mass index.[48]

The two types of regional fat distribution are depicted in Figure 29.5. The increased health risk from fat deposition in the abdominal area (**central** or **android-type obesity**), especially in the internal, visceral deposits, may be a result of this tissue's lively lipolysis in response to catecholamine stimulation. Lipids stored in this area are more responsive metabolically than those in the gluteal and femoral regions (**peripheral** or **gynoid-type obesity**) and, thus, more likely to enter into processes related to heart disease.[5, 6, 111, 127] Central fat deposition increases one's risk of hyperinsulinemia, insulin resistance, non-insulin-dependent diabetes, endometrial cancer, hypercholesterolemia, hypertension, and atherosclerosis.[40, 119]

To some extent, one's fat distribution pattern is an inherited characteristic governed by the regional activity of **lipoprotein lipase (LPL)**.[49] This rate-limiting enzyme facilitates triglyceride uptake and storage by the fat cell, or **adipocyte.** Variations in LPL activity not only contribute to fat distribution differences among people, put probably affect the changes in fat distribution that occur during pregnancy and middle age, and may be responsible for the observed lower visceral adipose tissue accumulation in blacks compared to whites.[34a] The sex differences in total body fat and fat distribution also are related to the larger amount of LPL possessed by females—the adipocytes of the hip, thigh, and breast region produce considerable LPL in the female, while in males, the abdominal adipocytes are active with this fat-storing enzyme.

ADIPOCYTE SIZE AND NUMBER: HYPERTROPHY VERSUS HYPERPLASIA

The size and number of adipocytes also help determine and classify obesity. Adipose tissue mass increases in two ways:

- Existing adipocytes become enlarged or filled with more lipid in a process called **fat cell hypertrophy**.
- The total number of adipocytes is increased in a process called **fat cell hyperplasia**.

One technique for studying adipose cellularity involves sucking small fragments of subcutaneous tissue into a syringe through a needle inserted directly into a fat depot. These tissue fragments usually are sampled from the back of the arm at the triceps, the subscapular region, the buttocks, and the lower abdomen. The tissue is then treated chemically so that the individual adipocytes can be isolated and counted. Once the number of adipocytes is determined for a known weight of fat tissue, the average quantity of lipid per cell is determined by dividing the lipid mass in the sample by the number of adipocytes present. If total body fat is known, a good estimate can then be made of the body's total number of adipocytes. For example, if a person weighs 88 kg and has 13% body fat, total fat mass equals 11.4 kg (0.13 × 88 kg). The total number of adipocytes in the body is determined by dividing 11.4 kg by the average content of lipid per cell. If the average adipocyte contained 0.60 μg of lipid, then there would be 19 billion adipocytes in the body (11.4 kg ÷ 0.6 μg).

Total cell number = Mass of body fat ÷ Lipid content per cell

In one of our laboratories, needle biopsy and photomicrographic techniques were used to extract and measure the average size of adipocytes at selected body sites. Figure 29.6 depicts adipocytes from the abdominal area of an endurance-trained athlete and a middle-aged subject. In the middle-aged subject, whose total fat mass was 17.02 kg (body mass of 89.1 kg and 19.1% body fat) with 0.73 μg of lipid per cell, the total number of adipocytes was estimated to be 23.3 billion (17.02 kg ÷ 0.73 μg).

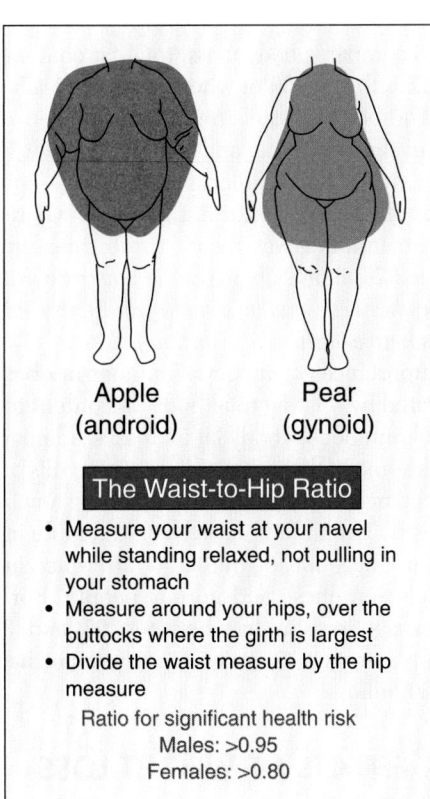

Apple
(android)

Pear
(gynoid)

The Waist-to-Hip Ratio

- Measure your waist at your navel while standing relaxed, not pulling in your stomach
- Measure around your hips, over the buttocks where the girth is largest
- Divide the waist measure by the hip measure

Ratio for significant health risk
Males: >0.95
Females: >0.80

FIGURE 29.5
Male (android)- and female (gynoid)-pattern obesity.

FIGURE 29.6

Top, Needle biopsy procedure to extract adipocytes of the upper buttocks region. The area is sterilized and anesthetized, and the biopsy needle is placed beneath the skin surface. Small tissue fragments are literally sucked from the site into the syringe. Photomicrographs are of the adipocytes biopsied from the buttocks of a physically active professor prior to and after 6 months of marathon training. The average adipocyte diameter was 8.6% smaller after training. On average, the volume of lipid in each cell decreased 18.2%. The large spherical structures in the background are lipid droplets. *Bottom,* Cross-section of human adipocytes magnified × 440. (From Geneser, F.: *Color Atlas of Histology.* Philadelphia, Lea & Febiger, 1985. Photomicrographs courtesy of P.M. Clarkson, Muscle Biochemistry Laboratory, University of Massachusetts, Amherst, MA.)

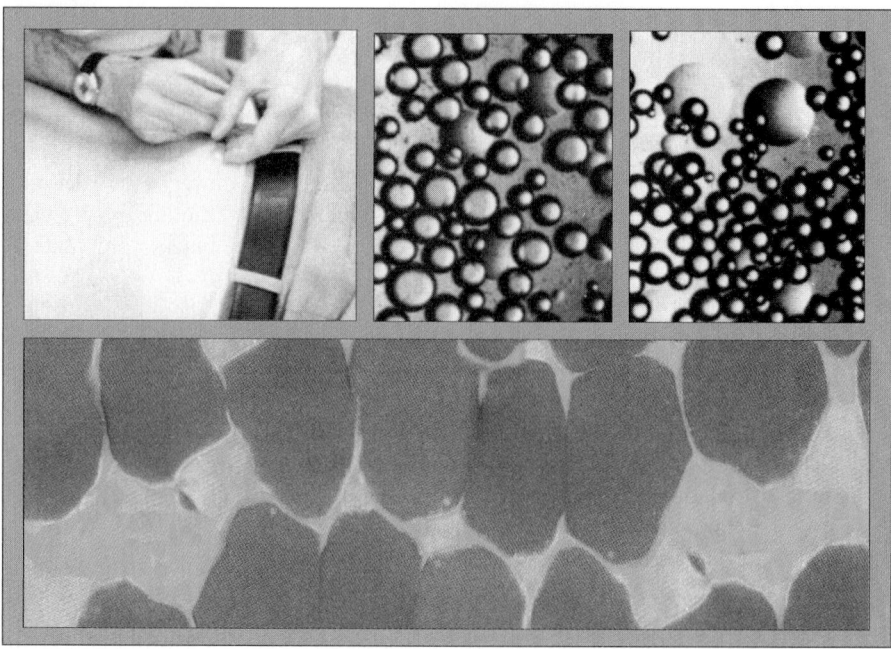

VARIETY OF HUMAN OBESITIES

Despite certain standards, it is not easy to distinguish the gradations and variations of obesity. Attempts have been made to describe obesity types based on the amount, distribution, and texture of adipose tissue.[35, 146] The idea of a classification schema is appealing because it permits quantification of the phenotype; it also allows for the evaluation of a variety of hormonal and biochemical correlates of each obesity type. Unfortunately, the term *obesity* is often used in a pejorative way that is not at all helpful in delineating its meaning: common adjectives include massive, morbid, severe, extreme, gross, and excessive. To avoid confusion, we will use the term **clinically severe obesity** to denote the obese condition in which total body fat exceeds 3 standard deviations above the mean value for percent body fat (30% body fat in males, 40% body fat in females). This level of body fat corresponds to a BMI of about 40 ("very high" category displayed in Figure 27.1).

Figure 29.7 presents six phenotypic patterns observed in female obesity (comparable data are unavailable for males). In addition, the photographic inserts complement several of the outline patterns and give examples of clinically severe obesity. The two panels at the bottom right illustrate the effects of a 35-kg weight loss over 15 months in a 49-year-old woman. Most of the weight lost was from the large abdominal panniculus, which was partially removed surgically. Note that even with a relatively large decrease in overall body mass, the pattern of the phenotype remains relatively invariant. Considerably more research in obesity classification is needed for men and women of all ages, particularly in conjunction with anthropometric, metabolic, biochemical, and genetic studies.

ADIPOSE CELLULARITY

COMPARISON OF CELLULARITY IN THE NORMAL AND OBESE

Figure 29.8 compares body mass, total fat content, and cellularity in 25 subjects, 20 of whom were clinically classified as obese. The body mass of the obese averaged more than twice that of the nonobese, and total fat content was nearly three times larger. For cellularity, the average lipid content per cell was about 50% larger in the obese, whereas the total adipocyte number was nearly three times greater (75 compared to 27 billion). *These results illustrate dramatically that cell number is the major structural difference in adipose tissue mass between the obese and nonobese.*

The importance of adipocyte number in obesity is further illustrated by relating total body fat content to both cell size and cell number. As body fat increases, adipocytes eventually reach some biologic upper limit. Once this occurs, cell number becomes the key factor determining any further extent of obesity. Even if adipocytes could double in size, this would still not account for the large difference in the total fat mass between obese and normal people. For comparison, an average person has between 25 and 30 billion adipocytes, whereas a severely obese person may have as many as 260 billion.[16]

EFFECTS OF WEIGHT LOSS

Figure 29.9 depicts the results of weight loss on the adipose tissue characteristics of 19 obese adults who reduced their body masses from 149 to 103 kg during the first stage of weight loss. The average adipocyte number before weight

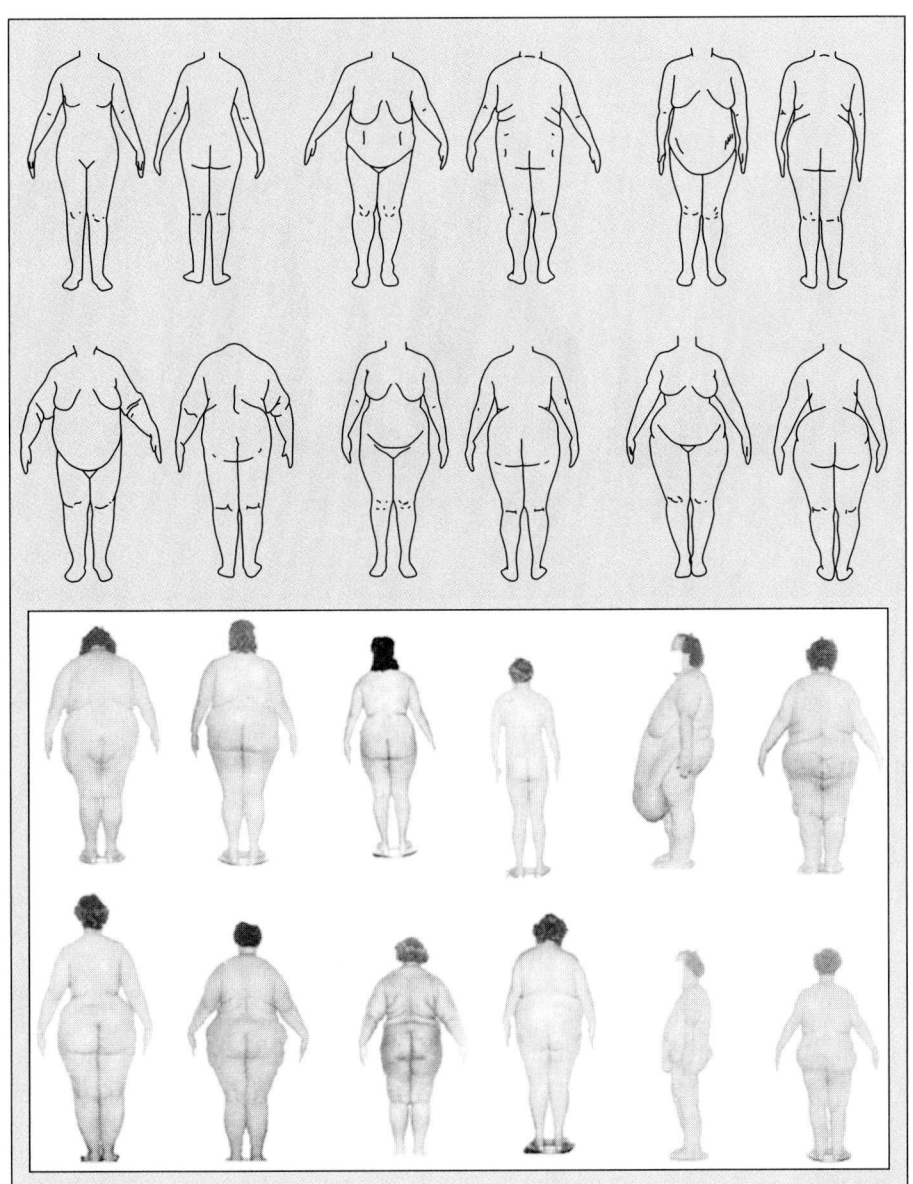

FIGURE 29.7
Variations in human obesity. Diagrams of patterns of female body form that illustrate the varieties of human obesity. The details of the rating profile used with this classification are presented in reference 35. The photographic inserts offer examples of several of the body patterns as well as intractable obesity, where the abdominal paniculus was estimated to weigh over 35 kg prior to weight loss *(two lower right panels)*. (Photographs and outline patterns courtesy of Leela S. Craig, M.D.)

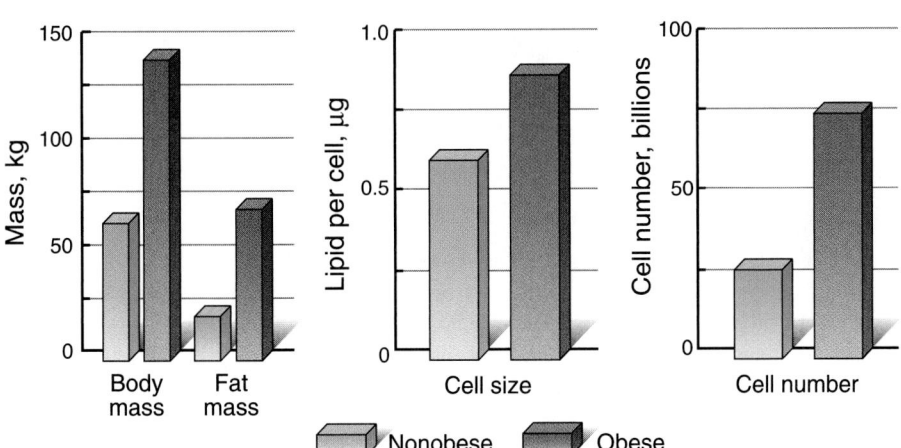

FIGURE 29.8
Comparison of body mass, total body fat, and adipocyte cell size and number in obese and nonobese subjects. (Modified from Hirsch, J., and Knittle, J.: Cellularity of obese and non-obese human adipose tissue. *Fed. Proc.*, 29:1518, 1970.)

FIGURE 29.9

Changes in adipose cellularity with weight reduction in obese subjects. (Data from Hirsch, J.: Adipose cellularity in relation to human obesity. In *Advances in Internal Medicine*. Vol. 17, G.H. Stollerman [Ed.], Chicago, Year Book, 1971.)

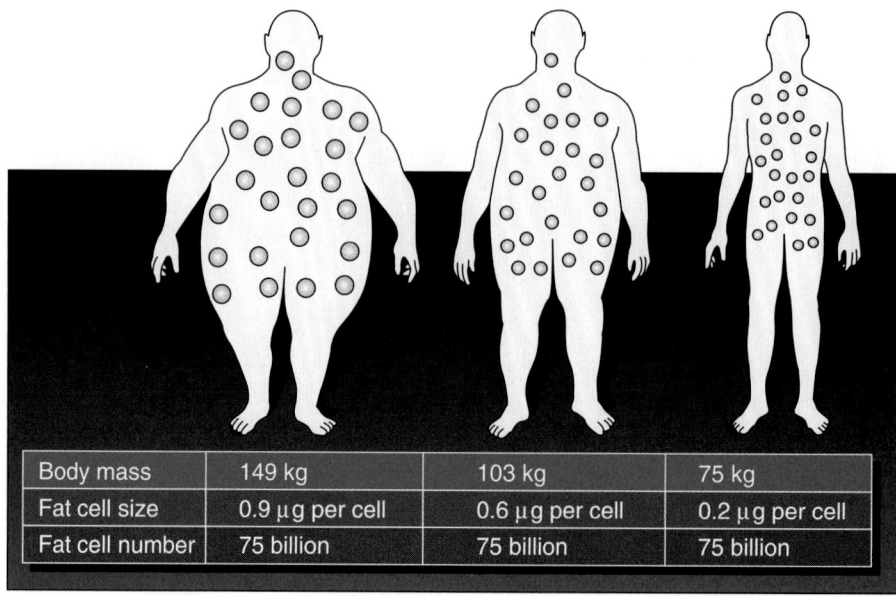

Body mass	149 kg	103 kg	75 kg
Fat cell size	0.9 µg per cell	0.6 µg per cell	0.2 µg per cell
Fat cell number	75 billion	75 billion	75 billion

reduction was 75 billion; this remained unchanged even after a 46-kg (101-lb) reduction. Adipocyte size, on the other hand, was reduced from 0.9 to 0.6 µg of lipid per cell, a decrease of 33%. When subjects attained normal body mass by losing an additional 28 kg, cell number remained unchanged, but cell size continued to shrink to about one-third the size of a normal, nonobese comparison group. As normal levels of body mass and body fatness were achieved, the adipocytes shrank and actually became smaller in size than those of the nonobese. *A shrinkage of adipocytes with no change in cell number is the major change in adipose cellularity following weight loss in adults.* These findings probably mean that formerly obese persons are not really "cured" of their obesity, at least in total number of adipocytes.

EFFECTS OF WEIGHT GAIN

An interesting series of studies has considered the dynamics of weight gain. In one study, adult male volunteers with an initial average body fat content of 15% deliberately increased their daily caloric intakes by three times normal, to about 7000 kcal for 40 weeks.[126] In a typical subject, body mass increased 25%, and percent body fat doubled from 14.6 to 28.2%. Of the 12.7 kg gained during the period of overeating, 10.5 kg was the result of increased body fat deposition. In a similar experiment with subjects who had no previous personal or family history of obesity, voluntary overeating caused an average increase in body mass of 16.4 kg.[118] A comparison of cell size and number before and after this 4-month experiment indicates that the average adipocyte increased substantially in size, with no change in cell number. When caloric intake was reduced and subjects achieved normal weight, total body fat declined, and the adipocytes reverted to their original size. *Generally, when*

adults gain fat as a result of overeating, existing adipocytes are being filled or enlarged rather than new ones being created.

The Possibility of Making New Ones? There is some indication that an extreme accumulation of body fat in adults may stimulate an increase in adipose cellularity. This is because there is an upper limit to adipocyte size beyond which hypertrophy fails to occur; this limit apparently is reached when the cell contains about 1.0 µg of lipid. At extremes of obesity (60% body fat: about 170% of normal weight), almost all of the adipocytes have attained their hypertrophic limits. In this situation, more cells may be recruited from the preadipocyte pool to increase cell number. *Thus, in maturity-onset severe obesity, in which the already fat adult becomes even fatter, hypercellularity may accompany the greatly increasing size of the existing adipocytes.*[15, 59] The increased cell number at this point would constitute a failure of adipocyte regulation, leading to further obesity.

ADIPOCYTE DEVELOPMENT

The growth and development of adipose tissue has been studied in animals and humans.

ANIMAL STUDIES

Extensive studies of adipose cellularity have been conducted with rats because these mammals have a relatively short life span, and various diet and exercise regimens can be studied during the growth cycle. Figure 29.10 illustrates the general upward-trending curves for body mass, fat mass, and adipocyte size and number in rats during the first 5 months of life. Note that cell number and cell size increase during weeks 6 through 15. As the animals become heavier and total body fat increases, there is a corresponding increase in adipocyte size only. The additional increase in body fat occurs because existing cells become filled with fat, not because new cells develop.

HUMAN STUDIES

Cell Size

Adipose cellularity was established for 34 infants and children ranging in age from a few days to 13 years.[60] Adipocyte size in newborn infants and children up to the age of 1 year was about one-fourth the size in adults; cell size tripled during the first 6 years, with little further increase until age 13. Although several studies have determined adipose cellularity in childhood and adolescence, there is still a scarcity of data on changes in adipocyte size between adolescence and adulthood.[27, 53] It generally is assumed that cell size increases during this growth period because the adipocytes of adults are significantly larger than those of adolescents.

Cell Number

Adipocytes increase in number rapidly during the first year of life, being about three times more numerous after 1 year than at birth. Most of the adipocytes existing before birth form during the last trimester of pregnancy. Beyond the age of 1 year, cell number increases gradually until about age 10. As with the increase in cell size, there is significant hyperplasia during the adolescent growth spurt; thereafter, cell number remains fairly stable. Percent body fat increases from about 16% of body mass at birth to between 24% and 30% over the first year.[36a] By age 6, body fat has decreased to about 14% of body mass in girls and 11% in boys. Thereafter, percent body fat progressively increases until, at age 11, it averages about 16% in boys and 27% in girls.

CAN ADIPOSE CELLULARITY BE MODIFIED?

It appears that certain behaviors can modify body fatness early in life. In humans, for example, maternal nutritional practices during pregnancy can affect the body composition of the developing fetus. A mother who gains more than 18

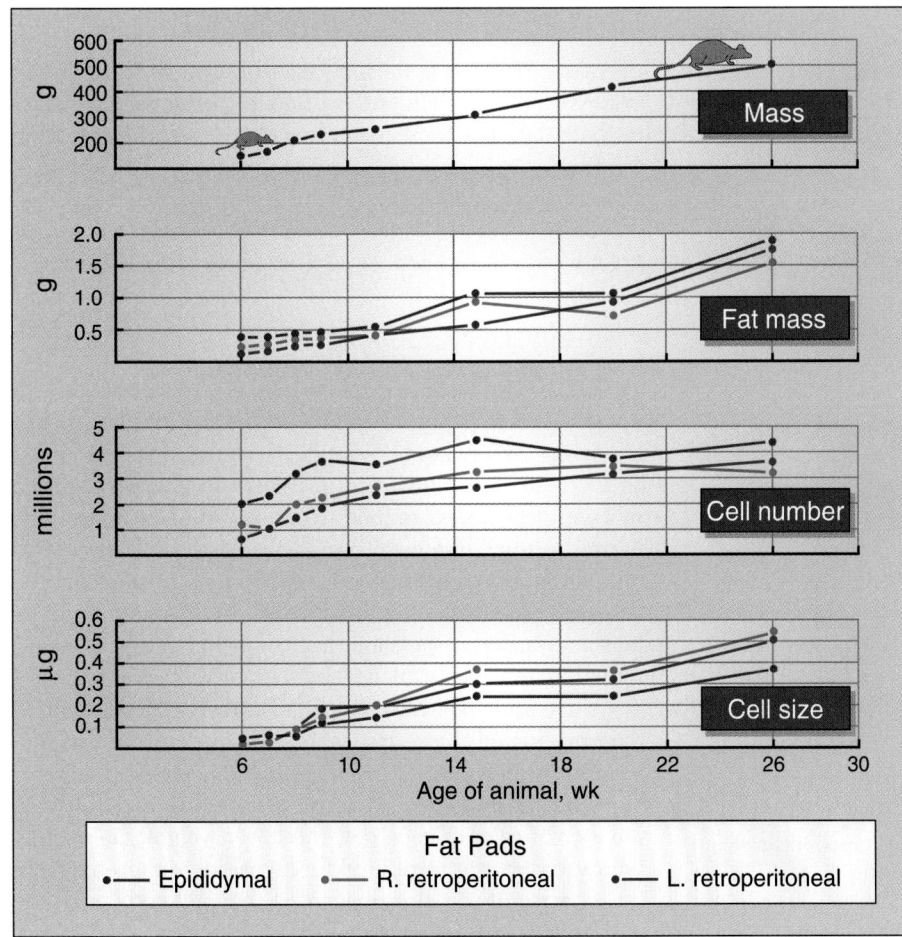

FIGURE 29.10

Changes in body mass, fat mass, and adipocyte cell number and size during the first 5 months of growth in rats. (From Hirsch, J., and Han, P.W.: Cellularity of rat adipose tissue: effects of growth, starvation, and obesity. *J. Lipid Res.*, 10:77, 1969.)

kg generally gives birth to a baby with a larger fatfold thickness than a woman who follows the recommended guidelines for weight gain during pregnancy.[143] Bottle feeding and early introduction of solid food also may be associated with childhood obesity. Conversely, breast feeding, which allows the infant to set the limits to food intake, and a delayed introduction to solid food may prevent overfeeding, the development of poor eating habits, and subsequent obesity.[74]

Research with animals suggests that alterations in adipocyte size and adipocyte number can be achieved in two ways: (*a*) modification of early nutrition, and (*b*) regular physical activity.

INFLUENCE OF NUTRITION

In one study of rats separated at birth, some mothers were "given" large litters of 22 animals and others smaller litters of four animals.[71] After weaning, at 21 days, all animals were given unlimited access to food. Subsamples of animals in each group were killed at 5, 10, 15, and 20 weeks of age. At weaning and after each subsequent 5-week period, the body masses of animals from the large (calorically deprived) litters were significantly lower than those of the other group. This suggested that early food deprivation caused a slowing in growth even though both groups of animals had free access to food after weaning.

Figure 29.11 shows that for cell size and number, the calorically deprived animals had fewer and smaller adipocytes at all age intervals than animals reared in small litters. At 5 and 10 weeks of age, the heights of the rectan-

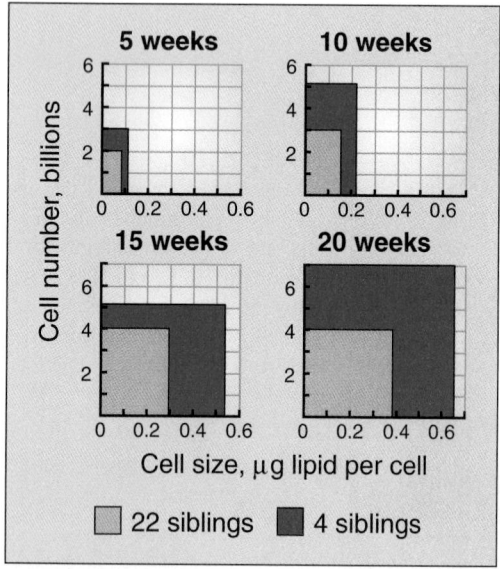

FIGURE 29.11
Changes in adipocyte size and number in rats raised in small and large litters. (Adapted from Knittle, J., and Hirsch, J.: Effect of early nutrition on the development of rat epididymal fat pads: cellularity and metabolism. *J. Clin. Invest.*, 467:2091, 1968.)

gles are greater than the bases, indicating that the adipocyte proliferation made a greater contribution to fat mass than did cell size. At the 15- and 20-week periods, the shape of the bar approaches a square, indicating that cell size played an increasingly important role in adipose tissue development. An interesting comparison is among animals raised in large and small litters. The blue area of the bar represents the fat depot of the well-fed animals raised in small litters; the orange area represents the depot for the calorically deprived animals; the difference in shading illustrates the difference in depot size between the two groups. By 15 weeks of age, the underfed group reached a definite plateau in adipocyte number, whereas cell number continued to increase in the small-litter animals. In both groups, cell size increased progressively during the experimental period. *These data suggest that there may be a critical time during the growth period when a permanent modification in adipose tissue cellularity can occur.*

Although extrapolation from animal data to humans is often difficult, some similarities in adipose tissue development between species are worth noting. As discussed previously, extremely obese humans have large numbers of adipocytes and, to a lesser extent, increased individual cell sizes. When these adults lose body fat, the adipocyte number remains unaltered, with the fat loss resulting from a reduction in cell size. This effect also occurs in adult rats. When these rats are deprived of food, weight loss can be attributed to adipocyte atrophy, with no change in cell number. As with adult humans, overfeeding of rats increases total body fat. The increase in body fat usually results from "stuffing" the individual adipocytes with lipid rather than from an increase in cell number. The exception occurs when adipocyte size reaches a maximum; adipose mass increases further with the additional proliferation of adipocytes.

INFLUENCE OF PHYSICAL ACTIVITY

Figure 29.12A–B summarizes the results of two studies with rats on the effects of exercise and food restriction early in life on body mass and body fat development throughout life. In the first study, illustrated in Figure 29.12A, young male rats with free access to food were forced to swim in plastic barrels for up to 6 hours, 6 days a week for 16 weeks.[98] Two other groups of rats remained sedentary: one group had free access to food, while the other was food-restricted to maintain body mass at the same lower level as the animals assigned to exercise.

The results were convincing. Animals given unlimited food but forced to exercise gained weight more slowly and had lower final body masses than their sedentary, freely eating counterparts. Because both groups consumed the same number of calories each day, the lower weight gain among the exercisers was attributed to the caloric requirements of the exercise. It was also shown that the total body fat of the exercisers was one-fourth that of the freely eating sedentary

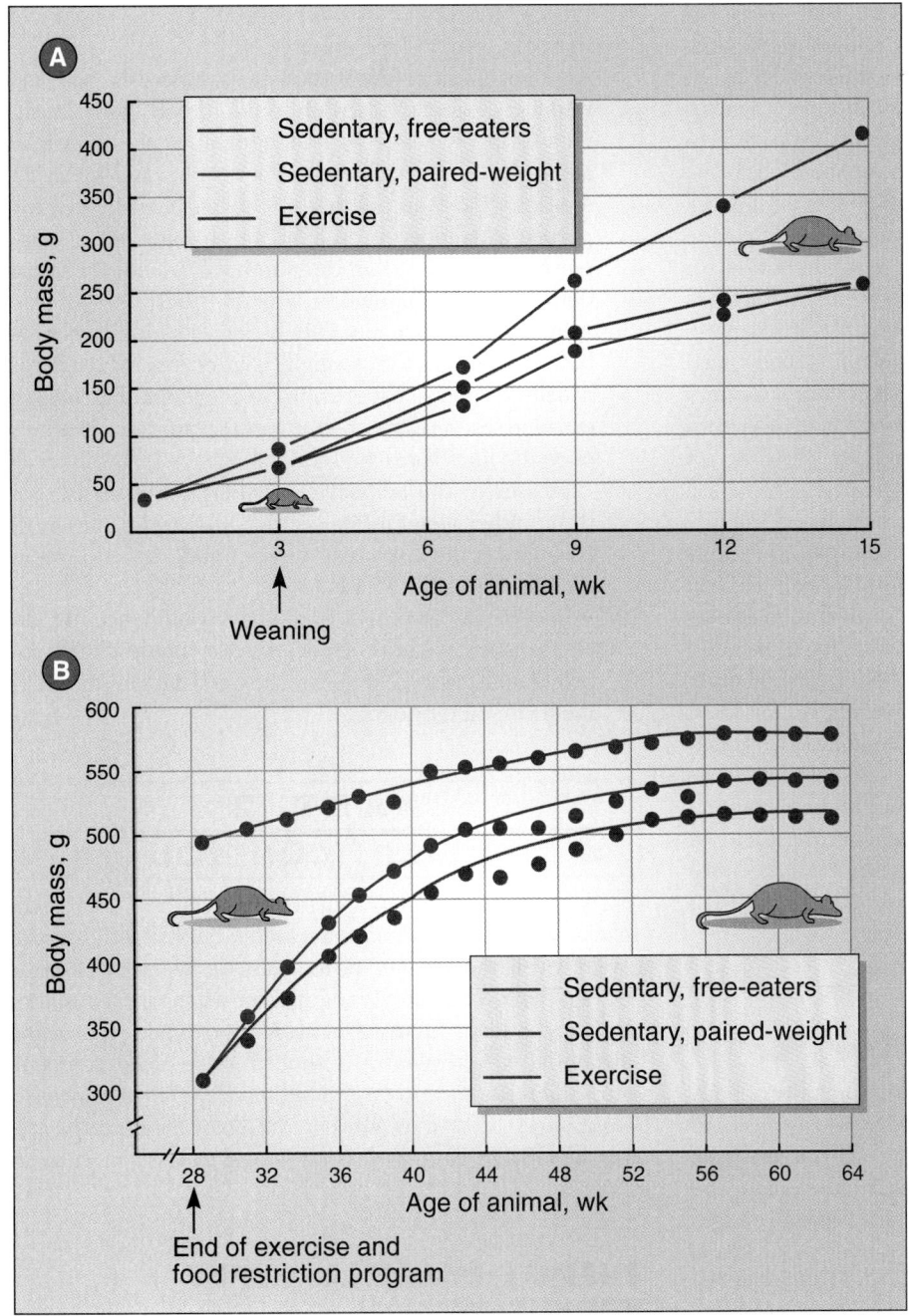

FIGURE 29.12
A, Effects of exercise and food restriction early in life on the body masses of rats up to 15 weeks. **B,** Effect of 28 weeks of exercise or food restriction on body masses of rats, followed by no exercise with unlimited access to food. (From Oscai, L., et al.: Effects of exercise and of food restriction on adipose tissue cellularity. *J. Lipid Res.,* 13:588, 1972; Oscai, L., et al.: Exercise or food restriction: effect on adipose tissue cellularity. *Am. J. Physiol.,* 277:901, 1974.)

group. This lesser body fat was the result of smaller cell size and cell number. In the sedentary, food-restricted group, total fat content was also lower than in the sedentary animals with free access to food. As happened with exercise, food restriction resulted in lower values for both adipocyte size and number. When body fat in the food-restricted and exercised animals was compared, the exercisers had fewer adipocytes and less fat per cell, even though the final body mass was about equal for both groups. The results demonstrated that exercise performed early during the growth of these animals depressed the development of adipocytes.

In a follow-up experiment, the fat-retarding effects of exercise or diet early in an animal's life were studied to determine whether either would result in less body fat accumulation throughout adulthood.[74, 99] Three similar groups of animals were again used. Exercise and food restriction were terminated after 28 weeks. Several animals from each group were then killed and compared for growth, total body fat, and adipocyte size and number. The remaining animals were subjected to 34 weeks of sedentary living with unlimited access to food. All animals were then killed and the groups were compared.

The data in Figure 29.12*B* indicate that the exercised animals had lower body mass at age 28 weeks than the sedentary free eaters. During the next 34 weeks of inactivity, the previously exercised animals continued to maintain this lower body mass, indicating that the exercise program performed earlier in life and then stopped led to the attainment of a lower body mass still evident into adulthood. As in the previous experiments, comparisons of adipocyte cell size and number at the end of the training period revealed that the exercisers had fewer and smaller adipocytes than either of the two sedentary groups. Furthermore, members of the exercise group had a lower final body mass and reduced total fat mass in later life than their sedentary counterparts, as well as significantly fewer adipocytes—even though the exercise period was followed by 34 weeks of inactivity.

Applied to humans, these findings raise the possibility that the introduction of prudent caloric intake and regular physical activity during the growth stage may help control the filling of existing adipocytes and the proliferation of new ones. Exercise and caloric restriction that begins later in life can certainly lead to a reduction in the body's total quantity of fat. As far as we know, it is only cell size, not cell number, that is reduced. If exercise or dietary intervention is discontinued, the existing adipose tissue mass is likely to increase again via expansion of the cellular volume. *Early prevention of obesity through proper exercise and diet, rather than the correction of existing obesity, may be the most effective method to curb the overfat condition so common in American children, teenagers, and adults.*

■ SUMMARY ■

1. The definition of obesity is an excessive quantity of body fat. There probably is no biological reason why men and women would get fatter as they grow older. If this is so, then the standards for overfatness in adult men and women could be based on the body fat levels of younger adults, namely, men—above 20%, women—above 30%.

2. Obesity has reached near epidemic proportions in the United States, with about one-third of all men and women being overweight (more than 20% above ideal body weight).

3. Genetic factors contribute about 25 to 30% to obesity. Genetic predisposition does not necessarily cause obesity; however, in the right environment, genetically susceptible individuals will gain weight, possibly lots of it.

4. Obesity should be viewed as a chronic disease because of the multiple health risks associated with a surprisingly low level of excess body fat. Weight loss in the obese significantly improves the health risk profile.

5. The patterning of fat on the body should be considered in evaluating the health risks of obesity. Fat distributed in the abdominal region (android-type obesity) poses a greater risk compared to fat deposited at the thighs and buttocks (gynoid-type obesity).

6. Another obesity classification is based on the size and number of adipocytes. Before adulthood, body fat increases in two ways: by enlargement of the individual adipocytes, termed fat cell hypertrophy, and by an increase in the total number of cells, termed fat cell hyperplasia. Adipocytes probably reach some biologic upper limit in size, so that cell number becomes the factor determining the ultimate extent of obesity.

7. Adipocyte number probably becomes stable sometime before adulthood; any weight gain or loss thereafter is usually related to hypertrophy of individual fat cells. In extreme cases, adipocyte number may increase in adults once the limit is reached for cell size.

8. Increases in the adipocyte number appear to involve three rather general time periods: the last trimester of pregnancy, the first year of life, and the adolescent growth spurt prior to adulthood.

9. Adipocyte development in animals is influenced by dietary restriction and regular exercise. These effects are prominent during early growth, when fat cell development can be retarded.

PART 2
WEIGHT CONTROL

In many adults, body mass fluctuates only slightly during a year, even though annual food intake averages close to 900 kg. This constancy is impressive when one considers that only a slight increase in daily food intake can cause substantial weight gain over time if there is no compensatory increase in energy expenditure. *If the total caloric intake ingested as food exceeds the daily energy expenditure, the excess calories will be stored as lipid in adipose tissue.*

ENERGY BALANCE: INPUT VERSUS OUTPUT

The energy balance equation states that body mass remains constant when caloric intake equals caloric expenditure. As shown in Figure 29.13, any chronic imbalance on either the energy output or input side of the equation causes the body mass to change.

There are three ways to "unbalance" the energy balance equation in the direction of weight loss:

• Reduce caloric intake below the daily energy requirements.

• Maintain normal caloric intake and increase energy expenditure through additional physical activity above the daily energy requirements.

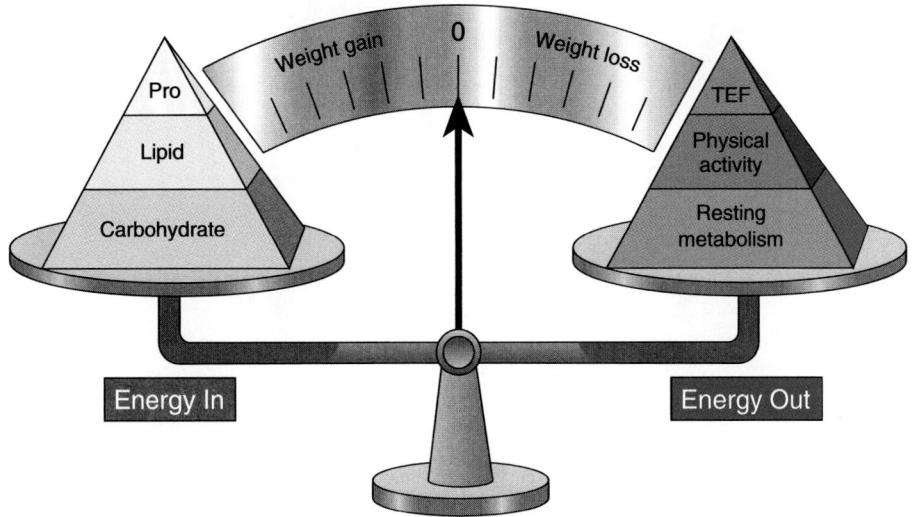

FIGURE 29.13
The energy balance equation (TEF refers to the thermic effect of food).

- Combine both methods by decreasing daily caloric intake and increasing daily energy expenditure.

When considering the sensitivity of overall energy balance as exhibited in the energy balance equation, we note that if caloric intake exceeds output by only 100 kcal per day, the surplus calories consumed in a year would be 365 days × 100 kcal, or 36,500 kcal. Because 0.45 kg (1.0 lb) of body fat contains about 3,500 kcal (each pound, or 454 g, of adipose tissue is about 87% lipid, or 395 g × 9 kcal · g^{-1} = 3,555 kcal per lb), this is equivalent to a yearly gain of about 4.7 kg of fat. On the other hand, if daily food intake is reduced by just 100 kcal and energy expenditure is increased 100 kcal by jogging 1 mile each day, then the yearly caloric deficit is equivalent to about 9.5 kg, or 21 lb, of body fat!

Note that the arithmetic for fat accumulation above is overly simplistic because the diet's composition influences the efficiency of how the body converts and stores excess calories as body fat.[125] Only about 3% of the calories in ingested lipid is required to convert these excess calories to stored body fat, whereas 25% of the calories in carbohydrate is "burned" in the conversion process. Simply stated, it is easier for the body to synthesize fat from dietary lipid than from an equivalent caloric excess in the form of carbohydrate. Consequently, shifting the diet's composition toward higher carbohydrate would result in less body fat gain, should a caloric excess occur.

DIETING FOR WEIGHT CONTROL

A prudent dietary approach to weight loss unbalances the energy balance equation by reducing daily energy intake 500 to 1000 kcal below daily energy expenditure. This relatively moderate reduction in food intake produces a greater weight loss in relation to the energy deficit than a more severe energy restriction.[135] Furthermore, people who create larger daily deficits to lose weight more rapidly are more likely to regain the weight than those who lose it slowly.[62] If an obese woman who normally consumes 2,800 calories daily and maintains body mass at 79.4 kg wishes to lose weight by dieting, she would maintain her regular physical activity but reduce daily food intake to 1800 calories to create a 1000-calorie deficit. In 7 days, the accumulated caloric deficit would equal 7000 calories, or the energy equivalent of 0.9 kg of body fat. Actually, considerably more than 0.9 kg would be lost during the first week of caloric restriction because, initially, the body's glycogen stores would be used to a greater extent in making up the energy deficit. This stored nutrient contains fewer calories per gram and much more water than stored lipid. For this reason, short periods of caloric restriction are often encouraging to the dieter but result in large percentages of water and carbohydrate loss per unit weight loss, with only a small decrease in body fat. Then, as weight loss continues, a larger proportion of body fat is used for the energy deficit created by food restriction. To reduce body fat an additional 1.4 kg, the reduced caloric intake of 1800 calories would have to be maintained for another 10.5 days; at this point, body fat theoretically would be reduced at a rate of 0.45 kg per every 3.5 days.

VERY DIFFICULT ON A LONG-TERM BASIS

A review of the scientific literature on weight loss reveals that initial success in modifying body composition has little relation to long-term success. Participants who remain in supervised weight-loss programs generally lose about 10% of their original body mass. The discouraging news is that, typically, one- to two-thirds of the lost weight is regained within a year, and almost all of it within 5 years.[12, 137] This has been pointed out in numerous follow-up studies of men and women who have participated in weight-reduction programs in which caloric intake was carefully regulated and

FIGURE 29.14

Percent of patients remaining at reduced weights at various time intervals following accomplished weight loss. *Solid line* represents 60 subjects with obesity onset before age 21; *broken line* represents 42 subjects with obesity onset after age 21. (From Johnson, D., and Drenick, E.J.: Therapeutic fasting in morbid obesity., *Arch. Intern. Med.*, 137:1381, 1977.)

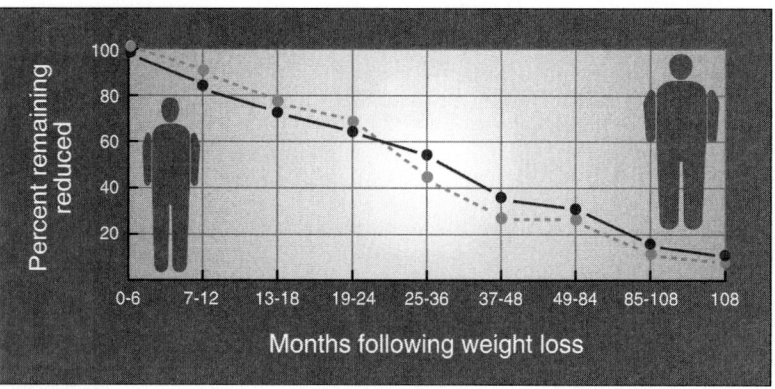

monitored. Over a 7.3-year follow-up of 121 patients, the tendency to regain weight was shown to be independent of length of the fast (up to 2 months), extent of weight loss (up to 41.4 kg), or age at the onset of obesity. Half of the subjects returned to their original weights within 2 to 3 years, and only seven patients remained at their reduced weights. Such statistics, illustrated in Figure 29.14, are discouraging and indicate that the long-term maintenance of a low-calorie diet is extremely difficult; it is particularly difficult in the relaxed atmosphere of one's home, where there is ready access to food and often little emotional support.

It also is difficult to initiate a physically active lifestyle even when some support is provided, but particularly so when support is withdrawn. Consider the following "practical" experiment, in which an intervention strategy was used in a natural environment in an attempt to augment physical activity.[29] Observations were made once a week for 8 weeks of the frequency with which those in the study either climbed stairs or used an escalator at a mall, train station, or bus terminal. Patrons were classified by sex, race (black/white), age (over 30/under 30 by visual inspection), and weight status (normal weight or overweight; designated overweight only when it was clearly the case). The numbers of steps required to climb were 30 steps at the shopping mall, 18 steps at the train station, and 24 steps at the bus station. During the intervention period, a large sign reading "Your heart needs exercise . . . here's your chance" was placed at the base of the stairs to encourage their use. Figure 29.15 indicates the percentage of patrons using the stairs before, during, and after the intervention. A total of 45,694 people were observed to use either the stairs or an adjacent escalator. It is evident that during the intervention period (when the signs were in place), there was almost a twofold increase in the percentage of people who climbed stairs (from 11.6% to 18.3%). When the sign was removed,

stair climbing decreased markedly to about 15% usage, but the level of use remained stable during a 1-month follow-up. Stair use decreased further, to 11.9%, at the 3-month follow-up. When the results were analyzed by age, degree of overweight status, sex, and race, it was discovered that overweight persons used the stairs significantly less than the normal-weight patrons, men used the stairs more than women (17.9% versus 13.8%), and white patrons used the stairs more than blacks during the intervention period; stair use declined more rapidly for blacks than for whites after the sign was removed. There were no differences in stair use by the younger or older men and women. The investigators commented that the most striking finding was the propensity for physical inactivity, as measured by limited stair use in the presence of an escalator. During both baseline periods, the average stair use was less than 10%! While the sign certainly was helpful in getting people to use the stairs, the overall participation rate really was not that large.

SETPOINT THEORY: A CASE AGAINST DIETING

One can crash off large amounts of weight in a relatively short time by simply not eating, but this success is short-lived, and eventually the urge to eat wins out and the weight is regained. The reason for this failure, it is argued, lies in "setpoints" that differ from what the dieter would like to have. The proponents of a **setpoint theory** argue that all people, fat or thin, have a well-regulated internal control mechanism, or setpoint, probably located deep within the brain's lateral hypothalamus[a], that drives the body to maintain a particular level of body weight or body fat.[69, 81] In a practical sense, this would be the body weight one would achieve when not counting calories. The problem is that we all have different setpoints, and various factors, such as the

---

[a]Recent research with mice indicates that the brain (perhaps via the hypothalamus) monitors the blood level of a hormone (leptin) secreted by the adipocytes to determine the quantity of body fat present.[53a, 102a] When levels of this hormone are low (perhaps because of hormone undersecretion), the body adjusts its metabolism to increase fat cell mass to maintain a constant level of this hormone (Refer to p. 605 and Figure 29.3.

drugs fenfluramine, amphetamine, and nicotine as well as exercise, may lower the particular setting—whereas dieting has no effect. Each time the level of body fat is reduced below a "natural" setpoint, the body makes internal adjustments to resist this change and conserve or replenish body fat. Even when a person attempts to gain weight above his or her normal level by overeating, the body resists this change by increasing resting metabolism.[61, 81, 154]

Resting Metabolism is Lowered

One well-documented change that occurs often during weight loss through dieting is a dramatic and sustained reduction in resting metabolism.[44, 81, 91] The decrease in resting metabolism exceeds the decrease attributable to the loss of either body mass or fat-free body mass—and with severe caloric restriction, the resting metabolism may become depressed as much as 45%! This calorie-sparing response is independent of the person's weight status or past dieting history. Metabolism becomes equally blunted in individuals attempting to lose weight, regardless of whether they have dieted before or whether they are fat or lean.[81] This greatly conserves energy and causes the diet to become progressively less effective despite a surprisingly low caloric intake. As a result, weight loss plateaus, and further weight loss is

considerably less than predicted from the mathematics of the restricted energy intake.

Figure 29.16 displays the results from a study of six obese men for whom body mass, resting oxygen uptake (minimal energy requirement), and caloric intake were carefully monitored for 31 days. During the pre-diet period, body mass and resting oxygen uptake remained stable with a daily food intake of 3500 kcal. Thereafter, the daily caloric intake was reduced markedly to 450 kcal. When the subjects switched to this low-calorie diet, both body mass and resting metabolism were lowered, but the percentage decline in metabolism was greater than the decrease in body mass. The dashed line represents the expected weight loss from the 450-calorie diet. The decline in resting metabolism actually conserved energy, causing the diet to become progressively less effective. More than half of the total weight loss occurred over the first 8 days of the diet, with the remaining weight loss occurring during the final 16 days. This plateauing of the theoretical weight-loss curve often leaves the dieter frustrated and discouraged.

Weight Cycling: Going No Place Fast

The futility of repeated cycles of weight loss and weight gain—the so-called off-and-on, or **yo-yo, effect**—occurs

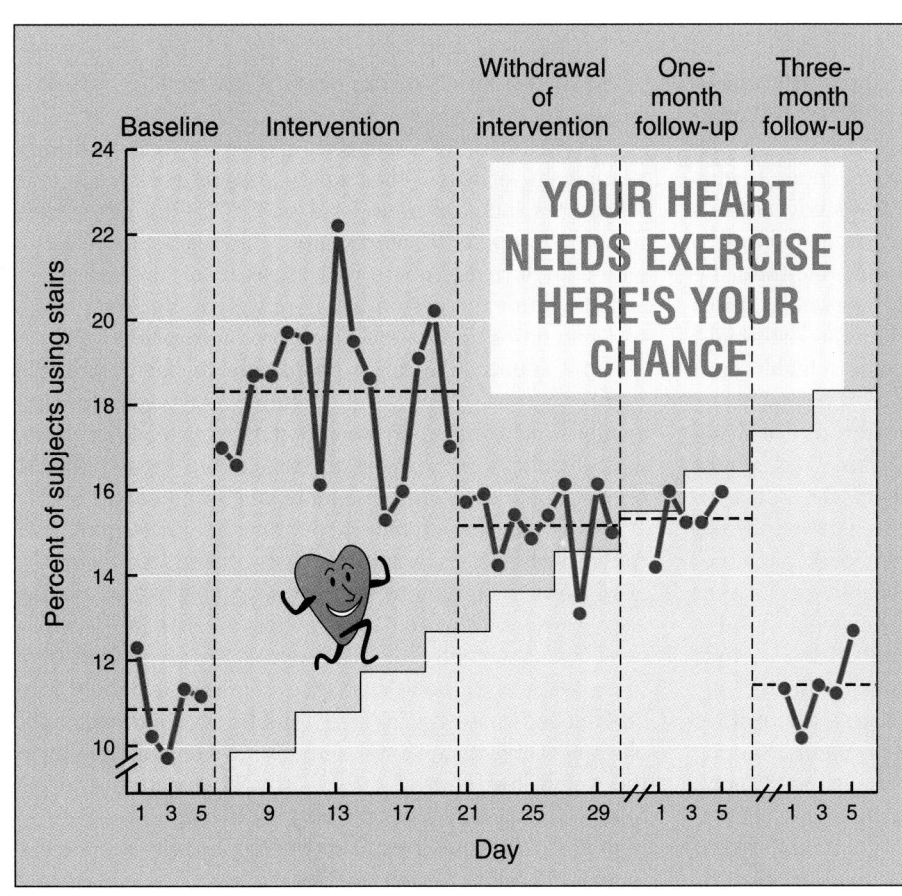

FIGURE 29.15
Percentage of subjects using the stairs before, during, and after an intervention consisting of a sign encouraging subjects to climb the stairs instead of taking the escalator. (Modified from Brownell, K.D., et al.: Evaluation and modification of exercise patterns in the natural environment. *Am. J. Psychol.*, 137:12, 1980.)

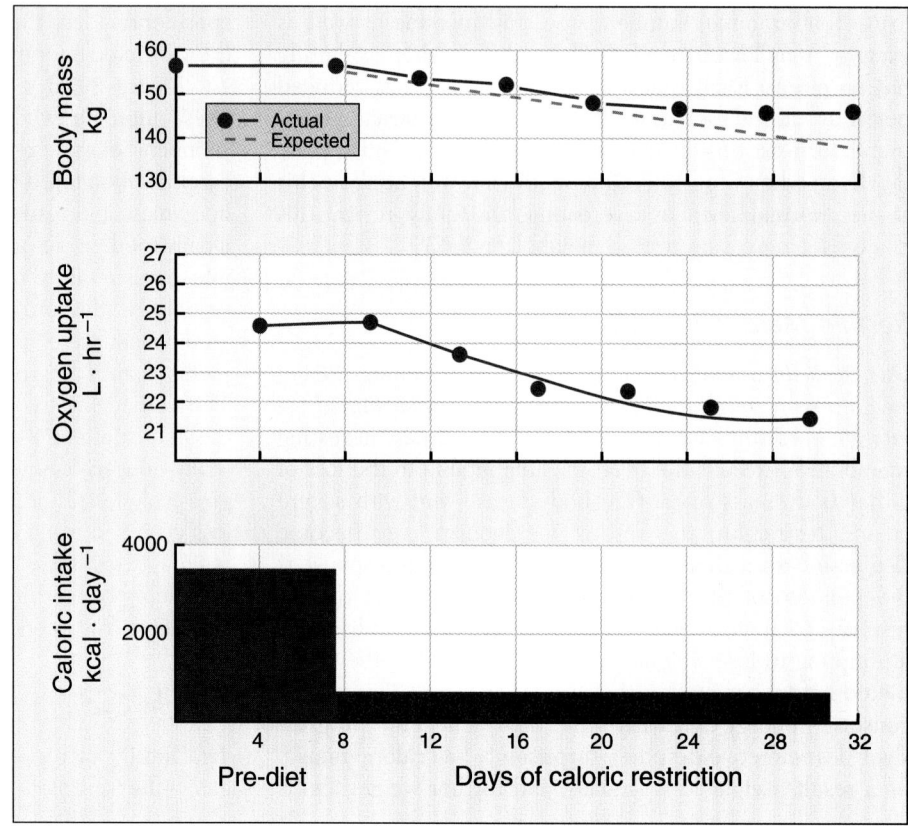

FIGURE 29.16

Effects of two levels of caloric intake on changes in body mass and resting oxygen uptake. Often the failure of the actual weight loss to keep pace with that predicted based on food restriction leaves the dieter frustrated and discouraged. (Adapted from Bray, G.: Effect of caloric restriction on energy expenditure in obese subjects. *Lancet*, 2:397, 1969.)

with animals in food efficiency studies that evaluate weight loss–weight gain in relation to ingested calories. Although significant controversy on the subject exists,[19, 87, 108, 157] some research indicates that weight gain occurs more readily with repeated cycles of weight loss. In one study, animals required twice the time to lose the same weight during a second period of caloric restriction and only one-third the time to regain it.[30] While simply being overweight raises the risk of heart disease, the failure to keep the lost weight off may pose an additional risk. Although a highly controversial topic, it has been observed that repeated bouts of weight loss and weight gain augment the risk of dying from a heart attack. In one study, this risk was almost 70% higher for those who took weight off and put it on again compared to people whose body weight stayed reasonably steady.[64] However, recent data from 6500 Japanese-American men who were originally healthy and never smoked revealed no ill effects in losing weight or in a repeated cycle of weight loss and regain.[63a] If it does turn out that weight cycling poses an additional health risk, one can only speculate on the potential for long-term negative effects from the repeated weight cycling so common among high school and collegiate wrestlers.[131] At this point, however, the health risks from obesity are far more conclusive than those from weight cycling. Therefore, obese people should not use a concern of the potential hazards

of yo-yo dieting as an excuse to abandon efforts to lose weight.[95]

There is further disconcerting news for those desiring a permanent fat loss. When obese people lose weight, the adipocytes increase their level of the fat-storing enzyme lipoprotein lipase.[68] Unfortunately, this adaptation makes it easier for formerly obese individuals to regain body fat—and the fatter the person is before weight loss, the greater the amount of lipoprotein lipase produced when weight is lost. In essence, the fatter people are to begin with, the more vigorously their bodies attempt to regain the lost weight. Such observations support the existence of a biologic feedback mechanism to explain the great difficulty obese people encounter in maintaining weight loss.[53a, 61, 158]

Although the setpoint theory may be unwelcome news to those who possess a setpoint that is tuned "too high," the good news, according to setpoint advocates, is that regular exercise may lower the setpoint toward a more desirable level.[43] Concurrently, regular exercise conserves and even increases fat-free body mass, raises resting metabolism (if fat-free body mass is increased), and brings about metabolic changes that facilitate lipid catabolism, all of which augment the weight loss effort.[58, 61, 81, 91, 148] As discussed in a subsequent section, in overweight men and women who exercise regularly, food intake tends to decline initially despite the increase in caloric output. Eventually, as an active lifestyle is maintained and body fat reserves decrease, caloric intake balances the daily energy requirements so that body mass is stabilized at a new, lower level.

EXTREMES OF DIETING

Professional organizations have voiced strong opposition to certain dietary practices, particularly the extremes of fasting and the low-carbohydrate, high-fat, and high-protein diets. These practices are particularly troublesome to those who work in the areas of sports medicine and athletics, where reports consistently document that athletes often exhibit bizarre and often pathogenic weight-control behaviors.[17, 140]

Ketogenic Diets

Ketogenic diets emphasize carbohydrate restriction while generally ignoring the total caloric content of the diet. Advocates of these diets maintain that with dietary restriction of carbohydrates, the body will mobilize significant lipids for energy. This generates excess plasma ketone bodies (byproducts of incomplete lipid breakdown resulting from inadequate carbohydrate catabolism) that supposedly suppress the appetite. The ketones lost in the urine represent unused energy, the elimination of which further facilitates the weight-loss effort. Some extremists maintain that this energy loss is so great, dieters can eat all they wish as long as carbohydrates are restricted. At best, the energy lost by urinary excretion of ketones probably equals only 100 to 150 calories a day.[4] This would account for a small weight loss of approximately 0.45 kg per month—not very appealing when the major source of food is a lipid intake that may be as high as 70% of the calories consumed. Also, any initial weight loss may be due largely to dehydration caused by an extra solute load on the kidneys, increasing the excretion of water. Such water loss is of no lasting significance in a program designed to reduce body fat. Low-carbohydrate diets can also potentially lead to a significant loss of lean tissue, as the body recruits amino acids in muscle to maintain blood glucose by gluconeogenesis. This is certainly an undesirable side effect of a diet designed to precipitate a body fat loss.

When compared to a standard, well-balanced, low-calorie diet, the ketogenic diet offers no advantage in facilitating a loss in body fat.[83] The diet is potentially hazardous in several ways. It can raise serum uric acid levels; alter electrolyte concentrations, initiating undesirable cardiac arrhythmias; cause acidosis; aggravate kidney problems because of the extra solute burden placed on the renal system; elevate blood lipids; deplete glycogen reserves to contribute to a fatigued state; and cause relative dehydration. The diet is definitely contraindicated during pregnancy because dietary carbohydrate is essential to fetal development.

High-Protein Diets

Various modifications of a high-protein diet are potentially dangerous. These diets have been extolled as "last chance diets" for the obese. It is argued that extremes of dietary protein cause suppression of the appetite through a reliance on lipid mobilization and subsequent ketone formation. It also is argued that the elevated thermic effect of dietary protein, along with its relatively low coefficient of digestibility, ultimately reduces the net calories available from this macronutrient compared to a well-balanced meal of equal caloric value. Although this point has some validity, many other factors must be considered in formulating a sound weight-loss program, including the potentially harmful strain on kidney and liver function and accompanying dehydration, electrolyte imbalance, and possible lean-tissue loss resulting from diets that are excessively high in protein and usually low in carbohydrate. When the protein is in liquid form, this "miracle liquid" often contains a blend of ground-up animal hooves and horns, and pigskin mixed in a broth with enzymes and tenderizers to "predigest" it. This protein blend often is not of the highest quality in its amino-acid mixture, and it is generally lacking in required vitamins and minerals.

Semistarvation Diets

A therapeutic fast, or **very-low-calorie diet (VLCD),** may be recommended in cases of severe clinical obesity, where body fat exceeds 40 to 50% of body mass.[2] Such diets are usually prescribed for up to 3 months, but only as "last resorts" prior to undertaking more extreme medical approaches such as various surgical treatments. This form of dieting must be closely supervised, usually in a hospital setting. The VLCD approach to weight loss is predicated on the hope that the severe restriction of food may break established dietary habits and, in turn, improve the long-term prospects for successful weight loss. These diets also may effect significant appetite depression, which could help the obese person comply with the diet plan.[150] Daily medications usually are prescribed, including calcium carbonate or antihistamines for nausea, bicarbonate of soda and potassium chloride to maintain consistency of body fluids, mouthwash and sugar-free chewing gum for bad breath (owing to a high level of ketones generated from lipid catabolism), and various bath oils for dry skin. *For most individuals, semistarvation is not an "ultimate diet" or proper approach to weight control.* If a person fasts even for several days and then attempts to exercise, deterioration in performance and fatigue are likely to occur. Because an adequate level of carbohydrates is not consumed, the glycogen-storage depots in the liver and muscles are reduced rapidly to low levels; this causes impairment in tasks requiring either a sustained muscular effort or a shorter term anaerobic power output. Furthermore, the success rate of prolonged fasting is poor. There is also the possibility that lean tissue loss may occur disproportionately from critical organs such as the heart.[149]

Table 29.2 summarizes the principles and main advantages and disadvantages of some of the popular dietary approaches to weight loss. Although most diets induce a weight loss during the first several weeks, much of the weight lost is body water. In addition, loss of lean tissue is usually significant with dieting only, especially in the early phase of very-low-calorie dieting.[18, 77] While it certainly is possible to lose significant weight through dieting, few people have been successful in altering their body size and composition on a long-term basis.

EXERCISE FOR WEIGHT CONTROL

The precise contributions of physical inactivity and excessive caloric intake to obesity are unclear. What is clear is that

TABLE 29.2
PRINCIPLES AND MAIN ADVANTAGES AND DISADVANTAGES OF SOME POPULAR WEIGHT-LOSS METHODS

Method	Principle	Advantages	Disadvantages	Comments
Surgical procedures	Alteration of the gastrointestinal tract changes capacity or amount of absorptive surface	Caloric restriction is less necessary	Risks of surgery and post-surgical complications can include death	Radical procedures include stapling of the stomach and removal of a section of the small intestine (a jejunoileal bypass)
Fasting	No energy input ensures negative energy balance	Weight loss is rapid (which may be a disadvantage) Exposure to temptation is reduced	Ketogenic A large portion of weight lost is from lean body mass Nutrients are lacking	Medical supervision is mandatory and hospitalization is recommended
Protein-sparing modified fast	Same as fasting except protein or protein with carbohydrate intake assumedly helps preserve lean body mass	Same as in fasting	Ketogenic Nutrients are lacking Some unconfirmed deaths have been reported, possibly from potassium depletion	Medical supervision is mandatory Popular presentation was made in Lin's *The Last Chance Diet*
One-food-centered diets	Low-caloric intake favors negative energy balance	Being easy to follow has initial psychologic appeal	Being too restrictive means that nutrients are probably lacking Repetitious nature may cause boredom	No food or food combination is known to "burn off" fat Examples include the grapefruit diet and the egg diet
Low-carbohydrate/high-fat diets	Increased ketone excretion removes energy-containing substances from the body Fat intake is often voluntarily decreased; a low caloric diet results	Inclusion of rich foods may have psychologic appeal Initial rapid loss of water may be an incentive	Ketogenic High-fat intake is contraindicated for heart and diabetes patients Nutrients are lacking	Popular versions have been offered by Taller and Atkins; some have been called the "Mayo," "Drinking Man's," and "Air Force" diets
Low-carbohydrate/high-protein diets	Low caloric intake favors negative energy balance		Expense and repetitious nature may make it difficult to sustain	If meat is emphasized, the diet becomes one that is high in fat The Pennington diet is an example
High-carbohydrate/low-fat diets	Low caloric intake favors negative energy balance	Wise food selections can make the diet nutritionally sound	Initial water retention may be discouraging	The Pritikin diet is an example

Modified and reprinted by permission from Reed, P.B.: *Nutrition: An Applied Science.* Copyright © 1980 by West Publishing Co. All Rights Reserved.

a sedentary lifestyle is an important factor in the weight-gaining process.

Not Simply a Problem of Gluttony. In the past, it was generally accepted that the obese condition was the result of an excessive food intake. Clearly then, the effective approach to weight loss would be some form of caloric restriction, that is, dieting. This view of obesity, however, is overly simplistic. *Available evidence indicates that excess weight gain often parallels reduced physical activity rather than increased caloric intake.* Among active young and middle-aged endurance-trained men, body fat was demonstrated as being inversely related to energy expenditure; no relationship existed between body fat and caloric intake.[88] Among the physically active, those who eat the most often weigh the least and are the most fit! In the United States, the caloric intake per person has steadily decreased over the past 100 years, yet body mass and body fat have increased steadily. Americans now eat 5 to 10% fewer calories than they did 20 years ago, yet the average body mass has steadily increased. Over the same period, there has been about a 4% decline in energy intake in children and adolescents, yet on the average, their body weights have continued to rise. If dieting were effective, a reduction in caloric intake would theoretically bring the national body weight to a lower, not higher, level!

Obese infants do not characteristically consume more calories than the recommended dietary standards.[11] In children aged 4 to 6 years, the daily energy expenditure averages 25% below the current recommendation for energy intake at this age. This blunted energy output is due primarily to a low level of daily physical activity.[33] More specifically, about 50% of boys and 75% of girls fail to engage in even moderate physical activity three or more times per week.[1, 144] Time-in-motion photography, used to document activity patterns of elementary school children, indicated that overweight children were considerably less active than their normal-weight peers, and that excess weight was not related to food intake. The caloric intake of obese high-school girls and boys is actually below that of their nonobese peers.[54, 65, 114] The observation that obese children often eat the same or even less than peers of average body weight is also true for adults as they become less active and slowly begin to add weight.[46, 128] *In fact, one is hard pressed to find evidence that groups of overweight individuals actually eat more, on average, than people of normal weight.* Consequently, further emphasizing a reduced caloric intake to effect a weight loss is neither prudent nor appropriate as the only method to combat the overfat condition.

Increased Energy Output Worth Considering. *It is increasingly clear that men and women with a physically active lifestyle, or those who become involved in endurance exercise programs, tend to maintain a desirable body composition.* Evidence is accumulating to support the contention that an increased level of regular physical activity may be more effective than dieting for long-term weight

control.[50, 137] Increased caloric expenditure through aerobic-type exercise is a significant option for unbalancing the energy balance equation to bring about both weight loss and a favorable modification in body composition.[8] This occurs with possibly less of the accumulation of central adipose tissue associated with aging.[13, 72, 107]

Two arguments have been raised against the exercise approach to weight loss. One is the belief that exercise inevitably causes an increase in appetite, so that any caloric deficit from exercising is rapidly made up by a proportionate increase in food intake. The second argument is that the calorie-burning effects of a normal bout of exercise are so small that they will not "dent" the body's fat reserves as significantly as starvation or semistarvation. We will take a closer look at these two misconceptions.

MISCONCEPTION 1: EXERCISE AND FOOD INTAKE

A delicate balance between energy intake and energy expenditure often is not maintained in sedentary people. This lack of precision in regulating food intake at the lower end of the physical activity spectrum may account for the "creeping obesity" observed in highly mechanized and technically advanced societies. On the other hand, in individuals who exercise on a regular basis, appetite control eventually falls within a "reactive zone," in which food intake is more readily matched to daily energy expenditure.

In considering the effects of exercise on appetite and food intake, a distinction should be made between the type and duration of the exercise. People such as lumberjacks, farm laborers, and endurance athletes who perform prolonged physical effort consume about twice the daily calories as their more sedentary counterparts. For example, endurance athletes such as marathon runners, cross-country skiers, and cyclists consume about 4000 to 5000 kcal a day, yet these men and women are among the leanest in the population! Obviously, this large caloric intake is required just to meet the energy requirements of training.

Regarding the energy intake of the overweight person, the apparent compensatory appetite-stimulating effect of only moderate physical activity is noticeably reduced in relation to the extra energy requirement of the exercise. To some extent, the larger energy reserve of the overweight person may ease that person's tolerance to a weight-loss program with exercise without the "obligatory" increase in caloric intake observed in a lean person.[67, 120, 130, 139]

MISCONCEPTION 2: CALORIC STRESS OF PHYSICAL ACTIVITY

A common misconception related to the role of exercise in weight loss concerns the quantity of calories typically burned. It is argued that an inordinate amount of exercise must be performed just to lose 0.45 kg of body fat, for example, chopping wood for 10 hours, playing golf for 20 hours, performing mild calisthenics for 22 hours, playing ping-pong for 28 hours, or playing volleyball for 32 hours. From a different perspective, however, if golf were played for only 2 hours per day (walking without cart, about 350 kcal), 2 days per week (700 kcal), it would take about 5 weeks to lose 0.45 kg of body fat. Assuming one could play year round, devoting 2 days per week to this form of exercise would result in a 4.5-kg yearly fat loss, provided food intake remains fairly constant. *The calorie-expending effects of exercise are cumulative: a caloric deficit of 3500 kcal is equivalent to a 0.45-kg body fat loss, regardless of whether the deficit occurs rapidly or systematically over time.*

In estimating the energy cost of various physical activities, the assumption is made that exercise energy expenditure is constant among people of a particular body size. In Chapter 8, we noted that the energy cost data for most physical activities were averages often based only on a few observations. A wide range of values is therefore possible because of individual differences in performance style and technique, environmental factors such as terrain, temperature, and wind resistance, and the intensity of participation. Consequently, the energy expenditure values of physical activities presented in Appendix D should not be viewed as constants. These are "average" values, applicable under "average" conditions, and applied to the "average" person of a given body mass. These values, however, do provide approximations of energy expenditure for establishing the caloric costs of diverse physical activities.

The Recovery "Afterglow." A controversy exists as to the quantitative significance, during weight loss, of excess postexercise oxygen consumption (EPOC) to the total energy expenditure of physical activity. During low to moderate submaximal exercise, as performed by most people who use exercise for weight control, the contribution of recovery metabolism—the so-called recovery "afterglow"—to total energy expenditure is probably quite small, averaging between 9 and 30 kcal for exercise durations less than 80 minutes.[26, 105]

EXERCISE IS EFFECTIVE

The effectiveness of regular exercise in achieving weight loss is linked to one's degree of obesity. Generally, persons who are obese lose weight and fat more readily with exercise than their counterparts of normal weight.[7] In addition, aerobic exercise, even without dietary restrictions, provides a significant positive "spin-off" because it favorably alters body composition (reduced body fat and maintenance or even a small increase in fat-free body mass) in the otherwise healthy person, the cardiac patient, and the physically challenged.[8, 23, 42, 97, 136] Even exercise programs that involve less energy-demanding conventional resistance training help maintain fat-free body mass during weight loss compared to programs relying solely on food restriction.[9] Because fat-

free body mass is metabolically more active than body fat, this conservation of lean tissue contributes to the maintenance of a high level of resting metabolism[39, 141, 142] and may enhance lipid oxidation during rest, thus lessening the age-associated increase in adiposity.[32]

(Note: This favorable effect of exercise, as compared to diet alone, on body composition changes during weight loss is not always observed. For example, among older obese men, equivalent reductions in fat and fat-free mass and changes in fat distribution have been observed regardless of whether weight loss was induced by hypocaloric diet therapy alone or combined with aerobic exercise training.[38])

When exercise is used for weight loss, factors such as frequency, intensity, duration, and the specific form of exercise must be considered. Continuous, big-muscle, aerobic activities having moderate to high caloric costs, such as walking, running, rope skipping, stair stepping, cycling, and swimming, are ideal. Many recreational sports and games also are effective in reducing body mass, although precise quantification and regulation of energy expenditure is difficult during such activities. Aerobic exercises also stimulate lipid metabolism, establish favorable blood pressure responses, and generally promote cardiovascular fitness. There generally is no selective effect of running, walking, or bicycling: each is equally effective in promoting fat loss.[106] An extra 300-kcal daily caloric expenditure induced by moderate jogging for 30 minutes, for example, causes a 0.45-kg fat loss in about 12 days. This represents a yearly caloric deficit equivalent to the energy in 13.6 kg of body fat.

A DOSE-RESPONSE RELATIONSHIP

The total energy expended in exercise is directly related, in a dose-response relationship, to the effectiveness of exercise in weight loss.[7] An overfat person who starts out with light exercise such as slow walking can accrue a considerable caloric expenditure simply by extending the exercise duration. This duration effect offsets the inability (and inadvisability) of the previously sedentary, obese person in beginning a program of more strenuous exercise. Also, the energy cost of weight-bearing exercise such as walking is proportional to body mass; thus, the overweight person expends considerably more calories in such exercise than someone of normal body mass.

The importance of exercise duration in weight loss was illustrated in a study of three groups of men who exercised for 20 weeks by walking and running for either 15, 30, or 45 minutes per session.[89] Compared to a sedentary control group, the three exercise groups significantly decreased in body fat, fatfolds, and waist girth. Comparisons between the three groups indicated that the 45-minute training group lost more body fat than either the 30- or 15-minute group. This extra fat loss was attributed to the greater caloric expenditure of the longer exercise period.

TABLE 29.3
EFFECTIVENESS OF REGULAR EXERCISE (16-WEEK WALKING PROGRAM) IN ELICITING CHANGES IN BODY COMPOSITION AND BLOOD LIPIDS IN SIX OBESE YOUNG ADULT MEN

Variable	Pre-Training[a]	Post-Training[a]	Difference
Body mass, kg	99.1	93.4	-5.7^b
Body density, g · mL^{-1}	1.044	1.056	$+0.012^b$
Body fat, %	23.5	18.6	-4.9^b
Fat mass, kg	23.3	17.4	-5.9^b
Fat-free body mass, kg	75.8	76.0	$+0.2$
Sum of fatfolds, mm	142.9	104.8	-38.1^b
HDL cholesterol, mg · 100 mL^{-1}	32	37	$+5.0^b$
HDL/LDL cholesterol	0.27	0.34	$+0.07^b$

From Leon, A.S., et al.: Effects of a vigorous walking program on body composition, and carbohydrate and lipid metabolism of obese young men. *Am. J. Clin. Nutr.*, 33:1776, 1979.
[a]Values are means.
[b]Statistically significant.

SOME GENERAL GUIDELINES FOR AN EXERCISE-WEIGHT LOSS PROGRAM

• Start slowly—*The initial stage of an exercise weight-loss program for a previously sedentary, overfat person should be developmental in nature and should not include an initial high total energy output.* During the initial stage, the individual should be urged to adopt long-term goals, personal discipline, and a restructuring of both eating and exercise behaviors.[86] It often is counterproductive to include unduly rapid training progressions because many obese men and women initially exhibit psychological resistance to increasing physical activity. During the first few weeks (or months), slow walking is replaced by intervals of walking and jogging that can eventually lead to continuous jogging. At least a 12-week time period is required before meaningful changes occur.[70] Behavioral changes should also be applied to a person's daily lifestyle. For example, walking or bicycling can replace the use of the automobile, stair climbing can replace the elevator, and manual tools can replace power tools.
• Table 29.3 illustrates the effectiveness of regular exercise on weight loss in six sedentary, obese young men who exercised 5 days per week for 16 weeks. The regimen consisted of 90 minutes of walking for each session.[82] The men lost an average of almost 6 kg of body fat, representing a decrease in percent body fat from 23.5 to 18.6%.

In addition, exercise capacity improved, as did the level of high-density lipoprotein cholesterol (15.6%) and the ratio of high-density to low-density lipoprotein cholesterol (25.9%).
• Regularity is the key—Exercise frequency is important when using exercise for weight reduction. It appears that at least 3 days of training per week is required to bring about meaningful changes in body composition through exercise—and more frequent exercise is even more effective.[3, 70] More than likely, this effect is the direct result of the added calorie burning required by the extra exercise. *Although the threshold exercise energy expenditure required for weight loss is probably highly individualized, it generally is recommended that each exercise session burn at least 300 kcal.* This can be achieved with 30 minutes of moderate to vigorous running, swimming, or bicycling, or walking for at least 60 minutes.

DIET PLUS EXERCISE: THE IDEAL COMBINATION

For moderately obese children and adults, combinations of regular aerobic exercise and diet (relatively more carbohydrate and less lipid) offer considerably more flexibility in achieving a negative caloric balance and accompanying body fat loss than either exercise alone or diet alone.[28, 42, 57, 70, 90, 109a, 149a] The addition of exercise to a program of weight control facilitates a longer-term maintenance of fat loss than does total reliance on food restriction.[31, 102] Table 29.4 summarizes the benefits of exercise when added to a weight-loss program.

How can an obese person using exercise and diet, while attempting to maintain a prudent weight loss of about 0.45 kg a week, reduce body mass by 9.1 kg (20 lb)? Under

TABLE 29.4
BENEFITS OF ADDING EXERCISE TO DIETARY RESTRICTION FOR WEIGHT LOSS

• Increases the overall size of the energy deficit
• Facilitates lipid mobilization and oxidation, especially from visceral adipose tissue depots
• Increases the relative loss of body fat by preserving the fat-free body mass
• By conserving and even increasing the fat-free body mass, may blunt the drop in resting metaboism that frequently accompanies weight loss
• Requires less reliance on caloric restriction to create energy deficit
• Contributes to the long-term success of the weight loss effort
• Provides unique and significant health-related benefits

these conditions, it would take 20 weeks to achieve the desired fat loss. Based on this goal, the weekly deficit would have to average 3500 calories, or a daily average of 500 calories. One-half hour of moderate exercise (about 350 "extra" calories) performed 3 days per week enhances the weekly deficit by 1050 calories. Consequently, the weekly caloric intake would have to be reduced by only 2400 calories (about 350 kcal a day) instead of 3500 calories to achieve the desired loss of 0.45 kg of body fat each week. If the number of exercise days is increased from 3 to 5, daily food intake need only be reduced by 250 calories. If the duration of the 5-day per week workouts is prolonged from 30 minutes to 1 hour, then no reduction in food intake is necessary to achieve a weight loss because the required deficit of 3500 kcal is created entirely through exercise.

If the intensity of the 1-hour exercise performed 5 days a week is then increased by only 10% (cycling at 22 mph instead of 20 mph; running a mile in 9 minutes instead of 10 minutes), the number of calories burned each week through exercise will increase by an additional 350 kcal (3500 kcal/week × 10%). This new weekly deficit of 3850 kcal, or 550 kcal per day, actually permits the "dieter" to **increase** daily food intake by 50 kcal and still lose 0.45 kg of fat each week!

Clearly, physical activity in combination with mild dietary restriction can be used to effectively unbalance the energy balance equation in the direction of weight loss.[23] This combined approach is much less likely to induce the feelings of intense hunger and psychological stress that occur when weight loss is attempted using caloric restriction exclusively. Of great significance is that both aerobic and resistance exercise protect against the loss in fat-free mass usually observed when weight loss is achieved through diet alone.[39, 42, 56, 101] This is true partly because exercise training enhances the mobilization and utilization of lipid from the body's adipose tissue depots.[112] In addition, exercise facilitates protein retention in skeletal muscle, while at the same time retarding its rate of breakdown. *These protein-sparing effects of regular exercise are part of the reason more weight lost is in the form of fat in a weight-reduction program.*

A Reality Check. Regardless of the approach taken, the difficulty in solving the overfat condition on a long-term basis is perhaps best summed up by this recent statement of the National Task Force on the Prevention and Treatment of Obesity: "Obese individuals who undertake weight loss efforts should be ready to commit to lifelong changes in their behavioral patterns, diet, and physical activity."[95]

SOME FACTORS THAT AFFECT WEIGHT LOSS

EARLY WEIGHT LOSS IS LARGELY WATER

Figure 29.17 shows the percentage composition in average daily weight loss of water, protein, and body fat, during

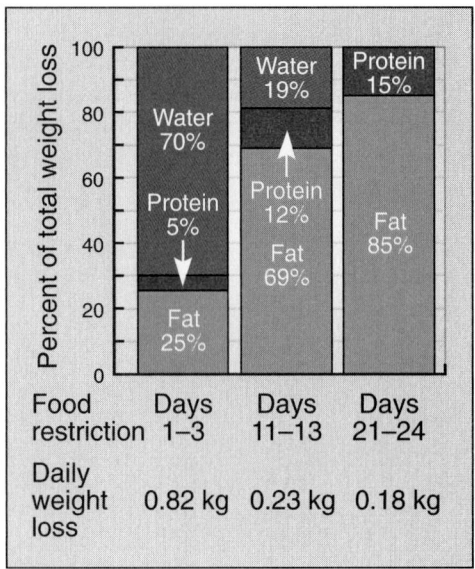

FIGURE 29.17

Percentage composition of weight loss at the start, middle, and end of 24 days of food restriction (1000-kcal daily intake) plus 2.5 hours of daily exercise. (From Grande, F.: Nutrition and energy balance in body composition studies. In *Techniques for Measuring Body Composition.* Washington, DC, National Academy of Sciences–National Research Council, 1961.)

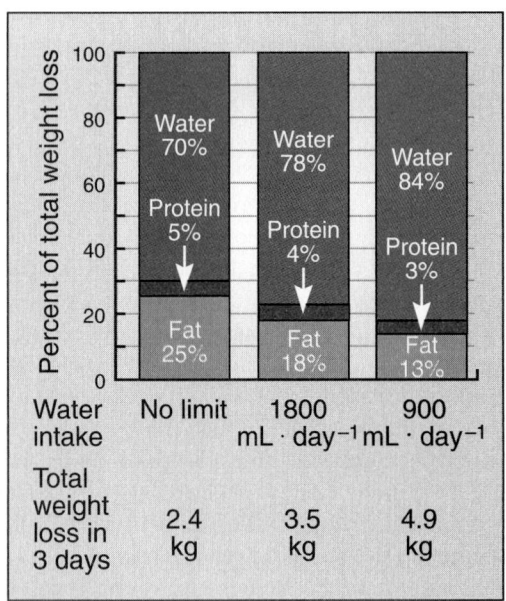

FIGURE 29.18

Percentage composition of weight loss during the first 3 days on a 1000-kcal diet with water intake either unrestricted or reduced to 1800 mL or 900 mL per day. (From Grande, F.: Nutrition and energy balance in body composition studies. In *Techniques for Measuring Body Composition.* Washington, DC, National Academy of Sciences–National Research Council, 1961.)

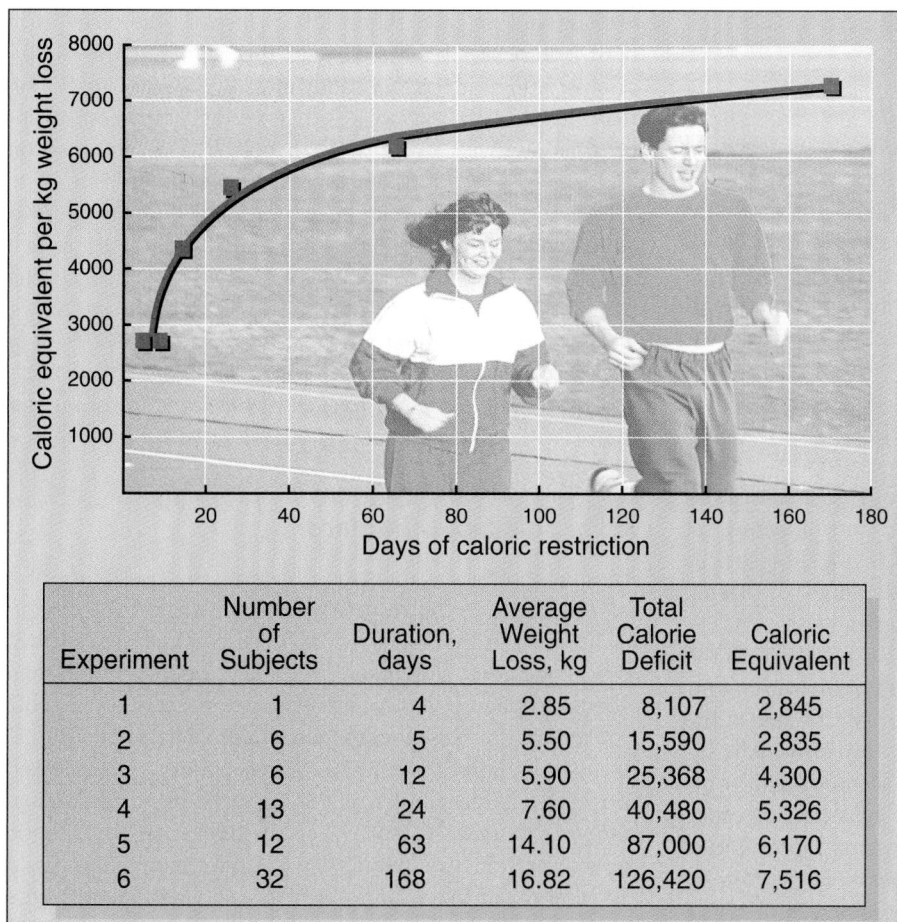

FIGURE 29.19
Caloric equivalent of weight loss in relation to the duration of caloric restriction. Each data point represents an experiment summarized in the accompanying legend. (From Grande, F.: Nutrition and energy balance in body composition studies. In *Techniques for Measuring Body Composition.* Washington, DC, National Academy of Sciences—National Research Council, 1961.)

Experiment	Number of Subjects	Duration, days	Average Weight Loss, kg	Total Calorie Deficit	Caloric Equivalent
1	1	4	2.85	8,107	2,845
2	6	5	5.50	15,590	2,835
3	6	12	5.90	25,368	4,300
4	13	24	7.60	40,480	5,326
5	12	63	14.10	87,000	6,170
6	32	168	16.82	126,420	7,516

24 days on a 1000-calorie, high-carbohydrate diet and 2.5 hours of prescribed exercise. During the first 3 days of energy deficit, 70% of the weight lost was water. This water loss became progressively less as the program continued, representing only 19% of the weight lost during days 11 to 13. At the same time, body fat loss accelerated from 25 to 69%. From days 21 to 24, 85% of the weight loss was the result of a reduction in body fat, with no further increase in water loss. The contribution of protein to weight loss increased from 5% initially, to 12% during days 11 to 13, to 15% by the end of the observation period.

MAINTAIN ADEQUATE HYDRATION

Figure 29.18 depicts the relationship between the proportion of water, protein, and fat lost and the amount of water consumed during the first few days of caloric restriction. The left bar is the same as that shown in Figure 29.17 for days 1 to 3, during which subjects had unlimited access to water. The middle bar represents data for six men who also subsisted on the 1000-calorie, high-carbohydrate diet, but with daily water intake restricted to 1800 mL. The bar at the right displays the compositional weight loss of six men who

consumed an identical diet but whose daily water intake was further reduced to 900 mL. Water restriction during the first 3 days significantly increased the proportion of body water lost and decreased the proportion of fat lost, especially in subjects who consumed the least water. Although more total weight was lost when daily water intake was reduced to 900 mL per day, this additional loss in body mass resulted solely from water loss. In essence, these men had become dehydrated. *Regardless of whether or not fluid intake was restricted, the total quantity of body fat lost was the same for all groups.*

LONGER-TERM DEFICIT PROMOTES FAT LOSS

Figure 29.19 illustrates an important concept: the caloric equivalent of the weight lost increases as the duration of caloric restriction is extended. More specifically, the caloric equivalent of weight loss more than doubles after 2 months on a diet compared to the first 5 days. *Thus, it is important to maintain a caloric deficit for an extended period because shorter periods of caloric restriction cause larger percentages of water and carbohydrate loss per unit weight reduction, with only minimal decreases in body fat.*

SPOT REDUCTION: DOES IT WORK?

The notion of spot reduction is based on the belief that an increase in a muscle's activity facilitates relatively greater lipid mobilization from the adipose tissue in proximity to the muscle. Therefore, by exercising a specific body area, more fat will be selectively reduced from that area than if exercise of the same caloric intensity is performed by a different muscle group. Advocates of spot reduction would recommend large numbers of sit-ups or side-bends for a person with excessive abdominal fat. Whereas the promise of spot reduction with exercise is attractive from an aesthetic and health-risk standpoint, a critical evaluation of the research does not support its use.[76, 96]

To examine the claims for spot reduction critically, comparisons were made of the girths and subcutaneous fat stores of the right and left forearms of high-caliber tennis players.[52] As expected, the girth of the dominant or playing arm was significantly larger than the nondominant arm because of a modest muscular hypertrophy associated with the exercise overload provided by playing tennis. Measurements of fatfold thickness, however, indicated no difference in the quantity of subcutaneous fat on the two forearms. Clearly, regular and prolonged exercise was not accompanied by reduced fat deposits in the playing arm. In another experiment, fat biopsies were taken at the abdominal, subscapular, and buttock sites before and after 27 days of sit-up exercise training.[66] The number of sit-ups was increased from 140 at the end of the first week to 336 on day 27. Following training, however, the adipocytes in the abdominal region were no smaller than those in the relatively unexercised buttocks or subscapular regions.

There is no doubt that the negative caloric balance created through regular exercise can significantly contribute to a reduction in total body fat. Exercise stimulates the mobilization of fatty acids through hormones delivered via the bloodstream that act on the fat depots throughout the body. The areas of greatest body fat concentration and/or lipid-mobilizing enzyme activity probably supply the greatest amount of this energy.[5, 41, 121] *There is no evidence that fatty acids are released to a greater degree from the fat pads directly over the active muscle.*

WHERE ON THE BODY DOES FAT REDUCTION OCCUR?

A question often asked concerning weight loss is, "Where on the body do changes occur when weight is lost?" To help answer this question, changes in body composition and body fat distribution were evaluated in 26 obese females, at successive 2.3-kg (5-lb) increments of weight loss, over a 14-week period.[70] Weight loss was induced by caloric restriction and a 45-minute, 3-day-per-week exercise program that included 15 minutes of general calisthenics and 30 minutes of

walking and jogging. Figure 29.20 displays the changes in body composition, fatfolds, and girths in the three subgroups, who reduced their body mass by 2.3, 4.5, and 9.1 kg, respectively. A 4.5-kg weight loss was accompanied by approximately twice the change in overall body composition than a loss of 2.3 kg. When weight loss doubled from 4.5 to 9.1 kg, the corresponding change in body composition was almost three times as much. For fat loss, there was approximately a twofold greater change in fatfolds and girths in the trunk region compared to the extremities. *These and other findings suggest a preferential mobilization and reduction of upper body subcutaneous and deep abdominal fat with exercise training instead of the loss of the more "resistant" fat in the gluteal and femoral regions.*[6, 37, 41, 73, 121]

A Possible Sex Difference?

Another interesting question concerns the possibility of a sex difference in the responsiveness of weight loss to regular exercise. A meta-analysis of 53 research studies on this topic concluded that men generally respond better than women to the weight-loss effects of exercise.[7] One possible explanation for this phenomenon may relate to the differences in body fat distribution between sexes. As discussed previously, fat distributed in the upper body and abdominal regions (central fat) displays a lively lipolysis to sympathetic nervous system stimulation and is preferentially mobilized for energy during exercise.[5, 121, 130, 151] Consequently, the greater distribution of upper body adipose tissue in men compared to women may contribute to their greater sensitivity to the weight-loss effects of regular exercise, particularly in the abdominal region. The final answer to this intriguing question awaits further research.

■ SUMMARY ■

1. There are three ways to unbalance the energy balance equation and bring about weight loss: (*a*) reduce energy intake to below daily energy expenditure, (*b*) maintain regular energy intake and increase energy output, and (*c*) combine both methods by decreasing energy intake and increasing energy expenditure.

2. Long-term maintenance of weight loss through dietary restriction is generally successful less than 20% of the time. Typically, one- to two-thirds of the lost weight is regained within a year, and almost all of it is regained within 5 years.

3. A caloric deficit of 3500 kcal created either through diet or exercise is the equivalent to the calories in 0.45 kg (1.0 lb) of adipose tissue.

4. Dieting for weight loss can be effective if done properly. The disadvantages of extremes of semistarvation, however, are significant and include a loss of fat-free body mass, lethargy, possible malnutrition and

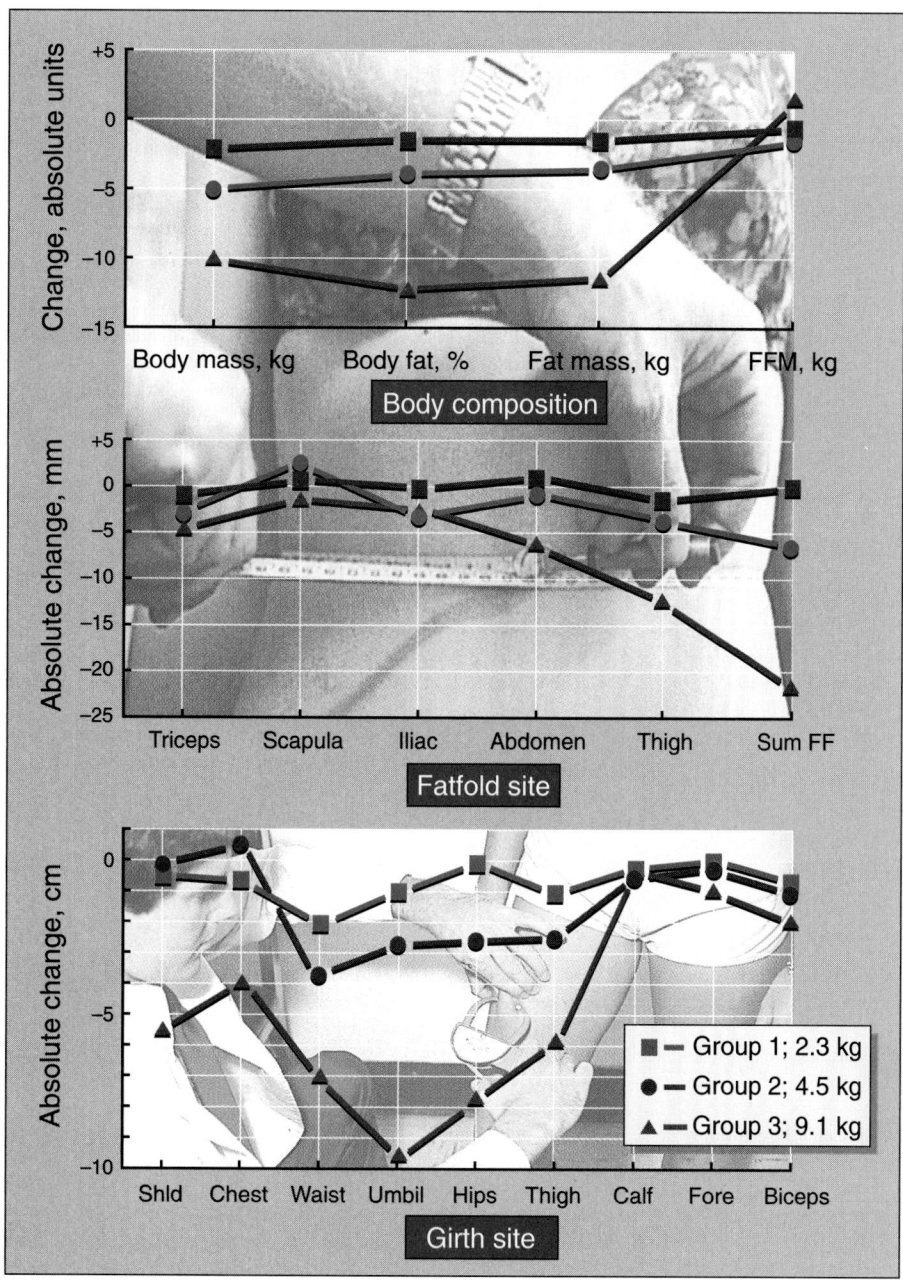

FIGURE 29.20

Changes in body composition *(top),* fatfolds *(middle),* and girths *(bottom)* with specified amounts of weight loss. The abbreviations for the girths are *Should,* shoulders; *Umbil,* umbilicus abdomen; *Fore,* forearm. The anatomic sites are those described in Appendix E. (Data are from reference 70.)

metabolic disorders, and a significant decrease in resting metabolism. Some of these factors actually conserve energy and cause dieting to be less effective.

5. Although controversy on the topic exists, repeated cycles of weight loss–weight gain may increase the body's ability to conserve energy. This "yo-yo" dieting may lead to a greater difficulty achieving weight loss with subsequent dieting; it also may facilitate regaining of the lost weight and pose an independent heart disease risk.

6. The calorie-burning effects of exercise are cumulative, so that over time, a little extra physical activity performed regularly has a dramatic effect. The precise role of exercise in appetite suppression or stimulation

is unclear, although a moderate increase in physical activity for obese men and women does not necessarily increase food intake. Over time, most athletes eventually consume enough calories to counterbalance the caloric expenditure of training—though many of these athletes are the leanest in the world.

7. A combination of exercise and diet offers a flexible and effective approach to weight loss. Exercise enhances the mobilization and utilization of lipids, thus enhancing fat loss. Regular exercise also retards lean tissue loss. Resistance exercise may even lead to an increase in fat-free body mass.

8. Rapid weight loss during the first few days of caloric deficit is the result primarily of a loss of body water and

stored glycogen. As weight loss continues, a greater loss of fat is exhibited per unit of weight lost.

9. Selective fat reduction at specific body areas through localized "spot exercise" is no more effective than more general physical activity.

10. The possible sex difference in the responsiveness of weight loss to exercise may relate to differences in body fat distribution. Fat deposited in the upper body and abdominal regions (male-pattern obesity) is highly responsive to neurohumoral stimulation. This depot of body fat is preferentially mobilized in exercise compared to fat deposited in gluteal and femoral regions (female-pattern obesity).

■ REFERENCES ■

1. Aaron, D.J., et al.: The epidemiology of leisure physical activity in an adolescent population. *Med. Sci. Sports Exerc.,* 25:847, 1993.

2. Alban, H.J., et al.: Metabolic response to low- and very-low-calorie diets. *Am. J. Clin. Nutr.,* 49:745, 1989.

3. American College of Sports Medicine: Position statement on proper and improper weight loss programs. *Med. Sci. Sports Exerc.,* 15:9, 1983.

4. American Medical Association: A critique of low-carbohydrate ketogenic weight and reduction regimens (a review of Dr. Atkins' diet revolution). *JAMA,* 224:1418, 1973.

5. Arner, P., et al.: Adrenergic regulation of lipolysis in situ at rest and during exercise. *J. Clin. Invest.,* 32:423, 1991.

6. Arner, P., et al.: Expression of lipoprotein lipase in different human subcutaneous adipose tissue regions. *J. Lipid Res.,* 32:423, 1991.

7. Ballor, D.L., and Keesey, R.E.: A meta-analysis of the factors affecting changes in body mass, fat mass and fat-free mass in males and females. *Int. J. Obes.,* 15:717, 1991.

8. Ballor, D.L., and Poehlman, E.T.: Exercise training enhances fat-free mass preservation during diet-induced weight loss: a meta-analytical finding. *Int. J. Obes.,* 18:35, 1994.

9. Ballor, D.L., et al.: Resistance weight training during caloric restriction enhances lean body weight maintenance. *Am. J. Clin. Nutr.,* 47:19, 1988.

10. Barlett, H.L., and Buskirk, E.R.: Body composition and the expiratory reserve volume in lean and obese men and women. *Int. J. Obesity,* 7:339, 1983.

11. Beaton, G., et al.: An examination of factors believed to be associated with infantile obesity. *Am. J. Clin. Nutr.,* 32:1997, 1979.

12. Begley, C.E.: Government should strengthen regulation in the weight loss industry. *J. Am. Diet. Assoc.,* 91:1255, 1991.

13. Bemben, M.G., et al.: Age-related patterns in body composition for men aged 20-79 yr. *Med. Sci. Sports Exerc.,* 27:264, 1995.

14. Björntorp, P.: Adipose tissue in obesity. In *Recent Advances in Obesity Research.* Vol. 4, J. Hirsch and T.B. Van Itallie (Eds.), London, Libby, 1985.

15. Björntorp, P.: Fat cells in obesity. In *Handbook of Eating Disorders.* K.D. Brownell and J.P. Foreyt (Eds.), New York, Basic Books, 1986.

16. Björntorp, P., et al.: Effect of an energy reduced dietary regimen in relation to adipose tissue cellularity in obese women. *Am. J. Clin. Nutr.,* 28:445, 1975.

17. Black, D.R., and Burckes-Miller, M.E.: Male and female college athletes: use of anorexia nervosa and bulimia nervosa weight loss methods. *Res. Q. Exer. Sport,* 59:252, 1988.

18. Blackburn, G.L., et al.: The very-low-calorie-diet: a weight reduction technique. In *Handbook of Eating Disorders.* K.D. Brownell and J.P. Foreyt (Eds.), New York: Basic Books, 1986.

19. Blackburn, G.L., et al.: Weight cycling: the experience of human dieters. *Am. J. Clin. Nutr.,* 49:1105, 1989.

20. Bouchard, C.: Genetics of obesity: overview and research directions. In *The Genetics of Obesity.* C. Bouchard (Ed.), Boca Raton, FL, CRC Press, 1994.

21. Bouchard, C., and Perusse, L.: Heredity and body fat. *Ann. Rev. Nutr.,* 8:259, 1988.

22. Bouchard, C., et al.: Inheritance of the amount and distribution of human body fat. *Int. J. Obes.,* 12:205, 1988.

23. Bouchard, C., et al.: Long-term exercise training with constant energy intake. 1: Effect on body composition and selected metabolic variables. *Int. J. Obesity,* 14:57, 1990.

24. Bouchard, C., et al.: The response to long term feeding in identical twins. *N. Engl. J. Med.,* 322:1477, 1990.

24a. Bouchard, C., et al.: The response to exercise with constant energy intake in identical twins. *Obes. Res.,* 2:400, 1994.

24b. Bouchard, C., et al.: Aims, design, and measurement protocol. *Med. Sci. Sports Exerc.,* 27:721, 1995.

25. Bray, G.A.: Effects of obesity on health and happiness. In *Handbook of Eating Disorders.* K.D. Brownell and J.B. Foreyt (Eds.), New York, Basic Books, 1986.

26. Brehm, B.A., and Gutin, B.: Recovery energy expenditure for steady state exercise in runners and nonexercisers. *Med. Sci. Sports Exerc.,* 18:205, 1986.

27. Brook, C.G.D., and Lloyd, J.K.: Adipose cell size and glucose tolerance in obese children and effects of diet. *Arch. Dis. Child.,* 48:301, 1973.

28. Brownell, K.D., and Kaye, K.S.: A school-based behavioral modification, nutrition education, and physical activity program for obese children. *Am. J. Clin. Nutr.,* 35:277, 1982.

29. Brownell, K.D., et al.: Evaluation and modification of exercise patterns in the natural envronment. *Am. J. Psychol.,* 137:12, 1980.

30. Brownell, K.D., et al.: The effects of repeated cycles of weight loss and regain in rats. *Physiol. Behav.,* 38:459, 1986.

31. Brownell, K.D., et al.: Understanding and preventing relapse. *Am. J. Psychol.,* 41:765, 1986

32. Calles-Escandón, J., et al.: Basal fat oxidation decreases with aging in women. *J. Appl. Physiol.,* 78:266, 1995.

33. Carpenter, W.H., et al.: Total energy expenditure in 4 to 6 year old children. *Am. J. Physiol.,* 27:E706, 1993.

34. Colditz, G.A.: Economic costs of obesity. *Am. J. Clin. Nutr,* 55:503S, 1992.

34a. Conway, J.M., et al.: Visceral adipose tissue differences in black and white women. *Am. J. Clin. Nutr.,* 61:765, 1995.

35. Craig, L.S., and Bayer, L.M.: Androgynic phenotypes in obese women. *Am. J. Phys. Anthrop.,* 26:23, 1967.

36. Dearborn, W.F., et al.: Data on the growth of public school children (from the materials of the Harvard Growth Study). *Monogr. Soc. Res. Child Dev.,* # (1), 1938.

36a. deBruin, N.C., et al.: Quantitative assessment of infant body fat by anthropometry and total-body electrical conductivity. *Am. J. Clin. Nutr.,* 61:279, 1995.

37. Dengel, D.R., et al.: Comparable effects of diet and exercise on body composition and lipoproteins in older men. *Med. Sci. Sports Exerc.,* 26:1307, 1994.

38. Dengel, D.R., et al.: Effects of weight loss by diet alone or combined with aerobic exercise on body composition in older obese men. *Metabolism,* 43:867, 1994.

39. Després, J-P.: Physical activity and adipose tissue. In *Physical Activity, Fitness, and Health.* C. Bouchard et al. (Eds.), Champaign, Ill., Human Kinetics, 1994.

40. Després, J-P., et al.: Regional distribution of body fat, plasma lipoproteins, and cardiovascular disease. *Atherosclerosis,* 10:497, 1990.

41. Després, J-P., et al.: Loss of abdominal fat and metabolic response to exercise training in obese women. *Am. J. Physiol.,* 261:E159, 1991.

42. DiPietro, L.: Physical activity, body weight, and adiposity: an epidemiologic perspective. *Exerc. Sport Sci. Rev.*, 23:275, 1995.

43. Donohoe, C.T., Jr., et al.: Metabolic consequences of dieting and exercise in the treatment of obesity. *J. Consult. Clin. Psychol.*, 52:829, 1984.

44. Elliot, D.L., et al.: Sustained depression of the resting metabolic rate after massive weight loss. *Am. J. Clin. Nutr.*, 49:93, 1989.

45. Emery, E.M., et al.: A review of the association between abdominal fat distribution, health outcome measures, and modifiable risk factors. *Am. J. Health Promotion*, 7:342, 1993.

46. Epstein, L.H., and Wing, R.R.: Aerobic exercise and weight. *Addictive Behaviors*, 5:371, 1980.

47. Felson, D.T., et al.: Weight loss reduces the risk for symptomatic knee osteoarthritis in women: the Framingham study. *Ann. Intern. Med.*, 116:535, 1992.

48. Folsom, R., et al.: Body fat distribution and 5-year risk of death in older women. *JAMA*, 269:483, 1993.

49. Forbes, G.B., et al.: Genetic factors in abdominal obesity, a risk factor for stroke. *N. Engl. J. Med.*, 318:1070, 1988.

50. French, S.A., et al.: Predictors of weight change over two years among a population of working adults: the Healthy Worker Project. *Int. J. Obes.*, 18:145, 1994.

51. Garn, S.M.: Continuities and changes in fatness from infancy through adulthood. *Curr. Probl. Pediatr.*, 15:1, 1985.

52. Gwinup, G., et al.: Thickness of subcutaneous fat and activity of underlying muscles. *Ann. Intern. Med*, 74:408, 1971.

53. Hagar, A., et al.: Adipose tissue cellularity in obese school girls before and after dietary treatment. *Am. J. Clin. Nutr.*, 31:68, 1978.

53a. Halaas, J.L., et al.: Weight-reducing effects of the plasma protein encoded by the *obese* gene. *Science*, 269:543, 1995.

54. Hampton, M.C., et al.: Caloric and nutrient intake of teenagers. *J. Am. Diet. Assoc.*, 50:385, 1987.

55. Heath, G.W., et al.: A physiological comparison of younger and older endurance-trained athletes. *J. Appl. Physiol.*, 51:634, 1981.

56. Hill, J.O., et al.: Effects of exercise and food restriction on body composition and metabolic rates in obese women. *Am. J. Clin. Nutr.*, 46:622, 1987.

57. Hill, J.O., et al.: Evaluation of an alternating-calorie diet with and without exercise in the treatment of obesity. *Am. J. Clin. Nutr.*, 50:248, 1989.

58. Hill, J.O., et al.: Exercise and moderate obesity. In *Physical Activity, Fitness, and Health*. C. Bouchard et al. (Eds.), Champaign, Ill., Human Kinetics, 1994.

59. Hirsch, J., and Batchelor, B.R.: Adipose tissue cellularity in human obesity. *Clin. Endocrinol. Metab.*, 5:299, 1976.

60. Hirsch, J., and Knittle, J.: Cellularity of obese and non-obese human adipose tissue. *Fed. Prod.*, 29:1518, 1970.

61. Hirsch, J., and Leibel, R.L.: New light on obesity. *N. Engl. J. Med.*, 318:509, 1988.

62. Hovell, M.F., et al.: Long term weight loss maintenance: assessment of behavioral and supplemental fasting regimen. *Am. J. Public Health*, 78:663, 1988.

63. Hubert, H.B., et al.: Obesity as an independent risk factor for cardiovascular disease: a 26-year follow-up of participants in the Framingham Heart Study. *Circulation*, 67:968, 1983.

63a. Iribarren, C., et al.: Association of weight loss and weight fluctuation with mortality among Japanese American men. *N. Engl. J. Med.*, 333:686, 1995.

64. Jeffrey, R., et al.: Weight cycling and cardiovascular risk factors in obese men and women. *Am. J. Clin. Nutr.*, 55:641, 1992.

65. Johnson, M.L., et al.: Relative importance of inactivity and overeating in energy balance in obese high school girls. *Am. J. Clin. Nutr.*, 44:779, 1986.

66. Katch, F.I., et al.: Effects of situp exercise training on adipose cell size and adiposity. *Res. Q. Exerc. Sport*, 55:242, 1984.

66a. Katzel, L.I., et al.: Effects of weight loss vs aerobic exercise training for coronary disease in healthy, obese, middle-aged and older men. *JAMA*, 274:1915, 1995.

67. Keim, N.L., et al.: The effect of exercise on energy intake and body composition in the overweight. *Int. J. Obes.*, 14:335, 1990.

68. Kern, P.A., et al.: The effects of weight loss on the activity and expression of adipose-tissue lipoprotein lipase in very obese humans. *N. Engl. J. Med.*, 322:1053, 1990.

69. Kessey, R.E.: A set-point theory of obesity. In *Handbook of Eating Disorders*. K.D. Brownell and J.P. Foreyt (Eds.), New York, Basic Books, 1986.

70. King, A.C., and Katch, F.I.: Changes in body density, fatfolds and girths at 2.3 kg increments of weight loss. *Hum. Biol.*, 58:708, 1986.

71. Knittle, J., and Hirsch, J.: Effect of early nutrition on the development of rat epididymal fat pads; cellularity and metabolism. *J. Clin. Invest.*, 47:2901, 1968.

72. Kohrt, W.M., et al.: Body composition of healthy sedentary and trained, young and older men and women. *Med. Sci. Sports Exerc.*, 24:832, 1992.

73. Kohrt, W.M., et al.: Exercise training improves fat distribution patterns in 60- to 70-year-old men and women. *J. Gerontol.*, 47:M99, 1992.

74. Kramer, M.S.: Do breast feeding and delayed introduction to solid food protect against subsequent obesity? *J. Pediatrics*, 98:883, 1981.

75. Krieger, D.R., and Landsberg, L.: Role of hormones in the etiology and pathogenesis of obesity. In *Obesity and Weight Control*. R.T. Frankel and M-U. Yang (Eds.), Rockville, Md., Aspen, 1988.

76. Krotkiewski, M., et al.: The effect of unilateral isokinetic strength training on local adipose and muscle tissue morphology, thickness and enzymes. *Eur. J. Appl. Physiol.*, 22:221, 1979.

77. Krotkiewski, M., et al.: Increased muscle dynamic endurance associated with weight reduction on a very-low-calorie diet. *Am. J. Clin. Nutr.*, 51:321, 1990.

78. Kuczmarski, R.J., et al.: Increasing prevalence of overweight among US adults. *JAMA*, 272:205, 1994.

79. Lee, I-M., and Paffenbarger, R.S., Jr.: Changes in body weight and longevity. *JAMA*, 268:2045, 1992.

80. Lee, I-M., et al.: Body weight and mortality. *JAMA*, 270:2823, 1993.

81. Leibel, R.L, et al.: Changes in energy expenditure resulting from altered body weight. *N. Engl. J. Med.*, 332:621, 1995.

82. Leon, A.S., et al.: Effects of a vigorous walking program on body composition, and carbohydrate and lipid metabolism of obese young men. *Am. J. Clin. Nutr.*, 32:1776, 1979.

83. Lewis, S.B., et al.: Effect of a diet's composition on metabolic adaptations to hypocaloric nutrition: comparison of high carbohydrate and high fat isocaloric diets. *Am. J. Clin. Nutr.*, 30:160, 1977.

84. Lissner, L., et al.: Variability of body weight and health outcomes in the Framingham population. *N. Engl. J. Med.*, 324:1839, 1991.

85. Manson, J.E., et al.: A prospective study of obesity and risk of coronary heart disease in women. *N. Engl. J. Med.*, 322:822, 1990.

85a. Manson, J.E., et al.: Body weight and mortality among women. *N. Engl. J. Med.*, 333:677, 1995.

86. McArdle, W.D., and Toner, M.M.: Application of exercise for weight control: the exercise prescription. In *Obesity and Weight Control*. R.T. Frankle and M-U. Yang (Eds.), Rockville, Md., Aspen, 1988.

87. Melby, C.L., et al.: Diet-induced weight loss and metabolic changes in obese women with high versus low prior weight loss/regain. *Nutr. Res.*, 11:971, 1991.

88. Meredith, C.N., et al.: Body composition and aerobic capacity in young and middle-aged endurance-trained men. *Med. Sci. Sports Exerc.*, 19:557, 1987.

89. Milesis, C.A., et al.: Effects of different durations of physical training on cardiorespiratory function, body composition and serum lipids. *Res. Q.*, 47:716, 1976.

90. Miller, W.C.: Diet composition, energy intake, and nutritional status in relation to obesity in men and women. *Med. Sci. Sports Exerc.*, 234:280, 1991.

91. Molé, P.A., et al.: Exercise reverses depressed metabolic rate produced by severe caloric restriction. *Med. Sci. Sports Exerc.*, 21:29, 1989.

92. Moore, L.L., et al.: Influence of parent's physical activity levels on young children. *J. Pediatr.*, 118:215, 1991.

93. Must, V., et al.: Long-term morbidity and mortality of overweight adolescents. *N. Engl. J. Med.*, 327:1350, 1992.

94. National Institutes of Health: *Health Implications of Obesity*, NIH Consensus Development Conference Statement, Vol. 5, No. 9. U.S. Government Printing Office, 1985.

95. National Task Force on the Prevention and Treatment of Obesity: Weight cycling. *JAMA*, 272:1196, 1994.

96. Noland, M., and Kearney, J.T.: Anthropometric and densitometric responses of women to specific and general exercise. *Res. Q.*, 49:322, 1978.

97. Olle, M.M., et al.: Body composition of sedentary and physically active spinal cord individuals estimated from total body electrical conductivity. *Arch. Phys. Med. & Rehab.*, 74:707, 1993.

98. Oscai, L., et al.: Effects of exercise and of food restriction on adipose tissue cellularity. *J. Lipid Res.*, 13:588, 1972.

99. Oscai, L., et al.: Exercise or food restriction: effect on adipose tissue cellularity. *Am. J. Physiol.*, 227:901, 1974.

100. Ostlund, R.E., et al.: The ratio of waist-to-hip circumference, plasma insulin level, and glucose intolerance as independent predictors of the HDL_2 cholesterol level in older adults. *N. Engl. J. Med.*, 332:229, 1990.

101. Pavlou, K.N., et al.: The effects of dieting and exercise on lean body mass, oxygen uptake, and strength. *Med. Sci. Sports Exerc.*, 17:446, 1985.

102. Pavlou, K.N., et al.: Exercise as an adjunct to weight loss and maintenance in moderately obese subjects. *Am. J. Clin. Nutr.*, 49:1115, 1989.

102a. Pellymounter, M.A., et al.: Effects of the *obese* gene product on body weight reduction in ob/ob mice. *Science*, 269:540, 1995.

103. Pi-Sunyer, F.X.: Medical hazards of obesity. *Ann. Intern. Med.*, 119:655, 1993.

104. Pi-Sunyer, F.X.: Obesity. In *Modern Nutrition in Health and Disease*. M.E. Shils et al. (Eds.), Philadelphia, Lea & Febiger, 1994.

105. Poehlman, E.T., et al.: The impact of exercise and diet restriction on daily energy expenditure. *Sports Med.*, 11:78, 1991.

106. Pollock, M.L., et al.: Effects of mode of training on cardiovascular function and body composition of adult men. *Med. Sci. Sports*, 7:139, 1975.

107. Prentice, A.M., et al.: Physiological responses to slimming. *Proc. Nutr. Soc.*, 50:441, 1991.

108. Prentice, A.M., et al.: Effects of weight cycling on body composition. *Am. J. Clin. Nutr.*, 56:209S, 1992.

109. Public Health Service: *Healthy People 2000: National Health Promotion and Disease Prevention Objectives*. Publication PHS 90-50212, Washington D.C., U.S. Dept. of Health and Human Services, 1990.

109a. Racette, S.B., et al.: Effects of aerobic exercise and dietary carbohydrate on energy expenditure and body composition during weight reduction in obese women. *Am. J. Clin. Nutr.*, 61:486, 1995.

110. Ravussin, E., et al.: Reduced rate of energy expenditure as a risk factor for body-weight gain. *N. Engl. J. Med.*, 318:467, 1988.

111. Rebuffé-Scrive, M., et al.: Metabolism of adipose tissue in intraabdominal depots in severely obese men and women. *Metabolism*, 39:1021, 1990.

112. Riviére, D., et al.: Lipolytic response of fat cells to catecholamines in sedentary and exercise trained women. *J. Appl. Physiol.*, 66:330, 1989.

113. Roberts, S.B., et al.: Energy expenditure and intake in infants born to lean and overweight mothers. *N. Engl. J. Med.*, 318:461, 1988.

114. Rolland-Cachera, M.F., and Bellisle, F.: No correlation between adiposity and food intake: why are working class children fatter? *Am. J. Clin. Nutr.*, 44:779, 1986.

115. Ross, J.G., and Pate, R.R.: The National Children and Youth Fitness Study. II: a summary of findings. *JOPERD*, 58:51, 1987.

116. Rossi, M., et al.: Cardiac autonomic dysfunction in obese subjects. *Clin. Sci.*, 76:567, 1989.

117. Rossner, S., and Hallberg, D.: Serum lipoproteins in massive obesity. *Acta Med. Scand.*, 204:103, 1978.

118. Salans, L.B., et al.: Experimental obesity in man: cellular character of the adipose tissue. *J. Clin. Invest.*, 50:1005, 1971.

119. Schapira, D.V., et al.: Upper-body fat distribution and endometrial cancer risk. *JAMA*, 266:1808, 1992.

120. Schutz, Y., et al.: Role of fat oxidation in the long-term stabilization of body weight in obese women. *Am. J. Clin. Nutr.*, 55:670, 1992.

121. Schwartz, R.S., et al.: The effect of intensive endurance exercise training on body fat distribution in young and older men. *Metabolism*, 40:545, 1991.

122. Segal, K.R., et al.: Body composition, not body weight, is related to cardiovascular disease risk factors and sex hormone levels in man. *J. Clin. Invest.*, 80:1050, 1987.

123. Shapira, D.V., et al.: Abdominal obesity and breast cancer risk. *Ann. Intern. Med.*, 112:182, 1990.

123a. Simoneau, J-A., and Bouchard, C.: Skeletal muscle metabolism and body fat content in men and women. *Obes. Res.*, 3:23, 1995.

124. Simopoulos, A.P.: Obesity and carcinogenesis: historical perspective. *Am. J. Clin. Nutr.*, 45:271, 1987.

125. Sims, E.A.H., and Danforth, E., Jr.: Expenditure and storage of energy in man (perspective). *J. Clin. Invest.*, 79:1019, 1987.

126. Sims, E.A.H., and Horton, E.S.: Endocrine and metabolic adaptation to obesity and starvation. *Am. J. Clin. Nutr.*, 21:1455, 1968.

127. Slyper, A.H., et al.: Low-density lipoprotein and atherosclerosis. *JAMA*, 272:305, 1994.

128. Spitzer, L., and Rodin, J.: Human eating behavior: A critical review of studies in normal weight and overweight individuals. *Appetite*, 2:293, 1981.

129. Stamler, R., et al.: Weight and blood pressure. Findings in hypertension screening of 1 million Americans. *JAMA*, 240:1607, 1978.

130. Staten, M.A.: The effect of exercise on food intake in men and women. *Am. J. Clin. Nutr.*, 53:27, 1991.

131. Steen, S.N., and Brownell, K.D.: Patterns of weight loss and regain in wrestlers: has the tradition changed? *Med. Sci. Sports Exerc.*, 22:762, 1990.

132. Stefanick, M.L.: Exercise and weight control. *Exerc. Sport Sci. Rev.*, 21:363, 1993.

133. Stern, J.S., et al.: Pancreatic insulin release and peripheral tissue resistance in Zucker obese rats fed high and low carbohydrate diets. *Am. J. Physiol.*, 228:543, 1975.

134. Stunkard, A.J.: An adoption study of human obesity. *N. Engl. J. Med.*, 314:193, 1986.

135. Sweeney, M.E., et al.: Severe vs moderate energy restriction with and without exercise in the treatment of obesity: efficiency of weight loss. *Am. J. Clin Nutr.*, 57:127, 1993.

136. Tanaka, K., et al.: Assessment of exercise-induced alterations in body composition of patients with coronary heart disease. *Eur. J. Appl. Physiol.*, 66:323, 1993.

137. Technology Assessment Conference Panel: Methods for voluntary weight loss and control. Technology Assessment Conference statement, *Ann. Intern. Med.*, 116:942, 1992.

138. Terry, R.B., et al.: Contributions of regional adipose tissue depots to plasma lipoprotein concentrations in overweight men and women: possible protective effects of thigh fat. *Metabolism*, 40:733, 1991.

139. Thompson, D.A., et al.: Acute effects of exercise intensity on appetite in young men. *Med. Sci. Sports Exerc.*, 20:227, 1988.

140. Thornton, J.S.: Feast or famine: eating disorders in athletes. *Phys. Sportsmed.,* 18:116, 1990.

141. Trembly, A., et al.: The effect of exercise training on resting metabolic rate in lean and moderately obese individuals. *Int. J. Obesity,* 10:511, 1986.

142. Trembly, A., et al.: Exercise training with constant energy intake. 2: Effect on glucose metabolism and resting energy expenditure. *Int. J. Obesity,* 14:75, 1990.

143. Udall, J.G., et al.: Interaction of maternal and neonatal obesity. *Pediatrics,* 62:17, 1978.

144. U.S. Centers for Disease Control: *Morbidity and Mortality Weekly Report,* 41:33, 1992.

145. Vaccaro, P., et al.: Body composition and physiological responses of Masters female swimmers 20 to 70 years of age. *Res. Q. Exerc. Sport,* 55:278, 1984.

146. Vague, J., et al.: The various forms of obesity. *Triangle. Sandoz J. Med. Sci.,* 13:41, 1974.

147. Van Itallie, T.B.: Health implications of overweight and obesity in the United States. *Ann. Intern. Med.,* 103:983, 1985.

148. VanDale, D., and Saris, W.H.M.: Repetitive weight loss and weight regain: effects on weight reduction, resting metabolic rate, and lipolytic activity before and after exercise and/or diet treatment. *Am. J. Clin. Nutr.,* 49:409, 1989.

149. Wadden, T.A.: Very low calorie diets: their efficacy, safety, and future. *Ann. Intern. Med.,* 99:675, 1983.

149a. Wadden, T.A.: Characteristics of successful weight loss maintenance. In *Obesity Treatment: Establishing Goals, Improving Outcomes, and Establishing the Research Agenda.* F.X. PiSunyer and D.B. Allison (Eds.), New York, Plenum Press, 1995.

150. Wadden, T.A., et al.: Less food, less hunger: reports of appetite and symptoms in a controlled study of a protein-sparing modified fast. *Int. J. Obesity,* 11:239, 1987.

151. Wahrenberg, H., et al.: Adrenergic regulation of lipolysis in human fat cells during exercise. *Eur. J. Clin. Invest.,* 21:534, 1991.

152. Warner, W.W.: The obese patient and anesthesia. *JAMA,* 205:102, 1968.

153. Weisinger, J.R., et al.: The nephrotic syndrome: a complication of massive obesity. *Ann. Intern. Med.,* 50:233, 1974.

154. Welle, S.L.: Some metabolic effects of overeating in man. *Am. J. Clin. Nutr.,* 44:718, 1986.

155. Willett, W.C., et al.: Weight, weight change, and coronary heart disease in women: risk within the "normal" weight range. *JAMA,* 273:461, 1995.

156. Williams, D.P., et al.: Body fatness and risk for elevated blood pressure, total cholesterol, and serum lipoprotein ratios in children and adolescents. *Am. J. Public Health,* 82:358, 1992.

157. Wing, R.R.: Weight cycling in humans: a review of the literature. *Ann. Behav. Med.,* 14:113, 1992.

158. Zhang, Y., et al.: Positional cloning of the mouse *obese* gene and its human homologue. *Nature,* 372:425, 1994.

Morris, J.N., et al. Coronary heart-disease and physical activity of work. *Lancet*, 265: 1053, 1953.

In the 1940s and 1950s, the epidemiology of coronary heart disease (CHD) did not include vigorous physical activity as a possible means of protection from early development of the disease. Morris and colleagues demonstrated an impressive link between higher levels of physical activity in specialized occupations and lower incidence of CHD. The researchers compiled statistics on CHD incidence for two large groups. The first sample consisted of 31,000 men, aged 35 to 64 years, em-

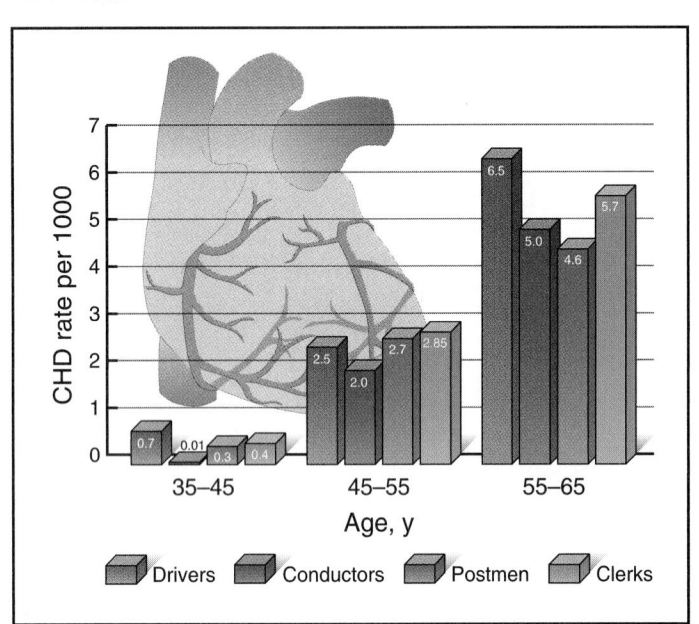

CHD incidence (rate per 1000) for drivers, conductors, postmen, and clerks. Note that within each age and job classification, the most active workers (conductors and postmen) had the lowest incidence of CHD.

ployed by the London Transport Authority. Job classifications included drivers and conductors of trams and trolley buses, and motormen and guards on the underground railway system. In these jobs, drivers and motormen were sedentary, while the conductors were physically active. The second sample included 110,000 postal workers and civil servants. The basic differences between these workers included the on-the-job physical require-

ments: the postmen were physically active delivering the mail, while civil servants (postal and telegraph officers, telephone operators, clerks) were sedentary in office jobs.

The figure shows the all-cause incidence (rate per 1000) for the first clinical episode of CHD determined from medical records that included angina pectoris, myocardial infarction, and death directly attributable to CHD. For the London Transport workers, 119 total CHD episodes (3.8% per 1000) occurred. In one-quarter of these episodes, death occurred within 3 days (34 of 119 cases); in 40%, death occurred within 3 months (49 of 119 cases). The pattern of CHD incidence differed between the conductors and the drivers: the drivers contracted the disease at a younger age than the conductors and had a higher total incidence (2.7 versus 1.9). The drivers had a rate of immediate mortality twice as high as that of the conductors. In contrast, angina occurred twice as frequently in the conductors (0.8 versus 0.4 per 1000). Overall, the conductors had less CHD than the drivers, and the disease appeared at a later age. Similarly to the transport workers, the total incidence of CHD and mortality for the physically active group of postmen was substantially less than for the sedentary group of clerks. The CHD incidence for postal workers and civil service clerks resembled that of the transport workers: the physically active group experienced less CHD that was less severe.

The researchers offered three possible explanations for the results. First, differences in "constitution" and physical activity preferences were such that the men "self-selected" themselves for the different jobs. Second, differences in the "mental strains" for the different jobs could affect CHD mortality. Third, the greater physical activity requirements of the job primarily caused the lower incidence of CHD. While all three explanations seemed plausible, the researchers hypothesized that differences in on-the-job physical effort provided protection against CHD. Cross-sectional and longitudinal research over the last 40 years confirms that increased physical activity confers a protective effect against CHD. In fact, a sedentary lifestyle now belongs to one of the four primary CHD risk factors along with cigarette smoking, hypertension, and hypercholesterolemia.

Physical Activity, Health, and Aging

Elderly persons represent the fastest growing segment of the American population; the average life expectancy for men and women is rapidly approaching 80 years. By the year 2020, approximately 20% of the population will be over 65 years of age, and approximately 1.3 million citizens will be 100 years or older by the year 2040. Despite this "graying" of America, evolution has not kept pace with automation, and humans have not adapted effectively to their sedentary lifestyles. Inadequate physical activity is responsible for approximately 30% of all deaths due to heart disease, colon cancer, and diabetes.[105] Beginning an active lifestyle could significantly reduce mortality from these ailments; the greatest benefits would be from strategies that get the population's most sedentary men and women into just light to moderate patterns of regular activity! Further good news is that at any age, behavioral changes such as becoming more physically active, quitting cigarette smoking, and controlling blood pressure act independently to delay all-cause mortality and extend life.[102] In this chapter, physical activity is explored as a health-related behavior with specific reference to aging and cardiovascular disease. Also presented are concepts about physical activity epidemiology and their application to health and longevity. A final section gives an overview of exercise stress testing and its role in formulating a prudent exercise prescription.

PART 1

PHYSICAL ACTIVITY IN THE POPULATION

PHYSICAL ACTIVITY EPIDEMIOLOGY

Epidemiology involves quantifying the various factors that determine the occurrence and patterns of diseases within a group. The ultimate goal is to generalize this information to a larger population to better understand, modify, or control a disease pattern or health problem.[82, 143] The specific field of **physical activity epidemiology** applies the general research strategies of epidemiology to study the association of physical activity as a health-related behavior with disease and other outcomes.[23]

TERMINOLOGY

Specific definitions are used in applications of physical activity epidemiology to characterize the behavioral patterns and outcomes of the groups under investigation. Examples of relevant terminology include the following:

- **Physical activity:** Any body movement produced by muscles that results in increased energy expenditure.
- **Exercise:** Physical activity that is planned, structured, repetitive, and purposeful.
- **Physical fitness:** A set of attributes that relate to one's ability to perform physical activity.
- **Health:** Physical, mental, and social well-being and not simply the absence of disease.
- **Health-related physical fitness:** Components of physical fitness that are associated with some aspect of good health and/or disease prevention (Fig. 30.1).[a]
- **Longevity:** Length of life.

Within this framework, physical activity is a generic term, of which exercise is the major component. Similarly, the definition of health focuses on the broad spectrum of well-being, which ranges from the complete absence of health (death) to the highest levels of physiological function. Although such definitions often challenge our ability to measure and quantify in an objective manner, they do offer the broad frame of reference to study the role of physical activity and exercise in health and disease.

[a]The trend in physical assessment during the past 20 years has been to deemphasize tests that stress motor performance and athletic fitness (i.e., tests of speed, power, balance, and agility). Focus is on those measures of fitness that assess functional capacity and reflect various aspects of overall good health and disease prevention.[13] The four components of health-related physical fitness most commonly evaluated are aerobic or cardiovascular fitness, body composition, abdominal muscular strength and endurance, and lower back and hamstring flexibility. An upper extremity measure of muscular strength also is often included in the fitness profile, although it is not related to health status in a direct way. A person's performance in each of these test items is not fixed: instead, status can be significantly improved through a program of regular exercise and weight control.

PARTICIPATION IN PHYSICAL ACTIVITY

More than 30 different methods have been used to assess physical activity, including direct and indirect calorimetry, self-reports and questionnaires, job classifications, survey procedures, physiological markers, behavioral observations, mechanical or electronic monitors, and dietary surveys. Each approach has unique advantages and disadvantages depending on the situation and the population studied. It has been difficult to obtain valid estimates of physical activity in large populations because such studies, by necessity, make use of self-reports of daily activity and exercise participation rather than direct monitoring or measurement.

The current status of participation in physical activity by adult Americans is not encouraging. According to data from the United States National Center for Health Statistics on the physical activity of noninstitutionalized adults aged 18 years and older, only 8.1% of men and 7.0% of women reported that they engaged in vigorous exercise on a regular basis. Regular but less intense activity was performed by 36.2% of the men and 31.5% of the women, indicating that only 44.3% men and 38.5% of women engage in some regular physical activity; the remaining 60% of American adults were completely sedentary.[24] A more recent analysis of self-reported leisure-time physical activity showed that 58.1% of adults reported irregular or no leisure-time physical activity; the percentage of adults who regularly exercised or played sports decreased significantly over a 5-year span among black, Hispanic, lower-income, and unemployed persons.[25]

The findings for exercise participation of more than 15,000 adults enrolled in exercise programs that included a variety of aerobic and muscle-strengthening activities are illustrated in Figure 30.2.[16] Participants' ages ranged from 19 to 64 years; subjects were placed into five age categories. A progressive decline occurred for participating in fitness activities with increasing age. A small percentage of each group exercised regularly; the smallest percentage of vigorous exercisers was among older individuals. A report complementing such discouraging findings revealed that only 14% of American adults expended more than 1,600 kcal per week in leisure-time physical activities and only 10% participated regularly in vigorous activities.[17]

At best, no more than 20% and possibly less than 10% of the adults in the United States (as well as in Australia, Canada, England) obtain sufficient regular physical activity of an intensity to impart discernible health and fitness benefits. Clearly, a real need to improve the physical activity profile of the population exists. With this in mind, the Public Health Service established *Healthy People 2000* objectives, which were designed to improve Americans' health status by reducing preventable death,

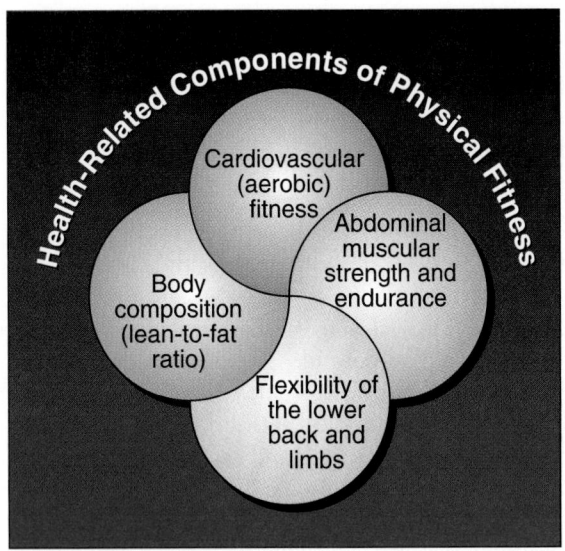

FIGURE 30.1
Health-related components of physical fitness.

FIGURE 30.2
Percentage of adults in the United States (grouped by age) who participate in fitness activities. (Courtesy of C. Brooks, Department of Sports Management and Communication, University of Michigan, Ann Arbor.)

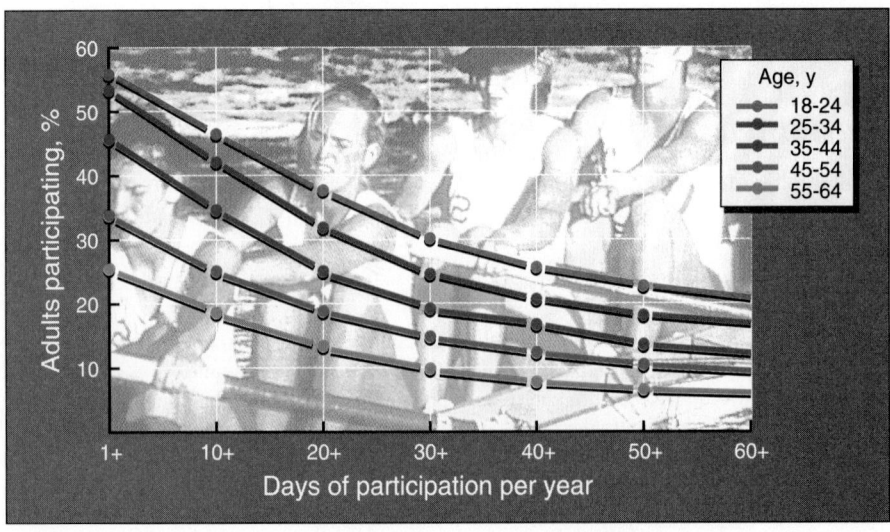

disability, and disease.[23a, 107] One of the important objectives focused on more involvement from individuals currently getting low to moderate levels of physical activity, with additional emphasis on development of muscular strength and flexibility.

IS EXERCISING SAFE?

The question of exercise safety was raised largely because of several well-publicized reports of sudden death during exercise.[80, 132, 144] In actuality, this rate has declined over the past 25 years despite an overall increase in exercise participation. In one report of cardiovascular episodes during 65 months, 2,935 exercisers recorded 374,798 hours of exercise that included 2,726,272 km of running and walking. There were no deaths during this time and only two nonfatal cardiovascular complications. This amounted to two complications per 100,000 hours of exercise for women and three complications for men. Although heavy physical exertion provides a small risk of sudden death during the activity (compared to resting for an equivalent time), especially for sedentary people, the longer-term health benefits of regular exercise far outweigh any potential for acute cardiovascular complications.[53, 95, 128a] Furthermore, considerably less risk of death exists during exercise among people who are regularly physically active.[132] The likelihood of an exercise catastrophe (e.g., cerebrovascular accident, aortic dissection and rupture, lethal arrhythmias, myocardial infarction) increases under the following conditions:[45, 150a]

- Family history of sudden death at young age.
- History of fainting or chest pain with exercise.
- Unaccustomed vigorous exercise.
- Exercise performed with accompanying psychological stress.

- Extremes of environmental temperature.
- Exercise involving a significant straining or static muscle action component.
- Exercising during viral infection or when not feeling well.

Perhaps not surprisingly, the most prevalent exercise complications are musculoskeletal in nature. In a longitudinal study of aerobic dance injuries in 351 participants and 60 instructors, 327 medical complaints were reported during nearly 30,000 hours of activity.[56] Only 84 of the injuries resulted in disability (2.8 per 1,000 person hours of participation), and only 2.1% of the injuries required medical attention. Age does not appear to affect the occurrence of orthopedic problems for exercise considered moderate in intensity and duration.[88] For running activities, the greatest orthopedic injury potential occurs in individuals who exercise for extended periods. In this regard, more certainly is not better.

One of the recurring themes in physical activity epidemiology includes the impact and interaction of aging and regular exercise on physical fitness, health risk, and actual disease, particularly cardiovascular disease. These interrelationships are explored in the sections that follow.

PART 2
AGING AND PHYSIOLOGIC FUNCTION

AGE TRENDS

As shown in Figure 30.3, physiologic and performance measures generally improve rapidly during childhood and reach a maximum between the late teens and 30 years

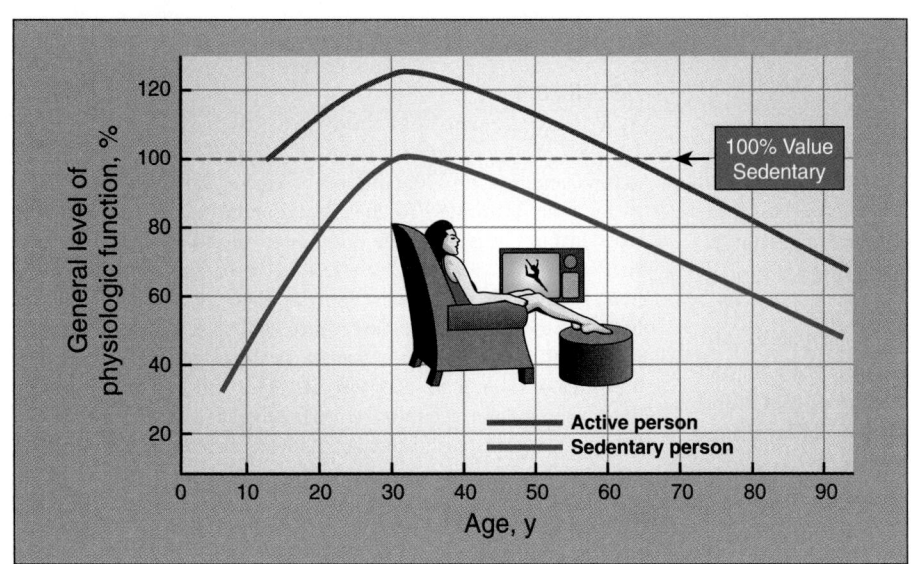

FIGURE 30.3
Generalized curve to illustrate changes in physiologic function with age. All of the comparisons are made against the 100% value achieved by the typical 20- to 30-year-old sedentary person.

of age. Functional capacity then declines with age; deterioration often varies widely at a particular age according to lifestyle characteristics.[68, 69] Although all physiologic measures generally do decline with age, not all decline at the same rate. Nerve conduction velocity, for example, declines only 10 to 15% from 30 to 80 years of age, whereas maximum breathing capacity at age 80 is approximately 40% that of a 30-year-old individual. In addition, some functions, such as heart rate, which shows very little if any aging effect at rest, usually show an appreciable decrement during maximal exercise. Furthermore, typical "aging effects" are greatly influenced by regular exercise. Aerobic capacity among the physically active, for example, is approximately 25% higher in each age category, so that an active 50-year-old man or woman often maintains the functional level of a 20-year-old. Because long-term exercise studies on the same subjects are scarce, the precise extent to which regular exercise participation alters the actual rate of decline in physiologic function or "overrides" deterioration in function truly due to aging is unknown. What is known is that there is an alarmingly large number of older men and women with such poor functional capacity that they cannot engage in relatively simple physical tasks or practice necessary personal hygiene skills without assistance.

Some Differences in Exercise Physiology Between Children and Adults. Some distinct differences between children and adults should be considered when evaluating the physiological and exercise performance responses of boys and girls.

- During weight-bearing exercise such as walking and running, the oxygen uptake of children ($mL \cdot kg^{-1} \cdot min^{-1}$) is 10 to 30% higher than adults at a designated submaximal pace. This lower economy, perhaps due to the shorter stride length and greater stride frequency of children, makes a standard walking or running pace physiologically more stressful (and performance scores poorer) for children than adults. This will be the case even though children generally have equal or somewhat higher aerobic capacities than adults.
- Because of their smaller body mass, children have lower absolute values ($L \cdot min^{-1}$) for aerobic capacity than adults (Fig. 30.4). Therefore, children will be disadvantaged when exercising against a standard external resistance that is not adjusted for body size (e.g., stationary cycling, arm cranking). This is because the fixed oxygen cost ($L \cdot min^{-1}$) of the exercise represents a greater percentage of the child's smaller absolute aerobic capacity. During weight-bearing exercise, on the other hand, energy cost directly relates to body mass so children are not disadvantaged by their smaller body size.
- Children do less well than adults on sprint tests of anaerobic power capacity. This is perhaps due to their inability to generate a high level of blood lactate (a marker for the glycolytic process) during exhaustive exercise. Also, their significantly lower intramuscular levels of the glycolytic enzyme phosphofructokinase compared to adults may contribute to their poorer anaerobic capacity.
- During submaximal exercise, children tend to breathe more (greater ventilatory equivalent) than adults at any level of oxygen uptake.
- Children, like adults, can adapt and significantly increase their muscle strength in response to resistance training. Unlike pubescent children and adults, however, prepubescent children have greater difficulty increasing muscle mass. This is probably due to the relatively low androgen levels in this age group.

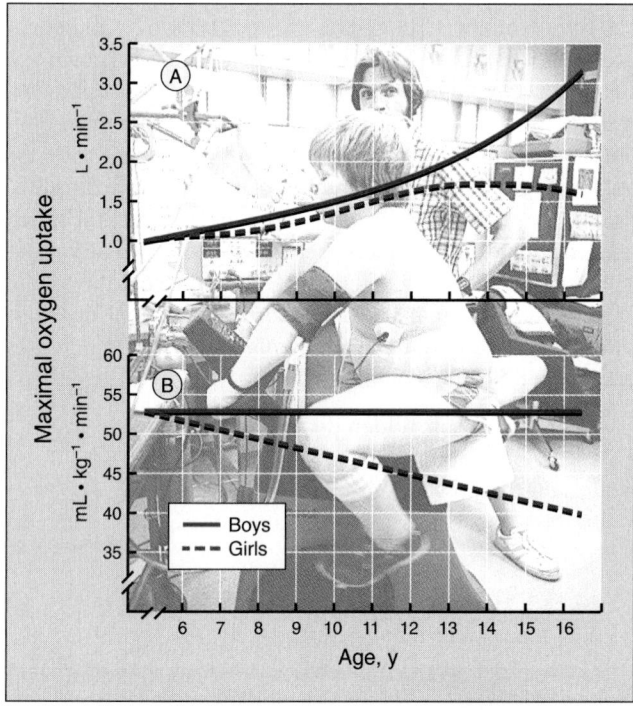

FIGURE 30.4

A, $\dot{V}O_2max$ ($L \cdot min^{-1}$) for boys and girls is similar until about 12 years of age; at age 14, $\dot{V}O_2max$ is approximately 25% higher in boys, and by age 16, the difference exceeds 50%. This difference is generally attributed to the development of a greater muscle mass in boys as well as sex differences in daily physical activity. **B,** For boys, $\dot{V}O_2max$ ($mL \cdot kg^{-1} \cdot min^{-1}$) remains level at approximately 52 ($mL \cdot kg^{-1} \cdot min^{-1}$) from 6 to 16 years of age; for females, the line slopes downward with age, reaching approximately 40 $mL \cdot kg^{-1} \cdot min^{-1}$ at 16 years of age, a value that is 32% below their male counterparts. This difference is probably due to the greater accumulation of body fat in females; this extra fat must be transported but does not contribute to an enhanced capacity for aerobic metabolism. (From Krahenbuhl, G.S., et al.: Developmental aspects of maximal aerobic power in children. In *Exercise and Sport Sciences Reviews.* Vol. 13. Edited by R.L. Terjung. New York, Macmillan, 1985.)

MUSCULAR STRENGTH

The highest strength levels for men and women are generally reached between the ages of 20 and 30 years, at the time when muscle cross-sectional area is usually the largest. Thereafter, strength in most muscle groups declines and progresses slowly at first and then more rapidly after middle age. Strength loss among elderly individuals is directly associated with their limited mobility and physical performance, as well as to increases in the incidence of accidents suffered by those with muscle weakness and poor balance.[18, 153]

Decrease in Muscle Mass. Normally, motor unit remodeling is a continual and natural process involving motor endplate repair and reconstruction. This occurs by selective denervation of muscle fibers, which is then followed by terminal sprouting of axons from adjacent motor units. It is speculated that in old age this process gradually deteriorates and leads to a **denervation muscle atrophy** and an irreversible degeneration of muscle fibers and endplate structures, especially in the type II muscle fibers.[18, 20, 47, 59] This leads to a progressive reduction in muscle cross section.

A 40 to 50% reduction in muscle mass between 25 and 80 years of age, due to motor unit losses and muscle fiber atrophy, is the primary factor responsible for the age-associated reduction in the contractile strength of muscle, even among healthy, active men and women.[12, 18, 38, 87] As shown in Figure 30.5A, the loss of muscle fibers, both type I and type II, becomes particularly apparent at approximately age 60. The loss of muscle volume (Fig. 30.5B) also is due to a reduced fiber size, particularly the fast-twitch fibers in the muscles of the lower extremities.[4, 146] This results in a proportionate increase in the area occupied by the slow-twitch or type I muscle fibers.

Strength Trainability Among Elderly Individuals. *The decrease in skeletal muscle mass and strength that occurs with aging is the combined result of progressive neuromotor processes and a decrease in the daily level of muscle loading.*[86] In older men and women, exercise training, particularly resistance training, facilitates protein synthesis and retention and blunts the "normal" and somewhat inevitable loss of muscle mass and strength with aging.[27, 33, 109, 131, 156] This is aptly illustrated in a study of healthy men between the ages of 60 and 72 years who trained for 12 weeks with standard-resistance exercise at loads equivalent to 80% of their dynamic muscle strength capacity (1-RM).[55] As shown in Figure 30.6, muscle strength increased progressively throughout training. By week 12, knee flexion strength had increased by 107% and knee extension strength had increased by 227%. This rate of improvement of approximately 5% per training session was similar to increases reported for young adults. These dramatic strength improvements were also accompanied by a significant hypertrophy of the fast- and slow-twitch muscle fibers. In another group of 70-year-old individuals who had resistance trained since age

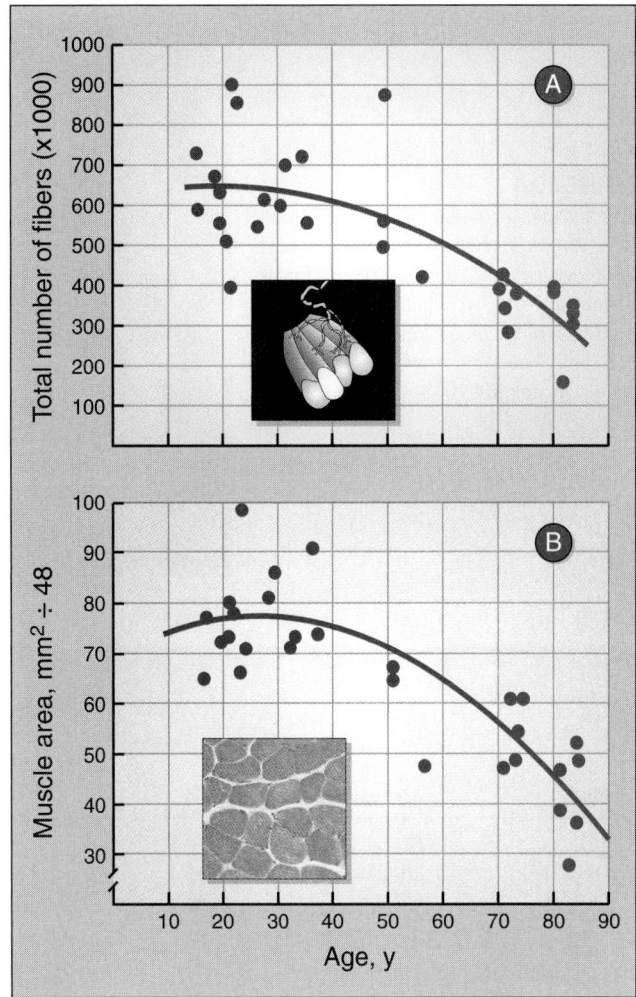

FIGURE 30.5

Relationship between age and **(A)** total number of muscle fibers and **(B)** muscle area. The reduction in muscle size begins at approximately 30 years of age, and by age 50, it is reduced by 10%. Thereafter, the decline in muscle area is more precipitous due largely to a decrease in the total number of muscle fibers. (From Lexell, J., et al.: What is the cause of the ageing atrophy? Total number, size, and proportion of different fiber types studied in whole vastus lateralis muscle from 15- to 83-year old men. *J. Neurol. Sci.*, 84:275, 1988.)

50, their muscle cross-sectional area and strength were equivalent to a group of 28-year-old students.[77] *Such findings clearly indicate an impressive plasticity in physiologic, structural, and performance characteristics among elderly individuals and that marked and rapid improvement can be achieved with vigorous training into the ninth decade of life.*[48] Improved muscle strength and overall fitness by regular exercise may also be the best way to reduce the incidence of orthopedic injury in older men and women.[107a, 115, 138]

Relevant literature on changes in muscle strength and size in older adults who participated in various programs of resistance training is summarized in Table 30.1. In most in-

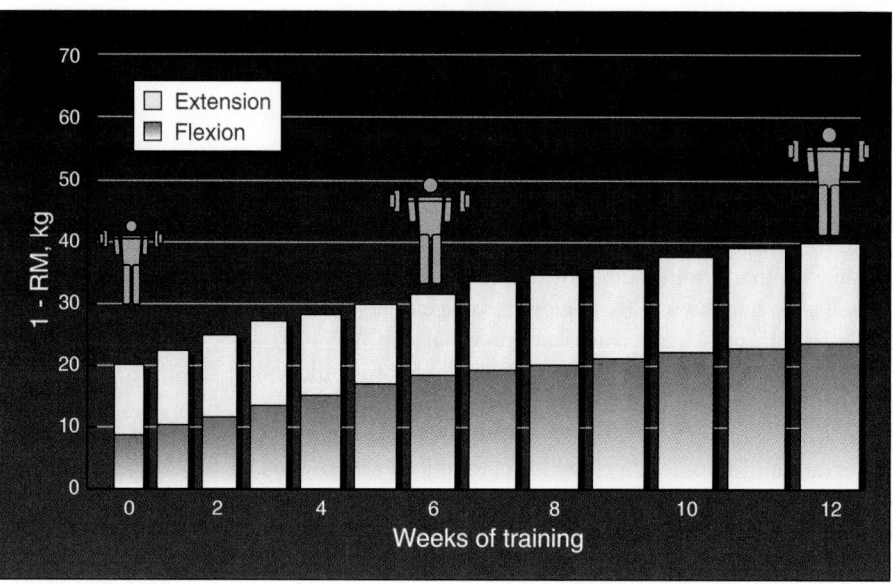

FIGURE 30.6

Weekly measurement of dynamic muscle strength (1-RM) of left knee extension (yellow) and flexion (red). (From Frontera, W.R., et al.: Strength conditioning in older men: skeletal muscle hypertrophy and improved function. *J. Appl. Physiol.*, 64:1038, 1988.)

TABLE 30.1
RESULTS FROM RESISTANCE TRAINING STUDIES IN OLDER INDIVIDUALS

Study	Age (y)	Sex	Training Type	Strength Gain (%)	Hypertrophy (%)
1	62–84	M + F	RT	57	NM
2	18–26	M	RT	30	9
	67–72	M	RT	22	NC
3	69–74	M	CT	9–22	NC
4	22–65	M	CT	3–8	19–20
5	63–84	F	RT	7–13	10
6	60–72	M	RT	9–19	9–12
1	62–84	M + F	Iso	45.8	NM
7	41–80	M	Iso	12–24	NM
8	20–26	F	Iso	95	NM
	65–73	F	Iso	72	NM
9	55–78	M + F	CV	1.9–13.4	NM
10	51–87	M	CV (6 wk)	6.4	NC
		M	CV (42 wk)	11.9	1.0
11	65	M + F	CV	5–13	NM
12	65	M	Hdr	15–132	NC

RT, resistance training; CT, circuit training; Iso, isometric training; CV, cardiovascular endurance training; Hdr, hydraulic resistance training; NC, no change; NM, not measured.

 1. Perkins, L.C., and Kaiser, H: *Phys. Ther. Rev.*, 41:633, 1961.
 2. Moritaini, T., and deVries, H.A.: *J. Gerontol.*, 35:672, 1980.
 3. Aniansson, A., and Gustafsson, E.: *Clin. Physiol.*, 1:87, 1981.
 4. Larsson, L.: *Med. Sci. Sports Exerc.*, 19:203, 1982.
 5. Aniansson, A., et al.: *Arch. Gerontol. Geriat.*, 3:229, 1984.
 6. Frontera, W.F., et al: *J. Appl. Physiol.*, 64:1038, 1988.
 7. Liemohm, W.P.: *Int. J. Aging Hum. Dev.*, 6:347, 1975.
 8. Kauffman, T.L.: *Arch. Phys. Med. Rehab.*, 66:223, 1985.
 9. Barry, A.J., et al.: *J. Gerontol.*, 21:192, 1966.
10. deVries, H.A.: *J. Gerontol.*, 25:325, 1970.
11. Sidney, L.H., et al.: *Am. J. Clin. Nutr.*, 30:326, 1977.
12. Becque, M.D.: Ph.D. Dissertation, University of Michigan, 1989.

stances, training responses were positive, and strength improvements ranged between 1.9 and 72% in individuals older than 60 years of age. Possible mechanisms to explain these often impressive training responses include the neural (motor unit recruitment and innervation pattern) and muscular (hypertrophy) factors previously discussed in Chapter 22. As in younger adults, the number of sets and repetitions and the intensity, duration, and frequency of training are crucial in determining strength adaptations in elderly individuals.

NEURAL FUNCTION

The cumulative effects of aging on central nervous system function are exhibited by a 37% decline in the number of spinal cord axons and a 10% decline in nerve conduction velocity.[8, 129] These changes may contribute to the age-related decrement in neuromuscular performance as assessed by both simple and complex reaction and movement times.[29, 135] When reaction time is partitioned into central processing time and muscle action time, it is the time required to detect a stimulus and process the information to produce the response that is affected most by the aging process. Because reflexes, such as the knee-jerk reflex, do not involve processing in the brain, they are less affected by aging than voluntary responses such as reaction and movement times.[30] As shown in Figure 30.7, movement times for simple and complex tasks were significantly slower for older subjects than for younger counterparts of the same level of daily activity. *In all instances, however, the active groups (whether young or old) moved significantly faster than a corresponding age group that was less physically active.* These observations suggest that an active lifestyle may positively affect neuromuscular functioning at any age. As with many other measures of physiologic function, older men who have remained active for 20 years or longer have reaction times that are equal to or faster than inactive men in their 20s.[136] It is tempting to speculate that the biologic aging of certain neuromuscular functions can be somewhat slowed by regular participation in physical activity.

PULMONARY FUNCTION

Both static and dynamic measures of lung function generally deteriorate with age. For example, there is a significant slowing of ventilation and gas exchange kinetics during the transition from rest to submaximal exercise.[6, 35] It is unknown whether regular exercise throughout one's lifetime can fully override this "aging" of pulmonary dynamics (or the uptake of oxygen by peripheral tissues). However, with aerobic training in elderly men, the kinetics of gas exchange were increased to a level that approached values reported in fit young adults.[5] Furthermore, older endurance-trained athletes have a greater pulmonary functional capacity than their sedentary peers. Values for vital capacity, total lung capacity, residual lung volume, maximum voluntary ventilation, $FEV_{1.0}$, and $FEV_{1.0}/FVC$ in athletes older than 60 years of age are consistently larger than expected based on their body size and significantly larger than those of sedentary, age-matched, healthy counterparts.[62] Such findings are encouraging because they indicate that a lifetime of regular physical activity may retard the decline in pulmonary function associated with aging.

CARDIOVASCULAR FUNCTION

Cardiovascular function and aerobic capacity are not immune from age-related effects.

Aerobic Capacity. Cross-sectional data indicate that the $\dot{V}O_2max$ declines between 0.4 and 0.5 mL · kg^{-1} (approximately 1%) each year in adults.[36, 69] Extrapolation of this average rate of decline reduces the aerobic capacity by age 100 to a level equivalent to the resting oxygen uptake.[12] This estimate may be somewhat severe because a clear difference exists in the age-related rate of decline in $\dot{V}O_2max$ between sedentary and active individuals.[117] Sedentary men and

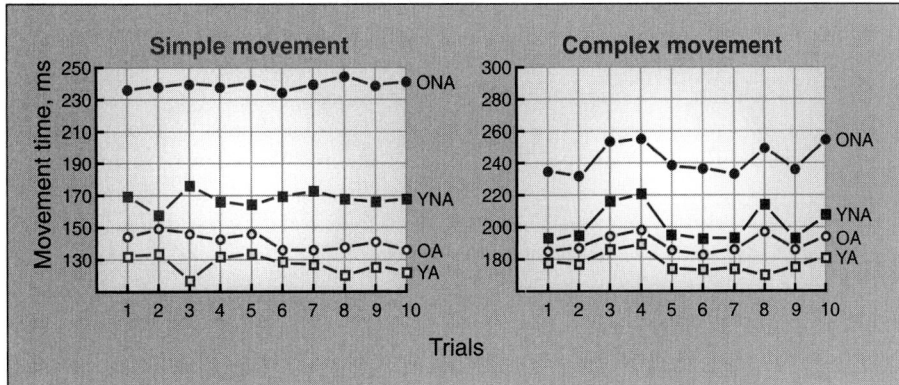

FIGURE 30.7

Simple and complex movement time in young active (YA), old active (OA), young nonactive (YNA), and old nonactive (ONA) subjects. Note that in both simple and complex movement tasks, the movement time is slower for the old and young nonactive individuals than in the young and old active individuals. (From Spirduso, W.W.: Reaction and movement time as a function of age and physical activity level. *J. Gerontol.*, 30:435, 1975.)

women have nearly a twofold faster rate of decline in $\dot{V}O_2$max as they age, and some research has actually shown no decline in aerobic capacity for individuals who have maintained relatively constant training during a 10-year period.[66, 73, 104] A recent study of a large cohort of men (who varied considerably in age, aerobic capacity, body composition, and lifestyle) revealed that if physical activity and body composition remain relatively stable over time, the expected yearly rate of decline in $\dot{V}O_2$max is approximately 0.25 mL $\cdot$ kg^{-1} $\cdot$ min^{-1}. In contrast, becoming overfat and sedentary accelerated this rate of decline.[69]

Many confounding factors influence the age-related decline in $\dot{V}O_2$max. Heredity undoubtedly plays an important role, as does the well-documented decrease in skeletal muscle mass.[49] It may be that the normal decline in aerobic capacity follows a two-component curve: one portion of the curve represents a faster rate of decline in sedentary adults from 20 to 30 years of age compared to adults who are physically active; thereafter, a slower rate of decline is observed for both groups.[19]

Central and Peripheral Function. For the active and sedentary person, the decline in aerobic capacity is influenced by age-related decrements in both central and peripheral physiologic functions linked to oxygen transport and utilization.[81, 111]

Heart Rate. No significant change in resting heart rate occurs with aging.[142] *However, one well-documented change in cardiovascular function with age is a decline in the maximum exercise heart rate.* This apparent age-effect is progressive with advancing years; it reflects reduced medullary outflow of sympathetic activity (β-adrenergic stimulation), which occurs to the same extent in both men and women.[60, 127] A rough approximation of the maximal heart rate with age is expressed by the following relationship:

$$\text{max HR (beats} \cdot \text{min}^{-1}\text{)} = 220 - \text{age (years)}$$

Cardiac Output. *Because of a lower maximum heart rate, maximum cardiac output generally is reduced with age.*[99] Contributing to this reduced capacity for blood flow is a reduction in the heart's stroke volume, which may account for as much as 50% of the age-related decline in $\dot{V}O_2$max. The decline in stroke volume reflects a reduced left ventricular systolic and diastolic contractile performance with aging, although for some active men and women contractile function is well maintained.[81, 150, 152] These healthy elderly individuals may compensate for their diminished heart rate response with an increased cardiac filling (end-diastolic volume) with a subsequent increase in stroke volume by the Frank-Starling mechanism.[49a, 114, 123]

Local Factors. Accompanying the age-related decrease in muscle mass is a reduction in peripheral blood flow capacity. This is probably the result of a decrease in the capillary-to-muscle fiber ratio and a reduction in arterial cross-sectional area.[31]

Lifestyle or Aging? The degree to which decrements in cardiovascular function are a direct result of the aging process or a lack of habitual physical activity has not been precisely determined. *Current knowledge, however, indicates that sedentary living may cause losses in functional capacity that are at least as great as the effects of aging itself.* In addition, there is a high degree of trainability among older men and women; skeletal muscle, substrate metabolism, and cardiovascular adaptations are similar to those of younger counterparts.[21, 32, 125, 140] Both low- and high-intensity regular exercise enables older individuals to retain cardiovascular functioning much above age-paired sedentary subjects of the same age.[7, 64, 94] When previously active middle-aged men followed a regular endurance exercise program over a 10-year period, the usual 9 to 15% decline in work capacity and maximal aerobic power was forestalled.[72] At age 55, these active men had maintained the same values for blood pressure, body mass, and $\dot{V}O_2$max as they had at 45 years of age.

Endurance Performance Capacity. Further evidence for the impressive effects of regular exercise on the preservation of cardiovascular function throughout life is seen when comparing the endurance performance of athletes of different ages. A plot of age-group, world-record marathon times, starting at age 4 for males and at age 5 for females and up to age 86 for males and age 80 for females, is presented in Figure 30.8. The world record of 2 hours, 7 minutes, 11 seconds by Carlos Lopes (age 37) of Portugal (recorded in April 1985) corresponds to a running speed of 4 minutes, 51 seconds per mile (12.4 mph). As can be seen, endurance performance sharply decreases in very young individuals and as people get older. Although from age 30 to 86 the performance decrement is progressive and considerable, the male 86-year-old world record time of 340.2 minutes corresponds to a pace of 12.9 minutes per mile, and the female 80-year-old world record time of 328.6 minutes corresponds to a pace of 12.5 minutes per mile. This running speed for 26.2 miles is truly remarkable for individuals in their ninth decade of life and attests to the tremendous cardiovascular capabilities of older men and women who continue to train on a regular basis as they grow older.

Aerobic Trainability Among Elderly Individuals. *Among healthy elderly individuals, exercise training can enhance the heart's systolic and diastolic properties and increase aerobic capacity to the same relative degree as in younger adults.*[41, 78, 85, 126, 142] For example, research has evaluated the contribution of training-induced increases in stroke volume and a-$\bar{v}$ O_2 difference to aerobic fitness improvements in healthy older men and women.[133] With 9 to 12 months of endurance training, $\dot{V}O_2$max increased 19% in men and 22% in women. These values are toward the high end of what is typically observed for younger adults. However, sex differences were apparent in aspects of the training response. For the men, the increased aerobic capacity was associated with a 15% larger maximum stroke volume (and corresponding increase in maximum cardiac output) and a 7% greater maximum a-$\bar{v}$ O_2 difference. For the women, the entire increase in $\dot{V}O_2$max was due solely to an expansion in the a-v̄ O_2 difference. This indicates that for older women, the increase in aerobic capacity with training depends on peripheral adaptations in the trained muscle. Further research is required to determine whether this lack of central circulatory adaptation to endurance training in postmenopausal women is a consistent finding and whether it is due to hormonal deficiencies in menopause.[134]

BODY COMPOSITION

After 35 years of age, men and women tend to progressively gain body fat until the fifth or sixth decade of life as shown in Figure 30.9. After 60 years of age, total body mass is reduced despite an increasing level of body fat. This is partly explained because in the upper age group, many of the

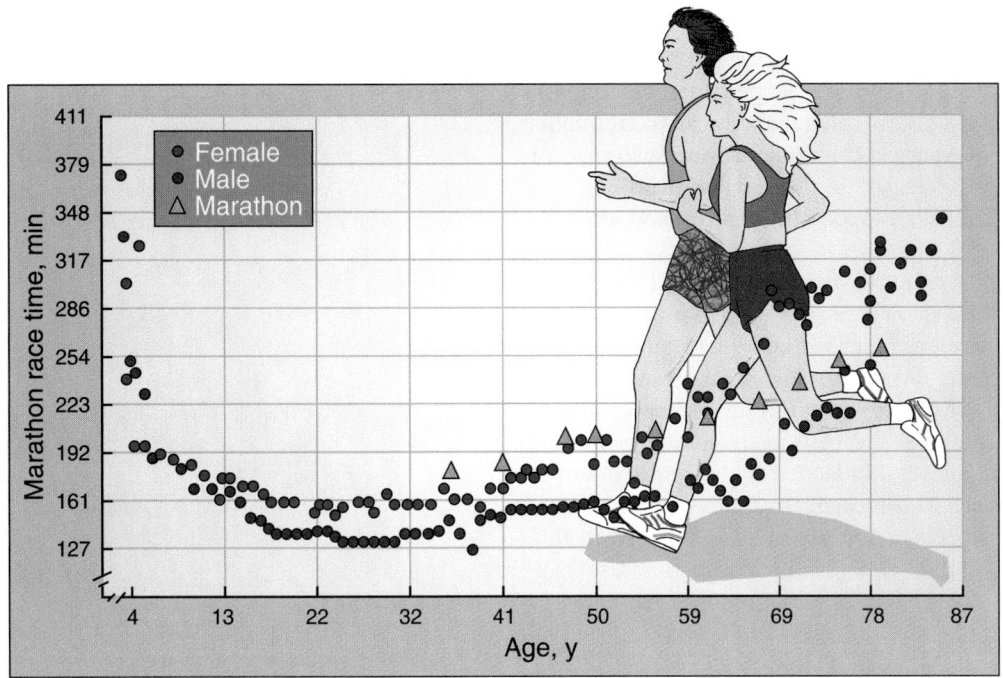

FIGURE 30.8

Plot of world record times for the marathon run by men and women of different ages. The yellow triangles represent the remarkable 50-year marathon achievements of the Greek runner Christos Vartzakis from 36 to 79 years of age. Over a 43-year span, this runner's mean velocity decreased by approximately 30% from 13.9 km · h⁻¹ at age 36 to 9.73 km · h⁻¹ at 79 years of age. Interestingly, his marathon time of 3 hours 56 minutes when he was 72 years old was faster than the average speed of master runners competing in the Basa Marathon Race who were about 40 years younger! (Data on Vartzakis courtesy of Dr. George Rontoyannis, Hellenic Sports Research Institute, Athens, Greece. Data originally published in: Rontoyannis, G.: Sixty-three years of competitive sport activity. Case study. *J. Sports Med. Phys. Fitness*, 32:331, 1992.)

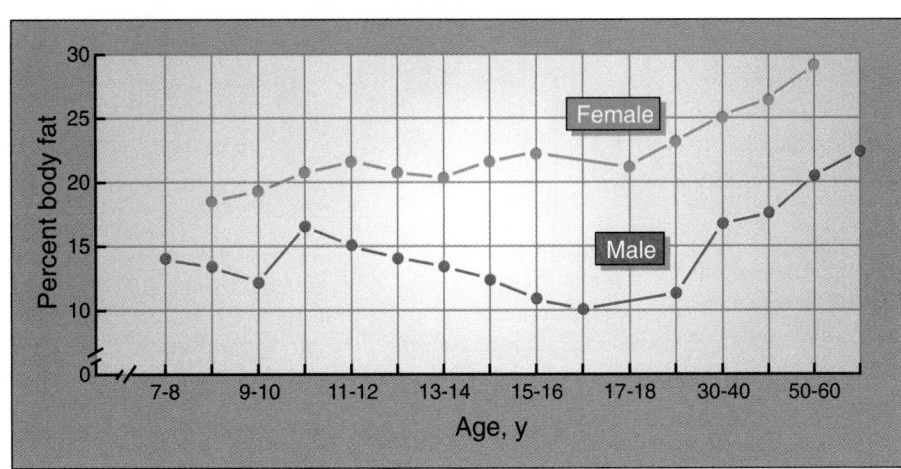

FIGURE 30.9

Body fat changes as a function of age. (From Parizkova, J., et al.: Body composition and exercise during growth and development. In *Physical Activity: Human Growth and Development*. Edited by G.L. Rarick. New York, Academic Press, 1974.)

grossly overweight people died and there were not many overweight subjects to be measured.

A major limitation of age-trend studies is that the same subjects are not followed over time; instead, different subjects in different age categories are evaluated at the same time. From these **cross-sectional** data, one attempts to generalize about expected age-related changes for an individual. Sometimes these generalizations are misleading. For example, today's 70- and 80-year-old individuals are generally shorter than 20-year-old college students. This observation does not necessarily mean that we get shorter as we grow older (although this does happen to some extent). Instead, the young adults of this generation are better nourished than their 80-year-old counterparts were at 20 years of age. For body fat changes, the limited **longitudinal** data from the same subjects support the trends noted in cross-sectional studies.[28]

Although it is common for most "normal" adults to grow fatter as they age, those who engage in heavy resistance training increase their lean body mass and decrease body fat. In Figure 30.10, an "older" resistance-trained athlete is shown; this figure demonstrates dramatically that it is possible to increase and then maintain a large muscle mass into late middle age. Indeed, it is a universal observation that individuals who engage in resistance training seem to defy certain aspects of the typical aging process. In this sport, there is certainly great truth to the axiom "Use it or lose it!"

BONE MASS

Osteoporosis is a major problem in aging, particularly among postmenopausal women. This condition results in a loss of bone mass as the aging skeleton becomes demineralized and porous. For people older than 60 years of age, these alterations in aging bone can reduce the bone mass by 30 to 50%. As discussed in Chapter 2, regular weight-bearing exercise may not only retard bone loss but can actually increase bone mass in elderly men and women.[110]

TRAINABILITY AND AGE

Regular moderate to vigorous physical activity produces physiologic improvements regardless of age. Of course, the magnitude of the changes depends on several factors, including initial fitness status, genetics, and the specific type of training. Concerning the age factor, it generally has been held that older individuals are not able to improve their strength and endurance capacity to the same extent as younger people.[120] The reasons for this blunted "trainability" were not well understood, although it was attributed to a general decline in neuromuscular function and an age-related impairment in the cellular capability for protein synthesis and chemical regulation.

Based on the significant research during the past 15 years on exercise and aging, a modification of the "classic" view of the improvement to be expected from physical conditioning for people of different ages is shown in Figure 30.11. When a healthy person, young or old, is given an appropriate training stimulus, large and rapid improvement in physiologic function occurs, often at the rate and magnitude that is **independent** of the person's age.[20, 27, 32, 55, 116] For ex-

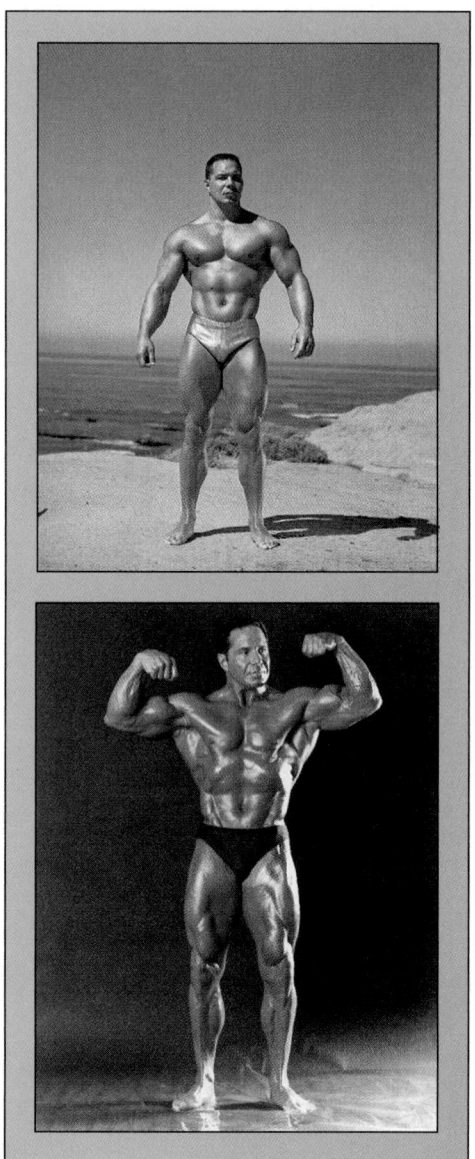

FIGURE 30.10

Fifty-three consecutive years of resistance training. Bill Pearl, currently 65 years of age, is one of the greatest body-building champions of all time. Holder of four Mr. Universe titles (1956, 1961, 1967, 1971), he still trains about 2.5 hours daily (beginning at 4:30 am). *Top,* 1967 Mr. Universe, age 37. *Bottom,* Last formal pose at age 59. (Photo courtesy of Bill Pearl.)

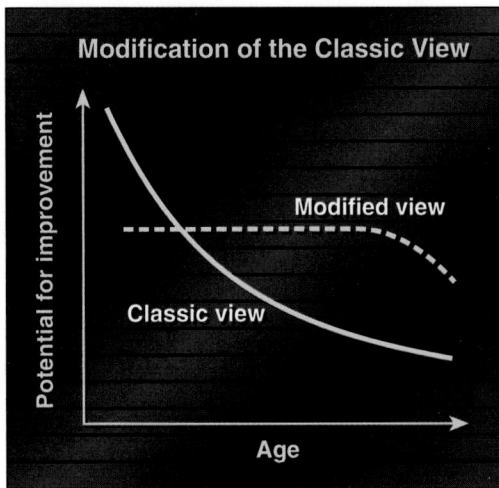

FIGURE 30.11

Traditional versus more current view of the improvement that might be expected with physical training related to age; a new look at some old beliefs.

ample, if the training stimulus is adequate, the skeletal muscles of older men and women adapt (fiber size, capillarization, glycolytic and respiratory enzymes) to specific endurance or resistance-training exercise in a manner similar to younger adults. These adaptations are particularly apparent with relatively intense training that is continuously adjusted to keep pace with training improvements. Healthy older adults show no negative metabolic or hormonal responses or maladaptations to regular exercise that would contraindicate participation in a standard training program.[61]

PART 3
PHYSICAL ACTIVITY, HEALTH, AND LONGEVITY

Because older fit individuals have many of the functional characteristics of younger people, it could be argued that improved physical fitness retards the aging process and thus offers some protection to health and possible longevity in later life.

EXERCISE AND LONGEVITY

In one of the first studies of the possibility that sport and regular exercise could prolong life, former Harvard oarsmen exceeded their predicted longevity by 5.1 years per man.[65] Other early studies showed similar but more modest results.[3] Much of this research, however, was plagued with methodological problems, including inadequate record keeping, small sample size, improper statistical

procedures for estimating expected longevity, and an inability to account for other important factors such as socioeconomic background, body type, tobacco use, and family background.

One group of researchers attempted to overcome many of these limitations in their study of the diseases and longevity of former college athletes.[96] No difference existed in the longevity of the ex-athletes compared to their nonathletic counterparts (Fig. 30.12). Some degree of equality in genetic background existed between the comparison groups because the average age at death was similar for the grandparents, parents, and siblings of the ex-athletes and nonathletes. These and more recent findings suggest that participation in athletics as a young adult does not necessarily ensure increased longevity.[15, 108] However, significant protection is provided for health and longevity if physical activity is maintained throughout life.[11, 11a, 121]

ENHANCED QUALITY TO A LONGER LIFE: A STUDY OF HARVARD ALUMNI

Research concerning the lifestyles and exercising habits of 17,000 Harvard alumni who entered college between 1916 and 1950 gives strong evidence that only **moderate** aerobic exercise, equivalent to jogging approximately 3 miles per day, promotes good health and may actually add years to life.[100] The results of these long-term studies can be summarized as follows:

Regular exercise countered the life-shortening effects of cigarette smoking and excess body mass. Even for people with hypertension, those who exercised regularly reduced their death rate by one-half. Even genetic tendencies toward early death were countered by regular exercise. For individuals who had one or both parents die before 65 years of age (a significant health risk), a lifestyle that included regular exercise reduced the risk of death by 25%. A 50% reduction in mortality rate was observed for those active men whose parents lived beyond 65 years.

As shown in Figure 30.13, the person who exercised more had an improved health profile. For example, the mortality rates were 21% lower for men who walked 9 or more miles per week than for men who walked 3 miles or less. Life expectancy was increased in men who performed the equivalent of light sport activity compared to men who remained sedentary. From the perspective of energy expenditure, the life expectancy of Harvard alumni increased steadily from an exercise energy expenditure of 500 kcal per week to 3,500 kcal, a value equivalent to 6 to 8 hours of strenuous weekly exercise. In addition, the active men lived an average of 1 to 2 years longer than sedentary classmates. Beyond weekly exercise of 3,500 kcal, there were no additional health or longevity benefits. When exercise was carried to extremes, the men had higher death rates than their more moderately active colleagues.

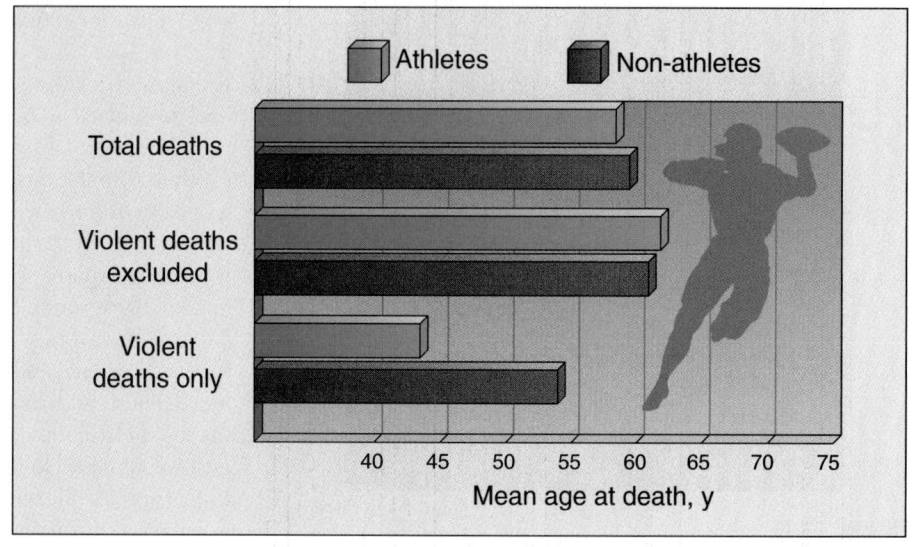

FIGURE 30.12
Age at death of athletes and nonathletes. None of the differences between the groups were statistically significant. (From Montoye, H.J., et al.: *The Longevity and Morbidity of College Athletes.* Indianapolis, IN, Phi Epsilon Kappa, 1957.)

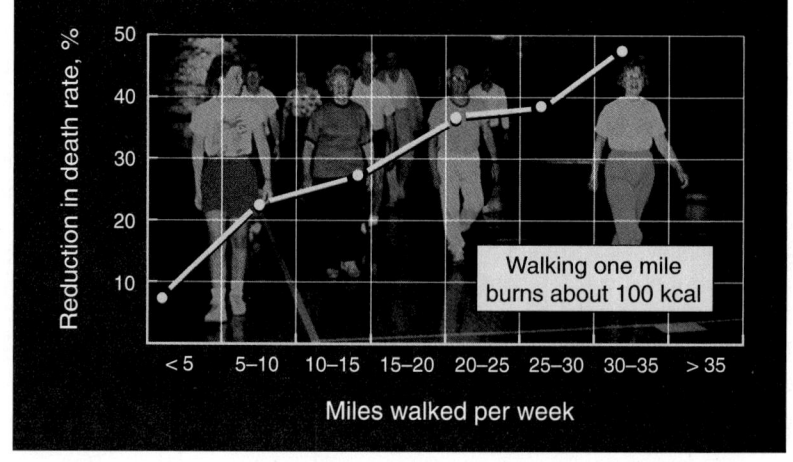

FIGURE 30.13
Reduced risk of death with regular exercise. (Adapted from Paffenbarger, R.S., Jr., et al.: Physical activity, all-cause mortality, and longevity of college alumni. *N. Engl. J. Med.,* 314:605, 1986.)

For Longevity, More Vigorous May Be Better. The previous research with Harvard alumni examined only the total amount of weekly physical activity, not its intensity, in relation to heart disease and mortality. Recent research with the same group of men indicates that vigorous regular exercise has the greatest effect in terms of extending life.[83a] Men who reported expending at least 1,500 kcal weekly in vigorous activities (i.e., physical activity of 6 times the resting metabolic rate [METs] or higher, such as jogging or walking briskly, lap swimming, singles tennis, fast cycling, or heavy yard chores for 45 minutes to an hour, 3 or 4 times a week) during the 20-year study period had a 25% lower death rate compared to the most sedentary men; the more active the men, the greater their life expectancies. The benefits of vigorous exercise were also seen in men who smoked or were overweight. The risk to longevity associated with a sedentary lifestyle was as great as smoking 1 pack of cigarettes per day or being 20% overweight.

EPIDEMIOLOGICAL EVIDENCE

A critique of 43 studies of the relationship between physical inactivity and coronary heart disease concluded that lack of regular exercise contributes to the heart disease process in a **cause-and-effect** manner; the sedentary person is almost twice as likely to develop heart disease as the most active individual.[106] *The strength of this protective association was essentially the same as that observed for hypertension, cigarette smoking, and high serum cholesterol.* In the researchers' opinion, this placed physical inactivity as the greater heart disease risk, considering that more people lead sedentary lifestyles than possessed one or more of the other risks. *From available data, it seems that if life-extending benefits of exercise exist, they are associated more with the prevention of early mortality than an improvement in overall life span.* Whereas the maximum life span may not be extended greatly, more active people tend to survive to a "ripe old age." Surprisingly, only light to moderate regular activity such as walking, gardening, stair climbing, and household chores is needed to achieve positive health benefits for previously sedentary men and women. This certainly is good news because it is these citizens who represent the largest percentage of the population and who are at the greatest risk.

IMPROVED FITNESS: A LITTLE GOES A LONG WAY

The findings of 30 years of research relating level of physical activity and physical fitness to selected chronic diseases or medical conditions are summarized in Table 30.2. Clearly, there is a strong association between regular physical activity and physical fitness and all causes of death; the greatest impact was noted for diseases of the cardiovascular system. An example of such research is a study of more than 13,000 men and women followed for an average of 8 years. Even a modest amount of regular exercise substantially reduced the risk of dying from heart disease, cancer, and other causes.[11, 22] This is one of the few studies that has directly examined fitness performance rather than verbal or written reports of regular physical activity habits. To isolate the effect of fitness, the study accounted for such factors as smoking, cholesterol and blood sugar levels, blood pressure, and family history of heart disease. Based on age-adjusted death rates per 10,000 person-years, death rates of the least fit group were more than three times that of the most fit individuals (Fig. 30.14). The most striking finding was that the greatest health benefit occurred in the group rated just above those in the most sedentary category. For men, the drop in death rate from the least fit category to the next fit category was more than 38 (64.0 vs. 25.5 deaths per 10,000 person-years), whereas the drop in mortality between the second group and the most fit group was only 7. Similar benefits occurred for women. To move from the most sedentary category to the next most fit (the change that produced the greatest health benefits) requires only moderate-intensity exercise such as walking briskly for 30 minutes several times a week.

Recent studies of Finnish men complement the above findings by demonstrating that leisure-time physical activity and aerobic capacity had an inverse, graded, and independent association with the risk of acute myocardial infarction.[71] Relatively low levels of both physical activity and fitness offered significant protection. For example, outwardly healthy middle-aged men with more than 2 hours of conditioning physical activity (walking, jogging, cross-country ski-ing, gymnastics) per week and men with a $\dot{V}O_2$max of at least 34 mL · kg^{-1} · min^{-1} (a relatively low aerobic capacity) had a 60% lower heart attack risk than the least active or least fit men. For a large group of middle-aged British men, regular physical activity also was protective from heart attack and stroke.[151] In the Finnish and British studies, engaging in just light to moderate regular exercise provided significant protection, although the greatest benefits were noted with more vigorous exercise.

TABLE 30.2
SUMMARY RESULTS OF STUDIES INVESTIGATING THE RELATIONSHIP BETWEEN PHYSICAL ACTIVITY OR PHYSICAL FITNESS AND SELECTED CHRONIC DISEASES OR CONDITIONS, 1963–1993

Disease or Condition	Number of Studies	Trends Across Activity or Fitness Categories and Strength of Evidence[a]
All-cause mortality	>10	↓↓↓
Coronary artery disease	>10	↓↓↓
Hypertension	5–10	↓↓
Obesity	>10	↓↓
Stroke	5–10	↓
Peripheral vascular disease	<5	→
Cancer		
Colon	>10	↓↓
Rectum	>10	→
Stomach	<5	→
Breast	<5	↓
Prostate	5–10	↓
Lung	<5	↓
Pancreas	<5	→
Noninsulin-dependent diabetes	<5	↓↓
Osteoarthritis	<5	→
Osteoporosis	5–10	↓↓
Functional capability	5–10	↓↓

From Blair, S.N.: Physical activity, physical fitness, and health. *Res. Q. Exerc. Sports:* 64: 365, 1993.
[a]→, No apparent difference in disease rates across activity or fitness categories; ↓, some evidence of reduced disease rates across activity or fitness categories; ↓↓, good evidence of reduced disease rates across activity or fitness categories, control of potential confounders, good methods, some evidence of biological mechanisms; ↓↓↓, excellent evidence of reduced disease rates across activity or fitness categories, good control of potential confounders, excellent methods, extensive evidence of biological mechanisms, relationship is considered causal.

FIGURE 30.14

Physical fitness and longevity: a little goes a long way. The greatest reduction in death rate risk occurs when going from the low fitness category to a moderate level of fitness. (From Blair, S.N., et al.: Physical fitness and all-cause mortality: a prospective study of healthy men and women. *JAMA*, 262:2395, 1989.)

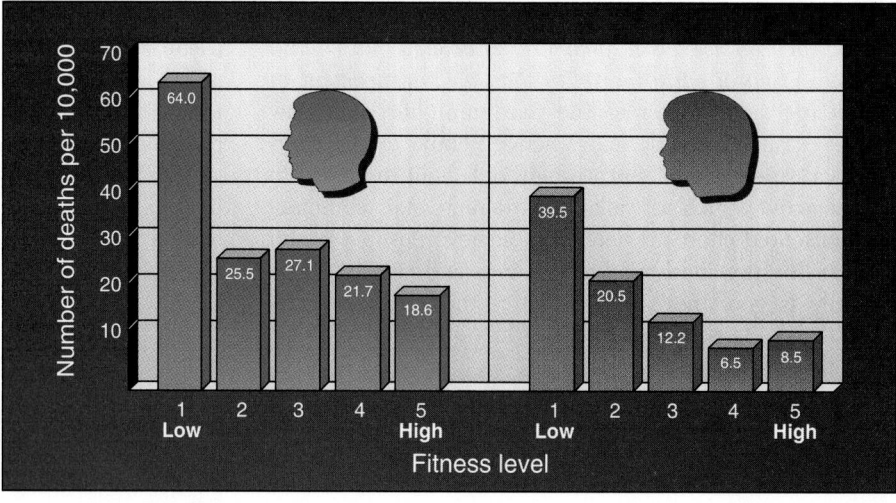

FIGURE 30.15

Adjusted relative risks (each relative risk is adjusted for age and all other variables in the figure) for CHD mortality by changes in lifestyle characteristics. The red bars represent men who initially had unfavorable characteristics (in 1962 or 1966) and at follow-up in 1977. The blue bars show the adjusted relative risks for men who made favorable changes on the variable of interest between baseline and follow-up. BMI, body mass index; Mod-Vig, moderately vigorous. (Modified from Blair, S. N.: Physical activity, physical fitness, and health. *Res. Q. Exerc. Sport*, 64:365, 1993; data from Paffenbarger, R.S., Jr., et al.: The association between changes in physical-activity level and other lifestyle characteristics with mortality among men. *N. Engl. J. Med.*, 328:538, 1993.)

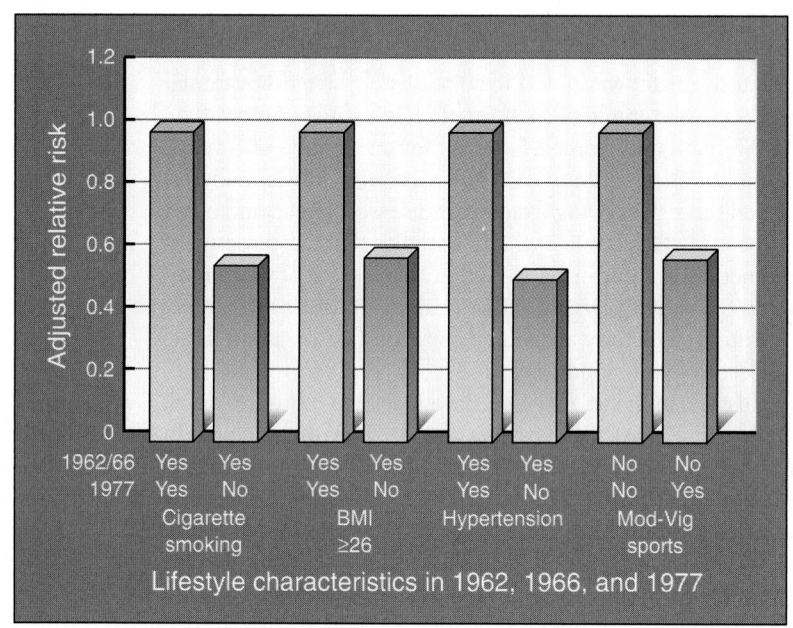

DOES A CHANGE IN FITNESS IMPROVE ONE'S HEALTH OUTLOOK?

Although it is well established that one's level of physical activity is associated with health risk, an important question is whether a sustained increase in regular activity reduces the risk of disease. To answer this question, previously sedentary, apparently healthy male Harvard alumni reported changes in their physical activity and other lifestyle habits over an 11- to 15-year period.[101] These changes were then related to mortality incidence as illustrated in Figure 30.15. Regardless of age, men who were initially sedentary but who adopted a more moderate to vigorous level of regular activity had a 51% lower risk of dying than men who chose to re-

main sedentary. For lifestyle change and heart disease mortality risk, becoming more physically active on a regular basis was of equal benefit in terms of risk reduction as quitting cigarette smoking, reducing body weight, or controlling blood pressure.

PART 4
CORONARY HEART DISEASE

Coronary heart disease (CHD) generally involves degenerative changes in the intima or inner lining of the larger arteries that supply the heart muscle or myocardium.

CHANGES ON THE CELLULAR LEVEL

The action and chemical modification of various compounds, including the oxidation of the cholesterol in low-density lipoproteins, initiates a complex process that ultimately causes bulging lesions in the arterial wall. The lesions initially take the form of fatty streaks, which are the first signs of atherosclerosis. With further damage and proliferation of underlying cells, the vessel becomes progressively congested with lipid-filled plaques, fibrous scar tissue, or both. This change progressively reduces the capacity for blood flow and causes the myocardium to become **ischemic**—that is, poorly supplied with oxygen due to reduced blood flow.

The progressive occlusion of an artery with a buildup of calcified fatty substances in the process of atherosclerosis is shown in Figure 30.16. In this degenerative process, which often begins early in life, the roughened, hardened lining of the coronary artery frequently causes the slowly flowing blood to clot. This blood clot (known as a **thrombus**) may plug one of the smaller coronary vessels. When this occurs, a portion of the heart muscle dies and the person is said to have suffered a heart attack or **myocardial infarction.** If the blockage is not too severe but blood flow is still reduced below the heart's requirement, the person may experience temporary chest pains termed **angina pectoris.** These pains usually are felt during exertion because increased physical activity causes the greatest demand for myocardial blood flow. Such anginal attacks provide painful and dramatic evidence of the importance of adequate oxygen supply to this vital organ.

STILL AN EPIDEMIC

Coronary artery disease has reached epidemic proportions throughout the United States and most technologically advanced societies. The percentage distribution of the leading causes of death in the United States is illustrated in Figure 30.17, *top.* CHD is responsible for more than 1.5 million myocardial infarctions and 90,000 strokes and causes more than 550,000 deaths annually (compared to 40,500 deaths from breast cancer and 40,000 deaths from lung cancer). Whereas CHD still remains the leading cause of death in the United States and the industrialized world (25% of all deaths versus 6% in less developed countries), the good news is that heart-disease deaths have declined more than one-third since 1970 (Fig. 30.17, *bottom*).

Almost all people show some evidence of coronary artery disease, and it can be severe in seemingly healthy young adults. The disease probably starts early in life because fatty streaks are common in the coronary arteries of children by 5 years of age. There seems to be little harm, however, unless there is a marked narrowing of the arteries. *At rest, the heart's blood supply becomes deficient only when obstruction of the coronary vessels reaches approximately 80%. At least 50 to 70% occlusion must take place before the disease can be detected clinically.* Generally, death from

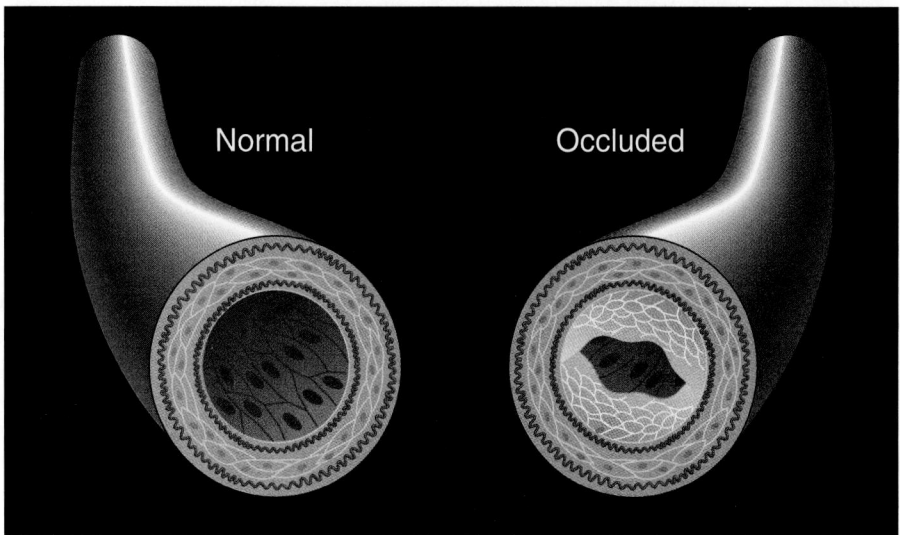

FIGURE 30.16

Left, Cross section of a normal coronary artery (magnification ×170). *Right,* Deterioration of a coronary artery resulting in deposits of fatty substances that roughen the vessel's center. Lipid-laden macrophage cells cluster under the endothelial lining to form a bulge (fatty streak) into the artery. This is the first overt sign of atherosclerotic change within the artery. Over time, there is a proliferation of smooth muscle cells that accumulate to narrow the lumen (center) of the artery. A clot forms and literally plugs the artery, depriving the heart muscle of normal blood flow through that region of the artery. When the artery occludes to approximately 75% of its normal diameter, the localized ischemia can result in a myocardial infarction or heart attack.

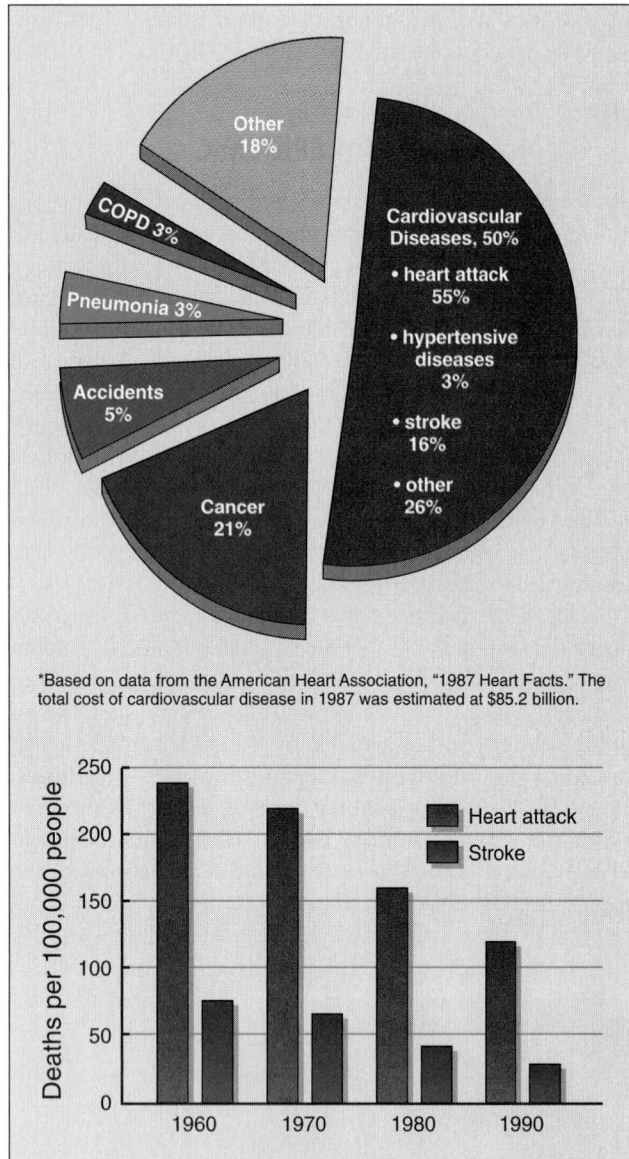

*Based on data from the American Heart Association, "1987 Heart Facts." The total cost of cardiovascular disease in 1987 was estimated at $85.2 billion.

FIGURE 30.17

Top, Leading causes of death in the United States. *Bottom,* Declining death rates from heart attacks and stroke between 1960 and 1990. (Data from National Center for Health Statistics and the American Heart Association.)

CHD occurs when there is advanced obstruction in several major vessels supplying the myocardium.

CORONARY HEART DISEASE RISK FACTORS

Significant information has been provided on the natural history and dynamics of heart disease. Various personal characteristics and environmental factors that are related to susceptibility to CHD have been identified during the past 30 years. The following is a list of the more frequently im-

plicated of these **risk factors** that identify men, women, and children at high or low risk for CHD.[59a, 98, 101, 141] It must be noted, however, that although the "modifiable" factors are associated with CHD, the associations do not necessarily infer causality. In some instances, it is unclear whether risk-factor modification offers effective protection from the disease. Until definite proof is demonstrated, however, it seems logical to assume that elimination or reduction of one or more risk factors will cause a corresponding decrease in the probability of contracting CHD.

Modifiable

- Diet
- Elevated blood lipids
- Hypertension
- Personality and behavior patterns
- Cigarette smoking
- High uric acid levels
- Sedentary lifestyle
- Pulmonary function abnormalities
- Obesity
- Diabetes mellitus
- Electrocardiogram (ECG) abnormalities
- Tension and stress
- Poor education

Nonmodifiable

- Age
- Sex
- Ethnic background
- Male pattern baldness
- Family history

It is difficult to determine quantitatively the importance of any single CHD risk factor in comparison to any other because many of the factors are interrelated (i.e., blood lipid abnormalities, diabetes, heredity, and obesity). One research study reported that men living in Ireland consumed more saturated fat than their blood brothers who lived in the United States, but the former had a much lower incidence of CHD.[148] This was attributed to higher physical activity levels of those living in Ireland. Similar findings for high saturated fat intake, high physical activity, and low incidence of CHD have been reported in Masai tribesmen of East Africa and farm laborers in Georgia.[89, 93]

AGE, SEX, AND HEREDITY

Age is a CHD risk factor largely because of its association with other risk factors such as hypertension, elevated blood lipids, and glucose intolerance. As shown in Figure 30.18, after age 35 in men and age 45 in women, the chances of dying from CHD increase progressively and dramatically.

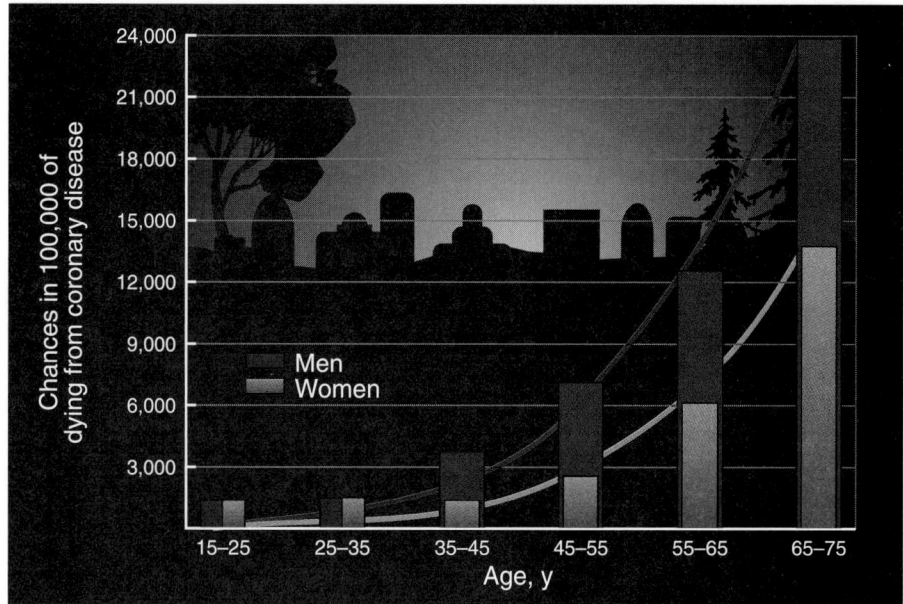

FIGURE 30.18
The chances of a single individual dying from coronary artery disease.

At most ages, women have lower risk of death from heart disease than men. For example, a middle-aged man has an approximately sixfold greater chance of dying from a heart attack compared to a woman. Despite this sex advantage, occurrence of heart disease in American women is still higher than in women in other countries. Speculation is that some of the CHD protection for women is provided by hormonal differences between the sexes, particularly differences related to levels of estrogen. Although the cause is not known, heart attacks that strike at an early age appear to run in families.

In the following sections, blood lipid abnormalities, obesity, cigarette smoking, and physical inactivity are examined. (Hypertension is discussed in Chapter 15.) These are listed as the "big four" heart-disease risks by the American Heart Association. Each is a potent CHD risk that can be modified by changes in lifestyle and health habits.[50]

BLOOD LIPID ABNORMALITIES

An increased lipid level in the blood is termed **hyperlipidemia,** which is a crucial factor in the initiation of the process of atherosclerosis. Table 30.3 presents levels of serum cholesterol above which young and older adults should seek advice on treatment; early treatment is desirable because there is a strong association between serum cholesterol as a young adult and cardiovascular disease in middle age.[76] Generally, a cholesterol level of 200 mg · dL^{-1} or lower is considered desirable.[58] A cholesterol value of 230 mg · dL^{-1} increases the risk of heart attack to about twice that of a person with 180 mg · dL^{-1}, and a value of 300 mg · dL^{-1} increases the risk fourfold.

TABLE 30.3
DESIRABLE LEVELS OF TOTAL CHOLESTEROL (MG · DL^{-1}), INCLUDING HDL AND LDL CHOLESTEROL, AND LEVELS ABOVE WHICH ADULTS SHOULD RECEIVE TREATMENT

Age (y)	Goal	Moderate Risk (75th percentile)	High Risk (90th percentile)
20–29	<180	>200	>220
30–39	<200	>220	>240
40 and over	<200	>240	>260

Undesirable Levels
HDL Cholesterol < 35 mg · dL^{-1}
LDL Cholesterol > 130 mg · dL^{-1}

Adapted from National Institutes of Health Consensus Development Conference Statement: Lowering blood cholesterol to prevent heart disease. *JAMA*, 253:2080, 1985.

Cholesterol and triglyceride are the two most common lipids associated with CHD risk. These lipids do not circulate freely in the blood plasma but are transported in combination with a carrier protein to form a **lipoprotein.** The four different lipoproteins, their approximate gravitational density, and percent composition in the blood are listed in Table 30.4. Serum cholesterol represents a composite of the total cholesterol contained in each of the different lipoproteins. Although it is proper to refer to hyperlipidemia, it is more meaningful to evaluate and discuss the different types of **hyperlipoproteinemia.** Overwhelming evidence links

TABLE 30.4
APPROXIMATE COMPOSITION OF LIPOPROTEINS IN THE BLOOD

	Chylomicrons	Very Low Density Lipoproteins (VLDL:Prebeta)	Low Density Lipoproteins (LDL:Beta)	High-Density Lipoproteins (HDL:Alpha)
Density, $g \cdot cm^{-3}$	0.95	0.95–1.006	1.006–1.019	1.063–1.210
Protein, %	0.5–1.0	5–15	25	45–55
Lipid, %	99	95	75	50
Cholesterol, %	2–5	10–20	40–45	18
Triglyceride, %	85	50–70	5–10	2
Phospholipid, %	3–6	10–20	20–25	30

high levels of blood lipids, especially low-density lipoproteins, with increased incidence of CHD. In many cases, raised levels of this lipoprotein are related to consumption of diets high in saturated fatty acids and cholesterol.

The distribution of cholesterol among the various lipoproteins is a more powerful predictor of heart disease than the total blood cholesterol (Fig. 30.19). Specifically, elevated levels of high-density lipoproteins (HDL) are associated with a lower heart disease risk, even among individuals with total cholesterol below 200 mg $\cdot$ dL^{-1}. Elevated levels of the low-density lipoproteins (LDL and VLDL), on the other hand, represent an increased CHD risk. An effective way to evaluate lipoprotein status is to divide total cholesterol by HDL cholesterol. This ratio is a superior measure of heart disease risk than either total cholesterol or LDL levels. *A ratio greater than 4.5 indicates a high heart-disease risk, whereas a ratio of 3.5 or lower is more optimal.*[90]

Although controversy exists regarding the precise role of lipoproteins in the heart-disease process, it is generally believed that the LDL and VLDL are means for transporting lipids throughout the body for delivery to the cells, including those of the smooth muscle walls of the arteries. When LDL cholesterol is oxidized, it becomes available for involvement in the arterial-clogging, plaque-forming process of atherosclerosis. Prevention of LDL oxidation, on the other hand, may slow the progression of this disease. In this regard, the potential benefit of dietary antioxidants such as vitamins C and E and β-carotene on heart-disease risk may lie in their role in blunting the oxidation of LDL cholesterol (refer to Chapter 2).

Whereas LDL is targeted for peripheral tissue and is associated with arterial damage, HDL facilitates reverse cholesterol transport by promoting the removal of cholesterol from peripheral tissues (including arterial walls) for transport to the liver for bile synthesis, where it is then excreted through the small intestine. There is considerable evidence to show a causal association between low levels of HDL cholesterol (and its subfractions) and the increased risk for developing CHD.[98]

Regular Exercise. Exercise has only a small effect on the level of LDL cholesterol when considering factors such as body composition and dietary lipid and cholesterol intake.[155] It is encouraging, however, that HDL levels are elevated in endurance athletes and are favorably altered in sedentary men and women of all ages who engage in either vigorous aerobic training or more moderate levels of regular exercise.[26, 39, 40] Exercise intensities required to produce changes in cardiovascular fitness are not necessary to favorably affect the lipoprotein profile. These favorable lipid alterations with aerobic exercise take place independently of changes in body mass. Such changes may be related to an enhanced triglyceride clearance from plasma in response to regular exercise.[119, 124, 145, 147] Even among trained endurance athletes, the variability in HDL cholesterol is quite high; in some runners, HDL cholesterol values are near the median value for the general population.[118] Moreover, no single factor—nutritional, body compositional, or related to the level of training—distinguishes runners with high HDL values from runners with lower values. This suggests that genetic factors may be the most important influence on blood lipid status. Generally, standard programs of resistance training have little or no effect on serum triglyceride, cholesterol, or lipoproteins. From a dietary perspective, substituting dietary protein from animal sources with protein from soybean sources significantly improves the cholesterol and lipoprotein profile, especially in persons with high levels of blood cholesterol.[2a] A moderate intake of alcohol (equivalent to about 2 oz or 30 mL of 90-proof alcohol, three 6-oz glasses of wine, or a bit less than three 12-oz cans of beer) reduces an otherwise healthy person's risk of heart attack. Although the protective mechanism is unclear, it may be because moderate alcohol intake increases HDL and its subfractions, particularly HDL$_2$ and HDL$_3$.[57] It is also postulated that certain components of red wine may inhibit the oxidation of LDL cholesterol, thus retarding the process of plaque formation.[55b] Excessive alcohol consumption, however, offers no lipoprotein benefit and greatly increases the risk of liver disease and cancer.[55a]

During the last three decades, there has been a substantial decline in serum cholesterol levels among United States adults, which coincides with a decrease in the national incidence of CHD. Despite this indication that public health programs are proving successful, approximately 30% of adults still require intervention for high cholesterol.[70]

OBESITY

Although excess body fat has received great notoriety as a CHD risk factor, its relationship is often codependent with other risks such as hypertension, elevated cholesterol, diabetes mellitus, and cigarette smoking.[67] Weight loss and accompanying body fat reduction, whether through diet or exercise, generally normalize cholesterol and triglyceride levels and have a beneficial effect on blood pressure and adult-onset diabetes. Although obesity may not be a primary CHD risk factor, its role cannot be denied as a secondary and contributing factor in heart disease and various other disease processes (see Chapter 29).

CIGARETTE SMOKING

Cigarette smoking may be one of the best predictors of CHD; the risk is directly related to the number of cigarettes smoked. The probability of death from heart disease for smokers is almost twice as great as for nonsmokers.[84] The Centers for Disease Control and Prevention estimates that every cigarette smoked steals 7 minutes from a smoker's life. This adds up to 5 million years of potential life Americans lose to cigarettes each year. The more one smokes (or is exposed to cigarette smoke), the deeper one inhales, and the stronger the cigarette in terms of tars and noxious by-products, the greater the CHD risk. The increased rate of death from heart disease among women in the United States almost parallels their increased consumption of cigarettes.[154] British researchers estimate that smokers in their 30s and 40s suffer five times as many heart attacks as nonsmokers in the same age range.[102a] When these relatively young smokers have a heart attack there is an 80% chance that cigarette smoking was the cause; the percent chance is nearly 70% for those in their 50s and 50% for those in their 60s and 70s. Also, smokers are nearly five times as likely to have a stroke as nonsmokers—and those who smoke 1 pack or more per day have an 11 times greater chance of suffering a specific type of sudden, deadly stroke that tends to strike younger men and women. Surprisingly, this CHD risk from smoking is associated with more deaths than the excess mortality of cigarette smokers due to lung cancer.

The smoking risk generally acts independently of other risk factors. At the same time, however, if other risk factors are present, cigarette smoking accentuates their influence. Cigarette smoking may facilitate heart disease through its effect on serum lipoproteins; individuals who smoke have lower levels of HDL cholesterol compared to nonsmokers. However, when smoking is stopped, the HDL and heart disease risk return to the levels of nonsmokers.[137]

PHYSICAL ACTIVITY

The consensus among the more recent prospective investigations is that regular physical activity protects against heart

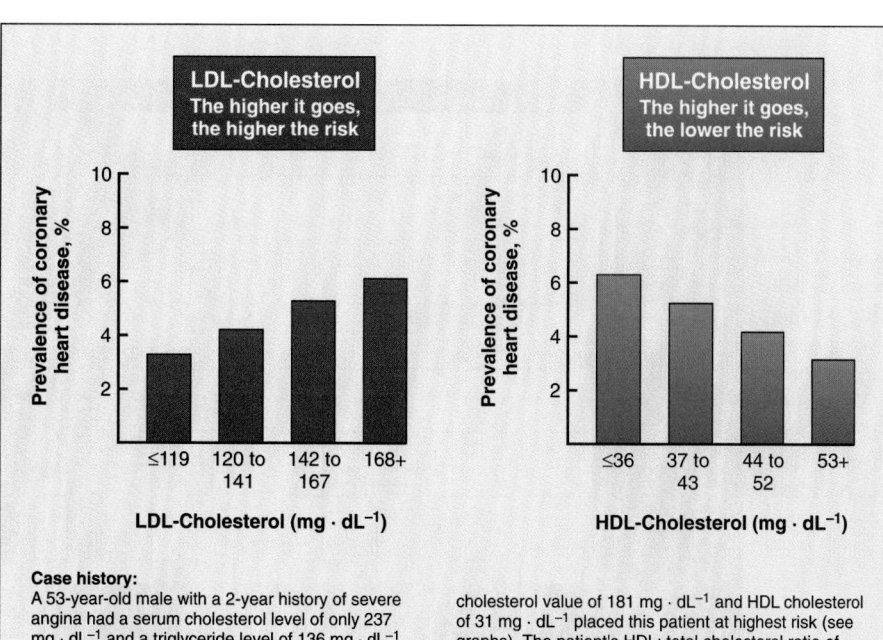

FIGURE 30.19
Coronary heart disease prevalence and lipoproteins. The risk increases as the LDL-cholesterol level increases; conversely, the risk decreases when the HDL-cholesterol level rises. (Courtesy of CPC Internal, Best Foods Division.)

Case history:
A 53-year-old male with a 2-year history of severe angina had a serum cholesterol level of only 237 mg · dL⁻¹ and a triglyceride level of 136 mg · dL⁻¹, both considered "normal". However, his LDL cholesterol value of 181 mg · dL⁻¹ and HDL cholesterol of 31 mg · dL⁻¹ placed this patient at highest risk (see graphs). The patient's HDL: total cholesterol ratio of 13% places him below the desired 20% "normal" ratio.

disease.[10, 97, 103] The relative risk of a fatal heart attack among sedentary individuals is approximately twice that of more active men and women. The maintenance of physical fitness throughout life also provides significant protection for CHD risk factors and the occurrence of actual disease.[1, 11, 42] It could be argued that one's level of physical fitness is more related to genetic factors and somewhat less to one's daily exercise patterns. Because fitness level is strongly related to a person's reported activity level, regular exercise may be even more important than genetics in determining physical fitness and its associated health benefits.

Mechanisms of Protection. Research on animals and humans indicates that regular aerobic exercise may operate against CHD in a variety of beneficial ways, including the following:

- Improves myocardial circulation and metabolism to protect the heart from hypoxic stress; this includes enhanced vascularization and modest increases in cardiac glycogen stores and glycolytic capacity that could be beneficial if there were a compromise in the heart's oxygen supply.[83]
- Enhances the mechanical properties of the myocardium to enable the exercise-trained heart to maintain or increase contractility during a specific challenge.[122]
- Establishes more favorable blood-clotting characteristics and other homeostatic mechanisms, with an increase in fibrinolysis and production of endothelial prostacyclin.[43, 139]
- Normalizes the blood lipid profile.[39, 46]
- Favorably alters heart rate and blood pressure so the work of the myocardium is significantly reduced at rest and during exercise.[100]
- Achieves a more desirable body composition and body fat distribution.[67, 74]

- Establishes a more favorable neural-hormonal balance to conserve oxygen for the myocardium, and improves the mixture of carbohydrates and lipids metabolized by the body.[106]
- Provides a favorable outlet and response pattern to psychological stress and tensions.[34, 130]

INTERACTION OF CHD RISK FACTORS

Many risk factors are associated with each other as well as with CHD itself. As shown in Figure 30.20, the interaction of three of the primary CHD risk factors when elevated in the same person most definitely magnifies their individual effects. With one risk factor, a 45-year-old man's chance of CHD during the year is approximately two times greater than a man with no risks. With three risk factors, this man's chance for angina, heart attack, or sudden death is five times higher than if he had no risk factors. An important consideration is that many of the CHD risks have a common root in behavioral patterns and, consequently, can be influenced by similar and in some cases identical interventions. For example, regular exercise exerts a positive influence on the risk factors of obesity, hypertension, diabetes, stress, and an elevated blood lipid profile.

RISK FACTORS IN CHILDREN

Multiple CHD risk factors are frequently observed in young children.[37] As shown in Table 30.5, in active and apparently healthy boys and girls aged 7 to 12 years, obesity and a family history of heart disease were the two most frequently occurring risk factors. A relatively large percentage of these children also showed abnormally high blood lipids. Of the total group,

FIGURE 30.20

Relation between a combination of abnormal risk factors (cholesterol higher than 250 mg/dL; systolic blood pressure higher than 160 mm Hg; smoking more than 1 pack of cigarettes per day) and incidence of coronary heart disease. (Adapted from Kannel, W.B., and Gordon, T.: *The Framingham Study: An Epidemiologic Investigation of Cardiovascular Disease.* Section 30. DHEW Publication #74-599. Washington, DC, National Institutes of Health, 1974.)

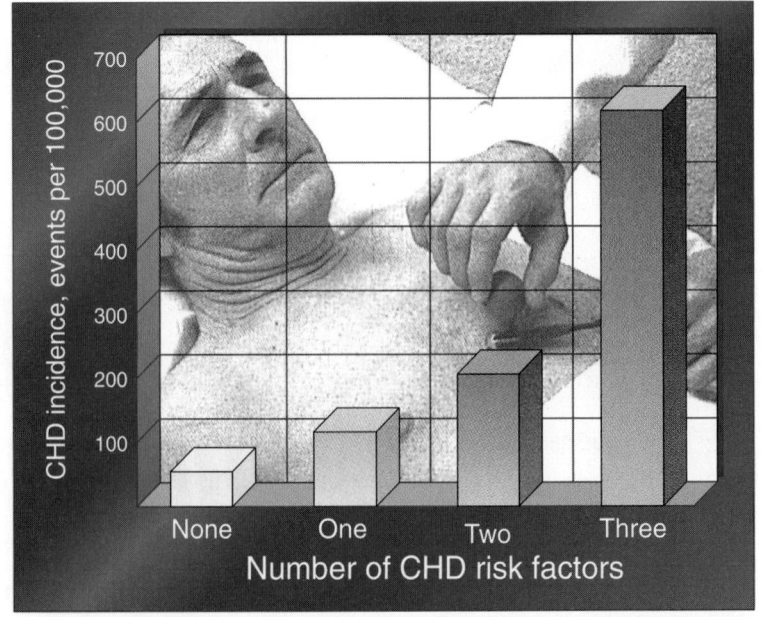

TABLE 30.5
PREVALENCE OF CHD RISK FACTORS IN BOYS AND GIRLS AGED 7 TO 12

	Prevalence				
Risk Factor	Male	Female	Total	N	Percent in Total Sample
Obesity (>20% body fat)	10	4	14	47	30
Low peak $\dot{V}O_2$ (<31 mL · kg^{-1} · min^{-1})	3	1	4	34	12
Elevated blood lipids					
Cholesterol (>200 mg · dL^{-1})	1	3	4	38	10
Triglycerides (>100 mg · dL^{-1})	4	3	7	38	18
Lipoprotein classification					
Type II	1	1	2	38	5
Type IV	4	3	7	38	18
Family history of CHD	7	5	12	47	26

From Gilliam, T., et al.: Prevalence of coronary heart disease risk factors in active children, 7 to 12 years of age. *Med. Sci. Sports*, 9:21, 1977.

65% had at least one or two risk factors, whereas 31% had three or more. As happens with adults, the association between body fatness and serum lipid levels becomes readily apparent in subjects classified as obese; the fattest children generally have the highest levels of cholesterol and triglycerides.

Because of the prevalence of CHD risk factors among preadolescents and adolescents, in addition to autopsy observations of young adults and children, it seems likely that heart disease has its origins in childhood. School-based programs aimed at reducing risk factors in adolescents are effective for increasing students' knowledge about risk factors and benefits of physical activity.[75] It remains to be seen whether the benefits from such "risk intervention" will improve a child's health outlook and can be carried into adulthood to improve overall health. Certainly, if regular physical activity can modify or at least stabilize the risk factor profile, then all children should be encouraged and taught to pursue active lifestyles.

Risk factor prevalence has also been evaluated for obese children or for children possessing one or more primary risk factors. In a sample of 62 obese children aged 10 to 15 years, only one child had just one CHD risk factor.[9] In the remaining group, 14% had two risk factors, 30% had three, 29% had four, 18% had five, and the remaining five children (8%) had six risk factors for heart disease. A subsample of these obese children then enrolled in a 20-week program to evaluate the effects of diet plus behavior therapy or regular exercise plus diet plus behavior therapy on the risk profile. No changes were noted in multiple-risk reduction in either the control or diet-plus-behavior group. In contrast, the children on exercise plus diet plus behavior therapy experienced a dramatic reduction in multiple risks (Fig. 30.21). These findings are encouraging because they show that a supervised program of moderate food restriction and exercise with behavior modification can reduce CHD risk factors in obese adolescents. The addition of regular ex-

ercise was the factor augmenting the effectiveness of this risk factor intervention.

CALCULATING THE RISK

Risk inventories or appraisals have been developed to quantify an individual's susceptibility to CHD. Most of these inventories assign point values to different aspects of lifestyle. Often, these values are arbitrary and are not based on actual risk (mortality or morbidity). Despite this limitation, such risk assignment is often valuable for screening in the overall assessment of current risk and lifestyle behaviors.

In Table 30.6, a popular risk inventory (**RISKO**) developed by the Michigan Heart Association is presented. To determine your own risk profile, study each risk factor and the accompanying numerical value that best describes your status. Find the box applicable to you and circle the number in it. For example, if you are 19 years old, circle the number 1 in the box labeled 10 to 20 years. After checking all the rows, add the circled numbers. The total number of points is your risk score; see footnote Table 30.6 for Relative Risk Category.

PART 5
PRUDENT PRE-EXERCISE EVALUATION

Vigorous aerobic exercise has a profound and positive effect on the functional capacity of the cardiovascular system. It also is generally accepted that this type of exercise can serve important protective and rehabilitative functions in the battle against heart disease. The potential therapeutic benefits of exercise, however, should be viewed in perspective. For a

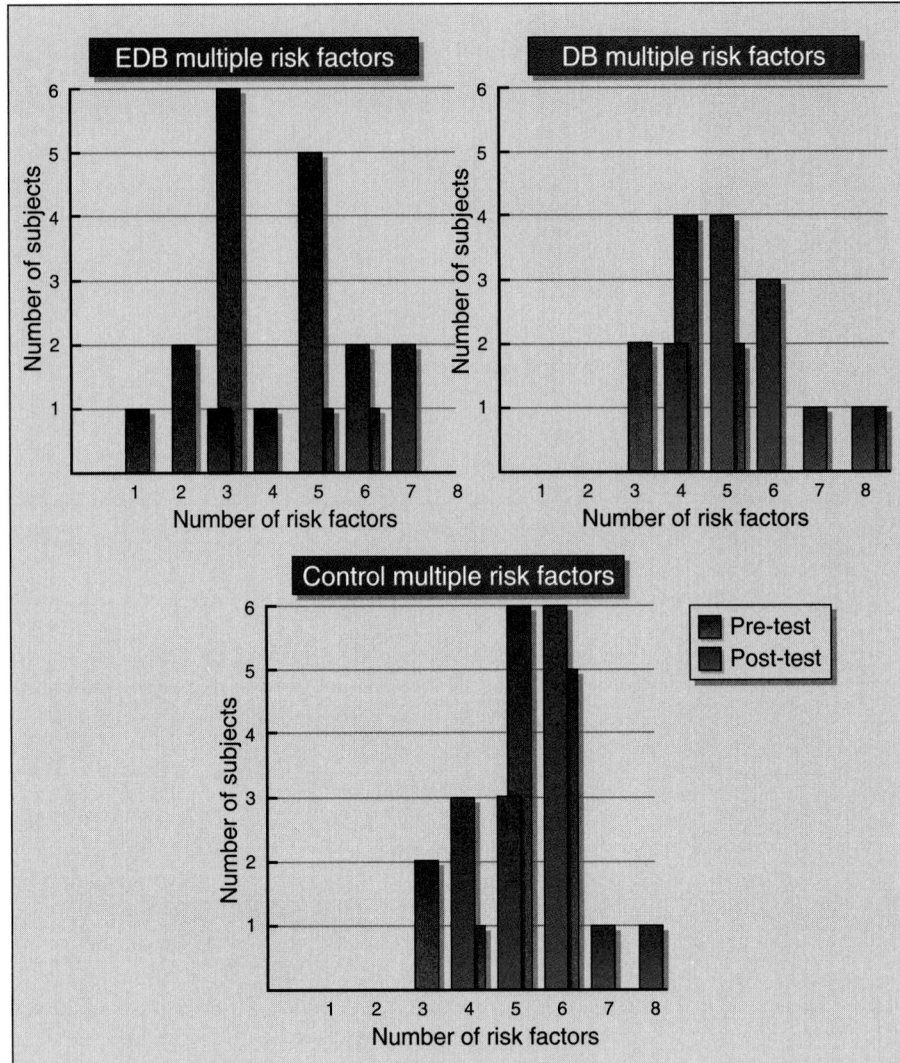

FIGURE 30.21
Multiple coronary heart disease risk factors for obese adolescents before and after treatment. DB, diet + behavior change group; EDB, exercise + diet + behavior change group. (From Becque, M.D., et al.: Coronary risk incidence of obese adolescents: reduction by exercise plus diet intervention. *Pediatrics*, 81:605, 1988.)

sedentary person with significant, undetected coronary heart disease, a sudden burst of strenuous exercise with its concomitant catecholamine release could impose an inordinate strain on the cardiovascular system. This risk can be reduced considerably with proper prior medical evaluation, which should minimally include a thorough personal health and family history and physical examination. The physical examination should emphasize signs and symptoms of cardiovascular disease and should include evaluation of blood pressure, resting 12-lead electrocardiogram, blood analysis, and possible cardiac murmurs and dysrhythmias, edema, chronic lung disease. For many people, an important part of the medical evaluation is the **exercise stress test**.

EXERCISE STRESS TESTING

The term "stress test" is generally used to describe the systematic use of exercise for two main purposes: (*a*) for ECG observations and (*b*) to evaluate the physiological adjustments to metabolic demands that exceed the resting requirement. The test can be a single-stage test such as the Master "2-step" bench stepping test, in which exercise intensity remains constant. However, multistage bicycle and treadmill tests are the most common means for exercise stress testing. These tests are **graded** for exercise intensity. They usually include at least several levels of 3 to 5 minutes of submaximal exercise and may bring the person to a self-imposed fatigue level. The graded nature of such testing allows exercise intensity to be increased in small increments to detect ischemic manifestations and rhythm disorders (e.g., anginal pain or ECG abnormalities). If heart disease is detected, a reliable and quantitative index of the person's level of functional impairment is then documented.[63] This enhances the objectivity of diagnosis and subsequent exercise prescription. For most screening purposes, the test need not be maximal, but it is desirable to bring a person to at least 85% of the age-predicted maximum heart rate.

TABLE 30.6
CHD RISK APPRAISAL, RISKO

Age	10 to 20	21 to 30	31 to 40	41 to 50	51 to 60	61 to 70 and over
	1	2	3	4	6	8
Heredity	No known history of heart disease	1 relative with cardiovascular disease over age 60	2 relatives with cardiovascular disease over age 60	1 relative with cardiovascular disease under age 60	2 relatives with cardiovascular disease under age 60	3 relatives with cardiovascular disease under age 60
	1	2	3	4	6	7
Weight	More than 5 lb below standard weight	−5 to +5 lb standard weight	6–20 lb overweight	21–35 lb overweight	36–50 lb overweight	51–65 lb overweight
	0	1	2	3	5	7
Tobacco smoking	Nonsmoker	Cigar and/or pipe	10 cigarettes or less per day	20 cigarettes per day	30 cigarettes per day	40 cigarettes per day or more
	0	1	2	4	6	10
Exercise	Intensive occupational and recreational exertion	Moderate occupational and recreational exertion	Sedentary work and intense recreational exertion	Sedentary occupational and moderate recreational exertion	Sedentary work and light recreational exertion	Complete lack of all exercise
	1	2	3	5	6	8
Cholesterol or fat % in diet	Cholesterol below 180 mg/dL Diet contains no animal or solid fats	Cholesterol 181–205 mg/dL Diet contains 10% animal or solid fats	Cholesterol 206–230 mg/dL Diet contains 20% animal or solid fats	Cholesterol 231-255 mg/dL Diet contains 30% animal or solid fats	Cholesterol 256-280 mg/dL Diet contains 40% animal or solid fats	Cholesterol 281–300 mg/dL Diet contains 50% animal or solid fats
	1	2	3	4	5	7
Blood pressure	100 systolic	120 systolic	140 systolic	160 systolic	180 systolic	200 or over systolic
	1	2	3	4	6	8
Sex	Female under age 40	Female aged 40–50	Female over age 50	Male	Stocky male	Bald stocky male
	1	2	3	4	6	7

Explanation of variables: *Heredity*—count parents, brothers, and sisters who have had a heart attack or stroke; *Smoking*—if you inhale deeply and smoke a cigarette way down, add one point to your score. Do not subtract because you think you do not inhale or smoke only a half inch on a cigarette; *Exercise*—lower your score one point if you exercise regularly and frequently; *Cholesterol/Saturated Fat Intake*—a cholesterol blood level is best. If you have not had a blood test recently, then estimate honestly the percentage of solid fats you eat. These are usually of animal origin (lard, cream, butter, and beef and lamb fat). If you eat much saturated fat, your cholesterol level will probably be high; *Blood Pressure*—if you have no recent reading but have passed an insurance or general medical examination, chances are you have a systolic blood pressure level of 140 or less; *Sex*—this takes into account the fact that men have from 6 to 10 times more heart attacks than women of child-bearing age. (Adapted from the Michigan Heart Association.) **Relative Risk Category:** 6–11, risk well below average; 12–17, risk below average; 18–24, average risk; 25–31, moderate risk; 32–40, high risk; 41–62, very high risk, see your physician.

A resting ECG should precede the exercise test to establish that the person can engage safely in subsequent graded exercise. The ECG at rest also provides the important baseline to compare exercise results. Stress testing is limited, however, by its inability to show the extent and specific location of the disease. Also, 25 to 40% of the people with relatively advanced CHD have a normal stress test. In reality, however, they have significant blockage in one or more coronary arteries.

WHY BE STRESS TESTED?

There are at least six reasons to include stress testing in an overall CHD evaluation:

- To establish a diagnosis of overt heart disease and to screen for possible "silent" coronary disease in seemingly healthy men and women. Approximately 30% of people with confirmed CHD have a normal ECG at rest. Approximately 70% of these abnormalities are uncovered with graded exercise testing.
- To reproduce and assess exercise-related chest symptoms. In many instances, individuals over 40 years of age suffer chest or related pain in the left shoulder or arm upon physical exertion. Proper ECG analysis during an exercise stress test helps identify myocardial abnormalities and provides a more precise diagnosis of exercise-induced pain.
- To screen candidates for preventive and cardiac rehabilitative exercise programs. Stress-test results provide the

framework to design an exercise program that is within a person's current functional capacity and health status. Repeated testing assesses progress and functional adaptations with regular exercise and determines the need for program modification.

- To detect an abnormal blood pressure response. It is not uncommon for an individual with normal resting blood pressure to show greater-than-normal increases in systolic blood pressure with exercise. Exercise hypertension may signify developing cardiovascular complications.
- To monitor the effectiveness of therapeutic interventions (drug, surgical, and dietary) designed to improve heart disease status and cardiovascular function. For example, the success of coronary bypass surgery can be detected by a patient's adjustment to exercise and ability to successfully reach a target exercise heart rate without complications.
- To define the functional aerobic capacity and evaluate its deviation from normal standards.

WHO SHOULD BE STRESS TESTED?

A classification system by age and health status for screening and supervisory procedures for use in exercise testing is shown in Table 30.7. These standards conform to policies and practices of the American College of Sports Medicine and the American Medical Association.[2] The prudent guidelines are as follows:

- If a person is younger than 35 years of age with no previous history of cardiovascular disease and no primary risk

---

TABLE 30.7
CLASSIFICATION BY AGE AND HEALTH STATUS FOR MEN AND WOMEN WHO REQUIRE DIFFERENT SCREENING AND SUPERVISORY PROCEDURES BEFORE AND DURING A STRESS TEST

Age (y)	Patient Health Status	Evaluation and Required Medical Clearance	12-Lead Restng ECG	Personnel Involved During Stress Test
<35	No known primary CHD risk factors;[a] may have secondary CHD risk factors[b]	During past 2 years, signed statement	Not required	No test required
35–40	No known primary CHD risk factors; may have secondary CHD risk factors	During past 2 years, signed statement	Required	Exercise technician; exercise physiologist; M.D. in area
>40	No known primary CHD risk factors; may have secondary CHD risk factors	During past 2 years, signed statement	Required	Exercise technician; exercise physiologist; M.D. in area
Any age	Documented CHD; hypertension; suspected CHD	During past 2 years, signed statement	Required	Exercise technician; exercise physiologist; M.D. conducting test

[a]Primary risk factors: Hypertension, hyperlipidemia, cigarette smoking, and physical inactivity.
[b]Secondary risk factors: Family history, obesity, and diabetes mellitus.

factors (and has had a medical evaluation within the past 2 years), it is generally acceptable to begin an exercise program without special medical clearance. These people may be stress tested for purposes of functional evaluation and for preparing the exercise prescription by a trained exercise specialist.

- If a person is younger than 35 years of age but has evidence of CHD or a significant combination of risk factors, he or she should be medically cleared before beginning an exercise program. Clearance should include a physician-supervised graded exercise test.

- For all adults older than 35 years of age, medical evaluation is advised before any major increase in exercise habits. This medical evaluation should include an ECG monitored before, during, and in recovery from a graded exercise test and supervised preferably by an internist or cardiologist.

EXERCISE-INDUCED INDICATORS OF CHD

Several clues to CHD become apparent during exercise because physical activity creates the greatest demand on coronary blood flow.

ANGINA PECTORIS

Approximately 30% of the initial manifestations of CHD take the form of chest-related pain called angina pectoris. This is a temporary but painful condition that indicates that coronary blood flow (oxygen supply) has momentarily reached a critically low level. This myocardial ischemia (usually the result of restricted coronary circulation caused by atherosclerosis) stimulates sensory nerves in the walls of the coronary arteries and myocardium. The resulting pain or discomfort is generally felt in the upper chest region, although it is frequently characterized by a sensation of pressure or constriction in the left shoulder, neck, jaw, or left arm. Many people also report sensations of "being smothered" during an angina episode. In addition to pain, cardiac performance also is impaired with angina. This depressed my-

ocardial function is accompanied by a reduced stroke volume and cardiac output and generally impaired contractility of the left ventricle. After a few minutes of inactivity, the pain usually subsides with no permanent damage to the heart muscle.

ELECTROCARDIOGRAPHIC DISORDERS

Alterations in the heart's normal pattern of electrical activity often indicate insufficient oxygen supply to the myocardium. These electrical "clues," however, are rarely observed until the metabolic (and blood flow) requirements are increased above the resting level.

The ECG tracing illustrated in Figure 30.22 is a plot of the dynamic electrical activity of the myocardium in millivolts (mV). Normal ECG paper is divided into 1-mm and 5-mm squares. Horizontally, each small square is equivalent to 0.04 seconds (with standard paper speed of 25 mm/s); each large square represents 0.2 seconds. On the vertical axis, a small square indicates a 0.1-mV deflection with a calibration of $10 \text{ mm} \cdot \text{mV}^{-1}$. One normal heart beat, or cardiac cycle, consists of five major electrical waves that are labeled P, Q, R, S, and T (Fig. 30.22A). The P wave is the electrical impulse or wave of depolarization associated with atrial contraction. The Q, R, and S waves are considered as a unit that represents the depolarization of the ventricles immediately before their physical contraction. Collectively, this is known as the QRS complex. The T wave is generated by the repolarization of the ventricles. Although it is not known why the S-T segment becomes depressed, this deviation from normal is closely correlated with other indicators of CHD including coronary artery narrowing. *Individuals with significant S-T-segment depression usually have severe and extensive obstruction in one or more coronary arteries.* In addition, the amount of S-T segment depression is related directly to the chances of dying from CHD. In one study, persons with 1- to 2-mm S-T segment depression during exercise had a 4.6-fold increase in mortality from CHD, whereas those with more than 2-mm depression had a 19.1-fold greater risk of death.[112]

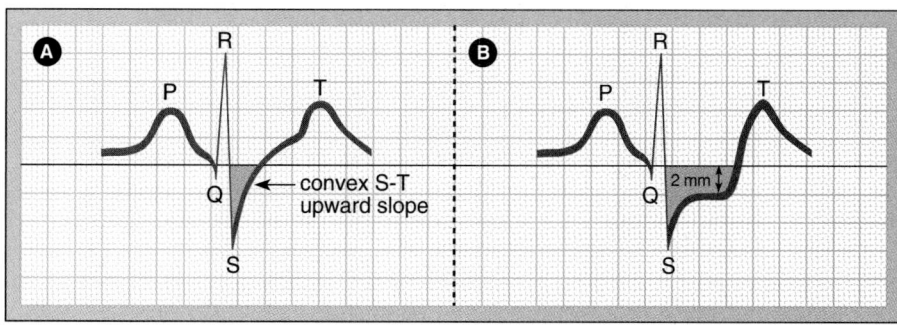

FIGURE 30.22

A, Tracing that illustrates the normal ECG complex. The arrow points to the slightly convex and upward sloping S-T segment. **B,** Tracing shows an abnormal horizontal S-T segment depression (shaded area) of 2 mm measured from a stable baseline.

CARDIAC RHYTHM ABNORMALITIES

Although exercise can induce abnormalities in the S-T segment of the ECG, it also provides an effective way to observe aspects of cardiac rhythm. One significant alteration in cardiac rhythm (arrhythmia) with exercise is the occurrence of a **premature ventricular contraction** or **PVC.** In this situation, the ventricles are not stimulated by the normal passage of the wave of depolarization through the atrioventricular node. Instead, portions of the ventricle become spontaneously depolarized. This disorganized electrical activity shows as an "extra" ventricular beat or QRS complex on the ECG that occurs without being preceded by a P wave, which indicates atrial depolarization.

Premature ventricular contractions in exercise generally herald the presence of severe ischemic atherosclerotic heart disease, often involving two or more major coronary vessels. This specific electrical instability of the myocardium during exercise has a greater predictive value than S-T segment depression for the diagnosis of CHD. The incidence of sudden death owing to **ventricular fibrillation** is generally about six to ten times as high in heart disease patients with frequent PVCs as in patients without this abnormality. With fibrillation, the ventricles are unable to contract in a unified manner. As a result, blood is not pumped effectively and cardiac output falls dramatically. Unless the normal ventricular rhythm is reestablished, the outcome is sudden death.

OTHER INDICES OF CHD

Two useful non-ECG indices of possible CHD are the blood pressure and heart rate responses to exercise.

- **Hypertensive response:** During a graded exercise test, there is a normal, progressive increase in systolic blood pressure from approximately 120 mm Hg to 160 to 190 mm Hg during peak exercise. The change in diastolic pressure is generally less than 10 mm Hg. For some individuals, however, exercise may cause the systolic blood pressure to rise well above 200 mm Hg, whereas the diastolic pressure can increase to 100 to 150 mm Hg. This abnormal hypertensive response can be a significant clue to cardiovascular disease.
- **Hypotensive response:** The inability of blood pressure to increase during exercise also may reflect cardiovascular malfunction. For example, failure of the systolic blood pressure to increase by at least 20 or 30 mm Hg during exercise testing may reflect diminished cardiac reserve.
- **Heart rate response:** A rapid, large increase in heart rate (tachycardia) early during exercise often is a harbinger of cardiac problems. Likewise, abnormally low exercise heart rates (bradycardia) may reflect unhealthy function of the heart's sinus node. Also, the inability of the heart rate to increase during exercise, especially when accompanied by extreme fatigue, may indicate cardiac strain and heart disease.

STRESS TEST PROTOCOLS

Many stress test protocols exist. In a national survey of 1,400 exercise stress test centers, 71% reported using the treadmill, 17% used the bicycle ergometer, and only 12% tested with step tests.[143] Of the treadmill tests, the Bruce protocol was used in 65.5% and the protocol designed by Balke was used in approximately 10%.

THE BRUCE AND BALKE TREADMILL TESTS

The Bruce and Balke graded exercise tests have been described in Chapter 11, p. 202. Each has advantages and disadvantages. For example, the Bruce test has a more abrupt increase in exercise intensity between stages. Although this may be beneficial for sensitivity to ischemic ECG responses (see p. 661), it also means the patient must tolerate the increased level of exercise. Both protocols start at relatively high levels of exercise for cardiac patients and thus have been modified. For the Bruce protocol, lower initial exercise levels were added, whereas a preliminary 2- to 3-minute stage (2 mph, 0% grade) was included in the Balke test.

The choice of a specific exercise test must be made based on the particular group to be evaluated for health, age, and fitness status. Generally, a stress test should start at a low level with increments in exercise intensity every 2 or 3 minutes. A warmup should be provided, either separately or incorporated into the test. The total duration of the test should be at least 8 minutes. A test that is much longer than 15 minutes is not needed, because most important cardiac and physiologic data can be obtained within this time.

BICYCLE ERGOMETER TESTS

Bicycle ergometers have distinct advantages for exercise stress testing. In contrast to the treadmill, power output on the ergometer is independent of the person's body mass and is easily calculated and regulated. Most ergometers are portable, safe, and relatively inexpensive. There are two different types of bicycle ergometers: (*a*) electrically braked ergometers and (*b*) weight-loaded, friction-type ergometers. With electrically braked ergometers, the preselected power output remains fixed within a range of pedaling frequencies. With weight-loaded ergometers, power output is directly related to the frictional resistance and rate of pedaling.

The same general guidelines used for treadmill testing apply to graded exercise on the bicycle ergometer. Power output on a bicycle ergometer is usually expressed in $kgm \cdot min^{-1}$ or watts ($1 W = 6.12 kgm \cdot min^{-1}$). Test protocols have 2- to 4-minute stages of graded exercise with an initial resistance between 0 and 15 or 30 watts; power output is generally increased in 15- to 30-watt increments per stage. Pedaling rate for weight-loaded ergometers is usually set at 50 or 60 revolutions per minute.

ARM-CRANK ERGOMETERS

Arm cranking also can be used for exercise stress testing. As discussed in Chapters 15 and 17, arm exercise results in lower $\dot{V}O_2$max values by as much as 30%, and maximum heart rate is generally 10 to 15 beats per minute lower compared to treadmill or bicycle exercise. In addition, blood pressure cannot be readily measured during arm-crank exercise. Furthermore, blood pressure, heart rate, and oxygen uptake values are higher during submaximal arm cranking compared to the same level of power output performed with the legs. Nevertheless, it is possible to use the same type of graded protocols developed for leg cycling tests when an evaluation of the patient's response to upper-body exercise is desired. Of course, the starting frictional resistance is less and the incremental power outputs must be adjusted accordingly.

OTHER EXERCISE DIAGNOSTIC TESTS

Although the conventional exercise ECG stress test has been used widely, it is not without limitations. As discussed on page 662, a significant number of patients can be misdiagnosed regarding the presence or absence of CHD by stress testing. This has led to the development of two other procedures that use radionuclide methods for detecting CHD. One of the methods, thallium-201 imaging, assesses myocardial perfusion at the small vessel level and the other, radionuclide angiocardiography, assesses coronary artery blood flow and ventricular function. Both of these techniques can be used during exercise.[52, 54]

GUIDELINES FOR STRESS TESTING

The following guidelines should be used for terminating a stress test. Each of the symptoms indicated generally reflects extreme cardiovascular strain, which could be dangerous to the patient.

- Repeated presence of PVCs.
- Progressive angina pain regardless of the presence or absence of ECG abnormalities.
- ECG changes that include the presence of S-T segment depression of 2 mm or more, continuous bigeminal or trigeminal ectopic ventricular complexes, and evidence of atrioventricular conduction disturbances (AV block).
- An extremely rapid increase in heart rate, which may reflect a severely compromised cardiovascular response.
- Failure of heart rate or blood pressure to increase with graded exercise, or a progressive drop in systolic blood pressure with increasing exercise intensity.

- An increase in diastolic pressure of 20 mm Hg or more or a rise above 110 mm Hg.
- Headache, blurred vision, pale and clammy skin, or extreme fatigue.
- Marked dyspnea (breathlessness) or cyanosis.
- Dizziness or near fainting.
- Nausea.

Persons who exhibit these responses during a stress test require further medical evaluation and should be excluded from unsupervised exercise programs pending such an evaluation. Patients who complete the stress test without an abnormal ECG response or other evidence of CHD can be medically cleared for unsupervised exercise that does not exceed the intensity of exercise reached during the stress test.

IS STRESS TESTING SAFE?

The yearly death rate during a stress test is between 2 and 12% for men who show clinical evidence of heart disease. Such broad variation in expected mortality is directly related to the number and severity of diseased coronary arteries. Generally, if a person has had a previous myocardial infarction or episode of angina, the risk of having another episode or dying is increased 10 to 30 times above normal. The elevated risk for death among heart disease patients raises some question as to the advisability of stress testing adults, especially patients who have had myocardial infarctions or who have demonstrated other heart disease symptoms or significant risk profiles.

Reports have indicated that in approximately 170,000 submaximum and maximum stress tests, only 16 high-risk but apparently healthy patients suffered coronary episodes during testing. This represented about one person per 10,000 or approximately 0.01% of the total group.[45, 113] A report of more than 9,000 stress tests showed no cardiovascular episodes for subjects with an elevated heart disease risk.[128] Other researchers have determined that the risk of having a coronary episode for healthy middle-aged adults during a maximum stress test was about 1 in 3,000.[92] The stress-test risk is generally about 6 to 12 times higher than normal for most middle-aged adults. For patients with documented CHD, the risk of a cardiovascular episode in stress testing may increase to as much as 30 to 60 times higher than normal. The American College of Sports Medicine lists specific absolute and relative contraindications for administering an exercise stress test.[2]

OUTCOMES OF A STRESS TEST

The value of a stress test depends on its ability to detect the existence of heart disease. More specifically, the **sensitivity** of a stress test refers to the percentage of people with actual disease who have an abnormal test result. No test is perfect for diagnosing heart disease. There are four possible outcomes from a graded exercise stress test:

- **True-Positive:** The test results are correct in diagnosing a person with heart disease (the test is successful).
- **False-Negative:** The test results are normal, but the person actually has heart disease (the test is unsuccessful—a person with heart disease goes undiagnosed).
- **True-Negative:** The test results are normal and the person does not have heart disease (the test is successful).
- **False-Positive:** The test results are abnormal but the person has no heart disease (the test is unsuccessful—a healthy person is diagnosed with heart disease).

It is estimated that false-negative results occur with stress testing 25% of the time and false-positive results occur 15% of the time.[44] Both a false-negative and a false-positive test can have dramatic ramifications, particularly a false-negative result. Whenever a stress test indicates the presence of heart disease, secondary tests such as thallium imaging or angiocardiography are performed to confirm the diagnosis. Similarly, because the result of a stress test is normal does not fully rule out the existence of heart disease. The predictive value of an abnormal stress test is much greater than the predictive value of a normal test.

EXERCISE PRESCRIPTION

Heart rate and oxygen uptake (or exercise intensity) data obtained during the stress test are used to formulate the exercise prescription. This is an individualized exercise program based on the person's current fitness and health status, with emphasis on intensity, frequency, duration, and type of exercise. Such an approach is important because many people who start exercising do not recognize their limitations and may exercise above a prudent level.

PRACTICAL ILLUSTRATION

A practical approach that permits the functional translation of treadmill or bicycle ergometer exercise test responses to the exercise prescription is illustrated in Figure 30.23.[51] The results depicted are for a male cardiac patient and were generated from an algorithm that used exercise test responses from the Bruce treadmill protocol for level-ground ambulation. During the Bruce test, the heart rate (A) was plotted as a function of time. A mathematical line of "best fit" was then applied to the heart rate data, and line B was drawn through the data points. A target zone for heart rate was calculated as 60 to 75% based on the maximum heart rate of 167 beats per minute (shaded portion, C). The individualized prescription is then detailed for pace (14.0 to 15.4 mi · min^{-1}, D) and METs (3.9 to 5.9 mL · kg^{-1} · min^{-1}, E). The acceptable range of exercise intensity in area C, based on heart rate response during the graded exercise test, includes the following recreational activities: bicycling, touch football, canoeing, alpine skiing, aerobics, volleyball, tennis and bad-minton, swimming, skating, and water-skiing. This quantitative method of exercise prescription may improve the effectiveness of the exercise prescription for the healthy previously sedentary individual, as well as the patient with known cardiovascular disease.

IMPROVEMENTS IN CHD PATIENTS

With a properly prescribed and monitored exercise program, many cardiac patients can safely improve their functional capacity to a degree comparable to a healthy person of the same age.[149] In some instances, even clinical symptoms such as ECG abnormalities are improved or even eliminated. This occurs because many individuals respond to exercise training with physiologic adjustments that actually reduce the work of the heart at any given external exercise load. For example, reduced exercise heart rate and blood pressure (two major determinants of myocardial workload and oxygen uptake) and improved myocardial contractility reduces myocardial effort. This delays the onset of anginal pain, allowing work of greater intensity and duration. For individuals whose occupations predominantly require arm work, this musculature should be exercised in training, because many of the benefits of physical conditioning are highly specific and generally are not transferable from one muscle group to another.

THE PROGRAM

Exercise programs for both prevention and rehabilitation are most effective when they are individualized. There is greater adherence to regimens of low- to moderate-intensity exercise than to programs of intense physical activity.[91] The exercises prescribed usually consist of rhythmic general movements that stimulate cardiovascular improvement such as walking, jogging, running, cycling, rope skipping, swimming, or dynamic calisthenics.

The guidelines for making decisions concerning frequency, duration, and intensity of training are discussed in Chapter 21. Ideally, the personalized exercise prescription should include a recommendation for weight loss and dietary modification (if necessary), warm-up and cool-down exercises, and a developmental flexibility and strength program. Some heart disease patients show a reduced heart rate response to exercise with a corresponding reduction in maximum heart rate. For these individuals, the use of target heart rates based on an age-predicted maximum for the general population will grossly overestimate the appropriate training intensity. This supports the wisdom of exercise stress testing each patient to a symptom-limited maximum and then formulating the exercise prescription from the actual heart rate data.

Level of Supervision. The American College of Sports Medicine has categorized several types of exercise

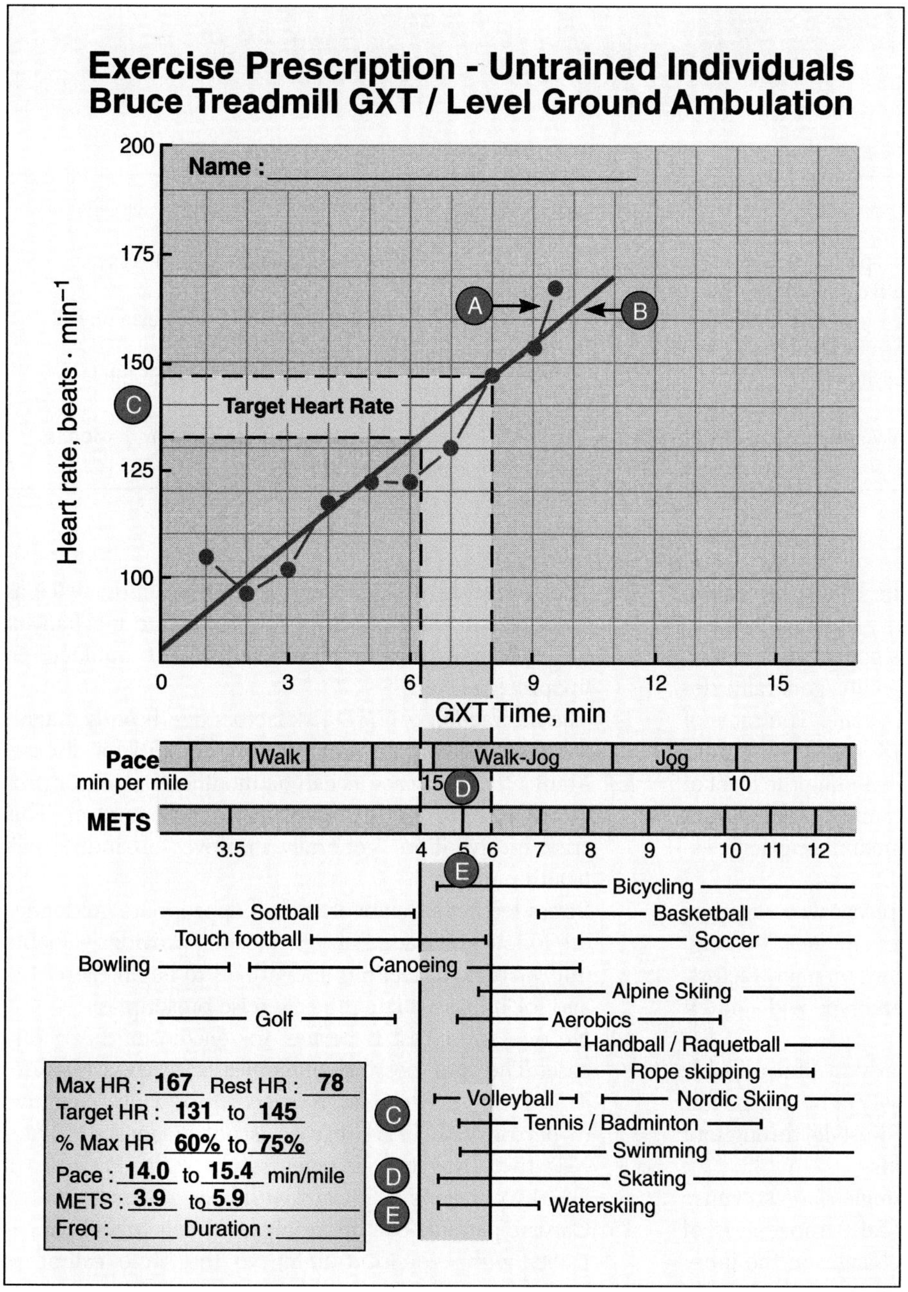

Exercise Prescription - Untrained Individuals
Bruce Treadmill GXT / Level Ground Ambulation

Name : _____

Heart rate, beats · min⁻¹

Target Heart Rate

GXT Time, min

Pace min per mile | Walk | Walk-Jog | Jog

METS 3.5 | 4 5 6 7 8 9 10 11 12

Bicycling
Basketball
Softball
Touch football
Soccer
Bowling — Canoeing
Alpine Skiing
Golf — Aerobics
Handball / Raquetball
Rope skipping
Volleyball — Nordic Skiing
Tennis / Badminton
Swimming
Skating
Waterskiing

Max HR : **167** Rest HR : **78**
Target HR : **131** to **145**
% Max HR **60%** to **75%**
Pace : **14.0** to **15.4** min/mile
METS : **3.9** to **5.9**
Freq :_____ Duration :_____

FIGURE 30.23
Exercise prescription based on functional translation algorithm for level ground ambulation. (Used with permission of Dr. Carl Foster, Department of Medicine, Cardiovascular Disease Section, Sinai Samaritan Center, Milwaukee, WI.)

programs with specific criteria for entry and supervision, as shown in Table 30.8. These programs are classified as **unsupervised** and **supervised** with four subdivisions of the supervised category. Unsupervised programs are for asymptomatic participants of any age with functional capacities of at least 8 METs with no known major risk factors. The supervised exercise programs are geared to people with different and specific needs. These include asymptomatic physically active or inactive persons of any age with CHD risk factors but no known disease (B-4) and symptomatic individuals,

(B1-3) including those with recent onset of CHD and those who report a change in disease status.

■ SUMMARY ■

1. Physical activity epidemiology evaluates the nature, extent, and demographics of exercise participation in a large population. These data often are linked to the occurrence of disease and other health-related outcomes.

TABLE 30.8
TYPES OF EXERCISE PROGRAMS RELATED TO PATIENT SYMPTOMS

Type	Participants	Entry MET Level	Supervision
A. Unsupervised	Asymptomatic	8+	None
B. Supervised			
1. Inpatient	All symptomatics—post myocardial infarction, postoperative, pulmonary disease	3	Supervised ambulatory therapy
2. Outpatient	All symptomatics—post myocardial infarction, postoperative pulmonary disease	3+	Exercise specialist, physician on call
3. In-Home	Symptomatic + asymptomatic	>3–5	Unsupervised; periodic hospital reevaluation
4. Community	Symptomatic + asymptomatic, 6–8 wk post infarct, 4–8 wk postoperative	>5	Exercise program director + exercise specialist

2. Only about 10 to 15% of adults in the United States obtain sufficient regular physical activity of an intensity to impart significant health and fitness benefits.

3. Physiologic and performance capability generally declines after approximately 30 years of age. The rates of decline in the various functions differ and are significantly influenced by many factors, including the level of physical activity. Regular physical training enables older persons to retain higher levels of functional capacity, especially cardiovascular function.

4. Regardless of age, regular vigorous physical activity produces measurable physiologic improvements. The magnitude of these improvements depends on many factors, including initial fitness status, age, and type and amount of training.

5. Participation in vigorous activity early in life probably contributes little to increased longevity or health in later life. However, a physically active lifestyle throughout life confers significant health benefits.

6. Coronary heart disease is the single largest cause of death in the Western world. The pathogenesis of this disease involves degenerative changes in the inner lining of the arterial wall that result in progressive occlusion.

7. Numerous factors have been identified that make individuals more susceptible to developing CHD. The major risk factors are age and sex, elevated blood lipids, hypertension, cigarette smoking, obesity, physical inactivity, diet, heredity, and ECG abnormalities during rest and exercise.

8. Generally, a cholesterol level of 200 mg · dL^{-1} or lower is considered desirable; many experts recommend lower values as being most healthful.

9. The distribution of the various lipoproteins, especially HDL and LDL cholesterol, is a more powerful predictor of heart disease risk than simply the total quantity of plasma cholesterol.

10. The risk of death from heart disease is almost twice as great for smokers as for nonsmokers. One mechanism for risk may be the adverse effects of smoking on lipoprotein levels.

11. The interaction of CHD risk factors significantly magnifies their individual effects on the possibility for disease.

12. Many CHD risk factors can be modified by proper programs of nutrition, exercise, and weight control. This "risk intervention" generally improves an individual's health outlook.

13. Stress testing is relatively safe if appropriate guidelines are followed. Graded exercise testing provides valuable information for clearing individuals to begin exercising and for individualizing the exercise prescription.

14. No one stress test is perfect for diagnosing heart disease. The four possible outcomes of a stress test are: True-Positive (the test is successful); False-Negative (a person with heart disease is not diagnosed); True-Negative (the test is successful); False-Positive (a healthy person is diagnosed with heart disease).

15. Cardiac patients can often improve their functional capacity with exercise training to the same extent as healthy people of the same age.

■ REFERENCES ■

1. Abbott, R.F., et al.: Cardiovascular risk factors and graded treadmill exercise endurance in healthy adults: the Framingham Offspring Study. *Am.J. Cardiol.,* 63:342, 1989.

2. American College of Sports Medicine: *Guidelines for Exercise, Testing and Prescription.* 4th ed. Philadelphia, Lea & Febiger, 1991.

2a. Anderson, J.W., et al.: Meta-analysis of the effects of soy protein intake on serum lipids. *N. Engl.J. Med.,* 333:276, 1995.

3. Andersen, W.G.: Further studies on the longevity of Yale athletes. *Med. Times,* 44:75, 1916.

4. Aniansson, A., et al.: Muscle morphology, enzymatic activity, and muscle strength in elderly men: a follow-up study. *Muscle Nerve,* 9:585, 1986.

5. Babcock, M.A., et al.: Effects of aerobic endurance training on gas exchange kinetics of older men. *Med. Sci. Sports Exerc.*, 26:447, 1994.

6. Babcock, M.A., et al.: Exercise on-transient gas exchange kinetics are slowed as a function of age. *Med. Sci. Sports Exerc.*, 26:440, 1994.

7. Badenhop, D.T., et al.: Physiological adjustments to higher- or lower-intensity exercise in elders. *Med. Sci. Sports Exerc.*, 15:496, 1983.

8. Barrett, J.H.: *Gerontological Psychology.* Springfield, IL, Charles C Thomas, 1972.

9. Becque, M.D., et al.: Coronary risk incidence of obese adolescents: reduction by exercise plus diet intervention. *Pediatrics*, 81:605, 1988.

10. Blair, S.N.: Physical activity, physical fitness, and health. *Res.Q. Exerc. Sport*, 64:365, 1993.

11. Blair, S.N., et al.: Physical fitness and all-cause mortality: a prospective study of healthy men and women. *JAMA*, 262:2395, 1989.

11a. Blair, S.N., et al.: Changes in physical fitness and all cause mortality: a prospective study of healthy and unhealthy men. *JAMA*, 273:1093, 1995.

12. Booth, F.W., et al.: Effect of aging on human skeletal muscle and motor function. *Med. Sci. Sports Exerc.*, 26:556, 1994.

13. Bouchard, C., and Shephard, R.J.: Physical activity, fitness, and health: the model and key concepts. In *Physical Activity, Fitness and Health.* Edited by C. Bouchard and R.J. Shepherd. Champaign, IL, Human Kinetics, 1994.

14. Bourey, R.E., and Santoro, S.A.: Interactions of exercise, coagulation, platets, and fibrinolysis—a brief review. *Med. Sci. Sports Exerc.*, 20: 439, 1988.

15. Brill, P.A., et al.: The impact of athleticism on exercise habits, physical fitness, and coronary heart disease risk factors in middle-aged men. *Res.Q. Exerc. Sport*, 60:209, 1989.

16. Brooks C.M.: Adult participation in physical activities requiring moderate to high levels of energy expenditure. *Phys. Sportsmed.*, 15:118, 1987.

17. Brooks, C.M.: Leisure time physical activity assessment of American adults through analysis of time diaries collected in 1981. *Am.J. Public Health*, 77:455, 1987.

18. Brooks, S.V., and Faulkner, J.A.: Skeletal muscle weakness in old age: underlying mechanisms. *Med. Sci. Sports Exerc.*, 26:432, 1994.

19. Buskirk, E.R., and Hodgson, J.L.: Age and aerobic power: The rate of change in men and women. *Fed. Proc.*, 46:1824, 1987.

20. Cartee, G.D.: Aging skeletal muscle: response to exercise. *Exerc. Sport Sci. Rev.*, 22:91, 1994.

21. Cartee, G.D.: Influence of age on skeletal muscle glucose transport and glycogen metabolism. *Med. Sci. Sports Exerc.*, 26:577, 1994.

22. Casazza, G.A., et al.: Exercise training and reduction in some coronary risk factors in female cigarette smokers. *Am.J. Cardiol.*, 75:85, 1995.

23. Casperson, C.J.: Physical activity epidemiology: concepts, methods, and applications to exercise science. In *Exercise and Sport Sciences Reviews.* Vol. 17. Edited by K.B. Pandolf. New York, Macmillan, 1989.

23a. Caspersen, C.J., and Merritt, R.K.: Physical activity trends among 26 states, 1986-1990. *Med. Sci. Sports Exerc.*, 27:713, 1995.

24. Caspersen C.J., et al.: Status of the 1990 physical fitness and exercise objectives—evidence from NHIS 1985. *Public Health Rep.*, 101:587, 1986.

25. Centers for Disease Control and Prevention. Prevalence of sedentary lifestyle. *MMWR Morb. Mortal. Wkly. Rep.*, 42:576, 1993.

26. Chandrashekar, Y., and Anand, L.C.: Exercise as a coronary protection process. *Am. Heart J.*, 122:1723, 1991.

27. Charette, S.L., et al.: Muscle hypertrophy response to resistance training in older women. *J. Appl. Physiol.*, 70:1912, 1991.

28. Chien, S., et al.: Longitudinal measurements of blood volume and essential body mass in human subjects. *J. Appl. Physiol.*, 39:818, 1975.

29. Clarkson, P.M.: The effect of age and activity level on simple and fractionated response time. *Eur.J. Appl. Physiol.*, 40:17, 1978.

30. Clarkson, P.M.: The relationship of age and level of physical activity with the fractionated components of patellar reflex time. *J. Gerontol.*, 3:650, 1978.

31. Coggan, A.R., et al.: Histochemical and enzymatic comparison of the gastrocnemius muscle of young and elderly men and women. *J. Gerontol. Biol. Sci.*, 46B:71, 1992.

32. Coggan, A.R., et al.: Skeletal muscle adaptations to endurance training in 60- to 70 yr-old men and women. *J. Appl. Physiol.*, 72:1780, 1992.

33. Cress, M.E., et al.: Effect of training on $\dot{V}O_2$max, thigh strength, and muscle morphology in septuagenarian women. *Med. Sci. Sports Exerc.*, 23:752, 1991.

34. Crews, D.J., and Landers, D.M.: A meta-analytic review of aerobic fitness and reactivity to psychosocial stressors. *Med. Sci. Sports Exerc.*, 19:S114, 1987.

35. Cunningham, D.A., et al.: Gas exchange dynamics with sinusoidal work in young and elderly women. *Respir. Physiol.*, 91:43, 1993.

36. Dehn, M.M., et al.: Longitudinal variations in maximal oxygen intake with age and activity. *J. Appl. Physiol.*, 33:805, 1972.

37. Després, J.-P., et al.: Physical activity and coronary heart disease risk factors during childhood and adolescence. In *Exercise and Sport Sciences Reviews.* Vol. 18. Edited by K.B. Pandolf and J.O. Holloszy. Baltimore, Williams & Wilkins, 1990.

38. Doherty, T.J., et al.: Effects of motor unit losses on strength in older men and women. *J. Appl. Physiol.*, 74:868,1993.

39. Duncan, J.J., et al.: Women walking for health and fitness: how much is enough? *JAMA*, 266:3295, 1992.

40. Durstine, J.L., and Haskell, W.L.: Effects of exercise training on plasma lipids and lipoproteins. *Exerc. Sport Sci. Rev.*, 22:477, 1994.

41. Ehsani, A.A., et al.: Exercise training improves left ventricular systolic function in older men. *Circulation*, 83:96, 1991.

42. Ekelund, L., et al. Physical fitness as a predictor of cardiovascular mortality in asymptomatic North American men: the Lipid Research Clinics mortality follow-up study. *N. Engl.J. Med.*, 319:1379, 1988.

43. El-Sayed, M.S.: Fibrinolytic activity and hemostatic parameter response after resistance exercise. *Med. Sci. Sports Exerc.*, 25:597, 1993.

44. Epstein, S.E.: Implications of probability analysis on the strategy used for non-invasive detection of coronary artery disease. *Am.J. Cardiol.*, 46:491, 1980.

45. Epstein, S.E., and Maron, B.J.: Sudden death and the competitive athlete: perspectives on preparticipation screening studies. *J. Am. Coll. Cardiol.*, 7:220, 1986.

46. Fang, C.-L., et al.: Exercise modality and selected coronary risk factors: a multivariate approach. *Med. Sci. Sports Exerc.*, 20:455, 1988.

47. Faulkner, J.A., et al.: Skeletal muscle weakness and fatigue in old age: underlying mechanisms. In *Annual Review of Gerontology and Geriatrics.* Edited by V.J. Cristofalo and M.P. Lawton. New York, Springer, 1991.

48. Fiatarone, M.A., et al.: Exercise training and nutritional supplementation for physical frailty in very elderly people. *N. Engl.J. Med.*, 330:1769, 1994.

49. Fleg, J.L., and Lakatta, E.G.: Role of muscle mass in the age-associated decrease in $\dot{V}O_2$max. *J. Appl. Physiol.*, 65:1147, 1988.

49a. Fleg, S.L., et al.: Impact of age on the cardiovascular response to dynamic upright exercise in healthy men and women. *J. Appl. Physiol.*, 78:890, 1995.

50. Fletcher, G.E., et al.: Benefits and recommendations for physical activity programs for all Americans: a statement for health professionals by the Committee on Exercise and Cardiac Rehabilitation for the Council on Clinical Cardiology. American Heart Association. *Circulation*, 86:340, 1992.

51. Foster, C.: Translation of exercise test responses to exercise prescription. In *Cardiac Rehabilitation and Clinical Exercise Programs: Theory and Practice.* Edited by N.B. Oldridge, et al. Ithaca, NY, Movement Publications, 1989.

52. Franklin, B.A., et al.: Additional diagnostic test: special populations. In *Resource Manual for Guidelines for Exercise Testing and Prescription.* Edited by S. Blair, et al. Philadelphia, Lea & Febiger, 1988.

53. Franklin, B.A., et al.: Exercise and cardiac complications: do the benefits outweigh the risks? *Phys. Sportsmed.*, 22(2): 56, 1994.

54. Froelicher, V.F.: *Exercise Testing and Training.* New York, LeJacq Publishing Co., 1983.

55. Frontera, W.R., et al.: Strength conditioning in older men: skeletal muscle hypertrophy and improved function. *J. Appl. Physiol.*, 64:1038, 1988.

55a. Fuchs, G.S., et al.: Alcohol consumption and mortality among women. *N. Engl.J. Med.*, 332:1245, 1995.

55b. Fuhrman, B., et al.: Consumption of red wine with meals reduces the susceptibility of human plasma and low-density lipoprotein to lipid peroxidation. *Am.J. Clin. Nutr.*, 61:549, 1995.

56. Garrick, J.G., et al.: The epidemiology of aerobic dance injuries. *Am.J. Sports Med.*, 14:67, 1986.

57. Gaziano, J.M., et al.: Moderate alcohol intake, increased levels of high-density lipoprotein and its subfractions, and decreased risk of myocardial infarction. *N. Engl.J. Med.*, 329:1829, 1993.

58. Goodman, D.S.: Report of National Cholesterol Education Program expert panel on detection, evaluation, and treatment of high cholesterol in adults. *Arch. Intern. Med.*, 148:36, 1988.

59. Grabner, M.D., and Enoka, R.A.: Changes in movement capabilities with aging. *Exerc. Sport Sci. Rev.*, 23:65, 1995.

59a. Gutin, B., et al.: Physical training, lifestyle education, and coronary risk factors in obese girls. *Med. Sci. Sports Exerc.*, 28:19, 1996.

60. Hagberg, J.M.: A hemodynamic comparison of young and old endurance athletes during exercise. *J. Appl. Physiol.*, 58:2041, 1985.

61. Hagberg, J.M., et al.: Metabolic responses to exercise in young and older athletes and sedentary men. *J. Appl. Physiol.*, 65:900, 1988.

62. Hagberg, J.M., et al.: Pulmonary function in young and older athletes and untrained men. *J. Appl. Physiol.*, 65:101, 1988.

63. Hanson, P.: Exercise testing and training in patients with chronic heart failure. *Med. Sci. Sports Exerc.*, 26:527, 1994.

64. Higginbotham, M.B., et al.: Physiologic basis for the age-related decline in aerobic work capacity. *Am.J. Cardiol.*, 57:1374, 1986.

65. Hill, A.B.: Cricket and its relation to the duration of life. *Lancet*, 2:949, 1927.

66. Holloszy, J.O., et al.: Health benefits of exercise in the elderly. *Med. Sci. Sports Exerc.*, 37:91, 1992.

67. Hubert, H.A., et al.: Obesity as an independent risk factor for cardiovascular disease. A 26-year follow-up of participants in the Framingham heart study. *Circulation*, 67:968, 1983.

68. Inbar, O., et al.: Normal cardiopulmonary responses during incremental exercise in 20- to 70-yr-old men. *Med. Sci. Sports Exerc.*, 26:538, 1994.

69. Jackson, A.S., et al.: Changes in aerobic power of men, ages 25-70 yr. *Med. Sci. Sports Exerc.*, 27:113, 1995.

70. Johnson, C.L., et al.: Declining serum total cholesterol levels among US adults. *JAMA*, 269:3002, 1993.

71. Kakka, T.A., et al.: Relation of leisure-time physical activity and cardiorespiratory fitness to the risk of acute myocardial infarction in men. *N. Engl.J. Med.*, 330:1549, 1994.

72. Kasch, F.W.: The effects of exercise on the aging process. *Phys. Sportsmed.*, 4:64, 1976.

73. Kasch, F.W., et al.: The effect of physical activity and inactivity on aerobic power in older men (a longitudinal study). *Phys. Sportsmed.*, 18:73, 1990.

74. Katch, F.I., and Katch, V.L.: Optimal health and body composition. In *Women and Exercise: Physiology and Sports Medicine.* Edited by M. Shangold and G. Mirkin. Philadelphia, F.A. Davis, 1988.

75. Killen, J.D., et al. Cardiovascular disease risk reduction for tenth graders. A multiple-factor school-based program. *JAMA*, 260:1728, 1988.

76. Klag, M.J., et al.: Serum cholesterol in young men and subsequent cardiovascular disease. *N. Engl.J. Med.*, 328:313, 1993.

77. Klitgaard, H., et al.: Function, morphology and protein expression of aging skeletal muscle: a cross-sectional study of elderly men with different training backgrounds. *Acta Physiol. Scand.*, 457(Suppl.):1, 1990.

78. Kohrt, W.M., et al.: Effects of gender, age, and fitness level on the response of $\dot{V}o_2$max to training in 60- to 71-yr-olds. *J. Appl. Physiol.*, 71:2004, 1991.

79. Kramsch, D.M., et al.: Reduction in coronary atherosclerosis by moderate conditioning exercise in monkeys on an atherogenic diet. *N. Engl.J. Med.*, 305:1483, 1981.

80. Kuller, L.H., et al.: Sudden death and the decline in coronary heart disease mortality. *J. Chron. Dis.*, 39:1001, 1986.

81. Lakatta, E.G.: Cardiovascular regulatory mechanisms in advanced age. *Physiol. Rev.*, 73:413, 1993.

82. Last, J.M.: *A Dictionary of Epidemiology.* New York, Oxford University Press, 1983.

83. Laughlin, M.H., et al.: Exercise training increases coronary transport reserve in miniature swine. *J. Appl. Physiol.*, 67:1140, 1989.

83a. Lee, I.-M., and Paffenbarger, R.S.: Exercise intensity and longevity in men: the Harvard Alumni Study. *JAMA*, 273:1179, 1995.

84. Levy, D., et al.: Stratifying the patient at risk from coronary disease: new insights from the Framingham Heart Study. *Am. Heart J.*, 119:712, 1990.

85. Levy, W.C., et al.: Endurance exercise training augments diastolic filling at rest and during exercise in healthy young and older men. *Circulation*, 88:116, 1993.

86. Lexell, J.: Ageing and human skeletal muscle: observations from Sweden. *Can. J. Appl. Physiol.*, 18:2, 1993.

87. Lexell, J., et al.: What is the cause of ageing atrophy? Total number, size, and proportion of different fiber types studied in whole vastus lateralis muscle from 15-to 83-year old men. *J. Neurol. Sci.*, 84:275, 1988.

88. Macera, C.A., et al.: Age, physical activity, physical fitness, body composition, and incidence of orthopedic problems. *Res.Q. Exerc. Sport*, 60:225, 1989.

89. Mann, G.V., et al: Physical fitness and immunity to heart disease in Masai. *Lancet*, 2:1308, 1965.

90. Manninen, V., et al.: Lipid alterations and decline in the incidence of coronary heart disease in the Helsinki Study. *JAMA*, 260:641, 1988.

91. Matsusaki, M., et al.: Influence of workload on the antihypertensive effect of exercise. *Clin. Exp. Pharmacol. Physiol.*, 19:471, 1992.

92. McDonough, J.R., and Bruce, R.A.: Maximal exercise testing in assessing cardiovascular function. *J.S.C. Med. Assoc.*, 65:26, 1969.

93. McDonough, J.R., et al.: Coronary heart disease among Negroes and Whites in Evans County, Georgia. *J. Chron. Dis.*, 18:443, 1965.

94. Meredith, C.N., et al.: Peripheral effects of endurance training in young and old subjects. *J. Appl. Physiol.*, 66:2844, 1989.

95. Mittleman, M.A., et al.: Triggering of acute myocardial infarction by heavy physical exertion. *N. Engl.J. Med.*, 329:1677, 1993.

96. Montoye, H.J., et al.: *The Longevity and Morbidity of College Athletes.* Indianapolis, Phi Epsilon Kappa, 1957.

97. Morris, J.N.: Exercise in the prevention of coronary heart disease: today's best bet in public health. *Med. Sci. Sports Exerc.*, 26:807, 1994.

98. NIH Consensus Conference. Triglyceride, high-density lipoprotein, and coronary heart disease. *JAMA*, 269:505, 1993.

99. Ogawa, T., et al.: Effects of aging, sex, and physical training on cardiovascular response to exercise. *Circulation*, 86:494, 1992.

100. Paffenbarger, R.S., Jr., et al.: Physical activity, all-cause mortality, and longevity of college alumni. *N. Engl.J. Med.*, 314:605, 1986.

101. Paffenbarger, R.S., Jr., et al.: The association between changes in physical-activity level and other lifestyle characteristics with mortality among men. *N. Engl.J. Med.*, 328:538, 1993.

102. Paffenbarger, R.S., Jr., et al.: Changes in physical activity and other lifeway patterns influencing longevity. *Med. Sci. Sports Exerc.*, 26:857, 1994.

102a. Parish, S., et al.: Cigarette smoking, tar yields, and non-fatal myocardial infarction: 14000 cases and 32000 controls. *Br. Med. J.*, 311:471, 1995.

103. Pate, R.R., et al.: Physical activity and public health: a recommendation from the Centers for Disease Control and Prevention and American College of Sports Medicine. *JAMA*, 273:402, 1995.

104. Pollock, M.L., et al.: Effect of age and training on aerobic capacity and body composition of master athletes. *J. Appl. Physiol.*, 62:625, 1987.

105. Powell, K.E., and Blair, S.N.: The public health burdens of sedentary living habits: theoretical but realistic estimates. *Med. Sci. Sports Exerc.*, 26:851, 1994.

106. Powell, K.E., et al.: Physical activity and the incidence of coronary heart disease. *Annu. Rev. Public Health*, 8:253, 1987.

107. Public Health Service. *Healthy People 2000: National Health Promotion and Disease Prevention Objectives*. US Dept. of Health and Human Services publication PHS 90-50212. Washington, DC, US Dept. of Health and Human Services, 1990.

107a. Province, M.A., et al.: The effects of exercise on falls in elderly patients: a preplanned meta-analysis of the FICSIT trials. *JAMA*, 273:1341, 1995.

108. Quinn, T.J., et al.: Caloric expenditure, life status, and disease in former male athletes and non-athletes. *Med. Sci. Sports Exerc.*, 22:742, 1990.

109. Rice, C.L., et al.: Strength training alters contractile properties of the triceps brachii in men aged 65-78 years. *Eur.J. Appl. Physiol.*, 66:275, 1993.

110. Rikli, R.E., and Mcmanis, B.G.: Effects of exercise on bone mineral content in postmenopausal women. *Res.Q. Exerc. Sport*, 61:243, 1990.

111. Rivera, A.M., et al.: Physiological factors associated with lower maximal oxygen consumption of master runners. *J. Appl. Physiol.*, 66:949, 1989.

112. Robb, G.P., and Marks, H.H.: Latent coronary artery disease determination, its presence and severity by the exercise electrocardiogram. *Am.J. Cardiol.*, 13:603, 1964.

113. Rochmis, P., and Blackburn, H.: Exercise tests. A survey of procedures, safety and litigation experience in approximately 170,000 tests. *JAMA*, 217:1060, 1971.

114. Rodenheffer, R.J., et al.: Exercise cardiac output is maintained with advancing age in healthy human subjects: cardiac dilation and increased stroke volume compensate for diminished heart rate. *Circulation*, 69:203, 1984.

115. Rogers, M.A., and Evans, W.J.: Changes in skeletal muscle with aging: effects of exercise training. *Exerc. Sport Sci. Rev.*, 21:65, 1993.

116. Rogers, M.A., et al.: Effect of 6 d of exercise training on responses to maximal and sub-maximal exercise in middle-aged man. *Med. Sci. Sports Exerc.*, 20:260, 1988.

117. Rogers, M.A., et al.: Decline in V̇o₂max with aging in master athletes and sedentary men. *J. Appl. Physiol.*, 68:2195, 1990.

118. Sady, S., et al.: Training, diet and physical characteristics of distance runners with low or high concentrations of high density lipoprotein cholesterol. *Atherosclerosis*, 53:273, 1984.

119. Sady, S.P., et al.: Elevated high-density lipoprotein cholesterol in endurance athletes is related to enhanced plasma triglyceride clearance. *Metabolism*, 37:568, 1988.

120. Saltin, B., et al.: Physical training in sedentary middle-aged and older men. II. Oxygen uptake, heart rate, and blood lactate concentration at submaximal and maximal exercise. *Scand.J. Clin. Lab. Invest.*, 24:323, 1969.

121. Sandvik, L., et al.: Physical fitness as a predictor of mortality among healthy, middle-aged Norwegian men. *N. Engl.J. Med.*, 328:533, 1993.

122. Scheuer, J.: Effects of physical training on myocardial vascularization and perfusion. *Circulation*, 66:491, 1982.

123. Schulman, S.P., and Gerstenblith, G.: Cardiovascular changes with aging. the response to exercise. *J. Cardiopulmonary Rehab.*, 9:12, 1989.

124. Schwartz, R.S., et al.: Effects of intensive endurance training on lipoprotein profiles in young and older men. *Metabolism*, 41:644, 1992.

125. Seals, D.R., et al.: Endurance training in older men and women. I. Cardiovascular responses to exercise. *J. Appl. Physiol.*, 57:1024, 1984.

126. Seals, D.R., et al.: Enhanced left ventricular performance in endurance trained older men. *Circulation*, 89:198, 1994.

127. Seals, D.R., et al.: Exercise and aging: autonomic control of the circulation. *Med. Sci. Sports Exerc.*, 26:568, 1994.

128. Sheffield, T., et al.: Safety of exercise testing volunteer subjects: the Lipid Research Clinics Prevalence Study experience. *J. Cardiopulmonary Rehab.*, 2:395, 1982.

128a. Shepard, R.J.: Exercise and sudden death: an overview. *Sport Sci. Rev.*, 4:1, 1995.

129. Shock, N.W.: Physical activity and the rate of aging. *Can. Med. Assoc.J.*, 96:836, 1967.

130. Shulhan, D., et al.: Phasic cardiac selectivity to psychological stress as a function of aerobic fitness level. *Psychophysiology*, 23:562, 1986.

131. Sipalä, S., and Suominen, H.: Effects of strength and endurance training on thigh and leg muscle mass and composition in elderly women. *J. Appl. Physiol.*, 78:334, 1995.

132. Siscovick, D.S., et al.: The incidence of primary cardiac arrest during vigorous exercise. *N. Engl.J. Med.*, 311:874, 1984.

133. Spina, R.J., et al.: Differences to cardiovascular adaptations to endurance exercise training between older men and women. *J. Appl. Physiol.*, 75:849, 1993.

134. Spina, R.J., et al.: Effect of exercise training on left ventricular performance in older women free of cardiopulmonary disease. *Am.J. Cardiol.*, 71:99, 1993.

135. Spirduso, W.W.: Reaction and movement time as a function of age and physical activity level. *J. Gerontol.*, 30:435, 1975.

136. Spirduso, W.W., and Clifford, P.: Replication of age and physical activity effects on reaction and movement time. *J. Gerontol.*, 33:26, 1978.

137. Stamford, B.A., et al.: Effects of smoking cessation on weight gain, metabolic rate, caloric consumption and blood lipids. *Am. J. Clin. Nutr.*, 43:486, 1986.

138. Stamford, B.A.: Exercise and the elderly. In *Exercise and Sport Sciences Reviews*. Edited by K.B. Pandolf. Vol. 16. New York, Macmillan, 1988.

139. Straton, J.R., et al.: Effects of physical conditioning on fibrinolytic variables and fibrinogen in young and old healthy adults. *Circulation*, 83:1692, 1991.

140. Straton, J.R., et al.: Cardiovascular responses to exercise: effects of aging. *Circulation*, 89:1648, 1994.

141. Sytkowski, P.A., et al.: Changes in risk factors and the decline in mortality from cardiovascular disease. *N. Engl.J. Med.*, 322:1635, 1990.

142. Tate, C.A., et al.: Mechanism for the responses of cardiac muscle to physical activity in old age. *Med. Sci. Sports Exerc.*, 26: 561, 1994.

143. Thacker, S.B., and Berkelman, R.L.: Public health surveillance in the United States. *Epidemiol. Rev.*, 10:164, 1988.

144. Thompson, P.D., et al.: Incidence of death during jogging in Rhode Island from 1975 through 1980. *JAMA*, 245:2535, 1982.

145. Thompson, P.D., et al.: Modest changes in high-density lipoprotein concentration with prolonged exercise training. *Circulation*, 78:25,1988.

146. Tomonaga, M.: Histochemical and ultrastructural changes in senile human skeletal muscle. *J. Am. Geriatr. Soc.*, 25:125, 1977.

147. Tran, Z.V., and Weltman, A.: Differential effects of exercise on serum lipids and lipoprotein levels seen with changes in body weight: a meta analysis. *JAMA*, 254:919, 1985.

148. Trulson, M.F., et al.: Comparisons of siblings in Boston and Ireland. *J. Am. Diet Assoc.*, 45:225, 1964.

149. Van Camp, S.P., and Peterson, R.A.: Cardiovascular complications of outpatient cardiac rehabilitation programs. *JAMA*, 256:1160, 1986.

150. Vanoverschelde, J.-L.J., et al.: Contribution of left ventricular diastolic function to exercise capacity in normal subjects. *J. Appl. Physiol.*, 74:2225, 1993.

150a. Vuori, I.M.: Sudden death and exercise: effects of age and type of activity. *Sport Sci. Rev.*, 4:46, 1995.

151. Wannamethee, G,, and Shaper, A.G.: Physical activity and stroke in British middle-aged men. *BMJ*, 304:597, 1992.

152. Weisfeldt, M.L., and Gerstenblith, G.: *Cardiovascular Aging and Adaptation to Disease in the Heart.* Edited by J.W. Hurst. New York, Macmillan, 1986.

153. Whipple, R.H., et al.: The relationship of knee and ankle weakness to falls in nursing home residents. *J. Am. Geriatr. Soc.*, 35:13, 1987.

154. Willett, W.C., et al.: Relative and absolute excess risks of coronary heart disease among women who smoke cigarettes. *N. Engl.J. Med.*, 317:1303, 1987.

155. Wood, P., et al.: The effects on plasma lipoproteins of a prudent weight-reducing diet, with or without exercise, in overweight men and women. *N. Engl.J. Med.*, 325:461, 1991.

156. Yarasheski, K.E., et al.: Acute effects of resistance exercise on muscle protein synthesis in young and elderly adults. *Am.J. Physiol.*, 65:E210, 1993.

Kavanagh, T., et al.: Marathon running after myocardial infarction. *JAMA* 229:1602, 1974.

In the late 1960s and early 1970s, few physicians prescribed regular exercise for patients recovering from a myocardial infarction (MI). Most heart specialists at that time believed that adopting a sedentary lifestyle after an MI "saved" the heart from further strain. The medical community did not appreciate that increased physical activity improved both functional capacity and long-term prognosis for the patient. Contrary to prevailing ideas about the benefits of exercise training, Kavanagh and colleagues investigated the clinical, physiological, and biochemical status of eight exercise-trained, post-MI patients (average age 42.9 years) prior to and following participation in the Boston Marathon.

The patients enrolled in a cardiac rehabilitation program and trained for the marathon in a project designed to assess the effects of an exhausting road race on adaptability in physiologic function. All patients had sustained a well-documented MI 1 to 4 years before beginning marathon training. Pretraining $\dot{V}O_2$max ranged from 21.4 to 31.8 mL · kg^{-1} · min^{-1} and increased after 8 to 12 months of training to a group average of 40.7 mL · kg^{-1} · min^{-1}. Training consisted mainly of slow long-distance running progressing to 45 miles weekly at a pace between 8.5 and 10.5 minutes per mile. Most of the training consisted of road work with periods of interval and Fartlek training. Medical personnel supervised all training sessions. Medical examinations took place 1 hour before and immediately after the marathon. Measurements included a brief questionnaire, body mass, blood pressure, 12-lead ECG, and blood and urine samples to evaluate sodium, potassium, chloride, bicarbonate, glucose, blood urea nitrogen (BUN), creatinine, creatine phosphokinase, and uric acid. At the time of the run, subjects were free from coronary complications, although one suffered from premature ventricular contractions (PVCs) at rest, and another experienced PVCs occasionally during exercise.

Seven of the eight men completed the marathon (the eighth man decided to stop at the halfway point) at an average speed of 5.4 mph (4 hours 55.8 minutes). They ran at 81% (33 mL · kg^{-1} min^{-1}) of their pre-race $\dot{V}O_2$max. Symptoms were remarkably few. Two men had no complaints, while the others reported general fatigue, slight nausea, stiffness, and muscle pain, leg and stomach cramps, and dehydration-symptoms not much different from those reported by the typical runner. The figure illustrates the percent changes in several variables after the race. Not unexpectedly, a significant loss occurred of 4.0 kg body mass (range of 3.2 to 4.8 kg). The runners lost an estimated 1.9 liters of water, which probably contributed to the symptoms of nausea, dizziness, and muscle pain. The concentrations of plasma sodium, chloride, BUN, and creatinine increased, whereas blood glucose (not indicated in the figure) remained unaltered at the end of the race. The ECG showed no deterioration after nearly 5 hours of running, and at 5 and 10 hours into recovery. Blood pressures decreased from pre- to post-race (118/65 to 108/60 mm Hg), but evidence of excessive fluid loss and dehydration concerned the doctors the most.

The results demonstrated convincingly that post-MI patients can successfully train and participate in exhausting physical activities with no apparent contraindications. The researchers concluded that strenuous physical training in most post-MI patients can play a useful role in rehabilitation from heart disease.

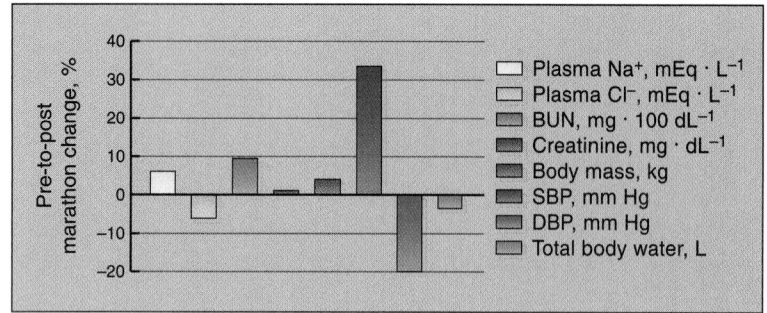

Changes in selected variables from before to immediately after running the marathon in men after rehabilitation from coronary heart disease. *Na* is serum sodium, milliequivalents per liter. *Cl* is serum chloride, milliequivalents per liter, *BUN* is blood urea nitrogen, milligrams per 100 mL; *Creat* is creatinine, milligrams per 100 mL; *SBP* is systolic blood pressure, millimeters of mercury; *DBP* is diastolic blood pressure, millimeters of mercury; *TBW* is total body water, liters.

Clinical Exercise Physiology for Cancer, Cardiovascular, and Pulmonary Rehabilitation

THE EXERCISE PHYSIOLOGIST IN THE CLINICAL SETTING

The **clinical exercise physiologist** has become part of a team approach to health care (Fig. 31.1) and is relied upon to assist in total patient care. In this setting, the exercise physiologist's primary focus is to help restore the patient's mobility and functional capacity by working closely with the physical therapist, occupational therapist, and physician. An expanded role for the exercise physiologist in clinical practice occurs because of the fundamental relationship between functional capacity and health. According to the World Health Organization (WHO), "health is a state of complete physical, mental and social well-being, not merely the absence of disease and infirmity."[27] It is helpful in this regard to define overall health as reflecting a person's ability to successfully complete physical tasks and to possess certain functional abilities. The measurement and demonstration of this functional ability provides an objective means to assess an individual's health status. Consequently, functional exercise capacity becomes an important part of being healthy.

The health continuum is illustrated in Figure 31.2. In this context, **disability** refers to an individual's diminished functional capacity, whereas *handicap* refers to a physical performance frame of reference defined by society.[13, 16] Individuals considered handicapped no longer perform tasks expected by society. Having a functional limitation, however, does not necessarily result in either disability or handicap.

SPORTS MEDICINE AND EXERCISE PHYSIOLOGY: A VITAL LINK

The traditional view of sports medicine concerns rehabilitating athletes from sports-related injuries. Sports medicine, viewed more broadly, relates to scientific and medical aspects of physical activity, physical fitness, and sports performance. Indeed, the WHO defines physical fitness and sports as the ability to perform muscular work satisfactorily.[19] This encompasses one's ability to perform physical activity at work, at home, or on the sports field. Therefore, sports medicine becomes closely linked to clinical exercise physiology, and the sports medicine profession becomes concerned with diverse populations. These populations include, at one extreme, the sedentary person who needs only a modest amount of physical exercise to reduce the risk of degenerative diseases and, at the other extreme, able-bodied and disabled athletes whose major focus is to enhance sports performance. The prescription of physical activity and athletic competition for the physically challenged is an important and growing area of interest in sports medicine and exercise physiology and provides new opportunities for research, clinical practice, and professional advancement.

Carefully prescribed, graded physical activity makes a significant, important, and immediate contribution to overall good health, life satisfaction, and life expectancy;[20] exercise physiologists assume important clinical positions in sports medicine by testing, diagnosing, and treating individuals with various types of physical disabilities.

PREVALENCE AND TYPES OF DISABILITIES

A variety of medical conditions adversely affect functional capacity and physical performance. Some disabilities occur at birth (e.g., deformed limbs, deafness, blindness, mental retardation, acquired diseases), whereas others occur during youth or young adulthood (e.g., injury-related disabilities, general diseases) or are acquired later in life (e.g., atherosclerosis, pulmonary and vascular diseases). The range of potential disabilities throughout one's life span truly is staggering, as evidenced by the expanding health-care industry.

FIGURE 31.1
The team approach in rehabilitation. Health-care professionals work cooperatively to improve a patient's functional ability.

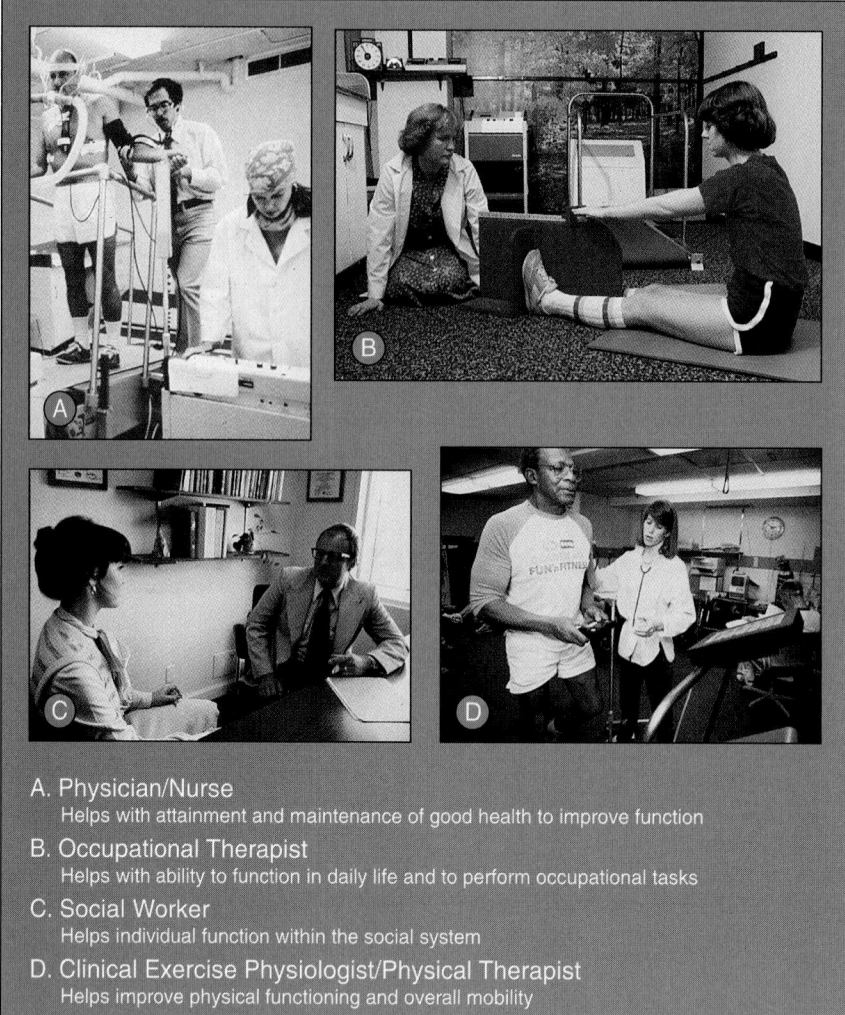

A. Physician/Nurse
Helps with attainment and maintenance of good health to improve function

B. Occupational Therapist
Helps with ability to function in daily life and to perform occupational tasks

C. Social Worker
Helps individual function within the social system

D. Clinical Exercise Physiologist/Physical Therapist
Helps improve physical functioning and overall mobility

FIGURE 31.2
Hierarchy of health status.

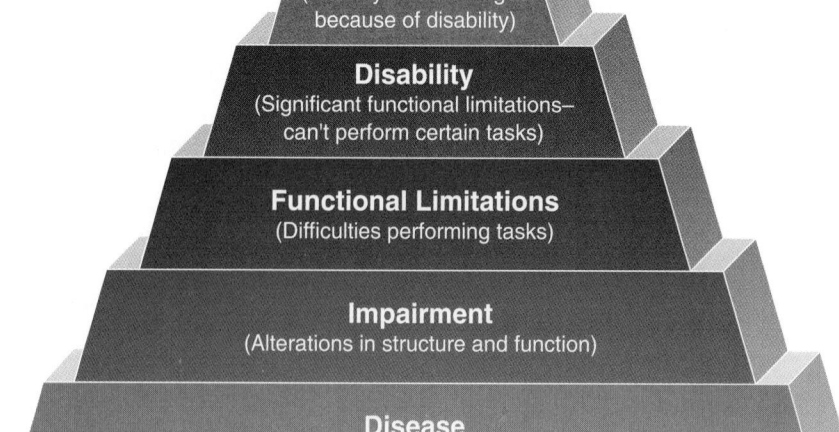

Handicap
(Socially disadvantaged because of disability)

Disability
(Significant functional limitations—can't perform certain tasks)

Functional Limitations
(Difficulties performing tasks)

Impairment
(Alterations in structure and function)

Disease
(Pathophysiology)

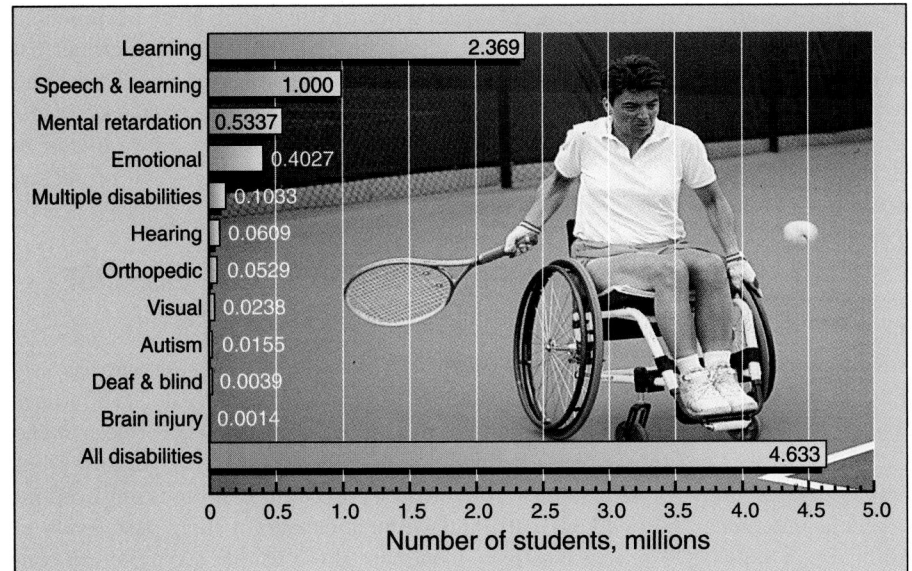

FIGURE 31.3
Prevalence of disabilities in students aged 6 to 21 years for the 1992-1993 school year. (Source: United States Department of Education. Office of Special Education Programs, Data Analysis System. 16th Annual Report to Congress, 1994.)

The prevalence of disabled school-aged individuals in United States public elementary schools is listed in Figure 31.3. Learning, speech and language, mental retardation, and emotional disturbances account for most disabilities.[23] Children with severe cardiovascular and pulmonary diseases are not included in the database because such children are not enrolled in school. Statistics regarding the exact prevalence of disabilities among individuals with a postsecondary school education are scarce, because different agencies define disabilities from either a legal, medical, or educational perspective. For many clinical conditions, a continuum ranges from mild to severe pathology. In some cases, disability does not parallel clinical severity, and many individuals are inflicted with multiple disabilities. Therefore, the overall proportion of the population with complete or partial disabilities is possibly much larger than currently estimated.

Another way of discerning the magnitude and impact of disabilities is to consider the increase in the number of health professionals. Enrollment in physical therapy programs in the United States is illustrated in Figure 31.4. During the last 15 years, the enrollment trend has not leveled off; in fact, there has been a 176% increase in the number of physical therapists in private offices and rehabilitation centers, with a projected growth rate of 88% through 2005.

In the following sections, the clinical applications of exercise physiology for the major areas of oncology, cardiovascular disease, and pulmonary system disabilities are presented. The focus is on these disabilities because they currently represent the areas of greatest involvement for the exercise physiologist.

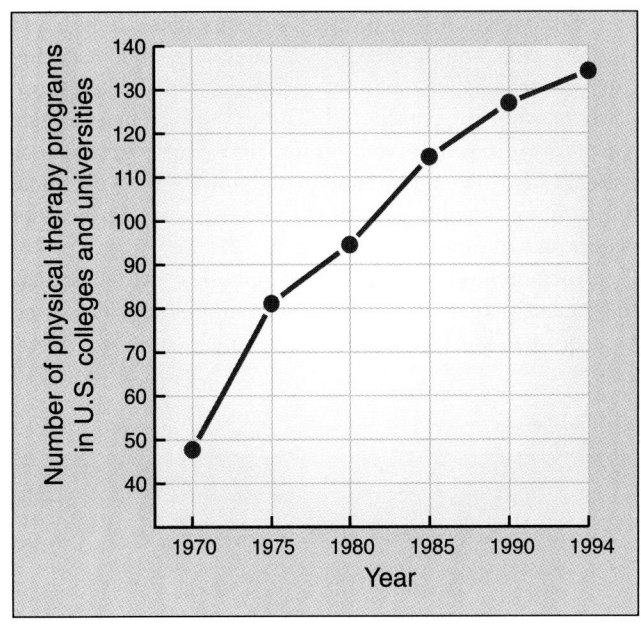

FIGURE 31.4
Increase in physical therapy programs in United States educational institutions from 1970 to 1994. (Source: Physical Therapy Association. Alexandria, VA, 1995.)

ONCOLOGY

Cancer is a group of diseases that is collectively characterized by uncontrolled growth and spread of abnormal cells. More than 100 different types of cancers exist, most of which occur in adults. Fifty percent of all adult cancers affect the breast, lung, bowel, and uterus. Cancer remains the second leading cause of death in the United States, and approximately one-third of the population has cancer of some type. In 1994 alone, 540,000 Americans died from cancer, and about 1.2 million new cases were diagnosed. Surprisingly, minorities (with their different cultural backgrounds and health and nutritional beliefs) consistently have higher rates of cancer. Cancer is the leading cause of death in young women between the ages of 25 and 44 years.[12] The estimated number of diagnosed cases of cancer per 1000 in the U.S. population, with functional limitations specific to various types of cancer, is listed in Table 31.1. The current population of more than 8 million cancer survivors (many of whom were diagnosed in the 1970s) points out the need for continued rehabilitative options in this important area of medicine.

For most cancer patients and survivors, loss of body mass and functional status are the most serious outcomes.[4] This loss of functional status includes difficulty in walking one block or more and serious fatigue that limits completion of even menial household chores. Approximately 75% of cancer survivors report extreme feelings of fatigue during radiotherapy or chemotherapy, which are generally associated with weight loss and decreased muscular strength and cardiovascular endurance.[6, 23] Maintaining and restoring function are challenges for the cancer survivor, even those patients who are considered "cured." Sufficient evidence warrants exercise intervention for cancer survivors, such as patients who have undergone mastectomy.[3, 12, 24] Nutritional intervention, combined with exercise, can help reduce the occurrence of other types of cancer.[5, 11, 14, 17, 22]

An increased level of regular physical activity assists the cancer patient in properly recuperating and returning to a normal lifestyle and in improving quality of life by increasing physical independence and level of function. General preventive and intervention goals for a cancer patient who faces sustained periods of inactivity, disuse, and bed rest are listed in Table 31.2. *The overall goal of the health-care team is to rehabilitate the patient to a level of function that allows return to work and pursuit of normal recreational activities.*

POSSIBLE MECHANISMS OF EXERCISE EFFECTS ON CANCER

Firm epidemiological evidence exists that regular exercise plays a significant role in reducing cancer risk. The findings of eight human and five animal studies of cancer occurrence and physical activity are listed in Table 31.3. All of the human studies were cross-sectional, in that they compared individuals with and without cancer to their past levels of physical activity. Generally, these studies attempted to control for factors such as age, nutritional and socioeconomic status, sex, and ethnic origin.

Several hypotheses can explain how regular exercise helps prevent cancer. A reduced cancer risk is mediated by regular exercise, which reduces levels of glucose and insulin and increases levels of corticosteroid hormones. Exercise also increases levels of anti-inflammatory cytokines and augments insulin-receptor expression in cancer-fighting T cells. It also is known that exercise increases interferon production, stimulates glycogen synthetase, augments leukocyte function, and improves the metabolism of ascorbic acid—all of which may blunt the formation of cancerous tumors. It has also been proposed that physical activity may exert beneficial effects on the process of provirus or oncogene activation. Physical activity also ap-

---

TABLE 31.1
ESTIMATED NUMBER OF PEOPLE BY AGE PER 1000 OF THE U.S. POPULATION WITH FUNCTIONAL LIMITATIONS FROM DIFFERENT TYPES OF CANCERS

Type of Cancer	All Ages	18	18–44	45–69	70–84	85+
Lung, broncial	125	—	4	81	39	2
Leukemia	58	9	7	29	13	1
Female breast	159	—	19	101	34	5
Genitourinary	173	2	20	96	48	8
Digestive	185	1	14	114	48	9
Skin	44	—	8	20	13	3
Bone	52	1	5	24	20	2

Age of Patient (y)

Data from Cole, T.M., and Edgerton, V.R.: Report on the task force on medical rehabilitation research. Hunt Valley, MD, Task Force Publications, 1990.

TABLE 31.2
TEN GENERAL TREATMENT GOALS OF CLINICAL EXERCISE PHYSIOLOGISTS FOR PATIENTS WITH DECONDITIONING, IMMOBILITY, OR DISUSE SYNDROMES

1. Improve patient's overall functional status
2. Improve active motion for nonrestrictive segments and joints
3. Prevent loss of flexibility by active motion and passive movements
4. Stimulate peripheral and central circulation through active motion exercise based on current functional level
5. Increase ventilatory function by use of systematic breathing exercises
6. Prevent thrombosis through physical activities
7. Prevent loss of motor control and muscle strength and endurance with resistance exercises
8. Reduce the rate of bone loss through weight-bearing aerobic and muscle-strengthening exercises
9. Through active aerobic and resistance exercise, slow the loss of fat-free body mass and subsequent reduction of BMR that accompanies deconditioning
10. Monitor signs of increased fatigue or weakness, lethargy, dyspnea, pallor, dizziness, claudication, or cramping during or following exercise

TABLE 31.3
PHYSICAL ACTIVITY AND THE DEVELOPMENT OF CANCER. REVIEW OF 13 STUDIES REPORTING THE RELATIONSHIP BETWEEN PHYSICAL ACTIVITY AND CANCER PROTECTION

Subjects[a]	Activity	Type of Cancer	Cancer Protection
Human (M + F)	Normal	Large bowel	Yes
Human (F)	Sports	Breast	Yes
Human (M)	Job	Colon	Yes
Human (M + F)	Job	Colon	Yes
Human (M + F)	Recreation	Left colon	Yes
Human (M)	Sports	Colon	Yes
Human (M)	Recreation	All-cause	Yes
Human (M + F)	Sports	All-cause	Yes
Animal	Voluntary	Mammary	Yes
Animal	Voluntary	Flank	Yes
Animal	Voluntary	Pancreas	Yes
Animal	Forced	Flank	No
Animal	Forced	Mammary	Yes

[a]All of the human studies surveyed individuals in different settings such as job, recreational, sports, and randomly from all settings (normal). Subjects were classified based on levels of physical activity, ranging from sedentary to very active. The recreation and sports studies included estimates of caloric expenditure during the day. Cancer protection was defined as relative risk or percent increase in the development of the disease. In each 12 of the 13 studies, increased protection was significantly different than a chance occurrence.

pears to enhance the volume and, to a lesser degree, the number of metastatic foci in the lungs of certain rodents fed high-lipid diets.[5] Although few human studies directly link increased physical activity to cancer prevention, the cross-sectional data shown in Table 31.3 certainly suggest such a link.

EXERCISE PRESCRIPTION AND CANCER

Evidence from studies of experimental animals, former athletes, people employed in active occupations, and those with an active recreational lifestyle suggests that physical activity plays an important role in cancer rehabilitation. There is less certainty, however, regarding the proper exercise prescription for cancer patients, and little research exists on the timing of exercise relative to the various phases of carcinogenesis. Therefore, it is difficult to determine when it is best to initiate exercise intervention. No information exists regarding proper doses of exercise or the corresponding responses of different cancers to exercise intervention among men and women of different ages. This uncertainty also applies to exercise

intensity and frequency. With such little objective information on exercise prescription and cancer rehabilitation, it is generally recommended that the exercise prescription be symptom-limited, progressive, and individualized. Ambulation of any kind is encouraged for the most sedentary and deconditioned patient. It does seem that there is a linear dose-response relationship, at least up to a point, between increased physical activity, health, and improved functional capacity.[12] Most sedentary adults will derive clinically significant health benefits by accumulating 30 minutes of daily walking (or an equivalent energy expenditure in other activities). The health benefits of physical activity are independent of whether the physical activity is sport, household, occupational, or recreational in nature.

Cancer patients are given a symptom-limited, graded exercise stress test (SLGXT), which serves as a basis for exercise prescription. Procedures for testing are the same as with healthy individuals, except that greater care is given to the patients' subjective feelings of fatigue. The exercise prescription is designed to produce ambulation if the patient has no specific contraindications to exercise. *Emphasis is placed on interval aerobic workouts rather than continuous exercise.* The prescription also should involve range of motion and flexibility exercises and other exercises to improve muscular strength and overall mobility (e.g., submaximal static exercises of the antigravity muscles, deep breathing exercises, and dynamic trunk rotation movements). In most cases, preference is for low-level exercise for short periods performed several times daily. Exercise progression and intensity are individualized, with initial work/rest ratios of 1:1 progressing to 2:1. Eventually, continuous exercise should be encouraged for as long as 10 to 15 minutes.

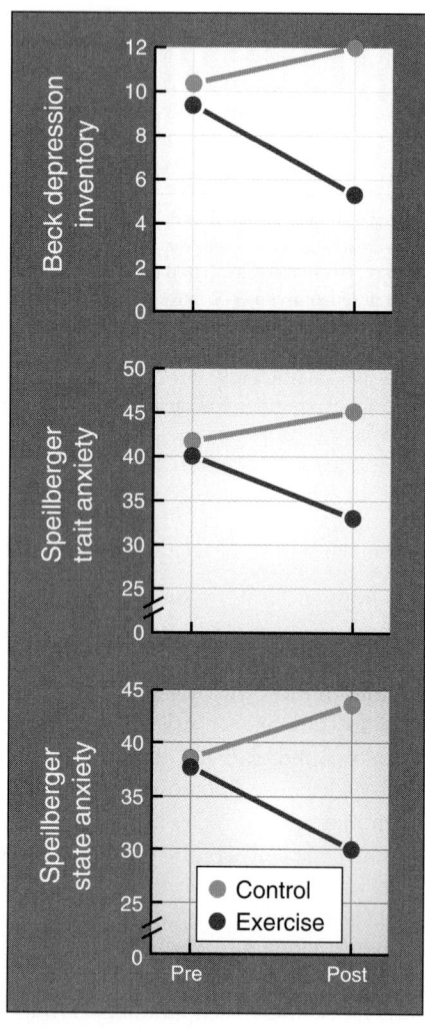

FIGURE 31.5
Effects of 10 weeks of moderate aerobic exercise on depression (*top*), trait (*middle*), and state anxiety (*lower*) in 28 women recovering from breast cancer surgery. (Data courtesy of M. Segar, Applied Physiology Laboratory, University of Michigan, Ann Arbor, MI, 1996.)

The Specific Case of Breast Cancer and Exercise. Carcinoma of the breast is one of the most common forms of cancer in white females aged 40 years and older. Approximately 183,000 new cases of breast cancer are diagnosed annually, which means that one of every nine females will have breast cancer at some time during her life, and there is a high rate of reoccurrence.[1] Breast cancer is the leading cause of death in women between the ages of 40 and 60 years. *The primary risk factors for breast cancer include a positive family history, as well as a personal history of cancer, first menstrual period at an early age, menopause at a late age, first childbirth after age 30 or no childbirth, and a high-fat diet.*

Although research on the role of exercise in breast cancer rehabilitation is limited, the available data suggest an important "psychologic" role for regular aerobic exercise and circuit resistance training. In a recent study from one of our laboratories, 28 patients recovering from breast cancer surgery enrolled in a 10-week aerobic circuit resistance training program to evaluate the effects of exercise on depression, self-esteem, and anxiety. The program was conducted 4 days per week and consisted of hydraulic resistance exercises performed in a 14-station aerobic exercise circuit. Exercise was self-paced and individualized to meet patient needs and fitness levels. The changes for depression (top graph), trait anxiety (middle), and state anxiety (bottom) are listed in Figure 31.5. Exercisers exhibited a 38% decrease in depression compared to a 13% increase for nonexercising controls also recovering from breast cancer surgery. The exercisers also exhibited a 16% decrease in trait anxiety and a 20% decrease in state anxiety compared to significant increases in both variables for the controls. These results demonstrate that exercise has a potent effect on psychosocial variables during breast cancer rehabilitation and that planned, moderate exercise is an important part of the total program of rehabilitation.

CARDIOVASCULAR DISEASES

OVERVIEW AND SCOPE OF CARDIOVASCULAR DISABILITIES

Heart disease is the leading cause of death in industrialized nations. Cardiovascular diseases account for more than 1 million deaths in the United States each year, and one in four Americans will have some form of cardiovascular disease in their lifetime. Fortunately, the rates of cardiovascular disease and death have declined during the last decade, due in part to the aggressive steps to reduce risk factors through early screening and implementation of cardiac prevention and rehabilitation programs.

In Chapters 17 and 21, the effects of regular exercise on cardiovascular function and exercise performance were

**TABLE 31.4
DIFFERENT CARDIAC DISEASES**

Diseases Affecting the Heart Muscle	Diseases Affecting Heart Valves	Diseases Affecting the Cardiac Nervous System
CHD	Rheumatic fever	Arrhythmias
Angina	Endocarditis	Tachycardia
Myocardial infarct	Mitral valve prolapse	Bradycardia
Pericarditis		
Congestive heart failure	Congenital deformations	
Aneurysms		

examined. In this chapter, the role of regular exercise on cardiovascular disease in the rehabilitation setting is discussed.

Aerobic exercise programs are implemented for cardiac patients, with consideration for the specific pathophysiology of the process, the mechanisms that may limit exercise capacity, and individual differences in functional ability. Three different categories of heart disease that lead to functional disability are listed in Table 31.4. By far, diseases of the myocardium are the most prevalent, particularly with advancing age. These diseases are generally referred to in one of the following terms: degenerative heart disease (DHD), athero-sclerotic cardiovascular disease, arterio-sclerotic cardiovascular disease, coronary artery disease (CAD), or coronary heart disease (CHD).[a]

DISEASES OF THE HEART MUSCLE

Recent advances in molecular biology have isolated a possible genetic link to CHD. The identified gene is on chromosome 19 near the gene related to the functioning of the low-density lipoprotein (LDL) receptor used to remove LDL cholesterol from the blood.[21] This gene, the **atherosclerosis susceptibility gene (ATHS)**, accounts for almost 50% of all cases of CHD.[15] The ATHS gene is believed to cause a set of characteristics that triple a person's risk of myocardial infarction. These characteristics include abdominal obesity, low levels of HDL cholesterol, and high levels of LDL cholesterol.

The pathogenesis of CHD probably follows this sequence:

1. Injury to endothelial cell wall.
2. Fibroblastic proliferation of the inner lining (intima) of the artery.

[a]The term CHD is used for consistency in presentation.

3. Accumulation of lipids at the junction of the arterial intima and middle lining, further obstructing blood flow.
4. Degeneration and formation of hyalin (a clear, homogeneous substance occurring in degeneration) in the intima.
5. Calcium deposition at edges of hyalinated area.

The major disorders caused by a reduced myocardial blood supply include angina pectoris, congestive heart failure, and myocardial infarction.

Angina Pectoris. Angina pectoris, characterized by acute chest pain, results from an imbalance between the work (oxygen demands) of the heart and its oxygen supply. Current theory suggests that anginal pain results from an accumulation of metabolites within an ischemic segment of the heart muscle. The sensation of angina pectoris includes squeezing, burning, and pressing or choking in the chest region and is often confused with the discomforts of simple heartburn (see Table 31.5). The duration of angina pain is usually 1 to 3 minutes. About one-third of individuals who suffer from angina die suddenly from a myocardial infarction.[16] Several types of angina exist, including chronic stable angina (often referred to as "walk-through" angina), which occurs at a predictable level of physical exertion and can be controlled with nitroglycerin.

The usual pattern of pain associated with an episode of acute angina pectoris is shown in Figure 31.6. Pain is present in the left shoulder or along the arm to the elbow. Occasionally, angina pain occurs in the back area of the left scapula along the spinal cord.

**TABLE 31.5
COMPARISON OF SYMPTOMS OF ANGINA AND HEARTBURN**

Angina	Heartburn
• Gripping, viselike feelings of pain or pressure behind the breast bone	• Frequent feeling of heartburn
• Paint that radiates to the neck, jaw, back, shoulders, or arms (usually left)	• Frequent use of antacids to relieve pain
• Toothache	• Heartburn wakes person up at night
• Burning indigestion	• Acid or bitter taste in mouth
• Shortness of breath	• Burning chest sensastion
• Nausea	• Discomfort after eating spicy food
• Frequent belching	• Difficulty in swallowing

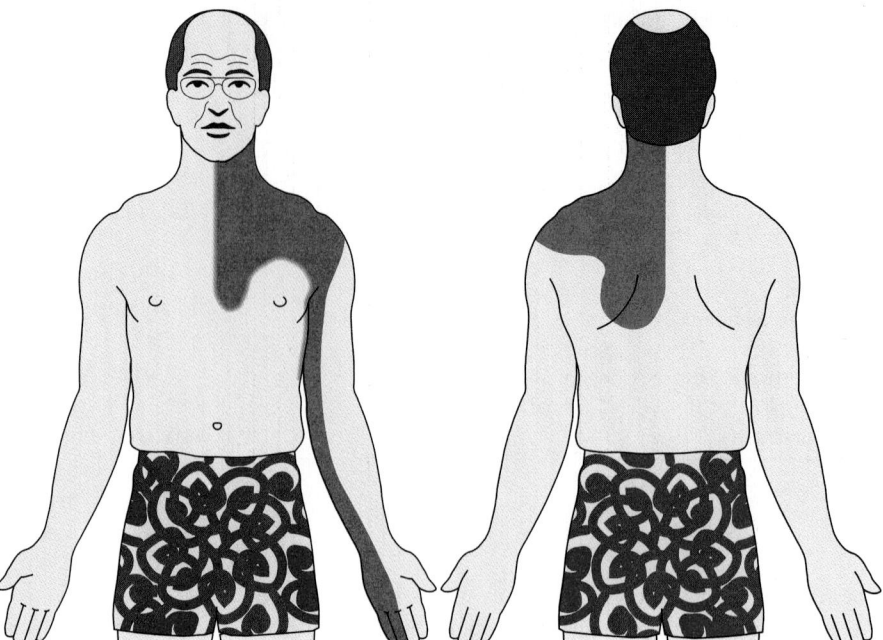

FIGURE 31.6
Locations of pain generally associated with angina pectoris.

Myocardial Infarction. Myocardial infarction (MI, heart attack, or **coronary occlusion**) results from an inadequate perfusion of blood in the coronary arteries or from an imbalance in myocardial oxygen demand in relation to oxygen supply during physical activity due to a significant reduction in the size of the coronary vasculature. A sudden occlusion results from a prior clot formation that developed from accumulation of plaque in one or more of the coronary vessels (see Chapter 30). The onset of an MI usually is preceded by severe fatigue for several days without specific pain. The diverse locations of the early warning signs of an MI are shown in Figure 31.7. During an MI, severe, unrelenting chest pain may last 30 minutes or longer and can persist for more than 1 hour.

Pericarditis. Pericarditis involves inflammation of the pericardium (the heart's outer lining or sac) and is classified as either acute or chronic (recurring or constrictive pericarditis). The symptoms of acute pericarditis vary but usually include chest pain, dyspnea, and an increase in resting heart rate and body temperature. Over time, the inflammation results in extreme chest pain due to fluid accumulation in the pericardial sac, which prevents the heart from fully expanding during diastole. The prognosis for acute viral pericarditis is excellent, whereas chronic pericarditis of a bacterial origin is more serious.

Congestive Heart Failure. Congestive heart failure (CHF or chronic decompensation) occurs when the heart is unable to pump an adequate supply of blood to meet the body's demands. The heart fails because of intrinsic myocardial disease or because of structural defects that result in inadequate pump performance. When this occurs, car-

diac output from the left ventricle is reduced and blood accumulates in the lungs. This results in shortness of breath and the eventual flooding of the pulmonary alveoli with blood, a condition referred to as "pulmonary congestion." Common CHF symptoms include dyspnea, coughing with large amounts of frothy blood-tinged sputum, pulmonary edema, general fatigue, and overall muscular weakness. Heart failure occurs from the right and left heart, each with different symptomatologies and prognoses depending on time of intervention.

Aneurysm. An aneurysm is an abnormal dilatation in the wall of an artery, vein, or the myocardium. Vascular aneurysms occur when a vessel wall becomes weakened from trauma, congenital vascular disease, infection, or atherosclerosis. These are identified as either "arterial" or "venous" and are classified according to the specific areas of the blood vessels inflicted (e.g., thoracic aneurysm). Most aneurysms are asymptomatic and are discovered during a routine chest x-ray. A common symptom of an aneurysm is chest pain with a specific, palpable, pulsating mass in the chest, abdomen, or lower back.

DISEASES AFFECTING THE HEART VALVES

Valvular problems related to heart valve abnormalities include the following:

- **Stenosis:** a narrowing or constriction that prevents heart valves from opening fully; may be caused by growths, scars, or abnormal deposits.

- **Insufficiency:** (also called regurgitation) occurs when the heart valve does not close properly and blood flows back into the heart chamber.
- **Prolapse:** only affects the mitral valve and occurs when enlarged valve leaflets bulge backward into the left atrium during the cardiac cycle.

Valvular abnormalities increase the work of the heart, requiring it to pump harder to force blood through a stenosed valve or to maintain cardiac output if blood seeps backward into one of the chambers. These conditions result from rheumatic fever, an infection by streptococcal bacteria that can be fatal or can lead to rheumatic heart disease, which causes valvular scarring and subsequent heart valve deformity. Fever and joint pain are the two most common symptoms of this valvular problem.

Endocarditis. Endocarditis, usually of bacterial origin, causes inflammation of the cardiac endothelium and results in damage to the tricuspid, aortic, or mitral valves. Patients initially have musculoskeletal symptoms, including arthritis, low back pain, and general weakness in one or several joints. Antibiotic drugs usually are used to treat this disease.

Congenital Malformations. Congenital malformations of the heart appear in one of every 100 births and include ventricular or atrial septal defects (hole between the ventricles and atria) and patent ductus arteriosus (shunt caused by an opening between the aorta and pulmonary artery). These defects require surgical repair.

Mitral Valve Prolapse. Mitral valve prolapse (MVP) occurs in about 10% of Americans and involves variations in either the shape or structure of the mitral valve. This defect has been called **floppy valve syndrome,** Barlow's syndrome, or the click-murmur syndrome. MVP usually is benign, but its diagnosis has increased in frequency over the last decade due to its association with endocarditis, atherosclerosis, and muscular dystrophy. MVP probably results from connective tissue abnormalities in the mitral valve leaflets. Sixty percent of patients with MVP have no symp-

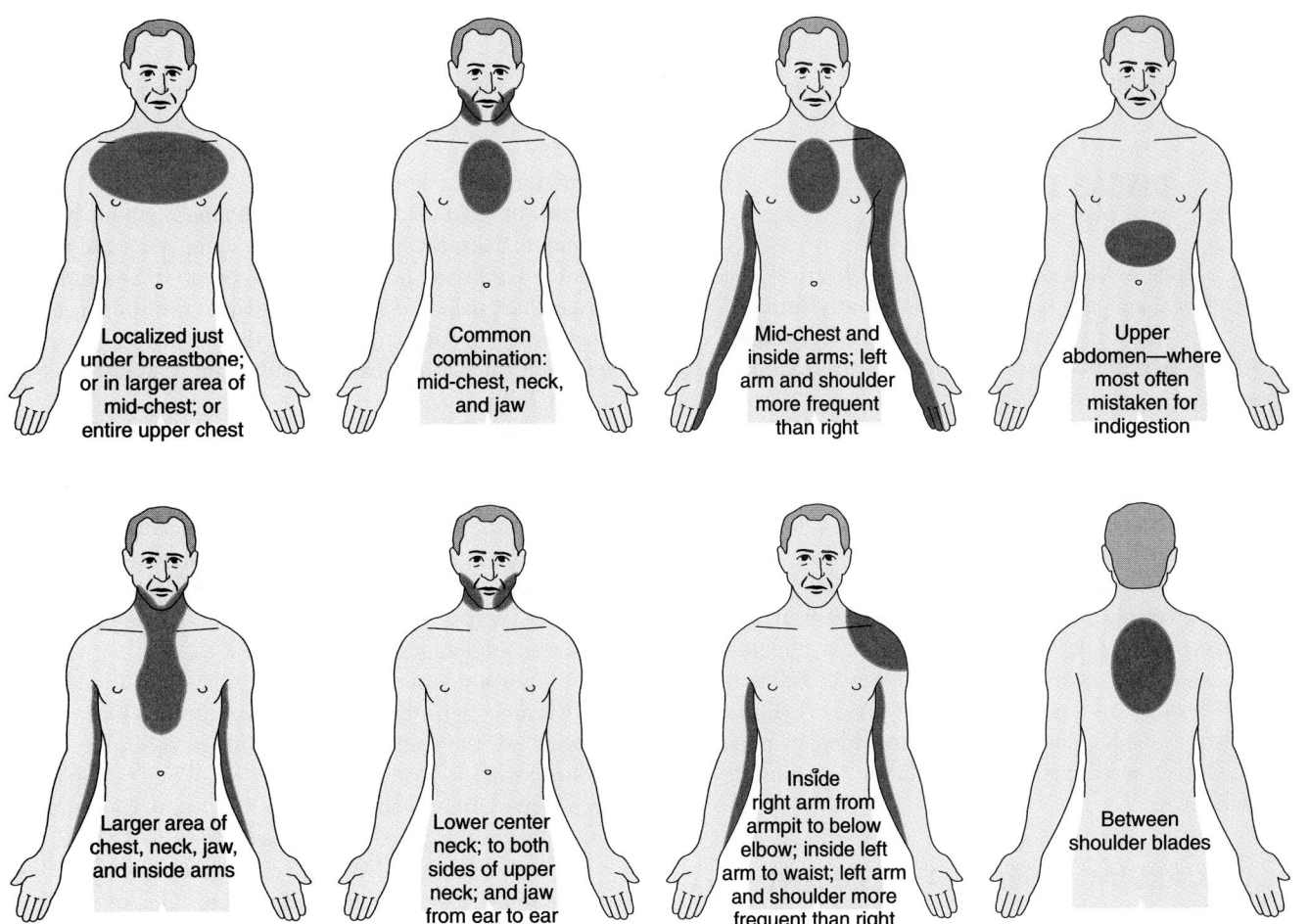

FIGURE 31.7
Location of early warning signs of myocardial infarction. Note the diverse locations for pain.

TABLE 31.6
DIAGNOSIS OF CHEST PAIN

Pain/Complaint/Findings	Possible Causes	Stimuli	Possible Pathology
Pressure, ache, tightness or burning in midsternum, left shoulder, arm; diaphoresis; nausea; vomiting; ST-segment changes	MI	Exertion; cold; smoking; heavy meal; fluid overload	CHD
Sharp pain worsens with inspiration, improves with sitting	Inflammation	Acute MI	Pericarditis
Chest tightness with breathlessness; low-grade fever	Infection	IV drug use; microbes	Myocarditis; Endocarditis
Sharp, stabbing pain, breathlessness, cough; loss of consciousness	Pulmonary	Recent surgery	Pulmonary embolism
Burning pain; indigestion relieved by antacids	Referred pain	Heavy meal, spicy food	Esophageal reflux
Angina pain, breathlessness, wide pulse pressure, ventricular hypertrophy on ECG	Ventricular outflow tract obstruction	Exertion; CHD	Aortic stenosis Mitral valve prolapse

toms, whereas 40% experience profound fatigue during exercise.

DISEASES OF THE CARDIAC NERVOUS SYSTEM

Cardiac diseases that affect the heart's electrical conduction system include **dysrhythmias (arrhythmias)** that cause the heart to beat too quickly **(tachycardia),** too slowly **(bradycardia),** or with extra beats **(extopic, extrasystole, or PVCs)** and possible subsequent fibrillation. Dysrhythmias usually lead to changes in circulatory dynamics resulting in hypotension (extremely low blood pressure), heart failure, and shock. They often occur after a stroke induced by increased physical exertion or other stress.

Sinus tachycardia is defined as a resting heart rate higher than 100 beats · min^{-1}, whereas bradycardia is defined as a resting heart rate lower than 60 beats · min^{-1}. Sinus bradycardia is normal in endurance athletes and young adults and is therefore considered to be asymptomatic. This form of bradycardia is a benign dysrhythmia and actually may be beneficial by producing a longer period of diastole and increasing ventricular filling time during the cardiac cycle.

CARDIAC DISEASE ASSESSMENT

The health-care team should review the patient's medical history, including physical examination, laboratory assessments, and pertinent physiological tests, before beginning an exercise intervention program. This clinical assessment is an important part of the rehabilitation process and provides the basis for an effective exercise prescription and intervention-rehabilitation program.

Patient History. A carefully obtained patient history documents the most common patient complaints and establishes the CHD risk profile. Because most CHD symptoms include chest pain, the differential diagnosis of this pain becomes a primary focus. A limited differential diagnosis of chest pain, including possible causes and pathogenesis, is listed in Table 31.6.

Physical Examination. The physician usually conducts the physical examination, which includes vital signs (body temperature, heart rate, breathing rate, and blood pressure), and shares the results with the health-care team. The resting heart rate is an important noninvasive measure to determine cardiovascular efficiency. Evidence of sinus tachycardia and increased breathing rate and systolic blood pressure can be indications to withhold exercise.

For purposes of prescribing exercise and identifying early warning signs, the clinical exercise physiologist must be aware of the patient's normal heart rate and blood pressure response to incremental exercise. For example, an increase in systolic blood pressure of 20 mm Hg or more in response to low-level physical activity (2 to 4 times the resting metabolic rate [METs]) can be a sign of cardiovascular impairment and can indicate an increase in myocardial oxygen demand, which suggests potential coronary ischemia. In contrast, a blunted systolic blood pressure response (hypotensive response) during low-level physical activity may indicate ventricular impairment, and at high levels of physical activity, a depressed response can be a significant risk for mortality. Patients who are unable to achieve systolic blood pressures higher than 140 mm Hg during maximal exercise may have significant dormant cardiac disease.

Heart Auscultation. Aspects of cardiac function can be evaluated by auscultation of heart sounds. The exercise physiologist should be familiar with the different abnormal heart sounds as well as how to listen for heart murmurs. Valvular diseases (e.g., MVP diagnosed by the classic click-murmur sounds) and congenital abnormalities (regurgitation sounds in ventricular septal defects) are easily diagnosed by auscultation.

Laboratory Tests. Laboratory studies of cardiac patients provide significant information to document the extent of CHD. These tests include the chest x-ray, electrocardiogram (ECG), blood lipid and lipoprotein analyses, and serum enzyme testing.

The chest x-ray reveals the size and shape of the heart and lungs, whereas the resting and exercise ECG are essen-tial to assess cardiac function in terms of electrical conductivity and myocardial oxygenation. Clinical exercise physiologists need considerable practice and experience reading and interpreting ECGs. The six different categories of ECG interpretations are listed in Table 31.7. The various ECG abnormalities and abnormal physiologic responses to exercise are discussed in Chapter 30.

Careful monitoring of ECG changes during exercise can target individuals with potential CHD for further evaluation. The more common ECG changes associated with CHD, compared to normal ECG responses during exercise in healthy individuals, are listed in Table 31.8.

Analysis of the blood lipid and lipoprotein profile usually is included as part of routine laboratory testing for CHD risk. Alterations in serum enzymes are often used to diagnose or rule out the existence of acute MI. When cell death (necrosis) or prolonged ischemia occurs, enzymes from the cardiac muscle leak into the blood because of the increased permeability of plasma membranes. This results in increased serum levels of three enzymes: creatine phosphokinase (**CPK**), lactate

---

TABLE 31.7
THE ECG IS INTERPRETED USING ONE OF SIX DIFFERENT CRITERIA

1. Measurements
   - Heart rate (atrial and ventricular)
   - PR interval (0.12 to 0.20 s)
   - QRS duration (0.06 to 0.10 s)
   - QT interval (HR dependent)
   - Frontal plane QRS Axis ($-30°$ to $+90°$)
2. Rhythm diagnosis
3. Conduction diagnosis
4. Wave form description
   - P wave (atrial enlargement)
   - QRS complex (ventricular hypertrophy, infarction)
   - ST segment (elevated or depressed)
   - T wave (flattened or inverted)
   - U wave (prominent or inverted)
5. ECG diagnosis
   - Within normal limits
   - Borderline abnormal
   - Abnormal
6. Comparison with previous ECG

From Fardy, P., and Yanowitz, F.G.: *Cardiac Rehabilitation, Adult Fitness and Exercise Testing.* Baltimore, Williams & Wilkins, 1996.

TABLE 31.8
NORMAL AND ABNORMAL ECG CHANGES DURING EXERCISE

Normal ECG Changes in Healthy Individuals[a]	Abnormal ECG Changes with CHD
1. Slight increase in P wave amplitude	1. Appearance of bundle branch block at a critical HR
2. Shortening of PR interval	2. Recurrent or multifocal PVCs during exercise and recovery
3. Shift to the right of QRS axis	3. Ventricular tachycardia
4. ST segment depression <1.0 mm	4. Appearance of brad-yarrhythmias, tach-yarrhythmias
5. Decreased T wave amplitude	5. ST segment depression/elevation of >1.0 mm 0.08 s after J point
6. Single or rare PVC during exercise and recovery	6. Exercise bradycardia
7. Single or rare PVCs or PACs	7. Submaximal exercise tachycardia
	8. Increase in frequency or severity of any known arrhythmia

[a]Abbreviations: PVC, premature ventricular contraction; PAC, premature atrial contraction.

dehydrogenase **(LDH),** and serum glutamic oxaloacetic transaminase **(SGOT).** Elevated levels of CPK reflect either skeletal or cardiac muscle necrosis. To pinpoint the source of the enzyme leak, electrophoresis or radio-immunoassay analysis of CPK separates this enzyme into three different isoenzymes: MM-isoenzyme, unique to skeletal muscle; BB-isoenzyme, specific to brain tissue; and MB-isoenzyme, specific for cardiac muscle necrosis. As with CPK, LDH can be fractionated into different iso-enzyme markers, one of which becomes elevated during an MI. The SGOT enzyme also is elevated following acute MI.

Noninvasive Physiological Tests. Specific cardiac dysfunction can be identified with different physiological tests using either **noninvasive** or **invasive** methods. Several noninvasive tests exist.

Echocardiography. Echocardiography uses pulses of reflected ultrasound to evaluate heart function and morphology; the anatomic components of the heart are identified, and their distances from the echo transducers are measured. This allows accurate estimation of the size of the various heart chambers and vessels as well as the thickness of the muscle itself. The echocardiogram has surpassed the ECG in recognizing chamber enlargement, myocardial hypertrophy, and other structural abnormalities. Echocardiograms also are used for diagnosing heart murmurs and evaluating valvular lesions and the extent of congenital heart diseases and cardiomyopathies.

Graded Exercise Stress Test. Part 5 of Chapter 30 presented a detailed discussion of the rationale for use of stress testing for apparently healthy individuals and those with CHD and outlined the various stress test protocols. *The main purpose of the graded exercise stress test (GXT) is to observe and evaluate the ECG under conditions that exceed resting requirements.* This enables the physician and exercise physiologist to confirm a diagnosis of CHD in patients with suspected angina or coronary insufficiency and to determine functional capacity in patients with known disease or after surgery or other interventional procedures.

Subjective and objective data collected during a GXT that form the basis of an exercise prescription are listed in Table 31.9. The exercise physiologist and cardiologist are the key health-care professionals who supervise the exercise test, interpret the data, and prepare the exercise prescription.

Invasive Physiological Tests. Invasive physiological tests provide information that is not obtainable through noninvasive procedures, including the extent, severity, and location of coronary atherosclerosis, the degree of ventricular dysfunction, and specific cardiac abnormalities.

Radionucleotide Studies. Radionucleotide studies involve injection of a radioactive isotope at rest and during exercise. The two types of radionucleotide procedures are

TABLE 31.9
DATA FROM AN EXERCISE STRESS TEST TO DIAGNOSE AND FORMULATE EXERCISE PRESCRIPTIONS

Subjective Data

Angina pain
Dyspnea ratings
Fatigue and weakness
Leg discomfort
Dizziness
Rating of perceived exertion (RPE)

Objective Data

- **Physical Examination Data**
  Breathing sounds
  Murmurs and gallops
  Blood pressure
  Pulmonary function tests (before or after exercise)
  Heart rate response
  Blood gas parameters

- **Physical Performance Data**
  Time on treadmill/cycle ergometer
  Maximum work or power output
  Rate-pressure product (RPP; HR × systolic blood pressure)

- **Electrocardiogram Data**
  ST segment changes
  Rate responses
  Dysrhythmias
  Conduction abnormalities

- **Cardiorespiratory Data**
  Lactate threshold
  Carbon dioxide output
  Minute ventilation
  Oxygen uptake
  Respiratory exchange ratio (R)

thallium imaging, which evaluates areas of myocardial blood flow and tissue perfusion to differentiate between a true and a false-positive S-T segment depression obtained by ECG evaluation, and **ventriculography,** which is an imaging procedure that provides information about the dynamics of left ventricular function.

Cardiac Catheterization. In cardiac catheterization, a fine tube or catheter is placed into a vein or artery and passed into the right or left side of the heart. Different pressure gradients are assessed at different locations within the heart, and blood is sampled directly from the ventricle or atria to determine the oxygen content of arterial and venous blood.

Coronary Angiography. Coronary angiography is an invasive method that provides an intracardiac x-ray when a radiopaque contrast medium is injected into the coronary blood vessels and its passage is viewed during the cardiac cycle. This technique is highly effective in assessing the extent of atherosclerosis and is the "gold standard" for calculating coronary blood flow; results are used as a baseline for all other test comparisons. Major drawbacks of this procedure are that it cannot show how readily blood flows within portions of the heart muscle and it cannot be performed during exercise.

CLASSIFICATION OF PATIENTS FOR CARDIAC REHABILITATION

In general, few symptoms are present in the early stages of CHD. As the disease progresses and coronary artery narrowing increases, clinical symptoms become evident and continue with progressive severity. The first sign of CHD often is slight angina pain accompanied by a decrease in functional capacity. With progression, this leads to ischemia, which may result in necrosis of myocardial tissue. In severe cases, the patient often experiences persistent chest pain, anxiety, nausea, vomiting, and dyspnea. If untreated, this can lead to weakening of the myocardium and eventual heart failure in which the cardiac output fails to meet the metabolic demands of the body. Often, pulmonary congestion increases (a persistent cough is a sign of congestive heart failure), and the patient coughs up blood. At this stage, the patient becomes dyspneic, even when sitting at rest, and may suffer a sudden mild to massive MI.

A system for classifying the functional and therapeutic characteristics in the various stages of heart disease is shown in Table 31.10. Such a classification system makes it possible to categorize patients for subsequent rehabilitation. It should be emphasized that there are large individual differences in symptoms, functional capacities, and appropriate rehabilitation requirements. Whenever a patient is referred for rehabilitation, it is important to make an appropriate classification based on all of the available medical screening information, including the most recently administered GXT.

**TABLE 31.10
FUNCTIONAL AND THERAPEUTIC
CLASSIFICATIONS OF HEART DISEASE**

Functional Capacity Classification

Class I: No limitation of physical activity. Ordinary physical activity does not cause undue fatigue, palpitation, dyspnea, or anginal pain

Class II: Slight limitation of physical activity. Comfortable at rest, but ordinary physical activity results in fatigue, palpitation, dyspnea, or anginal pain

Class III: Marked limitation of physical activity. Comfortable at rest, but less than ordinary activity causes fatigue, palpitation, dyspnea, or anginal pain

Class IV: Unable to carry on any physical activity without discomfort. Symptoms of cardiac insufficiency or of the anginal syndrome may be present even at rest. If any physical activity is undertaken, discomfort is increased

Therapeutic Classification

Class A: Physical activity need not be restricted

Class B: Ordinary physical activity need not be restricted, but unusually severe or competitive efforts should be avoided

Class C: Ordinary physical activity should be moderately restricted, and more strenuous efforts should be discontinued

Class D: Ordinary physical activity should be markedly restricted

Class E: Patient should be at complete rest and confined to bed or chair

From New York Heart Association.

PHASES OF CARDIAC REHABILITATION

After diagnosis and appropriate intervention (e.g., bypass surgery, angioplasty, or other intervention strategies), the cardiac patient is referred to the exercise physiologist for functional capacity testing and subsequent classification and rehabilitation.[8a] The rehabilitation program uses exercise applied under precise guidelines as a treatment modality with a low risk of complications. The five most important aspects for a successful cardiac rehabilitation program include the following:

1. Appropriate patient selection.
2. Concurrent medical, surgical, and pharmacological therapies.
3. Comprehensive patient education.
4. Appropriate exercise prescription.
5. Careful patient monitoring during rehabilitation.

As shown in Table 31.11, rehabilitation programs consist of three distinct phases, each with a different objective, different physical activities for the patient, and different levels of required supervision. Patients are required to complete a GXT with no symptoms before progressing to the next phase. These phases are sometimes classified as **inpatient, outpatient, in-home,** and **community** (see Table 30.8, Chapter 30, p. 664).

TABLE 31.11
CARDIAC REHABILITATION PROGRAMS

Phase	Duration	Treatment Objectives	Role of Exercise Physiologist	Patient Activities	Patient Education	Discharge
Phase I Hospital inpatient; usually follows surgery; usually coordinated with physician, physical therapist, and exercise physiologist	6 to 14 d; 1–7 d in ICU, 7–14 d in ward	1. Prevent the effects of bed rest and deconditioning 2. Reduce orthostatic hypotension 3. Maintain joint mobility	1. Supervise low level exercise 2. Monitor daily living activities 3. Evaluate heart rate and blood pressure responses	1. Range of motion (ROM) activities 2. Progressive ambulation, stair climbing 3. MET activities not to exceed 1-3 METs, or HR greater than 20 beats · min^{-1} > resting HR 4. Includes continuous ambulatory monitoring	1. Lifestyle education 2. Identifying personal risk factors	Before discharge patient completes low-level, symptom-limited GXT with no complications; purpose of GXT evaluates functional capacity and determines symptom-limited HR for Phase II prescription
Phase II Convalescent (outpatient) stage following hospital discharge; at a supervised cardiac rehab center (YMCA, hospital, or university center)	14 d to 12 wk post-coronary event; usually begins immediately after hospital discharge	1. Move from recuperation to improving functional capacity; promote return to normal daily activities 2. Promote positive lifestyle changes	1. Formulate exercise prescription based on GXT results 2. Monitor HR, BP, RPE, and determine energy expenditure during exercise 3. Ensure progression for discharge to Phase III	1. Individually prescribed progressive exercise using different modes (walking, cycling, arm exercise, circuit-resistance training, swimming) 2. Careful monitoring (including frequent GXT testing) during progressive increases in exercise intensity	1. Risk factor modification programs 2. Comprehensive patient and family education	Before discharge patient must complete a symptom limited maximal GXT without complications
Phase III Non–hospital-based community rehab program; patients may have finished a Phase I or II program, or may enter with no prior involvement; patients stable with decreasing or no angina, controlled arrhythmias, ability to self regulate exercise; minimal functional capacity (>6 METs)	4 to 6 months or longer; some patients may be in Phase III for 1 y or more	1. Maintenance of function 2. Compliance with an exercise program 3. Risk factor modification	1. Formulate exercise prescription based on GXT results 2. Monitor HR, BP, RPE, and sometimes energy expenditure during exercise 3. Ensure compliance 4. Help patients with self selection of different activities	1. Individually prescribed progressive exercise using a variety of modes (walking, cycling, arm exercise, circuit-resistance training, swimming) 2. Successfully completes maximal GXT	1. Maintenance of risk factor modification	Before discharge, patients complete symptom limited maximal GXT with no complications; patient resumes normal life

Patients are placed on a cardiac rehabilitation program partially based on level of CHD risk. An example of a three-level CHD risk classification system is presented in Table 31.12. The proper identification of CHD risk makes patient management easier and safer.

THE EXERCISE PRESCRIPTION

As reviewed in Part 5 of Chapter 30, the principles that govern exercise prescription are based on exercise **type, intensity, duration, frequency,** and **progression.** Prescribing exercise for the CHD patient requires particular concern for patient safety and involves vigilant and careful monitoring, especially for patients with moderate to high risk. The patient's clinical status and performance on the GXT determine the specifics of the exercise prescription. Any rhythmic activity that involves the large muscles of the body is appropriate. Most exercises are chosen on the basis of the patient's preference, skill requirement, potential carryover to the home environment, and availability of exercise equipment.

Determining the exercise intensity is the most difficult yet important aspect of the exercise prescription. The intensity must ensure that the proper percentage of the individual's functional capacity is achieved and maintained. Most exercise programs for cardiac rehabilitation begin with symptom-limited exercises in which the goal is simple ambulation (see Table 31.11). Initially, an intensity level between 50 and 60% of the subject's maximally achieved MET level on the GXT should be established. In some cases, a lower level of 20 to 40% of maximum is required as the target level.

In Chapter 30, a practical example of an exercise prescription based on percentage of maximum heart rate was illustrated (Fig. 30.23). Exercise can also be prescribed by the MET method. In this approach, the patient and exercise physiologist select activities for training with known energy expenditures that are within the patient's capability (determined from the GXT). For example, for a 50-year-old male whose maximum exercise level is 8 METs ($\dot{V}o_2max = 28$ mL $\cdot$ kg$^{-1} \cdot$ min$^{-1}/3.5$ mL $\cdot$ kg$^{-1} \cdot$ min$^{-1} = 8$ METs), the training intensity level for the exercise prescription corresponding to 60 to 70% of functional capacity would be 4.8 to 5.6 METs (8 METs $\times$ 0.60; 8 METs $\times$ 0.70). The data in Table 31.13 represent comparisons of exercise intensity and comparative MET levels for cycle ergometer and corresponding treadmill exercises for a 70-kg person. For example, for this person riding a stationary bike at 600 kg $\cdot$ m $\cdot$ min^{-1} (100 W) is the MET equivalent to walking on a treadmill at 3.0 mph with a 7.5% incline.

Exercise should begin with 5 to 15 minutes of light warmup stretching and range-of-motion activities, followed by several minutes of light to moderate cardiovascular warmup with rhythmic movements. The aerobic conditioning phase should progress in duration so individuals are eventually able to perform 30 to 45 minutes of continuous activity at the prescribed intensity. This is then followed by a 5- to 15-minute period of low-intensity, cool-down movements.

Most cardiac rehabilitation patients are able to tolerate exercising 3 days per week with no more than a 2-day lapse between exercise sessions. For the elderly individuals or those with low functional capacity (less than 5 METs), low-intensity exercise is recommended daily or twice daily.[25] As a patient's functional capacity improves, exercise intensity and duration can be progressively increased with little fear of complications. Updating the exercise prescription is usually based on the findings of a recently administered GXT.

TABLE 31.12
CLASSIFICATION OF CHD RISK BY SPECIFIC CHARACTERISTICS

CHD Risk Level	Characteristics
Low	1. Uncomplicated clinical symptoms 2. No evidence of MI 3. Functional capacity ≥ 7 METs 4. Normal left ventricular function 5. Absence of significant ventricular ectopy
Moderate	1. ST segment depression ≥ 2 mm, flat or downsloping 2. Reversible thallium defects 3. Moderate to good left ventricular function 4. Changing pattern, or new development of angina
High	1. Prior MI or infarct involving $\geq 35\%$ of left ventricle 2. Ejection fraction $\leq 35\%$ at rest 3. Fall in exercise SBP or failure of SBP to rise more than 10 mm Hg on GXT 4. Persistent or recurrent ischemic pain 24 h or more after hospital admission 5. Functional capacity ≤ 5 METs with hypotensive BP response, or ≥ 1 mm ST segment depression 6. Congestive heart failure 7. ≥ 2 mm ST segment depression at peak HR ≤ 135 beats $\cdot$ min^{-1} 8. High-grade ventricular ectopy

From *Guidelines for Cardiac Rehabilitation Programs. American Association of Cardiovascular and Pulmonary Rehabilitation.* Champaign, IL, Human Kinetics, 1991.

TABLE 31.13
ESTIMATED ENERGY EXPENDITURE AND POWER OUTPUT FOR A 70-KG PERSON DURING BICYCLE ERGOMETRY AND TREADMILL EXERCISE[a]

Bicycle Ergometry Power Output		Treadmill			Estimated Energy Expenditure	
$kg \cdot m \cdot min^{-1}$	Watts	Speed	% Grade	METs	$\dot{V}_{O_2}, mL \cdot kg^{-1} \cdot min^{-1}$	$kcal \cdot min^{-1}$
150	25	2.0	0	2.4	8.5	3.0
300	50	3.0	0	3.7	13.0	4.5
450	75	3.0	5.0	5.0	17.0	6.0
600	100	3.0	7.5	6.0	21.0	7.5
750	125	3.0	10.0	7.0	26.0	9.0
900	150	3.0	15.0	8.5	30.0	10.5
1050	175	4.0	14.0	10.0	36.0	12.0
1200	200	7.0	0	11.0	39.0	14.0
1350	225	4.0	18.0	12.0	43.0	15.0
1500	250	8.0	0	13.5	47.0	17.0
1650	275	3.5	26.0	14.5	51.0	18.0
1800	300	10.0	0	16.0	56.0	20.0

[a]Values for bicycle and treadmill equivalents are estimated for a 70-kg person only. The oxygen cost ($L \cdot min^{-1}$) of weight-supported stationary cycling at a particular power output is relatively fixed and independent of body mass. In contrast, the absolute oxygen cost of weight-bearing walking or running depends directly on body mass. Thus, considerable deviation from the equivalence values in the table will occur for individuals who are heavier or lighter than 70 kg. In such cases, another table must be constructed using appropriate but specific oxygen cost values for a particular mode of exercise and body mass. (Table values adapted from American College of Sports Medicine: *Guidelines for Exercise Testing and Prescription,* 5th ed. Baltimore, Williams & Wilkins, 1995, p. 275–282).

Along with an exercise prescription, two other important components of cardiac rehabilitation are patient education and appropriate drug intervention. It also is common to include family support counseling as part of a total program of rehabilitation. Successful rehabilitation is enhanced by positive family support. A trained social worker is often helpful in facilitating this aspect of the rehabilitative process.

Resistance Exercises Can Be Beneficial. As part of a comprehensive cardiac rehabilitation program, resistance-type exercises can restore and maintain muscular strength and help promote preservation of the fat-free mass. Because of the augmented blood pressure response with straining-type exercises, resistance training for the cardiac patient involves only light resistance (30 to 50% of dynamic muscle strength [1-RM]) with 12 to 15 repetitions. Progression should be slow, starting with one set and progressing to three sets by the end of rehabilitation.

CARDIAC MEDICATIONS

Knowledge of the physiologic effects of drug intervention allows the clinical exercise physiologist to accurately assess the patient's response during physical activity. An improvement in functional capacity may allow for alterations (decreases) in drug therapy. Patients should be aware of what drugs they are taking and the potential side effects of those drugs. The six classifications of common cardiac drugs, along with trade names, side effects, and possible effects on the exercise response, are presented in Table 31.14.

PULMONARY DISEASES

The exercise physiologist's involvement in treatment of patients with pulmonary disease is focused primarily on improving ventilation, decreasing the work of breathing, and increasing the overall level of functional capacity.[6a] The exercise physiologist interprets clinical information from the personal history, physical examination, pertinent laboratory data, and imaging studies. A disorder of the cardiovascular system most always affects pulmonary function and eventually results in accompanying pulmonary disabilities. Conversely, pulmonary disease is intimately related to cardiovascular complications.

Many diseases and disabilities of the pulmonary system require exercise rehabilitation. Pulmonary abnormalities

TABLE 31.14
CARDIAC MEDICATIONS: THEIR USE, SIDE EFFECTS, AND EFFECTS ON EXERCISE RESPONSE

Type/Trade Name	Use	Side Effects	Effects on Exercise Response
I. Anti-anginal Agents			
A. Nitroglycerin compounds [*Amyl nitrate; Isordil; Nitrostat*]	Smooth muscle relaxation; decrease cardiac output	Headache, dizziness, hypotension	Hypotension; increase exercise capacity
B. Beta blockers [*Inderal; Propranolol; Lopressor; Corgard; Biocadren*]	Block beta receptors; decrease sympathetic tone; decrease HR, contractility, BP	Bradycardia, heart block, insomnia, nausea, fatigue, weakness, increased cholesterol and blood sugar	Decrease HR; hypotension; decrease cardiac contractility
C. Calcium Antagonists [*Verapamil; Nifedipine; Procardia*]	Block influx of calcium; dilate coronary arteries; suppress dysrhythmias	Dizziness, syncope, flushing, hypotension headache, fluid retention	Hypotension
II. Antihypertensive Agents			
A. Diuretics [*Thiazides, Lasix, Aldactone*]	Inhibit NA$^+$ and CI$^-$ in kidney; increase excretion of sodium and water, and control high BP and fluid retention	Drowsiness, dehydration, electrolyte imbalance; gout, nausea, pain, hearing loss, elevated cholesterol and lipoproteins	Hypotension
B. Vasodilators [*Hydralazine, Captopril, Apresoline, Loniten, Minoxidil*]	Dilate peripheral blood vessels; used in conjunction with diuretics; decrease BP	Increase HR and contractility; headache, drowsiness, nausea, vomiting, diarrhea	
C. Drugs interfering with sympathetic nervous system [*Reserprine, Propranolol, Aldomet, Catapres, Minipress*]	Decrease BP, HR, and cardiac output by dilating blood vessels	Drowsiness, depression, sexual dysfunction, fatigue, dry mouth, stuffy nose, fever, upset stomach, fluid retention, weight gain	Hypotension
III. Digitalis Glycosides, Derivatives [*Digoxin, Lonoxin, Digitoxin*]	Strengthen heart's pumping force and decrease electrical conduction	Arrhythmias, heart block, altered ECG, fatigue, weakness, headache, nausea, vomiting	Increase exercise capacity; increase myocardial contractility
IV. Anticoagulant Agents [*Coumadin, Sodium Heparin, Aspirin, Persantine*]	Prevent blood clot formation	Easy bruising, stomach irritation, joint or abdominal pain, difficulty in swallowing, unexplained swelling, uncontrolled bleeding	
V. Antilipidemic Agents [*Cholestyramine, Lopid, Niacin, Atromid-S, Mevacor, Questran Zocor*]	Interfere with lipid metabolism and lowers cholesterol and low density lipoproteins	Nausea, vomiting, diarrhea, constipation, flatulence, abdominal discomfort, glucose intolerance	
VI. Antiarrhythmic Agents [*Cardioquin, Procaine, Quinidine Lidocaine, Dilantin, Propranolol, Bretylium tosylate, Verapamil*]	Alter conduction patterns throughout the myocardium	Nausea, palpitations, vomiting, rash, insomnia, dizziness, shortness of breath, swollen ankles, coughing up blood, fever, psychosis, impotence	Hypotension; decrease HR; decrease cardiac contractility

are commonly classified as either **obstructive** (normal air flow is impeded) or **restrictive** (various dimensions of air volume in the lungs are reduced). Although this is a convenient classification system, several pulmonary disorders can be indicative of both a restrictive and obstructive impairment.

RESTRICTIVE LUNG DYSFUNCTION

Restrictive lung dysfunction (RLD) is characterized by an abnormal reduction in pulmonary ventilation, along with diminished lung expansion and a decrease in the volume of air moved during tidal volume. Trauma or therapeutic interventions such as radiation trauma also can lead to the development of RLD.

There are three aspects of pulmonary ventilation: **lung compliance, lung volumes and capacities,** and the **work of breathing** involved in the genesis of RLD. Lung compliance refers to the change in lung volume in relation to pressure differentials and is a measure of the distensibility of the lungs, chest wall, or both. In RLD, the chest and lung tissues tend to stiffen and offer considerable resistance to expansion under normal pressure differentials. Because pulmonary compliance is decreased in RLD, resistance to lung expansion increases (decreased pulmonary compliance requires an increase in pressure to maintain adequate lung expansion and minute ventilation). This greatly increases the energy cost of normal ventilation. Eventually, RLD progresses to a point at which significant decreases in all lung volumes and capacities occur. Examples of typical lung volumes in different impairments associated with RLD are illustrated in Figure 31.8. Diminished inspiratory and expiratory reserve volumes occur under all conditions.

The major restrictive lung diseases, along with their causes, signs and symptoms, and suggested treatments, are listed in Table 31.15. Other known causes of RLD include rheumatoid arthritis, immunologic causes, massive obesity, diabetes mellitus, trauma from crash injuries, penetrating wounds, burns and other inhalation injuries, poisoning, and complications from drug therapy (including reactions to antibiotics and anti-inflammatory drugs).

CHRONIC OBSTRUCTIVE PULMONARY DISEASE

Chronic obstructive pulmonary disease (COPD), also termed chronic airflow limitations or CAL, is a group of diseases of the respiratory tract that produce an obstruction to airflow. This ultimately affects the lung's mechanical function, and gas exchange is compromised at the alveolar level. This disorder is the fifth leading cause of death and the second leading cause of morbidity in the United States. The natural history of COPD spans 20 to 50 years and is closely associated with a history of chronic cigarette smoking.

COPD usually is diagnosed by changes in pulmonary function tests, most notably a decrease in expiratory flow rates and an increase in residual lung volume. The classic symptoms of this disease include spontaneous spasms of the bronchial smooth muscle that result in a chronic cough, increased mucus production, inflammation and thickening of the mucosal lining of the bronchi and bronchioles, wheezing, and dyspnea upon physical exertion. The differences among the major COPD conditions are summarized in Table 31.16. Factors predisposing to COPD include chronic cigarette smoking, air pollution, occupational exposure to irritating dusts or gases, heredity, infection, allergies, aging, and drugs. *COPD rarely occurs in nonsmokers.* In all forms of COPD, the airways narrow to obstruct airflow in the lungs (see Table 31.16). This narrowing hinders ventilation by trapping air in the bronchioles and alveoli; in essence,

FIGURE 31.8
Example of lung volumes in different conditions of restrictive lung disease. Abbreviations: IRV, inspiratory reserve volume; FVC, forced vital capacity; ERV, expiratory reserve volume; RLV, residual lung volume; ALS, amyotrophic lateral sclerosis.

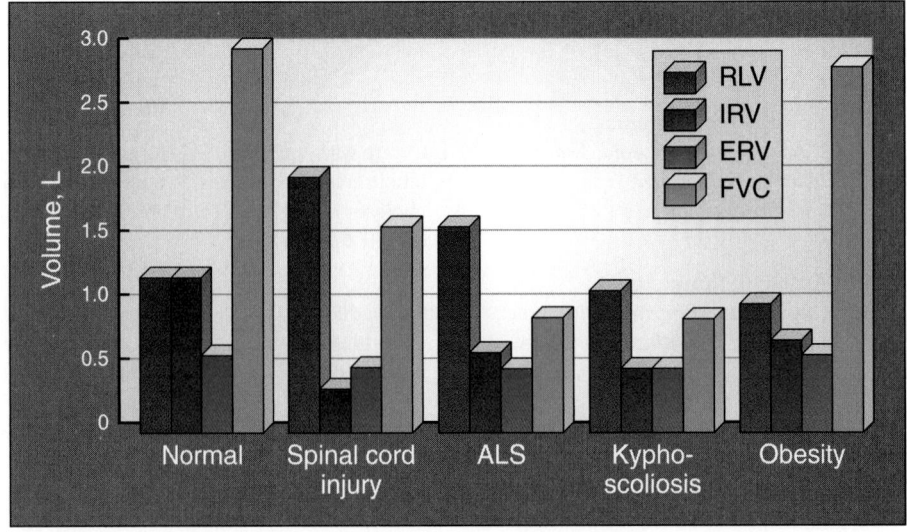

TABLE 31.15
RESTRICTIVE LUNG DISEASES

	Causes/Type	Etiology	Signs and Symptoms	Treatment
I.	**Maturational**			
	a. *Abnormal fetal lung development*	Premature birth; (hypoplasia-reduced lung tissue)	Asymptomatic; pulmonary insufficiency	No specific treatment
	b. *Respiratory distress syndrome* (hyaline membrane disease)	Insufficient maturation of lungs due to premature birth	↑ respiration rate; ↓ lung volumes; ↓ PaO$_2$; acidemia; rapid and labored respiration pressure	Treat mother prior to birth (corticosteroids); Hyperalimentation; continuous positive airway
	c. *Aging*	Aging and cumulative effects of pollution, noxious gas, inhaled drug use and cigarette smoking	↑ residual volume; ↓ vital capacity; repetitive periodic apnea	No specific treatment; increase physical activity
II.	**Pulmonary**			
	a. *Idiopathic pulmonary fibrosis* (IPF)	Unknown origin (perhaps viral or genetic)	↓ lung volumes; ↓ lung volumes; pulmonary hypertension; dyspnea; cough; weight loss, fatigue	Corticosteroids; maintain adequate nutrition and ventilation
	b. *Coal workers' pneumoconiosis*	Repeated inhalation of coal dust over 10–12 y	↓ TLC, VC, FRC; ↓ lung compliance; dyspnea; ↓ PaO$_2$; pulmonary hypertension; cough	Nonreversible, no known cure
	c. *Asbestosis*	Chronic exposure to asbestos	↓ lung volumes; abnormal x-ray; ↓ PaO$_2$; dyspnea on exertion, shortness of breath	Nonreversible, no known cure
	d. *Pneumonia*	Inflammatory process caused by various, bacteria, microbes, viruses	↓ lung volumes; abnormal x-ray; tachypneic dyspnea; high fever, chills, cough; pleuritic pain	Drug therapy (antibiotic)
	e. *Adult respiratory distress syndrome*	Acute lung injury (fat emboli, drowning, drug induced, shock, blood transfusion, pneumonia)	Abnormal lung function tests; PaO$_2$ < 60 mmHg; extreme dyspnea; cyanotic; headache; anxiety	Intubation and mechanical ventilation
	f. *Bronchogenic carcinoma*	Tobacco use	Variable depending on type and location of growth	Surgery, radiation, chemotherapy; specific drainage
	g. *Pleural effusions*	Accumulation of fluid within plueral space; heart failure; cirrhosis	Shortness of breath; pleuritic chest pain; ↓ PaO$_2$	
III.	**Cardiovascular**			
	a. *Pulmonary edema*	↑ pulmonary capillary hydrostatic pressure secondary to left ventricular failure	↑ respiration rate; ↓ lung volumes; ↓ PaO$_2$; arrhythmias; report feeling of suffocation, shortness of breath, cyanotic, cough	Drug therapy, diuretics; supplemental O$_2$
	b. *Pulmonary emboli*	Complications of venous thrombosis	↓ lung volumes; ↓ PaO$_2$; tachycardia; acute dyspnea, shortness of breath; syncope	Heparin therapy; mechanical ventilation

TABLE 31.15—continued

Causes/Type	Etiology	Signs and Symptoms	Treatment
IV. Neuromuscular			
a. *Spinal cord injury*	Trauma paralysis of respiratory muscles	↓ lung volumes; hypoxemia; fatigue; shortness of breath; inability to cough; ↓ voice volume	Active and passive chest wall stretching
b. *Amyotrophic lateral sclerosis*	Degenerative disease of nervous system	↓ lung volumes; ↓ maximum voluntary volume	No treatment except supportive therapy
c. *Poliomyelitis*	Viral infectious disease that attacks motor nerves	Paralysis of diaphragm; shortness of breath	No treatment except supportive therapy
d. *Guillain-Barré syndrome*	Demyelinating disease of motor neurons	Profound muscular weakness; ↓ lung volumes	Passive range of motion exercises; active exercise
e. *Neuromuscular diseases (myasthenia gravis, tetanus, muscular dystrophy)*	Diseases of neuromuscular system, genetic or other etiology resulting in chronic muscular weakness and wasting	Weakness, fatigue, loss of muscle function and strength, paralysis—will effect pulmonary system with eventual loss of function	Drugs; passive and active exercise; supportive therapy
V. Musculoskeletal			
a. *Diaphragmatic paralysis*	Loss or impairment of motor function of diaphragm muscle due to specific lesion	↓ lung volumes; dyspnea, shortness of breath	Not needed
b. *Kyphoscoliosis*	Excessive anteroposterior and lateral curvature of thoracic spine (cause unknown)	↓ lung volumes; exertional dyspnea	Use of orthotic devices; active exercise
c. *Ankylosing spondylitis*	Chronic inflammatory disease of spine (inherited)	Exertional dyspnea	No treatment

TABLE 31.16
DIFFERENCES AMONG THE MAJOR COPD DISEASES

Name	Area Affected	Result
Bronchitis	Membrane lining bronchial tubes	Inflammation of bronchial lining
Bronchiectasis	Bronchial tubes (bronchi or air passages)	Bronchial dilation with inflammation
Emphysema	Air spaces beyond terminal bronchioles (aleveoli)	Breakdown of alveolar walls; air spaces enlarged
Asthma	Bronchioles (small airways)	Bronchioles obstructed by muscle spasm; swelling of mucosa, thick secretions
Cystic fibrosis	Bronchioles	Bronchioles become obstructed and obliterated; plugs of mucus cling to airway walls leading to bronchitis, atelectasis, pneumonia, or pulmonary abscess

the result is an increase in the physiologic dead space. The obstruction increases the resistance to airflow (especially during expiration), hinders normal gas exchange, and reduces exercise capacity by increasing the energy cost of breathing and reduces ventilatory capacity.

In the following sections, discussion centers on three of the major COPD diseases: **chronic bronchitis, emphy-** **sema,** and **cystic fibrosis.** The obstructive conditions of **asthma** and **exercise-induced bronchospasm** are discussed in detail in Chapter 12.

Chronic Bronchitis. Acute bronchitis is an inflammation of the trachea and bronchi that is self-limiting and of short duration. In contrast, chronic bronchitis is associated with prolonged exposure to nonspecific irritants and is

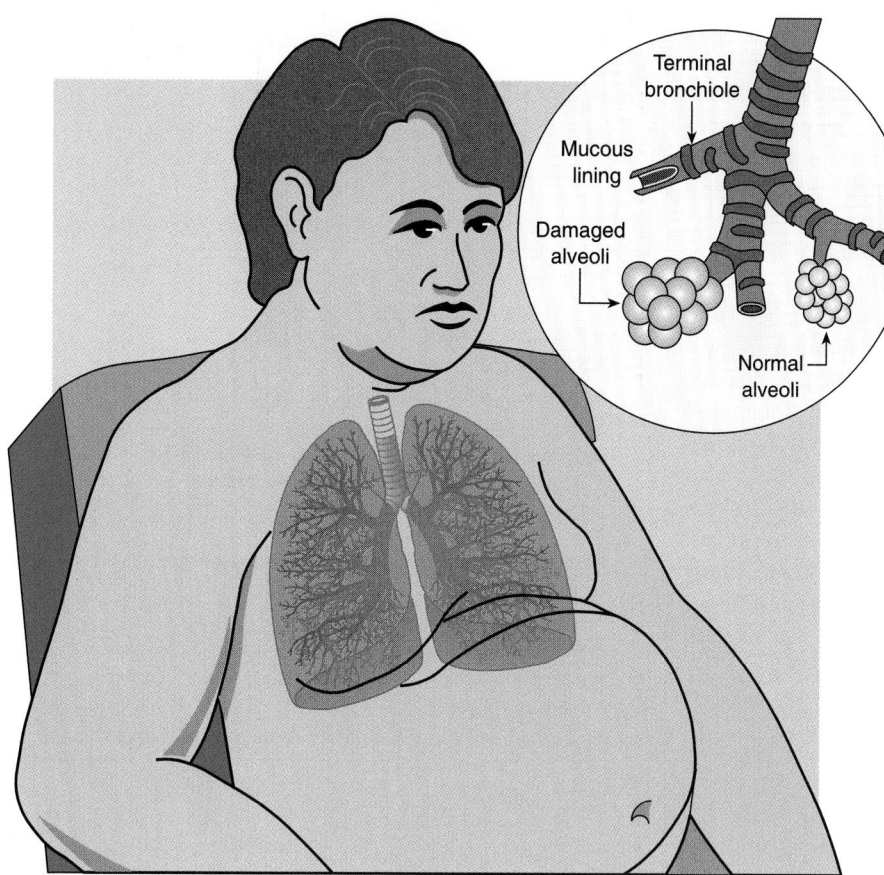

FIGURE 31.9

A person with chronic bronchitis usually develops cyanosis and pulmonary edema with the characteristic appearance known as the "Blue Bloater." The effects of chronic bronchitis displayed in the insert illustrate misshapen or large alveolar sacs with reduced space for oxygen and carbon dioxide exchange.

accompanied by increases in mucus secretion. Over time, the swollen mucus membranes and thick sputum obstruct the airways, causing wheezing and chronic coughing. Partial or complete blockage of the airways from mucus secretion causes insufficient arterial saturation and edema, which results in the patient's developing the characteristic look known as a "Blue Bloater" (Fig. 31.9). Chronic bronchitis develops slowly and worsens over time. Patients with chronic bronchitis usually have been long-term smokers. Functional capacity is low, and fatigue occurs readily with only moderate exercise. If left untreated, this disease can lead to death.

Emphysema. Emphysema is characterized by abnormal, permanent enlargement of air spaces distal to the terminal bronchioles. It is most common in chronic cigarette smokers. Emphysema can develop as a consequence of chronic bronchitis and is characterized by extreme dyspnea, hypercapnea, persistent cough, cyanosis, and digital clubbing (evidence of chronic hypoxemia; Fig. 31.10). Patients with emphysema have a low physical work capacity and exhibit extreme dyspnea upon physical exertion; they are often thin and lean forward with arms braced on the knees to support the shoulders and chest for easy breathing. The effects of trapped air and alveolar distension change the size and

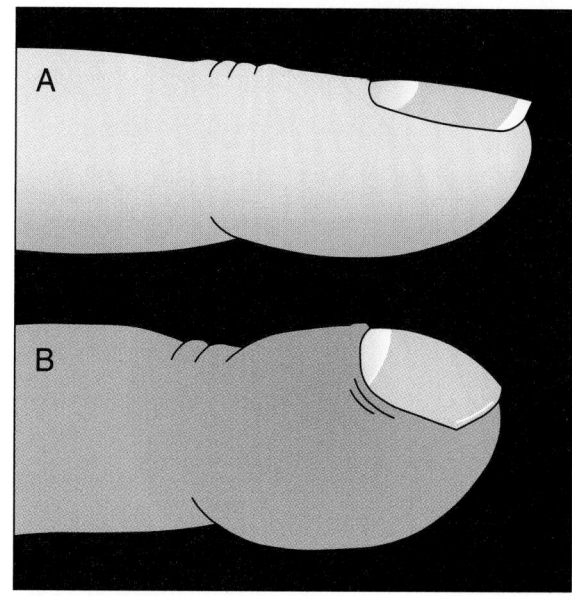

FIGURE 31.10

Normal digit configuration (**A**) and example of digital clubbing (**B**). Club fingers and toes indicate chronic tissue hypoxia, a common diagnosis in emphysema.

shape of the chest, causing the characteristic emphysemic "barrel chest" appearance (Fig. 31.11).

Although exercise will not improve pulmonary function for an individual with emphysema, it nevertheless enhances cardiovascular fitness and strengthens the respiratory muscles. Regular exercise also often improves the psychological mood of the patient.

Cystic Fibrosis. The term cystic fibrosis (CF) is derived from the diagnosis of cysts and scar tissue observed on the pancreas during autopsy of patients who have died from CF. Although pancreatic cysts and scar tissue often are present, they are not primary characteristics of the disease; however, the term "cystic fibrosis" has been retained.[16] Clinical signs and symptoms of CF are listed in Table 31.17. CF is a genetically inherited disease that is characterized by a thickening of the secretions of all exocrine glands (e.g., pancreatic, pulmonic, and gastrointestinal). This leads to obstruction in the pulmonary system, mainly in the lung tissue. CF is the most commonly inherited genetic disease in Caucasians and affects approximately 1 in 2000 white newborn infants in the United States. The

TABLE 31.17
CLINICAL SIGNS AND SYMPTOMS OF CYSTIC FIBROSIS AND RELATED PULMONARY INVOLVEMENT

Clinical Signs and Symptoms of Cystic Fibrosis (Early Stages)

- Persistent cough and wheezing
- Recurrent pneumonia
- Excessive appetite but poor weight gain
- Salty skin or sweat
- Bulky, foul-smelling stools (undigested lipids)

Clinical Signs and Symptoms of Cystic Fibrosis (Latter Stages)
With Pulmonary Involvement

- Tachypnea (rapid breathing)
- Sustained chronic cough with mucus production on vomiting
- Barrel chest
- Cyanosis and digital clubbing
- Exertional dyspnea with decreased exercise capacity
- Pneumothorax
- Right heart failure secondary to pulmonary hypertension

disease is inherited as a recessive trait (both parents must be carriers) and is always fatal. CF is rare among African-Americans and Asian-Americans. Approximately 5% (12 million) of Americans carry the gene for CF, which is located on chromosome 7.[8]

Diagnosis of CF is made by a positive sweat electrolyte (chloride) test. Patients with CF have a faulty copy of the gene that enable cells to construct a channel through which the chloride ion passes. Consequently, salt accumulates in the cell lining of the lungs and digestive tissue, making the surrounding mucus abnormally thick and salty. These mucus secretions obstruct ducts and passages in the pancreas, liver, and lungs and are the main features of CF.

Pulmonary involvement is the most common and severe manifestation of CF. Obstruction of the airways leads to a chronic state of hyperinflation. Over time, RLD becomes superimposed on the obstructive disease, leading to chronic hypoxia, hypercapnea, and acidosis. Pneumothorax and pulmonary hypertension eventually follow and lead to death.

Treatment of CF includes antibiotics, enzyme supplements, nutritional intervention, and frequent secretion removal. Many patients can also benefit from regular physical activity. Twenty minutes of aerobic exercise, for example, can replace one session of secretion removal in some children.[26, 28] It appears that the increased minute ventilation with aerobic exercise helps clear the airways of excessive se-

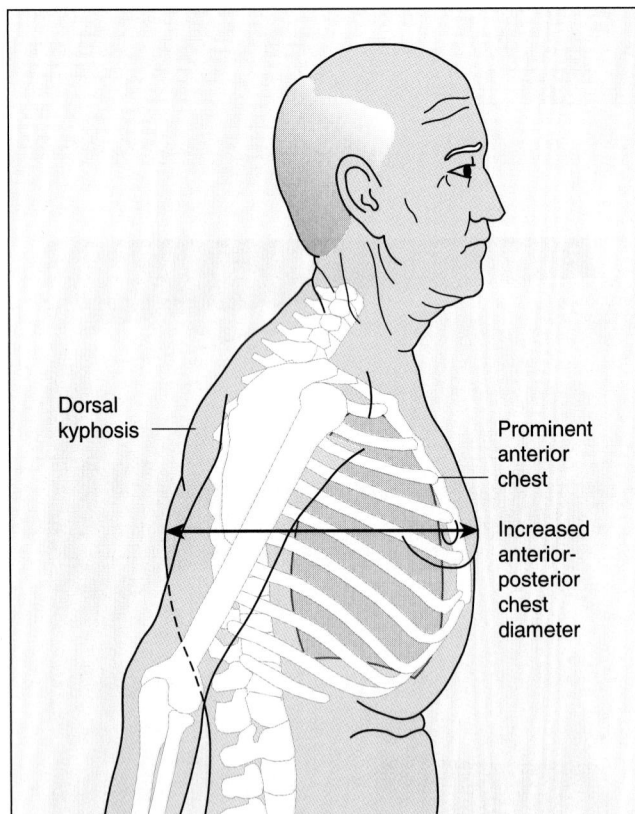

Dorsal kyphosis

Prominent anterior chest

Increased anterior-posterior chest diameter

FIGURE 31.11
Emphysema traps air in the lungs, making exhalation difficult. With time, changes occur in the physical features of the patient, hence the name "pink puffer."

cretions. It is suggested that an increase in fitness may play a role in delaying the crippling effects of CF.

PULMONARY ASSESSMENTS

The diagnosis of pulmonary disease involves several different objective measures. Although the pulmonary diagnosis is not performed by exercise physiologists, they nevertheless must understand the different tests and the results to assist in planning and implementing exercise intervention. Pulmonary assessments include chest imaging, flow and volume tests, blood gas analyses, and cytologic and hematologic tests.

Chest and lung imaging are by far the most popular pulmonary assessment techniques. These include the conventional x-ray, in which roentgen rays (named after Wilhelm Konrad Roentgen, who received the first Nobel Prize for physics in 1901 for discovering x-rays) penetrate the body to provide an image (called a **radiograph** or **roentgenogram**) of the chest's anatomy on film. This standard diagnostic tool is used to screen for abnormalities, to provide a baseline for subsequent assessments, and to monitor disease progression. The major objects visible on a chest radiograph are body fat, water, tissue, bone, and air space. Air in the lungs is of low density and thus allows greater roentgen ray penetration, which results in a dark image on the radiograph. At the other extreme is relatively dense bone, which allows fewer roentgen rays to penetrate its tissue and produces a white image on the radiograph. The chest x-ray usually is taken in posteroanterior (PA) and left lateral views. The left of Figure 31.12 is a normal chest

radiograph in the PA position. The right of Figure 31.12 is the same radiograph with the normal anatomic structures labeled. Specific lung lesions are assessed by observing abnormal densities from the radiograph.

Computed tomography (CT) scanning is probably the single greatest advance in radiography since the discovery of roentgen rays. This process uses a narrow beam of roentgen rays moving across the body in a way that successfully defines adjacent columns of tissue known as **translation.** Another pass of the beam is then made at a different angle and is known as **rotation.** The process is repeated many times with subsequent digitization of each analog image by a computer. The digital images are manipulated mathematically to produce a summated image for diagnostic interpretation.

Magnetic resonance imaging (MRI) involves the interaction of stimulated hydrogen nuclei and a strong magnetic field. An MRI scanner produces a gradient magnetic field in the scanned region of the body part. The hydrogen nuclei align with the magnetic field and resonate at a frequency proportional to the strength of the magnetic field. The stimulated nuclei emit a radio signal that is picked up by the MRI scanner and digitally recorded by a computer to produce an enhanced image. The use of MRI lung scans is limited, because large portions of the lung are of insufficient density to generate clear magnetic signals.

Static and dynamic tests of lung function with simple spirometry are discussed in Chapter 12. Carefully collected spirometric data such as forced vital capacity (FVC), forced expiratory volume in 1 second ($FEV_{1.0}$), maximum voluntary ventilation (MVV), peak expiratory flow (PEF), and tests of

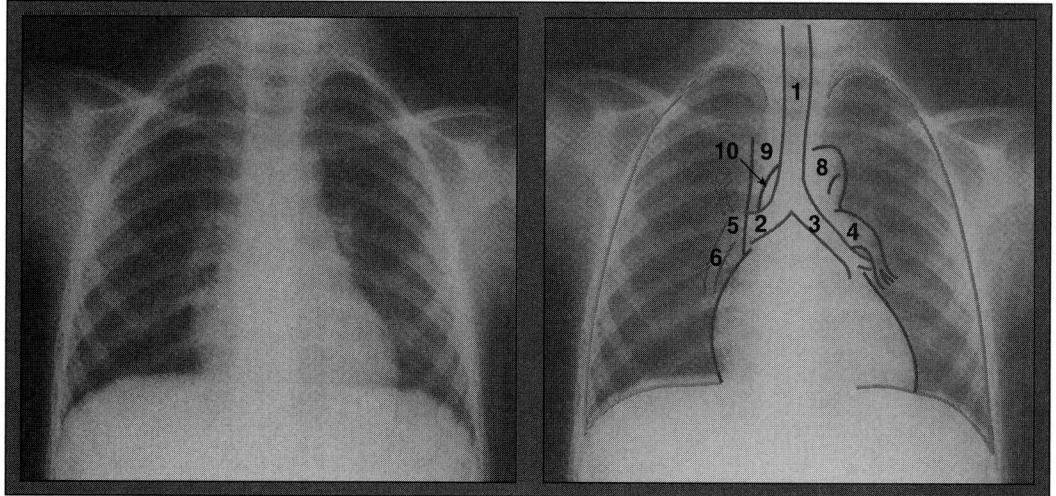

FIGURE 31.12
The chest x-ray. The left radiograph shows a normal chest x-ray in the PA view. The right radiograph shows labeling of the normal anatomic structures. 1, trachea; 2, right mainstem bronchus; 3, left mainstem bronchus; 4, left pulmonary artery; 5, pulmonary vein to the right upper lobe; 6, right interlobular artery; 8, aortic knob; 9, superior vena cava; 10, ascending aorta.

compliance are crucial in diagnosis of lung disease. To measure compliance, the patient swallows a balloon catheter. The catheter is positioned in the lower third of the esophagus and connected to a manometer to measure esophageal pressure. The relation of lung volume change to any change in pressure is then used to establish the curve for lung compliance.

Other useful functional tests include pulmonary diffusing capacity (DL or DLCO, expressed in milliliters per minute per millimeter of mercury), which measures the amount of gas entering the pulmonary blood per unit time per unit pressure differential across the alveolar-capillary membrane. Flow-volume loops are used to graphically represent the events occurring during forced inspiration and expiration. By recording the flow against volume on an X-Y recorder, it is possible to diagnose central or peripheral airway obstruction.

Blood gas analysis is crucial in the assessment of problems related to acid-base balance, ventilation, and the level of arterial oxygen saturation. Similarly, cytologic and hematologic tests are important in identifying organisms that cause disease.

PULMONARY REHABILITATION AND EXERCISE PRESCRIPTION

Despite the fact that COPD and RLD are two leading causes of morbidity and mortality in the United States, pulmonary rehabilitation programs have received considerably less attention than those for cardiovascular and musculoskeletal diseases. Perhaps the reason for this lack of emphasis on pulmonary rehabilitation has been the failure of such rehabilitation to markedly improve levels of pulmonary function or the failure to reverse the natural progression of these deadly diseases. Nevertheless, successful pulmonary rehabilitation can have marked, positive effects on exercise capacity, functional improvement in respiratory muscle function, improved psychological status, enhanced quality of life variables (e.g., self-esteem, and self-efficacy), reduced frequency of hospitalization, and attenuating disease progression. Within this framework, the major goals for pulmonary rehabilitation include the following:

- Improving health status.
- Improving respiratory symptoms (shortness of breath and cough).
- Recognizing early signs that require medical intervention.
- Decreasing frequency and severity of respiratory problems.
- Obtaining maximal arterial oxygen saturation.
- Improving daily functional capacity through improvement in muscular strength, joint flexibility, and cardiorespiratory endurance.
- Improving body composition to enhance functional capacity.
- Improving nutritional status.

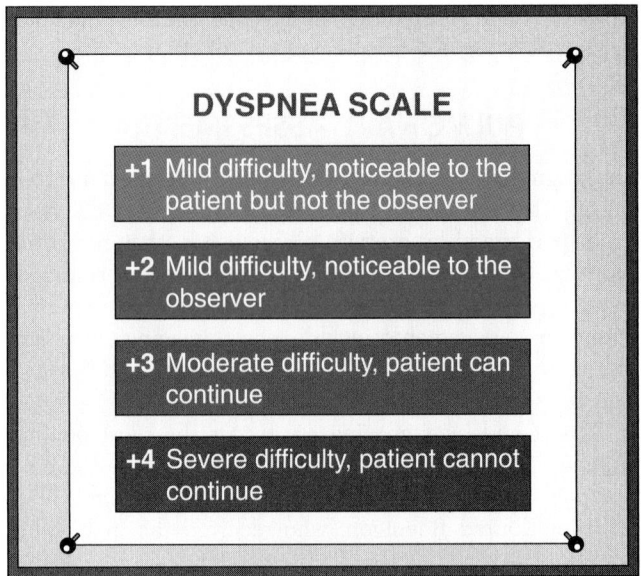

DYSPNEA SCALE

+1 Mild difficulty, noticeable to the patient but not the observer

+2 Mild difficulty, noticeable to the observer

+3 Moderate difficulty, patient can continue

+4 Severe difficulty, patient cannot continue

FIGURE 31.13
Dyspnea scale. Grading of subjective ratings of dyspnea intensity during exercise testing are graded on a scale of 1 to 4. Dyspnea usually accompanies poor exercise capacity and impaired systolic blood pressure response (or a rapidly decreasing systolic blood pressure).

The pulmonary rehabilitation program includes the following components: general care, pulmonary respiratory care, exercise and functional training, education, and psychosocial management. The exercise and functional training aspects of rehabilitation are particularly important to individuals with end-stage disease who have symptoms of weakness, fatigue, and severe dyspnea that profoundly limit physical activity. Physiological monitoring during rehabilitation training is important for these patients and includes measurement of heart rate, blood pressure, respiratory rate, arterial oxygen saturation by pulse oximetry, and dyspnea. Dyspnea monitoring involves a perceived dyspnea scale, much like the Borg scale for rating perceived exertion (Fig. 31.13). The following symptoms are sufficient to stop exercise: extreme shortness of breath, fatigue, palpitations, chest discomfort, or a decrease of 3 to 5% on pulse oximetry.

The exercise prescription is based on results of the pretraining GXT and spirometric analyses. Interpretation of the exercise stress test includes determining whether the test was terminated for cardiovascular or ventilatory endpoints, determining the difference between pre- and postexercise pulmonary function (e.g., a decrease of 10% in $FEV_{1.0}$ indicates the need for bronchodilator therapy before exercise), and determining the need for supplemental oxygen (e.g., a decrease in PaO_2 of more than 20 mm Hg or a PaO_2 of less than 55 mm Hg) during exercise.

Exercise prescription for patients with **mild lung disease** (shortness of breath with heavy exercise) can be the same as that used for normal subjects. For patients with **moderate lung disease** (shortness of breath with normal daily activities or clinical symptoms of RLD or COPD), exercise is usually performed at an intensity no greater than 75% of the ventilatory reserve, in the middle of the calculated training heart rate range (50 to 70% of age-predicted maximum), or at the point at which the patient becomes noticeably dyspneic. For most individuals, this corresponds to 40 to 85% of maximum MET level on a GXT. In this case, exercise duration usually is about 20 minutes, 3 times per week. If shorter exercise durations are needed (e.g., 5 to 15 minutes per session), the frequency of exercise should be increased to 5 to 7 days per week.

Patients with **severe lung disease** (shortness of breath during most daily activities, and FVC and $FEV_{1.0}$ below 55% of predicted values) require a modified approach to exercise testing and prescription. Usually low-level, discontinuous testing can be used starting at 2 to 3 METs with increments every 2 to 3 minutes. Exercise prescription is based on symptom-limited walking speeds and distances. Brief bouts of interval exercise are optimal for this population. Because the initial training prescription is low, patients should exercise a minimum of once per day. Minimal gains in exercise tolerance for these patients can be significant for improving functional capacity and quality of life indices.

For all pulmonary disease patients, exercise is essential for improving respiratory muscle function. There are two approaches for achieving this goal:

1. Providing resistance training for the ventilatory musculature by means of a continuous positive airway pressure device (CPAP). This overloads the muscles in a manner similar to progressive resistance exercise for other skeletal muscles.
2. Increasing the performance capacity of the respiratory muscles through regular and progressive exercise training.

PULMONARY MEDICATIONS

The several groups of pulmonary medications include bronchodilators, anti-inflammatory agents, decongestants, antihistamines, mucokinetic agents, respiratory stimulants, depressants, and paralyzing and antimicrobial agents. These drugs promote bronchodilatation, facilitate the removal of lung secretions, improve alveolar ventilation and arterial oxygenation, and optimize breathing patterns. The most common pulmonary drugs are listed in Table 31.18.

TABLE 31.18
MAJOR PULMONARY BRONCHODILATOR DRUGS: THEIR USES AND SIDE EFFECTS

Drug/Name	Action and Clinical Uses	Side Effects
Sympathomimetics Isoproterenol, Ephedrine, Bronkosol, Alupent, Brethine, Proventil, Ventolin	Decrease intracellular calcium; smooth muscle relaxation; bronchodilation	Tachycardia, palpitations, GI distress, nervousness, headache, dizziness
Methylxanthines Amnodur, Elixophyllin, Theodur, Choladril	Increase cAMP; block the decrease of cAMP	Agitation, hypotension, chest pain, nausea, tachycardia, palpitations, GI distress, nervousness, headache, dizziness
Alpha Sympatholytics	Block the decrease of cAMP; bronchodilation	Agitation, hypotension, chest pain, nausea, tachycardia, palpitations, GI distress, nervousness, headache, dizziness
Parasympatholytics Atrovent, Atropine sulfate	Block parasympathetic stimulation and prevents increases in cGMP; prevents bronchoconstriction	Central nervous system stimulation with low doses and depression with high doses; delirium, hallucinations, decreased GI activity
Glucocorticoids Prednisone, Cortisol, Azmacort, Vanceril	Decrease inflammatory response; bronchodilation	Obesity, growth suppression, hyperglycemia and diabetes, mood changes, irritability, or depression, thinning of skin, muscle wasting
Cromolyn sodium Intal, Fivent	Prevents influx of calcium ions, thus blocking mast cell release of mediators responsible for bronchoconstriction; bronchodilation	Throat irritation, hoarseness, dry mouth, cough, chest tightness, bronchospasm

■ SUMMARY ■

1. "Disability" refers to a diminished functional capacity, whereas "handicap" is a physical performance frame of reference defined by society. A person is considered handicapped when he or she can no longer perform expected tasks. However, loss of functional ability does not necessarily mean that a person is disabled or handicapped.

2. The number of health professionals seeking specialized training has paralleled the increase in the number of disabled persons in the United States.

3. There are more than 100 different types of cancers; the most prevalent are cancers of the breast, lung, bowel, and uterus.

4. Exercise plays an important role in cancer risk reduction, perhaps by increasing levels of anti-inflammatory cytokines and augmenting insulin receptor expression in the cancer-fighting T cells or exerting a positive effect on provirus and oncogene activation.

5. The exercise prescription for cancer patients must be symptom-limited, progressive, and individualized. For most patients, the goal of exercise prescription is to improve the level of ambulation.

6. For women recovering from breast cancer surgery, a carefully planned, moderate aerobic circuit resistance exercise program decreases depression and state and trait anxieties.

7. The major cardiovascular diseases either affect the heart muscle directly, the heart valves, or the neural regulation of cardiac function. Each of these disease categories has its own specific pathogenesis and intervention strategies.

8. Diseases of the myocardium include angina pectoris, myocardial infarction, pericarditis, congestive heart failure, and aneurysm.

9. Diseases affecting heart valves include stenosis, insufficiency (regurgitation), prolapse, and endocarditis. Congenital malformations include ventricular or atrial septal defects and patent ductus arteriosus, both of which require surgical repair.

10. Diseases of the heart's nervous system include different types of dysrhythmias, such as bradycardia and tachycardia.

11. Assessment of the cardiac patient includes a carefully obtained patient history, physical examination, heart auscultation to uncover murmurs and valvular problems, and laboratory tests (including a chest x-ray, ECG, blood lipid analyses, and certain serum enzyme testing).

12. The different physiological assessments for the CHD patient include noninvasive tests such as echocardiography, exercise stress testing, and ECG analysis and invasive testing such as radionucleotide (thallium) imaging, cardiac catheterization, and coronary angiography.

13. Based on diagnosis, patients are placed into different cardiac rehabilitation phases depending on the severity of disease and the degree of risk. The exercise prescription for the cardiac patient is based on intensity, type, frequency, duration, and the patient's initial functional capacity.

14. A wide variety of cardiac medications play an important role in the management of the cardiac patient. The clinical exercise physiologist should understand the actions of these drugs and their effects on the patient's response to exercise.

15. Two major categories of diseases of the pulmonary system are restrictive lung disease (RLD) and chronic obstructive lung disease (COPD). RLD relates to a variety of dysfunctions that culminate in a significantly increased resistance of the chest-lung inflation. COPD includes bronchitis, emphysema, asthma, exercise-induced bronchospasm, and cystic fibrosis. These diseases greatly affect expiratory flow capacity and ultimately impede the aeration process in the alveoli.

16. Assessment of pulmonary disease requires different diagnostic tools, including chest x-ray, CT scanning, MRI, and standard spirometric lung volume testing.

17. Exercise can be used effectively in managing various pulmonary diseases if close attention is given to exercise intensity, patient monitoring, and exercise progression.

■ REFERENCES ■

1. American Cancer Society: *Cancer Facts and Figures.* Atlanta, GA, American Cancer Society, 1995.
2. American College of Sports Medicine.: *Guidelines to Exercise Testing and Prescription.* 5th ed. Philadelphia, Lea & Febiger, 1995.
3. Bostwick, J.: Rehabilitation after mastectomy. *J. Med. Assoc. Ga.,* 76:336, 1987.
4. Brown, J.K.: Gender, age, usual weight loss, and tobacco use as predictors of weight loss in patients with lung cancer. *Oncol. Nurs. Forum,* 20:466, 1993.
5. Cohn, L.A., et al.: Voluntary exercise and experimental cancer. *Adv. Exp. Med. Biol.,* 322:41, 1992.
6. Cole, T.M., and Edgerton, V.R.: *Report on the Task Force on Medical Rehabilitation Research.* Hunt Valley, MD, Task Force Publications, 1990.
6a. Cooper, C.B.: Determining the role of exercise in patients with chronic pulmonary disease. *Med. Sci. Sports Exerc.,* 27:147, 1995.
7. Cronin, S.N.: Nursing care of clients with lower airway disorders. In *Luckmann and Soreensen's Medical Surgical Nursing.* 4th ed. Edited by J.M. Black and E. Matassain-Jacob. Philadelphia, W.B. Saunders, 1993.
8. Davis, P.B.: Cystic fibrosis: a major cause of obstructive airway disease in the young. In *Chronic Obstructive Pulmonary Disease.* Edited by N.S. Cherniack. Philadelphia, W.B. Saunders, 1991.
8a. Fardy, P.S., and Yanowitz, F.G.: *Cardiac Rehabilitation, Adult Fitness, and Exercise Testing.* Baltimore, Williams & Wilkins, 1996.
9. Floger, J.A.: *A Treatise of Asthma.* London, R. Wilkin, 1968.
10. Gilbert, I., et al.: Heat and water flux in the intrathoracic airways and exercised induced asthma. *J. Appl. Physiol.,* 63:1681, 1987.
11. Hegsted, D.M.: Exercise, calories, and fat: future challenges. *Adv. Exp. Med. Biol.,* 322:185, 1992.

12. Hicks, J.E.: Exercise for cancer patients. In *Therapeutic Exercise.* 5th ed. Edited by J.V. Basmajian and S.L. Wolf. Baltimore, Williams & Wilkins, 1990.

13. Jette, A.M.: State of the art in functional status assessment. In *Measurement in Physical Therapy.* Edited by J. Rothstein. New York, Churchill Livingstone, 1985.

14. Leis, H.P., Jr.: The relationship of diet to cancer, cardiovascular disease and longevity. *Int. Surg.,* 76:1, 1991.

15. Nishina, P.M., et al.: Linkage of atherogenic lipoprotein phenotype to the low density lipoprotein receptor locus on the short arm of chromosome 19. *Proc. Natl. Acad. Sci. U.S.A.,* 89:708, 1992.

16. O'Toole, M.: *Miller-Keane Encyclopedia and Dictionary of Medicine, Nursing and Allied Health.* 5th ed. Philadelphia, W.B. Saunders, 1992.

17. Paffenbarger, R.S., et al.: The influence of physical activity on the incidence of site-specific cancers in college alumni. *Adv. Exp. Med. Biol.,* 322:7, 1992.

18. Scano, G., et al.: Changes in ventilatory muscle function with negative pressure ventilation in patients with severe COPD. *Chest,* 97:322, 1990.

19. Shephard, R.J.: *Rapporteur: Meeting of Investigators on Exercise Tests in Relation to C-V Function.* New York, World Health Organization, 1994.

20. Stewart, N.: Value of sport in the rehabilitation of the physically disabled. *Can. J. Appl. Sport. Sci.,* 6:166, 1981.

21. Tas, J.: Genetic predisposition to coronary heart disease and gene for apolipoprotein CIII. *Lancet,* 337:113, 1991.

22. Uhlenbrock, G., and Oder, U.: Can endurance sports stimulate immune mechanisms against cancer and metastasis. *Int. J. Sports Med.,* 12(Suppl. 1):S63, 1991.

23. United States Department of Health and Human Services: *Healthy People 2000: National Health Promotion and Disease Prevention Objectives.* DHHS Publ. No. (PHS) 91-50212. Washington, DC, U.S. Government Printing Office, 1990.

24. Winningham, M.L., et al.: Effects of aerobic exercise on body weight and composition in patients with breast cancer on adjuvant chemotherapy. *Oncol. Nurs. Forum,* 16:683, 1989.

25. Wolf, E., and Hossack, H.: Guidlines for exercise training of elderly healthy individuals and elderly patients with coronary disease. *J. Cardiac Rehab.,* 9:40, 1989.

26. Wolff, R., et al.: Effects of exercise and eucapnic hyperventilation on bronchial clearance in man. *J. Appl. Physiol.,* 43:46, 1977.

27. World Health Organization: *The First Ten Years Of The World Health Organization.* Geneva, World Health Organization, 1958.

28. Zach, M., et al.: Cystic fibrosis: physical exercise versus chest physiotherapy. *Arch. Dis. Child.,* 57:587, 1982.

APPENDIXES

The Metric System and Conversion Constants in Exercise Physiology

Appendix A has three parts. Part 1 deals with the metric system, Part 2 discusses the Système International d'Unités (SI units), and Part 3 presents conversion factors for clinical hematology and clinical chemistry.

PART 1
THE METRIC SYSTEM

Most measurements in science are expressed in terms of the metric system. This system uses units that are related to one another by some power of 10. The prefix *centi-* means one-hundredth, *milli-* means one-thousandth, and the prefix *kilo-* is derived from a word that means one thousand. In the following sections, we show the relationship between metric units and English units of measurement that are relevant to the material presented in this book.

UNITS OF MASS (WEIGHT)

Use the following conversions for common units of mass (weight) and volume. For example, 1 ounce = 0.06 pound. Two ounces would therefore equal $2 \times 0.06 = 0.12$ pound, and 16 ounces = 0.96 pound (16×0.06).

UNITS OF MASS (WEIGHT)

Metric Unit	Equivalent Metric Units	Equivalent English Units
kilogram (kg)	1,000 g	35.3 oz;
	1,000,000 mg	2.2046 lb
gram (g)	0.001 kg	
	1,000 mg	0.353 oz
milligram (mg)	0.000001 kg	
	0.001	0.0000353 oz

UNITS OF LENGTH

Metric Unit	Equivalent Metric Units	Equivalent English Units
meter (m)	100 cm; 1000 mm	39.37 in;
		3.28 ft; 1.09 yd
centimeter (cm)	0.01 m; 10 mm	0.3937 in
millimeter (mm)	0.001 m; 0.1 cm	0.03937 in

UNITS OF VOLUME

Metric Unit	Equivalent Metric Units	Equivalent English Units
liter (L)	1000 mL	1.057 qt
milliliter (mL) or cubic centimeter (cc)	0.001 L	0.001057 qt

TEMPERATURE

To convert Fahrenheit to Celsius: $°C = (°F - 32) \div 1.8$
To convert Celsius to Fahrenheit: $°F = (1.8 \times °C) + 32$
On the Fahrenheit scale, water freezes at 32°F and boils at 212°F. On the Celsius scale, water freezes at 0°C and boils at 100°C.

UNITS OF SPEED

mph	$km \cdot hr^{-1}$	$m \cdot s^{-1}$	mph	$km \cdot hr^{-1}$	$m \cdot s^{-1}$
1	1.6	0.47	11	17.7	5.17
2	3.2	0.94	12	19.3	5.64
3	4.8	1.41	13	20.9	6.11
4	6.4	1.88	14	22.5	6.58
5	8.0	2.35	15	24.1	7.05
6	9.6	2.82	16	25.8	7.52
7	11.2	3.29	17	27.4	7.99
8	12.8	3.76	18	29.0	8.46
9	14.4	4.23	19	30.6	8.93
10	16.0	4.70	20	32.2	9.40

COMMON EXPRESSIONS OF WORK, ENERGY, AND POWER

Watts	Kilocalories (kcal)	Foot-Pounds (ft · lb)
1 watt = 0.73756 ft-lb $\cdot$ s^{-1}	1 kcal = 3086 ft-lb	1 ft $\cdot$ lb = 3.2389 $\times$ 10^{-3} kcal
1 watt = 0.01433 kcal $\cdot$ min^{-1}	1 kcal = 426.8 kg-m	1 ft $\cdot$ lb = 0.13825 kg-m
1 watt = 1.341 $\times$ 10^{-3} hp	1 kcal = 3087.4 ft-lb	1 ft $\cdot$ lb = 5.050
or 0.0013 hp	1 kcal = 1.5593	$\times$ 10^{-3} hp $\cdot$ h^{-1}
1 watt = 6.12 kg-m $\cdot$ min^{-1}	$\times$ 10^{-3} hp $\cdot$ h^{-1}	

TERMINOLOGY AND UNITS OF MEASUREMENT

The American College of Sports Medicine suggests that the following terminology and units of measurement be used in scientific endeavors to promote consistency and clarity of communication, and to avoid ambiguity. The terms defined below utilize the units of measurement of the Système International d'Unités (SI units).

Exercise: Any and all activity involving generation of force by the activated muscle(s) which results in disruption of a homeostatic state. In dynamic exercise, the muscle may perform shortening (concentric) contractions or be overcome by external resistance and perform lengthening (eccentric) contractions. When muscle force results in no movement, the contraction should be termed static or isometric.

Exercise intensity: A specific level of maintenance of muscular activity that can be quantified in terms of power (energy expenditure or work performed per unit of time), isometric force sustained, or velocity of progression.

Endurance: The time limit of a person's ability to maintain either a specific isometric force or a specific power level

involving combinations of concentric or eccentric muscular contractions.

Mass: A quantity of matter of an object, a direct measure of the object's inertia (note: mass = weight ÷ acceleration due to gravity; unit: gram or kilogram).

Weight: The force with which a quantity of matter is attracted toward Earth by normal acceleration of gravity (traditional unit: kilogram of weight).

Energy: The capability of producing force, performing work, or generating heat (unit: joule or kilojoule).

Force: That which changes or tends to change the state of rest or motion in matter (unit: newton).

Speed: Total distance traveled per unit of time (unit: meters per second).

Velocity: Displacement per unit of time A vector quantity requiring that direction be stated or strongly implied (unit: meters per second or kilometers per hour).

Work: Force expressed through a distance but with no limitation on time (unit: joule or kilojoule). Quantities of energy and heat expressed independently of time should also be presented in joules. The term "work" should *not* be employed synonymously with muscular exercise.

Power: The rate of performing work; the derivative of work with respect to time; the product of force and velocity (unit: watt). Other related processes such as energy release and heat transfer should, when expressed per unit of time, be quantified and presented in watts.

Torque: Effectiveness of a force to produce axial rotation (unit: newton · meter).

Volume: A space occupied, for example, by a quantity of fluid gas (unit: liter or milliliter). Gas volumes should be indicated as ATPS, BTPS, or STPD.

Amount of a substance: The amount of a substance is frequently expressed in moles. A mole is the quantity of a chemical substance that has a weight in mass units (e.g., grams) numerically equal to the molecular weight, or that in the case of a gas has a volume occupied by such a weight under specified conditions. One mole of a respiratory gas is equal to 22.4 liters at STPD.

PART 2
SI UNITS

The uniform numerical value system is known as the Système International d'Unités, or its abbreviation, SI. SI was developed through international cooperation to create a universally acceptable system of measurement. SI ensures that units of measurement are uniform in concept and style. The SI system permits quantities in common use to be more easily compared. Many scientific organizations endorse the concept of the SI, and leading journals in nutrition, health, and exercise science now require that laboratory data be presented in SI units. The information in this appendix has been summarized from a detailed description about the SI published in the following article:

Young DS: Implementation of SI units for clinical laboratory data. Style specifications and conversion tables. *Ann. Intern. Med.,* 106:114, 1987.

DEFINITIONS OF COMMON SI UNITS

Degree Celsius (°C)	The degree Celsius (centigrade) is equivalent to $K - 273.15$.
Radian (rad)	The radian is the plane angle between two radii of a circle which subtend on the circumference of an arc equal in length to the radius.
Joule (J)	The joule is the work done when the point of application of a force of one newton is displaced through a distance of one meter in the direction of the force. $1 J = 1 N \cdot m$.
Kelvin (K)	The kelvin is the fraction $1/273.16$ of the thermodynamic temperature of the triple point of water.
Kilogram (kg)	The kilogram is a unit of mass equal to the mass of the international prototype of the kilogram.
Meter (m)	The meter is the length equal to 1,650,763.73 wavelengths in vacuum of the radiation that corresponds to the transition between the levels $2p_{10}$ and $5d_5$ of the krypton 86 atom.
Newton (N)	The newton is that force which, when applied to a mass of one kilogram, gives it an acceleration of one meter per second squared. $1 N = 1 kg \cdot m/s^2$.
Pascal (Pa)	The pascal is the pressure produced by a force of one newton applied, with uniform distribution, over an area of one square meter. $1 Pa = 1 N/m^2$.
Second (s)	The second is the duration of 9,192,631,770 periods of the radiation that corresponds to the transition between the two hyperfine levels of the ground state of the cesium 133 atom.
Watt (W)	The watt is the power that in one second gives rise to the energy of one joule. $1 W = 1 J/s$.

BASE UNITS OF SI NOMENCLATURE

Physical Quantity	*Base Unit*	*SI Symbol*
Length	meter	m
Mass	kilogram	kg
Time	second	s
Amount of substance	mole	mol
Thermodynamic temperature	kelvin	K
Electric current	ampere	A
Luminous intensity	candela	cd

GENERAL SI STYLE GUIDLINES

Guidelines	Example	Incorrect Style	Correct Style
Lowercase letters are used for symbols or abreviations Exceptions:	kilogram	Kg	kg
	kelvin	k	K
	ampere	a	A
	liter	l	L
Symbols are not followed by a period Exception: end of sentence	meter	m.	m
	mole	mol.	mol
Symbols are not to be pluralized	kilograms	kgs	kg
	meters	ms	m
Names and symbols are not to be combined	force	kilogram · meter · s^{-2}	kg · m · s^{-2} kg · m/s^2
When numbers are printed, symbols are preferred		100 meters	100 m
		2 moles	2 mol
A space should be placed between number and symbol		50ml	50 mL
The product of units is indicated by a dot above the line		kg × m/s^2	kg · m · s^{-2} kg · m/s^2
Only one solidus (/) should be used per expression		mmol/L/s	mmol/(L · s)
A zero should be placed before the decimal		.01	0.01
Decimal numbers are preferable to fractions		¾	0.75
		75%	0.75
Spaces are used to separate long numbers Exception: optional with four-digit number		1,500,000	1 500 000
		1,000	1000 or 1 000

COMMON PREFIXES USED WITH SI UNITS OF MEASUREMENT

Prefix	Abbreviation	Multiplication factor
tera	T	$1,000,000,000,000 = 10^{12}$
giga	G	$1,000,000,000 = 10^{9}$
mega	M	$1,000,000 = 10^{6}$
kilo	k	$1,000 = 10^{3}$
hecto	h	$100 = 10^{2}$
deci	d	$0.1 = 10^{-1}$
centi	c	$0.01 = 10^{-2}$
milli	m	$0.001 = 10^{-3}$
micro	μ	$0.000,001 = 10^{-6}$
nano	n	$0.000,000,001 = 10^{-9}$
pico	p	$0.000,000,000,001 = 10^{-12}$

For SI units in exercise physiology, the term *body weight* is properly referred to as mass (kg), height should be referred to as stature (m), second is s, minute is min, hour is h, week is wk, month is mo, year is y, day is d, gram is g, liter is L, hertz is Hz, joule is J, kilocalorie is kcal, ohm is Ω, pascal is Pa, revolutions per minute is rpm, volt is V, and watt is W. These abbreviations or symbols are used for the singular or plural form.

CONVERSION FACTORS FOR USE IN THE EXERCISE SCIENCES

To Convert	Into	Multiply By	To Convert	Into	Multiply By
A			centimeters of mercury	feet of water	0.4461
ampere-hours	coulombs	3,600.0	centimeters of mercury	kilograms/square meter	136.0
ampere-hours	faradays	0.03731	centimeters of mercury	pounds/square foot	27.85
angstrom units	inches	3.937×10^{-9}			
angstrom units	meters	1×10^{-10}	centimeters of mercury	pounds/square inch	0.1934
angstrom units	micrometers	1×10^{-4}			
B			centimeters/ second	feet/minute	1.1969
BTU	ergs	1.0550×10^{-10}			
BTU	foot-pounds	778.3	centimeters/ second	feet/second	0.03281
BTU	gram-calories	252.0			
BTU	horsepower-hours	3.931×10^{-4}	centimeters/ second	kilometers/hour	0.036
BTU	joules	1,054.8			
BTU	kilogram-calories	0.2520	centimeters/ second	knots	0.1943
BTU	kilogram-meters	107.5			
BTU	kilowatt-hours	2.928×10^{-4}	centimeters/ second	meters/minute	0.6
BTU/hour	foot-pounds/ second	0.2162			
			centimeters/ second	miles/hour	0.02237
BTU/hour	gram-calorie/ second	0.0700	centimeters/ second	miles/minute	3.728×10^{-4}
BTU/hour	horsepower-hours	3.929×10^{-4}			
BTU/hour	watts	0.2931	centimeters/ second/second	feet/second/ second	0.03281
BTU/minute	foot-pound/ second	12.96			
			centimeters/ second/second	km/hour/second	0.036
BTU/minute	horsepower	0.02356			
BTU/minute	kilowatts	0.01757	centimeters/ second/second	meters/second/ second	0.01
BTU/minute	watts	17.57			
BTU/square foot/ minute	watts/square inch	0.1221	centimeters/ second/second	miles/hour/ second	0.02237
C			cubic centimeters	cubic feet	3.531×10^{-5}
calories, gram (mean)	BTU (mean)	3.9685×10^{-3}	cubic centimeters	cubic inches	0.06102
centigrade (celsius)	Fahrenheit	$(C° \times 9/5) + 32$	cubic centimeters	cubic meters	1×10^{-6}
centigrams	grams	0.01	cubic centimeters	cubic yards	1.308×10^{-6}
centiliters	fluid ounces (U.S.)	0.3382	cubic centimeters	gallons (U.S. liq.)	2.642×10^{-4}
centiliters	cubic inches	0.6103	cubic centimeters	liters	0.001
centiliters	drams	2.705	cubic centimeters	pints (U.S. liq.)	2.113×10^{-3}
centiliters	liters	0.01	cubic centimeters	quarts (U.S. liq.)	1.057×10^{-3}
centimeters	feet	3.281×10^{-2}	cubic feet	bushels (dry)	0.8036
centimeters	inches	0.3937	cubic feet	cubic centimeters	28,320.0
centimeters	kilometers	1×10^{-5}	cubic feet	cubic inches	1,728.0
centimeters	meters	0.01	cubic feet	cubic meters	0.02832
centimeters	miles	6.214×10^{-6}	cubic feet	cubic yards	0.03704
centimeters	millimeters	10.0	cubic feet	gallons (U.S. liq.)	7.48052
centimeters	mils	393.7	cubic feet	liters	28.32
centimeters	yards	1.094×10^{-2}	cu feet	pints (U.S. liq.)	59.84
centimeter-dynes	centimeter-grams	1.020×10^{-3}	cubic feet	quarts (U.S. liq.)	29.92
centimeter-dynes	meter-kilograms	1.020×10^{-8}	cubic feet/minute	cubic centimeters/ second	472.0
centimeter-dynes	pound-feet	7.376×10^{-8}			
centimeter-grams	centimeter-dynes	980.7	cubic feet/minute	gallons/second	0.1247
centimeter-grams	meter-kilograms	1×10^{-5}	cubic feet/minute	liters/second	0.4720
centimeter-grams	pound-feet	7.233×10^{-6}	cubic feet/minute	pounds of water/ minute	62.43
centimeters of mercury	atmospheres	0.01316			
			cubic feet/second	million gal/day	0.646317

CONVERSION FACTORS FOR USE IN THE EXERCISE SCIENCES—*continued*

To Convert	Into	Multiply By
cubic feet/second	gallons/minute	448.831
cubic inches	cubic centimeters	16.39
cubic inches	cubic feet	5.787×10^{-4}
cubic inches	cubic meters	1.639×10^{-4}
cubic inches	cubic yards	2.143×10^{-5}
cubic inches	gallons	4.329×10^{-3}
cubic inches	liters	0.01639
cubic inches	pints (U.S. liq.)	0.03463
cubic inches	quarts (U.S. liq.)	0.01732
cubic meters	bushels (dry)	28.38
cubic meters	cubic centimeters	1×10^{-6}
cubic meters	cubic feet	35.31
cubic meters	cubic inches	61,023.0
cubic meters	cubic yards	1.308
cubic meters	gallons (U.S. liq.)	264.2
cubic meters	liters	1,000.0
cubic meters	pints (U.S. liq.)	2,113.0
cubic meters	quarts (U.S. liq.)	1,057.0
cubic yards	cubic centimeters	7.646×10^{5}
cubic yards	cubic feet	27.0
cubic yards	cubic inches	46,656.0
cubic yards	cubic meters	0.7646
cubic yards	gallons (U.S. liq.)	202.0
cubic yards	liters	764.6
cubic yards	pints (U.S. liq.)	1,615.9
cubic yards	quarts (U.S. liq.)	807.9
cubic yards/minute	cubic ft/second	0.45
cubic yards/minute	gallons/second	3.367
cubic yards/minute	liters/second	12.74
D		
days	seconds	86,400.0
decigrams	grams	0.1
deciliters	liters	0.1
decimeters	meters	0.1
degrees (angle)	quadrants	0.01111
degrees (angle)	radians	0.01745
degrees (angle)	seconds	3,600.0
degrees/second	radians/second	0.01745
degrees/second	revolutions/minute	0.1667
degrees/second	revolutions/second	2.778×10^{-3}
dekagrams	grams	10.0
dekaliters	liters	10.0
dekameters	meters	10.0
drams	grams	1.7718
drams	ounces	0.0625
dyne/centimeter millimeter	ergs/square	0.01
dyne/square centimeter	atmospheres	9.869×10^{-7}

To Convert	Into	Multiply By
dyne/square centimeter	inches of mercury at 0°C	2.953×10^{-5}
dyne/square centimeter	inches of water at 4°C	4.015×10^{-4}
dynes	grams	1.020×10^{-3}
dynes	joules/centimeter	1×10^{-7}
dynes	jouls/meter (newtons)	1×10^{-5}
dynes	kilograms	1.020×10^{-6}
dynes	poundals	7.233×10^{-5}
dynes	pounds	2.248×10^{-6}
dynes/square centimeter	bars	1×10^{-6}
E		
ergs	BTU	9.480×10^{-11}
ergs	dyne-centimeters	1.0
ergs	foot-pounds	7.3670×10^{-8}
ergs	gram-calories	0.2389×10^{-7}
ergs	gram-centimeters	1.020×10^{-3}
ergs	horsepower hours	3.7250×10^{-14}
ergs	joules	1×10^{-7}
ergs	kilogram-calories	2.389×10^{-11}
ergs	kilogram-meters	1.020×10^{-8}
ergs	kilowatt-hours	0.2778×10^{-13}
ergs	watt-hours	0.2778×10^{-10}
ergs/second	BTU/minute	$5,688 \times 10^{-9}$
ergs/second	foot-pounds/minute	4.427×10^{-6}
ergs/second	foot-pounds/second	7.3756×10^{-8}
ergs/second	horsepower	1.341×10^{-10}
ergs/second	kilogram-calories/minute	1.433×10^{-9}
ergs/second	kilowatts	1×10^{-10}
F		
feet	centimeters	30.48
feet	kilometers	3.048×10^{-4}
feet	meters	0.3048
feet	miles (naut.)	1.645×10^{-4}
feet	miles (stat.)	1.894×10^{-4}
feet	millimeters	304.8
feet	mils	1.2×10^{4}
feet of water	atmospheres	0.02950
feet of water	inches of mercury	0.8826
feet of water	kilograms/sq centimeter	0.03048
feet of water	kilograms/square meter	304.8
feet of water	pounds/square foot	62.43
feet of water	pounds/square inch	0.4335
feet/minute	centimeters/second	0.5080
feet/minute	feet/second	0.01667
feet/minute	kilometers/hour	0.01829
feet/minute	meters/minute	0.3048
feet/minute	miles/hour	0.01136
feet/second	centimeters/second	30.48

CONVERSION FACTORS FOR USE IN THE EXERCISE SCIENCES—*continued*

To Convert	Into	Multiply By	To Convert	Into	Multiply By
feet/second	kilometers/hour	1.097	gallons/minute	cu feet/second	2.228×10^{-3}
feet/second	knots	0.5921	gallons/minute	liters/second	0.06308
feet/second	meters/minute	18.29	gallons/minute	cubic feet/hour	8.0208
feet/second	miles/hour	0.6818	grams	dynes	980.7
feet/second	miles/minute	0.01136	grams	grains	15.43
feet/second/ second	centimeters/second	30.48	grams	joules/centimeter	9.807×10^{-5}
feet/second/ second	kilometers/hour/ second	1.097	grams	joules/meter (newtons)	9.807×10^{-3}
feet/second/ second	meters/second/ second	0.3048	grams	kilograms	0.001
			grams	kilograms	0.001
feet/second/ second	miles/hour/second	0.6818	grams	milligrams	1,000.0
feet/100 feet	percent grade	1.0	grams	ounces (avoirdupois)	0.03527
foot-candles	lumens/square meter	10.764	grams	ounces (troy)	0.03215
foot-pounds	BTU	1.286×10^{-3}	grams	poundals	0.07093
foot-pounds	ergs	1.356×10^{7}	grams	pounds	2.205×10^{-3}
foot-pounds	gram-calories	0.3238	grams/ centimeter	pounds/inch	5.600×10^{-3}
foot-pounds	horsepower-hours	5.050×10^{-7}	grams/cubic centimeter	pounds/cubic foot	62.43
foot-pounds	joules	1.356			
foot-pounds	kilogram-calories	3.24×10^{-4}	grams/cubic centimeter	pounds/cubic inch	0.03613
foot-pounds	kilogram-meters	0.1383	grams/cubic centimeter	pounds/mil-foot	3.405×10^{-7}
foot-pounds	kilowatt-hours	3.766×10^{-7}			
foot-pounds/ minute	BTU/minute	1.286×10^{-3}	grams/liter	grains/gallon	58.417
foot-pounds/ minute	foot-pounds/ second	0.01667	grams/liter	pounds/1000 gallon	8.345
foot-pounds/ minute	horsepower	3.030×10^{-5}	grams/liter	pounds/cubic foot	0.062427
			grams/liter	parts/million	1,000.0
foot-pounds/ minute	kilogram-calories/ minute	3.24×10^{-4}	grams/square centimeter	pounds/square foot	2.0481
foot-pounds/ minute	kilowatts	2.260×10^{-5}	gram/calories	BTU	3.9683×10^{-3}
foot-pounds/ second	BTU/hour	4.6263	gram-calories	ergs	4.1868×10^{7}
			gram-calories	foot-pounds	3.0880
foot-pounds/ second	BTU/minute	0.07717	gram-calories	horsepower-hours	1.5596×10^{-6}
			gram-calories	kilowatt-hours	1.1630×10^{-6}
foot-pounds/ second	horsepower	0.818×10^{-3}	gram-calories	watt-hours	1.1630×10^{-3}
foot-pounds/ second	kilogram-calories/ minute	1.01945	gram-calories/ second	BTU/hour	14.286
foot-pounds/ second	kilowatts	1.356×10^{-3}	gram-centimeters	BTU	9.297×10^{-8}
G			gram-centimeters	ergs	980.7
gallons	cubic centimeters	3,785.0	gram-centimeters	joules	9.807×10^{-5}
gallons	cubic feet	0.1337	gram-centimeters	kilogram-calories	2.343×10^{-8}
gallons	cubic inches	231.0	gram-centimeters	kilogram-meters	1×10^{-5}
gallons	cubic meters	3.785×10^{-3}	**H**		
gallons	cubic yards	4.951×10^{-3}	horsepower	BTU/minute	42.44
gallons	liters	3.785	horsepower	foot-pound/ minute	33,000.0
gallons (liq. British imp.)	gallons (U.S. liq.)	1.20095	horsepower	foot-pound/ second	550.0
gallons (U.S.)	gallons (imp.)	0.83267	horsepower (metric) (542.5 foot-pounds/second)	horsepower (550 foot-pounds/ second)	0.9863
gallons of water	pounds of water	8.3453			

CONVERSION FACTORS FOR USE IN THE EXERCISE SCIENCES—*continued*

To Convert	Into	Multiply By	To Convert	Into	Multiply By
horsepower (550 foot/pounds/ second)	horsepower (metric) (542.5 foot-pounds/ second)	1.014	inches of water (at 4°C)	ounces/square inch	0.5781
horsepower	kilogram-calories/ minute	10.68	inches of water (at 4°C)	pounds/square foot	5.204
horsepower	kilowatts	0.7457	inches of water (at 4°C)	pounds/square inch	0.03613
horsepower	watts	745.7			
horsepower (boiler)	BTU/hour	33,479.0	**J**		
			joules	BTU	9.480×10^{-4}
horsepower (boiler)	kilowatts	9.803	joules	ergs	1×10^7
			joules	foot-pounds	0.7376
horsepower- hours	BTU	2,547.0	joules	kg-calories	2.389×10^{-4}
			joules	kg-meters	0.1020
horsepower- hours	ergs	2.6845×10^{13}	joules	watt-hours	2.778×10^{-4}
			joules/ centimeter	grams	1.020×10^4
horsepower- hours	foot-pounds	1.98×10^6	joules/ centimeter	dynes	1×10^7
horsepower- hours	gram-calories	641,190.0	joules/ centimeter	joules/meter (newtons)	100.0
horsepower- hours	joules	2.684×10^6	joules/ centimeter	poundals	723.3
horsepower- hours	kilogram-calories	641.1	joules/ centimeter	pounds	22.48
horsepower- hours	kilogram-meters	2.737×10^5	**K**		
horsepower- hours	kilowatt-hours	0.7457	kilograms	dynes	980,665.0
			kilograms	grams	1,000.0
hours	days	4.167×10^{-2}	kilograms	joules/centimeter	0.09807
hours	weeks	5.952×10^{-3}	kilograms	joules/meter (newtons)	9.807
I			kilograms	poundals	70.93
inches	centimeters	2.540	kilograms	pounds	2.205
inches	meters	2.540×10^{-2}	kilograms	tons (long)	9.842×10^{-4}
inches	miles	1.578×10^{-5}	kilograms	tons (short)	1.102×10^{-3}
inches	millimeters	25.40	kilograms/cubic meter	grams/cubic centimeter	0.001
inches	mils	1,000.0	kilograms/cubic meter	pounds/cubic foot	0.06243
inches	yards	2.778×10^{-2}			
inches of mercury	atmospheres	0.03342	kilograms/cubic meter	pounds/cubic inch	3.613×10^{-5}
inches of mercury	feet of water	1.133	kilograms/cubic meter	pounds/mil-foot	3.405×10^{-10}
inches of mercury	kilograms/square centimeter	0.03453	kilograms/ meter	pounds/foot	0.6720
inches of mercury	kilograms/square meter	345.3	kilograms/square centimeter	dynes	980,665.0
inches of mercury	pounds/square foot	70.73	kilograms/square centimeter	atmospheres	0.9678
inches of mercury	pounds/square inch	0.4912	kilograms/square centimeter	feet of water	32.81
inches of water (at 4°C)	atmospheres	2.458×10^{-3}	kilograms/square centimeter	inches of mercury	28.96
inches of water (at 4°C)	inches of mercury	0.07355	kilograms/square centimeter	pouns/square foot	2,048.0
inches of water (at 4°C)	kg/square centimeter	2.540×10^{-3}			

CONVERSION FACTORS FOR USE IN THE EXERCISE SCIENCES—*continued*

To Convert	Into	Multiply By	To Convert	Into	Multiply By
kilograms/square centimeter	pounds/square inch	14.22	kilowatts	foot-pounds/ minute	4.426×10^4
kilograms/square meter	atmospheres	9.678×10^{-5}	kilowatts	foot-pounds/ second	737.6
kilograms/square meter	bars	98.07×10^{-6}	kilowatts	horsepower	1.341
kilograms/square meter	feet of water	3.281×10^{-3}	kilowatts	kilogram-calories/ minute	14.34
kilograms/square meter	inches of mercury	2.896×10^{-3}	kilowatts	watts	1,000.0
kilograms/square meter	pounds/square foot	0.2048	kilowatt-hours	BTU	3,413.0
			kilowatt-hours	ergs	3.600×10^{13}
kilograms/square meter	pounds/square inch	1.422×10^{-3}	kilowatt-hours	foot-pounds	2.655×10^6
			kilowatt-hours	gram-calories	859,850.0
kilograms/square millimeter	kilograms/square meter	1×10^6	kilowatt-hours	horsepower-hours	1.341
			kilowatt-hours	joules	3.6×10^6
kilogram-calories	BTU	3.968	kilowatt-hours	kilogram-calories	860.5
kilogram-calories	foot-pounds	3,088.0	kilowatt-hours	kilogram-meters	3.671×10^5
kilogram-calories	horsepower-hours	1.560×10^{-3}	kilowatt-hours	pounds of water evaporated from and at 212°F	3.53
kilogram-calories	joules	4,186.0			
kilogram-calories	kilogram-meters	426.9			
kilogram-calories	kilojoules	4.186	kilowatt-hours	pounds of water raised from 62° to 212°F	22.75
kilogram-calories	kilowatt-hours	1.163×10^{-3}	**L**		
kilogram-meters	BTU	9.294×10^{-3}	liters	bushels (U.S. dry)	0.02838
kilogram-meters	ergs	9.804×10^7	liters	cubic centimeters	1,000.0
kilogram-meters	foot-pounds	7.233	liters	cubic feet	0.03531
kilogram-meters	joules	9.804	liters	cubic inches	61.02
kilogram-meters	kilogram-calories	2.342×10^{-3}	liters	cubic meters	0.001
kilogram-meters	kilowatt-hours	2.723×10^{-6}	liters	cubic yards	1.308×10^{-3}
kilolines	maxwells	1,000.0	liters	gallons (U.S. liq.)	0.2642
kiloliters	liters	1,000.0	liters	pints (U.S. liq.)	2.113
kilometers	centimeters	1×10^5	liters	quarts (U.S. liq.)	1.057
kilometers	feet	3,281.0	liters/minute	cubic feet/second	5.886×10^{-4}
kilometers	inches	3.937×10^4	liters/minute	gallons/second	4.403×10^{-3}
kilometers	meters	1,000.0	**M**		
kilometers	miles	0.6214	meters	centimeters	100.0
kilometers	millimeters	1×10^6	meters	feet	3.281
kilometers	yards	1,094.0	meters	inches	39.37
kilometers/hour	centimeters/ second	27.78	meters	kilometers	0.001
			meters	miles (nautical)	5.396×10^{-4}
kilometers/hour	feet/minute	54.68	meters	miles (statute)	6.214×10^{-4}
kilometers/hour	feet/second	0.9113	meters	millimeters	1,000.0
kilometers/hour	knots	0.5396	meters	yards	1.094
kilometers/hour	meters/minute	16.67	meters/minute	cms/second	1.667
kilometers/hour	miles/hour	0.6214	meters/minute	feet/minute	3.281
kilometers/hour/ second	centimeters/second/ second	27.78	meters/minute	feet/second	0.05468
			meters/minute	kilometers/hour	0.06
kilometers/hour/ second	feet/second/second	0.9113	meters/minute	knots	0.03238
			meters/minute	miles/hour	0.03728
kilometers/hour/ second	meters/second/ second	0.2778	meters/second	feet/minute	196.8
			meters/second	feet/second	3.281
kilometers/hour/ second	miles/hour/second	0.6214	meters/second	kilometers/hour	3.6
			meters/second	kilometers/minute	0.06
kilowatts	BTU/minute	56.92	meters/second	miles/hour	2.237

CONVERSION FACTORS FOR USE IN THE EXERCISE SCIENCES—*continued*

To Convert	Into	Multiply By	To Convert	Into	Multiply By
meters/second	miles/minute	0.03728	millimeters	centimeters	0.1
meters/second/second	centimeters/second/second	100.0	millimeters	feet	3.281×10^{-3}
			millimeters	inches	0.03937
meters/second/second	feet/second/second	3.281	millimeters	kilometers	1×10^{-6}
			millimeters	meters	0.001
meters/second/second	kilometers/hour/second	3.6	millimeters	miles	6.214×10^{-7}
			millimeters	mils	39.37
meters/second/second	miles/hour/second	2.237	millimeters	yards	1.094×10^{-3}
			minutes (angles)	degrees	0.01667
meter-kilograms	centimeter-dynes	9.807×10^{7}	minutes (angles)	quadrants	1.852×10^{-4}
meter-kilograms	centimeter-grams	1×10^{5}	minutes (angles)	radians	2.909×10^{-4}
meter-kilograms	pound-feet	7.233	minutes (angles)	seconds	60.0
miles (nautical)	feet	6,080.27	**N**		
miles (nautical)	kilometers	1.853	newtons	dynes	1×10^{5}
miles (nautical)	meters	1,853.0	**O**		
miles (nautical)	miles (statute)	1.1516	ohms (international)	ohms (absolute)	1.005
miles (nautical)	yards	2,027.0			
miles (statute)	centimeters	1.609×10^{5}	ohms	megohms	1×10^{-6}
miles (statute)	feet	5,280.0	ohms	microhms	1×10^{6}
miles (statute)	inches	6.336×10^{4}	ounces	drams	16.0
miles (statute)	kilometers	1.609	ounces	grains	437.5
miles (statute)	meters	1,609.0	ounces	grams	28.349527
miles (statute)	miles (nautical)	0.8684	ounces	pounds	0.0625
miles (statute)	yards	1,760.0	ounces	ounces (troy)	0.9115
miles/hour	centimeters/second	44.70	ounces	tons (long)	2.790×10^{-5}
			ounces	tons (metric)	2.835×10^{-5}
miles/hour	feet/minute	88.0	ounces (fluid)	cubic inches	1.805
miles/hour	feet/second	1.467	ounces (fluid)	liters	0.02957
miles/hour	kilometers/hour	1.609	ounces (troy)	grains	480.0
miles/hour	kilometers/minute	0.02682	ounces (troy)	grams	31.103481
miles/hour	knots	0.8684	ounces (troy)	ounces (avoirdupois)	1.09714
miles/hour	meters/minute	26.82			
miles/hour	miles/minute	0.1667	ounces (troy)	pennyweights (troy)	20.0
miles/hour/second	centimeters/second/second	44.70			
			ounces (troy)	pounds (troy)	0.08333
miles/hour/second	feet/second/second	1.467	ounces/square inch	dynes/square centimeter	4,309.0
miles/hour/second	kilometers/hour/second	1.609	ounces/square inch	pounds/square inch	0.0625
miles/hour/second	meters/second/second	0.4470	**P**		
			pints (liquid)	cubic centimeter	473.2
miles/minute	centimeters/second	2,682.0	pints (liquid)	cubic feet	0.01671
miles/minute	feet/second	88.0	pints (liquid)	cubic inches	28.87
miles/minute	kilometers/minute	1.609	pints (liquid)	cubic meters	4.732×10^{-4}
miles/minute	knots/minute	0.8684	pints (liquid)	cubic yards	6.189×10^{-4}
miles/minute	miles/hour	60.0	pints (liquid)	gallons	0.125
mil-feet	cubic inches	9.425×10^{-6}	pints (liquid)	liters	0.4732
milliers	kilograms	1,000.0	pints (liquid)	quarts (liquid)	0.5
millimicrons	meters	1×10^{-9}	pounds (avoirdupois)	ounces (troy)	14.5833
milligrams	grains	0.01543236			
milligrams	grams	0.001	pounds	drams	256.0
milligrams/liter	parts/million	1.0	pounds	dynes	44.4823×10^{4}
millihenries	henries	0.001	pounds	grains	7,000.0
milliliters	liters	0.001	pounds	grams	453.5924

CONVERSION FACTORS FOR USE IN THE EXERCISE SCIENCES—*continued*

To Convert	Into	Multiply By	To Convert	Into	Multiply By
pounds	joules/centimeter	0.04448	square centimeters	square meters	0.0001
pounds	joules/meter (newtons)	4.448	square centimeters	square miles	3.861×10^{-11}
			square centimeters	square millimeters	100.0
pounds	kilograms	0.4536			
pounds	ounces	16.0	square centimeters	square yards	1.196×10^{-4}
pounds	ounces (troy)	14.5833	square feet	acres	2.296×10^{-5}
pounds	poundals	32.17	square feet	circular mils	1.833×10^{8}
pounds	pounds (troy)	1.21528	square feet	square centimeters	929.0
pounds	tons (short)	0.0005	square feet	square inches	144.0
pounds of water	cubic inches	27.68	square feet	square meters	0.09290
			square feet	square miles	3.587×10^{-8}
pounds of water	gallons	0.1198	square feet	square millimeters	9.290×10^{4}
Q			square feet	square yards	0.1111
quarts (dry)	cubic inches	67.20	square inches	circular mils	1.273×10^{6}
quarts (liquid)	cubic centimeters	946.4	square inches	square centimeters	6.452
quarts (liquid)	cubic feet	0.03342	square inches	square feet	6.944×10^{-3}
quarts (liquid)	cubic inches	57.75	square inches	square millimeters	645.2
quarts (liquid)	cubic meters	9.464×10^{-4}			
quarts (liquid)	cubic yards	1.238×10^{-3}	square inches	square mils	1×10^{6}
quarts (liquid)	gallons	0.25	square inches	square yards	7.716×10^{-4}
quarts (liquid)	liters	0.9463	square kilometers	acres	247.1
R			square kilometers	square centimeters	1×10^{10}
radians	degrees	57.30	square kilometers	square feet	10.76×10^{6}
revolutions	degrees	360.0	square kilometers	square inches	1.550×10^{9}
revolutions	quadrants	4.0	square kilometers	square meters	1×10^{6}
revolutions	radians	6.283	square kilometers	square miles	0.3861
revolutions/minute	degrees/second	6.0	square kilometers	square yards	1.196×10^{6}
revolutions/minute	radians/second	0.1047	square meters	acres	2.471×10^{-4}
revolutions/minute	revolutions/second	0.01667	square meters	square centimeters	1×10^{4}
revolutions/minute/ minute	radians/second/ second	1.745×10^{-3}	square meters	square feet	10.76
			square meters	square inches	1,550.0
revolutions/minute/ minute	revolutions/ minute/second	0.01667	square meters	square miles	3.861×10^{-7}
			square meters	square millimeters	1×10^{6}
revolutions/minute/ minute	revolutions/ second/second	2.778×10^{-4}	square meters	square yards	1.196
			square miles	acres	640.0
revolutions/second	degrees/second	360.0	square miles	square feet	27.88×10^{6}
revolutions/second	radians/second	6.283	square miles	square kilometers	2.590
revolutions/second	revolutions/ minute	60.0	square miles	square meters	2.590×10^{6}
			square miles	square yards	3.098×10^{6}
revolutions/second/ second	radians/second/ second	6.283	square millimeters	circular mils	1,973.0
			square millimeters	square centimeters	0.01
revolutions/second/ second	revolutions/ minute/minute	3,600.0	square millimeters	square feet	1.076×10^{-5}
			square millimeters	square inches	1.550×10^{-3}
revolutions/second/ second	revolutions/ minute/second	60.0	square yards	acres	2.066×10^{-4}
			square yards	square centimeters	8,361.0
S			square yards	square feet	9.0
seconds (angle)	degrees	2.778×10^{-4}	square yards	square inches	1,296.0
seconds (angle)	minutes	0.01667	square yards	square meters	0.8361
seconds (angle)	quadrants	3.087×10^{-6}	square yards	square miles	3.228×10^{-7}
seconds (angle)	radians	4.848×10^{-6}	square yards	square millimeters	8.361×10^{5}
square centimeters	circular mils	1.973×10^{5}	**T**		
square centimeters	square feet	1.076×10^{-3}	temperature (°F) + 460	absolute temperature (°F)	1.0
square centimeters	square inches	0.1550			

CONVERSION FACTORS FOR USE IN THE EXERCISE SCIENCES—*continued*

To Convert	Into	Multiply By	To Convert	Into	Multiply By
temperature (°F) − 32	temperature (°C)	5/9	watts	kilowatts	0.001
temperature (°F) + 460	absolute temperature (°F)	1.0	watts (absolute)	BTU (mean)/ minute	0.056884
temperature (°F) − 32	temperature (°C)	5.9	watts (absolute)	joules/second	1.0
tons (metric)	kilograms	1,000.0	watt-hours	BTU	3.413
tons (metric)	pounds	2,205.0	watt-hours	ergs	3.60×10^{-10}
W			watt-hours	foot-pounds	2,656.0
watts	BTU/hour	3.4129	watt-hours	gram-calories	859.85
watts	BTY/minute	0.05688	watt-hours	horsepower-hours	1.341×10^{-3}
watts	ergs/second	107.0	watt-hours	kilogram-calories	0.8605
watts	foot-pounds/ minute	44.27	watt-hours	kilogram-meters	367.2
watts	foot-pounds/ second	0.7378	watt-hours	kilowatt-hours	0.001
watts	horsepower	1.341×10^{-3}	watts (international)	watts (absolute)	1.0002
watts	horsepower (metric)	1.360×10^{-3}	**Y**		
			yards	centimeters	91.44
watts	kilogram-calories/ minute	0.01433	yards	kilometers	9.144×10^{-4}
			yards	meters	0.9144
			yards	miles (nautical)	4.934×10^{-4}
			yards	mils (statute)	5.682×10^{-4}
			yards	millimeters	914.4

PART 3

CLINICAL HEMATOLOGY AND CLINICAL CHEMISTRY

SI CONVERSION TABLE FOR COMMON VALUES IN CLINICAL HEMATOLOGY AND CLINICAL CHEMISTRY

Component	Present Reference Intervals (Examples)	Present Unit	Conversion Factor	SI Reference Intervals	SI Unit Symbol	Significant Digits	Suggested Minimum Increment
Hemoglobin (B)							
Mass concentration							
—female	12.0–15.0	g/dL	10	120-150	g/L	XXX	1 g/L
—male	13.6–17.2	g/dL	10	136-172	g/L	XXX	1 g/L
Substance conc. Hb [Fe]							
—female	12.0–15.0	g/dL	0.6206	7.45–9.30	mmol/L	XX.XX	0.05 mmol/L
—male	13.6–17.2	g/dL	0.6206	8.45–10.65	mmol/L	XX.XX	0.05 mmol/L
Alkaline phosphatase (S)	30–120	U/L	0.01667	0.5–2.0	μkat/L	X.X	0.1 μkat/L
Amino acid nitrogen (P)	4.0–6.0	mg/dL	0.7139	2.9–4.3	mmol/L	X.X	0.1 mmol/L
Amino acid nitrogen (U)	50–200	mg/24 h	0.07139	3.6–14.3	mmol/d	X.X	0.1 mmol/d
Androstenedione (S)							
—male > 18 years	0.2–3.0	μg/L	3.492	0.5–10.5	mmol/L	XX.X	0.5 nmol/L
—female > 18 years	0.8–3.0	μg/L	3.492	3.0–10.5	nmol/L	XX.X	0.5 nmol/L
Bilirubin, total (S)	0.1–1.0	mg/dL	17.10	2–18	μmol/L	XX	2 μmol/L

SI CONVERSION TABLE FOR COMMON VALUES IN CLINICAL HEMATOLOGY AND CLINICAL CHEMISTRY—*continued*

Component	Present Reference Intervals (Examples)	Present Unit	Conversion Factor	SI Reference Intervals	SI Unit Symbol	Significant Digits	Suggested Minimum Increment
Calcium (S)							
—male	8.8–10.3	mg/dL	0.2495	2.20–2.50	mmol/L	X.XX	0.02 mmol/L
—female <50 y	8.8–10.0	mg/dL	0.2495	2.20–2.50	mmol/L	X.XX	0.02 mmol/L
—female >50 y	8.8–10.2	mg/dL	0.2495	2.20–2.56	mmol/L	X.XX	0.02 mmol/L
Calcium (U), normal diet	<250	mg/24 h	0.02495	<6.2	mmol/d	X.X	0.1 mmol/d
Cholesterol (P)							
—<29 years	<200	mg/dL	0.02586	<5.20	mmol/L	X.XX	0.05 mmol/L
—30–39 years	<225	mg/dL	0.02586	<5.85	mmol/L	X.XX	0.05 mmol/L
—40–49 years	<245	mg/dL	0.02586	<6.35	mmol/L	X.XX	0.05 mmol/L
—>50 years	<265	mg/dL	0.02586	<6.85	mmol/L	X.XX	0.05 mmol/L
Ferritin (S)	18–300	ng/mL	1.00	18–300	μg/L	XX0	10 μg/L
Glucose (P)—fasting	70–110	mg/dL	0.05551	3.9–6.1	mmol/L	XX.X	0.1 mmol/L
Hemoglobin (B)							
—male	14.0–18.0	g/dL	10.0	140–180	g/L	XXX	1 g/L
—female	11.5–15.5	g/dL	10.0	115–155	g/L	XXX	1 g/L
Insulin (P,S)	5–20	μU/mL	7.175	35–145	pmol/L	XXX	5 pmol/L
	5–20	mU/L	7.175	35–145	pmol/L	XXX	5 pmol/L
	0.20–0.84	μg/mL	172.2	35–145	pmol/L	XXX	5 pmol/L
Iron (S)							
—male	80–180	μg/dL	0.1791	14–32	μmol/L	XX	1 μmol/L
—female	60–160	μg/dL	0.1791	11–29	μmol/L	XX	1 μmol/L
Lipoproteins (P)							
Low density [LDL]— as cholesterol	50–190	mg/dL	0.02586	1.30–4.90	mmol/L	X.XX	0.05 mmol/L
High density [HDL]— as cholesterol							
Male	30–70	mg/dL	0.02586	0.80–1.80	mmol/L	X.XX	0.05 mmol/L
Female	30–90	mg/dL	0.02586	0.80–2.35	mmol/L	X.XX	0.05 mmol/L
Testosterone (P)							
—female	0.6	ng/mL	3.467	2.0	nmol/L	XX.X	0.5 nmol/L
—male	4.6–8.0	ng/mL	3.467	14.0–28.0	nmol/L	XX.X	0.5 nmol/L
Thyroid tests:							
Thyroid stimulating hormone [TSH] (S)	2–11	μU/mL	1.00	2–11	mU/L	XX	1 mU/L
Thyroxine [T$_4$] (S)	4.0–11.0	μg/dL	12.87	51–142	nmol/L	XXX	1 nmol/L
Thyroxine binding globulin [TBG] (S)—[as thyroxine]	12.0–28.0	μg/dL	12.87	150–360	nmol/L	XX0	1 nmol/L
Thyroxine, free (S)	0.8–2.8	ng/dL	12.87	10–36	pmol/L	XX	1 pmol/L
Triiodothyronine [T$_3$] (S)	75–220	ng/dL	0.01536	1.2–3.4	nmol/L	X.X	0.1 nmol/L
T$_3$ uptake (S)	25–35	%	0.01	0.25–0.35	1	0.XX	0.01
Tolbutamide (P)— therapeutic	50-120	mg/L	3.699	180–450	μmol/L	XX0	10 μmol/L
Transferrin (S)	170–370	mg/dL	0.01	1.70–3.70	g/L	X.XX	0.01 g/L
Triglycerides (P) [as triolein]	<160	mg/dL	0.01129	<1.80	mmol/L	X.XX	0.02 mmol/L
Vitamin A [retinol] (P,S)	10–50	μg/dL	0.03491	0.35–1.75	μmol/L	X.XX	0.05 μmol/L
Vitamin B$_1$ [thiamine hydrochloride] (U)	60–500	μg/24 h	0.002965	0.18–1.48	μmol/d	X.XX	0.01 μmol/d
Vitamin B$_2$ [riboflavin] (S)	2.6–3.7	μg/dL	26.57	70–100	nmol/L	XXX	5 nmol/L

SI CONVERSION TABLE FOR COMMON VALUES IN CLINICAL HEMATOLOGY AND CLINICAL CHEMISTRY—*continued*

Component	Present Reference Intervals (Examples)	Present Unit	Conversion Factor	SI Reference Intervals	SI Unit Symbol	Significant Digits	Suggested Minimum Increment
Vitamin B_6 [pyridoxal] (B)	20–90	ng/mL	5.982	120–540	nmol/L	XXX	5 nmol/L
Vitamin B_{12} [cyano-cobalamin] (P,S)	200–1000	pg/mL	0.7378	150–750	pmol/L	XX0	10 pmol/L
		ng/dL	7.378		pmol/L		
Vitamin C [ascorbic acid]	0.6–2.00	mg/dL	56.78	30–110	μmol/L	X0	10 μmol/L
Vitamin D_3							
[cholecalciferol] (P)	24–40	μg/mL	2.599	60–105	nmol/L	XXX	5 nmol/L
25 OH-cholecalciferol	18–36	ng/mL	2.496	45–90	nmol/L	XXX	5 mmol/L
Vitamin E [alpha-tocopherol] (P,S)	0.78–1.25	mg/dL	23.22	18–29	μmol/L	XX	1 μmol/L

Abbreviations: B, blood; P, plasma; S, serum; U, urine.

Nutritive Values for Common Foods, Alcoholic and Nonalcoholic Beverages, and Specialty and Fast-Food Items

This appendix has three parts. Part 1 lists nutritive values for common foods, Part 2 lists nutritive values for alcoholic and nonalcoholic beverages, and Part 3 presents nutritive values for specialty and fast-food items. The nutritive values of foods and alcoholic and nonalcoholic beverages are expressed in 1-ounce (28.4 g) portions so comparisons can readily be made between the different food categories. Thus, for example, the protein content of 1.55 g for 1 ounce of banana nut bread can be compared directly to the protein content of 6.28 g for 1 ounce of processed American cheese.

PART 1

NUTRITIVE VALUES FOR COMMON FOODS[a]

The foods are grouped into categories and are listed in alphabetical order within each category. The categories include breads, cakes and pies, cookies, candy bars, chocolate, desserts, cereals, cheese, fish, fruits, meats, eggs, dairy products, vegetables, and typical salad bar entries. An additional section labeled Variety consists of food items such as soups, sandwiches, salad dressings, oils, some condiments, and other "goodies." The nutritive value for each food is expressed per ounce or 28.4 g of that food item. The specific values for each food include the caloric content (kcal) for 1 ounce, protein, total fat, carbohydrate, calcium, iron, vitamin B_1, vitamin B_2, fiber content, and cholesterol.

---

[a] The information about the nutritive value of the foods was taken from a variety of sources. This includes primarily data from Watt, B.K., and Merrill, A.L.: *Composition of Foods—Raw, Processed and Prepared.* U.S. Department of Agriculture, Washington, DC, 1963; Adams, C, and Richardson, M.: *Nutritive Value of Foods.* Home and Garden Bulletin No. 72, rev, Washington, DC, U.S. Government Printing Office, 1981; and Pennington, J.A.T., and Church, H.N.: *Food Values of Portions Commonly Used,* 14th ed. New York, Harper & Row, 1985. Other sources include a comprehensive database on the Cyber mainframe computer at the University of Massachusetts, the consumer relations departments of manufacturers, and journal articles that evaluated specific foods items. *NA indicates data not available.*

BREADS

	kcal	Protein (g)	Fat (g)	CHO (g)	Ca (mg)	Fe (mg)	B₁ (mg)	B₂ (mg)	Fiber (g)	Cholesterol (mg)
Banana nut	91	1.55	4.00	12.7	10.0	0.470	0.054	0.046	0.66	18.3
Boston brown—canned	60	1.26	0.39	13.2	25.8	0.567	0.038	0.025	1.34	1.9
Cornmeal muffin—recipe	91	1.89	3.15	13.2	41.6	0.567	0.069	0.069	1.00	14.5
Croutons—dry	105	3.69	1.04	20.5	35.0	1.020	0.099	0.099	0.09	0
Cracked wheat	74	2.63	0.99	14.2	18.1	0.755	0.108	0.108	1.50	0
Cracked wheat—toast	88	3.00	1.17	16.9	21.6	0.899	0.100	0.128	1.82	0
French—chunk	81	2.67	1.10	14.3	31.6	0.875	0.130	0.097	0.57	0
Italian	78	2.55	0.25	16.0	4.7	0.756	0.116	0.066	0.47	0
Mixed grain	74	2.27	1.05	13.6	30.6	0.907	0.113	0.113	1.78	0
Mixed grain—toast	80	2.47	1.15	14.8	33.3	0.986	0.099	0.123	1.97	0
Oatmeal	74	2.37	1.25	13.6	17.0	0.794	0.130	0.075	1.10	0
Oatmeal—toast	80	2.47	1.36	14.8	18.5	0.863	0.110	0.081	1.20	0
Pita pocket	78	2.94	0.42	15.6	23.2	0.685	0.129	0.061	0.45	0
Pumpernickel	71	2.60	0.98	13.6	20.4	0.777	0.097	0.147	1.67	0
Pumpernickel—toast	78	2.86	1.08	15.0	22.5	0.857	0.088	0.162	1.87	0
Raisin—	77	2.15	1.12	15.0	28.4	0.879	0.093	0.176	0.68	0
Raisin—toasted	92	2.57	1.34	17.6	33.8	1.080	0.081	0.209	0.81	0
Rye—light	74	2.40	1.04	13.6	22.7	0.771	0.116	0.090	1.87	0
Rye—light—toast	84	2.73	1.18	15.5	25.8	0.876	0.107	0.103	2.15	0
Vienna	79	2.72	1.10	14.4	31.2	0.873	0.130	0.100	0.91	0
White	76	2.35	1.10	13.8	35.7	0.806	0.133	0.088	0.54	0
White—toast	84	2.67	1.26	15.7	40.6	0.915	0.121	0.103	0.64	0
Whole wheat	69	2.84	1.22	12.9	20.2	0.964	0.100	0.059	2.10	0
Whole wheat—toasted	79	3.42	1.47	14.4	22.5	1.090	0.090	0.066	2.74	0
Bread crumbs—dry grated	111	3.69	1.42	20.7	34.6	1.160	0.099	0.099	1.15	1.4
Bread crumbs—soft	76	2.35	1.10	13.9	35.9	0.806	0.134	0.088	0.54	0
Bread sticks wo/salt	109	3.40	0.82	21.3	7.9	0.255	0.017	0.020	0.43	0
Bread sticks w/salt	86	2.67	0.89	16.4	13.0	0.243	0.016	0.024	0.41	0

CAKES AND PIES

	kcal	Protein (g)	Fat (g)	CHO (g)	Ca (mg)	Fe (mg)	B₁ (mg)	B₂ (mg)	Fiber (g)	Cholesterol (mg)
Cakes										
Angel food cake	67	1.71	0.09	15.2	23.5	0.123	0.014	0.057	0	0
Boston cream pie	61	0.59	1.89	10.4	6.1	0.142	0.002	0.043	0	4.7
Carrot cake	103	1.05	5.32	13.2	6.9	0.304	0.030	0.035	0	14.6
Cheesecake	86	1.54	5.45	8.1	15.9	0.136	0.009	0.037	0	52.4
Choc cupcake/choc frosting	97	1.24	3.29	16.5	16.9	0.575	0.029	0.041	0	15.2
Coffee cake	91	1.78	2.70	14.8	17.3	0.480	0.054	0.059	0	18.5
Dark fruitcake	109	1.32	4.62	16.5	27.0	0.791	0.053	0.053	0	13.2
Gingerbread cake	91	1.15	2.86	15.2	12.2	0.706	0.042	0.038	0	7.8
Pound cake	113	1.89	4.72	14.2	18.9	0.472	0.047	0.057	0	30.2
Sheet cake—plain	104	1.32	3.96	15.8	18.1	0.429	0.046	0.049	0	20.1
Sheet cake—white frosting	104	0.94	3.28	18.0	14.3	0.281	0.030	0.037	0	16.4
Sponge cake	83	2.01	1.27	16.0	10.8	0.524	0.043	0.046	0	58.8
White cake/coconut	109	1.30	4.05	17.0	13.7	0.454	0.041	0.053	0	1.2

CAKES AND PIES—continued

	kcal	Protein (g)	Fat (g)	CHO (g)	Ca (mg)	Fe (mg)	B₁ (mg)	B₂ (mg)	Fiber (g)	Cholesterol (mg)
Cakes—cont'd										
White cake/white frosting	104	1.20	3.59	16.8	13.2	0.399	0.080	0.052	0	1.2
Yellow cake/chocolate frosting	101	1.03	4.48	15.9	9.5	0.509	0.020	0.058	0	15.6
Pies										
Apple pie	73	0.66	3.14	10.7	5.0	0.300	0.031	0.023	0	0
Apple pie—fried	85	0.73	4.67	10.7	4.0	0.312	0.030	0.020	0	4.7
Banana cream pie	46	0.90	1.85	6.7	21.0	0.156	0.022	0.042	0	2.2
Blueberry pie	68	0.72	3.05	9.9	4.7	0.377	0.031	0.025	0	0
Boston cream pie	61	0.59	1.89	10.4	6.1	0.142	0.002	0.043	0	4.7
Cherry pie	74	0.77	3.19	10.9	6.6	0.569	0.034	0.025	0	0
Cherry pie—fried	83	0.68	4.74	10.7	3.7	0.233	0.020	0.020	0	4.3
Chocolate cream pie	50	1.20	2.04	6.9	25.9	0.175	0.024	0.049	0	2.4
Coconut cream pie	57	1.03	2.79	7.2	24.0	0.198	0.021	0.042	0	2.5
Coconut custard pie	66	1.69	3.85	6.3	25.0	0.304	0.029	0.055	0	31.4
Cream pie	85	0.56	4.29	11.0	8.6	0.205	0.011	0.028	0	1.5
Custard pie	55	1.43	2.65	6.3	23.1	0.269	0.026	0.050	0	27.6
Lemon meringue pie	72	0.95	2.90	10.7	5.1	0.283	0.020	0.028	0	27.7
Mincemeat pie	70	0.65	2.13	12.8	6.9	0.360	0.028	0.024	0	0
Peach pie	73	0.63	3.14	10.9	4.8	0.340	0.031	0.028	0	0
Pecan pie	120	1.30	4.87	18.9	7.2	0.380	0.045	0.034	0	28.1
Pumpkin pie	52	1.28	2.23	7.3	30.0	0.373	0.019	0.042	0	15.5
Strawberry chiffon pie	65	0.85	3.46	8.0	7.7	0.254	0.022	0.023	0	7.1

COOKIES

	kcal	Protein (g)	Fat (g)	CHO (g)	Ca (mg)	Fe (mg)	B₁ (mg)	B₂ (mg)	Fiber (g)	Cholesterol (mg)
Animal cookies	120	1.90	2.89	22.0	3.0	0.918	0.080	0.130	0	0.1
Brownies w/nuts	135	1.84	8.93	15.6	12.8	0.567	0.070	0.070	0	25.5
Butter cookies	130	1.76	4.82	20.2	36.3	0.170	0.011	0.017	0	4.1
Fig bars	106	1.02	1.93	21.4	20.2	0.689	0.039	0.037	0	13.7
Lady fingers	102	2.19	2.19	18.3	11.6	0.515	0.019	0.039	0	101.0
Oatmeal raisin cookies	134	1.64	5.45	19.6	9.8	0.600	0.049	0.044	0	1.1
Peanut butter cookies	145	2.36	8.27	16.5	12.4	0.650	0.041	0.041	0	13.0
Sandwich type cookies	138	1.42	5.67	20.6	8.5	0.992	0.064	0.050	0	0
Shortbread cookies	137	1.77	7.09	17.7	11.5	0.709	0.089	0.080	0	23.9
Sugar cookies	139	1.18	7.09	18.3	29.5	0.532	0.053	0.035	0	17.1
Vanilla wafers	131	1.42	4.96	20.6	11.3	0.567	0.050	0.070	0	17.7

CANDY BARS

	kcal	Protein (g)	Fat (g)	CHO (g)	Ca (mg)	Fe (mg)	B₁ (mg)	B₂ (mg)	Fiber (g)	Cholesterol (mg)
Almond Joy	151	1.69	7.82	18.5	2.0	0.778	0	0	0	0
Sugar-coated almonds	146	3.10	9.12	14.6	39.6	0.775	0.042	0.156	0	0

CANDY BARS—*continued*

	kcal	Protein (g)	Fat (g)	CHO (g)	Ca (mg)	Fe (mg)	B₁ (mg)	B₂ (mg)	Fiber (g)	Cholesterol (mg)
Bittersweet chocolate	141	1.90	9.73	15.7	13.0	1.040	0.015	0.050	0	0
Caramel—plain or chocolate	115	1.00	2.99	22.0	41.9	0.399	0.010	0.050	0	1.0
Chocolate candy kisses	154	2.10	8.98	15.9	52.9	0.499	0.020	0.080	0	0
Chocolate-coated almonds	161	3.92	12.70	8.0	47.8	1.090	0.052	0.186	0	0
Chocolate-covered coconut	133	0.91	7.10	17.5	8.4	0.614	0.008	0.016	0	0
Chocolate-covered mints	116	0.50	2.99	23.0	16.0	0.299	0.010	0.020	0	0
Chocolate-covered peanuts	159	5.00	11.70	9.8	32.9	0.689	0.086	0.043	0	0
Chocolate-covered raisins	111	1.06	2.71	20.6	12.2	0.663	0.034	0.025	0	0
Chocolate fudge	115	0.56	2.78	21.0	22.0	0.299	0.010	0.030	0	1.0
Chocolate fudge with nuts	114	1.06	4.99	18.8	22.0	0.299	0.016	0.030	0	7.4
English toffee	195	0.89	16.90	9.8	0	0.177	0.470	0.044	0	0
Gum drops	98	0	0.20	24.8	2.0	0.100	0	0	0	0
Hard candy	109	0	0	27.6	6.0	0.100	0	0	0	0
Jelly beans	104	0	0.10	26.4	1.0	0.299	0	0	0	0
Kit Kat	138	1.98	7.25	16.5	42.9	0.369	0.020	0.073	0	0
Krackle	149	2.00	8.09	16.9	50.0	0.400	0.017	0.075	0	0
Malted milk balls	135	2.30	6.99	17.8	62.9	0	0	0	0	0
M&M's plain chocolate	140	1.95	6.08	19.5	46.7	0.449	0.015	0.073	0	0
M&M's peanut chocolate	144	3.23	7.25	16.5	35.4	0.402	0.016	0.056	0	0
Mars bar	136	2.27	6.24	17.0	48.2	0.312	0.014	0.093	0	0
Milk chocolate—plain	145	2.00	8.98	16.0	49.9	0.399	0.020	0.100	0	6.0
Milk chocolate w/almonds	150	2.90	10.40	15.0	60.9	0.559	0.030	0.130	0	4.5
Milk chocolate w/peanuts	155	4.89	11.70	10.0	31.9	0.679	0.112	0.065	0	3.0
Milk chocolate + rice cereal	140	2.00	6.99	18.0	47.9	0.200	0.010	0.080	0	6.0
Milky Way	123	1.53	4.25	20.3	40.6	0.232	0.013	0.070	0	6.6
Mr. Goodbar	151	3.62	9.05	13.9	39.2	0.567	0.030	0.072	0	4.2
Reese's peanut butter cup	151	3.65	9.07	13.9	21.7	0.430	0.020	0.032	0	1.6
Snickers	134	3.08	6.62	17.0	32.4	0.227	0.013	0.050	0	0
Vanilla fudge	118	0.70	3.15	22.0	29.9	0.030	0.006	0.025	0	10.0
Vanilla fudge with nuts	122	1.00	5.01	18.3	25.0	0.159	0.017	0.026	0	8.5

CHOCOLATE

	kcal	Protein (g)	Fat (g)	CHO (g)	Ca (mg)	Fe (mg)	B₁ (mg)	B₂ (mg)	Fiber (g)	Cholesterol (mg)
Baking chocolate	145	3.49	15.00	7.5	22.0	1.900	0.015	0.099	0	0
Bittersweet chocolate	141	1.90	9.73	15.7	13.0	1.040	0.015	0.050	0	0
Milk chocolate—plain	145	2.00	8.98	16.0	49.9	0.399	0.020	0.100	0	6.0
Semi-sweet chocolate chips	143	1.17	10.20	16.2	8.5	0.967	0.017	0.023	0	0
Dark chocolate—sweet	150	1.00	9.98	16.0	7.0	0.599	0.010	0.040	0	0
Chocolate cupcake/ chocolate frosting	97	1.24	3.29	16.5	16.9	0.575	0.029	0.041	0	15.2
Chocolate candy kisses	154	2.10	8.98	15.9	52.9	0.499	0.020	0.080	0	0
Chocolate chip cookies	122	1.54	5.94	18.9	11.0	0.540	0.068	0.155	0	3.4

CHOCOLATE—continued

	kcal	Protein (g)	Fat (g)	CHO (g)	Ca (mg)	Fe (mg)	B₁ (mg)	B₂ (mg)	Fiber (g)	Cholesterol (mg)
Chocolate coated almonds	161	3.92	12.70	8.0	47.8	1.090	0.052	0.186	0	0
Chocolate coated peanuts	159	5.00	11.70	9.8	32.9	0.689	0.086	0.043	0	0
Chocolate covered mints	116	0.50	2.99	23.0	16.0	0.299	0.010	0.020	0	0
Chocolate covered raisins	111	1.06	2.71	20.6	12.2	0.663	0.034	0.025	0	0
Chocolate cream pie	50	1.20	2.04	6.9	25.9	0.175	0.024	0.049	0	2.4
Chocolate fudge	115	0.56	2.78	21.0	22.0	0.299	0.010	0.030	0	1.0
Chocolate fudge with nuts	114	1.06	4.99	18.8	22.0	0.299	0.016	0.030	0	7.4
Cake flour-baked value	103	2.08	0.28	22.4	4.5	1.250	0.154	0.096	0	0
Reese's peanut butter cup	151	3.65	9.07	13.9	21.7	0.430	0.020	0.032	0	1.6
Chocolate pudding/recipe	42	0.88	1.25	7.3	27.3	0.142	0.005	0.039	0	4.3
Chocolate pudding instant	34	0.85	0.818	5.9	28.4	0.065	0.009	0.039	0	3.1

DESSERTS AND BREAKFAST PASTRIES

	kcal	Protein (g)	Fat (g)	CHO (g)	Ca (mg)	Fe (mg)	B₁ (mg)	B₂ (mg)	Fiber (g)	Cholesterol (mg)
Apple brown betty	43	0.30	1.60	7.40	5.4	0.130	0.016	0.012	0	3.8
Apple cobbler	55	0.53	1.74	9.57	8.8	0.206	0.023	0.019	0	0.3
Apple crisp	53	0.33	1.93	9.09	7.4	0.278	0.018	0.013	0	0
Apple dumpling	55	0.32	2.37	8.64	7.1	0.253	0.012	0.013	0	0
Banana nut bread	91	1.60	4.00	12.70	10.0	0.470	0.054	0.046	0	18.3
Bread + raisin pudding	60	1.20	2.47	8.54	27.7	0.304	0.030	0.048	0	24.4
Cheesecake	86	1.50	5.45	8.10	15.9	0.136	0.009	0.037	0	52.4
Cherry cobbler	44	0.53	1.37	7.52	8.5	0.391	0.019	0.021	0	0.3
Cherry & cream cheese torte	79	1.28	3.96	10.00	28.5	0.266	0.015	0.052	0	11.2
Vanilla milkshake	32	0.98	0.841	5.09	34.5	0.026	0.013	0.052	0	3.2
Cream puff w/custard fill	72	1.24	4.54	6.83	16.4	0.276	0.015	0.040	0	58.8
Chocolate eclair w/custard fill	79	1.20	4.43	8.96	18.6	0.258	0.019	0.041	0	50.4
Gelatin salad	17	0.43	0	3.99	0.5	0.024	0.002	0.002	0	0
Peach cobbler	28	0.50	1.35	7.96	7.6	0.197	0.018	0.017	0	0.3
Peach crisp	34	0.31	1.06	6.18	4.8	0.203	0.010	0.010	0	0
Crepe, unfilled	49	2.06	1.32	7.07	25.0	0.475	0.045	0.070	0.21	43.0
Pancakes—plain	63	2.10	2.10	9.45	28.4	0.525	0.063	0.074	0.42	16.8
Croissant	117	2.32	6.02	13.40	10.0	1.040	0.085	0.065	0.54	6.5
Danish pastry—plain	109	1.99	5.97	12.90	29.8	0.547	0.080	0.085	0	24.4
Danish pastry w/fruit	102	1.74	5.67	12.20	7.41	0.567	0.070	0.061	0	24.4
Doughnut—cake type	119	1.33	6.75	13.90	13.0	0.454	0.068	0.068	0	11.3
Doughnut—jelly filled	99	1.48	3.84	13.00	12.2	0.349	0.052	0.044	0	0
Doughnut—yeast-raised	111	1.89	6.28	12.30	8.0	0.661	0.132	0.057	0	9.9
Chocolate pudding	42	0.88	1.25	7.28	27.3	0.142	0.005	0.039	0	4.3
Tapioca pudding	38	1.43	1.44	4.85	29.7	0.120	0.012	0.052	0	27.3
Vanilla pudding	32	0.99	1.10	4.50	33.1	0.089	0.009	0.046	0	4.1
Chocolate pudding—instant	34	0.85	0.82	5.89	28.4	0.065	0.009	0.039	0	3.1
Rice pudding	33	0.86	0.86	5.80	28.6	0.107	0.021	0.039	0	3.2
Butterscotch pudding pop	47	1.19	1.29	7.80	37.8	0.020	0.015	0.055	0	0.5
Chocholate pudding pop	49	1.34	1.34	8.20	42.8	0.179	0.015	0.055	0	0.5
Vanilla pudding pop	46	1.19	1.29	7.80	37.8	0.020	0.015	0.055	0	0.5

CEREALS (WITHOUT MILK)

	kcal	Protein (g)	Fat (g)	CHO (g)	Ca (mg)	Fe (mg)	B₁ (mg)	B₂ (mg)	Fiber (g)	Cholesterol (mg)
All-Bran	70	3.99	0.50	21.0	23.00	4.49	0.369	0.429	8.490	0
Alpha Bits	111	2.20	0.60	24.6	7.99	1.80	0.399	0.399	0.650	0
Apple Jacks	110	1.50	0.10	25.7	2.99	4.49	0.399	0.399	0.200	0
Bran Buds	73	3.95	0.68	21.6	18.90	4.52	0.371	0.439	7.860	0
Bran Chex	90	2.95	0.81	22.6	16.80	4.51	0.347	0.150	5.200	0
Buc Wheats	110	2.00	1.00	24.0	59.90	8.09	0.674	0.764	2.000	0
C.W. Post—plain	126	2.54	4.44	20.3	13.70	4.50	0.380	0.438	0.643	0
C.W. Post w/raisins	123	2.45	4.05	20.3	14.00	4.51	0.358	0.413	0.660	0
Cap'n Crunch	120	1.46	2.60	22.9	4.60	7.53	0.506	0.544	0.709	0
Cap'n Crunchberries	118	1.46	2.35	23.0	8.91	7.32	0.478	0.543	0.324	0
Cap'n Crunch—peanut butter	125	2.03	3.64	21.5	5.67	7.37	0.486	0.567	0.324	0
Cheerios	110	4.24	1.77	19.4	47.30	4.44	0.394	0.394	3.000	0
Cocoa Krispies	109	1.50	0.39	25.2	4.73	1.81	0.394	0.394	0.354	0
Cocoa Pebbles	117	1.35	1.49	24.7	5.40	1.75	0.405	0.405	0.312	0
Corn Bran	98	1.97	1.02	23.9	32.30	9.60	0.299	0.551	5.390	0
Corn Chex	111	2.00	0.10	24.9	2.99	1.80	0.399	0.070	0.499	0
Corn flakes—Kellogg's	110	2.30	0.09	24.4	1.00	1.80	0.367	0.424	0.594	0
Corn flakes—Post Toasties	110	2.30	0.09	24.4	1.00	0.70	0.367	0.424	0.594	0
Corn grits—enriched yellow dry	105	2.49	0.33	22.5	0.55	1.10	0.182	0.107	3.270	0
Corn grits—enriched ckd	17	0.41	0.06	3.7	0.12	0.18	0.028	0.018	0.527	0
Cracklin' Oat Bran	108	2.60	4.16	19.4	18.90	1.80	0.378	0.425	4.280	0
Cream of Rice	15	0.24	0.01	3.3	0.93	0.05	0.012	0	0.163	0
Cream of Wheat	16	0.42	0.07	3.4	6.27	1.27	0.028	0.008	0.395	0
Crispy Wheat 'n Raisins	99	2.00	0.46	23.1	46.80	4.48	0.396	0.396	1.320	0
Farina—cooked	14	0.41	0.02	3.0	0.49	0.14	0.023	0.015	0.389	0
Fortified Oat Flakes	105	5.32	0.41	20.5	40.20	8.09	0.354	0.413	0.827	0
40% Bran Flakes—Kellogg's	91	3.60	0.54	22.2	13.80	8.14	0.369	0.430	0.850	0
40% Bran Flakes—Post	92	3.20	0.45	22.3	12.70	4.50	0.374	0.435	3.800	0
Froot Loops	111	1.70	1.00	25.0	2.99	4.49	0.399	0.399	0.299	0
Frosted Mini-Wheats	102	2.93	0.27	23.4	9.15	1.83	0.366	0.457	2.160	0
Frosted Rice Krispies	109	1.30	0.10	25.7	1.00	1.80	0.399	0.399	0.998	0
Fruit & Fiber w/apples	90	2.99	1.00	22.0	9.98	4.49	0.374	0.424	4.190	0
Fruit & Fiber w/dates	90	2.99	1.00	21.0	9.98	4.49	0.374	0.424	4.190	0
Fruitful Bran	92	2.50	0	22.5	8.34	6.75	0.313	0.354	4.170	0
Fruity Pebbles	115	1.10	1.50	24.4	2.99	1.80	0.399	0.399	0.226	0
Golden Grahams	109	1.60	1.09	24.1	17.40	4.50	0.363	0.436	1.670	0
Granola—homemade	138	3.49	7.69	15.6	17.70	1.12	0.170	0.072	2.970	0
Granola—Nature Valley	126	2.89	4.92	18.9	17.80	0.95	0.098	0.048	2.960	0
Grape Nuts	100	3.28	0.11	23.2	10.90	1.22	0.398	0.398	1.840	0
Grape Nuts Flakes	102	2.99	0.30	23.2	11.00	4.49	0.399	0.399	1.900	0
Honey & Nut Corn Flakes	113	1.80	1.50	23.3	2.99	1.80	0.399	0.399	0.299	0
Honey Bran	96	2.51	0.57	23.2	13.00	4.54	0.405	0.405	3.160	0
Honey Comb	111	1.68	0.52	25.3	5.15	1.80	0.387	0.387	0.387	0
Honey Nut Cheerios	107	3.09	0.69	22.8	19.80	4.47	0.344	0.430	0.790	0
King Vitamin	115	1.49	1.62	24.0	NA	17.10	0.124	1.430	0.135	0
Kix	109	2.49	0.70	23.3	34.80	8.06	0.398	0.398	0.398	0
Life	104	5.22	0.52	20.3	99.20	7.47	0.612	0.644	0.902	0
Lucky Charms	111	2.57	1.06	23.1	31.90	4.52	0.354	0.443	0.624	0
Malt-O-Meal	14	0.43	0.03	3.1	0.59	1.13	0.057	0.028	0.354	0
Maypo—cooked	1	0.02	0.01	0.1	0.52	0.04	0.003	0.003	0.012	0

CEREALS (WITHOUT MILK)—continued

	kcal	Protein (g)	Fat (g)	CHO (g)	Ca (mg)	Fe (mg)	B₁ (mg)	B₂ (mg)	Fiber (g)	Cholesterol (mg)
Nutri-Grain—barley	106	3.11	0.21	23.4	7.60	1.00	0.346	0.415	1.660	0
Nutri-Grain—corn	108	2.30	0.68	24.0	0.68	0.60	0.338	0.405	1.750	0
Nutri-Grain—rye	102	2.48	0.21	24.0	5.67	0.80	0.354	0.425	2.160	0
Nutri-Grain—wheat	102	2.45	0.32	24.0	7.73	0.80	0.387	0.451	1.800	0
Oatmeal—prepared	18	0.73	0.29	3.1	2.42	0.19	0.032	0.006	0.497	0
Rolled Oats	109	4.55	1.78	19.0	14.70	1.19	0.206	0.038	3.090	0
Instant Oatmeal w/apples	26	0.74	0.30	5.0	30.00	1.15	0.091	0.053	0.552	0
Instant Oatmeal w/bran & raisins	23	0.71	0.28	4.4	25.20	1.10	0.081	0.092	0.480	0
Instant Oatmeal w/maple	30	0.84	0.35	5.8	29.60	1.16	0.097	0.059	0.530	0
Instant Oatmeal w/cinnamon & spice	31	0.85	0.34	6.2	30.30	1.17	0.099	0.60	0.510	0
Instant Oatmeal w/raisins & spice	29	0.77	0.32	5.7	29.60	1.18	0.092	0.065	0.556	0
100% Bran	77	3.57	1.42	20.7	19.80	3.49	0.687	0.773	8.380	0
100% Natural	135	3.02	6.02	18.0	48.90	0.83	0.085	0.150	3.390	0
100% Natural—w/apples	130	2.92	5.32	19.0	42.80	0.79	0.090	0.158	1.300	0
100% Natural—w/raisins & dates	128	2.89	5.23	18.7	41.20	0.80	0.077	0.165	1.080	0
Product 19	108	2.75	0.17	23.5	3.44	18.00	1.460	1.720	0.369	0
Puffed Rice	111	1.79	0.20	25.5	2.03	0.30	0.030	0.028	0.227	0
Puffed Wheat	104	4.25	0.24	22.4	7.09	1.35	0.047	0.070	5.430	0
Quisp	117	1.42	2.08	23.6	8.50	5.96	0.510	0.718	0.378	0
Raisin Bran—Kellogg's	91	3.07	0.46	21.4	14.50	13.90	0.293	0.332	3.410	0
Raisin Bran—Post	86	2.68	0.55	21.4	13.70	4.56	0.373	0.430	3.190	0
Raisins, Rice & Rye	96	1.60	0.06	24.2	6.16	3.45	0.308	0.370	0.308	0
Ralston—cooked	15	0.62	0.09	3.2	1.57	0.18	0.022	0.020	0.370	0
Rice Chex	112	1.49	1.00	25.2	3.88	1.79	0.400	0.298	1.840	0
Rice Krispies	109	1.86	0.20	24.2	3.91	1.76	0.391	0.391	0.312	0
Roman Meal—dry	91	4.07	0.60	20.4	18.40	1.31	0.142	0.069	0.905	0
Roman Meal—cooked	17	0.77	0.11	3.9	3.45	0.25	0.028	0.014	0.877	0
Shredded Wheat	102	3.09	0.71	22.5	11.00	1.20	0.070	0.080	3.100	0
Shredded wheat	97	3.06	0.45	16.4	11.20	0.89	0.082	0.075	2.900	0
Special K	111	5.58	0.10	21.3	7.97	4.48	0.399	0.399	0.266	0
Sugar Corn Pops	108	1.40	0.10	25.6	0.10	1.80	0.399	0.399	0.100	0
Sugar Frosted Flakes	108	1.46	0.08	25.7	0.81	1.78	0.405	0.405	0.446	0
Sugar Smacks	106	2.00	0.50	24.7	2.99	1.80	0.369	0.429	0.319	0
Super Golden Crisp	106	1.80	0.26	25.6	6.01	1.80	0.344	0.430	0.430	0
Team	111	1.82	0.48	24.3	4.05	1.73	0.371	0.425	0.270	0
Total	105	2.84	0.60	22.3	172.00	18.00	1.460	1.720	2.060	0
Trix	108	1.50	0.40	24.9	5.99	4.49	0.399	0.399	0.184	0
Wheat & Raisin Chex	97	2.68	0.21	22.6	NA	4.04	0.263	0.315	1.890	0
Wheat Chex	104	2.77	0.68	23.3	11.00	4.50	0.370	0.105	2.100	0
Wheat germ—toasted	108	8.25	3.09	14.0	12.50	2.19	0.474	0.233	3.910	0
Wheat germ w/brown sugar, honey	107	6.19	2.30	17.2	8.98	1.93	0.349	0.180	3.390	0
Wheatena—cooked	16	0.58	0.13	3.4	1.28	0.16	0.002	0.006	0.385	0
Wheaties	99	2.74	0.51	22.6	43.00	4.50	0.391	0.391	2.540	0
Whole wheat berries	16	0.54	0.11	3.2	1.70	0.17	0.023	0.006	0.680	0
Whole wheat cereal—cooked	18	0.58	0.11	3.9	1.99	0.18	0.020	0.014	0.457	0

CHEESE

	kcal	Protein (g)	Fat (g)	CHO (g)	Ca (mg)	Fe (mg)	B_1 (mg)	B_2 (mg)	Fiber (g)	Cholesterol (mg)
American—processed	106	6.28	8.84	0.45	174	0.110	0.008	0.111	0	27.0
American cheese food—cold pack	94	5.23	6.78	2.36	145	0.240	0.009	0.274	0	18.0
American cheese spread	82	5.16	6.00	2.48	159	0.090	0.014	0.380	0	16.0
Blue	100	6.09	8.14	0.66	150	0.090	0.008	0.395	0	21.0
Brick	105	6.40	8.40	0.79	191	0.130	0.004	0.159	0	27.0
Brie	95	5.87	7.84	0.13	52	0.140	0.020	0.147	0	28.0
Camembert	85	5.60	6.86	0.13	110	0.094	0.008	0.138	0	20.0
Caraway	107	7.13	8.27	0.87	191	0.100	0.009	0.196	0	25.0
Cheddar	114	7.05	9.38	0.36	204	0.197	0.008	0.106	0	29.9
Cheshire	110	6.60	8.66	1.36	182	0.060	0.013	0.198	0	28.9
Colby	112	6.73	9.08	0.73	194	0.216	0.004	0.171	0	27.0
Cottage	29	3.54	1.20	0.76	17	0.040	0.006	0.115	0	4.2
Cottage—lowfat 2%	26	3.90	0.55	1.03	20	0.045	0.007	0.052	0	2.4
Cottage—lowfat 1%	21	3.51	0.29	0.77	18	0.040	0.006	0.115	0	1.3
Cottage—dry curd	24	4.89	0.12	0.52	9	0.065	0.007	0.004	0	2.0
Cottage—w/fruit	35	2.80	0.96	3.78	14	0.031	0.005	0.115	0	3.1
Cream	99	2.10	9.87	0.75	23	0.337	0.005	0.056	0	30.9
Edam	101	7.07	7.79	0.40	207	0.125	0.010	0.274	0	25.0
Feta	75	4.49	6.19	1.16	140	0.180	0.040	0.315	0	25.0
Fontina	110	7.25	8.62	0.44	156	0.060	0.006	NA	0	32.9
Gjetost	132	2.74	8.32	12.00	113	0.130	0.009	0.170	0	25.0
Gorgonzola	111	6.99	8.98	0	149	0.120	0.010	0.512	0	25.0
Gouda	101	7.06	7.72	0.63	198	0.070	0.009	0.232	0	31.9
Gruyere	117	8.44	9.05	0.10	286	0.060	0.017	0.095	0	30.9
Liederkranz	87	4.99	7.99	0	110	0.120	0.010	0.389	0	21.0
Limburger	93	5.67	7.59	0.14	141	0.040	0.023	0.227	0	26.0
Monterey jack	106	6.93	8.56	0.19	212	0.200	0.004	0.119	0	26.0
Mozzarella—skim, low moist	80	7.60	4.67	0.89	207	0.076	0.006	0.150	0	15.0
Mozzarella—whole milk, regular	80	5.50	5.75	0.63	147	0.050	0.004	0.106	0	22.0
Mozzarella—whole milk, moist	90	6.10	7.19	0.43	163	0.060	0.005	0.119	0	25.0
Muenster	104	6.40	8.42	0.32	203	0.125	0.004	0.178	0	27.0
Neufchatel	74	2.82	6.70	0.83	21	0.080	0.004	0.113	0	22.0
Parmesan—hard	111	10.00	7.30	0.91	335	0.230	0.010	0.453	0	19.0
Parmesan—grated	129	11.80	8.50	1.06	389	0.270	0.013	0.527	0	22.0
Pimento processed	106	6.26	8.82	0.49	174	0.120	0.008	0.404	0	27.0
Port du salut	100	6.73	7.99	0.16	84	0.140	0.004	0.151	0	34.9
Provolone	100	7.13	7.54	0.61	214	0.146	0.005	0.248	0	20.0
Ricotta—part skim	39	3.23	2.25	1.45	77	0.126	0.006	0.052	0	8.8
Ricotta—whole milk	49	3.19	3.68	0.86	59	0.108	0.004	0.024	0	14.3
Romano	110	9.00	7.63	1.03	301	0.230	0.010	0.339	0	28.9
Romano—grated	128	10.50	8.86	1.20	350	0.270	0.013	0.394	0	32.9
Roquefort	105	6.10	8.93	0.57	188	0.172	0.010	0.512	0	26.0
Swiss	107	8.03	7.79	0.96	272	0.050	0.006	0.074	0	26.0
Swiss processed	95	7.00	6.97	0.60	219	0.170	0.004	0.078	0	24.0

FISH

	kcal	Protein (g)	Fat (g)	CHO (g)	Ca (mg)	Fe (mg)	B_1 (mg)	B_2 (mg)	Fiber (g)	Cholesterol (mg)
Bass—freshwater raw	32	5.36	1.05	0	22.7	0.422	0.028	0.009	0	19.3
Bluefish—baked/broiled	45	7.43	1.42	0	2.6	0.174	0.022	0.030	0	17.9
Bluefish—fried in crumbs	58	6.44	2.78	1.33	2.3	0.151	0.017	0.023	0	17
Bluefish—raw	35	5.67	1.20	0	2.0	0.136	0.016	0.023	0	16.7
Carp—raw	36	5.05	1.59	0	11.6	0.352	0.013	0.011	0	18.7
Catfish—channel—raw	33	5.16	1.20	0	11.3	0.275	0.013	0.030	0	16.4
Cod—baked w/butter	37	6.46	0.94	0	5.7	0.139	0.025	0.022	0	17.0
Cod—batter-fried	56	5.56	2.92	2.13	22.7	0.142	0.011	0.011	0	15.6
Cod—baked/broiled	30	6.46	0.24	0	4.0	0.139	0.025	0.022	0	15.6
Cod—poached	29	6.24	0.24	0	4.0	0.139	0.025	0.022	0	15.6
Cod—steamed	29	6.24	0.24	0	4.0	0.139	0.025	0.022	0	15.9
Cod—smoked	22	5.19	0.17	0	4.0	0.113	0.023	0.020	0	14.2
Cod—Atlantic—raw	23	5.05	0.19	0	4.5	0.108	0.022	0.018	0	12.2
Cod liver oil	255	0	28.40	0	0	0	0	0	0	162.0
Eel—smoked	94	5.27	7.88	0.23	26.9	0.198	0.040	0.099	0	19.8
Haddock—breaded/fried	58	5.67	3.00	2.33	11.3	0.384	0.020	0.033	0.01	18.3
Haddock—smoked	33	7.14	0.27	0	13.9	0.397	0.013	0.014	0	21.8
Haddock—raw	22	5.36	0.20	0	9.4	0.298	0.010	0.010	0	16.2
Herring—pickled	74	4.03	5.10	2.73	21.8	0.346	0.010	0.039	0	3.7
Herring—smoked/ kippered	62	6.97	3.52	0	23.8	0.428	0.036	0.090	0	22.7
Herring—canned w/liquid	59	5.64	3.86	0	41.7	0.879	0.007	0.051	0	27.5
Mackerel—fried	49	7.00	2.35	0	4.3	0.445	0.045	0.116	0	19.8
Mackerel—Atlantic— baked/broiled	74	6.78	5.05	0	4.3	0.445	0.045	0.117	0	21.3
Mackerel—Atlantic—raw	58	5.27	3.94	0	3.4	0.462	0.050	0.088	0	19.8
Mackerel—Pacific—raw	45	6.12	2.84	0	2.3	0.567	0.043	0.096	0	22.7
Northern pike—raw	25	5.47	0.20	0	16.2	0.156	0.017	0.018	0	11.0
Ocean perch—breaded/ fried	62	5.34	3.67	2.33	30.7	0.400	0.033	0.037	0.03	15.3
Pollock—baked/broiled	28	6.60	0.31	0	19.3	0.149	0.014	0.057	0	19.8
Pollock—poached	36	6.60	0.31	0	17.0	0.149	0.010	0.050	0	19.8
Salmon—broiled/baked	61	7.74	3.10	0	2.0	0.157	0.061	0.048	0	24.7
Coho salmon—steamed/ poached	52	7.77	2.14	0	8.22	0.252	0.057	0.031	0	13.9
Smoked salmon— Chinook	33	5.17	1.22	0	03.0	0.240	0.007	0.029	0	6.7
Atlantic salmon— small can	36	5.05	1.62	0	3.1	0.204	0.057	0.097	0	17.0
Pink salmon—raw	33	5.64	0.98	0	11.3	0.218	0.040	0.057	0	14.7
Sardines	59	7.00	3.24	0	108.0	0.826	0.023	0.064	0	40.4
Sea trout steelhead—raw	30	4.73	1.02	0	4.8	0.077	0.023	0.057	0	23.5
Sea trout steelhead— cooked	37	6.07	1.42	0	5.7	0.088	0.024	0.064	0	32.3
Shad—baked with bacon	57	6.58	3.20	0	6.8	0.170	0.037	0.074	0	17.0
Smelt—rainbow—raw	28	4.99	0.69	0	17.0	0.255	0.016	0.034	0	19.8
Snapper—baked or broiled	36	7.46	0.49	0	11.3	0.068	0.015	0.021	0	13.3
Snapper—raw	28	5.81	0.38	0	9.1	0.051	0.013	0.017	0	10.5
Sole/flounder—baked w/butter	40	5.34	2.00	0	5.3	0.093	0.023	0.032	0	22.7
Sole/flounder—baked/ broiled	33	6.84	0.43	0	5.3	0.093	0.023	0.032	0	19.3

FISH—continued

	kcal	Protein (g)	Fat (g)	CHO (g)	Ca (mg)	Fe (mg)	B₁ (mg)	B₂ (mg)	Fiber (g)	Cholesterol (mg)
Sole/flounder—batter-fried	83	4.47	5.10	4.07	16.7	0.239	0.057	0.042	0.01	15.0
Sole/flounder—breaded/fried	53	4.96	2.55	2.54	11.3	0.128	0.037	0.034	0	15.0
Sole/flounder—steamed	26	5.67	0.33	0	4.5	0.079	0.017	0.027	0	14.7
Sole/flounder—raw	26	5.33	0.34	0	5.1	0.102	0.025	0.022	0	13.6
Lemon sole—raw	23	4.85	0.21	0	4.8	0.088	0.026	0.023	0	17.0
Lemon sole—fried w/crumbs	56	4.56	3.12	2.64	26.9	0.176	0.020	0.023	0	18.4
Lemon sole—steamed	26	5.84	0.26	0	6.0	0.147	0.026	0.026	0	17.0
Swordfish—raw	34	5.61	1.14	0	1.1	0.230	0.010	0.027	0	11.0
Swordfish—broiled/baked	44	7.20	1.46	0	1.7	0.295	0.012	0.033	0	14.2
Trout—baked/broiled	43	7.47	1.22	0	24.3	0.690	0.024	0.064	0	20.7
Tuna—oil pack	56	8.26	2.34	0	3.8	0.395	0.010	0.030	0	5.0
Tuna—water pack	37	8.38	0.14	0	3.4	0.409	0.010	0.033	0	16.0
Tuna—raw	31	6.63	0.27	0	4.5	0.207	0.123	0.013	0	12.8
Whiting—flour/bread-fried	54	5.13	1.56	1.98	11.3	0.198	0.023	0.020	0	18.4

FRUITS

	kcal	Protein (g)	Fat (g)	CHO (g)	Ca (mg)	Fe (mg)	B₁ (mg)	B₂ (mg)	Fiber (g)	Cholesterol (mg)
Apple w/peel	16	0.055	0.100	4.31	2.05	0.051	0.005	0.004	0.709	0
Apple slices w/peel—fresh	17	0.054	0.100	4.33	2.06	0.052	0.005	0.004	0.709	0
Apple juice—canned/bottled	13	0.017	0.032	3.32	1.94	0.105	0.006	0.005	0.034	0
Apple juice—frozen concentrate	47	0.144	0.105	11.60	5.78	0.258	0.003	0.015	0.089	0
Applesauce—sweetened	22	0.052	0.052	5.67	1.11	0.111	0.003	0.008	0.397	0
Apricot—fresh halves	14	0.397	0.110	3.15	4.02	0.154	0.009	0.011	0.538	0
Apricot halves—light syrup	18	0.150	0.013	4.67	3.34	0.110	0.005	0.006	0.319	0
Apricot nectar—canned	16	0.104	0.025	4.08	2.03	0.108	0.003	0.004	0.170	0
Avocado—average	46	0.563	0.340	2.10	3.07	0.284	0.030	0.035	2.720	0
Banana—fresh slices	26	0.293	0.136	6.63	1.74	0.088	0.013	0.028	0.578	0
Blackberries—canned	26	0.370	0.040	6.54	5.98	0.184	0.008	0.011	1.011	0
Blackberries—fresh	15	0.205	0.110	3.62	9.06	0.158	0.008	0.011	1.910	0
Blackberries—frozen	18	0.334	0.122	4.45	8.26	0.173	0.008	0.013	1.460	0
Blueberries—fresh	16	0.190	0.108	4.00	1.76	0.047	0.014	0.014	0.763	0
Blueberries-frozen unsweetened	14	0.119	0.181	3.46	2.19	0.051	0.009	0.010	0.658	0
Boysenberries—frozen	14	0.314	0.075	3.46	7.73	0.240	0.015	0.010	1.100	0
Sour cherries—frozen	13	0.260	0.124	3.13	3.66	0.150	0.012	0.010	0.384	0
Sweet cherries—fresh	20	0.340	0.272	4.69	4.10	0.110	0.014	0.017	0.430	0
Sweet cherries—frozen	25	0.325	0.037	6.34	3.39	0.099	0.008	0.013	0.224	0
Cranberries—whole—raw	14	0.110	0.057	3.58	2.09	0.057	0.009	0.006	1.190	0
Cranberry/apple juice	19	0.015	0.090	4.82	2.02	0.017	0.001	0.006	0.070	0
Cranberry juice cocktail	16	0.009	0.015	4.03	0.90	0.043	0.002	0.002	0.085	0
Date—whole—each	78	0.557	0.127	20.80	9.22	0.342	0.026	0.028	2.300	0

FRUITS—continued

	kcal	Protein (g)	Fat (g)	CHO (g)	Ca (mg)	Fe (mg)	B_1 (mg)	B_2 (mg)	Fiber (g)	Cholesterol (mg)
Figs—medium—fresh	21	0.215	0.085	5.44	10.20	0.102	0.017	0.014	1.050	0
Fig—dried—each	72	0.864	0.330	18.50	40.80	0.634	0.020	0.025	3.140	0
Fruit cocktail—heavy syrup	21	0.111	0.020	5.36	1.78	0.081	0.005	0.005	0.280	0
Fruit cocktail—light syrup	16	0.114	0.020	4.23	1.80	0.082	0.005	0.005	0.284	0
Grapefruit half—pink/red	9	0.157	0.028	2.18	3.00	0.034	0.010	0.006	0.369	0
Grapefruit half—white	10	0.195	0.029	2.38	3.36	0.017	0.010	0.006	0.368	0
Grapefuit sections/fresh	9	0.179	0.028	2.29	3.33	0.025	0.010	0.006	0.370	0
Grapefruit sections—canned	17	0.160	0.028	4.38	4.02	0.114	0.010	0.006	0.313	0
Grapefruit juice—fresh	11	0.142	0.029	2.60	2.53	0.056	0.011	0.006	0.113	0
Grapefruit juice—sweetened	13	0.164	0.026	3.15	2.27	0.102	0.011	0.007	0.076	0
Grapefruit juice—unsweetened	11	0.148	0.028	2.54	1.95	0.057	0.012	0.006	0.077	0
Grapefruit juice—frozen concentrate	41	0.548	0.137	9.86	7.67	0.140	0.041	0.022	0.383	0
Grapes—Thompson	20	0.188	0.163	5.03	3.01	0.073	0.026	0.016	0.333	0
Grape juice—bottled/canned	17	0.158	0.021	4.25	2.47	0.068	0.007	0.010	0.141	0
Grape juice—frozen concentrate	51	0.184	0.088	12.60	3.68	0.102	0.015	0.026	0.492	0
Grape juice—prep frozen	15	0.053	0.026	3.62	1.13	0.029	0.004	0.007	0.142	0
Kiwi fruit	17	0.280	0.127	4.22	7.46	0.112	0.007	0.015	0.962	0
Lemon—fresh wo/peel	8	0.313	0.083	2.64	7.33	0.171	0.011	0.006	0.582	0
Lemon juice—fresh	7	0.107	0.081	2.45	2.09	0.009	0.008	0.003	0.099	0
Lemon juice—bottled	6	0.114	0.081	1.84	3.02	0.036	0.012	0.003	0.085	0
Lime—fresh	9	0.199	0.055	2.99	9.30	0.169	0.008	0.006	0.228	0
Lime juice—fresh	8	0.124	0.029	2.56	2.54	0.009	0.006	0.003	0.113	0
Lime juice—bottled	6	0.115	0.115	1.84	3.46	0.069	0.009	0.001	0.099	0
Loganberries—fresh	20	0.430	0.088	3.69	8.50	0.181	0.014	0.010	1.760	0
Loganberries—frozen	16	0.430	0.089	3.68	7.33	0.181	0.014	0.010	1.760	0
Mango—fresh—slices	19	0.146	0.077	4.83	2.92	0.360	0.016	0.016	0.997	0
Mango—fresh—whole	19	0.145	0.078	4.82	2.88	0.356	0.016	0.016	1.010	0
Cantaloupe—cubes	10	0.250	0.079	2.37	3.19	0.060	0.006	0.006	0.284	0
Casaba melon—cubes	8	0.255	0.028	1.75	1.50	0.113	0.017	0.006	0.284	0
Honeydew melon—cubes	10	0.128	0.028	2.60	1.67	0.020	0.022	0.005	0.307	0
Melon balls—mixed—frozen	9	0.239	0.023	2.25	2.79	0.008	0.005	0.006	0.295	0
Mixed fruit—dried	69	0.697	0.139	18.20	10.60	0.767	0.012	0.045	1.220	0
Mixed fruit—frozen—thawed	28	0.397	0.052	6.87	2.04	0.079	0.005	0.010	0.386	0
Nectarine	14	0.267	0.129	3.34	1.25	0.044	0.005	0.012	0.554	0
Orange	13	0.266	0.035	3.33	11.30	0.029	0.025	0.011	0.680	0
Orange sections—fresh	13	0.266	0.035	3.34	11.30	0.029	0.025	0.011	0.680	0
Mandarin oranges—canned	17	0.113	0.011	4.61	2.03	0.101	0.015	0.012	0.478	0
Orange juice—fresh	13	0.199	0.057	2.95	3.09	0.057	0.025	0.008	0.113	0
Oranged juice—frozen concentrate	45	0.679	0.059	10.80	9.05	0.099	0.079	0.018	0.313	0

FRUITS—*continued*

	kcal	Protein (g)	Fat (g)	CHO (g)	Ca (mg)	Fe (mg)	B₁ (mg)	B₂ (mg)	Fiber (g)	Cholesterol (mg)
Orange juice—frozen	13	0.191	0.016	3.05	2.50	0.031	0.023	0.005	0.057	0
Papaya—whole fresh	11	0.173	0.040	2.78	6.71	0.028	0.008	0.009	0.482	0
Papaya—slices fresh	12	0.174	0.040	2.77	6.68	0.060	0.008	0.009	0.482	0
Papaya nectar—canned	16	0.049	0.043	4.12	2.72	0.098	0.002	0.001	0.170	0
Peaches—fresh	12	0.199	0.026	3.14	1.30	0.031	0.005	0.012	0.489	0
Peach slices—frozen/ thawed	27	0.177	0.037	6.80	0.91	0.105	0.004	0.010	0.467	0
Peach halves—heavy syrup	21	0.130	0.028	5.67	1.05	0.077	0.003	0.007	0.315	0
Peach halves—light syrup	15	0.126	0.010	4.13	1.05	0.101	0.002	0.007	0.402	0
Peach halves—dried	68	0.020	0.216	17.40	8.07	1.150	0	0.060	2.330	0
Peach nectar—canned	15	0.076	0.006	3.95	1.48	0.054	0	0.004	0.170	0
Pears—Bartlett	17	0.111	0.113	4.29	3.24	0.070	0.006	0.011	0.779	0
Pear halves—heavy syrup	21	0.057	0.036	5.42	1.44	0.061	0.004	0.006	0.395	0
Pear halves—light syrup	16	0.054	0.007	4.30	1.44	0.082	0.003	0.005	0.395	0
Pear nectar—canned	17	0.030	0.003	4.47	1.25	0.073	0	0.004	0.204	0
Pineapple slices—heavy syrup	22	0.098	0.034	5.72	3.91	0.108	0.025	0.007	0.270	0
Pineapple slices—light syrup	15	0.103	0.034	3.81	3.91	0.110	0.026	0.007	0.268	0
Pineapple—frozen sweetened	24	0.113	0.029	6.29	2.55	0.113	0.028	0.009	0.496	0
Pineapple juice—frozen concentrate	51	0.369	0.029	12.60	11.00	0.255	0.065	0.017	0.255	0
Plums	16	0.223	0.176	3.69	1.29	0.030	0.012	0.027	0.550	0
Plums—canned—heavy syrup	25	0.102	0.028	6.59	2.53	0.238	0.005	0.010	0.434	0
Plums—canned—light syrup	18	0.105	0.029	4.61	2.70	0.243	0.005	0.011	0.444	0
Prunes—dried	68	0.739	0.145	17.80	14.50	0.702	0.023	0.046	2.700	0
Prune juice—bottled	20	0.172	0.009	4.95	3.43	0.334	0.005	0.020	0.310	0
Raisins—seedless	85	0.914	0.130	22.50	13.90	0.594	0.044	0.025	1.670	0
Raspberries—fresh	14	0.256	0.157	3.27	6.22	0.162	0.009	0.026	1.770	0
Raspberries—canned w/liquid	26	0.235	0.034	6.62	2.99	0.120	0.006	0.009	1.200	0
Raspberries—frozen	29	0.197	0.044	7.42	4.30	0.184	0.005	0.013	1.300	0
Rhubarb—raw—diced	6	0.253	0.056	1.29	39.50	0.062	0.006	0.009	0.737	0
Rhubarb—cooked w/sugar	33	0.111	0.013	8.85	41.10	0.060	0.005	0.006	0.624	0
Strawberries—fresh	9	0.173	0.105	2.00	4.00	0.108	0.006	0.019	0.736	0
Strawberries—frozen	10	0.120	0.030	2.59	4.38	0.213	0.006	0.010	0.736	0
Tangerine—fresh	13	0.179	0.054	3.17	4.05	0.028	0.030	0.006	0.574	0
Tangerines—canned— light syrup	17	0.127	0.028	4.61	2.03	0.105	0.015	0.012	0.453	0
Watermelon	9	0.175	0.121	2.04	2.24	0.048	0.023	0.006	0.114	0

MEATS

	kcal	Protein (g)	Fat (g)	CHO (g)	Ca (mg)	Fe (mg)	B_1 (mg)	B_2 (mg)	Fiber (g)	Cholesterol (mg)
Beef chuck—pot roasted	108	7.20	8.64	0	3.67	0.840	0.020	0.065	0	29.0
Beef chuck—pot roasted lean	77	8.80	4.34	0	3.67	1.040	0.024	0.080	0	30.0
Beef round—pot roasted lean & fat	74	8.44	4.20	0	1.67	0.920	0.020	0.069	0	27.0
Beef round—pot roasted lean	63	8.97	2.74	0	1.33	0.980	0.021	0.074	0	27.0
Ground beef—lean	77	7.00	5.34	0	3.00	0.600	0.013	0.060	0	24.7
Ground beef—regular	82	6.67	5.94	0	3.00	0.700	0.010	0.053	0	25.3
Sirloin steak—lean	57	8.10	2.53	0	2.33	0.700	0.026	0.056	0	21.7
T-bone steak—lean & fat	92	6.80	6.97	0	2.67	0.720	0.026	0.059	0	23.7
Beef lunchmeat—thin-sliced	50	7.96	1.09	1.62	2.99	0.759	0.023	0.054	0	12.0
Beef lunchmeat—loaf/roll	87	4.06	7.42	0.82	2.99	0.659	0.030	0.062	0	18.0
Beef rib—oven roasted—lean	68	7.70	3.90	0	3.34	0.740	0.023	0.060	0	22.7
Beef round—oven roasted—lean	54	8.14	2.12	0	1.67	0.834	0.028	0.076	0	23.0
Beef rump roast—lean only	51	8.40	1.89	0	1.13	0.567	0.026	0.049	0	19.6
Beef brains—pan-fried	56	3.57	4.50	0	2.67	0.630	0.037	0.074	0	566.0
Beef heart	47	8.17	1.59	0.12	1.67	2.130	0.040	0.436	0	54.7
Beef kidney	41	7.23	0.97	0.27	5.00	2.070	0.054	1.150	0	110.0
Beef liver—fried	61	7.57	2.27	2.23	3.00	1.780	0.060	1.170	0	137.0
Beef tongue—cooked	80	6.27	5.87	0.09	2.00	0.960	0.009	0.009	0	30.4
Beef tripe—raw	28	4.14	1.12	0	36.00	0.553	0.002	0.047	0	26.9
Beef tripe—pickled	17	3.29	0.40	0	25.00	0.389	0	0.028	0	15.0
Corned beef—canned	71	7.67	4.24	0	5.67	0.590	0.006	0.042	0	24.3
Corned beef hash—canned	49	2.35	1.29	2.82	3.74	0.567	0.016	0.052	0.153	17.0
Beef—dried/cured	47	8.24	1.10	0.44	2.00	1.280	0.050	0.230	0	45.9
Beef & vegetable stew	26	1.85	1.27	1.74	3.36	0.336	0.017	0.020	0.393	8.2
Beef stew—canned	22	1.64	0.88	2.06	2.66	0.368	0.008	0.014	0.150	1.7
Burrito—beef & bean	63	3.40	2.84	6.48	26.70	0.437	0.042	0.047	0.810	8.4
Tostada w/beans & beef	49	2.72	3.06	2.98	27.50	0.319	0.012	0.036	0.583	9.1
Beef + macaroni + tomato	24	1.25	0.73	3.16	3.81	0.300	0.024	0.021	0.291	2.8
Beef enchilada	69	3.09	3.26	3.69	60.20	0.418	0.017	0.039	0.465	8.9
Frankfurter—beef	92	3.20	8.36	0.68	3.48	0.378	0.014	0.029	0	13.4
Frankfurter—beef & pork	91	3.20	8.26	0.73	2.98	0.328	0.056	0.034	0	14.4
Beef pot pie—frozen	52	1.99	2.73	4.77	2.42	0.436	0.022	0.018	0.109	5.0
Beef pie—recipe	70	2.84	4.05	5.27	3.92	0.513	0.039	0.039	0.155	5.7
Beef taco	75	4.94	4.80	3.67	30.90	0.469	0.010	0.049	0.407	16.2
Chicken meat—all-fried	62	8.67	2.59	0.48	4.86	0.383	0.024	0.056	0.002	26.5
Chicken meat—all-roasted	54	8.20	2.10	0	4.25	0.342	0.020	0.050	0	25.3
Chicken meat—all-stewed	50	7.74	1.90	0	4.05	0.330	0.014	0.046	0	23.5
Boned chicken w/broth	47	6.17	2.26	0	3.99	0.439	0.004	0.037	0	17.6
Chicken—dark meat—fried	68	8.22	3.30	0.74	5.06	0.423	0.026	0.070	0.002	27.3
Chicken—dark meat—roasted	58	7.76	2.75	0	4.25	0.377	0.020	0.064	0	26.3
Chicken—dark meat—stewed	55	7.37	2.55	0	4.05	0.385	0.016	0.057	0	24.9

MEATS—continued

	kcal	Protein (g)	Fat (g)	CHO (g)	Ca (mg)	Fe (mg)	B₁ (mg)	B₂ (mg)	Fiber (g)	Cholesterol (mg)
Chicken—light meat—fried	54	9.31	1.57	0.12	4.45	0.322	0.020	0.036	0	25.3
Chicken—light meat—roasted	49	8.77	1.28	0	4.25	0.302	0.018	0.033	0	23.9
Chicken—light meat—stewed	45	8.18	1.17	0	3.64	0.265	0.012	0.033	0	21.7
Chicken breast—no skin	47	8.80	0.99	0	4.29	0.295	0.020	0.032	0	24.0
Chicken breast meat—stewed	43	8.20	0.86	0	3.58	0.250	0.012	0.034	0	21.8
Chicken drumstick—batter fried	76	6.22	4.45	2.36	4.73	0.382	0.032	0.061	0.008	24.4
Chicken drumstick—roasted	61	7.69	3.16	0	3.27	0.376	0.020	0.061	0	26.2
Chicken wing—batter-fried	92	5.64	6.19	3.10	5.79	0.365	0.030	0.043	0.012	22.6
Chicken wing—flour-fried	91	7.40	6.28	0.67	4.43	0.354	0.017	0.039	0.009	23.0
Chicken wing—roasted	83	7.48	5.53	0	4.17	0.359	0.012	0.037	0	24.2
Chicken gizzards—simmered	44	7.73	1.04	0.32	2.58	1.180	0.008	0.070	0	54.9
Chicken hearts—simmered	52	7.49	2.23	0.03	5.27	2.560	0.017	0.206	0	68.7
Chicken livers—simmered	44	6.90	1.55	0.25	4.05	2.400	0.043	0.496	0	179.0
Chicken roll—light meat	45	5.52	2.08	0..69	11.90	0.274	0.018	0.037	0	13.9
Chicken frankfurter	73	3.67	5.52	1.93	27.00	0.567	0.019	0.033	0	28.4
Chicken a la king	54	3.12	3.93	1.93	14.70	0.289	0.012	0.049	0.154	25.6
Chicken + noodles	43	2.60	2.13	3.07	3.07	0.278	0.006	0.020	0.142	12.2
Chicken chow mein	29	2.60	1.25	1.13	6.58	0.284	0.009	0.026	0.466	8.5
Chicken curry	26	2.21	1.53	0.64	2.52	0.170	0.009	0.019	0.033	5.3
Chicken frankfurter	72	3.67	5.52	1.93	27.00	0.567	0.019	0.033	0	28.4
Chicken pot pie—frozen	53	1.84	2.84	5.08	3.70	0.382	0.020	0.020	0.210	4.9
Chicken roll—light meat	45	5.52	2.08	0.69	11.90	0.274	0.018	0.037	0	13.9
Chicken salad w/celery	97	3.82	8.90	0.47	5.92	0.239	0.012	0.028	0.109	17.3
Chicken patty sandwich	79	4.48	4.06	6.10	7.95	0.338	0.052	0.047	0.244	12.3
Chicken broth—from dry	2	0.16	0.13	0.17	1.74	0.009	0	0.004	0.001	0.1
Chicken broth—from cube	2	0.11	0.04	0.18	0.04	0.014	0.001	0.003	0	0.1
Chicken noodle soup	9	0.48	0.29	1.10	2.00	0.092	0.006	0.007	0.085	0.8
Tostada w/beans/chicken	45	3.50	2.06	3.38	29.30	0.305	0.013	0.034	0.668	9.6
Chicken taco	63	5.60	3.03	3.67	31.60	0.237	0.014	0.043	0.407	16.5
Chicken enchilada	64	3.38	2.48	3.69	60.50	0.359	0.018	0.036	0.465	9.1
Turkey dark meat—roasted	53	8.10	2.05	0	9.11	0.662	0.018	0.070	0	24.0
Turkey white meat—roasted	44	8.48	0.91	0	5.47	0.380	0.017	0.037	0	19.6
Turkey breast—barbecued	40	6.39	1.40	0	2.00	0.120	0.010	0.030	0	16.0
Turkey gizzards	46	8.34	1.10	0.17	4.32	1.540	0.009	0.093	0	65.6
Turkey hearts	50	7.58	1.73	0.58	3.72	1.950	0.019	0.250	0	64.0
Turkey livers	48	6.80	1.69	0.97	3.02	2.210	0.015	0.404	0	177.0
Turkey loaf	31	6.38	0.45	0	2.00	0.113	0.011	0.030	0	11.6
Turkey roll	41	5.27	2.03	0.15	11.40	0.358	0.025	0.064	0	11.9
Turkey bologna	56	3.86	4.27	0.27	23.40	0.432	0.015	0.047	0	28.0
Turkey frankfurter	64	4.05	5.22	0.42	36.50	0.485	0.023	0.050	0	24.6
Turkey ham	36	5.37	1.49	0.42	2.49	0.776	0.020	0.075	0	15.9
Turkey pastrami	37	5.22	1.75	0.43	2.49	0.403	0.022	0.075	0	14.9
Turkey salami	55	4.62	3.89	0.15	5.47	0.463	0.029	0.075	0	22.9
Turkey pot pie—frozen	51	1.80	2.75	4.65	7.79	0.256	0.020	0.020	0.110	2.4

EGGS

	kcal	Protein (g)	Fat (g)	CHO (g)	Ca (mg)	Fe (mg)	B₁ (mg)	B₂ (mg)	Fiber (g)	Cholesterol (mg)
Egg white, cooked	13	2.68	0	0.33	3.20	0.008	0.002	0.072	0	0
Egg yolk, cooked	108	4.76	8.73	0.07	44.40	1.620	0.044	0.121	0	355.0
Egg, fried in butter	56	3.54	3.45	0.38	15.70	0.536	0.018	0.148	0	129.0
Egg, hard cooked	40	3.52	2.79	0.34	13.80	0.474	0.014	0.132	0	113.0
Egg, poached	40	3.50	2.79	0.34	13.80	0.474	0.014	0.132	0	113.0
Egg, scrambled milk + butter	40	2.88	2.57	0.61	23.90	0.412	0.013	0.106	0	93.9
Egg raw—large	40	3.52	2.79	0.34	13.80	0.474	0.017	0.139	0	113.0
Egg white—raw	13	2.68	0	0.33	3.20	0.008	0.002	0.075	0	0
Egg yolk, raw	108	4.76	8.73	0.07	44.40	1.620	0.051	0.126	0	355.0
Egg substitute, frozen	45	3.20	3.15	0.91	20.80	0.562	0.034	0.110	0	0.5
Egg substitute, powder	125	15.60	3.66	6.12	90.70	0.879	0.062	0.493	0	162.0

DAIRY PRODUCTS

	kcal	Protein (g)	Fat (g)	CHO (g)	Ca (mg)	Fe (mg)	B₁ (mg)	B₂ (mg)	Fiber (g)	Cholesterol (mg)
Milk—1% lowfat	12	0.93	0.30	1.36	34.9	0.014	0.011	0.047	0	1.16
Milk—2% lowfat	14	0.94	0.56	1.36	34.5	0.012	0.011	0.047	0	2.56
Milk—skim	10	0.97	0.05	1.38	34.9	0.012	0.010	0.040	0	0.46
Milk—whole	17	0.93	0.95	1.32	33.8	0.014	0.010	0.046	0	3.83
Buttermilk	12	0.94	0.25	1.35	33.0	0.014	0.010	0.044	0	1.04
Milk—instant nonfat dry	102	9.96	0.21	14.80	349.0	0.088	0.117	0.496	0	5.00
Canned skim milk— evaporated	22	2.11	0.06	3.22	82.0	0.078	0.013	0.088	0	1.11
Canned whole milk— evaporated	38	1.91	2.20	2.81	73.9	0.054	0.014	0.090	0	8.33
Carob flavor mix—powder	106	0.47	0.05	26.50	0	1.300	0.002	0	4.020	0
Chocolate milk—1%	18	0.92	0.28	2.96	32.5	0.068	0.010	0.047	0.425	0.79
Chocolate milk—2%	20	0.91	0.57	2.95	32.2	0.068	0.010	0.046	0.425	1.93
Chocolate milk—whole	24	0.90	0.96	2.94	31.8	0.068	0.010	0.046	0.425	3.52
Hot cocoa—with whole milk	25	1.03	1.03	2.93	33.8	0.088	0.012	0.049	0.340	3.74
Instant breakfast w/2% milk	25	1.52	0.47	3.50	31.0	0.807	0.040	0.048	0	1.82
Instant breakfast w/1% milk	23	1.51	0.25	3.50	31.3	0.807	0.040	0.048	0	1.00
Instant breakfast w/skim milk	22	1.55	0.04	3.50	31.4	0.804	0.039	0.041	0	0.40
Instant breakfast w/whole milk	28	1.51	0.82	3.47	30.4	0.807	0.040	0.047	0	3.33
Egg nog	38	1.08	2.12	3.84	36.8	0.057	0.010	0.054	0	16.60
Kefir	20	1.13	0.55	1.07	42.6	0.060	0.055	0.054	0	1.22
Malt powder—chocolate flavored	107	1.49	1.08	24.80	17.6	0.648	0.049	0.057	0.540	1.35
Malted milk powder	117	3.12	2.30	21.50	85.0	0.209	0.143	0.260	0.405	5.40
Malted milk drink— chocolate	25	1.00	0.95	3.19	32.5	0.064	0.014	0.047	0.043	3.64

DAIRY PRODUCTS—*continued*

	kcal	Protein (g)	Fat (g)	CHO (g)	Ca (mg)	Fe (mg)	B_1 (mg)	B_2 (mg)	Fiber (g)	Cholesterol (mg)
Chocolate milkshake	36	0.96	1.05	5.80	32.0	0.088	0.016	0.069	0.035	3.70
Strawberry milkshake	32	0.95	0.80	5.35	32.0	0.030	0.013	0.055	0.024	3.10
Vanilla milkshake	32	0.98	0.84	5.09	34.5	0.026	0.013	0.052	0.019	3.20
Ovaltine powder—chocolate flavored	102	2.00	0.85	23.70	134.0	6.190	0.719	0.772	0.013	0
Ovaltine powder—malt flavored	104	2.53	0.24	23.60	106.0	5.820	0.772	1.010	0.040	0
Ovaltine drink—chocolate flavored	24	1.02	0.94	3.12	41.9	0.510	0.067	0.104	0.001	3.53
Ovaltine drink—malt flavored	24	1.06	0.89	3.10	39.7	0.480	0.072	0.124	0.003	3.53
Milk—goat	20	1.00	1.17	1.27	37.9	0.014	0.014	0.039	0	3.25
Milk—sheep	31	1.70	1.99	1.52	54.8	0.028	0.018	0.100	0	0
Milk—soybean	9	0.78	0.54	0.51	1.2	0.163	0.046	0.020	0	0
Ice cream—regular-vanilla	57	1.02	3.05	6.76	37.5	0.026	0.011	0.070	0	12.60
Ice cream—rich-vanilla	67	0.79	4.54	6.13	28.9	0.019	0.008	0.054	0	16.90
Ice cream—soft-serve	62	1.15	3.69	6.28	38.7	0.070	0.013	0.073	0	25.00
Creamsicle ice cream bar	44	0.52	1.33	7.56	19.8	0	0.009	0.034	0	0
Drumstick ice cream bar	88	1.23	4.68	10.20	31.7	0.047	0.009	0.043	0	0
Fudgesicle ice cream bar	35	1.48	0.08	7.22	50.0	0.039	0.012	0.070	0	0
Ice milk	40	1.12	1.22	6.28	38.0	0.039	0.016	0.075	0	3.90
Ice milk—soft serve—3% fat	36	1.30	0.75	6.22	44.4	0.045	0.019	0.088	0	2.10
Yogurt—coffee-vanilla	24	1.40	0.35	3.90	48.5	0.020	0.012	0.057	0	1.42
Yogurt—lowfat with fruit	29	1.24	0.31	5.37	43.0	0.020	0.010	0.050	0	1.25
Yogurt—lowfat-plain	18	1.49	0.43	2.00	51.8	0.022	0.012	0.060	0	1.75
Yogurt—nonfat milk	16	1.62	0.05	2.17	56.5	0.025	0.014	0.066	0	0.50
Yogurt—whole milk	17	0.98	0.92	1.32	34.3	0.014	0.008	0.040	0	3.68

VEGETABLES

	kcal	Protein (g)	Fat (g)	CHO (g)	Ca (mg)	Fe (mg)	B_1 (mg)	B_2 (mg)	Fiber (g)	Cholesterol (mg)
Alfalfa sprouts	9	1.13	0.200	1.07	9.5	0.272	0.021	0.036	1.030	0
Artichoke hearts—marinated	28	0.680	0.250	2.18	6.5	0.270	0.010	0.029	1.780	0
Asparagus—raw spears	6	0.865	0.063	1.05	6.4	0.193	0.032	0.035	0.395	0
Asparagus—canned spears	5	0.606	0.184	0.70	3.9	0.177	0.017	0.025	0.454	0
Bamboo shoots—sliced—raw	8	0.738	0.088	1.47	3.8	0.143	0.043	0.020	0.738	0
Bamboo shoots—sliced, canned	5	0.489	0.113	0.91	2.2	0.090	0.007	0.007	0.706	0
Bean sprouts—fresh raw	9	0.861	0.050	1.68	3.8	0.258	0.024	0.035	0.736	0
Bean sprouts—boiled	6	0.576	0.025	1.19	3.4	0.185	0.014	0.029	0.572	0
Bean sprouts—stir fried	14	1.220	0.059	3.00	3.7	0.549	0.040	0.050	0.777	0
Black beans—cooked	37	2.500	0.152	6.72	7.8	0.593	0.069	0.017	2.540	0

VEGETABLES—continued

	kcal	Protein (g)	Fat (g)	CHO (g)	Ca (mg)	Fe (mg)	B_1 (mg)	B_2 (mg)	Fiber (g)	Cholesterol (mg)
Green beans—raw uncooked	9	0.515	0.034	2.02	10.6	0.363	0.024	0.030	0.644	0
Green beans—fresh— cooked	10	0.535	0.082	2.24	13.2	0.363	0.021	0.027	0.737	0
Green beans—frozen— cooked	8	0.386	0.038	1.73	12.8	0.233	0.014	0.021	0.880	0
Green beans—canned/ drained	6	0.326	0.028	1.28	7.6	0.256	0.004	0.016	0.378	0
Red kidney beans—dry	94	6.690	0.234	16.90	40.5	2.330	0.150	0.062	6.160	0
Lima beans—dry large	96	6.080	0.194	18.00	22.9	2.130	0.144	0.057	8.600	0
Lima beans—fresh— cooked	35	1.930	0.090	6.70	9.0	0.695	0.040	0.027	2.670	0
Lima beans—dry small	98	5.790	0.397	18.20	18.4	2.270	0.136	0.048	8.500	0
Lima beans—canned/ drained	27	1.530	0.100	5.20	8.0	0.487	0.010	0.013	2.420	0
Beans/w/franks—canned	40	1.900	1.860	4.37	13.6	0.490	0.016	0.016	1.950	1.7
Pork & beans—canned	32	1.500	0.413	5.95	17.4	0.470	0.013	0.017	1.560	1.9
Navy beans—dry, cooked	40	2.460	0.162	7.77	19.9	0.703	0.057	0.017	2.490	0
Pinto beans—dry, cooked	39	2.320	0.148	7.28	13.6	0.741	0.053	0.026	3.230	0
Refried beans—canned	30	1.770	0.303	5.24	13.2	0.500	0.014	0.016	2.470	0
Soybeans—dry	118	10.400	5.650	8.55	78.5	4.450	0.248	0.247	1.570	0
White beans—dry	95	5.990	0.334	17.70	36.0	2.190	0.210	0.059	0.766	0
White beans—dry, cooked	40	2.550	0.182	7.32	20.7	0.808	0.067	0.017	2.230	0
Yellow wax beans—raw	9	0.515	0.034	2.02	10.6	0.294	0.024	0.030	0.644	0
Yellow wax beans—raw	10	0.535	0.082	2.24	13.2	0.363	0.021	0.027	0.726	0
Yellow wax beans—frozen	8	0.386	0.038	1.73	12.8	0.233	0.014	0.021	0.880	0
Beets—cooked	9	0.300	0.014	1.90	3.1	0.176	0.009	0.004	0.539	0
Beets—pickled slices	18	0.227	0.028	4.63	3.1	0.116	0.006	0.014	0.587	0
Broccoli—raw chopped	8	0.844	0.097	1.49	13.5	0.251	0.019	0.034	0.934	0
Broccoli—raw spears	8	0.845	0.098	1.49	13.5	0.250	0.018	0.034	0.935	0
Broccoli—frozen cooked spears	8	0.879	0.034	1.51	14.5	0.173	0.015	0.023	0.826	0
Brussels sprouts—raw	12	0.960	0.084	2.54	11.6	0.396	0.039	0.026	1.260	0
Brussels sprouts—cooked	11	1.090	0.145	2.45	10.2	0.342	0.030	0.023	1.220	0
Brussels sprouts—frozen cooked	12	1.030	0.112	2.36	7.0	0.210	0.029	0.032	1.230	0
Cabbage—raw, shredded	7	0.340	0.049	1.52	13.0	0.162	0.015	0.009	0.680	0
Cabbage—cooked	6	0.272	0.070	1.35	9.5	0.110	0.016	0.016	0.661	0
Bok choy—raw, shredded	4	0.425	0.057	0.62	30.0	0.227	0.011	0.020	0.486	0
Bok choy—cooked	3	0.442	0.045	0.51	26.3	0.295	0.009	0.018	0.454	0
Red cabbage—raw	8	0.393	0.073	1.74	14.6	0.142	0.018	0.009	0.648	0
Red cabbage—cooked	6	0.299	0.057	1.32	10.6	0.102	0.010	0.006	1.567	0
Carrot—whole, raw	12	0.291	0.055	2.87	7.5	0.142	0.028	0.017	1.906	0
Carrot—grated, raw	12	0.289	0.052	2.88	7.7	0.142	0.027	0.016	0.907	0
Carrots—sliced, cooked	13	0.309	0.050	2.97	8.7	0.176	0.010	0.016	0.992	0
Carrots—frozen, cooked	10	0.338	0.031	2.34	8.2	0.136	0.008	0.010	1.050	0
Carrots—canned, drained	7	0.183	0.054	1.57	7.4	0.181	0.005	0.009	0.435	0
Carrot juice	11	0.267	0.041	2.63	6.7	0.130	0.026	0.015	0.385	0
Cauliflower—raw	7	0.561	0.051	1.39	7.9	0.164	0.022	0.016	0.720	0
Cauliflower—cooked	7	0.530	0.050	1.31	7.8	0.119	0.018	0.018	0.622	0

VEGETABLES—continued

	kcal	Protein (g)	Fat (g)	CHO (g)	Ca (mg)	Fe (mg)	B₁ (mg)	B₂ (mg)	Fiber (g)	Cholesterol (mg)
Cauliflower—frozen, cooked	5	0.457	0.061	1.06	4.9	0.116	0.010	0.015	0.535	0
Celery—raw—chopped	5	0.189	0.033	1.03	10.4	0.137	0.009	0.009	0.472	0
Swiss chard—raw	5	0.510	0.057	1.06	14.5	0.510	0.011	0.025	0.512	0
Swiss chard—cooked	6	0.533	0.023	1.17	16.5	0.642	0.010	0.024	0.616	0
Collards—fresh	5	0.445	0.062	1.07	33.0	0.299	0.009	0.018	0.590	0
Collards—fresh, cooked	4	0.313	0.043	0.75	22.0	0.116	0.005	0.012	0.798	0
Collards—frozen, cooked	10	0.840	0.115	2.02	59.5	0.317	0.013	0.033	0.794	0
Corn—kernels raw	24	0.913	0.335	5.38	0.6	0.147	0.057	0.017	1.220	0
Corn on the cob—cooked	31	0.943	0.363	7.14	0.6	0.173	0.061	0.020	1.190	0
Corn—cooked from frozen	23	0.857	0.020	5.80	0.6	0.085	0.020	0.020	1.190	0
Corn—canned, drained	23	0.743	0.283	5.26	1.4	0.142	0.009	0.014	0.398	0
Corn—canned cream style	21	0.494	0.119	5.14	0.9	0.108	0.007	0.015	0.354	0
Cucumber slices w/peel	4	0.153	0.037	0.82	4.0	0.079	0.009	0.006	0.329	0
Eggplant—cooked	8	0.236	0.066	1.88	1.7	0.099	0.022	0.006	1.060	0
Escarole/curly endive—chopped	5	0.354	0.057	0.95	14.7	0.235	0.023	0.022	0.369	0
Garbanzo/chickpeas—dry	103	5.470	1.720	17.20	29.9	1.770	0.135	0.060	5.390	0
Garbanzo/chickpeas—cooked	47	2.500	0.735	7.78	13.8	0.819	0.033	0.018	1.920	0
Jerusalem artichoke—raw	22	0.567	0.004	4.95	4.0	0.964	0.057	0.017	0.369	0
Kale—fresh, chopped	14	0.935	0.198	2.84	38.0	0.482	0.031	0.037	1.650	0
Kohlrabi—raw slices	8	0.482	0.028	1.76	6.9	0.113	0.014	0.006	0.405	0
Kohlrabi—cooked	8	0.510	0.030	1.96	7.0	0.113	0.011	0.006	0.395	0
Leeks—chopped raw	17	0.425	0.085	4.00	16.7	0.594	0.017	0.008	0.668	0
Leeks—cooked, chopped	9	0.230	0.057	2.16	8.5	0.310	0.007	0.006	0.927	0
Lentils—dry	96	7.960	0.273	16.20	14.6	2.550	0.135	0.069	3.400	0
Lentils—cooked from dry	33	2.560	0.106	5.73	5.3	0.944	0.048	0.020	1.430	0
Lentils—sprouted, raw	30	2.540	0.156	6.30	7.0	0.909	0.065	0.036	1.150	0
Lettuce—butterhead	4	0.367	0.062	0.66	9.5	0.085	0.017	0.017	0.397	0
Lettuce—iceberg	4	0.286	0.054	0.59	5.4	0.142	0.013	0.009	0.347	0
Lettuce—romaine	5	0.459	0.057	0.67	10.2	0.312	0.028	0.028	0.482	0
Mushrooms—raw sliced	7	0.593	0.119	1.32	1.4	0.352	0.029	0.127	0.508	0
Mushrooms—cooked	8	0.614	0.134	1.46	1.7	0.494	0.020	0.085	0.625	0
Mushrooms—canned, drained	7	0.530	0.082	1.40	3.1	0.224	0.017	0.063	0.596	0
Mustard greens—fresh	7	0.764	0.057	1.39	29.4	0.414	0.023	0.031	0.764	0
Mustard greens—cooked	4	0.640	0.068	0.60	21.0	0.316	0.012	0.018	0.587	0
Okra pods—cooked	9	0.530	0.048	2.04	17.9	0.128	0.037	0.016	0.624	0
Okra slices—cooked	11	0.589	0.085	2.32	27.1	0.190	0.028	0.035	0.709	0
Onions—chopped, raw	10	0.335	0.074	2.07	7.1	0.105	0.017	0.003	0.454	0
Onion slices—raw	10	0.335	0.074	2.08	7.2	0.105	0.017	0.003	0.454	0
Onion—dehydrated flakes	91	2.530	0.122	23.70	72.9	0.446	0.022	0.018	2.510	0
Onion rings—frozen, heated	115	1.520	7.570	10.80	8.8	0.482	0.079	0.040	0.240	
Parsley—freeze dried	81	8.910	1.420	11.90	40.5	15.200	0.304	0.648	22.000	0
Parsley—fresh chopped	9	0.624	0.085	1.96	36.9	1.760	0.023	0.031	1.550	0
Parsnips—sliced raw	21	0.341	0.085	5.09	10.0	0.167	0.026	0.014	1.280	0
Fresh peas—uncooked	23	1.530	0.113	4.10	7.0	0.416	0.075	0.037	1.380	0
Peas—cooked	24	1.520	0.060	4.43	7.8	0.438	0.073	0.042	1.360	0
Peas—frozen, cooked	22	1.460	0.078	4.04	6.7	0.443	0.080	0.050	1.280	0
Peas—edible pods—fresh	12	0.794	0.057	2.15	12.1	0.589	0.043	0.023	0.794	0
Split peas—dry	97	6.970	0.328	17.10	15.5	1.250	0.206	0.061	4.030	0

VEGETABLES—continued

	kcal	Protein (g)	Fat (g)	CHO (g)	Ca (mg)	Fe (mg)	B₁ (mg)	B₂ (mg)	Fiber (g)	Cholesterol (mg)
Peas + carrots—frozen, cooked	14	0.875	0.120	2.87	6.4	0.266	0.064	0.020	1.170	0
Green chili pepper—raw	11	0.557	0.057	2.68	5.0	0.340	0.026	0.026	0.504	0
Red chili peppers—raw/ chopped	11	0.567	0.057	2.68	4.9	0.340	0.026	0.026	0.454	0
Jalapeno peppers—canned chopped	7	0.225	0.170	1.39	7.5	0.792	0.008	0.014	0.850	0
Baked potato with skin	31	0.653	0.028	7.16	2.8	0.386	0.030	0.009	0.660	0
Baked potato—flesh only	26	0.556	0.029	6.10	1.5	0.100	0.030	0.006	0.436	0
Potato skin—oven baked	56	1.220	0.029	13.20	9.8	1.080	0.035	0.034	1.130	0
Potato + peel— microwaved	30	0.692	0.028	6.83	3.1	0.350	0.034	0.009	0.660	0
Peeled potato—boiled	24	0.485	0.029	5.67	2.1	0.088	0.028	0.005	0.426	0
French fries—oven heated	63	0.980	2.480	9.64	2.3	0.380	0.035	0.009	0.567	0
French fries—frozen— vegetable oil	90	1.140	4.690	11.20	5.7	0.215	0.050	0.008	0.567	0
Cottage-fried potatoes	62	0.975	2.320	9.64	2.8	0.425	0.034	0.009	0.567	0
Hash-brown potatoes	30	0.343	1.980	3.02	1.1	0.115	0.010	0.003	0.567	0
Mashed potatoes prep/ milk	22	0.548	0.166	4.98	7.4	0.077	0.025	0.011	0.405	0.5
Mashed potatoes—milk & margarine	30	0.533	1.200	4.74	7.3	0.074	0.024	0.014	0.405	0.5
Potato pancakes	88	1.730	4.700	9.85	7.8	0.451	0.039	0.035	0.563	34.7
Potatoes au gratin mix	26	0.653	1.170	3.65	23.5	0.090	0.006	0.023	0.487	1.4
Scalloped potatoes— recipe	24	0.813	1.040	3.05	16.2	0.163	0.020	0.026	0.289	3.4
Potato chips	148	1.590	10.000	14.70	7.0	0.339	0.040	0.006	1.360	0
Potato flour	100	2.260	0.226	22.60	9.3	4.880	0.119	0.040	0.317	0
Pumpkin—canned	10	0.311	0.080	2.28	7.4	0.394	0.007	0.015	0.519	0
Red radishes	4	0.170	0.151	1.01	5.7	0.082	0.001	0.013	0.624	0
Rutabaga—cooked cubes	10	0.314	0.053	2.19	12.0	0.133	0.020	0.010	0.434	0
Sauerkraut—canned liquid	5	0.258	0.040	1.21	8.7	0.417	0.006	0.006	0.529	0
Soybeans—mature, raw	37	3.700	1.900	3.17	19.4	0.599	0.096	0.033	0.656	0
Spinach—cooked from fresh	7	0.843	0.074	1.06	38.4	1.010	0.027	0.067	0.702	0
Summer squash—raw slices	6	0.334	0.061	1.23	5.7	0.130	0.018	0.010	0.425	0
Zucchini squash—cooked	5	0.181	0.014	1.11	3.6	0.099	0.012	0.012	0.567	0
Acorn squash—boiled/ mashed	10	0.190	0.023	2.49	7.5	0.159	0.028	0.002	0.680	0
Butternut squash/baked— cube	12	0.256	0.026	2.97	11.6	0.170	0.020	0.005	0.794	0
Spaghetti squash—baked/ boiled	8	0.187	0.073	1.83	6.0	0.095	0.010	0.006	0.794	0
Winter squash—boiled	10	0.319	0.050	2.40	5.2	0.136	0.018	0.006	0.794	0
Sweet potato—baked in skin	29	0.487	0.032	6.89	8.0	0.129	0.020	0.036	0.850	0
Candied sweet potatoes	39	0.246	0.920	7.91	7.3	0.324	0.005	0.012	0.545	0
Tofu (soybean curd)	22	2.290	1.360	0.53	29.7	1.520	0.023	0.015	0.343	0
Tomato—fresh whole	6	0.251	0.060	1.23	2.1	0.136	0.017	0.014	0.415	0
Tomatoes—whole canned	6	0.265	0.070	1.22	7.4	0.171	0.013	0.009	0.298	0

VEGETABLES—*continued*

	kcal	Protein (g)	Fat (g)	CHO (g)	Ca (mg)	Fe (mg)	B₁ (mg)	B₂ (mg)	Fiber (g)	Cholesterol (mg)
		Protein (g)	Fat (g)	CHO (g)	Ca (mg)	Fe (mg)	B_1 (mg)	B_2 (mg)	Fiber (g)	Cholesterol (mg)
Tomato sauce—canned	9	0.376	0.047	2.04	3.9	0.218	0.019	0.016	0.425	0
Tomato paste—canned	24	1.070	0.249	5.33	9.9	0.848	0.044	0.054	1.210	0
Tomato juice—canned	5	0.215	0.017	1.20	2.6	0.164	0.013	0.009	0.220	0
Turnip cubes—raw	8	0.255	0.028	1.76	8.5	0.085	0.011	0.009	0.587	0
Mixed vegetables—frozen, cooked	17	0.812	0.043	3.70	7.2	0.232	0.020	0.034	1.120	0
Vegetable juice cocktail	6	0.178	0.026	1.29	3.1	0.119	0.012	0.008	0.178	0
Water chestnuts—raw	30	0.398	0.027	6.77	3.2	0.170	0.040	0.057	0.869	0
Watercress—fresh	3	0.650	0.033	0.37	33.4	0.050	0.025	0.033	0.719	0
White yams—raw	34	0.438	0.049	7.90	8.7	0.153	0.032	0.009	0.822	0

SALAD BAR

	kcal	Protein (g)	Fat (g)	CHO (g)	Ca (mg)	Fe (mg)	B_1 (mg)	B_2 (mg)	Fiber (g)	Cholesterol (mg)
Alfalfa sprouts	8.59	1.130	0.196	1.070	9.45	0.272	0.021	0.036	1.030	0
Artichoke hearts, marinated	28.00	0.680	2.250	2.180	6.50	0.270	0.010	0.029	1.780	0
Asparagus	6.35	0.867	0.062	1.050	6.35	0.193	0.032	0.035	0.432	0
Avocado	45.70	0.563	4.340	2.100	3.07	0.284	0.030	0.035	2.720	0
Bacon, regular	163.00	8.640	14.000	0.164	2.98	0.482	0.195	0.080	0	23.9
Bean sprouts	8.50	0.861	0.050	1.680	3.82	0.258	0.024	0.035	0.7365	0
Beets	8.67	0.300	0.013	1.900	3.00	0.176	0.009	0.004	0.567	0
Beets, canned, diced	9.00	0.260	0.040	2.040	4.34	0.517	0.003	0.012	0.590	0
Broccoli, raw	7.73	0.844	0.097	1.490	13.50	0.251	0.019	0.034	0.934	0
Cabbage	6.48	0.340	0.049	1.520	13.00	0.162	0.015	0.009	0.680	0
Cabbage, red	7.70	0.393	0.073	1.740	14.60	0.142	0.018	0.009	0.648	0
Carrots, grated	12.40	0.289	0.052	2.880	7.73	0.142	0.027	0.016	0.907	0
Cauliflower	6.80	0.561	0.051	1.390	7.94	0.164	0.022	0.016	0.720	0
Celery	4.54	0.189	0.030	1.030	10.40	0.137	0.009	0.009	0.472	0
Chicken salad	96.70	3.820	8.900	0.469	5.92	0.239	0.012	0.028	0.109	17.3
Crab, cooked	23.90	5.050	0.561	0.140	12.90	0.104	0.012	0.044	0	18.0
Croutons, dry bread cubes	105.00	3.690	1.040	20.500	35.00	1.020	0.099	0.099	0.085	0
Cucumber slices	3.69	0.153	0.037	0.824	3.99	0.079	0.009	0.006	0.329	0
Egg, chopped	40.40	3.520	2.790	0.338	13.80	0.475	0.014	0.133	0	113
Escarole/curly endive	4.82	0.354	0.057	0.953	14.70	0.235	0.023	0.022	0.369	0
Garbanzo/chickpeas, cooked	46.50	2.500	0.735	7.780	13.80	0.819	0.033	0.018	1.920	0
Green pepper, sweet	6.80	0.244	0.130	1.500	1.70	0.357	0.024	0.014	0.454	0
Ham salad	51.50	5.000	3.000	0.880	2.00	0.280	0.244	0.072	0	16
Ham, minced	74.20	4.620	5.860	0.526	2.70	0.216	0.203	0.054	0	20.2
Leeks	17.30	0.425	0.085	4.000	16.70	0.594	0.017	0.008	0.688	0
Lettuce, butterhead	3.69	0.366	0.062	0.658	9.47	0.085	0.017	0.017	0.370	0
Lettuce, iceberg	3.69	0.287	0.054	0.592	5.37	0.142	0.013	0.009	0.370	0
Lettuce, loose leaf	5.11	0.369	0.085	0.992	19.20	0.397	0.014	0.023	0.391	0
Lettuce, Romaine	4.54	0.459	0.057	0.673	10.20	0.312	0.028	0.028	0.482	0
Lobster meat	27.80	5.800	0.168	0.364	17.20	0.111	0.020	0.019	0	20.3

SALAD BAR—*continued*

	kcal	Protein (g)	Fat (g)	CHO (g)	Ca (mg)	Fe (mg)	B_1 (mg)	B_2 (mg)	Fiber (g)	Cholesterol (mg)
Mushrooms, raw	7.09	0.593	0.119	1.320	1.42	0.352	0.029	0.127	0.508	0
Onions	9.57	0.335	0.074	2.070	7.09	0.105	0.017	0.003	0.454	0
Parmesan cheese, grated	129.00	11.800	8.500	1.060	389.00	0.270	0.013	0.109	0	22.0
Peas, cooked	22.30	1.460	0.078	4.040	6.73	0.443	0.080	0.050	1.280	0
Sesame seed kernels, dried	167.00	7.480	15.500	2.660	37.20	2.210	0.204	0.024	1.950	0
Shrimp, boiled	28.00	5.930	0.306	0	11.00	0.876	0.009	0.009	0	55.3
Spinach, fresh	6.23	0.810	0.099	0.992	28.00	0.770	0.022	0.054	0.947	0
Sunflower seeds, dry	162.00	6.460	14.000	5.320	32.90	1.920	0.650	0.070	1.970	0
Tomatoes	5.51	0.252	0.061	1.230	1.89	0.135	0.017	0.014	0.416	0
Tuna salad	53.00	4.550	2.630	2.670	4.84	0.282	0.009	0.019	0.340	3.73
Turkey meat	41.30	5.270	2.030	0.149	11.40	0.358	0.025	0.064	0	11.9

VARIETY

	kcal	Protein (g)	Fat (g)	CHO (g)	Ca (mg)	Fe (mg)	B_1 (mg)	B_2 (mg)	Fiber (g)	Cholesterol (mg)
Chips & crackers										
Doritos—nacho flavor	139	2.20	6.79	18.00	17.0	0.399	0.040	0.030	1.10	0
Doritos—taco flavor	140	2.60	6.59	17.60	44.9	0.699	0.080	0.090	1.10	0
Potato chips—sour cream & onion	153	2.40	9.48	14.60	21.0	0.474	0.040	0.055	1.35	1.0
Wheat cracker—thin	124	3.19	4.96	17.70	10.6	1.060	0.142	0.106	1.84	0
Whole wheat crackers	124	3.19	5.32	17.70	10.6	1.850	0.070	0.106	2.94	0
Condiments										
Catsup	30	0.52	0.11	7.17	6.2	0.228	0.026	0.020	0.45	0
Mustard	21	1.34	1.25	1.81	23.8	0.567	0.024	0.057	0.11	0
Soy sauce	14	1.46	0.02	2.40	4.7	0.567	0.014	0.036	0	0
Deli meats										
Bologna—beef	89	3.32	8.04	0.56	3.7	0.394	0.016	0.036	0	16.0
Bratwurst	92	4.05	7.90	0.84	13.8	0.292	0.070	0.064	0	17.8
Keilbasa sausage	88	3.76	7.70	0.61	12.0	0.414	0.064	0.061	0	18.5
Knockwurst sausage	87	3.37	7.88	0.05	2.9	0.258	0.097	0.040	0	16.3
Liverwurst	93	4.00	8.10	0.63	7.9	1.810	0.077	0.291	0	44.1
Pepperoni sausage	140	5.94	12.50	0.80	2.8	0.397	0.09	0.07		9.79
Polish sausage	92	3.99	8.13	0.46	3.0	0.409	0.142	0.042	0	20.0
Salami—beef	72	4.17	5.69	0.70	2.47	0.567	0.036	0.073	0	17.3
Salami—pork & beef	72	3.94	5.70	0.64	3.68	0.755	0.068	0.106	0	18.5
Salami—turkey	55	4.62	3.89	0.15	5.47	0.463	0.029	0.075	0	22.9
Salami—dry—beef & pork	120	6.49	9.75	0.74	2.84	0.425	0.170	0.082	0	22.7
Turkey pastrami	37	5.22	1.75	0.43	2.49	0.403	0.022	0.075	0	14.9
Mexican foods										
Beef taco	75.2	4.94	4.80	3.67	30.9	0.469	0.01	0.049	0.407	16.2
Beef enchilada	69.0	3.09	3.26	3.69	60.2	0.418	0.017	0.039	0.465	8.93
Cheese enchilada	78.0	3.12	4.2	3.78	108.0	0.324	0.015	0.050	0.465	10.2
Chicken enchilada	63.6	3.38	2.48	3.69	60.5	0.359	0.018	0.036	0.465	9.10
Corn tortilla, enriched, regular	61.4	1.89	0.964	12.30	39.7	0.567	0.047	0.028	2.27	0

VARIETY—*continued*

	kcal	Protein (g)	Fat (g)	CHO (g)	Ca (mg)	Fe (mg)	B₁ (mg)	B₂ (mg)	Fiber (g)	Cholesterol (mg)
Mexican Foods—*continued*										
Corn torilla, enriched, thin	61.0	1.64	0.95	12.30	39.8	0.567	0.046	0.028	2.26	0
Corn tortilla, fried	82.2	2.08	2.84	12.30	39.7	0.567	0.047	0.028	2.27	0
Enchirito	60.4	3.15	2.75	3.31	51.5	0.410	0.015	0.037	0.748	9.18
Flour tortilla	84	2.07	2.15	15.50	17.0	0.440	0.102	0.062	0.800	0
Refried beans, canned	30.3	1.77	0.303	5.24	13.2	0.500	0.014	0.016	2.47	0
Nuts & seeds										
Almonds—dried, chopped	167	5.65	14.80	5.78	75.5	1.040	0.060	0.220	3.36	0
Almonds—whole toasted	167	5.77	14.40	6.48	80.0	1.400	0.037	0.170	3.99	0
Sunflower seeds—dry	162	6.46	14.00	5.32	32.9	1.920	0.650	0.070	1.97	0
Oils & shortening										
Cocoa butter oil	251	0	28.40	0	0	0	0	0	0	0
Corn oil	251	0	28.40	0	0	0.001	0	0	0	0
Cottonseed oil	251	0	28.40	0	0	0	0	0	0	0
Olive oil	251	0	28.40	0	0.1	0.109	0	0	0	0
Palm oil	251	0	28.40	0	0.1	0.003	0	0	0	0
Palm kernel oil	251	0	28.40	0	0	0	0	0	0	0
Peanut oil	251	0	28.40	0	0	0.008	0	0	0	0
Safflower oil	251	0	28.40	0	0	0	0	0	0	0
Sesame oil	250	0	28.40	0	0	0	0	0	0	0
Soybean oil	251	0	28.40	0	0	0.007	0	0	0	0
Sunflower oil	251	0	28.40	0	0	0	0	0	0	0
Walnut oil	251	0	28.40	0	0	0	0	0	0	0
Wheat germ oil	250	0	28.40	0	0	0	0	0	0	0
Vegetable shortening	251	0	28.40	0	0	0	0	0	0	0
Pasta & noodles										
Spaghetti, cooked firm, hot	41	1.42	0.142	8.53	3.1	0.454	0.051	0.028	0.482	0
Spaghetti, cooked tender, hot	31	1.01	0.111	6.48	3.0	0.405	0.04	0.022	0.425	0
Whole wheat spaghetti, cooked	35	1.53	0.113	7.49	4.3	0.244	0.048	0.020	1.040	0
Spaghetti + sauce + cheese, canned	22	0.68	0.227	4.42	4.5	0.318	0.040	0.032	0.284	0.3
Spaghetti + sauce + cheese, homemade	30	1.02	1.02	4.20	9.07	0.260	0.028	0.020	0.284	0.9
Spaghetti + sauce + meat, canned	30	1.36	1.13	4.42	6.01	0.374	0.017	0.020	0.312	2.6
Spaghetti + sauce + meat, homemade	38	2.17	1.37	4.46	14.20	0.423	0.029	0.034	0.314	10.2
Spaghetti sauce, homemade	23	0.77	1.25	2.95	6.70	0.380	0.026	0.017	0.343	0
Spaghetti sauce, canned	31	0.52	1.35	4.52	7.97	0.184	0.016	0.017	0.343	0
Spaghetti meat sauce,	30	1.03	1.30	3.72	4.95	0.385	0.028	0.022	0.193	2.3
Spaghetti sauce, dry, packet	79	1.70	0.28	18.20	48.20	0.765	NA	0.162	0.057	0
Spaghetti sauce + mushrooms, packet	85	2.84	2.55	13.90	113.00	0.510	NA	0.136	0.085	0
Egg noodles, cooked	35	1.17	0.35	6.60	3.19	0.400	0.039	0.023	0.624	8.9

VARIETY—continued

	kcal	Protein (g)	Fat (g)	CHO (g)	Ca (mg)	Fe (mg)	B₁ (mg)	B₂ (mg)	Fiber (g)	Cholesterol (mg)
Pasta & noodles—continued										
Chow mein noodles, dry	139	3.72	6.93	16.40	8.82	0.252	0.032	0.019	1.100	3.2
Spinach noodles, dry	108	3.97	1.08	20.20	11.60	1.290	0.278	0.133	1.930	0
Spinach noodles, cooked	32	1.13	0.36	5.97	3.37	0.429	0.043	0.027	0.569	0
Chicken + noodles, recipe	43	2.60	2.13	3.07	3.07	0.278	0.006	0.020	0.142	12.2
Chicken + noodles, frozen	32	2.17	1.30	2.49	15.70	0.393	0.009	0.018	0.022	8.0
Noodles-ramen-beef, cooked	28	0.76	0.94	4.17	NA	NA	NA	NA	0.500	NA
Noodles, ramen, chicken, cooked	25	0.76	0.85	3.63	NA	NA	NA	NA	0.512	NA
Noodles, ramen, oriental	26	0.74	1.07	3.83	NA	NA	NA	NA	0.512	NA
Lasagna, frozen entree	38	2.32	1.71	2.61	34.00	0.343	0.026	0.045	0.194	12.4
Pizza										
Pizza—cheese	69	3.54	2.13	9.21	52.00	0.378	0.080	0.069	0.510	13.2
Pizza—mozzarella	80	7.60	4.67	0.89	207.00	0.076	0.006	0.097	0	15.0
Pizza—Canadian bacon	52	6.82	2.36	0.38	3.00	0.229	0.231	0.055	0	16.3
Pizza—pepperoni	140	5.94	12.50	0.81	2.80	0.397	0.090	0.070	0	9.8
Pizza—onion	10	0.34	0.07	2.07	7.10	1.105	0.017	0.003	0.450	0
Popcorn										
Popcorn—plain, air popped	106	3.50	1.42	21.30	3.50	0.709	0.106	0.035	4.600	0
Popcorn—cooked in oil/salted	142	2.32	7.99	15.50	7.70	0.696	0.026	0.052	3.090	0
Popcorn—syrup-coated	109	1.60	0.81	24.30	1.60	0.405	0.106	0.016	0.810	0
Rice										
Brown—dry	102	2.13	0.54	21.90	9.04	0.510	0.096	0.014	0.965	0
Brown—cooked	34	0.709	0.17	7.23	3.40	0.170	0.026	0.006	0.483	0
White—regular, dry	103	1.90	0.11	22.80	6.74	0.828	0.125	0.009	0.340	0
White—regular, cooked	31	0.567	0.03	6.86	2.84	0.397	0.03	0.003	0.102	0
White—converted, dry	105	2.10	0.15	23.00	17.00	0.828	0.124	0.010	0.624	0
White—converted, cooked	30	0.599	0.02	6.60	5.35	0.227	0.03	0.003	0.180	0
White—instant, dry	106	2.13	0.06	23.40	1.42	1.300	0.125	0.008	0.737	0
White—instant, prepared	31	0.624	0.03	6.86	0.85	0.227	0.037	0.003	0.216	0
Wild—cooked	26	1.02	0.06	5.39	1.42	0.312	0.031	0.045	0.709	0
Rice bran	78	3.77	5.44	14.40	21.50	5.500	0.64	0.070	6.150	0
Rice polish	75	3.43	3.62	16.40	19.40	4.560	0.521	0.051	0.680	0
Salad dressings										
Blue cheese salad dressing	143	1.37	14.80	2.09	22.90	0.057	0.003	0.028	0.020	7.6
Caesar's salad dressing	126	2.66	12.70	0.67	44.40	0.239	0.007	0.025	0.050	33.9
French dressing	150	0.16	16.00	1.81	3.55	0.113	0	0	0.220	0
Italian dressing—low calorie	15	0.02	1.18	1.37	0.59	0.059	0	0	0.080	1.7

VARIETY—*continued*

	kcal	Protein (g)	Fat (g)	CHO (g)	Ca (mg)	Fe (mg)	B₁ (mg)	B₂ (mg)	Fiber (g)	Cholesterol (mg)
Salad dressings—*continued*										
Mayonnaise	203	0.31	22.60	0.77	5.67	0.168	0.005	0.012	0	16.8
Imitation mayonnaise	66	0	5.67	3.78	0	0	0	0	0	7.6
Ranch salad dressing	104	0.86	10.70	1.31	28.40	0.075	0.010	0.040	0	11.1
Russian salad dressing	140	0.45	14.50	3.00	5.44	0.174	0.014	0.014	0.080	18.4
1000 island dressing	107	0.26	10.10	4.30	3.52	0.170	0.006	0.009	0.060	7.3
1000 island dressing— low calorie	45	0.22	3.00	4.58	3.12	1.174	0.006	0.008	0.340	3.4
Vinegar & oil dressing	124	0	14.20	0	0	0	0	0	0	0
Salads, prepared										
Chicken salad w/celery	97	3.82	8.90	0.47	5.92	0.239	0.012	0.028	0.110	17.3
Cole slaw	20	0.36	0.74	3.52	12.80	0.166	0.019	0.017	0.570	2.3
Egg salad	68	2.91	6.01	0.45	14.50	0.525	0.019	0.070	0	97.4
Ham salad spread	62	2.46	4.39	3.01	2.24	0.168	0.123	0.034	0.030	10.4
Macaroni salad—no cheese	75	0.54	6.66	3.52	5.50	0.229	0.020	0.014	0.270	4.9
Potato salad w/mayo + eggs	41	0.76	2.32	3.16	5.44	0.185	0.022	0.017	0.420	19.3
Tuna salad	53	4.55	2.53	2.67	4.84	0.282	0.009	0.019	0.340	3.7
Waldorf salad	85	0.72	8.33	2.62	8.82	0.196	0.020	0.013	0.720	4.3
Sandwiches										
Avocado & cheese— white	64	2.02	4.00	5.39	43.1	0.418	0.057	0.059	0.98	4.4
Avocado & cheese— whole wheat	62	2.14	3.97	5.24	37.8	0.477	0.047	0.05	1.76	4.3
BLT —whole wheat	68	2.49	3.77	6.45	11.4	0.570	0.077	0.043	1.55	4.1
BLT—white	70	2.30	3.77	6.70	18.2	0.489	0.092	0.055	0.43	4.2
Grilled cheese—wheat	91	4.22	5.37	7.10	87.4	0.565	0.057	0.076	1.59	11.8
Grilled cheese— part WW	95	4.39	5.82	6.59	103.0	0.526	0.067	0.093	0.61	13.3
Grilled cheese—white	97	4.22	5.79	6.88	103.0	0.441	0.068	0.092	0.30	13.3
Chicken salad—wheat	80	3.00	4.25	8.13	14.7	0.679	0.066	0.046	1.88	6.2
Chicken salad—white	85	2.83	4.63	8.05	22.7	0.552	0.080	0.060	0.39	7.1
Corn dog	84	2.55	5.10	6.97	8.7	0.495	0.072	0.043	0.03	9.5
Corned beef & swiss on rye	83	5.26	4.59	4.90	63.8	0.768	0.044	0.078	0.97	16.4
English muffin (egg/ cheese/bacon)	74	3.70	3.70	6.37	40.5	0.637	0.095	0.103	0.32	43.8
Egg salad—wheat	79	2.60	4.56	7.44	17.0	0.744	0.063	0.059	1.67	48.8
Egg salad—soft white	83	2.41	4.90	7.25	24.5	0.636	0.075	0.074	0.30	41.6
Ham—rye bread	59	3.84	2.09	6.10	12.0	0.474	0.182	0.073	1.24	7.1
Ham—whole wheat	59	3.79	2.04	6.84	12.4	0.617	0.164	0.060	1.54	6.1
Ham—soft white	61	3.74	2.08	6.60	18.6	0.504	0.186	0.073	0.29	6.7
Ham & swiss—rye	68	4.65	3.23	5.08	63.5	0.389	0.147	0.079	0.99	10.8
Ham & cheese— wheat	67	4.20	3.23	5.72	40.5	0.527	0.136	0.066	1.27	9.7
Ham & cheese—soft white	69	4.20	3.36	5.43	48.0	0.428	0.152	0.078	0.23	10.6
Ham salad—wheat	75	2.45	4.02	7.83	11.5	0.569	0.104	0.045	1.52	5.6
Ham salad—white	78	2.25	4.26	7.71	17.5	0.454	0.119	0.057	0.28	6.2
Hotdog/frankfurter & bun	87	2.80	5.10	7.04	19.6	0.570	0.095	0.062	0.40	7.6

VARIETY—*continued*

	kcal	Protein (g)	Fat (g)	CHO (g)	Ca (mg)	Fe (mg)	B₁ (mg)	B₂ (mg)	Fiber (g)	Cholesterol (mg)
Sandwiches—*continued*										
Patty melt—gound beef/rye	91	5.09	6.07	3.96	36.5	0.533	0.040	0.072	0.81	17.1
Peanut butter & jam—whole wheat	92	3.40	3.85	12.30	15.4	0.751	0.070	0.045	2.29	0
Peanut butter & jam—white	98	3.29	4.14	12.80	23.4	0.632	0.085	0.059	0.85	0
Reuben grilled	58	3.43	3.38	3.53	43.6	0.633	0.030	0.052	0.80	10.4
Roast beef—whole wheat	64	4.00	2.52	6.71	12.3	0.760	0.061	0.054	1.53	6.2
Roast beef—white	67	3.97	2.63	6.46	18.5	0.665	0.072	0.066	0.27	6.9
Tuna salad—wheat	72	3.29	3.29	8.03	13.0	0.667	0.057	0.040	1.74	5.5
Tuna salad—white	76	3.18	3.47	7.92	19.6	0.555	0.068	0.052	0.44	6.2
Turkey—whole wheat	62	4.09	2.33	6.67	11.6	0.554	0.056	0.044	1.53	6.0
Turkey—white	64	4.07	2.42	6.41	17.8	0.435	0.066	0.055	0.27	6.7
Turkey & ham—rye	58	3.74	2.12	6.18	12.3	0.743	0.060	0.079	1.23	8.4
Turkey & ham— whole wheat	59	3.71	2.07	6.90	12.6	0.846	0.060	0.064	1.54	7.2
Turkey & ham—white	60	3.65	2.10	6.67	18.8	0.762	0.071	0.078	0.28	8.0
Turkey & ham & cheese on rye	68	4.22	3.46	5.04	44.2	0.616	0.050	0.083	0.99	12.1
Turkey & ham & cheese—wheat	67	4.14	3.25	5.77	40.5	0.716	0.051	0.070	1.27	10.6
Turkey & ham & cheese—white	69	4.13	3.38	5.48	48.3	0.636	0.059	0.082	0.23	11.6
Sauces										
Bordelaise sauce	24	0.33	1.46	1.10	3.80	0.179	0.008	0.010	0.01	3.8
Hot chili sauce, red pepper	5	0.25	0.17	1.10	2.51	0.137	0.003	0.026	2.29	0
Teriyaki sauce	24	1.69	0.09	4.52	6.30	0.488	0.008	0.020	0	0
Seafood										
Anchovy—raw	37	5.78	1.37	0	41.7	0.921	0.016	0.073	0	19.6
Frog legs—raw meat	21	4.65	0.085	0	5.1	0.539	0.040	0.070	0	14.2
Lobster meat— cooked	28	5.80	0.17	0.36	17.2	0.111	0.020	0.019	0	20.3
Scampi—fried in crumbs	69	6.07	3.49	3.26	19.0	0.357	0.037	0.039	0.04	50.2
Shrimp—boiled	28	5.93	0.31	0	11.0	0.876	0.009	0.009	0	55.3
Squid (calamari)— fried in flour	50	5.10	2.12	2.20	11.0	0.287	0.016	0.130	0	73.7
Soups										
Cream of celery	20	0.38	1.27	2.00	9.04	0.141	0.007	0.011	0.09	3.2
Chicken, chunky	20	1.43	0.75	1.95	2.71	0.195	0.010	0.020	0.03	3.4
Chicken + dumpling	23	1.30	1.28	1.39	3.34	0.144	0.004	0.017	0.10	7.6
Chicken gumbo	13	0.60	0.32	1.89	5.53	0.201	0.006	0.009	0.05	0.9
Chicken-noodle— chunky	14	1.50	0.70	0.24	2.84	0.170	0.009	0.020	0.09	2.1
Chili with beans	32	1.62	1.56	3.38	13.20	0.973	0.014	0.030	0.91	4.8
Clam chowder— New England	19	1.08	0.75	1.90	21.40	0.169	0.008	0.027	0.11	2.5
Minestrone—chunky	15	0.60	0.33	2.45	7.20	0.209	0.006	0.014	0.12	0.6
Cream of mushroom	29	0.46	2.15	2.10	7.23	0.119	0.007	0.019	0.06	0.4
Mushroom—barley	14	0.43	0.51	1.69	2.82	0.113	0.006	0.020	0.17	0

VARIETY—continued

	kcal	Protein (g)	Fat (g)	CHO (g)	Ca (mg)	Fe (mg)	B₁ (mg)	B₂ (mg)	Fiber (g)	Cholesterol (mg)
Soups—continued										
Onion—canned	13	0.87	0.40	1.89	6.10	0.156	0.008	0.006	0.11	0
Oyster stew	14	0.49	0.89	0.94	4.96	0.227	0.005	0.008	0	3.1
Pea—prepared w/milk	27	1.40	0.79	3.59	19.30	0.224	0.017	0.030	0.07	2.0
Cream of potato	17	0.39	0.53	2.59	4.52	0.107	0.008	0.008	0.10	1.5
Split pea + ham	22	1.31	0.47	3.17	3.90	0.253	0.014	0.011	0.19	0.8
Tomato—canned	19	0.47	0.43	3.75	3.05	0.396	0.020	0.011	0.11	0
Tomato-beef-noodle	32	1.00	0.97	4.78	3.95	0.252	0.019	0.020	0.03	0.9
Tomato bisque prepared w/milk	22	0.71	0.75	3.32	21.00	0.099	0.013	0.030	0.01`	2.5
Turkey—chunky	16	1.23	0.53	1.69	6.00	0.229	0.010	0.029	0.12	1.1
Turkey noodle	16	0.88	0.45	1.95	2.60	0.212	0.017	0.014	0.03	1.1
Cream vegetable— dry mix	126	2.27	6.84	14.80	1.42	0.539	1.470	0.127	0.22	1.2
Vegetable	16	0.49	0.45	2.77	4.96	0.249	0.012	0.010	0.37	0
Miscellanous										
Garlic cloves	42	1.80	0.14	9.38	51.30	0.482	0.057	0.030	0.47	0
Gelatin salad/desert	17	0.43	0	3.99	0.50	0.024	0.002	0.002	0.02	0
Quiche lorraine	97	2.09	7.73	4.67	34.00	0.226	0.018	0.052	0.09	45.9
Spinach souffle	45	2.29	3.84	0.59	47.90	0.279	0.019	0.064	0.79	38.4

PART 2

NUTRITIVE VALUES FOR ALCOHOLIC AND NONALCOHOLIC BEVERAGES

The nutritive values for alcoholic and nonalcoholic beverages are expressed in 1-ounce (28.4-g) portions. We have also included the nutritive values for the minerals calcium, iron, magnesium, phosphorus, and potassium and the vitamins thiamine, riboflavin, niacin, and cobalamin. The alcoholic beverages contain no cholesterol or fat.

ALCOHOLIC BEVERAGES (1 OUNCE)

				Minerals					Vitamins			
	kcal	Protein (g)	CHO (g)	Ca (mg)	Fe (mg)	Mg (mg)	P (mg)	K (mg)	B₁ (mg)	B₂ (mg)	Niacin (mg)	B₁₂ (mg)
Beer, regular	12	0.072	1.1	1.4	0.009	1.83	3.50	7.09	0.002	0.007	0.128	0.005
Beer, light	8	0.057	0.4	1.4	0.011	1.42	3.44	5.13	0.003	0.008	0.111	0.002
Brandy	69	0	10.6	2.5	0.012		1.01	1.01	0.002	0.002	0.004	0
Champagne	22	0.043	0.6	1.6	0.093	2.40	1.90	22.60	0	0.003	0.019	0
Dessert wine, dry	36	0.057	1.2	2.3	0.068	2.55	2.55	26.20	0.005	0.005	0.060	0
Dessert wine, sweet	44	0.057	3.3	2.3	0.057	2.55	2.64	26.20	0.005	0.005	0.060	0
Gin, rum, vodka, scotch, whiskey, 80 proof	64	0	0	0	0.010	0	0	1.01	0	0	0	0
Gin, rum, vodka, scotch, whiskey, 86 proof	71	0	0	0	0.012	0	1.16	0.55	0.002	0.002	0.004	0

ALCOHOLIC BEVERAGES (1 OUNCE)—*continued*

| | kcal | Protein (g) | CHO (g) | Minerals | | | | | Vitamins | | | |
				Ca (mg)	Fe (mg)	Mg (mg)	P (mg)	K (mg)	B₁ (mg)	B₂ (mg)	Niacin (mg)	B₁₂ (mg)
Gin, rum, vodka, scotch, whiskey, 90 proof	74	0	0	0	0.010	0	0	0.86	0	0	0	0
Sherry, dry	28	0.024	0.3	2.1	0.052	1.96	2.60	17.80	0.002	0.002	0.024	0
Sherry, medium	40	0.066	2.3	2.3	0.071	2.27	1.89	23.60	0.002	0.008	0.035	0
Vermouth, dry	34	0.028	1.6	2.0	0.096	1.42	1.89	11.30	NA	NA	0.011	0
Vermouth, sweet	44	0.014	4.5	1.7	0.099	1.13	1.65	8.50	NA	NA	0.011	0
Wine, dry white	19	0.029	0.2	2.6	0.093	2.62	1.67	17.40	0	0.001	0.019	0
Wine, medium white	19	0.028	0.2	2.5	0.085	3.03	3.84	22.60	0.001	0.001	0.019	0
Wine, red	20	0.055	0.5	2.2	0.122	3.60	3.84	31.50	0.001	0.008	0.023	0.004
Wine, rosé	20	0.055	0.4	2.4	0.108	2.74	4.08	28.10	0.001	0.004	0.020	0.002
Creme de menthe	105	0	11.8	0	0.023	0	0	0	0	0	0.001	0
Bloody mary	22	0.153	0.9	1.9	0.105	2.10	4.02	41.40	0.010	0.006	0.123	0
Bourbon and soda	26	0	0	1.0	0.244	0.24	0.48	0.48	0	0	0.005	0
Daiquiri	52	0	1.9	0.9	0.043	0.47	1.89	6.14	0.004	0.	0.012	0
Manhattan	64	0	0.9	0.5	0.025	0.01	1.99	7.46	0.003	0.001	0.026	0
Martini	63	0	0.1	0.4	0.024	0.40	0.81	5.26	0	0	0.004	0
Pina colada	53	0.120	8.0	2.2	0.062		2.01	20.10	0.008	0.004	0.033	0
Screwdriver	23	0.160	2.5	2.1	0.023	2.26	3.86	43.30	0.018	0.004	0.046	0
Tequila	31	0.099	2.4	1.7	0.077	1.98	2.80	29.30	0.010	0.005	0.054	0
Tom collins	16	0.013	0.4	1.3	NA	0.38	0.12	2.30	0	0	0.004	0
Whiskey sour	42	0	3.7	0.3	0.021	0.26	1.60	5.08	0.003	0.002	0.006	0
Coffee + cream liqueur	93	0.784	5.9	4.2	0.036	0.60	13.90	9.05	0	0.016	0.022	0
Coffee liqueur	95	0	13.3	0.5	0.016	0.54	1.64	8.18	0.001	0.003	0.040	0

NONALCOHOLIC BEVERAGES (1 OUNCE)

| | kcal | Protein (g) | CHO (g) | Minerals | | | | | Vitamins | | | |
				Ca (mg)	Fe (mg)	Mg (mg)	P (mg)	K (mg)	B₁ (mg)	B₂ (mg)	Niacin (mg)	B₁₂ (mg)
Hot cocoa with whole milk	25	1.030	2.9	33.8	0.088	6.350	30.60	54.400	0.012	0.049	0.041	0.099
Cocoa mix + water— diet	7	0.561	1.3	13.3	0.110	4.870	19.80	59.800	0.006	0.030	0.024	0
Coffee—brewed	0.2	0.016	0.1	0.5	0.113	1.590	0.32	15.400	0	0.002	0.063	0
Coffee—instant dry powder	1.4	0.016	0.3	0.8	0.019	1.100	2.05	67.70	0	0	0.061	0
Coffee—capuchino	9.2	0.059	1.6	1.0	0.022	1.330	3.84	17.600	0	0	0.048	0
Coffee—Swiss mocha	7.7	0.078	1.3	1.1	0.036	1.360	4.37	17.900	0	0	0.039	0
Coffee whitener—												
nondairy,	38.5	0.284	3.2	2.6	0.009	0.060	18.20	54.1	0	0	0	0
liquid powder	155	1.360	15.6	6.3	0.326	1.200	120.00	230.0	0	0.047	0	0
Cola beverage, regular	12	0	3.0	0.7	0.009	0.230	3.52	0.306	0	0	0	0
Diet cola— w/aspartame	0	0	0	1.0	0.009	0.319	2.40	0	0.001	0.007	0	0
Club soda	0	0	0	1.4	0.012	0.319	0	0.479	0	0	0	0

NONALCOHOLIC BEVERAGES (1 OUNCE)—*continued*

	kcal	Protein (g)	CHO (g)	Minerals					Vitamins			
				Ca (mg)	Fe (mg)	Mg (mg)	P (mg)	K (mg)	B₁ (mg)	B₂ (mg)	Niacin (mg)	B₁₂ (mg)
Cream soda	15	0	3.8	1.5	0.015	0.229	0	0.306	0	0	0	0
Diet soda-avg assorted	0	0	0.0	1.1	0.011	0.200	3.03	0.559	0	0	0	0
Egg nog—commercial	38	1.080	3.8	36.8	0.057	5.250	31.00	46.900	0.010	0.054	0.030	0.127
Five Alive citrus	13	0.135	3.1	1.7	0.021	1.950	2.70	34.000	0.015	0.003	0.060	0
Fruit flavored soda pop	13	0	3.2	1.1	0.020	0.305	0.15	1.520	0	0	0.002	0
Fruit punch drink—canned	13	0.015	3.4	2.1	0.058	0.610	0.31	7.160	0.006	0.006	0.006	0
Gatorade	5	0	1.3	2.8	NA	NA	0	2.840	NA	NA	NA	0
Ginger ale	10	0.008	2.5	0.9	0.051	0.232	0.08	0.387	0	0	0	0
Grape soda carbonated	12	0	3.2	0.9	0.024	0.305	0	0.229	0	0	0	0
Kool-Aid w/ NutraSweet	0	0	0	0	0	0.028	0	0	0	0	0	0
Kool-Aid w/sugar added	12	0	3.0	0	0	0	0	0	0	0	0	0
Lemon-lime soda	12	0	3.0	0.7	0.019	0.154	0.08	0.308	0	0	0.004	0
Lemonade drink from dry	11	0	2.9	7.6	0.016	0.322	3.65	3.540	0	0	0.004	0
Lemonade frozen conc	51	0.078	13.3	1.9	0.205	1.420	2.46	19.200	0.007	0.027	0.020	0
Limeade frozen conc	53	0.052	14.0	1.4	0.029	7.800	1.69	16.800	0.003	0.003	0.028	0
Chocolate milkshake	36	0.962	5.8	32.0	0.088	4.700	28.90	56.800	0.016	0.069	0.046	0.097
Strawberry milkshake	32	0.952	5.4	32.0	0.030	3.600	28.40	51.700	0.013	0.055	0.050	0.088
Vanilla milkshake	32	0.982	5.1	34.5	0.026	3.500	29.00	49.300	0.013	0.052	0.052	0.101
Orange drink/ carbonated	14	0	3.5	1.5	0.018	0.305	0.31	0.686	0	0	0	0
Pepper-type soda	12	0	2.9	0.9	0.010	0.077	3.16	0.154	0	0	0	0
Root beer	12	0.008	3.0	1.5	0.014	0.306	0.15	0.230	0	0	0	0
Pineapple grapefruit drink	13	0.068	3.3	2.0	0.087	1.700	1.59	17.500	0.009	0.005	0.076	0
Pineapple orange drink	14	0.352	3.3	1.5	0.076	1.590	1.13	13.200	0.009	0.005	0.059	0
Tang orange juice crystals	13	0.170	0.06	3.1	4.57	0.002	0.02	0.008	0	0	0	0
Tonic water/Quinine water	10	0	2.5	0.4	0.019	0.077	0	0.077	0	0	0	0
Tea-brewed	0	0.001	0.1	0	0.006	0.796	0.16	10.500	0	0.004	0.012	0
Herbal tea, brewed	0	0	0	0.6	0.022	0.319	0	2.390	0.003	0.001	0	0
Perrier water	0	0	0	3.8	0	0.148	0	0	0	0	0	0
Poland Springs bottled water	0	0	0	0.4	0.001	0.239	0	0	0	0	0	0

Note: Alcoholic beverages contain no fat or cholesterol; light beer contains 0.5 g fiber and regular beer contains 1.2 g fiber per 8 oz. serving. All of the other nonmixed alcoholic beverages have no fiber.

Note: Other nonalcoholic beverages are listed in the sections on fruits and vegetables.

PART 3

NUTRITIVE VALUES FOR SPECIALTY AND FAST-FOOD ITEMS

Nutrient information was kindly provided by the manufacturer or its representative, and is reproduced as presented in their literature. Unlike Parts 1 and 2, nutritive values are not given for 1-ounce portions but for the actual amounts of the foods as sold commercially. To make a direct comparison of the kcal values and the various nutrients, we recommend that the weight of the food and its nutrients be expressed relative to 1-ounce (28.4-g) portions.

ARBY'S

Food Item	Serving Size (g)	kcal	Protein (g)	Fat (g)	CHO (g)
Bacon Cheddar Deluxe	225	561	28	34	78
Baked Potato Plain	312	291	8	1	0
Beef 'n Cheddar	190	490	24	21	51
Chicken Breast Sandwich	210	592	28	27	57
Chocolate Shake	300	384	9	11	32
French Fries	71	211	2	8	6
Hot Ham 'n Cheese Sandwich	161	353	26	13	50
Jamocha Shake	305	424	8	10	31
Junior Roast Beef	86	218	12	8	22
King Roast Beef	192	467	27	19	49
Potato Cakes	85	201	2	14	13
Regular Roast Beef	147	353	22	15	32
Super Roast Beef	234	501	25	22	40
Superstuffed Potato Broccoli and Cheddar	340	541	13	22	24
Superstuffed Potato Deluxe	312	648	18	38	72
Superstuffed Potato Mushroom and Cheese	300	506	16	22	21
Superstuffed Potato Taco	425	619	23	27	145
Turkey Deluxe	197	375	24	17	39
Vanilla Shake	250	295	8	10	30

Source: Arby's Inc. Nutritional information provided by Consumer Affairs, Arby's Inc., Atlanta, GA, 1986.

BURGER KING

Food Item	Serving Size (g)	kcal	Pro-tein (g)	Total Carbo-hydrate (g)	Total Fat (g)	Choles-terol (mg)	Sodium (mg)	Dietary Fiber (g)	Percentage of U.S. RDA*			
									Vit A	Vit C	Ca	Fe
Burgers												
Whopper sandwich	270	640	27	45	39	90	870	3	10	15	8	25
Whopper with cheese sandwich	294	730	33	46	46	115	1300	3	15	15	25	25
Double Whopper sandwich	351	870	46	45	56	170	940	3	10	15	8	40
Double Whopper with cheese sandwich	375	960	52	46	63	195	1360	3	15	15	25	40
Whopper Jr. sandwich	168	420	21	29	24	60	570	2	4	8	6	20
Whopper Jr. with cheese sandwich	180	460	23	29	28	75	780	2	8	8	15	20
Hamburger	129	330	20	28	15	55	570	1	2	0	4	15
Cheeseburger	142	380	23	28	19	65	780	1	6	0	15	15
Double cheese-burger	213	600	41	29	36	135	1040	1	8	0	20	25
Double cheese-burger with bacon	221	640	44	29	39	145	1220	1	8	0	20	25
Sandwich/Side Orders												
BK Big Fish sandwich	255	720	25	59	43	60	1090	2	2	2	6	20
BK Broiler Chicken sandwich	248	540	30	41	29	80	480	2	4	10	4	30
Chicken sandwich	229	700	26	54	43	60	1400	2	°	°	10	20
Chicken Tenders (6 piece)	88	250	16	14	12	35	530	2	°	°	°	4
Broiled Chicken salad†	302	200	21	7	10	60	110	3	100	25	15	20
Garden salad†	215	90	6	7	5	15	110	3	110	50	15	6
Side salad†	133	50	3	4	3	5	55	2	50	20	6	2
French fries (medium, salted)	116	400	5	43	20	0	240	3	°	4	°	6
Onion rings	124	310	4	41	14	0	810	5	°	°	°	°
Dutch apple pie	113	310	3	39	15	0	230	2	°	10	°	8
Drinks												
Vanilla shake (medium)	284	310	9	53	7	20	230	1	6	6	30	°
Chocolate shake (medium)	284	310	9	54	7	20	230	3	6	°	20	10
Chocolate shake (medium, syrup added)	341	460	11	87	7	20	300	1	6	6	30	°
Strawberry shake (medium, syrup added)	341	430	9	83	7	20	260	1	6	6	30	°

BURGER KING—continued

Food Item	Serving Size (g)	kcal	Pro- tein (g)	Total Carbo- hydrate (g)	Total Fat (g)	Choles- terol (mg)	Sodium (mg)	Dietary Fiber (g)	Vit A	Vit C	Ca	Fe
Drinks—continued												
Coca-Cola Classic (medium)	22 (FL OZ)	260	0	70	0	0	@	0	°	°	°	°
Diet Coke (medium)	22 (FL OZ)	1	0	<1	0	0	@	0	°	°	°	°
Sprite (medium)	22 (FL OZ)	260	0	66	0	0	@	0	°	°	°	°
Tropicana orange juice	311	140	2	33	0	0	0	0	0	100	0	0
Coffee	355	5	0	1	0	0	5	0	°	°	°	°
Milk—2% low fat	244	120	8	12	5	20	120	0	10	4	30	°
Breakfast												
Croissan'wich with bacon, egg and cheese	118	350	15	18	24	225	790	<1	8	°	15	10
Croissan'wich with sausage, egg and cheese	159	530	20	21	41	255	1000	<1	8	°	15	15
Croissan'wich with ham, egg and cheese	144	350	18	19	22	230	1390	<1	8	°	15	10
French toast sticks	141	500	4	60	27	0	490	1	°	°	6	15
Hash browns	71	220	2	25	12	0	320	2	10	8	°	2
A.M. Express grape jam	12	30	0	7	0	0	0	0	0	0	0	0
A.M. Express strawberry jam	12	30	0	8	0	0	5	0	0	0	0	0
Condiments/ Toppings												
Processed American cheese	25	90	6	0	8	25	420	0	6	°	15	°
Lettuce	21	0	0	0	0	0	0	0	°	°	°	°
Tomato	28	5	0	1	0	0	0	0	2	8	°	°
Onion	14	5	0	1	0	0	0	0	°	°	°	°
Pickles	14	0	0	0	0	0	140	0	0	0	0	0
Ketchup	14	15	0	4	0	0	180	0	4	°	°	°
Mustard	3	0	0	0	0	0	40	0	0	0	0	0
Mayonnaise	28	210	0	<1	23	20	160	0	°	°	°	°
Tartar sauce	28	180	0	0	19	15	220	0	°	°	°	°
Land O' Lakes whipped classic blend	10	65	0	0	7	0	75	0	8	°	°	°
Bull's Eye barbecue sauce	14	20	0	5	0	0	140	0	°	°	°	2
Bacon bits	3	15	1	0	1	5	0	0	°	°	°	°
Croutons	7	30	<1	4	1	0	75	0	°	°	°	°

BURGER KING—*continued*

Food Item	Serving Size (g)	kcal	Protein (g)	Total Carbohydrate (g)	Total Fat (g)	Cholesterol (mg)	Sodium (mg)	Dietary Fiber (g)	Percentage of U.S. RDA★			
									Vit A	Vit C	Ca	Fe
Burger King Salad Dressings												
Thousand Island dressing	30	140	0	7	12	15	190	<1	30	°	°	°
French dressing	30	140	0	11	10	0	190	0	15	°	°	°
Ranch dressing	30	180	<1	2	19	10	170	<1	°	°	°	°
Bleu cheese dressing	30	160	2	1	16	30	260	<1	°	°	°	°
Reduced calorie light Italian dressing#	30	15	0	3	0.5	0	50	0	°	°	°	°
Dipping Sauces												
A.M. Express dip	28	80	0	21	0	0	20	0	°	°	°	°
Honey dipping sauce	28	90	0	23	0	0	10	0	°	°	°	°
Ranch dipping sauce	28	170	0	2	17	0	200	0	°	°	°	°
Barbecue dipping sauce	28	35	0	9	0	0	400	0	2	2	°	°
Sweet & sour dipping sauce	28	45	0	11	0	0	50	0	°	°	°	°

Source: From Burger King Corporation, Miami, FL, 1996. For additional information, call 1-800-937-1800.

† = Without dressing   @ = Depends on the water supply   ° = Less than 2% of the U.S. RDA

★ = Values for vitamins A and C and minerals calcium and iron represent percent daily values based on a 2,000 calorie diet   # = Regular Italian dressing—150 calories—16 grams (g) Fat.

— = Negligible.

DAIRY QUEEN

Food Item	Serving Size (g)	Description	kcal	Protein (g)	Fat (g)	CHO (g)	Ca (mg)	Fe (mg)	Vitamin A (IU)	Vitamin C (mg)	Vitamin B₁ (mg)	Vitamin B₂ (mg)
Banana Split	383		540	9	11	103	—	—	—	—	—	—
Big Brazier	213	deluxe	470	28	24	36	111	5.2	—	<2.5	0.34	0.37
Big Brazier	184	regular	184	27	23	37	113	5.2	—	<2.0	0.37	0.39
Big Brazier	213	w/cheese	553	32	30	38	268	5.2	495	<2.3	0.34	0.53
Blizzard Banana Split	—	regular	763	—	—	—	—	—	—	—	—	—
Blizzard Banana Split	—	large	1333	—	—	—	—	—	—	—	—	—
Blizzard chocolate sandwich cookies	—	regular	600	—	—	—	—	—	—	—	—	—
Blizzard chocolate sandwich cookies	—	large	1050	—	—	—	—	—	—	—	—	—

DAIRY QUEEN—continued

Food Item	Serving Size (g)	Description	kcal	Protein (g)	Fat (g)	CHO (g)	Ca (mg)	Fe (mg)	Vitamin A (IU)	Vitamin C (mg)	Vitamin B₁ (mg)	Vitamin B₂ (mg)
Blizzard German chocolate	—	regular	794	—	—	—	—	—	—	—	—	—
Blizzard German chocolate	—	large	1460	—	—	—	—	—	—	—	—	—
Blizzard, Heath	—	regular	824	—	—	—	—	—	—	—	—	—
Blizzard, Heath	—	large	1212	—	—	—	—	—	—	—	—	—
Blizzard, M&M	—	regular	766	—	—	—	—	—	—	—	—	—
Blizzard, M&M	—	large	1154	—	—	—	—	—	—	—	—	—
Brazier cheese dog	113		330	15	19	24	168	1.6	—	—	—	0.18
Brazier chili dog	128		330	13	20	25	86	2.0	—	11.0	0.15	0.23
Brazier dog	99		273	11	15	23	75	1.5	—	11.0	0.12	0.15
Brazier french fries	71	regular	200	2	10	25	tr	0.4	tr	3.6	0.06	tr
Brazier french fries	113	large	320	3	16	40	tr	0.4	tr	4.8	0.09	0.03
Brazier onion rings	85		300	6	17	33	20	0.4	tr	2.4	0.09	tr
Brazier regular	106		260	13	9	28	70	3.5	—	<1.0	0.28	0.26
Brazier w/cheese	121		318	18	14	30	163	3.5	—	<1.2	0.29	0.29
Buster Bar	149		460	10	29	41	—	—	—	—	—	—
Chicken sandwich	220		670	29	41	46	—	—	—	—	—	—
Cone	213	large	340	9	10	57	—	—	—	—	—	—
Cone	142	regular	240	6	7	38	—	—	—	—	—	—
Cone	85	small	140	3	4	22	—	—	—	—	—	—
Dairy Queen Parfait	284		460	10	11	81	300	1.8	400	tr	0.12	0.43
Dilly Bar	85		240	4	15	22	100	0.4	100	tr	0.06	0.17
Dilly Bar	85		210	3	13	21	—	—	—	—	—	—
Dipped, cone	234	large	510	9	24	64	—	—	—	—	—	—
Dipped, cone	156	regular	340	6	16	42	—	—	—	—	—	—
Dipped, cone	92	small	190	3	9	25	—	—	—	—	—	—
Double Delight	255		490	9	20	69	—	—	—	—	—	—
Double hamburger	210		530	36	28	33	—	—	—	—	—	—
Double w/cheese	239		650	43	37	34	—	—	—	—	—	—
Chocolate dipped cone	234	large	450	10	20	58	300	0.4	400	tr	0.12	0.51
Chocolate dipped cone	156	medium	300	7	13	40	200	0.4	300	tr	0.09	0.34
Chocolate dipped cone	78	small	150	3	7	20	100	tr	100	tr	0.03	0.17
Chocolate malt	588	large	840	22	28	125	600	5.4	750	6.0	0.15	0.85
Chocolate malt	418	medium	600	15	20	89	500	3.6	750	3.6	0.12	0.60
Chocolate malt	241	small	340	10	11	51	300	1.8	400	2.4	0.06	0.34
Chocolate sundae	248	large	400	9	9	71	300	1.8	400	tr	0.09	0.43
Chocolate sundae	184	medium	300	6	7	53	200	1.1	300	tr	0.06	0.26

DAIRY QUEEN—continued

Food Item	Serving Size (g)	Description	kcal	Protein (g)	Fat (g)	CHO (g)	Ca (mg)	Fe (mg)	Vitamin A (IU)	Vitamin C (mg)	Vitamin B₁ (mg)	Vitamin B₂ (mg)
Chocolate sundae	106	small	170	4	4	30	100	0.7	100	tr	0.03	0.17
Cone	213	large	340	10	10	52	300	tr	400	tr	0.15	0.43
Cone	142	medium	230	6	7	35	200	tr	300	tr	0.09	0.26
Cone	71	small	110	3	3	18	100	tr	100	tr	0.03	0.14
Float	397		330	6	8	59	200	tr	100	tr	0.12	0.17
Freeze	397		520	11	13	89	300	tr	200	tr	0.15	0.34
Sandwich	60		140	3	4	24	60	0.4	100	tr	0.03	0.14
Fiesta sundae	269		570	9	22	84	200	tr	200	tr	0.23	0.26
Fish sandwich	170		400	20	17	41	60	1.1	tr	tr	0.15	0.26
Fish sandwich w/cheese	177		440	24	21	39	150	0.4	100	tr	0.15	0.26
Float	397		410	5	7	82	—	—	—	—	—	—
Freeze	397		500	9	12	89	—	—	—	—	—	—
French fries	71	regular	200	2	10	25	—	—	—	—	—	—
French fries	113	large	320	3	16	40	—	—	—	—	—	—
Frozen dessert	113		180	4	6	27	—	—	—	—	—	—
Hot dog	100		280	11	16	21	—	—	—	—	—	—
Hot dog w/cheese	114		330	15	21	21	—	—	—	—	—	—
Hot dog w/chili	128		320	13	20	23	—	—	—	—	—	—
Hot Fudge brownie delight	266		600	9	25	85	—	—	—	—	—	—
Malt	588	large	1060	20	25	187	—	—	—	—	—	—
Malt	418	regular	760	14	18	134	—	—	—	—	—	—
Malt	291	small	520	10	13	91	—	—	—	—	—	—
Mr. Misty	439	large	340	0	0	84	—	—	—	—	—	—
Mr. Misty	330	regular	250	0	0	63	—	—	—	—	—	—
Mr. Misty	248	small	190	0	0	48	—	—	—	—	—	—
Mr. Misty float	404		440	6	8	85	200	tr	120	tr	0.12	0.17
Mr. Misty float	411		390	5	7	74	—	—	—	—	—	—
Mr. Misty freeze	411		500	9	12	91	—	—	—	—	—	—
Mr. Misty Kiss	89		70	0	0	17	—	—	—	—	—	—
Onion rings	85		280	4	16	31	—	—	—	—	—	—
Parfait	283		430	8	8	76	—	—	—	—	—	—
Peanut Buster Parfait	305		740	16	34	94	—	—	—	—	—	—
Shake	588	large	990	19	26	168	—	—	—	—	—	—
Shake	418	regular	710	14	19	120	—	—	—	—	—	—
Shake	291	small	490	10	13	82	—	—	—	—	—	—
Single hamburger	148		360	21	16	33	—	—	—	—	—	—
Single w/cheese	162		410	24	20	33	—	—	—	—	—	—
Strawberry shortcake	312		540	10	11	100	—	—	—	—	—	—
Sundae	248	large	440	8	10	78	—	—	—	—	—	—
Sundae	177	regular	310	5	8	56	—	—	—	—	—	—
Sundae	106	small	190	3	4	33	—	—	—	—	—	—
Super Brazier	298		783	53	48	35	282	7.3	—	<3.2	0.39	0.69
Super Brazier chili dog	210		555	23	33	42	158	4.0	—	18.0	0.42	0.48

DAIRY QUEEN—*continued*

Food Item	Serving Size (g)	Description	kcal	Protein (g)	Fat (g)	CHO (g)	Ca (mg)	Fe (mg)	Vitamin A (IU)	Vitamin C (mg)	Vitamin B₁ (mg)	Vitamin B₂ (mg)
Super Brazier dog	182		518	20	30	41	158	4.3	tr	14.0	0.42	0.44
Super Brazier dog w/cheese	203		593	26	36	43	297	4.4	—	14.0	0.43	0.48
Super hot dog	175		520	17	27	44	—	—	—	—	—	—
Super hot dog w/cheese	196		580	22	34	45	—	—	—	—	—	—
Super hot dog w/chili	218		570	21	32	47	—	—	—	—	—	—
Triple hamburger	272		710	51	45	33	—	—	—	—	—	—
Triple w/cheese	301		820	58	50	34	—	—	—	—	—	—

Source: International Dairy Queen, Inc., Minneapolis, MN, 1982. Nutritional information reviewed and edited by Dr. David J. Aulik in cooperation with Raltech Scientific Services.

JACK IN THE BOX

Menu Item	Serving Size (g)	Calories (per serving)	Protein (g)	Fat (g)	Carbo-hydrates (g)	Percentage of U.S. RDA			
						Calcium	Iron	Vitamin A	Vitamin C
Sandwiches									
Beef Gyro	260	620	27	32	55	8	30	4	15
Chicken Fajita Pita	189	290	24	8	29	25	15	10	10
Chicken sandwich	160	400	20	18	38	15	10	4	0
Chicken supreme	245	620	25	36	48	20	15	10	4
Country fried steak sandwich	153	450	14	25	42	6	15	2	8
Fish supreme	245	590	22	32	51	20	20	10	8
Grilled chicken fillet	211	430	29	19	36	15	35	6	10
Smoked chicken cheddar & bacon	223	540	30	30	37	30	15	10	15
Sourdough ranch chicken sandwich	225	490	29	21	45	—	10	—	0
Spicy crispy chicken sandwich	224	560	24	27	55	10	15	4	8
Hamburgers									
Hamburger	97	280	13	11	31	10	15	2	2
Cheeseburger	110	330	16	15	32	20	15	6	2
Double cheeseburger	152	450	24	24	35	25	20	10	0
Jumbo Jack	229	560	26	32	41	10	25	4	10
Jumbo Jack with cheese	242	610	29	36	41	20	30	6	10
Bacon bacon cheeseburger	242	710	35	45	41	25	30	8	15
Grilled sourdough burger	223	670	32	43	39	20	25	15	10
Ultimate cheeseburger	280	830	47	57	33	30	35	15	0
¼ lb. burger	172	510	26	27	39	15	20	6	0
The Colossus burger	272	940	52	60	48	30	35	10	6
Teriyaki Bowls									
Chicken Teriyaki bowl	440	580	28	1.5	115	10	10	110	15
Beef Teriyaki bowl	440	580	28	3	124	15	25	100	10
Soy sauce	9	5	**	0	**	0	0	0	0

JACK IN THE BOX—*continued*

Menu Item	Serving Size (g)	Calories (per serving)	Protein (g)	Fat (g)	Carbo-hydrates (g)	Percentage of U.S. RDA			
						Calcium	Iron	Vitamin A	Vitamin C
Breakfast									
Breakfast Jack	121	300	18	12	30	20	15	8	15
Pancake platter	231	610	15	22	87	10	10	8	10
Sausage crescent	156	580	22	43	28	15	15	10	0
Scrambled egg platter	213	560	18	32	50	15	25	15	15
Scrambled egg pocket	183	430	29	21	31	20	20	20	0
Sourdough breakfast sandwich	147	380	21	20	31	25	20	15	15
Supreme crescent	153	530	23	33	34	15	20	15	20
Hash browns	57	160	1	11	14	0	2	0	10
Country Crock Spread	5	25	0	3	0	0	2	4	0
Grape jelly	14	40	0	0	9	0	0	0	0
Pancake syrup	42	120	0	0	30	0	0	0	0
Salads									
Chef salad	324	320	19	30	9	35	15	90	35
Taco salad	397	470	23	34	30	40	25	30	15
Side salad	111	50	3	7	°°	6	0	60	15
Bleu cheese dressing	70	260	22	°°	14	0	0	0	0
Buttermilk house dressing	70	360	36	°°	8	0	0	0	0
Low calorie Italian dressing	70	25	2	°°	2	0	0	0	0
Thousand Island dressing	70	310	30	°°	12	0	0	0	0
Mexican Food									
Taco	78	190	11	7	15	10	6	0	0
Super taco	126	280	17	12	22	15	10	0	4
Guacamole	25	50	4	°°	3	°	°	2	70
Salsa	28	10	0	0	2	°	°	2	°
Sides & Desserts									
Seasoned curly fries	109	360	5	20	39	2	8	0	8
Small french fries	68	220	3	11	28	0	4	0	30
Regular french fries	109	350	4	17	45	0	6	0	40
Jumbo fries	123	400	5	19	51	0	8	0	45
Onion rings	103	380	5	23	38	2	10	0	4
Sesame breadsticks	16	70	2	2	12	0	0	0	0
Tortilla chips	28	140	2	6	18	0	0	0	0
Hot apple turnover	110	350	3	19	48	0	10	0	15
Cheesecake	99	310	8	18	29	10	2	0	0
Chocolate chip cookie dough cheesecake	102	360	7	18	44	15	6	6	0
Cinamon Churritos	75	330	3	21	34	2	30	0	0
Finger Foods									
Egg rolls-3 piece	165	440	3	24	54	8	15	0	6
Egg rolls-5 piece	285	750	5	41	92	15	20	0	10
Chicken strips (breaded)-4 piece	112	290	25	13	18	0	4	0	0
Chicken strips (breaded)-6 piece	177	450	39	20	28	0	6	0	0
Chicken Taquitos-5 piece	136	350	19	15	34	15	10	4	2
Chicken Taquitos-8 piece	218	560	30	25	54	20	15	8	4
Barbeque sauce	28	45	1	0	11	0	0	0	0
Buttermilk house sauce	25	130	°°	13	3	0	°	0	2
Hot sauce	13	5	°°	0	1	0	0	0	0
Sweet & sour sauce	28	40	°°	0	11	0	0	0	0

JACK IN THE BOX—*continued*

Menu Item	Serving Size (g)	Calories (per serving)	Protein (g)	Fat (g)	Carbo-hydrates (g)	Percentage of U.S. RDA Calcium	Iron	Vitamin A	Vitamin C
Drinks									
Orange juice	183	80	1	0	20	2	2	8	160
Lowfat milk (2%)	244	120	8	5	12	30	0	10	4
Vanilla milk shake (regular)	304	350	9	7	62	30	0	0	0
Chocolate milk shake (regular)	322	330	11	7	59	35	4	0	0
Strawberry milk shake (regular)	298	330	9	7	60	30	0	0	0
Iced tea (small)	16	0	0	0	0	0	0	0	0
Coffee (small)	8	5	0	0	1	0	0	0	0

Source: Jack In The Box; nutritional information provided by Foodmaker, Inc., San Diego, CA.

KENTUCKY FRIED CHICKEN

Food Item	Serving Size (g)	kcal	Protein (g)	CHO (g)	Fat (g)	Cholesterol (mg)	Vit A (mg)	Vit C (mg)	Thia (mg)	Ribo (mg)	Nia (mg)	Ca (mg)	Fe (mg)
Original Recipe Chicken													
Wing	55	178	12.2	6.0	11.7	64	<100	<1.0	0.03	0.08	3.7	47.9	1.2
Side breast	90	267	18.8	10.8	16.5	77	<100	<1.0	0.06	0.13	6.9	68.0	1.2
Center breast	115	283	27.5	8.8	15.3	93	<100	<1.0	0.09	0.17	11.5	68.0	1.0
Drumstick	57	146	13.1	4.2	8.5	67	<100	<1.0	0.05	0.12	3.2	21.2	1.1
Thigh	104	294	17.9	11.1	19.7	123	104	<1.0	0.08	0.30	5.5	65.1	1.3
Extra Tasty Crispy Chicken													
Wing	65	254	12.4	9.3	18.6	67	<100	<1.0	0.04	0.06	3.3	17.8	0.6
Side breast	110	343	21.7	14.0	22.3	81	<100	<1.0	0.09	0.10	8.5	30.4	0.8
Center breast	135	342	33.0	11.7	19.7	114	<100	<1.0	0.11	0.13	13.1	33.3	0.8
Drumstick	69	204	13.6	6.1	13.9	71	<100	<1.0	0.06	0.12	3.7	12.9	0.7
Thigh	119	406	20.0	14.4	29.8	129	131	<1.0	0.10	0.21	6.5	49.0	1.2
Kentucky Nuggets	16	46	2.8	2.2	2.9	11.9	<100	<1.0	<0.01	0.03	1.00	2.4	0.1
Barbeque sauce	28.3	35	0.3	7.1	0.6	<1.0	<370	<1.0	<0.01	0.01	0.19	6.1	0.2
Sweet 'n sour	28.3	58	0.1	13.0	0.6	<1.0	<100	<1.0	<.01	0.02	0.04	4.7	0.2
Honey	14.2	49	0.0	12.1	<0.01	<1.0	<100	<1.0	<0.01	0.00	0.04	0.6	0.1
Mustard	28.3	36	0.9	6.1	0.9	<1.0	<100	<1.0	<0.01	0.01	0.16	10.2	0.3
Chicken Littles	47	169	5.7	13.8	10.1	18	<100	<1.0	0.16	0.12	2.2	22.6	1.7
Buttermilk biscuits	65	235	4.5	28.0	11.7	1	<100	<1.0	0.24	0.19	2.6	95.0	1.6
Mashed potatoes w/gravy	98	71	2.4	11.7	1.6	<1	<100	<1.0	<0.01	0.04	1.2	21.8	0.04
French fries	77	244	3.2	31.1	11.9	2	<100	15.7	0.15	0.05	2.0	12.5	0.06
Corn on the cob	143	176	5.1	31.9	3.1	<1	272	2.3	0.14	0.11	1.8	7.2	0.08
Cole slaw	91	119	1.5	13.2	6.6	5	310	21.5	0.03	0.03	0.2	32.8	0.02
Colonel's Chicken sandwich	166	482	20.8	38.6	27.3	47	<100	<1.0	0.38	0.27	11.1	46.1	1.3

Source: Public Affairs Department, KFC Corporation, Louisville, KY.

LONG JOHN SILVER'S

Food Item	Serving Size (g)	Description	kcal	Protein (g)	Fat (g)	CHO (g)
3 Pc. Nugget dinner		6 chicken nuggets, Fryes, slaw	699	23	45	54
Apple pie	113		280	2	11	43
Barbecue sauce	34		45	0	0	11
Battered shrimp dinner		6 battered shrimp, Fryes, slaw	771	17	45	60
Bleu cheese dressing	45		225	4	23	3
Breaded clams			465	13	25	46
Breaded fish sandwich platter		Fish sandwich, Fryes, slaw	835	30	42	84
Breaded oysters		6 pieces	460	14	19	58
Breaded shrimp platter		Breaded shrimp, Fryes, slaw, 2 hush puppies	962	20	57	93
Cherry pie	113		294	3	11	46
Chicken planks		4 pieces	458	27	23	35
Clam chowder	187		128	7	5	15
Clam dinner		Clams, Fryes, slaw	955	22	58	100
Cole slaw			138	1	8	16
Cole slaw, drained on fork	98		182	1	15	11
Combo salad		4.25 oz. seafood salad, 2 oz salad shrimp, 6 oz lettuce, 2.4 oz tomato, 1 pkg crackers	397	27	29	21
Corn on the cob	150	1 ear	176	5	4	29
Fish & Chicken		1 fish, 2 tender chicken planks, Fryes, slaw	935	36	55	73
Fish & Fryes		3 fish, Fryes	853	43	48	64
Fish & Fryes		2 pc fish, Fryes	651	30	36	53
Fish & More		2 fish, Fryes, slaw, 2 hush puppies	978	34	58	92
Fish w/batter		2 pieces	319	19	19	19
Fish w/batter		3 pieces	477	28	28	28
Four nuggets and Fryes			427	16	24	39
Fryes	85		247	4	12	31
Fryes			275	4	15	32
Honey-Mustard sauce	35		56	—	—	14
Hush Puppies	47	2 pieces	145	3	7	18
Hush Puppies		3 pieces	158	1	7	20
Kitchen–breaded fish (three piece dinner)		3 kitchen breaded fish, Fryes, slaw, 2 hush puppies	940	35	52	84

LONG JOHN SILVER'S—*continued*

Food Item	Serving Size (g)	Description	kcal	Protein (g)	Fat (g)	CHO (g)
Kitchen–breaded (two piece dinner)		2 kitchen-breaded fish, Fryes, slaw, 2 hush puppies	818	26	46	76
Lemon Meringue pie	99		200	2	6	37
Ocean chef salad		6 oz lettuce, 1.25 oz shrimp, 2 oz seafood blend, 2 tomato wedges, ¾ oz cheese	229	27	8	13
Ocean scallops		6 pieces	257	10	12	27
One fish and Fryes			449	16	24	42
One fish, two nuggets, and Fryes			539	23	30	46
Oyster dinner		6 oysters, Fryes, slaw	789	17	45	78
Pecan pie	113		446	5	22	59
Peg leg w/batter		5 pieces 514	25	33	30	
Pumpkin pie	113		251	4	11	34
Reduced calorie Italian dressing	49		20	0	1	3
Scallop dinner		6 scallops, Fryes,	747	17	45	66
Sea salad dressing	45		220	4	21	5
Seafood platter shrimp, 2 scallops, Fryes, slaw		1 fish, 2 battered	976	29	58	85
Seafood salad		5.6 oz seafood salad, 6 oz lettuce, 2.4 oz tomato	426	19	30	22
Shrimp & Fish dinner		1 fish, 3 battered shrimp, Fryes, slaw, 2 hush puppies	917	27	55	80
Shrimp salad shrimp, 6 oz lettuce, 2.4 oz tomato		4.5 oz salad	203	28	3	16
Shrimp w/batter		5 pieces	269	9	13	31
Sweet-n-sour sauce	30		—	—	—	—
Tartar sauce	30		117	—	11	5
Tender chicken plank dinner		3 chicken planks, Fryes, slaw	885	32	51	72
Tender chicken plank dinner		4 chicken planks, Fryes, slaw	1037	41	59	82
Thousand Island dressing	48		223	—	22	8

LONG JOHN SILVER'S—continued

Food Item	Serving Size (g)	Description	kcal	Protein (g)	Fat (g)	CHO (g)
Three piece fish dinner		3 fish, Fryes, slaw, 2 hush puppies	1180	47	70	93
Treasure chest		2 pc fish, 2 peg legs	467	25	29	27
Two planks and Fryes			551	22	28	51

Source: Long John Silver's Seafood Shoppes; sampling and nutrient analysis conducted independently by the Department of Nutrition and Food Science, University of Kentucky, April 10, 1986.

MCDONALD'S

Menu Item	Serving Size	Calories	Protein (g)	Carbo-hydrates (g)	Total Fat (g)	Choles-terol (mg)	Sodium (mg)	Dietary Fiber (g)	Percentage of U.S. RDA			
									Vitamin A	Vitamin C	Calcium	Iron
Sandwiches												
Hamburger	160 g	270	12	34	10	30	520	2	2	4	15	15
Cheeseburger	120 g	320	15	35	14	45	750	2	6	4	15	15
Quarter Pounder	172 g	420	23	37	21	70	690	2	4	4	15	25
Quarter Pounder with cheese	200 g	530	28	38	30	95	1160	2	10	4	15	25
McLean deluxe	214 g	350	24	38	12	60	800	3	8	15	15	25
McLean deluxe with cheese	228 g	400	27	39	17	70	1040	3	10	15	15	25
Big Mac	216 g	530	25	47	28	80	960	3	6	4	20	25
Filet-O-Fish	143 g	360	14	40	16	35	690	2	2	°	10	10
McGrilled chicken Classic	189 g	260	24	33	4	45	500	2	4	8	10	10
McChicken sandwich	190 g	510	17	44	30	50	820	2	2	2	15	15
French Fries												
Small French fries	68 g	210	3	26	10	0	135	2	°	15	°	2
Large French fries	147 g	450	6	57	22	0	290	5	°	30	2	6
Super Size French fries	176 g	540	8	68	26	0	350	6	°	35	2	8
Chicken McNuggets/Sauce												
Chicken McNuggets (4 piece)	73 g	200	12	10	12	40	350	0	°	°	°	4
Chicken McNuggets (6 piece)	109 g	300	19	16	18	65	530	0	°	°	2	6
Chicken McNuggets (9 piece)	165 g	450	28	24	27	95	800	0	°	°	2	8
Hot Mustard (1 pkg)	28 g	60	1	7	3.5	5	240	<1	°	°	°	4
Barbeque sauce (1 pkg)	28 g	45	0	10	0	0	250	0	°	6	°	°
Sweet 'n sour sauce (1 pkg)	28 g	50	0	11	0	0	140	0	6	°	°	°
Honey (1 pkg)	14 g	45	0	12	0	0	0	0	°	°	°	°
Honey mustard (1 pkg)	14 g	50	0	3	4.5	10	85	0	°	°	°	°
Salads												
Chef salad	313 g	210	19	9	11	180	730	2	90	35	16	10
Fajita chicken salad	285 g	160	20	9	6	65	400	3	160	50	4	10

MCDONALD'S—continued

Menu Item	Serving Size	Calories	Pro-tein (g)	Carbo-hydrate (g)	Total Fat (g)	Choles-terol (mg)	Sodium (mg)	Dietary Fiber (g)	Vitamin A	Vitamin C	Calcium	Iron
Salads—cont'd												
Garden salad	234 g	80	6	7	4	140	60	2	60	35	6	8
Side salad	139 g	45	3	4	2	70	35	1	50	20	4	4
Croutons (1 pkg)	11 g	50	1	7	1.5	0	125	0	°	°	2	2
Bacon bits (1 pkg)	3 g	15	1	0	1	5	90	0	°	°	°	°
Salad Dressings												
Bleu cheese (1 pkg)	60 g	190	2	8	17	30	650	0	2	°	6	2
Ranch (1 pkg)	60 g	230	1	10	21	20	550	0	°	2	4	°
1000 Island	63 g	190	1	16	13	25	510	1	2	2	2	2
Lite Vinaigrette (1 pkg)	62 g	50	0	9	2	0	240	0	6	6	°	°
Red French reduced calorie (1 pkg)	68 g	160	0	23	8	0	490	0	4	6	°	°
Breakfast												
Egg McMuffin	137 g	290	17	27	13	235	730	1	10	2	15	15
Sausage McMuffin	112 g	360	13	26	23	45	750	1	4	°	15	10
Sausage McMuffin with Egg	163 g	440	19	27	29	255	820	1	10	°	15	15
English muffin	55 g	140	4	25	2	0	220	1	°	°	10	8
Sausage biscuit	119 g	430	10	32	29	35	1130	1	°	°	8	15
Sausage biscuit with egg	170 g	520	16	33	35	245	1220	1	6	°	10	15
Bacon, egg & cheese biscuit	152 g	450	17	33	27	240	1340	1	10	°	10	15
Biscuit	76 g	260	4	32	13	0	840	1	°	°	6	10
Sausage	43 g	170	6	0	16	35	290	0	°	°	°	2
Scrambled eggs (2)	102 g	170	13	1	12	425	190	0	10	°	6	6
Hash browns	53 g	130	1	14	8	0	330	1	°	4	°	2
Hotcakes (plain)	150 g	310	9	53	7	15	610	2	°	°	10	15
Hotcakes (margarine 2 pats & syrup)	222 g	580	9	100	16	15	760	2	8	°	10	15
Cheerios (1 pkg)	19 g	70	2	15	1	0	180	2	15	15	2	25
Wheaties (1 pkg)	23 g	80	2	18	0.5	0	160	2	15	15	4	30
Muffins/Danish												
Fat free apple bran muffin	70 g	170	4	38	0	0	200	1	°	°	4	6
Apple danish	105 g	360	5	51	16	40	290	1	10	°	8	6
Cheese danish	105 g	410	7	47	22	70	340	0	15	°	8	6
Cinnamon Raisin danish	105 g	430	5	56	22	50	280	1	10	°	10	8
Raspberry danish	105 g	400	5	58	16	45	300	1	10	°	8	6
Desserts/Shakes												
Vanilla lowfat frozen yogurt cone	90 g	120	4	24	0.5	5	85	0	°	2	15	2
Strawberry lowfat frozen yogurt sundae	178 g	240	6	51	1	5	115	1	°	2	20	2
Hot caramel lowfat frozen yogurt sundae	182 g	310	7	63	3	5	200	1	2	2	25	°
Hot fudge sundae	179 g	290	8	54	5	5	190	2	°	2	25	4
Nuts (sundaes)	7 g	40	2	2	3.5	0	0	0	°	°	°	°
Baked apple pie	77 g	260	3	34	13	0	200	<1	°	40	2	6
McDonaldland cookies (1 pkg)	56 g	260	4	41	9	0	270	1	°	°	°	10
Vanilla shake—small	414 mL	340	11	62	5	25	220	0	4	6	40	2

MCDONALD'S—*continued*

Menu Item	Serving Size	Calories	Pro-tein (g)	Carbo-hydrate (g)	Total Fat (g)	Choles-terol (mg)	Sodium (mg)	Dietary Fiber (g)	Percentage of U.S. RDA			
									Vitamin A	Vitamin C	Calcium	Iron
Desserts/Shakes—*continued*												
Chocolate shake—small	414 mL	340	12	64	5	25	300	1	4	6	45	4
Strawberry shake—small	414 mL	340	12	63	5	25	220	0	4	10	40	4
Milk/Juices												
1% lowfat milk (8 fl oz)	1 crtn.	100	8	13	2.5	10	115	0	10	4	30	°
Orange juice (6 fl oz)	177 mL	80	1	20	0	0	20	0	2	90	2	2
Apple juice (6 fl oz)	177 mL	80	0	20	0	0	0	0	°	°	°	2

Source: McDonald's Corporation. Oak Brook, IL 60521. (708) 575-3663. 1996.

° = less than 2% of the U.S. RDA

PIZZA HUT

Food Item (1 slice)	kcal	Protein (g)	Fat (g)	CHO (g)	Ca (mg)	Fe (mg)	Vitamin A (IU)	Vitamin C (mg)	Vitamin B_1 (mg)	Vitamin B_2 (mg)
Thick 'n' chewy, beef	620	38	20	73	400	7.2	750	<1.2	0.68	0.60
Thick 'n' chewy, cheese	560	34	14	71	500	5.4	1000	<1.2	0.68	0.68
Thick 'n' chewy, pepperoni	560	31	18	68	400	5.4	1250	3.6	0.68	0.68
Thick 'n' chewy, pork	640	36	23	71	400	7.2	750	1.2	0.90	0.77
Thick 'n' chewy, supreme	640	36	22	74	400	7.2	1000	9.0	0.75	0.85
Thick 'n' crispy, beef	490	29	19	51	350	6.3	750	<1.2	0.30	0.60
Thick 'n' crispy, cheese	450	25	15	54	450	4.5	750	<1.2	0.30	0.51
Thick 'n' crispy, pepperoni	430	23	17	45	300	4.5	1000	<1.2	0.30	0.51
Thick 'n' crispy, pork	520	27	23	51	350	6.3	1000	<1.2	0.38	0.68
Thick 'n' crispy, supreme	510	27	21	51	350	7.2	1250	2.4	0.38	0.68

Source: Research 900 and Pizza Hut, Inc., Wichita, KS.

ROY ROGERS

Food Item	Serving Size (g)	kcal	Protein (g)	Fat (g)	CHO (g)
Apple danish	71	249	4.5	11.6	31.6
Bacon cheeseburger	180	581	32.3	39.2	25.0
Biscuit	63	231	4.4	12.1	26.2
Breakfast crescent sandwich	127	401	13.3	27.3	25.3
Breakfast crescent sandwich w/bacon	133	431	15.4	29.7	25.5
Breakfast crescent sandwich w/ham	165	557	19.8	41.7	25.3
Breakfast crescent sandwich w/sausage	162	449	19.9	29.4	25.9
Breast & wing	196	604	43.5	36.5	25.4

ROY ROGERS—*continued*

Food Item	Serving Size (g)	kcal	Protein (g)	Fat (g)	CHO (g)
Brownie	64	264	3.3	11.4	37.3
Caramel sundae	145	293	7.0	8.5	51.5
Cheese danish	71	254	4.9	12.2	31.4
Cheeseburger	173	563	29.5	37.3	27.4
Cherry danish	71	271	4.4	14.4	31.7
Chicken breast	144	412	33.0	23.7	16.9
Chocolate shake	319	358	7.9	10.2	61.3
Cole slaw	99	110	1.0	6.9	11.0
Crescent roll	70	287	4.7	17.7	27.2
Egg and biscuit platter	165	394	16.9	26.5	21.9
Egg and biscuit platter w/bacon	173	435	19.7	29.6	22.1
Egg and biscuit platter w/ham	200	442	23.5	28.6	22.5
Egg and biscuit platter w/sausage	203	550	23.4	40.9	21.9
French fries	85	268	3.9	13.5	32.0
Hamburger	143	456	23.8	28.3	65.6
Hot chocolate	8 oz	123	3.0	2.0	22.0
Hot fudge sundae	151	337	6.5	12.5	53.3
Hot topped potato plain	227	211	5.9	0.2	47.9
Hot topped potato w/bacon 'n cheese	248	397	17.1	21.7	33.3
Hot topped potato w/broccoli 'n cheese	312	376	13.7	18.1	39.6
Hot topped potato w/oleo	236	274	5.9	7.3	47.9
Hot topped potato w/sour cream 'n chives	297	408	7.3	20.9	47.6
Hot topped potato w/taco beef 'n cheese	359	463	21.8	21.8	45.0
Large fries	113	357	5.3	18.4	42.7
Large roast beef	182	360	33.9	11.9	29.6
Large roast beef w/cheese	211	467	39.6	20.9	30.3
Leg	53	140	11.5	8.0	5.5
Macaroni	100	186	3.1	10.7	19.4
Milk	8 oz	150	8.0	8.2	11.4
Orange juice	8 oz	99	1.5	0.2	22.8
Orange juice	8 oz	136	2.0	0.3	31.3
Pancake platter (w/syrup, butter)	165	452	7.7	15.2	71.8
Pancake platter (w/syrup, butter) w/bacon	173	493	10.4	18.3	72.0
Pancake platter (w/syrup, butter) w/ham	200	506	14.3	17.3	72.4

ROY ROGERS—*continued*

Food Item	Serving Size (g)	kcal	Protein (g)	Fat (g)	CHO (g)
Pancake platter (w/syrup, butter) w/sausage	203	608	14.2	29.6	71.8
Potato salad	100	107	2.0	6.1	10.9
Roast beef sandwich	154	317	27.2	10.2	29.1
Roast beef sandwich w/cheese	182	424	32.9	19.2	29.9
RR bar burger	208	611	36.1	39.4	28.0
Salad bar 1,000 Island	2 T	160	NA	16.0	4.0
Salad bar bacon 'n tomato	2 T	136	NA	12.0	6.0
Salad bar bacon bits	1 T	24	4.0	1.0	38.0
Salad bar blue cheese dressing	2 T	150	2.0	16.0	2.0
Salad bar cheddar cheese	¼ cup	112	5.8	9.0	0.8
Salad bar Chinese noodles	¼ cup	55	1.5	2.8	6.5
Salad bar chopped eggs	2 T	55	4.0	4.0	0.7
Salad bar croutons	2 T	132	5.5	0	31.0
Salad bar cucumbers	5–6 slices	4	NA	0	1.0
Salad bar green peas	¼ cup	7	0.5	0	1.2
Salad bar green peppers	2 T	4	0.3	0	1.0
Salad bar lettuce	1 cup	10	NA	0	4.0
Salad bar lo-cal Italian	2 T	70	NA	6.0	2.0
Salad bar macaroni salad	2 T	60	1.0	3.6	6.2
Salad bar mushrooms	¼ cup	5	0.5	0	0.7
Salad bar potato salad	2 T	50	1.0	3.0	5.5
Salad bar ranch	2 T	155	NA	14.0	4.0
Salad bar shredded carrots	¼ cup	12	0.6	0	24.0
Salad bar sliced beets	¼ cup	16	0.5	0	3.8
Salad bar sunflower seeds	2 T	101	4.0	9.0	5.0
Salad bar tomatoes	3 slices	20	0.8	0	4.8
Strawberry shake	312	315	7.6	10.2	49.4
Strawberry shortcake	205	447	10.1	19.2	59.3
Strawberry sundae	142	216	5.7	7.1	33.1
Thigh	98	296	18.4	19.5	11.7
Thigh & leg	151	436	29.9	27.5	17.2
Vanilla shake	306	306	8.0	10.7	45.0
Wing	52	192	10.5	12.8	8.5

Source: Roy Rogers Restaurants, Marriott Corporation, Washington, DC. Nutritional data furnished by Lancaster Laboratories, 1985.

TACO BELL

Food Item	kcal	Protein (g)	Fat (g)	Calories From Fat	Saturated Fat	Cholesterol (mg)	Na (mg)	Percent U.S. RDA Ca	Fe
Tacos & Tostadas									
Chicken soft taco	223	14	10	90	4	58	553	6	8
Soft taco	223	12	11	100	5	32	539	5	10
Soft taco supreme	268	13	15	140	8	47	551	8	11
Steak soft taco	217	12	9	80	4	31	569	5	6
Taco	180	10	11	100	5	32	276	8	5
Taco supreme	225	11	15	130	7	47	287	10	6
Tostada	242	9	11	100	4	14	593	17	8
Burritos									
7 layer burrito	485	15	21	190	8	28	1115	25	25
Bean burrito	391	13	12	110	4	5	1138	19	20
Beef burrito	432	22	19	170	8	57	1303	16	22
Big beef burrito supreme	525	25	25	220	11	72	1418	20	25
Burrito supreme	443	18	19	170	9	47	1184	20	21
Chicken burrito	345	17	13	110	5	57	854	14	14
Chicken burrito supreme	520	27	23	200	9	125	1130	15	50
Chili cheese burrito	391	17	18	160	9	47	980	30	17
Combo burrito	412	17	16	140	6	32	1221	17	21
Steak burrito supreme	500	26	23	200	11	75	1350	20	15
Specialty Items									
Beef MexiMelt	262	13	14	130	7	38	711	23	8
Cinnamon twists	139	1	6	50	0	0	189	°	2
Mexican pizza	574	19	38	340	12	50	1003	31	25
Nachos	345	7	18	160	6	9	398	23	4
Nachos BellGrande	633	22	34	300	12	49	952	36	20
Nachos supreme	364	12	18	160	5	17	470	19	15
Pintos 'n cheese	190	9	9	80	4	14	640	15	7
Taco salad	838	31	55	490	16	79	1132	25	34
Side Orders & Condiments									
Green sauce	4	0	0	0	0	0	136	°	°
Guacamole	36	0	3	30	1	0	132	4	°
Hot taco sauce	2	0	0	0	0	0	91	°	°
Milk taco sauce	0	0	0	0	0	0	6	°	°
Nacho cheese sauce	51	2	4	40	2	4	196	6	°
Picante sauce	3	0	0	0	0	0	132	2	0
Pico de Gallo	6	0	0	0	0	0	65	°	°
Ranch dressing	136	1	14	130	3	20	330	2	°
Red sauce	10	0	0	0	0	0	261	°	°
Salsa	27	1	0	0	0	0	709	5	3
Seasoned rice	110	2	3	30	1	5	230	°	8
Sour cream	44	1	4	40	3	15	11	2	°

Source: Taco Bell Corporation, Irvine, CA. 1996.

° = trace

WENDY'S

Food Item	Serving Size (g)	kcal	Protein (g)	CHO (g)	Fat (g)	Cholesterol (mg)	Percentage of U.S. RDA						
							Vit A (mg)	Vit C (mg)	Thia (mg)	Ribo (mg)	Nia (mg)	Ca (mg)	Fe (mg)
Sandwiches													
½ lb. hamburger patty	74	180	19	—	12	65	—	—	4	—	20	—	20
Plain single	126	340	24	30	15	65	—	—	25	20	30	10	30
Single with everything	210	420	25	35	21	70	5	15	25	20	30	10	30
Wendy's Big Classic	260	570	27	47	33	90	10	20	30	25	35	15	35
Jr. Hamburger	111	260	15	33	9	34	2	4	25	20	20	10	20
Jr. cheeseburger	125	310	18	33	13	34	2	4	25	50	20	10	20
Jr. bacon cheeseburger	155	430	22	32	25	50	2	15	30	50	25	10	20
Jr. Swiss deluxe	163	360	18	34	18	40	4	10	25	60	20	20	20
Kids' meal hamburger	104	260	15	32	9	35	2	2	25	20	20	10	20
Kids' meal cheeseburger	116	300	18	33	13	35	2	2	25	50	20	10	20
Grilled chicken fillet	70	100	18	—	3	55	—	—	4	4	35	—	6
Grilled chicken sandwich	175	340	24	36	13	60	2	8	30	25	50	10	20
Chicken breast fillet	99	220	21	11	10	55	—	—	8	8	60	—	70
Chicken sandwich	219	430	26	41	19	60	2	8	30	25	70	10	80
Chicken club sandwich	205	506	30	42	25	70	2	15	35	30	80	10	80
Fish fillet sandwich	170	460	18	42	25	55	2	2	40	35	20	10	15
Kaiser bun	65	200	6	37	3	10	—	—	25	20	10	10	10
White bun	56	160	5	30	3	tr	—	—	20	20	10	10	10
Sandwich Toppings													
American cheese slice	18	70	4	—	6	15	6	—	—	4	—	12	—
Bacon	6	30	2	—	3	5	—	4	4	—	2	—	—
Ketchup	14	17	—	4	—	NA	4	4	—	—	—	—	—
Lettuce	10	1	—	—	—	0	—	—	—	—	—	—	—
Mayonnaise	13	90	—	—	10	10	—	—	—	—	—	—	—
Mustard	5	4	—	—	—	0	—	—	—	—	—	—	—
Onion	10	4	—	—	—	0	—	—	—	—	—	—	—
Pickles	14	2	—	—	—	0	—	—	—	—	—	—	—
Tomatoes	21	4	—	—	—	0	—	6	—	—	—	—	—
Honey mustard	14	71	—	4	6	5	—	—	—	—	—	—	—
Tartar sauce	21	120	—	—	14	15	—	—	15	10	—	—	—
Superbar—Pasta													
Alfredo sauce	56	35	1	5	1	tr	—	—	—	—	—	6	—
Fettucini	56	190	4	27	3	10	—	—	10	6	6	—	6
Garlic toast	18.3	70	2	9	3	tr	4	—	6	2	2	2	2
Pasta medley	56	60	2	9	2	tr	6	15	6	4	4	—	4
Rotini	56	90	3	15	2	tr	—	—	6	4	6	—	4
Spaghetti sauce	56	28	—	7	0	tr	—	—	—	—	—	—	—
Spaghetti meat sauce	56	60	4	8	2	10	4	4	—	2	4	—	4
Garden Spot Salad Bar													
Alfalfa sprouts	28	8	1	1	0	0	—	4	—	2	—	—	—
Applesauce, chunky	28	22	—	6	—	0	—	—	—	—	—	—	—
Bacon bits	14	40	5	—	14	10	—	2	6	4	6	—	—
Bananas	28	26	—	7	—	0	—	4	—	2	—	—	—
Breadsticks	7.5	30	1	5	1	0	—	—	2	2	2	2	2
Broccoli	43	12	1	2	0	0	6	65	2	2	—	2	2
Cantaloupe	57	20	—	5	0	0	20	30	—	—	—	—	—
Carrots	27	12	—	2	0	0	80	4	2	—	—	—	—
Cauliflower	57	14	1	3	0	0	—	70	4	2	2	2	2
Cheddar chips	28	160	3	12	12	5	—	—	2	—	4	6	2
Cheese, shredded (imitation)	28	90	6	1	6	tr	4	—	—	15	—	20	—
Chicken salad	56	120	7	4	8	tr	—	4	—	4	6	—	2
Chives	28	71	6	18	1	0	195	313	15	25	8	25	30
Chow mein noodles	14	74	1	8	4	0	—	—	6	4	4	—	4

WENDY'S—continued

Food Item	Serving Size (g)	kcal	Protein (g)	CHO (g)	Fat (g)	Cholesterol (mg)	Percentage of U.S. RDA Vit A (mg)	Vit C (mg)	Thia (mg)	Ribo (mg)	Nia (mg)	Ca (mg)	Fe (mg)
Garden Spot Salad Bar—continued													
Cole slaw	57	70	—	8	5	5	4	25	—	—	—	2	—
Cottage cheese	105	108	13	3	4	15	6	—	—	10	—	6	—
Croutons	14	60	2	8	3	—	—	—	4	4	4	—	4
Cucumbers	14	2	—	—	0	0	—	—	—	—	—	—	—
Eggs (hard cooked)	20	30	3	—	2	90	4	—	—	6	—	—	—
Garbanzo beans	28	46	3	8	1	0	—	—	2	—	—	—	6
Green peas	28	21	1	4	0	0	4	8	6	2	—	—	2
Green peppers	37	10	—	2	0	0	2	60	2	—	—	—	—
Honeydew melon	57	20	—	5	0	0	—	25	2	—	2	—	—
Jalapeno peppers	14	2	—	—	0	0	—	—	—	—	—	—	—
Lettuce—iceberg	55	8	—	1	0	0	2	4	2	—	—	—	2
Lettuce—romaine	55	9	1	1	0	0	15	20	4	4	—	2	4
Mushrooms	17	4	—	—	0	0	—	—	—	4	4	—	—
Olives, black	28	35	—	2	3	0	—	—	—	—	—	2	4
Oranges	56	26	—	7	0	0	—	50	4	—	—	2	—
Parmesan cheese	28	130	12	1	9	20	6	—	—	6	—	40	—
Parmesan cheese (imitation)	28	80	9	4	3	tr	20	—	—	—	—	50	—
Pasta salad	57	35	2	6	—	0	—	—	—	2	2	—	2
Peaches	57	31	—	8	0	0	2	2	—	—	2	—	—
Pepperoni, sliced	28	140	5	2	12	35	—	—	160	4	10	—	2
Pineapple chunks	100	60	—	16	0	0	—	15	6	—	—	—	2
Potato salad	57	125	—	6	11	10	—	10	2	—	2	—	2
Pudding—butterscotch	57	90	1	11	4	tr	—	—	—	—	—	6	2
Pudding—chocolate	57	90	—	12	4	tr	—	—	2	2	—	15	2
Red onions	9	2	—	—	0	0	—	—	—	—	—	—	—
Red peppers, crushed	28	120	5	15	4	0	200	15	10	15	20	2	15
Seafood salad	56	110	4	7	7	tr	—	2	—	2	—	20	2
Strawberries	56	17	—	4	0	0	—	50	—	2	—	—	—
Sour topping	28	58	—	2	5	0	—	—	—	—	—	—	—
Sunflower seeds & raisins	28	140	5	6	10	0	—	—	30	4	6	2	10
Three bean salad	57	60	1	13	—	—	4	—	—	—	—	—	2
Tomatoes	28	6	—	1	0	0	2	10	—	—	—	—	—
Tuna salad	56	100	8	4	6	tr	—	4	—	4	25	—	2
Turkey ham	28	35	5	—	1	15	—	—	—	4	6	—	4
Watermelon	57	18	—	4	0	0	2	10	4	—	—	—	—
Salad Dressings													
Blue cheese	15	9	—	—	10	10	—	—	—	—	—	—	—
Celery seed	15	70	—	3	6	5	—	—	—	—	—	—	—
French	15	60	—	4	6	0	—	—	—	—	—	—	—
French, sweet red	15	70	—	5	6	0	—	—	—	—	—	—	—
Hidden Valley ranch	15	50	—	—	6	5	—	—	—	—	—	—	—
Italian Caesar	15	80	—	—	9	5	—	—	—	—	—	—	—
Italian, golden	15	45	—	3	4	0	—	—	—	—	—	—	—
Salad oil	28	250	0	0	28	0	—	—	—	—	—	—	—
Thousand island	15	70	—	2	7	5	—	—	—	—	—	—	—
Wine, vinegar	15	2	—	—	0	0	—	—	—	—	—	—	—
Red. Cal. bacon & tomato	15	45	—	3	4	—	—	—	—	—	—	—	—
Reduced calorie Italian	15	25	—	2	2	0	—	—	—	—	—	—	—
Prepared Salads													
Chef salad	331	180	15	10	9	120	110	110	15	25	6	25	15
Garden salad	277	102	7	9	5	0	110	110	10	20	6	20	10
Taco salad	791	660	40	46	37	35	80	80	30	45	25	80	35

WENDY'S—*continued*

Food Item	Serving Size (g)	kcal	Protein (g)	CHO (g)	Fat (g)	Cholesterol (mg)	Percentage of U.S. RDA						
							Vit A (mg)	Vit C (mg)	Thia (mg)	Ribo (mg)	Nia (mg)	Ca (mg)	Fe (mg)
Superbar—Mexican Fiesta (where available)													
Cheese sauce	56	39	1	5	2	tr	—	—	—	—	—	6	—
Picante sauce	56	18	—	4	—	NA	10	30	2	—	2	—	2
Refried beans	56	70	4	10	3	tr	—	—	4	2	—	2	6
Rice, Spanish	56	70	2	13	1	tr	6	—	45	—	8	4	10
Taco chips	40	260	4	40	10	0	—	—	2	4	—	8	4
Taco meat	56	110	10	4	7	25	—	—	8	6	10	4	10
Taco sauce	28	16	—	3	—	tr	4	2	—	—	—	—	—
Taco shells	11	45	—	6	3	0	—	—	—	—	—	—	—
Tortilla, flour	37	110	3	19	3	NA	—	—	4	2	2	8	2
French fries (small) 3.2 oz°°	91	240	3	33	12	0	—	10	10	2	10	—	4
Chili (regular) 9 oz	255	220	21	23	7	45	15	15	8	10	10	8	35
Cheddar cheese, shredded	28	110	7	1	10	30	10	—	—	6	—	20	—
Sour cream	28	60	1	1	6	10	6	—	—	2	—	4	—
Crispy chicken nuggets (6)	93	280	14	12	20	50	—	—	6	6	30	4	4
Nuggets sauces													
Barbeque	28	50	—	11	—	0	6	—	—	—	—	—	4
Honey	14	45	—	12	—	0	—	—	—	—	—	—	—
Sweet & sour	28	45	—	11	—	0	—	—	—	—	—	—	2
Sweet mustard	28	50	—	9	1	0	—	—	—	—	—	—	—
Hot Stuffed Baked Potatoes													
Plain	250	270	6	63	—	0	—	50	20	6	20	2	20
Bacon & cheese	362	520	20	70	18	20	10	60	35	15	35	8	24
Broccoli & cheese	350	400	8	58	16	tr	14	60	20	10	20	10	15
Cheese	318	420	8	66	15	10	10	50	20	100	20	6	20
Chili & cheese	403	500	15	71	18	25	15	60	20	100	25	8	28
Sour cream & chives	323	500	8	67	23	25	50	75	20	10	20	10	20
Beverages													
Frosty, small°°°	243	400	8	59	14	50	10	—	8	30	2	30	6
Cola, small	8°	100	0	25	0	0	—	—	—	—	—	—	—
Lemon-lime soft drink, small	8°	100	0	24	0	0	—	—	—	—	—	—	—
Diet cola	8°	1	0	—	0	0	—	—	—	—	—	—	—
Coffee	6°	2	0	—	0	0	—	—	—	—	—	—	—
Decaf coffee	6°	2	0	—	0	0	—	—	—	—	—	—	—
Hot chocolate	6°	110	2	22	1	tr	—	—	—	8	—	6	2
Lemonade	8°	90	0	24	0	0	—	15	—	4	—	—	2
Choc milk	8°	160	7	24	5	15	15	4	6	20	—	25	4
Milk, 2%	8°	110	8	11	4	20	10	4	6	20	—	30	—
Tea (hot or ice)	6°	1	0	0	0	0	—	—	—	—	—	—	—
Chocolate chip cookie	64	275	3	40	13	15	2	—	8	8	6	2	8

Source: Consumer Relations, Wendy's International, Dublin, OH.

°Fluid ounces.

°°To determine nutritional information for a large order of Fries, multiply figures by 1.3; Biggie Fries, multiply by 1.87; large Chili, multiply by 1.5; 9-piece Nuggets, multiply by 1.5; 20-piece Nuggets, multiply by 3.3.

°°°To determine nutritional information for a medium Frosty, multiply figures by 1.3; large Frosty, multiply by 1.7. For medium soft drink, multiply by 1.5; large soft drink, multiply by 2. For Biggie soft drink, multiply by 3.5.

Metabolic Computations in Open-Circuit Spirometry

STANDARDIZING GAS VOLUMES: ENVIRONMENTAL FACTORS

Gas volumes obtained during physiologic measurements are usually expressed in one of three ways: *ATPS, STPD,* or *BTPS.*

ATPS refers to the volume of gas at the specific conditions of measurement, which are therefore at Ambient Temperature (273°K + ambient temperature°C), ambient Pressure, and Saturated with water vapor. Gas volumes collected during open-circuit spirometry and pulmonary function tests are measured initially at ATPS.

The volume of a gas varies, however, depending on its temperature, pressure, and content of water vapor, even though the absolute number of gas molecules remains constant. These environmental influences are summarized as follows:

Temperature: The volume of a gas varies *directly* with temperature. Increasing the temperature causes the molecules to move more rapidly; the gas mixture expands, and the volume increases proportionately *(Charles' law).*

Pressure: The volume of a gas varies *inversely* with pressure. Increasing the pressure on a gas forces the molecules closer together, causing the volume to decrease in proportion to the increase in pressure *(Boyle's law).*

Water vapor: The volume of a gas varies depending on its water vapor content. The volume of a gas is greater when the gas is saturated with water vapor than it is when the same gas is dry (i.e., contains no moisture).

These three factors—temperature, pressure, and the relative degree of saturation of the gas with water vapor—must be considered, especially when gas volumes are to be compared under different environmental conditions and used subsequently in metabolic and physiologic calculations. The standards that provide the frame of reference for expressing a volume of gas are either STPD or BTPS.

STPD refers to the volume of a gas expressed under Standard conditions of Temperature (273°K or 0°C), Pressure (760 mm Hg), and Dry (no water vapor). Ex-

pressing a gas volume STPD, for example, makes it possible to evaluate and compare the volumes of expired air measured while running in the rain at high altitude, along a beach in the cold of winter, or in a hot desert environment below sea level. *In all metabolic calculations, gas volumes are always expressed at STPD.*

1. To reduce a gas volume to standard temperature (ST), the following formula is applied:

$$\text{Gas volume ST} = V_{ATPS} \times \frac{273°K}{273°K + T°C} \qquad (1)$$

where T°C = temperature of the gas in the measuring device and 273°K = absolute temperature Kelvin, which is equivalent to 0°C.

2. The following equation is used to express a gas volume at standard pressure (SP):

$$\text{Gas volume SP} = V_{ATPS} \times \frac{P_B}{760 \text{ mm Hg}} \qquad (2)$$

where P_B = ambient barometric pressure in mm Hg and 760 = standard barometric pressure at sea level, mm Hg.

TABLE C.1
VAPOR PRESSURE (P_{H_2O}) OF WET GAS AT TEMPERATURES NORMALLY ENCOUNTERED IN THE LABORATORY

T (°C)	P_{H_2O} (mm Hg)	T (°C)	P_{H_2O} (mm Hg)
20	17.5	31	33.7
21	18.7	32	35.7
22	19.8	33	37.7
23	21.1	34	39.9
24	22.4	35	42.2
25	23.8	36	44.6
26	25.2	37	47.1
27	26.7	38	49.7
28	28.4	39	52.4
29	30.0	40	55.3
30	31.8		

3. To reduce a gas to standard dry (SD) conditions, the effects of water vapor pressure at the particular environmental temperature must be subtracted from the volume of gas. Because expired air is 100% saturated with water vapor, it is not necessary to determine its percent saturation from measures of relative humidity. The vapor pressure in moist or completely humidified air at a particular ambient temperature can be obtained in Table C.1 and is expressed in mm Hg. This vapor pressure (P_{H_2O}) is then subtracted from the ambient barometric pressure (P_B) to reduce the gas to standard pressure dry (SPD) as follows:

$$\text{Gas volume SPD} = V_{ATPS} \times \frac{P_B - P_{H_2O}}{760} \qquad (3)$$

TABLE C.2
FACTORS TO REDUCE MOIST GAS TO A DRY GAS VOLUME AT 0° C AND 760 mm Hg

Barometric Reading	Temperature (°C)																	
	15	16	17	18	19	20	21	22	23	24	25	26	27	28	29	30	31	32
700	0.855	851	847	842	838	834	829	825	821	816	812	807	802	797	793	788	783	778
702	857	853	849	845	840	836	832	827	823	818	814	809	805	800	795	790	785	780
704	860	856	852	847	843	839	834	830	825	821	816	812	807	802	797	792	787	783
706	862	858	854	850	845	841	837	832	828	823	819	814	810	804	800	795	790	785
708	865	861	856	852	848	843	839	834	830	825	821	816	812	807	802	797	792	787
710	867	863	859	855	850	846	842	837	833	828	824	819	814	809	804	799	795	790
712	870	866	861	857	853	848	844	839	836	830	826	821	817	812	807	802	797	792
714	872	868	864	859	855	851	846	842	837	833	828	824	819	814	809	804	799	794
716	875	871	866	862	858	853	849	844	840	835	831	826	822	816	812	807	802	797
718	877	873	869	864	860	856	851	847	842	838	833	828	824	819	814	809	804	799
720	880	876	871	867	863	858	854	849	845	840	836	831	826	821	816	812	807	802
722	882	878	874	869	865	861	856	852	847	843	838	833	829	824	819	814	809	804
724	885	880	876	872	867	863	858	854	849	845	840	835	831	826	821	816	811	806
726	887	883	879	874	870	866	861	856	852	847	843	838	833	829	824	818	813	808
728	890	886	881	877	872	868	863	859	854	850	845	840	836	831	826	821	816	811
730	892	888	884	879	875	871	866	861	857	852	847	843	838	833	828	823	818	813
732	895	890	886	882	877	873	868	864	859	854	850	845	840	836	831	825	820	815
734	897	893	889	884	880	875	871	866	862	857	852	847	843	838	833	828	823	818
736	900	895	891	887	882	878	873	869	864	859	855	850	845	840	835	830	825	820
738	902	898	894	889	885	880	876	871	866	862	857	852	848	843	838	833	828	822
740	905	900	896	892	887	883	878	874	869	864	860	855	850	845	840	835	830	825
742	907	903	898	894	890	885	881	876	871	867	862	857	852	847	842	837	832	827
744	910	906	901	897	892	888	883	878	874	869	864	859	855	850	845	840	834	829
746	912	908	903	899	895	890	886	881	876	872	867	862	857	852	847	842	837	832
748	915	910	906	901	897	892	888	883	879	874	869	864	860	854	850	845	839	834
750	917	913	908	904	900	895	890	886	881	876	872	867	862	857	852	847	842	837
752	920	915	911	906	902	897	893	888	883	879	874	869	864	859	854	849	844	839
754	922	918	913	909	904	900	895	891	886	881	876	872	867	862	857	852	846	841
756	925	920	916	911	907	902	898	893	888	883	879	874	869	864	859	854	849	844
758	927	923	918	914	909	905	900	896	891	886	881	876	872	866	861	856	851	846
760	930	925	921	916	912	907	902	898	893	888	883	879	874	869	864	859	854	848
762	932	928	923	919	914	910	905	900	896	891	886	881	876	871	866	861	856	851
764	936	930	926	921	916	912	907	903	898	893	888	884	879	874	869	864	858	853
766	937	933	928	924	919	915	910	905	900	896	891	886	881	876	871	866	861	855
768	940	935	931	926	922	917	912	908	903	898	893	888	883	878	873	868	863	858
770	942	938	933	928	924	919	915	910	905	901	896	891	886	881	876	871	865	860

ATPS→STPD

By combining equations (1) and (3), any volume of moist air can be converted to STPD as follows:

$$\text{Gas volume STPD} = V_{ATPS}\left(\frac{273}{273 + T°C}\right)\left(\frac{P_B - P_{H_2O}}{760}\right) \quad (4)$$

Fortunately, these computations need not be carried out, because the appropriate *STPD correction factors* have already been calculated for moist gas in the range of temperatures and pressures ordinarily encountered in most laboratories. These factors are presented in Table C.2. Multiplying any gas volume ATPS by the appropriate correction factor gives the same gas volume STPD that would be obtained if values for the ambient temperature, barometric pressure, and water vapor pressure were substituted in equation (4).

The term *BTPS* refers to a volume of a gas expressed at *Body Temperature* (usually 273°K + 37°C or 310°K), ambient *Pressure* (whatever the barometer reads), and *Saturated* with water vapor with a partial pressure of 47 mm Hg at 37°C. Conventionally, pulmonary physiologists express lung volumes such as vital capacity, inspiratory and expiratory capacity, residual lung volume, and the dynamic measures of lung function such as maximum breathing capacity at body temperature and moist, or BTPS. The following equation converts a gas volume ATPS to BTPS:

Gas volume BTPS =

$$V_{ATPS}\left(\frac{P_B - P_{H_2O}}{P_B - 47 \text{ mm Hg}}\right)\left(\frac{310}{273 + T°C}\right) \quad (5)$$

As was the case with the correction to STPD, appropriate BTPS *correction factors* are available for converting a moist gas volume at ambient conditions to a volume BTPS. These BTPS factors for a broad range of ambient temperatures are presented in Table C.3. These factors have been computed assuming a barometric pressure of 760 mm Hg,

ATPS → BTPS

TABLE C.3
BTPS FACTORS

T (°C)	BTPS[a]	T (°C)	BTPS
20	1.102	29	1.051
21	1.096	30	1.045
22	1.091	31	1.039
23	1.085	32	1.032
24	1.080	33	1.026
25	1.075	34	1.020
26	1.068	35	1.014
27	1.063	36	1.007
28	1.057	37	1.000

[a]Body temperature, ambient pressure, and saturated with water vapor.

and small deviations (±10 mm Hg) from this pressure introduce only a minimal error.

CALCULATION OF OXYGEN UPTAKE

In determining oxygen uptake by open-circuit spirometry, we are interested in knowing how much oxygen has been removed from the *inspired air*. Because the composition of inspired air remains relatively constant ($CO_2 = 0.03\%$, $O_2 = 20.93\%$, $N_2 = 79.04\%$), it is possible to determine how much oxygen has been removed from the inspired air by measuring the amount and composition of the expired air. When this is done, the expired air contains more carbon dioxide (usually 2.5 to 5.0%), less oxygen (usually 15.0 to 18.5%), and more nitrogen (usually 79.04 to 79.60%). It should be noted, however, that nitrogen is inert in terms of metabolism; any change in its concentration in expired air reflects the fact that the number of oxygen molecules removed from the inspired air is not replaced by the same number of carbon dioxide molecules produced in metabolism. This results in the volume of expired air (V_E, STPD) being unequal to the inspired volume (V_I, STPD). For example, if the respiratory quotient is less than 1.00 (i.e., less CO_2 produced in relation to O_2 consumed), and 3 liters of air are inspired, *less* than 3 liters of air will be expired. In this case, the nitrogen concentration is higher in the expired air than in the inspired air. This is not to say that nitrogen has been produced, only that nitrogen molecules now represent a larger percentage of V_E compared to V_I. In fact, V_E differs from V_I in direct proportion to the change in nitrogen concentration between the inspired and expired volumes. Thus, V_I can be determined from V_E using the relative change in nitrogen in an equation known as the *Haldane transformation*.

$$V_I, \text{STPD} = V_E, \text{STPD} \times \frac{\%N_2E}{\%N_2I} \quad (6)$$

where $\%N_2I = 79.04$ and $\%N_2E =$ percent nitrogen in expired air computed from gas analysis as $[(100 - (\%O_2E + \%CO_2)]$.

The volume of O_2 in the inspired air ($V_{O_2}I$) can then be determined as follows:

$$V_{O_2}I = V_I \times \%O_2I \quad (7)$$

Substituting equation (6) for V_I,

$$V_{O_2}I = V_E \times \frac{\%N_2E}{79.04\%} \times \%O_2I \quad (8)$$

where $\%O_2I = 20.93\%$

The amount or volume of oxygen in the expired air ($V_{O_2}E$) is computed as

$$V_{O_2}E = V_E \times \%O_2E \quad (9)$$

where %O_2E is the fractional concentration of oxygen in expired air determined by gas analysis (chemical or electronic methods).

The amount of O_2 removed from the inspired air each minute ($\dot{V}O_2$) can then be computed as follows:

$$\dot{V}O_2 = (\dot{V}I \times \%O_2I) - (\dot{V}E \times \%O_2E) \tag{10}$$

By substitution

$$\dot{V}O_2 = \left\{\left[\left(\dot{V}E \times \frac{\%N_2E}{79.04\%}\right) \times 20.93\%\right] - (\dot{V}E \times \%O_2E)\right\} \tag{11}$$

where $\dot{V}O_2$ = volume of oxygen consumed per minute, expressed in milliliters or liters, and $\dot{V}_E$ = expired air volume per minute expressed in milliliters or liters.
Equation (11) can be simplified to:

$$\dot{V}O_2 = \dot{V}_E\left[\left(\frac{\%N_2E}{79.04\%} \times 20.93\%\right) - \%O_2E\right] \tag{12}$$

The final form of the equation is:

$$\dot{V}O_2 = \dot{V}E[(\%N_2E \times 0.265) - \%O_2E] \tag{13}$$

The value obtained within the brackets in equations (12) and (13) is referred to as the *true O_2*; this represents the "oxygen extraction" or, more precisely, the percentage of oxygen consumed for any volume of air *expired*.

Although equation (13) is the equation used most widely to compute oxygen uptake from measures of expired air, it is also possible to calculate $\dot{V}O_2$ from direct measurements of both $\dot{V}I$ and $\dot{V}E$. In this case, the Haldane transformation is not used, and oxygen uptake is calculated directly as

$$\dot{V}O_2 = (\dot{V}I \times 20.93) - (\dot{V}E \times \%O_2E) \tag{14}$$

In situations in which only $\dot{V}I$ is measured, the $\dot{V}E$ can be calculated from the Haldane transformation as

$$\dot{V}E = \dot{V}I \frac{\%N_2I}{\%N_2E}$$

By substitution in equation (14), the computational equation is:

$$\dot{V}O_2 = \dot{V}I\left[\%O_2I - \left(\frac{\%N_2I}{\%N_2E} \times \%O_2E\right)\right] \tag{15}$$

CALCULATION OF CARBON DIOXIDE PRODUCTION

The carbon dioxide production per minute ($\dot{V}CO_2$) is calculated as follows:

$$\dot{V}CO_2 = \dot{V}_E(\%CO_{2_E} - \%CO_2I) \tag{16}$$

where %CO_{2_E} = percent carbon dioxide in expired air determined by gas analysis, and %CO_2I = percent carbon

dioxide in inspired air, which is essentially constant at 0.03%.
The final form of the equation is:

$$\dot{V}CO_2 = \dot{V}E(\%CO_2E - 0.03\%) \tag{17}$$

CALCULATION OF RESPIRATORY QUOTIENT

The respiratory quotient (RQ) is calculated in one of two ways:

1. $$RQ = \dot{V}CO_2/\dot{V}O_2 \tag{18}$$

   or

2. $$RQ = \frac{(\%CO_2E - 0.03\%)}{\text{"true" } O_2} \tag{19}$$

SAMPLE METABOLIC CALCULATIONS

The following data were obtained during the last minute of a steady-rate, 10-minute treadmill run performed at 6 miles per hour at a 5% grade.

$\dot{V}E$: 62.1 liters, ATPS
Barometric pressure: 750 mm Hg
Temperature: 26°C
%O_2 expired: 16.86 (O_2 analyzer)
%CO_2 expired: 3.60 (CO_2 analyzer)
%N_2 expired: [100 − (16.86 + 3.60)] = 79.54

Determine the following:

1. $\dot{V}E$, STPD
2. $\dot{V}O_2$, STPD
3. $\dot{V}CO_2$ STPD
4. RQ
5. kcal · min^{-1}

1. $\dot{V}E$, STPD (use equation 4 or STPD correction factor in Table C.2).

$$\dot{V}E, STPD = \dot{V}E, ATPS\left(\frac{273}{273 + T°C}\right)\left(\frac{P_B - P_{H_2O}}{760}\right)$$

$$= 62.1\left(\frac{273}{299}\right)\left(\frac{750 - 25.2}{760}\right)$$

$$= 62.1 (0.913 \times 0.954)$$

$$= 54.07 \text{ liters} \cdot \text{min}^{-1}$$

2. $\dot{V}O_2$, STPD (use equation 13)

$$\dot{V}O_2, STPD = \dot{V}E, STPD [(\%N_2E \times 0.265) - \%O_2E]$$

$$= 54.07 [(0.7954 \times 0.265) - 0.1686]$$

$$= 54.07 (0.0422)$$

$$= 2.281 \text{ liters} \cdot \text{min}^{-1}$$

3. $\dot{V}_{CO_2}$, STPD (use equation 17)

$$\dot{V}_{CO_2}, \text{STPD} = \dot{V}_E, \text{STPD} (CO_2E - 0.03\%)$$
$$= 54.07 (0.0360 - 0.0003)$$
$$= 54.07 (0.0357)$$
$$= 1.930 \text{ liters} \cdot \text{min}^-$$

4. RQ (use equation 18 or 19)

$$RQ = \dot{V}_{CO_2}/\dot{V}_{O_2}$$

$$= \frac{1.930 \text{ liters } CO_2/\text{min}}{2.281 \text{ liters } O_2/\text{min}}$$

$$= 0.846$$

or

$$RQ = \frac{(\%CO_2E - 0.03\%)}{\text{"true" } O_2}$$

$$= \frac{3.60 - .03}{4.22}$$

$$= 0.846$$

Because the exercise was performed in a steady rate of aerobic metabolism, the obtained RQ of 0.846 can be applied in Table 8.1 (p. 147) to obtain the appropriate caloric transformation. In this way, the exercise oxygen uptake can be transposed to kcal of energy expended per minute as follows:

5. Energy expenditure (kcal · min^{-1}) = $\dot{V}_{O_2}$ (liters · min^{-1}) × caloric equivalent per liter O_2 at the given steady-rate RQ

$$\text{Energy expenditure} = 2.281 \times 4.862$$

$$= 11.09 \text{ kcal} \cdot \text{min}^{-1}$$

Assuming that the RQ value reflects the nonprotein RQ, a reasonable estimate of both the percentage and quantity of lipid and carbohydrate metabolized during each minute of the run can be obtained from Table 8.1 (p. 147).

Percentage kcal derived from lipid = 50.7%
Percentage kcal derived from carbohydrate = 49.3%
Grams of lipid utilized = 0.267 g per liter of oxygen or approximately 0.61 g per minute (0.267 × 2.281 L O_2)

Grams of carbohydrate utilized = 0.580 g per liter of oxygen or approximately 1.36 g per minute (0.580 × 2.281 L O_2)

WEIR FACTORS TO ESTIMATE ENERGY EXPENDITURE

In 1949, J. Weir presented a simple and accurate method for calculating caloric expenditure from ventilation and expired oxygen percentage. Weir's calculations assumed a protein content of the diet of 12.5%.

The formula for calculating kcal · min^{-1} from $\dot{V}_E$, STPD and O_2E is:

$$\text{kcal} \cdot \text{min}^{-1} = \dot{V}_E, \text{STPD} \times 1.044 - (0.0499 \times \%O_2E)$$

Example: $\dot{V}_E$, STPD = 50 L · min^{-1}; O_2E = 16.0%
kcal · min^{-1} = 50 L · min^{-1} 1.044 − (0.0499 × 16.0)
kcal · min^{-1} = 50 L · min^{-1} × 0.2456
kcal · min^{-1} = 12.28

The factor $1.044 - (0.0499 \times \%O_2E)$, termed the "Weir factor," can be determined for any value of O_2E. The Weir factors for different expired oxygen percentages are shown in the table below. To use the table, find the expired oxygen percentage and corresponding Weir factor. Multiply the Weir factor by the $\dot{V}_E$, STPD to obtain the caloric expenditure. (Reference: Weir, J.B. deV.: New methods for calculating metabolic rate with special reference to protein metabolism. *J. Physiol.*, 109:1, 1949.

CALCULATION OF ENERGY EXPENDITURE BY USE OF THE WEIR FACTORS[a]

%O_2E	Weir Factor	%O_2E	Weir Factor
14.50	.3205	17.00	.1957
.60	.3155	.10	.1907
.70	.3105	.20	.1857
.80	.3055	.30	.1807
.90	.3005	.40	.1757
15.00	.2955	.50	.1707
.10	.2905	.60	.1658
.20	.2855	.70	.1608
.30	.2805	.80	.1558
.40	.2755	.90	.1508
.50	.2705	18.00	.1468
.60	.2556	.30	.1308
.70	.2606	.20	.1368
.80	.2556	.30	.1308
.90	.2506	.40	.1268
16.00	.2456	.50	.1208
.10	.2406	.60	.1168
.20	.2366	.70	.1109
.30	.2306	.80	.1068
.40	.2256	.90	.1009
.50	.2206	19.00	.0969
.60	.2157	.10	.0909
.70	.2107	.20	.0868
.80	.2057	.30	.0809
.90	.2007	.40	.0769
		.50	.0710

[a]The Weir factor is computed as $1.044 - (0.0499 \times \%O_2E)$. Use this calculation for accurate determination of the Weir factor if the O_2E is not shown in the table. The accuracy of the computation of kcal is within ±1% of actual values when the subject has a steady-rate $\dot{V}_{O_2}$ and the diet averages about 12.5% protein.

Energy Expenditure in Household, Occupational, Recreational, and Sports Activities[a, b]

HOW TO USE APPENDIX D

Refer to the column that comes closest to your present body mass. Multiply the number in this column by the number of minutes you spend in an activity. Suppose that an individual weighing 62.3 kg (137 lb) spends 30 minutes playing a casual game of billiards. To determine the energy cost of participation, multiply the caloric value per minute (2.6 kcal) by 30 to obtain the 30-minute gross expenditure of 78 kcal. If the same individual does aerobic dance for 45 minutes, the **gross** (value includes resting energy expenditure) energy expended would be calculated as 6.4 kcal × 45 minutes, or 288 kcal.

[a] All values for energy expenditure are in kilocalories per minute.
[b] Copyright © 1996 by Frank I. Katch, Victor L. Katch, and William D. McArdle, and Fitness Technologies, Inc., P.O. Box 430, Amherst, MA 01004. No part of this appendix may be reproduced in any manner without written permission from the copyright holders.

YOUR BODY WEIGHT

Activity	kg lb	47 104	50 110	53 117	56 123	59 130	62 137	65 143	68 150
Archery		3.1	3.3	3.4	3.6	3.8	4.0	4.2	4.4
Backpacking									
without load		5.7	6.1	6.4	6.8	7.1	7.5	7.9	8.2
with 11 pound load		6.1	6.5	6.8	7.2	7.6	8.0	8.4	8.8
with 22 pound load		6.6	7.0	7.4	7.8	8.3	8.7	9.1	9.5
with 44 pound load		7.0	7.4	7.8	8.2	8.7	9.1	9.6	10.0
Badminton									
leisure		4.6	4.9	5.1	5.4	5.7	6.0	6.3	6.6
tournament		7.0	7.3	7.7	8.1	8.6	9.0	9.4	9.9
Baking, general (F)		1.6	1.8	1.9	2.0	2.1	2.2	2.3	2.4
Baseball									
fielder		2.8	3.0	3.2	3.4	3.6	3.8	4.0	4.1
pitcher		4.2	4.5	4.8	5.0	5.3	5.6	5.9	6.2
Basketball									
competition		7.1	7.4	7.9	8.3	8.7	9.2	9.6	10.1
practice		6.5	6.9	7.3	7.7	8.1	8.6	9.0	9.4
Baton twirling		6.3	6.8	7.3	7.6	8.1	8.5	8.9	9.3
Billiards ("pool")		2.0	2.1	2.2	2.4	2.5	2.6	2.7	2.9
Bookbinding		1.8	1.9	2.0	2.1	2.2	2.4	2.5	2.6
Bowling		4.4	4.8	5.2	5.4	5.7	6.0	6.3	6.6
Boxing									
in ring, match		10.4	11.1	11.8	12.4	13.1	13.8	14.4	15.1
sparring, practice		6.5	6.9	7.3	7.7	8.1	8.6	9.0	9.4
Calisthenics, warm-ups		3.4	3.7	4.0	4.2	4.4	4.7	4.9	5.1
Canoeing									
leisure (2.5 mph)		2.1	2.2	2.3	2.5	2.6	2.7	2.9	3.0
racing ("fast")		4.8	5.2	5.5	5.8	6.1	6.4	6.7	7.0
Car washing		3.3	3.5	3.7	3.9	4.1	4.3	4.5	4.8
Card playing		1.2	1.3	1.3	1.4	1.5	1.6	1.6	1.7
Carpentry, general		2.4	2.6	2.8	2.9	3.1	3.2	3.4	3.5
Carpet sweeping (F)		2.2	2.3	2.4	2.5	2.7	2.8	2.9	3.1
Carpet sweeping (M)		2.3	2.4	2.5	2.7	2.8	3.0	3.1	3.3
Circuit resistance training									
Free weights		4.0	4.3	4.5	4.8	5.0	5.3	5.5	5.8
Hydra-Fitness		6.2	6.6	7.0	7.4	7.8	8.2	8.6	9.0
Nautilus		4.3	4.6	4.9	5.2	5.5	5.8	6.0	6.3
Universal		5.3	5.8	6.2	6.5	6.9	7.2	7.5	7.9
Cleaning (F)		2.9	3.1	3.3	3.5	3.7	3.8	4.0	4.2
Cleaning (M)		2.7	2.9	3.1	3.2	3.4	3.6	3.8	3.9
Coal mining									
drilling coal, rock		4.4	4.7	5.0	5.3	5.5	5.8	6.1	6.4
erecting supports		4.1	4.4	4.7	4.9	5.2	5.5	5.7	6.0
shoveling coal		5.1	5.4	5.7	6.0	6.4	6.7	7.0	7.3
Cooking (F)		2.1	2.3	2.4	2.5	2.7	2.8	2.9	3.1
Cooking (M)		2.3	2.4	2.5	2.7	2.8	3.0	3.1	3.3
Cricket									
batting		3.9	4.2	4.4	4.6	4.9	5.1	5.4	5.6
bowling		4.2	4.5	4.8	5.0	5.3	5.6	5.9	6.1
fielding		3.7	3.9	4.1	4.3	4.8	4.8	5.0	5.3

Note: Symbols (M) and (F) denote experiments for males and females, respectively.

| 71 | 74 | 77 | 80 | 83 | 86 | 89 | 92 | 95 | 98 |
157	163	170	176	183	190	196	203	209	216
4.6	4.8	5.0	5.2	5.4	5.6	5.8	6.0	6.2	6.4
8.6	9.0	9.3	9.7	10.0	10.4	10.8	11.1	11.5	11.9
9.2	9.5	9.9	10.3	10.7	11.1	11.5	11.9	12.3	12.6
9.9	10.4	10.8	11.2	11.6	12.0	12.5	12.9	13.3	13.7
10.4	10.9	11.3	11.8	12.2	12.6	13.1	13.5	14.0	14.4
6.9	7.2	7.5	7.8	8.1	8.3	8.6	8.9	9.2	9.5
10.4	10.8	11.2	11.6	12.1	12.5	12.9	13.4	13.8	14.3
2.5	2.6	2.7	2.8	2.9	3.0	3.1	3.2	3.3	3.4
4.3	4.5	4.7	4.9	5.1	5.2	5.4	5.6	5.8	6.0
6.4	6.7	7.0	7.2	7.5	7.8	8.0	8.3	8.6	8.9
10.5	10.9	11.4	11.8	12.3	12.7	13.1	13.6	14.0	14.5
9.8	10.2	10.6	11.0	11.5	11.9	12.3	12.7	13.1	13.5
9.5	9.7	9.9	10.1	10.4	10.6	10.8	11.0	11.2	11.4
3.0	3.1	3.2	3.4	3.5	3.6	3.7	3.9	4.0	4.1
2.7	2.8	2.9	3.0	3.2	3.3	3.4	3.5	3.6	3.7
6.9	7.2	7.5	7.7	8.1	8.4	8.6	8.9	9.2	9.5
15.8	16.4	17.1	17.8	18.4	19.1	19.8	20.4	21.1	21.8
9.8	10.2	10.6	11.0	11.5	11.9	12.3	12.7	13.1	13.5
5.3	5.5	5.8	6.0	6.2	6.5	6.7	6.9	7.1	7.3
3.1	3.3	3.4	3.5	3.7	3.8	3.9	4.0	4.2	4.3
7.3	7.6	7.9	8.2	8.5	8.9	9.2	9.5	9.8	10.1
5.0	5.2	5.5	5.7	5.7	5.9	6.1	6.3	6.5	6.9
1.8	1.9	1.9	2.0	2.1	2.2	2.2	2.3	2.4	2.5
3.7	3.8	4.0	4.2	4.3	4.5	4.6	4.8	4.9	5.1
3.2	3.3	3.5	3.6	3.7	3.9	4.0	4.1	4.3	4.4
3.4	3.6	3.7	3.8	4.0	4.1	4.3	4.4	4.6	4.7
6.1	6.3	6.6	6.8	7.1	7.4	7.6	7.9	8.1	8.4
9.4	9.7	10.2	10.5	10.9	11.4	11.7	12.1	12.5	12.9
6.6	6.8	7.1	7.4	7.7	8.0	8.2	8.5	8.8	9.1
8.3	8.6	8.9	9.3	9.6	10.0	10.3	10.7	11.0	11.4
4.4	4.6	4.8	5.0	5.1	5.3	5.5	5.7	5.9	6.1
4.1	4.3	4.5	4.6	4.8	5.0	5.2	5.3	5.5	5.7
6.7	7.0	7.2	7.5	7.8	8.1	8.4	8.6	8.9	9.2
6.2	6.5	6.8	7.0	7.3	7.6	7.8	8.1	8.4	8.6
7.7	8.0	8.3	8.6	9.0	9.3	9.6	9.9	10.3	10.6
3.2	3.3	3.5	3.6	3.7	3.9	4.0	4.1	4.3	4.4
3.4	3.6	3.7	3.8	4.0	4.1	4.3	4.4	4.6	4.7
5.9	6.1	6.4	6.6	6.9	7.1	7.4	7.6	7.9	8.1
6.4	6.7	6.9	7.2	7.5	7.7	8.0	8.3	8.6	8.8
5.6	5.9	6.2	6.5	6.8	7.1	7.4	7.7	8.0	8.3

YOUR BODY WEIGHT—*continued*

Activity	kg lb	47 104	50 110	53 117	56 123	59 130	62 137	65 143	68 150
Croquet		2.8	3.0	3.1	3.3	3.5	3.7	3.8	4.0
Cycling									
leisure, 5.5 mph		3.0	3.2	3.4	3.6	3.8	4.0	4.2	4.4
leisure, 9.4 mph		4.8	5.0	5.3	5.6	5.9	6.2	6.5	6.8
racing, fast		8.0	8.5	9.0	9.5	10.0	10.5	11.0	11.5
Dancing									
aerobic, easy		4.3	4.8	5.2	5.6	5.9	6.2	6.4	6.7
aerobic, medium		4.8	5.2	5.5	5.8	6.1	6.4	6.7	7.0
aerobic, intense		6.3	6.7	7.1	7.5	7.9	8.3	8.7	9.2
ballroom		2.4	2.6	2.7	2.9	3.0	3.2	3.3	3.5
choreographed		5.0	5.2	5.5	5.8	6.1	6.4	6.7	7.0
"twist," "lambada"		8.0	8.4	8.9	9.4	9.9	10.4	10.9	11.4
modern		3.4	3.6	3.8	4.0	4.3	4.5	4.7	4.9
Digging trenches		6.8	7.3	7.7	8.1	8.6	9.0	9.4	9.9
Drawing (standing)		1.7	1.8	1.9	2.0	2.1	2.2	2.3	2.4
Eating (sitting)		1.1	1.2	1.2	1.3	1.4	1.4	1.5	1.6
Electrical work		2.7	2.9	3.1	3.2	3.4	3.6	3.8	3.9
Farming									
barn cleaning		6.3	6.8	7.2	7.6	8.0	8.4	8.8	9.2
driving harvester		1.9	2.0	2.1	2.2	2.4	2.5	2.6	2.7
driving tractor		1.8	1.9	2.0	2.1	2.2	2.3	2.4	2.5
feeding cattle		4.2	4.3	4.5	4.8	5.0	5.3	5.5	5.8
feeding animals		3.1	3.3	3.4	3.6	3.8	4.0	4.2	4.4
forking straw bales		6.7	6.9	7.3	7.7	8.1	8.6	9.0	9.4
milking by hand		2.5	2.7	2.9	3.0	3.2	3.3	3.5	3.7
milking by machine		1.1	1.2	1.2	1.3	1.4	1.4	1.5	1.6
shoveling grain		4.2	4.3	4.5	4.8	5.0	5.3	5.5	5.8
Fencing									
competition		7.2	7.6	8.1	8.5	9.0	9.4	9.9	10.8
practice		3.6	3.9	4.2	4.4	4.6	4.9	5.1	5.3
Field hockey		6.5	6.7	7.1	7.5	7.9	8.3	8.7	9.1
Fishing		3.0	3.1	3.3	3.5	3.7	3.8	4.0	4.2
Food shopping (F)		3.0	3.1	3.3	3.5	3.7	3.8	4.0	4.2
Football, competition		6.2	6.6	7.0	7.4	7.8	8.2	8.6	9.0
Forestry									
ax chopping, fast		14.0	14.9	15.7	16.6	17.5	18.4	19.3	20.2
ax chopping, slow		4.0	4.3	4.5	4.8	5.0	5.3	5.5	5.8
barking trees		5.8	6.2	6.5	6.9	7.3	7.6	8.0	8.4
carrying logs		8.7	9.3	9.9	10.4	11.0	11.5	12.1	12.6
felling trees		6.2	6.6	7.0	7.4	7.8	8.2	8.6	9.0
hoeing		4.2	4.6	4.8	5.1	5.4	5.6	5.9	6.2
planting by hand		5.1	5.5	5.8	6.1	6.4	6.8	7.1	7.4
sawing by hand		5.7	6.1	6.5	6.8	7.2	7.6	7.9	8.3
sawing, power		3.5	3.8	4.0	4.2	4.4	4.7	4.9	5.1
stacking firewood		4.2	4.4	4.7	4.9	5.2	5.5	5.7	6.0
trimming trees		6.1	6.5	6.8	7.2	7.6	8.0	8.4	8.8
weeding		3.4	3.6	3.8	4.0	4.2	4.5	4.7	4.9
Frisbee		4.7	5.0	5.3	5.5	5.9	6.2	6.4	6.8
Furriery		3.9	4.2	4.4	4.6	4.9	5.1	5.4	5.6

| 71 | 74 | 77 | 80 | 83 | 86 | 89 | 92 | 95 | 98 |
157	163	170	176	183	190	196	203	209	216
4.2	4.4	4.5	4.7	4.9	5.1	5.3	5.4	5.6	5.8
4.5	4.7	4.9	5.1	5.3	5.5	5.7	5.9	6.1	6.3
7.1	7.4	7.7	8.0	8.3	8.6	8.9	9.2	9.5	9.8
12.0	12.5	13.0	13.5	14.0	14.5	15.0	15.5	16.1	16.6
6.9	7.2	7.5	7.8	8.1	8.4	8.8	9.1	9.4	9.7
7.3	7.6	7.9	8.2	8.5	8.9	9.2	9.5	9.8	10.1
9.6	10.0	10.4	10.8	11.2	11.6	12.0	12.4	12.8	13.2
3.6	3.8	3.9	4.1	4.2	4.4	4.5	4.7	4.8	5.0
7.3	7.6	7.9	8.2	8.5	8.9	9.2	9.5	9.8	10.1
11.9	12.4	12.9	13.4	13.9	14.4	15.0	15.5	16.0	16.5
5.1	5.3	5.6	5.8	6.0	6.2	6.4	6.7	6.9	7.1
10.3	10.7	11.2	11.6	12.0	12.5	12.9	13.3	13.8	14.2
2.6	2.7	2.8	2.9	3.0	3.1	3.2	3.3	3.4	3.5
1.6	1.7	1.8	1.8	1.9	2.0	2.0	2.1	2.2	2.3
4.1	4.3	4.5	4.6	4.8	5.0	5.2	5.3	5.5	5.7
9.6	10.0	10.4	10.8	11.2	11.6	12.0	12.4	12.8	13.2
2.8	3.0	3.1	3.2	3.3	3.4	3.6	3.7	3.8	3.9
2.6	2.7	2.8	3.0	3.1	3.2	3.3	3.4	3.5	3.6
6.0	6.3	6.5	6.8	7.1	7.3	7.6	7.8	8.1	8.3
4.6	4.8	5.0	5.2	5.4	5.6	5.8	6.0	6.2	6.4
9.8	10.2	10.6	11.0	11.5	11.9	12.3	12.7	13.1	13.5
3.8	4.0	4.2	4.3	4.5	4.6	4.8	5.0	5.1	5.3
1.6	1.7	1.8	1.8	1.9	2.0	2.0	2.1	2.2	2.3
6.0	6.3	6.5	6.8	7.1	7.3	7.6	7.8	8.1	8.3
11.2	11.7	12.1	12.6	13.1	13.5	14.0	14.4	14.9	15.5
5.6	5.8	6.1	6.3	6.5	6.8	7.0	7.2	7.4	7.7
9.5	9.9	10.3	10.7	11.1	11.5	11.9	12.3	12.7	13.1
4.4	4.6	4.8	5.0	5.1	5.3	5.5	5.7	5.9	6.1
4.4	4.6	4.8	5.0	5.1	5.3	5.5	5.7	5.9	6.1
9.4	9.8	10.2	10.6	11.0	11.4	11.7	12.1	12.5	12.9
21.1	22.0	22.9	23.8	24.7	25.5	26.4	27.3	28.2	29.1
6.0	6.3	6.5	6.8	7.1	7.3	7.6	7.8	8.1	8.3
8.7	9.1	9.5	9.8	10.2	10.6	10.9	11.3	11.7	12.1
13.2	13.8	14.3	14.9	15.4	16.0	16.6	17.1	17.7	18.2
9.4	9.8	10.2	10.6	11.0	11.4	11.7	12.1	12.5	12.9
6.5	6.7	7.0	7.3	7.6	7.8	8.1	8.4	8.6	8.9
7.7	8.1	8.4	8.7	9.0	9.4	9.7	10.0	10.4	10.7
8.7	9.0	9.4	9.8	10.1	10.5	10.9	11.2	11.6	12.0
5.3	5.6	5.8	6.0	6.2	6.5	6.7	6.9	7.1	7.4
6.2	6.5	6.8	7.0	7.3	7.6	7.8	8.1	8.4	8.6
9.2	9.5	9.9	10.3	10.7	11.1	11.5	11.9	12.3	12.6
5.1	5.3	5.5	5.8	6.0	6.2	6.4	6.6	6.8	7.1
7.1	7.4	7.7	8.0	8.2	8.5	8.8	9.1	9.4	9.7
5.9	6.1	6.4	6.6	6.9	7.1	7.4	7.6	7.9	8.1

YOUR BODY WEIGHT—*continued*

Activity	kg lb	47 104	50 110	53 117	56 123	59 130	62 137	65 143	68 150
Gardening									
digging		5.9	6.3	6.7	7.1	7.4	7.8	8.2	8.6
hedging		3.3	3.9	4.1	4.3	4.5	4.8	5.0	5.2
mowing		5.3	5.6	5.9	6.3	6.6	6.9	7.3	7.6
raking		2.5	2.7	2.9	3.0	3.2	3.3	3.5	3.7
Golf		4.0	4.3	4.5	4.8	5.0	5.3	5.5	5.8
Gymnastics		3.0	3.3	3.5	3.7	3.9	4.1	4.3	4.5
Handball		6.9	7.2	7.7	8.1	8.5	9.0	9.4	9.8
Horse-grooming		6.0	6.4	6.8	7.2	7.6	7.9	8.3	8.7
Horseback riding									
galloping		6.4	6.9	7.3	7.7	8.1	8.5	8.9	9.3
trotting		5.2	5.5	5.8	6.2	6.5	6.8	7.2	7.5
walking		1.9	2.1	2.2	2.3	2.4	2.5	2.7	2.8
Horseshoes		3.3	3.4	3.5	3.7	3.9	4.1	4.3	4.5
Housework									
mopping floors		2.8	3.1	3.3	3.5	3.7	3.8	4.0	4.2
dusting		3.0	3.3	3.4	3.6	3.8	4.0	4.2	4.4
laundry		3.1	3.4	3.5	3.7	3.9	4.1	4.3	4.5
washing windows		3.2	3.5	3.6	3.8	4.0	4.2	4.4	4.6
vacuuming		3.0	3.3	3.4	3.6	3.8	4.0	4.2	4.4
Hunting		4.1	4.4	4.7	4.9	5.2	5.5	5.7	6.0
Ice hockey		7.4	7.7	8.2	8.6	9.1	9.6	10.0	10.5
Ironing clothes		1.6	1.7	1.7	1.8	1.9	2.0	2.1	2.2
Judo		9.2	9.8	10.3	10.9	11.5	12.1	12.7	13.3
Jumping rope									
70 per min		7.6	8.1	8.6	9.1	9.6	10.0	10.5	11.0
80 per min		7.7	8.2	8.7	9.2	9.7	10.2	10.7	11.2
125 per min		8.3	8.9	9.4	9.9	10.4	11.0	11.5	12.0
145 per min		9.3	9.9	10.4	11.0	11.6	12.2	12.8	13.4
Karate		9.5	9.8	10.3	10.9	11.5	12.1	12.7	13.3
Kendo		9.3	9.7	10.2	10.8	11.4	12.0	12.6	13.2
Knitting, sewing		1.1	1.1	1.2	1.2	1.3	1.4	1.4	1.5
Lacrosse		7.0	7.4	7.9	8.3	8.7	9.2	9.6	10.1
Locksmith		2.8	2.9	3.0	3.2	3.4	3.5	3.7	3.9
Lying at ease		1.0	1.1	1.2	1.2	1.3	1.4	1.4	1.5
Machine-tooling									
machining		2.3	2.4	2.5	2.7	2.8	3.0	3.1	3.3
operating lathe		2.5	2.6	2.8	2.9	3.1	3.2	3.4	3.5
operating punch press		4.2	4.4	4.7	4.9	5.2	5.5	5.7	6.0
tapping and drilling		3.2	3.3	3.4	3.6	3.8	4.0	4.2	4.4
welding		2.4	2.6	2.8	2.9	3.1	3.2	3.4	3.5
working sheet metal		2.3	2.4	2.5	2.7	2.8	3.0	3.1	3.3
Marching, rapid		6.7	7.1	7.5	8.0	8.4	8.8	9.2	9.7
Mountain climbing		7.4	7.9	8.4	8.9	9.4	9.9	10.3	10.8
Motorcycle riding		6.5	6.9	7.3	7.7	8.1	8.5	8.9	9.3

| 71 | 74 | 77 | 80 | 83 | 86 | 89 | 92 | 95 | 98 |
157	163	170	176	183	190	196	203	209	216
8.9	9.3	9.7	10.1	10.5	10.8	11.2	11.6	12.0	12.3
5.5	5.7	5.9	6.2	6.4	6.6	6.9	7.1	7.3	7.5
8.0	8.3	8.6	9.0	9.3	9.6	10.0	10.3	10.6	11.0
3.8	4.0	4.2	4.3	4.5	4.6	4.8	5.0	5.1	5.3
6.0	6.3	6.5	6.8	7.1	7.3	7.6	7.8	8.1	8.3
4.7	4.9	5.1	5.3	5.5	5.7	5.9	6.1	6.3	6.5
10.3	10.7	11.2	11.5	12.0	12.5	12.9	13.3	13.7	14.2
9.1	9.5	9.9	10.2	10.6	11.0	11.4	11.8	12.2	12.5
9.7	10.1	10.6	11.0	11.4	11.8	12.2	12.6	13.0	13.4
7.8	8.1	8.5	8.8	9.1	9.5	9.8	10.1	10.5	10.8
2.9	3.0	3.2	3.3	3.4	3.5	3.6	3.8	3.9	4.0
4.7	4.9	5.1	5.3	5.5	5.7	5.9	6.1	6.3	6.5
4.4	4.6	4.8	5.0	5.2	5.4	5.6	5.8	6.0	6.2
4.6	4.7	4.9	5.1	5.3	5.5	5.7	5.9	6.1	6.3
4.7	4.9	5.1	5.3	5.5	5.7	5.9	6.1	6.3	6.5
4.8	5.0	5.2	5.4	5.6	5.8	6.0	6.2	6.4	6.6
4.6	4.8	5.0	5.2	5.4	5.6	5.8	6.0	6.2	6.4
6.2	6.5	6.7	7.0	7.2	7.5	7.8	8.0	8.2	8.5
11.0	11.5	12.0	12.5	13.1	13.6	14.1	14.6	15.1	15.7
2.3	2.4	2.5	2.6	2.7	2.8	2.9	3.0	3.1	3.2
13.8	14.4	15.0	15.6	16.2	16.8	17.4	17.9	18.5	19.1
11.5	12.0	12.5	13.0	13.4	13.9	14.4	14.9	15.4	15.9
11.6	12.1	12.6	13.1	13.6	14.1	14.6	14.6	15.6	16.1
12.6	13.1	13.6	14.2	14.7	15.2	15.8	16.3	16.8	17.3
14.0	14.6	15.2	15.8	16.4	16.9	17.5	18.1	18.7	19.3
13.8	14.4	15.0	15.6	16.2	16.8	17.4	17.9	18.5	19.1
13.7	14.3	14.9	15.5	16.1	16.7	17.3	17.8	18.4	19.0
1.6	1.6	1.7	1.8	1.8	1.9	2.0	2.0	2.1	2.2
10.4	10.7	11.0	11.2	11.5	11.8	12.1	12.4	12.7	13.0
4.0	4.2	4.4	4.6	4.7	4.9	5.1	5.2	5.4	5.6
1.6	1.6	1.7	1.8	1.8	1.9	2.0	2.0	2.1	2.2
3.4	3.6	3.7	3.8	4.0	4.1	4.3	4.4	4.6	4.7
3.7	3.8	4.0	4.2	4.3	4.5	4.6	4.8	4.9	5.1
6.2	6.5	6.8	7.0	7.3	7.6	7.8	8.1	8.4	8.6
4.6	4.8	5.0	5.2	5.4	5.6	5.8	6.0	6.2	6.4
3.7	3.8	4.0	4.2	4.3	4.5	4.6	4.8	4.9	5.1
3.4	3.6	3.7	3.8	4.0	4.1	4.3	4.4	4.6	4.7
10.1	10.5	10.9	11.4	11.8	12.2	12.6	13.1	13.5	13.9
11.3	11.7	12.2	12.7	13.2	13.7	14.1	14.6	15.0	15.6
9.7	10.1	10.5	10.9	11.3	11.7	12.1	12.5	12.9	13.3

YOUR BODY WEIGHT—*continued*

Activity	kg lb	47 104	50 110	53 117	56 123	59 130	62 137	65 143	68 150
Music playing									
accordion (sitting)		1.5	1.6	1.7	1.8	1.9	2.0	2.1	2.2
cello (sitting)		2.0	2.1	2.2	2.3	2.4	2.5	2.7	2.8
conducting		1.9	2.0	2.1	2.2	2.3	2.4	2.5	2.7
drums (sitting)		3.1	3.3	3.5	3.7	3.9	4.1	4.3	4.5
flute (sitting)		1.7	1.8	1.9	2.0	2.1	2.2	2.3	2.4
horn (sitting)		1.4	1.5	1.5	1.6	1.7	1.8	1.9	2.0
organ (sitting)		2.6	2.7	2.8	3.0	3.1	3.3	3.4	3.6
piano (sitting)		1.9	2.0	2.1	2.2	2.4	2.5	2.6	2.7
trumpet (standing)		1.5	1.6	1.6	1.7	1.8	1.9	2.0	2.1
violin (sitting)		2.2	2.3	2.4	2.5	2.7	2.8	2.9	3.1
woodwind (sitting)		1.5	1.6	1.7	1.8	1.9	2.0	2.1	2.2
Paddleball		8.5	8.9	9.4	10.0	10.5	11.0	11.6	12.1
Paddle tennis		8.4	8.6	9.1	9.6	10.1	10.7	11.1	11.7
Painting									
inside projects		1.6	1.7	1.8	1.9	2.0	2.1	2.2	2.3
outside projects		3.7	3.9	4.1	4.3	4.5	4.8	5.0	5.2
scraping		3.1	3.2	3.3	3.5	3.7	3.9	4.1	4.3
Planting seedings		3.3	3.5	3.7	3.9	4.1	4.3	4.6	4.8
Plastering		3.7	3.9	4.1	4.4	4.6	4.8	5.1	5.3
Printing press work		1.7	1.8	1.9	2.0	2.1	2.2	2.3	2.4
Racquetball		8.4	8.9	9.4	10.0	10.5	11.0	11.6	12.1
Roller skating, leisure		5.3	5.8	6.2	6.5	6.9	7.3	7.3	8.0
Rope jumping									
110 rpm		6.7	7.1	7.5	7.9	8.4	8.8	9.2	9.7
120 rpm		6.4	6.8	7.3	7.7	8.1	8.5	8.9	9.3
130 rpm		6.0	6.4	6.8	7.1	7.5	7.7	8.3	8.7
Rowing									
machine, moderate		5.7	6.0	6.3	6.7	7.0	7.4	7.7	8.1
machine, race pace		8.6	8.9	9.4	10.0	10.5	11.0	11.6	12.1
skull, leisure		4.7	5.0	5.3	5.5	5.9	6.2	6.4	6.8
skull, race pace		8.7	8.9	9.4	10.0	10.5	11.0	11.6	12.1
Running, cross-country		7.8	8.2	8.6	9.1	9.6	10.1	10.6	11.1
Running, on flat surface									
11 min, 30 s per mile		6.3	6.8	7.2	7.6	8.0	8.4	8.8	9.2
9 min per mile		9.1	9.7	10.2	10.8	11.4	12.0	12.5	13.1
8 min per mile		9.8	10.8	11.3	11.9	12.5	13.1	13.6	14.2
7 min per mile		10.7	12.2	12.7	13.3	13.9	14.5	15.0	15.6
6 min per mile		11.8	13.9	14.4	15.0	15.6	16.2	16.7	17.3
5 min, 30 s per mile		13.6	14.5	15.3	16.2	17.1	17.9	18.8	19.7
Sailing, leisure		2.1	2.2	2.3	2.5	2.6	2.7	2.9	3.0
Scrubbing floors		5.1	5.5	5.8	6.1	6.4	6.8	7.1	7.4
Scuba diving		10.9	11.2	11.5	11.8	12.1	12.4	12.7	13.0
Shoe repair, general		2.2	2.3	2.4	2.5	2.7	2.8	2.9	3.1
Sitting quietly		1.0	1.1	1.1	1.2	1.2	1.3	1.4	1.4
Skateboarding		5.6	5.8	6.2	6.5	6.9	7.2	7.5	7.9
Skiing, hard snow									
level, moderate speed		5.6	6.0	6.3	6.7	7.0	7.4	7.7	8.1
level, walking speed		6.7	7.2	7.6	8.0	8.4	8.9	9.3	9.7
uphill, "fast" speed		12.9	13.7	14.5	15.3	16.2	17.0	17.8	18.6

| 71 | 74 | 77 | 80 | 83 | 86 | 89 | 92 | 95 | 98 |
157	163	170	176	183	190	196	203	209	216
2.3	2.4	2.5	2.6	2.7	2.8	2.8	2.9	3.0	3.1
2.9	3.0	3.2	3.3	3.4	3.5	3.6	3.8	3.9	4.0
2.8	2.9	3.0	3.1	3.2	3.4	3.5	3.6	3.7	3.8
4.7	4.9	5.1	5.3	5.5	5.7	5.9	6.1	6.3	6.6
2.5	2.6	2.7	2.8	2.9	3.0	3.1	3.2	3.3	3.4
2.1	2.1	2.2	2.3	2.4	2.5	2.6	2.7	2.8	2.8
3.8	3.9	4.1	4.2	4.4	4.6	4.7	4.9	5.0	5.2
2.8	3.0	3.1	3.2	3.3	3.4	3.6	3.7	3.8	3.9
2.2	2.3	2.4	2.5	2.6	2.7	2.8	2.9	2.9	3.0
3.2	3.3	3.5	3.6	3.7	3.9	4.0	4.1	4.3	4.4
2.3	2.4	2.5	2.6	2.7	2.8	2.8	2.9	3.0	3.1
12.6	13.2	13.7	14.2	14.8	15.3	15.8	16.4	16.9	17.4
12.2	12.7	13.2	13.7	14.2	14.2	15.2	15.8	16.3	16.8
2.4	2.5	2.6	2.7	2.8	2.9	3.0	3.1	3.2	3.3
5.5	5.7	5.9	6.2	6.4	6.6	6.9	7.1	7.3	7.5
4.5	4.7	4.9	5.0	5.2	5.4	5.6	5.8	6.0	6.2
5.0	5.2	5.4	5.6	5.8	6.0	6.2	6.4	6.7	6.9
5.5	5.8	6.0	6.2	6.5	6.7	6.9	7.2	7.4	7.6
2.5	2.6	2.7	2.8	2.9	3.0	3.1	3.2	3.3	3.4
12.6	13.2	13.7	14.2	14.8	15.3	15.8	16.4	16.9	17.4
8.3	8.6	9.0	9.3	9.7	10.1	10.4	10.8	11.1	11.4
10.1	10.5	10.5	11.3	11.8	12.2	12.6	13.1	13.5	13.9
9.8	10.1	10.6	10.9	11.4	11.8	12.2	12.6	13.0	13.4
9.1	9.4	9.8	10.2	10.6	11.0	11.3	11.7	12.1	12.5
8.5	8.9	9.3	9.7	10.1	10.6	11.1	11.6	12.1	12.6
12.6	13.2	13.7	14.2	14.8	15.3	15.8	16.4	16.9	17.4
7.2	7.6	8.0	8.4	8.8	9.2	9.6	10.0	10.4	10.8
12.6	13.2	13.7	14.2	14.8	15.3	15.8	16.4	16.9	17.4
11.6	12.1	12.6	13.0	13.5	14.0	14.5	15.0	15.5	16.0
9.6	10.0	10.5	10.9	11.3	11.7	12.1	12.5	12.9	13.3
13.7	14.3	14.9	15.4	16.0	16.6	17.2	17.8	18.3	18.9
14.8	15.4	16.0	16.5	17.1	17.7	18.3	18.9	19.4	20.0
16.2	16.8	17.4	17.9	18.5	19.1	19.7	20.3	20.8	21.4
17.9	18.5	19.1	19.6	20.2	20.8	21.4	22.0	22.5	23.1
20.5	21.4	22.3	23.1	24.0	24.9	25.7	26.6	27.5	28.3
3.1	3.3	3.4	3.5	3.7	3.8	3.9	4.1	4.2	4.3
7.7	8.1	8.4	8.7	9.0	9.4	9.7	10.0	10.4	10.7
13.3	13.6	13.9	14.2	14.5	14.8	15.1	15.4	15.7	16.0
3.2	3.3	3.5	3.6	3.7	3.9	4.0	4.1	4.3	4.4
1.5	1.6	1.6	1.7	1.7	1.8	1.9	1.9	2.0	2.1
8.3	8.6	8.9	9.3	9.6	10.0	10.3	10.7	11.0	11.4
8.4	8.8	9.2	9.5	9.9	10.2	10.6	10.9	11.3	11.7
10.2	10.6	11.0	11.4	11.9	12.3	12.7	13.2	13.6	14.0
19.5	20.3	21.1	21.9	22.7	23.6	24.4	25.2	26.0	26.9

YOUR BODY WEIGHT—*continued*

| Activity | kg | 47 | 50 | 53 | 56 | 59 | 62 | 65 | 68 |
	lb	104	110	117	123	130	137	143	150
Skiing, soft snow									
leisure (F)		4.6	4.9	5.2	5.5	5.8	6.1	6.4	6.7
leisure (M)		5.2	5.6	5.9	6.2	6.5	6.9	7.2	7.5
Skindiving									
considerable motion		13.0	13.8	14.6	15.5	16.3	17.1	17.9	18.8
moderate motion		9.7	10.3	10.9	11.5	12.2	12.8	13.4	14.0
Snorkeling		4.3	4.6	4.9	5.2	5.5	5.8	6.0	6.3
Snowshoeing, soft snow		7.8	8.3	8.8	9.3	9.8	10.3	10.8	11.3
Snowmobiling		3.4	3.7	4.0	4.2	4.4	4.7	4.9	5.1
Soccer		6.5	6.8	7.3	7.7	8.1	8.5	8.9	9.3
Softball		3.3	3.5	3.7	3.9	4.1	4.3	4.5	4.7
Squash		10.0	10.6	11.2	11.9	12.5	13.1	13.8	14.4
Standing quietly (M)		1.3	1.4	1.4	1.5	1.6	1.7	1.8	1.8
Steel mill, working in									
fettling		4.3	4.5	4.7	5.0	5.3	5.5	5.8	6.1
forging		4.7	5.0	5.3	5.6	5.9	6.2	6.5	6.8
hand rolling		6.4	6.9	7.3	7.7	8.1	8.5	8.9	9.3
merchant mill rolling		6.8	7.3	7.7	8.1	8.6	9.0	9.4	9.9
removing slag		8.4	8.9	9.4	10.0	10.5	11.0	11.6	12.1
tending furnace		5.9	6.3	6.7	7.1	7.4	7.8	8.2	8.6
tipping molds		4.3	4.6	4.9	5.2	5.4	5.7	6.0	6.3
Surfing		3.9	4.1	4.3	4.5	4.8	5.0	5.3	5.5
Stock clerking		2.5	2.7	2.9	3.0	3.2	3.3	3.5	3.7
Swimming, fitness swims									
back stroke		7.9	8.5	9.0	9.5	10.0	10.5	11.0	11.5
breast stroke		7.6	8.1	8.6	9.1	9.6	10.0	10.5	11.0
butterfly			8.6	9.1	9.6	10.1	10.7	11.1	11.7
crawl, fast		7.3	7.8	8.3	8.7	9.2	9.7	10.1	10.6
crawl, slow		6.0	6.4	6.8	7.2	7.6	7.9	8.3	8.7
side stroke		5.7	6.1	6.5	6.8	7.2	7.6	7.9	8.3
treading, fast		8.0	8.5	9.0	9.5	10.0	10.5	11.1	11.6
treading, normal		2.9	3.1	3.3	3.5	3.7	3.8	4.0	4.2
Table tennis (ping pong)		3.2	3.4	3.6	3.8	4.0	4.2	4.4	4.6
Tailoring									
cutting		2.0	2.1	2.2	2.3	2.4	2.5	2.7	2.8
hand-sewing		1.5	1.6	1.7	1.8	1.9	2.0	2.1	2.2
machine-sewing		2.2	2.3	2.4	2.5	2.7	2.8	2.9	3.1
pressing		2.9	3.1	3.3	3.5	3.7	3.8	4.0	4.2
Tennis									
competition		6.9	7.3	7.8	8.2	8.7	9.1	9.5	9.9
recreational		5.1	5.5	5.8	6.1	6.4	6.8	7.1	7.4
Typing									
electric (computer)		1.3	1.4	1.4	1.5	1.6	1.7	1.8	1.8
manual		1.5	1.6	1.6	1.7	1.8	1.9	2.0	2.1
Volleyball									
competition		5.9	7.3	7.8	8.2	8.7	9.1	9.5	10.0
recreational		2.4	2.5	2.7	2.8	3.0	3.1	3.3	3.4

71 157	74 163	77 170	80 176	83 183	86 190	89 196	92 203	95 209	98 216
7.0	7.3	7.5	7.8	8.1	8.4	8.7	9.0	9.3	9.6
7.9	8.2	8.5	8.9	9.2	9.5	9.9	10.2	10.5	10.9
19.6	20.4	21.3	22.1	22.9	23.7	24.6	25.4	26.2	27.0
14.6	15.2	15.9	16.5	17.1	17.7	18.3	19.0	19.6	20.2
6.6	6.8	7.1	7.4	7.7	8.0	8.2	8.5	8.8	9.1
11.8	12.3	12.8	13.3	13.8	14.3	14.8	15.3	15.8	16.3
5.3	5.5	5.8	6.0	6.2	6.5	6.7	6.9	7.1	7.3
9.8	10.1	10.6	10.9	11.4	11.8	12.2	12.6	13.0	13.4
4.9	5.1	5.3	5.5	5.7	5.9	6.1	6.3	6.5	6.7
15.1	15.7	16.3	17.0	17.6	18.2	18.9	19.5	20.1	20.8
1.9	2.0	2.1	2.2	2.2	2.3	2.4	2.5	2.6	2.6
6.3	6.6	6.9	7.1	7.4	7.7	7.9	8.2	8.5	8.7
7.1	7.4	7.7	8.0	8.3	8.6	8.9	9.2	9.5	9.8
9.7	10.1	10.6	11.0	11.4	11.8	12.2	12.6	13.0	13.4
10.3	10.7	11.2	11.6	12.0	12.5	12.9	13.3	13.8	14.2
12.6	13.2	13.7	14.2	14.8	15.3	15.8	16.4	16.9	17.4
8.9	9.3	9.7	10.1	10.5	10.8	11.2	11.6	12.0	12.3
6.5	6.8	7.1	7.4	7.6	7.9	8.2	8.5	8.7	9.0
5.7	6.0	6.3	6.5	6.8	7.0	7.2	7.4	7.6	7.9
3.8	4.0	4.2	4.3	4.5	4.6	4.8	5.0	5.1	5.3
12.0	12.5	13.0	13.5	14.0	14.5	15.0	15.5	16.1	16.6
11.5	12.0	12.5	13.0	13.4	13.9	14.4	14.9	15.4	15.9
12.2	12.7	13.2	13.7	14.2	14.2	15.2	15.8	16.3	16.8
11.1	11.5	12.0	12.5	12.9	13.4	13.9	14.4	14.8	15.3
9.1	9.5	9.9	10.2	10.6	11.0	11.4	11.8	12.2	12.5
8.7	9.0	9.4	9.8	10.1	10.5	10.9	11.2	11.6	12.0
12.1	12.6	13.1	13.6	14.1	14.6	15.1	15.6	16.2	16.7
4.4	4.6	4.8	5.0	5.1	5.3	5.5	5.7	5.9	6.1
4.8	5.0	5.2	5.4	5.6	5.8	6.1	6.3	6.5	6.7
2.9	3.0	3.2	3.3	3.4	3.5	3.6	3.8	3.9	4.0
2.3	2.4	2.5	2.6	2.7	2.8	2.8	2.9	3.0	3.1
3.2	3.3	3.5	3.6	3.7	3.9	4.0	4.1	4.3	4.4
4.4	4.6	4.8	5.0	5.1	5.3	5.5	5.7	5.9	6.1
10.2	10.6	11.1	11.5	11.9	12.4	12.8	13.2	13.7	14.1
7.7	8.1	8.4	8.7	9.0	9.4	9.7	10.0	10.4	10.7
1.9	2.0	2.1	2.2	2.2	2.3	2.4	2.5	2.6	2.6
2.2	2.3	2.4	2.5	2.6	2.7	2.8	2.9	2.9	3.0
3.6	3.7	3.9	4.0	4.2	4.3	4.5	4.6	4.8	4.9
10.5	10.9	11.4	11.8	12.3	12.7	13.1	13.6	14.0	14.5

YOUR BODY WEIGHT—*continued*

Activity	kg lb	47 104	50 110	53 117	56 123	59 130	62 137	65 143	68 150
Walking, leisure outdoors									
asphalt road		3.8	4.0	4.2	4.5	4.7	5.0	5.2	5.4
fields and hillsides		3.9	4.1	4.3	4.6	4.8	5.1	5.3	5.6
grass track		3.8	4.1	4.3	4.5	4.8	5.0	5.3	5.5
plowed field		3.6	3.9	4.1	4.3	4.5	4.8	5.0	5.2
Walking, treadmill level									
2.0 mph		2.4	2.6	2.8	3.0	3.1	3.3	3.4	3.6
2.5 mph		3.0	3.2	3.4	3.6	3.8	4.0	4.2	4.4
3.0 mph		3.6	3.8	4.0	4.2	4.4	4.6	4.8	5.0
3.5 mph		4.0	4.3	4.6	4.8	5.1	5.3	5.6	6.1
4.0 mph		4.6	4.9	5.2	5.4	5.7	6.0	6.3	6.6
Wallpapering		2.3	2.4	2.5	2.7	2.8	3.0	3.1	3.3
Water polo, recreation		7.0	7.4	7.7	8.1	8.5	8.9	9.3	9.7
Water polo, competition		9.4	9.9	10.4	11.0	11.5	12.0	12.5	13.1
Water-skiing		5.6	6.0	6.4	6.7	7.1	7.5	7.8	8.2
Watch repairing		1.2	1.3	1.3	1.4	1.5	1.6	1.6	1.7
Whitewater rafting, recreational		4.1	4.4	4.6	4.9	5.2	5.4	5.7	6.0
Window cleaning		2.9	3.0	3.1	3.3	3.5	3.7	3.8	4.0
Wind surfing		3.3	3.5	3.7	3.9	4.1	4.3	4.6	4.8
Wrestling, competition		9.1	9.7	10.3	10.8	11.4	12.0	12.6	13.2
Writing (sitting)		1.4	1.5	1.5	1.6	1.7	1.8	1.9	2.0
Yoga		2.9	3.1	3.3	3.5	3.7	3.8	4.0	4.2

| 71 | 74 | 77 | 80 | 83 | 86 | 89 | 92 | 95 | 98 |
157	163	170	176	183	190	196	203	209	216
5.7	5.9	6.2	6.4	6.6	6.9	7.1	7.4	7.6	7.8
5.8	6.1	6.3	6.6	6.8	7.1	7.3	7.5	7.8	8.0
5.8	6.0	6.2	6.5	6.7	7.0	7.2	7.5	7.7	7.9
5.5	5.7	5.9	6.2	6.4	6.6	6.9	7.1	7.3	7.5
3.7	3.9	4.1	4.2	4.4	4.5	4.7	4.9	5.0	5.2
4.5	4.7	4.9	5.1	5.3	5.5	5.7	5.9	6.1	6.3
5.3	5.5	5.7	5.9	6.2	6.5	6.7	6.9	7.1	7.3
6.1	6.4	6.6	6.9	7.1	7.4	7.7	7.9	8.2	8.4
6.9	7.2	7.5	7.8	8.1	8.4	8.7	8.9	9.2	9.5
3.4	3.6	3.7	3.8	4.0	4.1	4.3	4.4	4.6	4.7
10.1	10.5	10.9	11.3	11.7	12.1	12.5	12.9	13.3	13.7
13.6	14.1	14.7	15.2	15.7	16.3	16.8	17.3	17.9	18.4
8.7	9.1	9.4	9.8	10.1	10.5	10.9	11.2	11.6	12.0
1.8	1.9	1.9	2.0	2.1	2.2	2.2	2.3	2.4	2.5
6.2	6.5	6.7	7.0	7.3	7.5	7.8	8.1	8.3	8.6
4.2	4.4	4.5	4.7	4.9	5.1	5.3	5.4	5.6	5.8
5.0	5.2	5.4	5.6	5.8	6.0	6.2	6.4	6.7	6.9
13.8	14.3	14.9	15.5	16.1	16.7	17.2	17.8	18.4	19.0
2.1	2.1	2.2	2.3	2.4	2.5	2.6	2.7	2.8	2.8
4.4	4.6	4.8	5.0	5.1	5.3	5.5	5.7	5.9	6.1

Body Composition[a]

This appendix contains the age- and sex-specific equations to predict body fat percentage based on three girth measurements. There are four charts, one each for young and older men and women. In our experience, it is important to calibrate the tape measure prior to its use. Use a meter stick as the standard and check the markings on the cloth tape at 10-cm increments. A cloth tape is preferred over a metal one because there is little skin compression when applying a cloth tape to the skin's surface at a relatively constant tension.

To use the charts, measure the three girths at the sites indicated in Figure 27.8. The anatomic landmarks and procedures are explained. The specific equation to predict percent body fat with its corresponding constant is presented at the bottom of each of the four charts (Charts E.2 to E.5).

CHART E.1
BODY SITES MEASURED BY THE CIRCUMFERENCE METHOD

Age (years)	Sex	Site Measured		
		A	B	C
18–26	M	Right upper arm	Abdomen	Right forearm
	F	Abdomen	Right thigh	Right forearm
27–50	M	Buttocks	Abdomen	Right forearm
	F	Abdomen	Right thigh	Right calf

CHART E.2
CONVERSION CONSTANTS TO PREDICT PERCENT BODY FAT FOR YOUNG MEN

Upper Arm			Abdomen			Forearm		
in	cm	Constant A	in	cm	Constant B	in	cm	Constant C
7.00	17.78	25.91	21.00	53.34	27.56	7.00	17.78	38.01
7.25	18.41	26.83	21.25	53.97	27.88	7.25	18.41	39.37
7.50	19.05	27.76	21.50	54.61	28.21	7.50	19.05	40.72
7.75	19.68	28.68	21.75	55.24	28.54	7.75	19.68	42.08
8.00	20.32	29.61	22.00	55.88	28.87	8.00	20.32	43.44
8.25	20.95	30.53	22.25	56.51	29.20	8.25	20.95	44.80
8.50	21.59	31.46	22.50	57.15	29.52	8.50	21.59	46.15
8.75	22.22	32.38	22.75	57.78	29.85	8.75	22.22	47.51
9.00	22.86	33.31	23.00	58.42	30.18	9.00	22.86	48.87
9.25	23.49	34.24	23.25	59.05	30.51	9.25	23.49	50.23
9.50	24.13	35.16	23.50	59.69	30.84	9.50	24.13	51.58
9.75	24.76	36.09	23.75	60.32	31.16	9.75	24.76	52.94
10.00	25.40	37.01	24.00	60.96	31.49	10.00	25.40	54.30
10.25	26.03	37.94	24.25	61.59	31.82	10.25	26.03	55.65
10.50	26.67	38.86	24.50	62.23	32.15	10.50	26.67	57.01

CHART E.2—continued

	Upper Arm			Abdomen			Forearm	
in	*cm*	*Constant A*	*in*	*cm*	*Constant B*	*in*	*cm*	*Constant C*
10.75	27.30	39.79	24.75	62.86	32.48	10.75	27.30	58.37
11.00	27.94	40.71	25.00	63.50	32.80	11.00	27.94	59.73
11.25	28.57	41.64	25.25	64.13	33.13	11.25	28.57	61.08
11.50	29.21	42.56	25.50	64.77	33.46	11.50	29.21	62.44
11.75	29.84	43.49	25.75	65.40	33.79	11.75	29.84	63.80
12.00	30.48	44.41	26.00	66.04	34.12	12.00	30.48	65.16
12.25	31.11	45.34	26.25	66.67	34.44	12.25	31.11	66.51
12.50	31.75	46.26	26.50	67.31	34.77	12.50	31.75	67.87
12.75	32.38	47.19	26.75	67.94	35.10	12.75	32.38	69.23
13.00	33.02	48.11	27.00	68.58	35.43	13.00	33.02	70.59
13.25	33.65	49.04	27.25	69.21	35.76	13.25	33.65	71.94
13.50	34.29	49.96	27.50	69.85	36.09	13.50	34.29	73.30
13.75	34.92	50.89	27.75	70.48	36.41	13.75	34.92	74.66
14.00	35.56	51.82	28.00	71.12	36.74	14.00	35.56	76.02
14.25	36.19	52.74	28.25	71.75	37.07	14.25	36.19	77.37
14.50	36.83	53.67	28.50	72.39	37.40	14.50	36.83	78.73
14.75	37.46	54.59	28.75	73.02	37.73	14.75	37.46	80.09
15.00	38.10	55.52	29.00	73.66	38.05	15.00	38.10	81.45
15.25	38.73	56.44	29.25	74.29	38.38	15.25	38.73	82.80
15.50	39.37	57.37	29.50	74.93	38.71	15.50	39.37	84.16
15.75	40.00	58.29	29.75	75.56	39.04	15.75	40.00	85.52
16.00	40.64	59.22	30.00	76.20	39.37	16.00	40.64	86.88
16.25	41.27	60.14	30.25	76.83	39.69	16.25	41.27	88.23
16.50	41.91	61.07	30.50	77.47	40.02	16.50	41.91	89.59
16.75	42.54	61.99	30.75	78.10	40.35	16.75	42.54	90.95
17.00	43.18	62.92	31.00	78.74	40.68	17.00	43.18	92.31
17.25	43.81	63.84	31.25	79.37	41.01	17.25	43.81	93.66
17.50	44.45	64.77	31.50	80.01	41.33	17.50	44.45	95.02
17.75	45.08	65.69	31.75	80.64	41.66	17.75	45.08	96.38
18.00	45.72	66.62	32.00	81.28	41.99	18.00	45.72	97.74
18.25	46.35	67.54	32.25	81.91	42.32	18.25	46.35	99.09
18.50	46.99	68.47	32.50	82.55	42.65	18.50	46.99	100.45
18.75	47.62	69.40	32.75	83.18	42.97	18.75	47.62	101.81
19.00	48.26	70.32	33.00	83.82	43.30	19.00	48.26	103.17
19.25	48.89	71.25	33.25	84.45	43.63	19.25	48.89	104.52
19.50	49.53	72.17	33.50	85.09	43.96	19.50	49.53	105.88
19.75	50.16	73.10	33.75	85.72	44.29	19.75	50.16	107.24
20.00	50.80	74.02	34.00	86.36	44.61	20.00	50.80	108.60
20.25	51.43	74.95	34.25	86.99	44.94	20.25	51.43	109.95
20.50	52.07	75.87	34.50	87.63	45.27	20.50	52.07	111.31
20.75	52.70	76.80	34.75	88.26	45.60	20.75	52.70	112.67
21.00	53.34	77.72	35.00	88.90	45.93	21.00	53.34	114.02
21.25	53.97	78.65	35.25	89.53	46.25	21.25	53.97	115.38
21.50	54.61	79.57	35.50	90.17	46.58	21.50	54.61	116.74
21.75	55.24	80.50	35.75	90.80	46.91	21.75	55.24	118.10
22.00	55.88	81.42	36.00	91.44	47.24	22.00	55.88	119.45
			36.25	92.07	47.57			
			36.50	92.71	47.89			
			36.75	93.34	48.22			
			37.00	93.98	48.55			
			37.25	94.61	48.88			
			37.50	95.25	49.21			
			37.75	95.88	49.54			

CHART E.2—continued

Upper Arm			Abdomen			Forearm		
in	cm	Constant A	in	cm	Constant B	in	cm	Constant C
			38.00	96.52	49.86			
			38.25	97.15	50.19			
			38.50	97.79	50.52			
			38.75	98.42	50.85			
			39.00	99.06	51.18			
			39.25	99.69	51.50			
			39.50	100.33	51.83			
			39.75	100.96	52.16			
			40.00	101.60	52.49			
			40.25	102.23	52.82			
			40.50	102.87	53.14			
			40.75	103.50	53.47			
			41.00	104.14	53.80			
			41.25	104.77	54.13			
			41.50	105.41	54.46			
			41.75	106.04	54.78			
			42.00	106.68	55.11			

Note: Percent Fat = Constant A + Constant B − Constant C − 10.2

CHART E.3
CONVERSION CONSTANTS TO PREDICT PERCENT BODY FAT FOR OLDER MEN

Buttocks			Abdomen			Forearm		
in	cm	Constant A	in	cm	Constant B	in	cm	Constant C
28.00	71.12	29.34	25.50	64.77	22.84	7.00	17.78	21.01
28.25	71.75	29.60	25.75	65.40	23.06	7.25	18.41	21.76
28.50	72.39	29.87	26.00	66.04	23.29	7.50	19.05	22.52
28.75	73.02	30.13	26.25	66.67	23.51	7.75	19.68	23.26
29.00	73.66	30.39	26.50	67.31	23.73	8.00	20.32	24.02
29.25	74.29	30.65	26.75	67.94	23.96	8.25	20.95	24.76
29.50	74.93	30.92	27.00	68.58	24.18	8.50	21.59	25.52
29.75	75.56	31.18	27.25	69.21	24.40	8.75	22.22	26.26
30.00	76.20	31.44	27.50	69.85	24.63	9.00	22.86	27.02
30.25	76.83	31.70	27.75	70.48	24.85	9.25	23.49	27.76
30.50	77.47	31.96	28.00	71.12	25.08	9.50	24.13	28.52
30.75	78.10	32.22	28.25	71.75	25.29	9.75	24.76	29.26
31.00	78.74	32.49	28.50	72.39	25.52	10.00	25.40	30.02
31.25	79.37	32.75	28.75	73.02	25.75	10.25	26.03	30.76
31.50	80.01	33.01	29.00	73.66	25.97	10.50	26.67	31.52
31.75	80.64	33.27	29.25	74.29	26.19	10.75	27.30	32.27
32.00	81.28	33.54	29.50	74.93	26.42	11.00	27.94	33.02
32.25	81.91	33.80	29.75	75.56	26.64	11.25	28.57	33.77
32.50	82.55	34.06	30.00	76.20	26.87	11.50	29.21	34.52
32.75	83.18	34.32	30.25	76.83	27.09	11.75	29.84	35.27
33.00	83.82	34.58	30.50	77.47	27.32	12.00	30.48	36.02
33.25	84.45	34.84	30.75	78.10	27.54	12.25	31.11	36.77
33.50	85.09	35.11	31.00	78.74	27.76	12.50	31.75	37.53

CHART E.3—*continued*

	Buttocks			Abdomen			Forearm	
in	*cm*	*Constant A*	*in*	*cm*	*Constant B*	*in*	*cm*	*Constant C*
33.75	85.72	35.37	31.25	79.37	27.98	12.75	32.38	38.27
34.00	86.36	35.63	31.50	80.01	28.21	13.00	33.02	39.03
34.25	86.99	35.89	31.75	80.64	28.43	13.25	33.65	39.77
34.50	87.63	36.16	32.00	81.28	28.66	13.50	34.29	40.53
34.75	88.26	36.42	32.25	81.91	28.88	13.75	34.92	41.27
35.00	88.90	36.68	32.50	82.55	29.11	14.00	35.56	42.03
35.25	89.53	36.94	32.75	83.18	29.33	14.25	36.19	42.77
35.50	90.17	37.20	33.00	83.82	29.55	14.50	36.83	43.53
35.75	90.80	37.46	33.25	84.45	29.78	14.75	37.46	44.27
36.00	91.44	37.73	33.50	85.09	30.00	15.00	38.10	45.03
36.25	92.07	37.99	33.75	85.72	30.22	15.25	38.73	45.77
36.50	92.71	38.25	34.00	86.36	30.45	15.50	39.37	46.53
36.75	93.34	38.51	34.25	86.99	30.67	15.75	40.00	47.28
37.00	93.98	38.78	34.50	87.63	30.89	16.00	40.64	48.03
37.25	94.61	39.04	34.75	88.26	31.12	16.25	41.27	48.78
37.50	95.25	39.30	35.00	88.90	31.35	16.50	41.91	49.53
37.75	95.88	39.56	35.25	89.53	31.57	16.75	42.54	50.28
38.00	96.52	39.82	35.50	90.17	31.79	17.00	43.18	51.03
38.25	97.15	40.08	35.75	90.80	32.02	17.25	43.81	51.78
38.50	97.79	40.35	36.00	91.44	32.24	17.50	44.45	52.54
38.75	98.42	40.61	36.25	92.07	32.46	17.75	45.08	53.28
39.00	99.06	40.87	36.50	92.71	32.69	18.00	45.72	54.04
39.25	99.69	41.13	36.75	93.34	32.91	18.25	46.35	54.78
39.50	100.33	41.39	37.00	93.98	33.14			
39.75	100.96	41.66	37.25	94.61	33.36			
40.00	101.60	41.92	37.50	95.25	33.58			
40.25	102.23	42.18	37.75	95.88	33.81			
40.50	102.87	42.44	38.00	96.52	34.03			
40.75	103.50	42.70	38.25	97.15	34.26			
41.00	104.14	42.97	38.50	97.79	34.48			
41.25	104.77	43.23	38.75	98.42	34.70			
41.50	105.41	43.49	39.00	99.06	34.93			
41.75	106.04	43.75	39.25	99.69	35.15			
42.00	106.68	44.02	39.50	100.33	35.38			
42.25	107.31	44.28	39.75	100.96	35.59			
42.50	107.95	44.54	40.00	101.60	35.82			
42.75	108.58	44.80	40.25	102.23	36.05			
43.00	109.22	45.06	40.50	102.87	36.27			
43.25	109.85	45.32	40.75	103.50	36.49			
43.50	110.49	45.59	41.00	104.14	36.72			
43.75	111.12	45.85	41.25	104.77	36.94			
44.00	111.76	46.12	41.50	105.41	37.17			
44.25	112.39	46.37	41.75	106.04	37.39			
44.50	113.03	46.64	42.00	106.68	37.62			
44.75	113.66	46.89	42.25	107.31	37.87			
45.00	114.30	47.16	42.50	107.95	38.06			
45.25	114.93	47.42	42.75	108.58	38.28			
45.50	115.57	47.68	43.00	109.22	38.51			
45.75	116.20	47.94	43.25	109.85	38.73			
46.00	116.84	48.21	43.50	110.49	38.96			
46.25	117.47	48.47	43.75	111.12	39.18			
46.50	118.11	48.73	44.00	111.76	39.41			
46.75	118.74	48.99	44.25	112.39	39.63			

CHART E.3—continued

Buttocks			Abdomen			Forearm		
in	cm	Constant A	in	cm	Constant B	in	cm	Constant C
47.00	119.38	49.26	44.50	113.03	39.85			
47.25	120.01	49.52	44.75	113.66	40.08			
47.50	120.65	49.78	45.00	114.30	40.30			
47.75	121.28	50.04						
48.00	121.92	50.30						
48.25	122.55	50.56						
48.50	123.19	50.83						
48.75	123.82	51.09						
49.00	124.46	51.35						

Note: Percent Fat = Constant A + Constant B − Constant C − 15.0

CHART E.4
CONVERSION CONSTANTS TO PREDICT PERCENT BODY FAT FOR YOUNG WOMEN

Abdomen			Thigh			Forearm		
in	cm	Constant A	in	cm	Constant B	in	cm	Constant C
20.00	50.80	26.74	14.00	35.56	29.13	6.00	15.24	25.86
20.25	51.43	27.07	14.25	36.19	29.65	6.25	15.87	26.94
20.50	52.07	27.41	14.50	36.83	30.17	6.50	16.51	28.02
20.75	52.70	27.74	14.75	37.46	30.69	6.75	17.14	29.10
21.00	53.34	28.07	15.00	38.10	31.21	7.00	17.78	30.17
21.25	53.97	28.41	15.25	38.73	31.73	7.25	18.41	31.25
21.50	54.61	28.74	15.50	39.37	32.25	7.50	19.05	32.33
21.75	55.24	29.08	15.75	40.00	32.77	7.75	19.68	33.41
22.00	55.88	29.41	16.00	40.64	33.29	8.00	20.32	34.48
22.25	56.51	29.74	16.25	41.27	33.81	8.25	20.95	35.56
22.50	57.15	30.08	16.50	41.91	34.33	8.50	21.59	36.64
22.75	57.78	30.41	16.75	42.54	34.85	8.75	22.22	37.72
23.00	58.42	30.75	17.00	43.18	35.37	9.00	22.86	38.79
23.25	59.05	31.08	17.25	43.81	35.89	9.25	23.49	39.87
23.50	59.69	31.42	17.50	44.45	36.41	9.50	24.13	40.95
23.75	60.32	31.75	17.75	45.08	36.93	9.75	24.76	42.03
24.00	60.96	32.08	18.00	45.72	37.45	10.00	25.40	43.10
24.25	61.59	32.42	18.25	46.35	37.97	10.25	26.03	44.18
24.50	62.23	32.75	18.50	46.99	38.49	10.50	26.67	45.26
24.75	62.86	33.09	18.75	47.62	39.01	10.75	27.30	46.34
25.00	63.50	33.42	19.00	48.26	39.53	11.00	27.94	47.41
25.25	64.13	33.76	19.25	48.89	40.05	11.25	28.57	48.49
25.50	64.77	34.09	19.50	49.53	40.57	11.50	29.21	49.57
25.75	65.40	34.42	19.75	50.16	41.09	11.75	29.84	50.65
26.00	66.04	34.76	20.00	50.80	41.61	12.00	30.48	51.73
26.25	66.67	35.09	20.25	51.43	42.13	12.25	31.11	52.80
26.50	67.31	35.43	20.50	52.07	42.65	12.50	31.75	53.88
26.75	67.94	35.76	20.75	52.70	43.17	12.75	32.38	54.96
27.00	68.58	36.10	21.00	53.34	43.69	13.00	33.02	56.04
27.25	69.21	36.43	21.25	53.97	44.21	13.25	33.65	57.11
27.50	69.85	36.76	21.50	54.61	44.73	13.50	34.29	58.19

CHART E.4—continued

Abdomen			Thigh			Forearm		
in	cm	Constant A	in	cm	Constant B	in	cm	Constant C
27.75	70.48	37.10	21.75	55.24	45.25	13.75	34.92	59.27
28.00	71.12	37.43	22.00	55.88	45.77	14.00	35.56	60.35
28.25	71.75	37.77	22.25	56.51	46.29	14.25	36.19	61.42
28.50	72.39	38.10	22.50	57.15	46.81	14.50	36.83	62.50
28.75	73.02	38.43	22.75	57.78	47.33	14.75	37.46	63.58
29.00	73.66	38.77	23.00	58.42	47.85	15.00	38.10	64.66
29.25	74.29	39.10	23.25	59.05	48.37	15.25	38.73	65.73
29.50	74.93	39.44	23.50	59.69	48.89	15.50	39.37	66.81
29.75	75.56	39.77	23.75	60.32	49.41	15.75	40.00	67.89
30.00	76.20	40.11	24.00	60.96	49.93	16.00	40.64	68.97
30.25	76.83	40.44	24.25	61.59	50.45	16.25	41.27	70.04
30.50	77.47	40.77	24.50	62.23	50.97	16.50	41.91	71.12
30.75	78.10	41.11	24.75	62.86	51.49	16.75	42.54	72.20
31.00	78.74	41.44	25.00	63.50	52.01	17.00	43.18	73.28
31.25	79.37	41.78	25.25	64.13	52.53	17.25	43.81	74.36
31.50	80.01	42.11	25.50	64.77	53.05	17.50	44.45	75.43
31.75	80.64	42.45	25.75	65.40	53.57	17.75	45.08	76.51
32.00	81.28	42.78	26.00	66.04	54.09	18.00	45.72	77.59
32.25	81.91	43.11	26.25	66.67	54.61	18.25	46.35	78.67
32.50	82.55	43.45	26.50	67.31	55.13	18.50	46.99	79.74
32.75	83.18	43.78	26.75	67.94	55.65	18.75	47.62	80.82
33.00	83.82	44.12	27.00	68.58	56.17	19.00	48.26	81.90
33.25	84.45	44.45	27.25	69.21	56.69	19.25	48.89	82.98
33.50	85.09	44.78	27.50	69.85	57.21	19.50	49.53	84.05
33.75	85.72	45.12	27.75	70.48	57.73	19.75	50.16	85.13
34.00	86.36	45.45	28.00	71.12	58.26	20.00	50.80	86.21
34.25	86.99	45.79	28.25	71.75	58.78			
34.50	87.63	46.12	28.50	72.39	59.30			
34.75	88.26	46.46	38.75	73.02	59.82			
35.00	88.90	46.79	29.00	73.66	60.34			
35.25	89.53	47.12	29.25	74.29	60.86			
35.50	90.17	47.46	29.50	74.93	61.38			
35.75	90.80	47.79	29.75	75.56	61.90			
36.00	91.44	48.13	30.00	76.20	62.42			
36.25	92.07	48.46	30.25	76.83	62.94			
36.50	92.71	48.80	30.50	77.47	63.46			
36.75	93.34	49.13	30.75	78.10	63.98			
37.00	93.98	49.46	31.00	78.74	64.50			
37.25	94.61	49.80	31.25	79.37	65.02			
37.50	95.25	50.13	31.50	80.01	65.54			
37.75	95.88	50.47	31.75	80.64	66.06			
38.00	96.52	50.80	32.00	81.28	66.58			
38.25	97.15	51.13	32.25	81.91	67.10			
38.50	97.79	51.47	32.50	82.55	67.62			
38.75	98.42	51.80	32.75	83.18	68.14			
39.00	99.06	52.14	33.00	83.82	68.66			
39.25	99.69	52.47	33.25	84.45	69.18			
39.50	100.33	52.81	33.50	85.09	69.70			
39.75	100.96	53.14	33.75	85.72	70.22			
40.00	101.60	53.47	34.00	86.36	70.74			

Note: Percent Fat = Constant A + Constant B − Constant C − 19.6

CHART E.5
CONVERSION CONSTANTS TO PREDICT PERCENT BODY FAT FOR OLDER WOMEN

Abdomen			Thigh			Forearm		
in	cm	Constant A	in	cm	Constant B	in	cm	Constant C
25.00	63.50	29.69	14.00	35.56	17.31	10.00	25.40	14.46
25.25	64.13	29.98	14.25	36.19	17.62	10.25	26.03	14.82
25.50	64.77	30.28	14.50	36.83	17.93	10.50	26.67	15.18
25.75	65.40	30.58	14.75	37.46	18.24	10.75	27.30	15.54
26.00	66.04	30.87	15.00	38.10	18.55	11.00	27.94	15.91
26.25	66.67	31.17	15.25	38.73	18.86	11.25	28.57	16.27
26.50	67.31	31.47	15.50	39.37	19.17	11.50	29.21	16.63
26.75	67.94	31.76	15.75	40.00	19.47	11.75	29.84	16.99
27.00	68.58	32.06	16.00	40.64	19.78	12.00	30.48	17.35
27.25	69.21	32.36	16.25	41.27	20.09	12.25	31.11	17.71
27.50	69.85	32.65	16.50	41.91	20.40	12.50	31.75	18.08
27.75	70.48	32.95	16.75	42.54	20.71	12.75	32.38	18.44
28.00	71.12	33.25	17.00	43.18	21.02	13.00	33.02	18.80
28.25	71.75	33.55	17.25	43.81	21.33	13.25	33.65	19.16
28.50	72.39	33.84	17.50	44.45	21.64	13.50	34.29	19.52
28.75	73.02	34.14	17.75	45.08	21.95	13.75	34.92	19.88
29.00	73.66	34.44	18.00	45.72	22.26	14.00	35.56	20.24
29.25	74.29	34.73	18.25	46.35	22.57	14.25	36.19	20.61
29.50	74.93	35.03	18.50	46.99	22.87	14.50	36.83	20.97
29.75	75.56	35.33	18.75	47.62	23.18	14.75	37.46	21.33
30.00	76.20	35.62	19.00	38.26	23.49	15.00	38.10	21.69
30.25	76.83	35.92	19.25	48.89	23.80	15.25	38.73	22.05
30.50	77.47	36.22	19.50	49.53	24.11	15.50	39.37	22.41
30.75	78.10	36.51	19.75	50.16	24.42	15.75	40.00	22.77
31.00	78.74	36.81	20.00	50.80	24.73	16.00	40.64	23.14
31.25	79.37	37.11	20.25	51.43	25.04	16.25	41.27	23.50
31.50	80.01	37.40	20.50	52.07	25.35	16.50	41.91	23.86
31.75	80.64	37.70	20.75	52.70	25.66	16.75	42.54	24.22
32.00	81.28	38.00	21.00	53.34	25.97	17.00	43.18	24.58
32.25	81.91	38.30	21.25	53.97	26.28	17.25	43.81	24.94
32.50	82.55	38.59	21.50	54.61	26.58	17.50	44.45	25.31
32.75	83.18	38.89	21.75	55.24	26.89	17.75	45.08	25.67
33.00	83.82	39.19	22.00	55.88	27.20	18.00	45.72	26.03
33.25	84.45	39.48	22.25	56.51	27.51	18.25	46.35	26.39
33.50	85.09	39.78	22.50	57.15	27.82	18.50	46.99	26.75
33.75	85.72	40.08	22.75	57.78	28.13	18.75	47.62	27.11
34.00	86.36	40.37	23.00	58.42	28.44	19.00	48.26	27.47
34.25	86.99	40.67	23.25	59.05	28.75	19.25	48.89	27.84
34.50	87.63	40.97	23.50	59.69	29.06	19.50	49.53	28.20
34.75	88.26	41.26	23.75	60.32	29.37	19.75	50.16	28.56
35.00	88.90	41.56	24.00	60.96	29.68	20.00	50.80	28.92
35.25	89.53	41.86	24.25	61.59	29.98	20.25	51.43	29.28
35.50	90.17	42.15	24.50	62.23	30.29	20.50	52.07	29.64
35.75	90.80	42.45	24.75	62.86	30.60	20.75	52.70	30.00
36.00	91.44	42.75	25.00	63.50	30.91	21.00	53.34	30.37
36.25	92.07	43.05	25.25	64.13	31.22	21.25	53.97	30.73
36.50	92.71	43.34	25.50	64.77	31.53	21.50	54.61	31.09
36.75	93.35	43.64	25.75	65.40	31.84	21.75	55.24	31.45
37.00	93.98	43.94	26.00	66.04	32.15	22.00	55.88	31.81
37.25	94.62	44.23	26.25	66.67	32.46	22.25	56.51	32.17
37.50	95.25	44.53	26.50	67.31	32.77	22.50	57.15	32.54

CHART E.5—*continued*

Abdomen			Thigh			Forearm		
in	*cm*	*Constant A*	*in*	*cm*	*Constant B*	*in*	*cm*	*Constant C*
37.75	95.89	44.83	26.75	67.94	33.08	22.75	57.78	32.90
38.00	96.52	45.12	27.00	68.58	33.38	23.00	58.42	33.26
38.25	97.16	45.42	27.25	69.21	33.69	23.25	59.05	33.62
38.50	97.79	45.72	27.50	69.85	34.00	23.50	59.69	33.98
38.75	98.43	46.01	27.75	70.48	34.31	23.75	60.32	34.34
39.00	99.06	46.31	28.00	71.12	34.62	24.00	60.96	34.70
39.25	99.70	46.61	28.25	71.75	34.93	24.25	61.59	35.07
39.50	100.33	46.90	28.50	72.39	35.24	24.50	62.23	35.43
39.75	100.97	47.20	28.75	73.02	35.55	24.75	62.86	35.79
40.00	101.60	47.50	29.00	73.66	35.86	25.00	63.50	36.15
40.25	101.24	47.79	29.25	74.29	36.17			
40.50	102.87	48.09	29.50	74.93	36.48			
40.75	103.51	48.39	29.75	75.56	36.79			
41.00	104.14	48.69	30.00	76.20	37.09			
41.25	104.78	48.98	30.25	76.83	37.40			
41.50	105.41	49.28	30.50	77.47	37.71			
41.75	106.05	49.58	30.75	78.10	38.02			
42.00	106.68	49.87	31.00	78.74	38.33			
42.25	107.32	50.17	31.25	79.37	38.64			
42.50	107.95	50.47	31.50	80.01	38.95			
42.75	108.59	50.76	31.75	80.64	39.26			
43.00	109.22	51.06	32.00	81.28	39.57			
43.25	109.86	51.36	32.25	81.91	39.88			
43.50	110.49	51.65	32.50	82.55	40.19			
43.75	111.13	51.95	32.75	83.18	40.49			
44.00	111.76	52.25	33.00	83.82	40.80			
44.25	112.40	52.54	33.25	84.45	41.11			
44.50	113.03	52.84	33.50	85.09	41.42			
44.75	113.67	53.14	33.75	85.72	41.73			
45.00	114.30	53.44	34.00	86.36	42.04			

Note: Percent Fat = Constant A + Constant B − Constant C − 18.4

Frequently Cited Journals in Exercise Physiology

Exercise physiology encompasses numerous scientific areas of inquiry. The following list of journals (with their common abbreviations) can be particularly useful in library searches on various topics of interest.

FREQUENTLY CITED JOURNALS IN EXERCISE PHYSIOLOGY

Journal	Abbreviation	Journal	Abbreviation
Acta Medica Scandinavica	Acta Med Scand	Canadian Journal of Applied Physiology	Can J Appl Physiol
Acta Physiologica Scandinavica	Acta Physiol Scand	Canadian Journal of Applied Sports Sciences	Can J Appl Sport Sci
American Journal of Clinical Nutrition	Am J Clin Nutr	Canadian Medical Association Journal	Can Med Assoc J
American Heart Journal	Am Heart J	Circulation Research	Circ Res
American Journal of Anatomy	Am J Anat	Circulation: Journal of the American Heart Association	Circulation
American Journal of Cardiology	Am J Cardiol		
American Journal of Epidemiology	Am J Epidemiol	Clinical Biomechanics	Clin Biomech
American Journal of Human Biology	Am J Hum Biol	Clinical Chemistry	Clin Chem
American Journal of Obstetrics and Gynecology	Am J Obstet Gynecol	Clinical Science	Clin Sci
		Clinical Sports Medicine	Clin Sports Med
American Journal of Physical Anthropology	Am J Phys Anthropol	Diabetes	Diabetes
		Diabetologia	Diabetologia
American Journal of Physics	Am J Physics	Endocrinology	Endocrinology
American Journal of Physiology	Am J Physiol	Ergonomics	Ergonomics
American Journal of Public Health	Am J Public Health	European Journal of Applied Physiology	Eur J Appl Physiol
American Journal of Sports Medicine	Am J Sports Med	Exercise Immunology Review	Exerc Immun Rev
		Experientia	Experientia
Annals of Human Biology	Ann Hum Biol	Experimental Brain Research	Exp Brain Res
Annals of Internal Medicine	Ann Intern Med	FASEB Journal	FASEB J
Appetite	Appetite	Fertility and Sterility	Fertil Steril
Archives of Environmental Health	Arch Environ Health	Geriatrics	Geriatrics
		Growth	Growth
Atherosclerosis	Atherosclerosis	Human Biology	Hum Biol
Aviation and Space Environmental Medicine	Aviat Space Environ Med	Human Movement Science	Hum Mov Sci
		International Journal of Obesity	Int J Obes
Brain: Journal of Neurology	Brain	International Journal of Sports Medicine	Int J Sports Med
British Heart Journal	Br Heart J		
British Journal of Nutrition	Br J Nutr	International Journal of Sport Nutrition	IJSN
British Journal of Sports Medicine	Br J Sports Med		
British Medical Journal	Br Med J	International Journal for Vitamin and Nutrition Research	Int J Vitam Nutr Res

FREQUENTLY CITED JOURNALS IN EXERCISE PHYSIOLOGY—*continued*

Journal	Abbreviation	Journal	Abbreviation
Journal of Aging and Physical Activity	J Aging Phys Act	JAMA (Journal of the American Medical Association)	JAMA
Journal of Applied Physiology	J Appl Physiol	Journal of Sports Medicine	J Sports Med
Journal of Biological Chemistry	J Biol Chem	Lancet	Lancet
Journal of Biomechanics	J Biomech	Medicine and Science in Sports and Exercise	Med Sci Sports Exerc
Journal of Bone and Joint Surgery	J Bone Joint Surg		
Journal of Clinical Endocrinology and Metabolism	J Clin Endocrinol Metab	Muscle and Nerve	Muscle Nerve
		Nature	Nature
Journal of Clinical Investigation	J Clin Invest	Neuroscience Letters	Neurosci Lett
Journal of Gerontology	J Gerontol	New England Journal of Medicine	N Engl J Med
Journal of Human Movement Studies	J Hum Mov Stud	Nutrition Abstracts and Reviews	Nutr Abstr Rev
		Nutrition and Metabolism	Nutr Metab
Journal of Laboratory and Clinical Medicine	J Lab Clin Med	Nutrition Reviews	Nutr Rev
		Pediatric Exercise Science	Pediatr Exerc Sci
Journal of Lipid Research	J Lipid Res	Pediatrics	Pediatrics
Journal of Neurophysiology	J Neurophysiol	Physical Therapy Reviews	Phys Ther Rev
Journal of Nutrition	J Nutr	Physician and Sportsmedicine	Physician Sportsmed
Journal of Parenteral and Enteral Nutrition	JPEN	Physiological Reviews	Physiol Rev
		Preventive Medicine	Prev Med
Journal of Pediatrics	J Pediatr	Proceedings of the Nutrition Society	Proc Nutr Soc
Journal of Physical and Medical Rehabilitation	J Phys Med Rehabil		
		Psychosomatic Medicine	Psychosom Med
Journal of Physiology	J Physiol	Public Health Reports	Public Health Rep
Journal of Sport and Exercise Psychology	J Sport Exerc Psychol	Radiology	Radiology
		Research Quarterly for Exercise and Sports	Res Q Exerc Sport
Journal of Sport Psychology	J Sport Psychol		
Journal of Sports Medicine and Physical Fitness	J Sports Med Phys Fitness	Scandinavian Journal of Sports Science	Scand J Sports Sci
Journal of Strength and Conditioning Research	JSCR	Science	Science
		Scientific American	Sci Am
Journal of the American Dietetic Association	J Am Diet Assoc	Sports Medicine	Sports Med
		Sport Science Review	Sport Sci Rev

Useful Tables and Computations in Exercise Physiology

WATER DENSITY–TEMPERATURE CORRECTION FACTORS FOR USE IN BODY VOLUME DETERMINATIONS BY HYDROSTATIC WEIGHING

Temperature, °C	Density	Temperature, °C	Density
4	1.00000	31	0.99537
10	0.99973	32	0.99505
15	0.99913	33	0.99473
20	0.99823	34	0.99440
25	0.99707	35	0.99406
26	0.99681	36	0.99371
27	0.99654	37	0.99336
28	0.99626	38	0.99299
29	0.99595	39	0.99262
30	0.99567	40	0.99224

PROCEDURE TO CALIBRATE TREADMILL ELEVATION[a]

The calibration procedures described below use a simple carpenter's level and square.

1. Use a carpenter's level to make sure that the treadmill is level, and check the zero on the grade meter under these conditions (with the treadmill electronics "on"). If the meter does not read zero, follow instructions to make the adjustment (usually the small screw on the face of the meter).

2. Elevate the treadmill so that the percent grade meter reads approximately 20%. Measure the exact incline of the treadmill as shown in Figure G.1. When the bubble of the level is exactly in the center of the tube, the "rise"

[a]From Howley ET. The exercise testing laboratory. In Blair SN et al. (eds.): *Resource Manual for Guidelines for Exercise Testing and Prescription.* Philadelphia, Lea & Febiger, 1988.

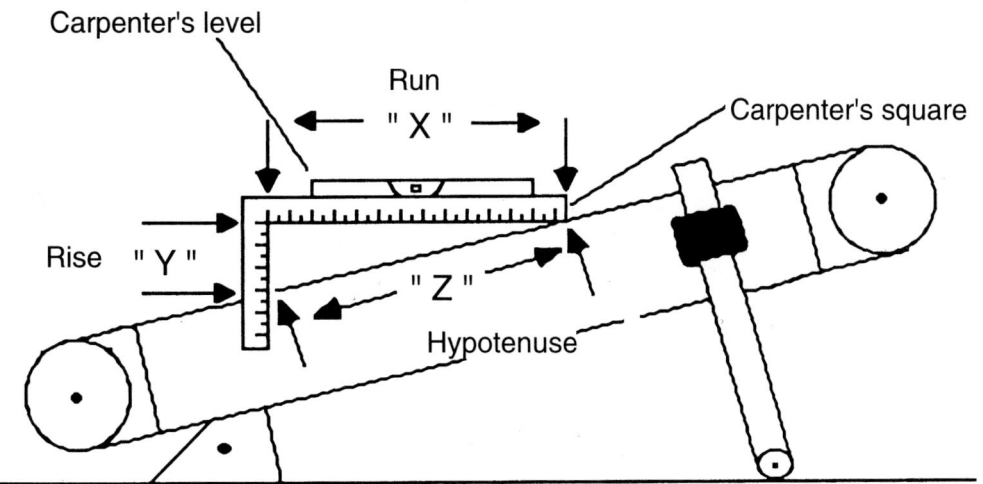

Grade = Tangent θ = Rise (" Y ") ÷ Run (" X ")

Grade = Sine θ = Rise (" Y ") ÷ Hypotenuse (" Z ")

FIGURE G.1

Calibration of grade by tangent method (rise ÷ run) with carpenter's square and level.

measurement is obtained. Calculate the grade as the "rise" over the "run" (tangent θ), and adjust the treadmill meter to read that exact grade. For example, if the rise is 4.5 in. to the 22.5 in. of the run, the fractional grade is:

$$\text{Grade} = \text{tangent } \theta = \text{rise} \div \text{run}$$
$$= 4.5 \text{ in.} \div 22.5 \text{ in.} = 0.20 = 20\%$$

3. Repeat this process at grades between 0° and 20° (0 to 34%) to make sure the meter is correct.

This "rise over the run" method is a typical engineering method for calculating grade—the vertical rise divided by the horizontal run. This method gives the tangent of the angle (the opposite side divided by the horizontal distance, as shown in Fig. G.1). Although this tangent method is not exactly correct, it is a good approximation for grades less than 20% or 12°.

The "correct" method expresses grade as the sine of the angle (sin θ), in which sin θ equals the vertical rise (opposite side) over the hypotenuse [sin θ = rise ÷ hypotenuse (see Fig. G.1)]. This method should be used to calculate very steep grades (greater than 20%). The vertical rise can be calculated very simply for a treadmill with a fixed rear axle. Simply measure the change in the height of the front axle above the horizontal (rise). Divide this value by the axle-to-axle length (hypotenuse), and the quotient is the grade, expressed as a fraction (Fig. G.2).

For the large treadmill with movable rear and front axles, the vertical rise is equal to the sum of the rise of the front axle and the drop of the rear axle. When this total is divided by the axle-to-axle length, the quotient is the grade, expressed as a fraction. For example, if the front axle height is 0.327 m on the level (0% grade) and 0.612 m at the unknown grade, then the front axle rise is 0.612 − 0.327 = 0.285 m. Similarly, if the rear axle height is 0.324 m at 0% grade and 0.299 m at the unknown grade, the drop is 0.025 m. The total vertical rise then is equal to the "rise" plus "drop" or 0.285 + 0.025 = 0.31 m. If the

axle-to-axle length (hypotenuse) is 2.095 m, then the grade can be calculated as:

$$\text{Grade} = \text{total rise} \div \text{hypotenuse}$$
$$= 0.31 \text{ m} \div 2.095 \text{ m} = 0.148 = 14.8\%$$

SPEED CONVERSIONS AMONG KILOMETERS PER HOUR, MILES PER HOUR, AND METERS PER SECOND[a]

$km \cdot h^{-1}$	mph	$m \cdot s^{-1}$	$km \cdot h^{-1}$	mph	$m \cdot s^{-1}$
10	6.22	2.78	200	124	55.6
20	12.4	5.56	220	137	61.1
30	18.7	8.34	240	149	66.7
40	24.9	11.1	260	162	72.2
50	31.1	13.9	280	174	77.8
60	37.4	16.7	300	187	83.3
70	43.6	19.4	320	199	88.9
80	49.8	22.2	340	211	94.5
90	56.0	25.0	360	224	100.0
100	62.2	27.8	380	236	105.6
120	74.7	33.3	400	249	111.1
140	87.1	38.9	420	261	116.7
160	99.5	44.5	440	271	122.2
180	112	50.0	460	286	133.4

[a]Consult Appendix A, Part 2 for additional conversions.

EQUATIONS FOR ESTIMATING OXYGEN UPTAKE DURING LEG AND ARM ERGOMETRY AND STEPPING[a, b]

Leg cycle ergometry (appropriate for power outputs between 300, and 1200 $kg \cdot m \cdot min^{-1}$)

1. R = 3.5 $mL \cdot kg^{-1} \cdot min^{-1}$ × body mass in kg
   - multiplication by body mass converts $mL \cdot kg^{-1} \cdot min^{-1}$ into $mL \cdot min^{-1}$
2. H = 0
   - there is no horizontal component for this activity
3. V = 2.0 × power output ($kg \cdot m \cdot min^{-1}$)
   - 2.0 is the regression constant for converting $kg \cdot m \cdot min^{-1}$ to $mL \cdot min^{-1}$
   - $kg \cdot m \cdot min^{-1}$ = kg (or kp) of resistance × meters per pedal revolution × pedal rate rev $\cdot min^{-1}$
     - kg is the resistance or "tension" setting on the ergometer

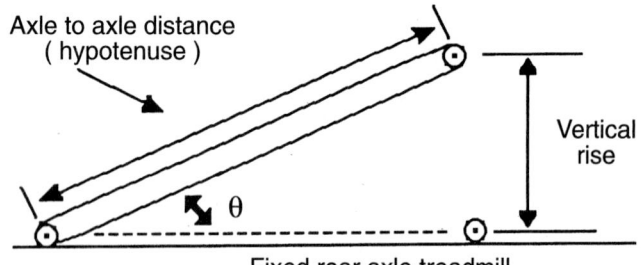

Axle to axle distance (hypotenuse)

Vertical rise

θ

Fixed rear axle treadmill

Grade = Sine θ = Rise ÷ Hypotenuse

FIGURE G.2
Calibration of grade for fixed rear axle treadmill by sine method (rise ÷ hypotenuse).

[a]From American College of Sports Medicine: *ACSM's Guidelines for Exercise Testing and Prescription*, 5th ed. Baltimore, Williams & Wilkins, 1995, pp. 282–283.
[b]R, resting $\dot{V}O_2$; H, horizontal component; V, vertical component.

- meters per pedal revolution is a function of the ergometer being used
  - $= 6$ m $\cdot$ rev^{-1} for Monark™ ergometers
  - $= 3$ m $\cdot$ rev^{-1} for Tunturi™ and BodyGuard™ ergometers
- pedal rate must be known
  - typically 50 or 60 rpm for untrained cyclists
  - can use 80 rpm or greater for trained cyclists
  - electronic ergometers control power output independent of pedal rate
4. $\dot{V}_{O_2}$ (in mL/min) $= R + H + V$, where H is 0

Arm ergometry (appropriate for power outputs between 150 and 750 kg $\cdot$ m $\cdot$ min^{-1})
1. $R = 3.5$ mL $\cdot$ kg^{-1} $\cdot$ min^{-1} $\times$ body mass in kg
   - multiplication by body mass converts mL $\cdot$ kg^{-1} $\cdot$ min^{-1} to mL $\cdot$ min^{-1}
2. $H = 0$
   - there is no horizontal component for this activity
3. $V = 3.0 \times$ power output (kg $\cdot$ m $\cdot$ min^{-1})
   - 3.0 is the regression constant for converting kg $\cdot$ m $\cdot$ min^{-1} to mL $\cdot$ min^{-1}
   - kg $\cdot$ m $\cdot$ min^{-1} = kg (or kp) of resistance $\times$ meters per crank revolution $\times$ cranking rate (rev $\cdot$ min^{-1})

- kg is the resistance or "tension" setting on the ergometer
- meters per pedal revolution is a function of the ergometer being used
  - $= 2.4$ m $\cdot$ rev^{-1} for Monark™ arm ergometers
- arm cranking rate must be known
- typically 50 or 60 rpm
4. $\dot{V}_{O_2}$ (mL $\cdot$ min^{-1}) $= R + H + V$, where H is 0

Stepping (appropriate for power outputs between 300 and 1200 kg $\cdot$ m $\cdot$ min^{-1})
1. R is already included in the H and V components of this equation
2. $H = 0.35 \times$ (steps per minute)
   - 0.35 is the regression constant for converting steps/min to mL $\cdot$ kg^{-1} $\cdot$ min^{-1}
3. V
   - for stepping up and down $= 2.4 \times$ steps $\cdot$ min^{-1}
   - for stepping up only $= 1.8 \times$ steps $\cdot$ min^{-1} $\times$ m $\cdot$ step^{-1}
   - for stepping down only $= 0.6 \times$ steps $\cdot$ min^{-1} $\times$ m $\cdot$ step^{-1}
   - note that step height is in meters (m)
4. $\dot{V}_{O_2}$ (mL $\cdot$ kg^{-1} $\cdot$ min^{-1}) $= R + H + V$, where R is 0

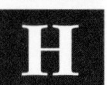
Selected American College of Sports Medicine Position Stands

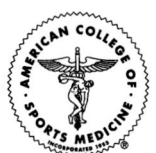

SUMMARY

American College of Sports Medicine Position Stand on Osteoporosis and Exercise. *Med. Sci. Sports Exerc.*, Vol. 27, No. 4, pp. i–vii, 1995. Osteoporosis is a disease characterized by low bone mass and microarchitectural deterioration of bone tissue leading to enhanced bone fragility and a consequent increase in fracture risk. Both men and women are at risk for osteoporotic fractures. However, as osteoporosis is more common in females and more exercise-related research has been directed at reducing the risk of osteoporotic fractures in women, this Position Stand applies specifically to women. Factors that influence fracture risk include skeletal fragility, frequency and severity of falls, and tissue mass surrounding the skeleton. Prevention of osteoporotic fractures, therefore, is focused on the preservation or enhancement of the material and structural properties of bone, the prevention of falls, and the overall improvement of lean tissue mass. The load-bearing capacity of bone reflects both its material properties, such as density and modulus, and the spatial distribution of bone tissue. These features of bone strength are all developed and maintained in part by forces applied to bone during daily activities and exercise. Functional loading through physical activity exerts a positive influence on bone mass in humans. The extent of this influence and the types of programs that induce the most effective osteogenic stimulus are still uncertain. While it is well-established that a marked decrease in physical activity, as in bedrest for example, results in a profound decline in bone mass, improvements in bone mass resulting from increased physical activity are less conclusive. Results vary according to age, hormonal status, nutrition, and exercise prescription. An apparent positive effect of activity on bone is more marked in cross-sectional studies than in prospective studies. Whether this is an example of selection bias or differences in the intensity and duration of the training programs is uncertain at this time. It has long been recognized that

changes in bone mass occur more rapidly with unloading than with increased loading. Habitual inactivity results in a downward spiral in all physiologic functions. As women age, the loss of strength, flexibility, and cardiovascular fitness leads to a further decrease in activity. Eventually older individuals may find it impossible to continue the types of activities that provide an adequate load-bearing stimulus to maintain bone mass. Fortunately, it appears that strength and overall fitness can be improved at any age through a carefully planned exercise program. Unless the ability of the underlying physiologic systems essential for load-bearing activity are restored, it may be difficult for many older women to maintain a level of activity essential for protecting the skeleton from further bone loss. For the very elderly or those experiencing problems with balance and gait, activities that might increase the risk of falling should be avoided. There is no evidence at the present time that exercise alone or exercise plus added calcium intake can prevent the rapid decrease in bone mass in the immediate postmenopausal years. Nevertheless, all healthy women should be encouraged to exercise regardless of whether the activity has a marked osteogenic component in order to gain the other health benefits that accrue from regular exercise. Based on current research, it is the position of the American College of Sports Medicine that: 1. Weight-bearing physical activity is essential for the normal development and maintenance of a healthy skeleton. Activities that focus on increasing muscle strength may also be beneficial, particularly for nonweight-bearing bones. 2. Sedentary women may increase bone mass slightly by becoming more active but the primary benefit of the increased activity may be in avoiding the further loss of bone that occurs with inactivity. 3. Exercise cannot be recommended as a substitute for hormone replacement therapy at the time of menopause. 4. The optimal program for older women would include activities that improve strength, flexibility, and coordination that may indirectly, but effectively, decrease the incidence of osteoporotic fractures by lessening the likelihood of falling.

INTRODUCTION

When force is applied to bone, the bone bends or is temporarily deformed. The extent of that deformation is measured as strain and depends on the magnitude and direction of the force, the distance from the point of application of the force to the axis of bending (lever arm), and the moment of inertia of the bone. Regulation of bone strength is a function of the mechanical forces or loads to which the respective bones of the skeleton are exposed.

The response of bone to mechanical loads is immediate, specific to the bone under load, and involves both cellular and tissue reactions. Mechanical loads stimulate bone cells within the loaded region to deform, increase their synthesis of PGI_2 (prostacyclin), PGE_2 (prostaglandin E_2), G6PD (glucose-6-phosphate dehydrogenase), and increase their synthesis of RNA within minutes of loading.[23, 60, 61, 68, 69, 85, 86] Thus, a cascade of events within the osteoblasts and osteocytes occurs in response to changes in bone strain, reflecting an adaptation to the imposed loading environment. It has been suggested that a mechanosensory mechanism exists, either within the bone cell or within the extracellular matrix of bone, that senses change in bone strain and then orchestrates the subsequent cascade of events.[16, 27, 86] It has further been proposed that the specific response to any bone strain is dependent upon the relationship of that strain to the strain thresholds for that bone.[26] Frost[26] has suggested that there exists a minimum effective strain for both modeling and remodeling such that bone strains falling between these threshold values will generally result in no net change in bone mass. Bone strains exceeding the minimum effective strain for modeling (MESm) will result in a net increase in bone mass, while strains falling below the minimum effective strain for remodeling (MESr) will result in increased bone remodeling and a net decrease in bone mass.[26, 27, 96] Although some evidence exists to support this proposal, experimental verification has yet to be presented.

ANIMAL MODEL STUDIES

The primary mechanical variables associated with the regulation of bone mass are: strain magnitude, strain rate, and the number of loading cycles. Due to the difficulties inherent in manipulating these variables and directly measuring their effect on bone in humans, animal models have been developed for the purpose of determining the mechanisms underlying the response of bone to mechanical stimulation. The models used most frequently in studies of bone biology include the rat, rooster, turkey, dog, and pig. As with all animal models, however, extrapolation to the human physiological system should be done with careful consideration of the differences between species.

External loading models. Using these models the primary mechanical variables can be manipulated *in vivo* and the response of bone studied in a unique and controlled manner. Results demonstrate a linear increase in bone mass with an increase in strain magnitude from 1000 to 4000 microstrain (strain is a measure of bone deformation).[69] In addition, the rate of change in bone strain during loading is positively related to the adaptive response.[57] Specifically, at high strain magnitudes (e.g., 2000 microstrain) relatively few loading cycles are required to stimulate a bone response; once the threshold for stimulation is achieved, no

measurable advantages to the properties of bone are derived through further increasing the rate of stimulation.[77, 78] Static loading of bone has been shown to provide significantly less stimulation to bone than dynamic loading.[34, 39–41] Based on these results and others, Whalen and Carter[103] have developed a theoretical model suggesting strain magnitude to be the most important variable for generating an adaptive response in bone, with number of loading cycles also an important factor that probably increases in significance when strain magnitudes are low.

The external loading models result in rapid bone formation at strains well below peak physiological levels for the specific animal model. This bone formation may be due to the application of force to bones in a unique and nonphysiological pattern so that the axis or direction of bending differs from that derived through normal locomotive patterns.[9, 41, 57, 60, 76, 77, 78, 85, 86] As the bone is not accustomed to this bending pattern, the bone initiates an adaptive response.

Underloading models. Studies looking at the effect of loads below the threshold for remodeling have typically used the rat, although one of the original studies used the beagle dog.[2, 94, 97] As for all other species, growing rats require mechanical forces for normal bone growth and development. Adult rats require mechanical loading for maintenance of normal structural and functional bone integrity. When these forces are removed from rat bones, as in hindlimb suspension, immobilization due to bandaging, neurotomy, or tenotomy, bone mass, bone cortical area and thickness, trabecular volume, and bone mechanical competence significantly decrease in comparison to age matched controls.[43–45, 82, 99, 102] In fact, the tissue dynamic changes associated with the underloaded condition correspond closely to the changes in bone properties measured in association with hypoestrogenism (e.g., menopause, ovariectomy). There is an initial rapid loss of bone mass (transient phase), followed by a new steady state (adapted phase). The duration of these phases is dependent upon the age of the animal, the type of bone (trabecular vs cortical), and the load-bearing capabilities of the bone under study.[2, 43, 44, 97] Strenuous treadmill running for approximately 60 min each day does not provide sufficient mechanical stimulation to offset the bone loss associated with underloading (or hypoestrogenism) in carefully controlled studies.[29, 102] With calcium deficiency the effects of unloading are exacerbated.[42, 101]

The effects of weightlessness in space flight are similar to those observed using other methods of unloading. In the absence of gravitational forces young rats show suppressed periosteal growth, lower cross-sectional area, reduced trabecular bone volume, depressed longitudinal growth, and decreased mechanical properties.[22, 33, 83, 84, 98, 108] Losses in bone mass occur primarily in the weight-bearing bones of the skeleton. As with other methods of unloading, these changes occur as a result of decreased osteoblastic activity combined with normal osteoclastic resorption.

Increased physical activity models. Unfortunately, the most frequently used method of increasing the physical activity patterns of animal models is to use running and other forms of aerobic exercise rather than designing studies to specifically overload the skeletal system. Bone mass and strength should be tested after weight-lifting in models such as those used for inducing muscle hypertrophy.[95]

Results of running training studies on bone material and structural properties in animal models have been equivocal, some showing increases in bone mass and others showing no change or decreases in bone material properties.[6, 8, 24, 25, 29, 35, 46, 49, 65, 79, 81, 87, 93, 107, 109] One of the primary limitations in studying changes in bone properties as a function of aerobic training protocols is the unavoidable but generally ignored systemic effects such programs have and their potential for either potentiating or diminishing the benefits of mechanical loading on bone.[24, 109]

Other confounding variables in these study designs include failure to control for growth, training durations that do not consider the length of the resorption-formation cycle for both cortical and trabecular bone; differences in body mass between control and exercising animals, and requiring nocturnal animals (e.g., the rat) to exercise under some form of artificial lighting. These and other confounding factors have limited the extent to which conclusions can be drawn regarding the effect of running and/or swimming[94] on bone properties.

HUMAN STUDIES

The types of programs that induce the best osteogenic stimulus and the extent of their influence are still controversial. Research has focused on the role of physical activity in maximizing bone mass during childhood and the early adult years, maintaining bone mass during the premenopausal years, and preventing or attenuating bone loss in the postmenopausal years. The success of the activity has been judged primarily by measuring changes in bone mass. Bone mass is expressed either as bone mineral content (BMC) or as bone mineral density (BMD). The two most common measurement techniques are dual energy x-ray absorptiometry (DEXA), which provides an areal density, $g \cdot cm^{-2}$, and computed tomography (CT), which provides a volumetric density, $mg \cdot cm^{-3}$. Although bone strength depends upon both the amount of mineral in bone and the macro- and microarchitecture of bone, only the mineral component of bone strength can be measured noninvasively in humans. The skeletal regions assessed most frequently to measure a training effect are those susceptible to the more serious osteoporotic fractures, the lumbar vertebrae, proximal femur (hip), and forearm.

Few investigators have considered the role of the principles that have been shown to affect the response of other physiologic systems to training. The following principles should be considered in evaluating the results of any training study:

Principle of specificity. The major impact of the activity should be at the site where BMD is being measured as the response to loading appears to be a localized effect.

Principle of overload. To effect change in bone mass, the training stimulus must exceed the normal loading.

Principle of reversibility. The positive effect of a training program on bone will be lost if the program is discontinued.

Principle of initial values. Those with the lowest levels of BMD have a greater capacity for percent improvement in training studies; those with average or above average bone mass have the least.

Principle of diminishing returns. Each person has an individual biological ceiling that determines the extent of a possible training effect. As this ceiling is approached, gains in bone mass will slow and eventually plateau.

ROLE OF PHYSICAL ACTIVITY IN MAXIMIZING BONE MASS

A primary factor associated with the risk of osteoporotic fractures is the "peak" bone mass developed during childhood and the early adult years. The age at which peak bone mass is attained appears to differ for cortical and trabecular bone. Several cross-sectional studies[10, 47, 73] have suggested that trabecular bone loss may begin as early as the third decade whereas cortical bone may increase or remain constant until the fifth decade.[50] A more recent longitudinal study[70] suggests that both cortical and trabecular bone mass may continue to increase slightly in healthy young women until an age of approximately 28 yr. Cross-sectional studies of young women report that active women and athletes who participate in weight-bearing activities have higher bone mass at the lumbar spine and femoral neck than sedentary controls.[30, 31, 74, 106] Weight-bearing is a key factor in this relationship. Studies[31, 74] that have examined female collegiate swimmers have reported lower vertebral BMD when compared with other athletes and controls. It is speculated that this finding is due to the nonweight-bearing nature of swimming. Consequently, nonweight-bearing activities such as swimming and cycling have not been promoted for increasing BMD.

An area of recent interest has been the relationship between muscle strength, muscle mass, and BMD. Among nonathletic young women, an independent, positive association has been reported between muscle strength and BMD.[63, 90] The relationship is independent of height and body weight. In some cases, BMD was predicted by muscle groups in the region of bone mass measurement (i.e., quadriceps and femur), although at the lumbar spine, muscle groups distant from the site (elbow flexors, forearm flexors) predicted BMD. It appears that overall strength is the key factor as strength in one area typically reflects strength in other regions of the body. While it has long been accepted that women with higher body weight have a greater BMD, this relationship was assumed to be a function of the heavier load on the skeleton. However, early studies did not investigate the relative contribution of the fat or lean component to this relationship. Most, but not all, recent work suggests that muscle mass makes a more important contribution to BMD than fat mass.[2, 72, 91, 92, 100]

The few prospective intervention studies[70, 88] in young adult women have shown little or no increase in BMD with increased activity. Snow-Harter et al.[88] trained young women for 8 months either by weight training or running. There was a slight positive effect of physical activity in a group of free-living young women over a span of 2 yr, but the contribution to the change in BMD was less than 3%. However, their data did indicate that bone mass could increase during the third decade. Mazess and Barden[51] in a nonintervention study divided women by quartiles of activity and found no difference in BMD at the spine, hip, or wrist. It would appear that normal active young women are either at or near their biological limit for BMD or that a greater training stimulus is required for a significant gain in bone mass.

Not all active young women profit fully from their activity. Women endurance athletes who experience a disruption in menstrual cycles and become hypoestrogenic lose bone despite regularly exercising at high intensity.[19–21, 48] Bone loss in this population is particularly striking at the lumbar spine[19, 48] but other regions that include more cortical bone may also be affected.[54] This profile of altered skeletal status may predispose these women to a higher incidence of stress fractures and to a risk of premature osteoporotic fractures.[53]

ROLE OF PHYSICAL ACTIVITY IN THE MATURE ADULT YEARS

Although cross-sectional data indicates a slow but continuous loss of trabecular bone mineral density beginning prior to or in the third decade,[89] the decrease in cortical bone appears minimal until the menopause.[50] Epidemiological data, from the normative data bases of three manufacturers of dual energy x-ray absorptiometry machines which measure bone density, indicate a change of about −7% in lumbar BMD from peak bone mass to age 50[18] but about −16% in the femoral neck. It is important to identify any combination of factors that can maintain or increase bone density during these years as a higher BMD at menopause may reduce the risk of osteoporotic fractures in the future.

There is some evidence from cross-sectional studies that physical activity may attenuate or prevent bone loss during this period.[1, 11] Moreover, a few studies[64, 91, 92] have shown that women with greater muscle strength and muscle mass have higher BMD.

Two longitudinal studies that have included premenopausal women between 30 and 50 yr provide mixed

results for exercise as an intervention therapy to offset age-related bone loss. Both studies used weight training as an intervention. While one study[28] reported a small non-significant increase in lumbar spine BMD (0.8%), the other investigation[75] observed a significant decline (−4%) in bone mass at this site. The lack of a positive effect may have been due to measurement error, an inadequate training stimulus, or a decrease in time spent in other activities during the training period. This is an important area of investigation and more studies need to be conducted in this age group with detailed attention to appropriate exercise prescription.

ROLE OF EXERCISE IN THE POSTMENOPAUSAL YEARS

Menopause is a time in which trabecular bone loss accelerates and cortical bone loss becomes apparent[89] as endogenous levels of gonadal hormones, estrogen and progesterone, decrease markedly. Both cross-sectional and longitudinal studies that have examined physical activity in this population report BMD values that vary according to mode, intensity, and estrogen status, but all are lower when compared with those of young women.

Two cross-sectional studies of masters runners report lumbar spine density between 9.2% and 35% higher compared with matched controls[38, 52] while another reports no difference.[36] In all cases the BMD of the older runners was well below that of the younger group. There has been only one study of masters swimmers, which reported no significant difference between swimmers vs controls, but did find a higher BMD in swimmers using estrogen than swimmers not using estrogen.[58] Both the running and swimming studies included some women on estrogen replacement therapy but still reported values below those of young women. Consequently, neither activity appears to protect the lumbar vertebrae from bone loss following menopause.

The few longitudinal studies in the postmenopausal population do not allow decisive conclusions due to the wide variation in exercise prescriptions, sites of measurement, and BMD results. Vertebral bone mass changes over time range from −12% to +8% and apply mainly to women who are not taking estrogen. In general, results from research examining walking intervention programs demonstrate that this activity, commonly prescribed to postmenopausal women, does not prevent bone loss.[12, 55, 80, 104] Other studies that included activities of higher intensity and the addition of muscle building exercises report a more positive skeletal response.[1, 5, 13, 14, 17, 37, 56, 62, 67] Increasing activity in this age group with an appropriate exercise prescription may slow bone loss even if there is no significant increase in BMD.

The relationships among bone mass and muscle strength and/or mass are not as robust for postmenopausal women compared with premenopausal women. Although muscle mass has been shown to correlate with BMD in postmenopausal women by some investigators,[2, 7, 64, 91, 100] the positive associations between muscle strength and bone mass are stronger in premenopausal women compared with postmenopausal women regardless of estrogen status.[64, 91] At least two studies[71] have reported that fat mass was more strongly associated with BMD in postmenopausal women. This may be due to the forces on bone during weight-bearing activity and/or conversion of androgens to estrogens in fat tissue in this age group. Both possibilities require further study.

To date, there is no evidence that exercise alone can replace the bone loss associated with the low reproductive hormones that accompany menopause. However, there are two reports suggesting that exercise combined with hormone replacement therapy may have an osteogenic effect.[56, 66]

Physical Activity and Fractures

Osteoporotic fractures are associated with low bone mass and occur most often at three skeletal sites.[3] Fractures of the vertebrae and distal radius (forearm) typically are the first to occur. Hip fractures (neck and intertrochanteric areas of the femur) occur later in life as a result of falls and are related not only to bone mass but to other factors such as decreased balance, reduced soft tissue in the hip region, and poor muscle strength and power in the lower extremities.

Epidemiological studies agree that women who have been able to maintain higher levels of physical activity have a lower incidence of hip fractures.[4, 15, 59, 105] Factors such as frequent muscle loading, faster walking speeds, more productive activity, increased participation in outdoor activities, and greater time standing and moving about were all associated with a reduced fracture incidence in these studies. Whether the reduction in risk was due to the activity or whether nonactive women represent the frail elderly is not known. Longitudinal research that documents physical activity patterns, bone mass measurements, and fractures needs to be conducted to further the knowledge in this area.

CONCLUSION

While weight-bearing activity is essential for the normal development and maintenance of a healthy skeleton, physical activity cannot be recommended as a substitute for hormone replacement therapy at the time of menopause. A general activity program emphasizing strength, flexibility, coordination, and cardiovascular fitness may indirectly reduce the risk for osteoporotic fractures by decreasing the risk of falling and by enabling older women to remain active, thereby avoiding loss of bone through inactivity.

This pronouncement was written for the American College of Sports Medicine by: Barbara L. Drinkwater, Ph.D., FACSM (chair); Susan K. Grimston, Ph.D., FACSM; Diane M. Raab-Cullen, Ph.D.; and Christine M. Snow-Harter, Ph.D., FACSM.

The pronouncement was reviewed for the American College of Sports Medicine by members-at-large, the Pronouncements Committee, and by Gail P. Dalsky, Ph.D., Robert P. Heaney, M.D., Thomas A. Lloyd, Ph.D., and Robert Marcus, M.D.

■ REFERENCES ■

1. Aloia, J.F., S.H. Cohn, J.A. Ostuni, R. Cane, and K. Ellis. Prevention of involutional bone loss by exercise. *Ann. Intern. Med.* 89:356–358, 1988.
2. Aloia, J.F., D.M. McGowan, A.N. Vaswani, P. Ross, and S.H. Cohen. Relationship of menopause to skeletal and muscle mass. *Am. J. Clin. Nutr.* 53:1378–1383, 1991.
3. Arnold, J.S. Amount and quality of trabecular bone in osteoporotic vertebral fractures. *Clin. Endocrinol. Metab.* 2:221–238, 1973.
4. Astrom, J., S. Ahnqvist, J. Veertema, and B. Jonsson. Physical activity in women sustaining fracture of the neck of the femur. *J. Bone Joint Surg.* 69-B:381–383, 1987.
5. Ayalon, J., A. Simkin, I. Leichter, and S. Raifmann. Dynamic bone loading exercises for postmenopausal women. Effect on the density of the distal radius. *Arch. Phys. Med Rehabil.* 68:280–283, 1987.
6. Bauer, K.D. and P. Griminger. Long-term effects of activity and of calcium and phosphorus intake on bones and kidneys of female rats. *J. Nutr.* 113:2111–2121, 1983.
7. Bevier, W., R.A. Wiswell, G. Pyka, et al. Relationship of body composition, muscle strength and aerobic capacity to bone mineral density in older men and women. *J. Bone Miner. Res.* 4:421–432, 1989.
8. Beyer, R.E., J.C. Huang, and G.B. Wilshire. The effects of endurance exercise on bone dimensions, collagen, and calcium in the aged male rat. *Exp. Gerontol.* 20:315–323, 1985.
9. Biewener, A.A., S.M. Swartz, and J.E. Bertram. Bone modeling during growth: dynamic strain equilibrium in the chick tibiotarsus. *Calcif. Tissue Int.* 39:390–395, 1986.
10. Birkenhager-Frenkel, D.H., P. Courpron, E.A. Hupscher, et al. Age-related changes in cancellous bone structure. *Bone Miner.* 4:197–216, 1988.
11. Brewer, V., B.M. Meyer, M.S. Keele, S.J. Upton, and R.D. Hagan. Role of exercise in prevention of involutional bone loss. *Med. Sci. Sports Exerc.* 15:445–449, 1983.
12. Cavanaugh, D.J. and C.E. Cann. Brisk walking does not stop bone loss in postmenopausal women. *Bone.* 9:201–204, 1988.
13. Chow, R., J.E. Harrison, and C. Notarius. Effect of two randomised exercise programmes on bone mass of healthy postmenopausal women. *Br. Med. J.* 295:1441–1444, 1987.
14. Chow, R., J.E. Harrison, C.F. Brown, and V. Hajek. Physical fitness effect on bone mass in postmenopausal women. *Arch. Phys. Med. Rehabil.* 67:231–234, 1986.
15. Cooper, C., D.J.P. Barker, and C. Wickham. Physical activity, muscle strength, and calcium intake in fracture of the proximal femur in Britain. *Br. Med. J.* 297:1443–1446, 1988.
16. Cowin, S.C., L. Moss-Salentijn, and M.L. Moss. Candidates for the mechanosensory system in bone. *J. Biomech. Eng.* 113:191–197, 1991.
17. Dalsky, G., K.S. Stocke, A.A. Eshani, E. Slatopolsky, W.C. Lee, and S.J. Birge. Weight-bearing exercise training and lumbar bone mineral content in postmenopausal women. *Ann. Intern. Med.* 108:824–828, 1988.
18. Drinkwater, B.L. Exercise in the prevention of osteoporosis. In: *Osteoporosis, Proceedings,* C. Christiansen and B. Riis (Eds.). Rodovre, Denmark: Osteopress Aps., 1993, pp. 105–108.

19. Drinkwater, B.L., K. Nilson, C.H. Chesnut III, J. Bremner, S. Shainholtz, and M.B. Southworth. Bone mineral content of amenorrheic and eumenorrheic athletes. *N. Engl. J. Med.* 311:277–281, 1984.

20. Drinkwater, B.L., B. Bruemmer, and C.H. Chesnut III. Menstrual history as a determinant of current bone density in young athletes. *JAMA* 263:545–548, 1990.

21. Drinkwater, B.L., K. Nilson, S. Ott, and C.H. Chesnut III. Bone mineral density after resumption of menses in amenorrheic women. *JAMA* 256:380–382, 1986.

22. Duke, P., G. Durnova, and D. Montufar-Solis. Histomorphometric and electron microscope analysis of tibial epiphyseal plates from Cosmos 1887 rats. *FASEB J.* 4:41–46, 1990.

23. El Haj, A.J., L. Minter, S.C.F. Rawlinson, R. Suswillo, and L.E. Lanyon. Cellular responses to mechanical loading in vitro. *J. Bone Miner. Res.* 5:923–932, 1990.

24. Forwood, M.R. and A. W. Parker. Repetitive loading, in vivo, of the tibiae and femora of rats: effects of repeated bouts of treadmill-running. *Bone Miner.* 13:35–46, 1991.

25. Forwood, M.R. and A.W. Parker. Effects of exercise on bone growth: mechanical and physical properties studied in the rat. *Clin. Biomech.* 2:185–190, 1987.

26. Frost, H.M. Structural adaptations to mechanical usage (SATMU). Redefining Wolff's Law. *Anat. Rec.* 226:403–422, 1990.

27. Frost, H.M. The mechanostat: a proposed pathogenic mechanism of osteoporosis and the bone mass effects of mechanical and nonmechanical agents. *Bone Miner.* 2:73–85, 1987.

28. Gleeson, P.B., E. J. Protas, A.D. LeBlanc, B.S. Schneider, and H.J. Evans. Effects of weight training on bone mineral density in premenopausal women. *J. Bone Miner. Res.* 5:153–158, 1990.

29. Grimston, S.K., A. Andersen, and H.J. Evans. Effects of chronic exercise and flurbiprofen on oophorectomy-induced osteopenia in the rat. *J. Bone Miner. Res.* 7(Suppl.):259, 1992.

30. Heinrich, C.H., S.B. Going, R.W. Parmenter, C.D. Perry, T.W. Boyden, and T.G. Lohman. Bone mineral content of cyclically menstruating female resistant and endurance trained athletes. *Med. Sci. Sports Exerc.* 22:558–563, 1990.

31. Jacobsen, P.C., W. Beaver, S.A. Grubb, T.N. Taft, and R.V. Talmadge. Bone density in women: college athletes and older athletic women. *J. Orthop. Res.* 2:328–332, 1984.

32. Jaworski, Z. F.G., M. Liskova-Kiar, and H.K. Uhtoff. Effect of long-term immobilization on the pattern of bone loss in older dogs. *J. Bone Joint Surg.* 62B:104–110, 1980.

33. Jee, W.S.S., T.J. Wronski, E.R.K. Morey, et al. Effects of spaceflight on trabecular bone in rats. *Am. J. Physiol.* 244:R310–R314, 1983.

34. Keller, T.S. and D.M. Spengler. Regulation of bone stress and strain in the immature and mature rat femur. *J. Biomech.* 22(11/2):1115–1127, 1989.

35. Kiiskinen, A. Physical training and connective tissues in young mice—physical properties of Achilles tendons and long bones. *Growth* 41:123–137, 1977.

36. Kirk, S. C.F. Sharp, N. Elbaum, D.B. Endres, S.M. Simons, J.G. Mohler, and R. K. Rude. Effect of long-distance running on bone mass in women. *J. Bone Miner. Res.* 4:515–522, 1989.

37. Krolner, B., B. Toft, S.P. Nielsen, and E. Tondevold. Physical exercise as prophylaxis against involutional vertebral bone loss: a controlled trial. *Clin. Sci.* 64:541–546, 1983.

38. Lane, N.E., D. Block, H. Jones, et al. Long distance running, osteoporosis and osteo-arthritis. *JAMA* 255:1147–1151, 1986.

39. Lanyon, L.E. Control of bone architecture by functional load bearing. *J. Bone Miner. Res.* 7:S369–375, 1992.

40. Lanyon, L.E. and C.T. Rubin. Static versus dynamic loads as an influence on bone remodeling. *J. Biomech.* 17:897–905, 1984.

41. Lanyon, L.E., A.E. Goodship, C.J. Pye, and H. MacFie. Mechanically adaptive bone remodeling. A quantitative study on functional adaptation in the radius following ulna osteotomy in sheep. *J. Biomech.* 15:767–781, 1982.

42. Lanyon, L.E., C.T. Rubin, and G. Baust. Modulation of bone loss during calcium insufficiency. *Calcif. Tissue Int.* 38:209–216, 1986.

43. Li, X.J., W.S.S. Jee, S.Y. Chow, and D.M. Woodbury. Adaptation of cancellous bone to aging and immobilization in the rat: a single photon absorptiometry and histomorphometry study. *Anat. Rec.* 227:291–297, 1990.

44. Li, X.J. and W.S.S. Jee. Adaptation of diaphyseal structure to aging and decreased mechanical loading in the adult rat: a single photon absorptiometry and histomorphometry study. *Anat. Rec.* 229:291–297, 1991.

45. Lindgren, J.U. Studies of the calcium accretion rate of bone during immobilization in intact and thyroparathyroidectomized adult rats. *Calcif. Tissue Res.* 22:41–47, 1976.

46. Loitz, B.J. and R.F. Zernicke. Strenuous exercise-induced remodelling of mature bone: relationship between in vivo strains and bone mechanics. *J. Exp. Biol.* 170:1–18, 1992.

47. Marcus, R., J. Kosek, A. Pfefferbaum, and S. Horning. Age-related loss of trabecular bone in premenopausal women: a biopsy study. *Calcif. Tissue Int.* 35:406–409, 1983.

48. Marcus, R., C. Cann, P. Madvig, et al. Menstrual function and bone mass in elite women distance runners: Endocrine and metabolic features. *Ann. Intern. Med.* 102:158–163, 1985.

49. Matsuda, J.J., R.F. Zernicke, A.C. Vailas, V.A. Pedrini, A. Pedrini-Mille, and J.A. Maynard. Structure and mechanical adaptation of immature bone to strenuous exercise. *J. Appl. Physiol.* 60:2028–2034, 1986.

50. Mazess, R.B. On aging bone loss. *Clin. Orthop. Relat. Res.* 165:239–252, 1982.

51. Mazess, R.B. and H.S. Barden. Bone density in premenopausal women: aspects of age, dietary intake, physical activity, smoking, and birth control pills. *Am. J. Clin. Nutr.* 53:132–142, 1991.

52. Michel, B.A., D.A. Bloch, and J.F. Fires. Weight-bearing exercise, overexercise, and lumbar bone density over age 50 years. *Arch. Intern. Med.* 149:2325–2329, 1989.

53. Myburgh, K., J. Hutchins, A.B. Fataar, et al. Low bone density is an etiologic factor for stress fractures in athletes. *Ann. Intern. Med.* 113:754–759, 1990.

54. Myburgh, K.H., L.K. Bachrach, B. Lewis, K. Kent, and R. Marcus. Low bone mineral density at axial and appendicular sites in amenorrheic athletes. *Med. Sci. Sports Exerc.* 25:1197–1202, 1993.

55. Nelson, M.E., E.C. Fisher, F.A. Dilmanian, G.E. Dallal, and W.J. Evans. A 1-year walking program and increased calcium in postmenopausal women: effects on bone. *Am. J. Clin. Nutr.* 53:1304–1311, 1991.

56. Notelovitz, M., D. Martin, T. Tesar, L. McKenzie, and C. Fields. Estrogen therapy and variable resistance weight training increases bone mineral in surgically menopausal women. *J. Bone Miner. Res.* 6:583–590, 1991.

57. O'Connor, J.A., L.E. Lanyon, and H. MacFie. The influence of strain rate on adaptive bone remodeling. *J. Biomech.* 15:767–781, 1982.

58. Orwoll, E.S., J. Ferar, S.K. Oviatt, M.R. McClung, and K. Huntington. The relationship of swimming exercise to bone mass in men and women. *Arch. Intern. Med.* 149:2197–2200, 1989.

59. Paganini-Hill, A., A. Chao, R.K. Ross, and B. Henerson. Exercise and other factors in the prevention of hip fracture: the Leisure World Study. *Epidemiology* 2:16–25, 1991.

60. Pead, M., T.M. Skerry, and L.E. Lanyon. Direct transformation from quiescence to formation in the adult periosteum following a single brief period of loading. *J. Bone Miner. Res.* 3:647–656, 1988.

61. Pead, M.J., R. Suswillo, T.M. Skerry, S. Vedi, and L.E. Lanyon. Increased (3H)uridine levels in osteocytes following a single short period of dynamic loading in vivo. *Calcif. Tissue Int.* 43:92–97, 1988.

62. Peterson, S.E., M.D. Peterson, G. Raymond, C. Gilligan, M.M. Checovich, and E.L. Smith. Muscular strength and bone density with weight training in middle-aged women. *Med. Sci. Sports Exerc.* 23:499–504, 1991.

63. Pocock, N., J.A. Eisman, T. Gwinn, et al. Muscle strength, physical fitness and weight but not age, predict femoral neck bone mass. *J. Bone Miner. Res.* 4:441–4418, 1989.

64. Pocock, N., J.A. Eisman, T. Gwinn, et al. Muscle strength, physical fitness and weight but not age predict femoral neck bone mass. *J. Bone Miner. Res.* 4:441–446, 1989.

65. Pohlman, R.L., L.A. Darby, and A.J. Lechner. Morphometry and calcium contents in appendicular and axial bones of exercised ovariectomized rats. *J. Appl. Physiol.* 248:R12–R17, 1985.

66. Prince, R., M. Smith, I.M. Dick, R.I. Price, P.G. Webb, K. Henderson, and M. M. Harris. Prevention of osteoporosis: a comparative study of exercise, calcium supplementation, and hormone-replacement therapy. *N. Engl. J. Med.* 325:1189–1195, 1991.

67. Pruitt, L., R.D. Jackson. R.L. Bartels, and H.J. Lehnhard. Weight training effects on bone mineral density in early postmenopausal women. *J. Bone Miner. Res.* 7:179–186, 1992.

68. Raab, D.M., E.L. Smith, T.D. Crenshaw, and D.P. Thomas. Bone mechanical properties after exercise training in young and old rats. *J. Appl. Physiol.* 68:130–134, 1990.

69. Rawlinson, S.C.F., A. . El Haj, S.L. Minter, A. Bennet, A. Tavares, and L.E. Lanyon. Load-related release of prostaglandins in cores of cancellous bone in culture—a role for prosacyclin in adaptive bone remodeling. *J. Bone Miner. Res.* 6:1345–1351, 1991.

70. Recker, R.R., K.M. Davies, S.M. Hinders, R.P. Heaney, M.R. Stegman, and D.B. Kimmel. Bone gains in young adult women. *JAMA* 268:2403–2408, 1992.

71. Reid, I.R., R. Ames, M.C. Evans, et al. Determinants of total body and regional bone mineral density in normal postmenopausal women: a key role for fat mass. *J. Clin. Endocrinol. Metab.* 75:45–51, 1992.

72. Reid, I.R., L.D. Plank, and M.C. Evans. Fat mass is an important determinant of whole body bone density in premenopausal women but not in men. *J. Clin. Endocrinol. Metab.* 75:779–782, 1992.

73. Riggs, B.L., H.W. Wahner, W.L. Dann, R.B. Mazess, and K.P. Offord. Differential changes in bone mineral density of the appendicular and axial skeleton with aging. *J. Clin. Invest.* 67:328–335, 1981.

74. Risser, W.L., E.J. Lee, A. LeBlanc, H.B. Poindexter, J.M. H. Risser, and V. Schneider. Bone density in eumenorrheic female college athletes. *Med. Sci. Sports Exerc.* 22:570–574, 1990.

75. Rockwell, J.C., A.M. Sorensen, S. Baker, D. Leahey, J.L. Stock, J. Michaels, and D.T.B. Weight training decreases vertebral bone density in premenopausal women: a prospective study. *J. Clin. Endocrinol. Metab.* 71:988–993, 1990.

76. Rubin, C.T. and L.E. Lanyon. Limb mechanics as a function of speed and gait: a study of functional strains in the radius and tibia of horse and dog. *J. Exp. Biol.* 101:187–211, 1982.

77. Rubin, C.T. and L.E. Lanyon. Regulation of bone formation by applied dynamic loads. *J. Bone Joint Surg.* 66:397–402, 1984.

78. Rubin, C.T. and L.E. Lanyon. Regulation of bone mass by mechanical strain magnitude. *Calcif. Tissue Int.* 37:411–417, 1985.

79. Salem, G.J., K.C. Li, R.F. Zernicke, and R.J. Barnard. Exercise related adaptation in geometry and mechanical properties of immature rat tibia and vertebra. *Proc XII International Congress of Biomechanics, UCLA, California, Abst.* 353:1989.

80. Sandler, R.B., J.A. Cauley, D.L. Hom, D, Sashin, and A.M. Kriska. The effects of walking on the cross-sectional dimensions of the radius in postmenopausal women. *Calcif. Tissue Int.* 41:65–69, 1987.

81. Saville, P. and M. Whyte. Muscle and bone hypertrophy. Positive effect of running exercise in the rat. *Clin. Orthop.* 65:81–88, 1969.

82. Shaw, S.R., R.F. Zernicke, A.C. Vailas, et al. Mechanical, morphological and biomechanical adaptation of bone and muscle to hindlimb suspension. *J. Biomech.* 20:225–234, 1987.

83. Shaw, S.R., A.C. Vailas, R.E. Gindeland, et al. Effects of 1-wk spaceflight on morphological and mechanical properties of growing bone. *Am. J. Physiol.* 254:R78–R83, 1988.

84. Simmons, D., M. Grynpas, and G. Rosenberg. Maturation of bone and dentin matrices in rats flown on the soviet biosatellite Cosmos 1887. *FASEB J.* 4:29–33, 1990.

85. Skerry, T.M., L. Bitensky, J. Chayen, and L.E. Lanyon. Early strain-related changes in enzyme activity in osteocytes following bone loading in vivo. *J. Bone Min. Res.* 4:783–788, 1989.

86. Skerry, T.M., L. Bitensky, J. Chayen, and L.E. Lanyon. Loading-related reorientation of bone proteoglycans. A strain memory in bone tissue? *J. Orthop. Res.* 6:547–552, 1988.

87. Smith, R. and I. Saville. Bone breaking stress as a function of weight bearing in bipedal rats. *Am. J. Phys. Anthropol.* 25:159–165, 1966.

88. Snow-Harter, C., M.L. Bouxsein, B.T. Lewis, D.R. Carter, and R. Marcus. Effects of resistance and endurance exercise on bone mineral status of young women: a randomized exercise intervention trial. *J. Bone Miner. Res.* 7:761–769, 1992.

89. Snow-Harter, C. and R. Marcus. Exercise, bone mineral density, and osteoporosis. In: *Exercise and Sport Science Reviews,* Vol. 19. Baltimore: Williams & Wilkins, 1991, pp. 351–388.

90. Snow-Harter, C., M. Bouxsein, B.T. Lewis, S. Charette, P. Weinstein, and R. Marcus. Muscle strength as a predictor of bone mineral density in young women. *J. Bone Miner. Res.* 5:589–595, 1990.

91. Snow-Harter, C., M. Wegner, T. Robinson, J. Shaw, and A. Shelley. Determinants of femoral neck BMD in pre- and postmenopausal women. *Med. Sci. Sports Exerc.* 25:S856, 1993.

92. Sowers, M.R., A. Kshirsager, M.M. Crutchfield, and S. Updike. Joint influence of fat and lean body composition compartments on femoral bone mineral density in premenopausal women. *Am. J. Epidemiol.* 136:257–265, 1992.

93. Steinberg, M.E. and J. Trueta. Effects of activity on bone growth and development in the rat. *Clin. Orthop. Relat. Res.* 156:52–60, 1981.

94. Swissa-Sivan, A. Simkin, I. Leichter, et al. Effect of swimming on bone growth and development in young rats. *Bone Miner.* 7:91–106, 1989.

95. Tamaki, T., S. Uchiyama, and S. Nakano. A weightlifting exercise model for inducing hypertrophy in the hindlimb muscles of rats. *Med. Sci. Sports Exerc.* 24:881–886, 1992.

96. Uhtoff, H.K. and Z.F.G. Jaworski. Bone loss in response to long-term immobilization. *J. Bone Joint Surg.* 60B:420–429, 1978.

97. Uhtoff, H.K., G. Sekaly, and Z.R.G. Jaworski. Effect of long term nontraumatic immobilization on metaphyseal spongiosa in young adult and old beagle dogs. *Clin. Orthop. Rel. Res.* 192:278–283, 1985.

98. Vailas, A., R.F. Zernicke, R. Grindeland, et al. Effects of spaceflight on rat humorous geometry, biomechanics, and biochemistry. *FASEB J.* 4:47–54, 1990.

99. Wakley, G.K., B.L. Baum, K.S. Hannon, and R.T. Turner. The effect of tamoxifen on the osteopenia induced by sciatic neurectomy in the rat: a histomorphometric study. *Calcif. Tissue Int.* 43:383–388, 1988.

100. Wegner, M., C. Snow-Harter, T. Robinson, J. Shaw, and A. Shelley. Lean mass, not fat mass, independently predicts whole body mineral density in postmenopausal women. *Med. Sci. Sports Exerc.* 25:S854, 1993.

101. Weinreb, M., B.A. Rodan, and D.D. Thompson. Immobilization-related bone loss in the rat is increased by calcium deficiency. *Calcif. Tissue Int.* 48:93–100, 1991.

102. Weinreb, M., G.A. Rodan, and D.D. Thompson. Osteopenia in the immobilized rat hind limb is associated with increased bone resorption and decreased bone formation. *Bone* 10:187–194, 1989.

103. Whalen, R.T. and D.R. Carter. Influence of physical activity on the regulation of bone density. *J. Biomech.* 21:825–837, 1988.

104. White, M.K., R.B. Martin, R.A. Yeater, R.L. Butcher, and E.L. Radin. The effects of exercise on the bones of postmenopausal women. *Int. Orthop.* 7:209–214, 1984.

105. Wickam, C.A.C., K. Walsh, C. Cooper, et al. Dietary calcium, physical activity, and risk of hip fracture: a prospective study. *Br. Med. J.* 299:889–892, 1989.

106. Wolman, R.L., L. Faulman, P. Clark, R. Hesp, and M.G. Harries. Different training patterns and bone mineral density of the femoral shaft in elite, female athletes. *Ann. Rheum. Dis.* 50:487–489, 1991.

107. Woo, S. L.–Y., S.C. Kuel, D. Amiel, et al. The effect of physical training on the properties of long bone: a study of Wolff's law. *J. Bone Joint Surg.* 63A:780–787, 1981.

108. Wronski, T.J., E.R. Mary-Holten, S.B. Doty, et al. Histomorphometric analysis of rat skeleton following spaceflight. *Am. J. Physiol.* 252: R252–R255, 1987.

109. Yeh, J.K. and J.F. Aloia. Effect of physical activity on calciotropic hormones and calcium balance in the rat. *Am. J. Physiol.* 258:E263–268, 1990.

PART 2

ACSM POSITION STAND ON PHYSICAL ACTIVITY, PHYSICAL FITNESS, AND HYPERTENSION[b]

SUMMARY

American College of Sports Medicine Position Stand: "PHYSICAL ACTIVITY, PHYSICAL FITNESS, AND HYPERTENSION." *Med. Sci. Sports Exerc.*, Vol. 25, No. 10, pp. i–x, 1993. Hypertension is present in epidemic proportions in adults of industrialized societies and is associated with a markedly increased risk of developing numerous cardiovascular pathologies. There is a continuing debate as to the efficacy of aggressive pharmacological therapy in individuals with mild to moderate elevations in blood pressure. This has led to a search for nonpharmacological therapies, such as exercise training, for these individuals. The available evidence indicates that endurance exercise training by individuals at high risk for developing hypertension will reduce the rise in blood pressure that occurs with time. Thus, it is the position of the American College of Sports Medicine that endurance exercise training is recommended as a nonpharmacological strategy to reduce the incidence of hypertension in susceptible individuals. A large number of studies indicate that endurance exercise training will elicit a 10 mm Hg average reduction in both systolic and diastolic blood pressures in individuals with mild essential hypertension (blood pressures 140–180/90–105 mm Hg). Endurance exercise training also has the capacity to improve other risk factors for cardiovascular disease in hypertensive individuals. Endurance exercise training appears to elicit even greater reductions in blood pressure in patients with secondary hypertension due to renal dysfunction. The mode (large muscle activities), frequency (3–5 d · wk^{-1}), duration (20–60 min), and intensity (50–85% of maximal oxygen uptake) of the exercise recommended to achieve this effect are generally the same as those prescribed for developing and maintaining cardiovascular fitness in healthy adults. Exercise training at somewhat lower intensities (40–70% $\dot{V}O_{2max}$) appears to lower blood pressure as much, or more,

than exercise at higher intensities, which may be important in specific hypertensive populations. Physically active and fit individuals with hypertension have markedly lower rates of mortality than sedentary, unfit hypertensive individuals. Thus, it seems reasonable to recommend exercise as the initial treatment strategy for individuals with mild to moderate essential hypertension. A follow-up period should assess the efficacy of the patient's exercise program, and adjunct therapies should be implemented according to the individual patient's blood pressure and CAD risk factor goals. Individuals with more marked elevations in blood pressure (> 180/105 mm Hg) should add endurance exercise training to their treatment regimen only after initiating pharmacologic therapy. Resistive, or strength, exercise training is not recommended to lower blood pressure in individuals with hypertension when done as their only form of exercise training. It is recommended when included as one component of a well-rounded fitness program, such as circuit training done in conjunction with endurance exercise training. Exercise testing is not advocated to determine normotensive individuals with an exaggerated exercise blood pressure response who might be at high risk of developing hypertension in the future. However, if exercise test results are available, they can be used to provide some indication of risk stratification and the need for appropriate lifestyle behavior counselling that might ameliorate this risk.

INTRODUCTION

Hypertension, defined as a blood pressure above 140/90 mm Hg, is present in 17% of adults according to the National Health and Nutrition Examination Survey[94]. However, hypertension prevalence rates rise sharply with age and are also generally higher in men than in women and in blacks than in whites[59]. At least 90% and probably as much as 95% of all hypertension is of unknown cause, i.e., primary or essential[59]. Despite tremendous increases in the recognition and treatment of hypertension over the past 25 yr,[9, 25] the incidence of hypertension has not decreased[26]. This Position Stand primarily addresses the effect of exercise training on individuals with hypertension and on those individuals at an increased risk of developing hypertension. In addition, this Position Stand also addresses the role of exercise testing in predicting those individuals at higher risk of developing hypertension in the future.

HYPERTENSION AND PREMATURE MORTALITY AND MORBIDITY

Men and women with blood pressures exceeding 160/95 mm Hg have a 150–300% higher annual incidence rate for coronary artery disease (CAD), congestive heart failure, intermittent claudication, and stroke than their normotensive peers[58]. Women appear to tolerate increased blood pressures better than men as they have substantially lower incidence rates for these four cardiovascular pathologies than men with comparable blood pressures[58]. On the other hand,

---

[b]"Physical Activity, Physical Fitness, and Hypertension" © 1993 American College of Sports Medicine (*Med. Sci. Sports Exerc.*, 25:10, 1993, pp. i–x).

black hypertensives have higher death rates than whites with the same blood pressure[59]. Older individuals also have a substantially greater risk of a cardiovascular event than younger persons with the same elevation in blood pressure[59], indicating that an increase in blood pressure should not be accepted as an inconsequential concomitant of the aging process.

The dramatic benefits derived from aggressive pharmacological therapy for individuals with marked elevations in blood pressure were first demonstrated over 20 yr ago in the Veterans Administration Cooperative Study on individuals with diastolic blood pressures of 115–129 mm Hg[115], where 40% of patients receiving a placebo experienced a cardiovascular event compared with only 3% of patients receiving antihypertensive medications over the same time period. Numerous other trials have continued to demonstrate the dramatic benefits of pharmacological therapy in individuals with marked elevations in blood pressure[59].

Individuals with mild hypertension (140–160/90–105 mm Hg) are also at a greater risk of developing future cardiovascular morbidity[58]. However, there is a continuing debate as to the efficacy of aggressive pharmacological therapy to reduce their cardiovascular risks, perhaps because of deleterious side effects of medications on other risk factors for CAD[59, 68]. This debate has led to a search for nonpharmacological therapies, such as exercise training, for individuals with mild hypertension. Exercise training has also been proposed as a strategy to reduce the likelihood of a high-risk individual developing hypertension and to reduce mortality in individuals initiating an exercise program even if they remain hypertensive. In addition, exercise testing has been advocated as a means to identify normotensive individuals who may have a greater risk for developing hypertension in the future.

EXERCISE TESTING AND THE PREDICTION OF THE DEVELOPMENT OF HYPERTENSION

Over 50 yr ago the blood pressure responses of pre-hypertensive individuals to local cold[51] and mental tests[70] were found to be higher than those of individuals at lower risk for the future development of hypertension. Although most studies have shown that normotensive individuals with a family history of hypertension have more marked pressor responses to dynamic and isometric exercise than individuals without such a history[10, 76, 119], other studies have not reported such differences[cf., 106, 107]. Several longitudinal studies indicate that normotensive individuals with a hypertensive response to exercise have an increased risk of developing hypertension in the future[20, 54, 69, 73, 103]. These reports vary in the type of population studied, the mode of exercise testing, the definition of a hypertensive response to exercise, and the length of follow-up. Nevertheless, results are consistent with a two- to threefold increase in risk for developing

hypertension in individuals with an exaggerated blood pressure response to exercise. The sensitivity and specificity of exercise hypertension to predict future hypertension at rest are modest[10], but these terms are usually discussed in reference to a diagnostic test where high values are required to have confidence in a definitive diagnosis. Screening tests to predict future disease or death have lower sensitivity and specificity than diagnostic tests, but screening is still useful to identify groups at risk. Thus, mass exercise testing is not recommended to identify future hypertensive individuals. However, if exercise test results are available, individuals with exercise blood pressure responses above the 85th or 90th percentile should be counselled about their increased risk for developing hypertension at rest in the future and given appropriate advice regarding health habits that might ameliorate that increased risk.

EXERCISE AND PREVENTION OF HYPERTENSION

Studies in animals. In animal models it is important to differentiate those animals that become hypertensive because of genetic influences [spontaneously hypertensive (SH) rats] from those that become hypertensive as a result of interventions such as hormonal injections (deoxycorticosterone), salt intake, or arterial constriction (two kidney-one clip). In the former, blood pressure is elevated because of interactions between genetic factors and the maturation process, whereas in the latter it is generally the magnitude and duration of the intervention that determines the rise in pressure. In general, the rise in blood pressure seen over time in SH rats is attenuated when they undergo exercise training during maturation, although the attenuation will not maintain their resting blood pressures within the normotensive range[108]. This effect of training is seldom found in rat models of renal hypertension and is variable in salt-sensitive rats[106, 107]. However, in these animal models the peripheral vasculature and renal structural changes that develop with hypertension are major and may totally eliminate the possibility of any physiological intervention maintaining a normotensive state.

Training intensity also appears to be an important consideration in SH rats because when the intensity exceeds 75% of their maximal oxygen consumption ($\dot{V}O_{2max}$), higher rather than lower resting systolic blood pressures result[108, 113]. On the other hand, when exercise intensity is 40–70% $\dot{V}O_{2max}$, lower resting pressures are found for trained SH rats[108, 109].

Studies in humans. Six of 13 epidemiological studies reviewed in 1972 showed somewhat lower blood pressures in active compared with sedentary individuals[77]. The remaining seven cross-sectional studies in this review by Montoye et al.[77] generally found no differences in blood pressure between active individuals and their less active peers. Reaven et al.[90] recently reported that in women a significant inverse relationship exists between physical activity and blood pressure, that the most active women had systolic and diastolic blood pressures 9–24 and 3–13 mm Hg lower, respectively, than the least active women, and that this relationship persisted after correcting for differences in body mass index. In the Tecumseh Community Health Study[77], the blood pressure of adult males was inversely related to occupational and leisure physical activity habits; however, the absolute difference in blood pressure was only 2–3 mm Hg between the most and least active men.

In more recent longitudinal studies, University of Pennsylvania alumni who played intramural sports less than 5 hr · wk^{-1} were found to be 32% more likely to bdevelop hypertension during 22–31 yr of follow-up than those who played sports more than 5 hr · wk^{-1}; similar results were evident when athletes and nonathletes were compared[81]. Follow-up surveys of this population indicated that participation in light or moderate activity later in life did not alter the incidence of hypertension, but alumni who had subsequently engaged in vigorous activity had a 19–29% lower rate of developing hypertension[83]. Harvard alumni who did not participate in vigorous sports had a 35% higher incidence of hypertension during a 6–10 yr follow-up period[84]. At the Institute for Aerobics Research in Dallas, physically unfit individuals, assessed by the results of treadmill exercise tests relative to age- and sex-specific norms, were 52% more likely than fit individuals to develop hypertension during a 4-yr follow-up period[13].

The first and only long-term primary prevention trial found that 75% of hypertension-prone men and women 30–44 yr of age in an exercise and dietary intervention increased their reported physical activity, and improved their exercise tolerance more than hypertension-prone controls[101]. The incidence of new hypertension in this intervention group (8.8%) was 54% lower than the incidence in the control group (19.2%) over the 5-yr duration of the trial. However, since this trial combined several interventions it was not possible to assess the independent contribution of exercise toward lowering the incidence of hypertension.

Thus, recent large, long-term studies that allow for control of potentially confounding variables support the concept that regular exercise and increased aerobic fitness levels ($\dot{V}O_{2max}$) reduce an individual's risk of developing hypertension. However, most of these investigations studied white, middle-class males and little information is available for women, minorities, and other demographic groups.

EFFECT OF EXERCISE ON INDIVIDUALS WITH HYPERTENSION

Studies in animals. There have been very few studies in which hypertension was established before the animals began training. In SH rats older than 40 wk of age, moderate intensity exercise training for several months maintained resting blood pressure at their initial value, whereas SH rats not undergoing training exhibited a gradual increase in pressure over the same time[117]. However, the available data on exercise training in animals do not convincingly support the concept that exercise training will lower blood pressures in those with established hypertension.

Studies in humans. Forty studies published prior to 1992 in the English literature have assessed the blood pressure-lowering effects of endurance exercise training on individuals with essential hypertension[2, 5, 7, 8, 14–16, 18, 19, 22–24, 27, 29, 32, 36, 38, 44, 47, 49, 50, 55, 56, 62, 64, 66, 67, 74, 78, 79, 92, 93, 95–97, 102, 114, 116–118]. All 1574 subjects enrolled in these studies initially had systolic hypertension (systolic blood pressure ≥ 140 mm Hg) while 755 subjects (48%) initially also had diastolic hypertension (diastolic blood pressure ≥ 90 mm Hg). Seventy-two percent of the groups in these studies that initially had systolic hypertension elicited significant decreases in systolic blood pressure as a result of endurance exercise training. Their training-induced reduction in systolic blood pressure averaged approximately 11 mm Hg from an initial systolic pressure of 153 mm Hg. Seventy-seven percent of the groups that initially had diastolic hypertension in these studies reduced their diastolic pressure significantly with endurance exercise training. Their reduction in diastolic blood pressure with exercise training averaged approximately 9 mm Hg from an initial value of 99 mm Hg. Thus, these data indicate that endurance exercise training lowers casual systolic and diastolic blood pressure measured in the laboratory or in a clinic setting by approximately 10 mm Hg in the large majority of individuals with mild elevations in blood pressure.

Four studies in individuals with hypertension have assessed the impact of exercise training on the ambulatory blood pressures measured while they took part in their usual daily activities[14, 36, 98, 100]. Two of these studies found no changes in either casual or ambulatory pressures as a result of endurance exercise training[14, 36]. The two remaining studies[98, 100] reported significant reductions in both casual and ambulatory blood pressures with exercise training in individuals with hypertension. However, the significant reduction in ambulatory blood pressure was generally only evident during the daytime hours, and the magnitude of the reduction was generally less than that observed in casual blood pressure. Thus, future studies must continue to assess the impact of exercise training on ambulatory blood pressure in individuals with hypertension, especially in light of the fact that ambulatory blood pressure is more indicative of their future prognosis[89].

Roughly half of the 40 investigations that have assessed the impact of endurance exercise training on individuals with hypertension studied only men and only two studies reported data from women separately. However, no studies that have compared men and women have found gender-related differences in the blood pressure changes elicited with exercise training[32, 44, 47, 97, 116]. This would also appear to be the case in numerous other studies that included hypertensive men and women and made no specific mention of gender-related differences in blood pressure reductions elicited by endurance exercise training[2, 7, 8, 14, 18, 23, 24, 27, 36, 38, 64, 66, 78, 79, 114, 117, 118].

The subjects in these 40 studies ranged in age from 15–79 yr. The one study in adolescent hypertensives reported reductions in systolic blood pressure, and in diastolic blood pressure in those with diastolic hypertension[44], that approximated 10 mm Hg, even though their initial pressures were lower than those in older hypertensives. Studies that have assessed the blood pressure-lowering effects of endurance exercise training programs longer than 3 months in hypertensive men and women over the age of 60 yr generally report reductions in blood pressure similar in magnitude to those elicited in younger hypertensives[18, 24, 32, 47]. The only races studied extensively have been Caucasians and Asians.

The few studies that are available generally indicate that the blood pressure-lowering effect of exercise training is also evident and quantitatively similar in patients taking antihypertensive medications[2, 19, 24, 47, 62]; rat models of hypertension undergoing exercise training generally require less than normal amounts of anti-hypertensive medications[108]. Thus, although the data support the general conclusion that endurance exercise training lowers blood pressure in individuals with essential hypertension, extrapolations of this conclusion to specific hypertensive populations and situations are, except for white middle-aged men and women, almost universally based on the results of single, or at best very few, studies.

A number of recent studies[24, 47, 55, 64, 66, 93, 97, 114] have reported that training at 40–70% $\dot{V}O_{2max}$ had the same, or greater, blood pressure-lowering effect as higher intensity training. Along these lines, it has also been shown that SH rats had lower blood pressures than nonexercising age-matched controls only if they trained at 40–70% $\dot{V}O_{2max}$[108, 109]. Thus, it appears that moderate-intensity training may elicit as great or greater reductions in blood pressure as higher intensity training; this may be especially important in specific populations of hypertensive individuals, such as the elderly, as acute cardiovascular and musculoskeletal risks will be reduced.

Most studies have found that blood pressure was reduced early (3 wk to 3 months) after the initiation of exercise training, and that up to 9 months of additional training failed to elicit further reductions in blood pressure[66, 93, 114]. However, it was recently reported that older hypertensives who decreased their blood pressure significantly with 3 months of moderate-intensity training reduced both their systolic and diastolic blood pressures further with an additional 6 months of training[47]. In a previous review[41], the reduction in diastolic blood pressure was found to be related to the length of the training, whereas the reduction in systolic pressure was not. Thus, although it appears that blood pressure may be reduced early after the initiation of an endurance exercise training program, it does not appear that

prolonging such training beyond 3 months will result in further decreases in blood pressure, though this may not be the case with more moderate training intensities. However, those investigations that have had individuals with hypertension stop training indicate that their blood pressure returns to initial untrained levels[44, 93, 100]. Thus, although more prolonged training may not bring about further reductions in blood pressure in individuals with hypertension, the blood pressure-lowering effect of exercise training is evident only as long as a regular endurance exercise training program is maintained.

It has been proposed that some specific subsets of hypertensive individuals might not lower their blood pressure in response to endurance exercise training. Recent studies and reviews have reported that overweight hypertensives[41], those with high initial plasma renin levels[66, 114], low norepinephrine levels[29], high cardiac output[64], high serum sodium to potassium ratios[64], or those taking nonselective beta-blockade medications[2] show either no, or attenuated, blood pressure-lowering responses to endurance exercise training. However, this attenuated blood pressure-lowering response is not consistent in other studies that have investigated these specific subgroups of hypertensives[24, 44, 47, 62]. A recent study reported that hypertensive subjects with hypertensive exercise blood pressure responses did not change their systolic blood pressure and actually increased their diastolic blood pressure significantly (from 87–92 mm Hg) in response to exercise training[5]. However, in the same study[5], hypertensives with normal blood pressure responses to exercise decreased their systolic and diastolic blood pressure significantly. This is the only study to report a significant increase in resting blood pressure in a group of hypertensive individuals as a result of exercise training. Finally, a recent review[41] indicated that in previous studies the magnitude of the reductions in systolic and diastolic blood pressure elicited with endurance exercise training were somewhat correlated to the initial diastolic blood pressure (r = 0.34 and 0.46, respectively) but not to the initial systolic blood pressure.

Thus, there is minimal definitive evidence to support the conclusion that certain subsets of individuals with essential hypertension do not lower their blood pressure in response to endurance exercise training. However, in view of the recent report of strikingly different blood pressure responses to exercise training between hypertensives with normal vs exaggerated blood pressure responses to maximal exercise, further investigation is warranted.

Another important consideration for hypertensive individuals is the possibility that endurance exercise training may elicit other potential benefits in addition to lowering their blood pressure. The incidence of other modifiable CAD risk factors, including obesity, abnormal plasma lipoprotein-lipid profiles, insulin resistance, and glucose intolerance, is also more prevalent in hypertensive individuals[60, 104]. Endurance exercise training, in addition to reducing blood pressure in hypertensive individuals, also improves glucose intolerance and insulin resistance[52], obesity and caloric balance[17], and plasma lipoprotein-lipid profiles[121] in healthy individuals. Furthermore, some of these beneficial training-induced adaptations have also already been demonstrated in individuals with essential hypertension[15, 38, 62, 97, 102, 116, 118]. These positive effects of exercise training are in contrast to the known deleterious side effects of many of the antihypertensive medication on CAD risk factors[58]. Preliminary research suggests that certain antihypertensive drug therapies such as beta-blockers may offset or negate the exercise training-induced increase in HDL-cholesterol levels[30]. However, the interactive effects of exercise and specific drug therapies on other CAD risk factors are largely unknown.

Studies in humans with secondary hypertension. Few studies have assessed the impact of exercise training on patients with secondary hypertension, probably because most of these patients have an underlying etiology that should be treated directly by standard medical, pharmacological, and surgical interventions. However, some patients with end-stage renal disease have endocrine abnormalities that maintain or exacerbate their hypertension even after their excess fluid volume is removed by dialysis. Two studies have reported that exercise training in end-stage renal disease patients decreases their systolic and diastolic blood pressures 2–3 times more than the reductions generally achieved in patients with essential hypertension, i.e., 20–30 mm Hg, and results in substantial reductions in the required dosages of their antihypertensive medications[43, 85]. Another study also found that a small number of patients with hypertension secondary to renal dysfunction decreased their blood pressures with exercise training to a greater extent than those with essential hypertension[19]. Therefore, it appears that patients with secondary forms of hypertension related to renal dysfunction can also reduce their blood pressure with endurance exercise training, and to an even greater extent than individuals with essential hypertension.

Death rates, fitness and hypertension. A strong inverse gradient for age-adjusted all-cause mortality exists across physical activity strata in Harvard alumni[82]. Hypertensive University of Pennsylvania alumni who engaged in vigorous sports had a 37% lower age-adjusted all-cause death rate than sedentary hypertensive alumni[83]. Additional studies have shown that morbidity and mortality rates are also inversely related to physical fitness status in hypertensive individuals[12, 53, 87]. More recently in one study, fit hypertensive individuals were shown to have a 60% lower mortality rate than their unfit normotensive peers, and that the increased mortality associated with hypertension was completely overcome by fitness[11]. Although more research is clearly needed, especially in women, minorities, and other demographic groups, the existing studies support the conclusion that physical activity, and the resultant increased physical fitness, is an effective secondary intervention therapy in hypertensive individuals.

Relative effectiveness of nonpharmacological therapies. A review of weight loss studies[59] found average reductions of 15 and 10 mm Hg in systolic and diastolic blood pressure, respectively, as a result of a 10-kg average weight loss. A recent review concluded that reducing dietary sodium intake by 80 meq $\cdot$ d^{-1} was associated with a 5 and 3 mm Hg reduction in systolic and diastolic blood pressure, respectively, and that increasing dietary potassium intake by the same amount resulted in average reductions of 8 and 4 mm Hg for systolic and diastolic blood pressures, respectively[59]. Thus, overweight individuals who undergo a substantial weight loss elicit a reduction in blood pressure only slightly greater than that observed with endurance exercise training. However, altering sodium and potassium intake alone has a smaller effect on blood pressure than endurance exercise training[59].

The other nonpharmacologic therapies proposed to induce an antihypertensive effect are behavioral modalities, such as relaxation and biofeedback. A review of 15 studies of the effect of biofeedback training, many of which lacked appropriate control groups, indicated that it reduces systolic and diastolic blood pressure by an average of 12 and 5 mm Hg, respectively, whereas relaxation techniques may be somewhat more effective with reductions averaging 18 and 11 mm Hg for systolic and diastolic blood pressure, respectively[99]. However, the addition of appropriate control groups in recent studies appears to have diminished the favorable effect of relaxation and biofeedback interventions to levels lower than those attained by endurance exercise training[37, 71].

SAFETY OF ENDURANCE EXERCISE

Hemodynamic responses. In unmedicated hypertensive individuals, acute exercise generally elicits a normal rise in systolic blood pressure from baseline levels, though the response may be exaggerated or diminished in certain patients[88, 120]. However, because of their elevated baseline levels, the absolute levels of systolic blood pressure during exercise are usually higher in hypertensive persons. Furthermore, hypertensive persons may not change, or may even slightly increase, their diastolic blood pressure during incremental exercise probably as a result of an impaired vasodilatory response[88]. On the other hand, recent studies have demonstrated that individuals with essential hypertension can exhibit 10–20 mm Hg reductions in systolic blood pressure for 1–3 hr following 30–45 min of moderate-intensity exercise[46, 61]. There is also some indication that this response may persist for up to 9 hr following acute exercise in individuals with hypertension[86]. This response appears to be mediated by a transient decrease in stroke volume and, hence, cardiac output, perhaps due to a decrease in venous return, rather than a peripheral vasodilation that persists after the cessation of exercise[46, 80].

In view of the higher levels of blood pressure induced by exercise in individuals with hypertension, it has been postulated that they are at greater risk for sudden cardiac death or hemorrhagic stroke. However, at present there is no convincing evidence to substantiate this assumption in humans[35, 88], even though in young and mature stroke-prone SH rats moderate-intensity endurance exercise training increased the incidence of cerebrovascular lesions[110]. Thus, it seems prudent to avoid an excessive rise in blood pressure during exercise training and, in patients with target organ involvement (e.g., left ventricular hypertrophy), to impose some restrictions on participation in vigorous exercise[35]. The facts that high blood pressure is a major risk factor for CAD, which is by far the leading cause of sudden death during exercise, and the impaired coronary vasodilatory capacity in patients with left ventricular hypertrophy may provoke myocardial ischemia, even in the absence of severe CAD, should also be considered when prescribing exercise for hypertensive patients.

Interaction between exercise and medication. Antihypertensive medications do not preclude participation in endurance exercise. Although most antihypertensive drugs do not substantially alter the blood pressure response to endurance exercise, they do lower resting blood pressure and thus, the absolute level attained[21, 88]. Beta-blockers, however, can attenuate the magnitude of the rise in systolic blood pressure during endurance exercise as well as resting blood pressure. Consequently, they may be considered as the antihypertensive agents of greatest potential benefit to hypertensive persons who have an excessive rise in systolic blood pressure during dynamic exercise. Unfortunately, the usefulness of beta-blockers, especially nonselective ones, is often considerably limited by a concomitant impairment of exercise tolerance in persons without myocardial ischemia[40] and the possibility that they may blunt the exercise training-induced lowering of blood pressure[2] and the exercise training-induced increases in HDL-cholesterol[30] in hypertensive individuals. Therefore, unless beta-blocker therapy is specifically indicated, other agents with more favorable side effect profiles should be considered for such patients. In this regard, angiotensin-converting enzyme inhibitors, calcium channel blockers, and alpha-blockers are especially well suited for persons with uncomplicated essential hypertension and physically active lifestyles[3, 40]. Irrespective of the drugs prescribed, the physician and patient should be aware of their interaction with exercise and whether any special precautions are needed[35].

Safety and effects of resistive exercise training. Patients with high blood pressure have traditionally been discourage from participating in resistive training for fear of precipitating a cerebrovascular event or imposing an excessive demand on an already-compromised myocardium. Such fears have arisen largely as a result of the marked pressor response elicited during acute high-intensity resistive exercise[34, 72]. However, studies investigating the impact of chronic resistive training on resting blood pressure have, in fact, not documented such an adverse effect. On the contrary, although considerable additional research is needed, the result of some[42, 50, 62, 65], but not all[6, 14, 24], studies suggest that resistive training, especially circuit weight training, may lower resting blood pressure.

Experimental evidence on the effects of acute and chronic resistive training on the risk for cerebrovascular complications in humans with high blood pressure is not available. Recently stroke-prone hypertensive rats were found to not increase their development of cerebrovascular lesions with long-term resistive exercise training[111]. Although considerable further research is required before these findings can be extrapolated to humans with high blood pressure, they do indicate that resistive training may not necessarily increase the risk for cerebrovascular lesions.

Resistive training produces concentric left ventricular hypertrophy in some individuals. In hypertensive patients, concentric left ventricular hypertrophy is associated with an accentuated risk of cardiovascular events even in the absence of other CAD risk factors[28]. In general, the magnitude of cardiac hypertrophy is smaller than the hypertrophy produced by chronic hypertension, perhaps in part due to the mild to moderate and intermittent nature of the pressure overload associated with resistive training compared with the chronic elevated pressure state associated with hypertension. In fact, resistive training is typically characterized by normal diastolic function, in contrast to what occurs with pathologic concentric hypertrophy. Thus, although the eccentric hypertrophy elicited by endurance training is seemingly more desirable, resistive training does not appear to produce any adverse effects on left ventricular function[31, 39].

POTENTIAL MECHANISMS UNDERLYING THE ANTIHYPERTENSIVE EFFECT OF EXERCISE TRAINING

At present the mechanisms by which exercise training decreases blood pressure in hypertensive individuals are unclear. This effect is probably not mediated by a single mechanism, and for the different types of hypertension or in heterogeneous hypertensive populations, different mechanisms are possible. The blood pressure-lowering effect of exercise is, however, independent of decreases in body weight and body fat[2, 5, 7, 15, 16, 22, 24, 29, 44, 55, 64, 74, 78, 97, 102, 114].

In most individuals with long-standing hypertension, total peripheral resistance (TPR) is usually increased at rest[1]. However, in the limited number of studies in humans that have measured cardiovascular hemodynamics, reductions in both cardiac output and TPR have been observed after training[41, 107]. Recently, trained SH rats were shown to have a lower cardiac output and blood pressure at rest than their sedentary strain-matched counterparts, although their TPR was actually increased[109].

The sympathetic nervous system (SNS) is believed to play a central role in essential hypertension[1, 75], and there is evidence that the decrease in pressure with exercise training in some hypertensives is associated with a decrease in plasma norepinephrine levels[29, 47, 66, 114]. This effect may be especially important in hypertensives who have high plasma norepinephrine levels at rest, where the reduction in blood pressure elicited with endurance exercise training was significantly correlated to the changes in plasma norepinephrine levels[29]. In addition, chemically sympathectomized SH rats have been shown to undergo less of a rise in blood pressure with exercise training than their treatment-matched sedentary counterparts[112]. The fact that not all studies have found a decrease in plasma norepinephrine with training[23, 24, 45] does not rule out SNS involvement as plasma norepinephrine levels are only an indirect estimate of SNS activity and small, but potentially important, training-induced decreases in peripheral SNS activity may not be detectable by measuring plasma norepinephrine levels[33].

Conversely the lowering of blood pressure with exercise training could be due to an increase in circulating vasodilator substances. However, except for a suggested role for endorphins[105], there are no consistent data indicating that the blood pressure-lowering effect of exercise training is mediated by compounds such as prostaglandins, kinins, adenosine, dopamine, or atrial natriuretic factor.

Recently, hyperinsulinemia secondary to insulin resistance has been proposed as a potential mechanism responsible for the development of hypertension and the increased incidence of diabetes, upper body obesity, hypertriglyceridemia, and CAD that occur in hypertensive individuals[91]. However, although it is known that exercise training can ameliorate an individual's hyperinsulinemic state[52], no studies have yet assessed if this mechanism is involved in the blood pressure-lowering effect of endurance exercise training.

The kidney, because of its ability to regulate body sodium, and thus plasma volume and cardiac output, is believed to play a dominant role in maintaining the increased blood pressure in essential hypertension[48]. Thus, exercise training may lower blood pressure by altering renal function[63]. Although acute exercise influences various hormones that may influence renal sodium metabolism (e.g., renin, angiotensin, aldosterone, atrial natriuretic factor, prostaglandins, and insulin[122]) there are no consistent data implicating these compounds in the blood pressure-lowering effect of endurance exercise training.

CONCLUSIONS

The American College of Sports Medicine makes the following recommendations regarding exercise testing and exercise training of persons with hypertension:

1. Mass exercise testing is not advocated to determine those individuals at high risk for developing hypertension at rest in the future as a result of an exaggerated exercise blood pressure response. However, if exercise test results are available and an individual has an exercise blood pressure response above the 85th percentile, this information does provide some indication of risk stratification for that patient and the necessity for appropriate lifestyle behavior counselling to ameliorate this increased risk.

2. Endurance exercise training by individuals who are at high risk for developing hypertension will reduce the rise in blood pressure that occurs with time, thus justifying its use as a nonpharmacological strategy to reduce the incidence of hypertension in susceptible individuals.

3. Endurance exercise training will elicit an average reduction of 10 mm Hg for both systolic and diastolic blood pressures in individuals with mild essential hypertension (blood pressures in the range of 140–180/90–105 mm Hg). Endurance exercise training appears to elicit even greater reductions in blood pressure in patients with secondary hypertension due to renal dysfunction. The mode (large muscle activities), frequency (3–5 d · wk^{-1}), duration (20–60 min), and intensity of exercise (50–85% of maximal oxygen uptake) recommended are generally the same as those outline in the previous Position Stand of the American College of Sports Medicine entitled "The Recommended Quality and Quantity of Exercise for Developing and Maintaining Cardiorespiratory and Muscular Fitness in Healthy Adults" (4). Exercise training at somewhat lower intensities (40–70% $\dot{V}O_{2max}$) appears to lower blood pressure as much, or more, than exercise at higher intensities, which may be especially important in specific hypertensive populations, such as the elderly. Physically active and aerobically fit patients with hypertension have markedly lower rates of mortality than sedentary, unfit hypertensive individuals, probably because exercise training also improves a number of other cardiovascular disease risk factors. In concurrence with the Joint National Committee's Recommendations for the Treatment of Essential Hypertension[57] and based on the high number of exercise-related health benefits and low risk for morbidity/mortality, it seems reasonable to recommend exercise as part of the initial treatment strategy for individuals with mild to moderate essential hypertension. A follow-up period should assess the efficacy of the patient's exercise program, and adjunct therapies should be implemented according to the individual patient's blood pressure and CAD risk factor goals.

4. Individuals with more marked elevations in blood pressure (>180/105) should add endurance exercise training to their treatment regimen only after initiating pharmacologic therapy, as it may reduce their blood pressure further, allow them to decrease their antihypertensive medications, and attenuate their risk for premature mortality.

5. Resistive, or strength, training is not recommended as the only form of exercise training for hypertensive indi-

viduals as, with the exception of circuit weight training, it has not consistently been shown to lower blood pressure. Thus, resistive exercise training is recommended when done as one component of a well-rounded fitness program, but not when done independently.

■ACKNOWLEDGMENTS■

This pronouncement was written for the American College of Sports Medicine by: James M. Hagberg, Ph.D., FACSM (Chair); Steven N. Blair, P.E.D., FACSM; Ali A. Ehasani, M.D.; Neil F. Gordon, M.D., Ph.D., FACSM; Norman Kaplan, M.D.; Charles M. Tipton, Ph.D., FACSM; and Edward J. Zambraski, Ph.D., FACSM.

This pronouncement was reviewed for the American College of Sports Medicine by: College Members-at-Large; the Pronouncements Committee; and by John J. Duncan, Ph.D.; William L. Haskell, Ph.D., FACSM; Ralph S. Paffenbarger, Jr., M.D., FACSM; and Douglas R. Seals, Ph.D., FACSM.

■REFERENCES■

1. Abboud, F.M. Sympathetic nervous system in hypertension. *Hypertension* 4(Suppl. II):II208–II225, 1982.
2. Ades, P.A., P. G. S. Gunther, W. L. Meyer, T. C. Gibson, J. Maddalena, and T. Orfeo. Cardiac and skeletal muscle adaptations to training in systemic hypertension and effect of beta blockade (metoprolol or propranolol). *Am. J. Cardiol.* 66:591–596, 1990.
3. American College of Sports Medicine. *Guidelines for Exercise Testing and Prescription.* Lea and Febiger: Philadelphia, 1991, pp. 150–154.
4. American College of Sports Medicine Position Stand. The recommended quantity and quality of exercise for developing and maintaining cardiorespiratory and muscular fitness in healthy adults. *Med. Sci. Sports Exercise.* 22:265–274, 1990.
5. Attina, D.A., G. Giuliano, G. Arcangeli, R. Musante, and V. Cupelli. Effects of one year of physical training on borderline hypertension: an evaluation by bicycle ergometer exercise testing. *J. Cardiovasc. Pharmacol.* 8 (Suppl. 5):S145–S147, 1986.
6. Baechle, T.R. Effects of heavy resistance weight training on arterial blood pressure and other selected measures in normotensive and borderline hypertensive college men. In: *Sports Medicine,* Vol. 5, F. Landry and W. A. R. Orban (Eds.). Miami, FL: Symposia Specialists: 1978, pp. 169–176.
7. Baglivo, H., G. Fabregues, H. Burrieza, R. C. Esper, M. Talarico, and R. J. Esper. Effect of moderate physical training on left ventricular mass in mild hypertensive persons. *Hypertension* 15(Suppl. I):I153–I156, 1990.
8. Barry, A.C., J.W. Daly, E.D.R. Pruett, et al. The effects of physical conditioning on older individuals. I. Work capacity, circulatory-respiratory function, and work electrocardiogram. *J. Gerontol.* 21:182–191, 1966.
9. Baum, C., D.L. Kennedy, M.B. Forbes, and J. K. Jones. Drug use and expenditures in 1982. *JAMA* 253:382–386, 1985.
10. Benbassat, J. and P. F. Froom. Blood pressure response to exercise as a predictor of hypertension. *Arch. Int. Med.* 146:2053–2055, 1986.
11. Blair, S.N., H.W. Kohl III, R.S. Paffenbarger Jr., D.G. Clark, K.H. Cooper, and L.W. Gibbons. Physical fitness and all-cause mortality: a prospective study of healthy men and women. *JAMA* 262:2395–2401, 1989.
12. Blair, S.N., H.W. Kohl III, C.E. Barlow, and L. W. Gibbons. Physical fitness and all-cause mortality in hypertensive men. *Ann. Med.* 23:307–312, 1991.
13. Blair, S.N., N.N. Goodyear, L.W. Gibbons, and K.H. Cooper. Physical fitness and incidence of hypertension in healthy normotensive men and women. *JAMA* 252:487–490, 1984.
14. Blumenthal, J.A., W.C. Siegel, and M. Appelbaum. Failure of exercise to reduce blood pressure in patients with mild hypertension. *JAMA* 266:2098–2104, 1991.
15. Bonnano, J.A. and J.E. Lies. Effects of physical training on coronary risk factors. *Am. J. Cardiol.* 33:760–763, 1974.
16. Boyer, J.L. and F.W. Kasch. Exercise therapy in hypertensive men. *JAMA* 211:1668–1671, 1970.
17. Bray, G.A. Exercise and obesity. In: *Exercise, Fitness, and Health.* C. Bouchard, R.J. Shephard, T. Stephens, J.R. Sutton, and B.D. McPherson. (Eds.). Champaign, IL: Human Kinetics Press, 1988, pp. 497–510.
18. Buccola, V. A. and W. J. Stone. Effects of jogging and cycling programs on physiological and personality variables in aged men. *Res. Q.* 46:134–139, 1975.
19. Cade, R., D. Mars, H. Wagemaker, et al. Effect of aerobic exercise training on patients with systemic arterial hypertension. *Am. J. Med.* 77:785–790, 1984.
20. Chaney, R.H. and R.K. Eyman. Blood pressure at rest and maximal dynamic and isometric exercise as predictors of systemic hypertension. *Am. J. Cardiol.* 62:1058–1061, 1988.
21. Chick, T.W., A.K. Halperin, and E.M. Gacek. Effect of antihypertensive medications on exercise performance: a review. *Med. Sci. Sports Exercise* 20:447–454, 1988.
22. Choquette, G. and R.J. Ferguson. Blood pressure reduction in borderline hypertensives following physical training. *Can. Med. Assoc. J.* 108:699–703, 1973.
23. Cleroux, J., F. Peronnet, and J. De Champlain. Effects of exercise training on plasma catecholamines and blood pressure in labile hypertensive subjects. *Eur. J. Appl. Physiol.* 56:550–554, 1987.
24. Cononie, C.C., J.E. Graves, M.L. Pollock, M.I. Phillips, C. Sumners, and J.M. Hagberg. Effect of exercise training on blood pressure in 70–79 year old men and women. *Med. Sci. Sports Exerc.* 23:505–511, 1991.
25. Cypress, B. K. NCHS Advance Data, No. 80, July 22, 1982, Vital and Health Statistics of the National Center for Health Statistics. U.S. Department of Health and Human Services.
26. Dannenberg, A.L., R.J. Garrison, and W.B. Kannel. Incidence of hypertension in the Framingham Study. *Am. J. Public Health* 78:676–679, 1988.
27. DePlaen, J.F. and J.M. Detry. Hemodynamic effects of physical training in established arterial hypertension. *Acta Cardiol.* 35:179–188, 1980.
28. DiPette, D.J. and E.D. Frohlich. Cardiac involvement in hypertension. *Am. J. Cardiol.* 61:67H–72H, 1988.
29. Duncan, J.J., J.E. Farr, J. Upton, R.D. Hagan, M.E. Oglesby, and S.N. Blair. The effects of aerobic exercise on plasma catecholamines and blood pressure in patients with mild essential hypertension. *J. Am. Med. Assoc.* 254:2609–2613, 1985.
30. Duncan, J.J., H. Vandrager, J.E. Farr, H.W. Kohl, and N.F. Gordon. Effect of intrinsic sympathomimetic activity on serum lipids during exercise training in hypertensive patients receiving chronic beta-blocker therapy. *J. Cardiopulmon. Rehabil.* 9:110–114, 1989.
31. Effron, M.D. Effects of resistive training on left ventricular function. *Med. Sci. Sports Exerc.* 21:694–697, 1989.
32. Emes, C.G. The effects of a regular program of light exercise on seniors. *Int. J. Sports Med. Phys. Fitness* 19:185–190, 1979.
33. Esler, M., G. Jennings, P. Korner, I. Willett, F. Dudley, G. Hasking, W. Anderson, and G. Lambert. Assessment of human sympathetic nervous system activity from measurements of norepinephrine turnover. *Hypertension* 11:3–20, 1988.

34. Fleck, S.J. Cardiovascular adaptations to resistance training. *Med. Sci. Sports Exerc.* 20:S146–S151, 1988.

35. Frohlich, E.D., D.T. Lowenthal, H.S. Miller, T. Pickering, and W.B. Strong. Task Force IV: Systemic arterial hypertension. *J. Am. Coll. Cardiol.* 6:1218–1221, 1985.

36. Gilders, R.M., C. Voiner, and G.A. Dudley. Endurance training and blood pressure in normotensive and hypertensive adults. *Med. Sci. Sports Exercise* 21:629–636, 1989.

37. Glasgow, M.S., K.R. Gaardner, and B.T. Engel. Behavioral treatment of high blood pressure. II. Acute and sustained effects of relaxation and systolic blood pressure feedback. *Psychosom. Med.* 44:155–170, 1982.

38. Gleichmann, U.M. H.-H. Philippi, S.I. Gleichmann, et al. Group exercise improves patient compliance in mild to moderated hypertension. *J. Hypertens.* 7(Suppl. 3):S77–S80, 1989.

39. Gordon, N.F., C.B. Scott, W.J. Wilkinson, J.J. Duncan, and S.N. Blair. Exercise and mild essential hypertension: recommendations for adults. *Sports Med.* 10:390–404, 1990.

40. Gordon, N.F. and J.J. Duncan. Effect of beta-blockers on exercise physiology: implications for exercise training. *Med. Sci. Sports Exerc.* 23:668–676, 1991.

41. Hagberg, J.M. Exercise, fitness, and hypertension, In: *Exercise, Fitness, and Health,* C. Bouchard, R.J. Shephard, T. Stephens, J.R. Sutton, and B.D. McPherson (Eds.). Champaign, IL: Human Kinetics Press, 1988, pp. 455–466.

42. Hagberg, J.M., A.A. Ehsani, D. Goldring, A. Hernandez, D.R. Sinacore, and J.O. Holloszy. Effect of weight training on blood pressure and hemodynamics in hypertensive adolescents. *J. Pediatr.* 104:147–151, 1984.

43. Hagberg, J.M., A.P. Goldberg, A.A. Ehsani, G.W. Heath, J.A. Delmez, and H.R. Harter. Exercise training improves hypertension in hemodialysis patients. *Am. J. Nephrol.* 3:209–212, 1983.

44. Hagberg, J.M., D. Goldring, A.A. Ehsani, et al. Effect of exercise training on the blood pressure and hemodynamic features of hypertensive adolescents. *Am. J. Cardiol.* 52:763–768, 1983.

45. Hagberg, J.M., D. Goldring, G.W. Heath, A.A. Ehsani, A. Hernandez, and J.O. Holloszy. Effect of exercise training on plasma catecholamines and hemodynamics of adolescent hypertensives during rest, submaximal exercise, and orthostatic stress. *Clin. Physiol.* 4:117–124, 1984.

46. Hagberg, J.M., S.J. Montain, and W.H. Martin. Blood pressure and hemodynamic responses after exercise in older hypertensives. *J. Appl. Physiol.* 63:270–276, 1987.

47. Hagberg, J.M., S.J. Montain, W.H. Martin, and A.A. Ehsani. Effect of exercise training on 60–69 year old persons with essential hypertension. *Am. J. Cardiol.* 64:348–353, 1989.

48. Hall, J.E., L. Mizelle, D.A. Hildebrandt, and M.W. Brands. Abnormal pressure natriuresis: a cause or consequence of hypertension? *Hypertension* 15:547–559, 1990.

49. Hanson, J.S. and W.H. Nedde. Preliminary observations on physical training for hypertensive males. *Circ. Res.* 27(Suppl. 1):49–53, 1970.

50. Harris, K.A. and R.G. Holly. Physiological response to circuit weight training in borderline hypertensive subjects. *Med. Sci. Sports Exercise.* 19:246–252, 1987.

51. Hines, E.A. Significance of vascular hyperreaction as measured by the cold pressor test. *Am. Heart J.* 20:408–416, 1940.

52. Holloszy, J.O., J. Schultz, J. Kusnierkiewicz, J.M. Hagberg, and A.A. Ehsani. Effects of exercise on glucose tolerance and insulin resistance. *Acta Med. Scand. Suppl.* 711:55–65, 1987.

53. Hossack, K.F., R.A. Bruce, and T.A. Derouen. Evaluation of hypertensive males for primary coronary heart disease events using conventional risk factors and maximal exercise testing. *Clin Cardiol.* 3:229–235, 1980.

54. Jackson, A.S., W.G. Squires, G. Grimes, and E.F. Beard. Prediction of future resting hypertension from exercise blood pressure. *J. Cardiac Rehabil.* 3:263–268, 1983.

55. Jo, Y., M. Arita, A. Baba, et al. Blood pressure and sympathetic activity following responses to aerobic exercise in patients with essential hypertension. *Clin. Exp. Hypertens. Theor. Pract.* A11(Suppl. 1): 411–417, 1989.

56. Johnson, W.P. and J.A. Grover. Hemodynamic and metabolic effects of physical training in four patients with essential hypertension. *Can. Med. Assoc. J.* 96:842–846, 1967.

57. Joint National Committee on Detection, Evaluation, and Treatment of High Blood Pressure, 1988 Report. *Arch. Int. Med.* 148:1023–1038, 1988.

58. Kannel, W.B., J.T. Doyle, A.M. Ostfeld, et al. Original resources for primary prevention of atherosclerotic diseases. *Circulation* 70:157A–205A, 1984.

59. Kaplan, N. *Clinical Hypertension,* 5th Ed. Baltimore: Williams and Wilkins, 1990, pp. 3–5, 17, 138, 149–153, 165–171.

60. Kaplan, N.M. The deadly quartet: upper-body obesity, glucose intolerance, hypertriglyceridemia, and hypertension. *Arch. Intern. Med.* 149:1514–1520, 1989.

61. Kaufman, F.L., R.L. Hughson, and J.P. Schaman. Effect of exercise on recovery blood pressure in normotensive and hypertensive subjects. *Med. Sci. Sports Exerc.* 19:17–20, 1987.

62. Kelemen, M.H., M.B. Effron, S.A. Valenti, and K.J. Stewart. Exercise training combined with antihypertensive drug therapy. *JAMA* 263:2766–2771, 1990.

63. Kenney, W.L. and E.J. Zambraski. Physical activity in human hypertension—a mechanisms approach. *Sports Med.* 1:459–473, 1984.

64. Kinoshita, A., H. Urata, Y. Tanabe, M. Ikeda, H. Tanaka, M. Shindo, and K. Arakawa. What types of hypertensives respond better to mild exercise therapy? *J. Hypertens.* 6(Suppl. 4):S631–S633, 1988.

65. Kiveloff, B. and O. Huber. Brief maximal isometric exercise in hypertension. *J. Am. Geriatr. Soc.* 19:1006–1009, 1971.

66. Kiyonaga, A., K. Arakawa, H. Tanaka, and M. Shindo. Blood pressure and hormonal responses to aerobic exercise. *Hypertension* 7:125–131, 1985.

67. Kukkonen, K., R. Rauramaa, E. Voutilainen, and E. Lansimies. Physical training of middle-aged men with borderline hypertension. *Ann. Clin. Res.* 14(Suppl. 34):139–145, 1982.

68. Kuller, L.H., S.B. Hulley, J.D. Cohen, and J. Neaton. Unexpected effects of treating hypertension in men with ECG abnormalities: a critical analysis. *Circulation* 73:114–123, 1986.

69. Lauer, R.M., T.L. Burns, L.T. Mahoney, and C.M. Tipton. Blood pressure in children. In: *Perspectives in Exercise Science and Sports Medicine.* C.V. Gisolfi and D.R. Lamb (Eds.). Indianapolis: Benchmark Press, 2:431–463, 1989.

70. Levy, R.L., C.C. Hillman, W.D. Stroud, and P.D. White. Transient hypertension: its significance in terms of later development of sustained hypertension and cardiovascular-renal diseases. *JAMA* 126:829–833, 1944.

71. Luborsky, L., P. Crits-Christoph, J.P. Brady, et al. Behavioral versus pharmacological treatments for essential hypertension—a needed comparison. *Psychosom. Med.* 44:203–213, 1982.

72. MacDougall, J.D., D. Tuxen, D.G. Sale, J.R. Moroz, and J.R. Sutton. Arterial blood pressure response to heavy resistance exercise. *J. Appl. Physiol.* 58:785–790, 1985.

73. Mahoney, L.T., R.M. Scheiken, W.R. Clarke, and R.M. Lauer. Left ventricular mass and exercise responses predict future blood pressure: the Muscatine study. *Hypertension* 12;206–213, 1988.

74. Martin, J.E., P.M. Dubbert, and W.C. Cushman. Controlled trial of aerobic exercise in hypertension. *Circulation* 81:1560–1567, 1990.

75. Michel, M.C., O.E. Brodde, and P.A. Insel. Peripheral adrenergic receptors in hypertension. *Hypertension* 16:107–120, 1990.

76. Molineux, D. and A. Steptoe. Exaggerated blood pressure responses to submaximal exercise in normotensive adolescents with a family history of hypertension. *J. Hypertens.* 6:261–265, 1988.

77. Montoye, H.J., H.L. Metzner, and J. B. Keller. Habitual physical activity and blood pressure. *Med. Sci. Sports* 4:175–181, 1972.

78. Nelson, L., M.D. Esler, G.L. Jennings, and P.I. Korner. Effect of changing levels of physical activity on blood pressure and haemodynamics in essential hypertension. *Lancet* 2:473–476, 1986.

79. Nomura, G., E. Kumagai, K. Midorikawa, T. Kitano, H. Tashiro, and H. Toshima. Physical training in essential hypertension: along and in combination with dietary salt restriction. *J. Cardiac Rehabil.* 4:469–475, 1984.

80. Overton, M.J., M.J. Joyner, and C.M. Tipton. Reductions in blood pressure after acute exercise by hypertensive rats. *J. Appl. Physiol.* 64:742–747, 1988.

81. Paffenbarger, R.S. Jr. Energy imbalance and hypertension risk. In: *Diet and Exercise: Synergism in Health Maintenance*, P.L. White and T. Mondeika (Eds.). Chicago: American Medical Association, 1982, pp. 115–125.

82. Paffenbarger, R.S. Jr., R.T. Hyde, A.L. Wing, and C.C. Hsieh. Physical activity, all-cause mortality, and longevity of college men. *N. Engl. J. Med.* 314:605–613, 1986.

83. Paffenbarger, R.S. Jr., D.L. Jung, R.W. Leung, and R.T. Hyde. Physical activity and hypertension in college alumni, *Ann. Med.* 23:319–327, 1991.

84. Paffenbarger, R.S. Jr., A.L. Wing, R.T. Hyde, and D.L. Jung. Physical activity and incidence of hypertension in college alumni. *Am. J. Epidemiol.* 117:245–257, 1983.

85. Painter, P.L., J.N. Nelson-Worrel, M.M. Hill, D.R. Thronbery, W.R. Schelp, A.R. Harrington, and A.B. Weinstein. Effects of exercise training during hemodialysis. Nephron 43:87–92, 1986.

86. Pescatello, L.S., A.E. Fargo, CN. Leach, and H.H. Scherzer. Short-term effect of dynamic exercise on arterial blood pressure. *Circulation* 83:1557–1561, 1991.

87. Peters, R.K., L.D. Cady Jr., D.P. Bischoff, L. Bernstein, and M.C. Pike. Physical fitness and subsequent myocardial infarction in healthy workers. *JAMA* 249:3052–3056, 1983.

88. Pickering, T.G. Pathophysiology of exercise hypertension. *Herz* 12:119–124, 1987.

89. Pickering, T.G. and R.B. Devereux. Ambulatory monitoring of blood pressure as a predictor of cardiovascular risk. *Am. Heart J.* 114:925–928, 1987.

90. Reaven, P.D., E. Barrett-Connor, and S. Edelstein. Relation between leisure-time physical activity and blood pressure in older women. *Circulation* 83:559–565, 1991.

91. Reaven, G.M. Role of insulin resistance in human disease. *Diabetes* 37:1595–1607, 1988.

92. Ressl, J., J. Chrastek, and R. Jandova. Haemodynamic effects of physical training in essential hypertension. *Cardiologica* 32:121–133, 1977.

93. Roman, O., A.L. Camuzzi, E. Villalon, and C. Klenner. Physical training program in arterial hypertension: a long-term prospective follow-up. *Cardiology* 67:230–243, 1981.

94. Rowland, M. and J. Roberts. NCHS Advance Data, No. 84, October 8, 1982, Vital and Health Statistics of the National Center for Health Statistics. U.S. Department of Health and Human Services.

95. Rudd, J.L. and W.C. Day. A physical fitness program for patients with hypertension. *J. Am. Geriatr. Soc.* 15:373–379, 1967.

96. Sannerstedt, R., H. Wasir, R. Henning, and L. Werko. Systemic haemodynamics in mild arterial hypertension before and after physical training. *Clin. Sci. Mol. Med.* 45:145s–149s, 1973.

97. Sasaki, J., H. Urata, Y. Tanabe, et al. Mild exercise therapy increases serum high density lipoprotein$_2$ cholesterol levels in patients with essential hypertension. *Am. J. Med. Sci.* 297:220–223, 1989.

98. Seals, D.R. and M.J. Reiling. Effect of regular exercise on 24-hr arterial pressure in older hypertensive humans. *Hypertension* 18:583–592, 1991.

99. Shapiro, A.P., G.E. Schwartz, D.C.E. Ferguson, D.P. Redmond, and S.M. Weiss. Behavioral methods in the treatment of hypertension: a review of their clinical status. *Am. Int. Med.* 86:626–636, 1977.

100. Somers, V.K., J. Conway, J. Johnston, and P. Sleight. Effects of endurance exercise training on baroreflex sensitivity and blood pressure in borderline hypertension. *Lancet* 337:1363–1368, 1991.

101. Stamler, R., J. Stamler, F.C. Gosch, J. Civinelli, J. Fishman, A. Mcdonald, and A.R. Dyer. Primary prevention of hypertension by nutritional-hygienic means: final report of a randomized clinical trial. *JAMA* 262:1801–1807, 1989.

102. Tanabe, Y., J. Sasaki, H. Urata, et al. Effect of mild aerobic exercise on lipid and apolipoprotein levels in patients with essential hypertension. *Jpn. Heart J.* 29:199–206, 1988.

103. Tanji, J.L., J.J. Champlin, G.Y. Wong, E.Y. Lew, T.C. Brown, and E.A. Amsterdam. Blood pressure recovery curves after submaximal exercise: a predictor of hypertension at 10 yr follow-up. *Am. J. Hypertens.* 2:135–138, 1989.

104. Teuscher, A., M. Egger, and J.B. Herman. Diabetes and hypertension: blood pressure in clinical diabetic patients and a control population. *Arch. Intern. Med.* 149:1945–1949, 1989.

105. Thoren, P., J.S. Floras, P. Hoffman, and D.R. Seals. Endorphins and exercise: physiological mechanisms and clinical implications. *Med. Sci. Sports Exerc.* 22:417–428, 1990.

106. Tipton, C.M. Exercise, training, and hypertension. In: *Exercise and Sport Science Reviews*, R. Terjung (Ed.). Lexington, MA: DC Heath, pp. 245–306, 1984.

107. Tipton, C.M. Exercise, training, and hypertension: an update. In: *Exercise and Sport Science Reviews*, Vol. 19, J.O. Holloszy (Ed.). Baltimore: Williams and Wilkins, 1991, pp. 447–505.

108. Tipton, C.M., R.D. Matthes, K.D. Marcus, K.A. Rowlett, and J.R. Leininger. Influences of exercise intensity, age, and medication on resting blood pressure in SHR populations. *J. Appl. Physiol.* 55:1305–1310, 1983.

109. Tipton, C.M., L.A. Sebastian, J. M. Overton, C.R. Woodman, and S.B. Williams. Chronic exercise and its hemodynamic influences on resting blood pressure of hypertensive rats. *J. Appl. Physiol.* 71:2206–2210, 1991.

110. Tipton, C.M., S. McMahon, J.R. Leininger, E.L. Pauli, and C. Lauber. Exercise training and incidence of cerebrovascular lesions in stroke-prone spontaneously hypertensive rats. *J. Appl. Physiol.* 68:1080–1085, 1990.

111. Tipton, C.M., S. McMahon, E.M. Youmans, et al. Response of hypertensive rats to acute and chronic conditions of static exercise. *Am. J. Physiol.* 254:H592–H598, 1988.

112. Tipton, C.M., M.S. Sturek, R.A. Oppliger, R.D. Matthes, J.M. Overton, and J.G. Edwards. Responses of SHR to combinations of chemical sympathectomy, adrenal demedullation, and training. *Am. J. Physiol.* 247:H109–H118, 1984.

113. Tomanek, R.J., C.V. Gisolfi, C.A. Bauer, and P.J. Palmer. Coronary vasodilator reserve, capillarity, and mitochondria in trained hypertensive rats. *J. Appl. Physiol.* 64:1170–1185, 1988.

114. Urata, H., Y. Tanabe, A. Kiyonaga, et al. Antihypertensive and volume-depleting effects of mild exercise on essential hypertension. *Hypertension* 9:245–252, 1987.

115. Veterans Administration Cooperative Study Group on Antihypertensive A. Effects of treatment on morbidity in hypertension: results in patients with diastolic blood pressures averaging 115 through 129 mm Hg. *JAMA* 202:116–122, 1967.

116. Weber, F., R.J. Barnard, and D. Roy. Effects of a high complex-carbohydrate, low-fat diet and daily exercise on individuals 70 years and older. *J. Gerontol.* 38:155–161, 1986.

117. Westheim, A., K. Simonsen, O. Schamaun, E.K. Qvigstad, P. Staff, and P. Teisberg. Effect of exercise training in patients with essential hypertension. Proceedings of the 10th Scandinavian Congress of Cardiology. *Acta Med. Scand. Suppl.* 712:99–103, 1986.

118. Westheim, A., K. Simonsen, O. Schamaun, O. Muller, O. Stokke, and P. Teisberg. Effect of exercise training in patients with essential hypertension. *J. Hypertens.* 3(Suppl. 3): S479–S481, 1985.

119. Wilson, M.F., B.H. Sung, G.A. Pincomb, and W.R. Lovallo. Exaggerated pressure response to exercise in men at risk for systemic hypertension. *Am. J. Cardiol.* 66:731–736, 1990.

120. Wong, H.E., I.S. Kasser, and R.A. Bruce. Impaired maximal exercise performance with hypertensive cardiovascular disease. *Circulation* 39:633–638, 1969.

121. Wood, P.D. and M.L. Stefanick. Exercise, fitness, and atherosclerosis, In: *Exercise, Fitness, and Health,* C. Bouchard, R.J. Shephard, T. Stephens, J.R. Sutton, and B.D. McPherson (Eds.). Champaign, IL: Human Kinetics Press, 1988, pp. 409–423.

122. Zambraski, E.J. Renal regulation of fluid homeostasis during exercise. In: *Perspectives in Exercise Science and Sports Medicine (Vol. 3), Fluid Homeostasis during Exercise,* C.V. Gisolfi and D.R. Lamb (Eds.). Carmel, IN: Benchmark Press, 1990, pp. 247–280.

PART 3

ACSM POSITION STAND ON EXERCISE AND FLUID REPLACEMENT[c]

SUMMARY

American College of Sports Medicine. Position Stand on Exercise and Fluid Replacement. *Med. Sci. Sports Exerc.,* Vol. 28, No. 1, pp. i–vii, 1966. It is the position of the American College of Sports Medicine that adequate fluid replacement helps maintain hydration and, therefore, promotes the health, safety, and optimal physical performance of individuals participating in regular physical activity. This position statement is based on a comprehensive review and interpretation of scientific literature concerning the influence of fluid replacement on exercise performance and the risk of thermal injury associated with dehydration and hyperthermia. Based on available evidence, the American College of Sports Medicine makes the following general recommendations on the amount and composition of fluid that should be ingested in preparation for, during, and after exercise or athletic competition:

1) It is recommended that individuals consume a nutritionally balanced diet and drink adequate fluids during the 24-h period before an event, especially during the period that includes the meal prior to exercise, to promote proper hydration before exercise or competition.

2) It is recommended that individuals drink about 500 ml (about 17 ounces) of fluid about 2 h before exercise to promote adequate hydration and allow time for excretion of excess ingested water.

3) *During* exercise, athletes should start drinking early and at regular intervals in an attempt to consume fluids at a rate sufficient to replace all the water lost through sweating (i.e., body weight loss), or consume the maximal amount that can be tolerated.

4) It is recommended that ingested fluids be cooler than ambient temperature [between 15° and 22°C (59° and 72°F)] and flavored to enhance palatability and promote fluid replacement. Fluids should be readily available and served in containers that allow adequate volumes to be ingested with ease and with minimal interruption of exercise.

5) Addition of proper amounts of carbohydrates and/or electrolytes to a fluid replacement solution is recommended for exercise events of duration greater than 1 h since it does not significantly impair water delivery to the body and may enhance performance. During exercise lasting less than 1 h, there is little evidence of physiological or physical performance differences between consuming a carbohydrate-electrolyte drink and plain water.

6) During intense exercise lasting longer than 1 h, it is recommended that carbohydrates be ingested at a rate of 30–60 $g \cdot h^{-1}$ to maintain oxidation of carbohydrates and delay fatigue. This rate of carbohydrate intake can be achieved without compromising fluid delivery by drinking 600–1200 $ml \cdot h^{-1}$ of solutions containing 4%–8% carbohyadrates ($g \cdot 100\ ml^{-1}$). The carbohydates can be sugars (glucose or sucrose) or starch (e.g., maltodextrin).

7) Inclusion of sodium (0.5–0.7 $g \cdot l^{-1}$ of water) in the rehydration solution ingested during exercise lasting longer than 1 h is recommended since it may be advantageous in enhancing palatability, promoting fluid retention, and possibly preventing hyponatremia in certain individuals who drink excessive quantities of fluid. There is little physiological basis for the presence of sodium in an oral rehydration solution for enhancing intestinal water absorption as long as sodium is sufficiently available from the previous meal.

INTRODUCTION

Disturbances in body water and electrolyte balance can adversely affect cellular as well as systemic function, subsequently reducing the ability of humans to tolerate prolonged exercise. Water lost during exercise-induced sweating can lead to dehydration of both intracellular and extracellular fluid compartments of the body. Even a small amount of dehydration (1% body weight) can increase cardiovascular strain as indicated by a disproportionate elevation of heart rate during exercise, and limit the ability of the body to transfer heat from contracting muscles to the skin surface where heat can be dissipated to the environment. Therefore, consequences of body water deficits can increase the probability for impairing exercise performance and developing heat injury.

[c]"Exercise and Fluid Replacement" © 1996 American College of Sports Medicine (*Med. Sci. Sports Exerc.,* 28:1, 1995, pp. i–vii).

The specific aim of this position statement is to provide appropriate guidelines for fluid replacement that will help avoid or minimize the debilitating effects of water and electrolyte deficits on physiological function and exercise performance. These guidelines will also address the rationale for inclusion of carbohydrates and electrolytes in fluid replacement drinks.

HYDRATION BEFORE EXERCISE

Fluid replacement following exercise represents hydration prior to the next exercise bout. Any fluid deficit prior to exercise can potentially compromise thermoregulation during the next exercise session if adequate fluid replacement is not employed. Water loss from the body due to sweating is a function of the total thermal load that is related to the combined effects of exercise intensity and ambient conditions (temperature, humidity, wind speed).[62, 87] In humans, sweating can exceed 30 g · min⁻¹ (1.8 kg · h⁻¹).[2, 31] Water lost with sweating is derived from all fluid compartments of the body, including the blood (hypovolemia),[72] thus causing an increase in the concentration of electrolytes in the body fluids (hypertonicity).[85] People who begin exercise when hypohydrated with concomitant hypovolemia and hypertonicity display impaired ability to dissipate body heat during subsequent exercise.[26, 28, 61, 85, 86] They demonstrate a faster rise in body core temperature and greater cardiovascular strain.[28, 34, 82, 83] Exercise performance of both short duration and high power output, as well as prolonged moderate intensity endurance activities, can be impaired when individuals begin exercise with the burden of a previously incurred fluid deficit,[1, 83] an effect that is exaggerated when activity is performed in a hot environment.[81]

During exercise, humans typically drink insufficient volumes of fluid to offset sweat losses. This observation has been referred to as "voluntary dehydration".[33, 77] Following a fluid volume deficit created by exercise, individuals ingest more fluid and retain a higher percentage of ingested fluid when electrolyte deficits are also replaced.[71] In fact, complete restoration of a fluid volume deficit cannot occur without electrolyte replacement (primarily sodium) in food or beverage.[39, 89] Electrolytes, primarily sodium chloride, and to a lesser extent potassium, are lost in sweat during exercise. The concentration of Na^+ in sweat averages ~50 mmol · l⁻¹ but can vary widely (20-100 mmol · l⁻¹) depending on the state of heat acclimation, diet, and hydration.[6] Despite knowing the typical electrolyte concentration of sweat, determination of a typical amount of total electrolyte loss during thermal or exercise stress is difficult because the amount and composition of sweat varies with exercise intensity and environmental conditions. The normal range of daily U.S. intake of sodium chloride (NaCl) is 4.6 to 12.8 g (~80-220 mmol) and potassium (K^+) is 2–4 g (50–100 mmol).[63] Exercise bouts that produce electrolyte losses in the range of normal daily dietary intake are easily

replenished within 24 h following exercise and full rehydration is expected if adequate fluids are provided. When meals are consumed, adequate amounts of electrolytes are present so that the composition of the drink becomes unimportant. However, it is important that fluids be available during meal consumption since most persons rehydrate primarily during and after meals. In the absence of meals, more complete rehydration can be accomplished with fluids containing sodium than with plain water.[32, 55, 71]

To avoid or delay the detrimental effects of dehydration during exercise, individuals appear to benefit from fluid ingested prior to competition. For instance, water ingested 60 min before exercise will enhance thermoregulation and lower heart rate during exercise.[34, 56] However, urine volume will increase as much as 4 times that measured without preexercise fluid intake. Pragmatically, ingestion of 400–600 ml of water 2 h before exercise should allow renal mechanisms sufficient time to regulate total body fluid volume and osmolality at optimal preexercise levels and help delay or avoid detrimental effects of dehydration during exercise.

FLUID REPLACEMENT DURING EXERCISE

Without adequate fluid replacement during prolonged exercise, rectal temperature and heart rate will become more elevated compared with a well-hydrated condition.[13, 19, 29, 54] The most serious effect of dehydration resulting from the failure to replace fluids during exercise is impaired heat dissipation, which can elevate body core temperature to dangerously high levels (i.e., >40°C). Exercise-induced dehydration causes hypertonicity of body fluids and impairs skin blood flow,[26, 53, 54, 65] and has been associated with reduced sweat rate,[26, 85] thus limiting evaporative heat loss, which accounts for more than 80% of heat loss in a hot-dry environment. Dehydration (i.e., 3% body weight loss) can also elicit significant reduction in cardiac output during exercise since a reduction in stroke volume can be greater than the increase in heart rate.[53, 80] Since a net result of electrolyte and water imbalance associated with failure to adequately replace fluids during exercise is an increased rate of heat storage, dehydration induced by exercise presents a potential for the development of heat-related disorders,[24] including potentially life-threatening heat stroke.[88, 92] It is therefore reasonable to surmise that fluid replacement that offsets dehydration and excessive elevation in body heat during exercise may be instrumental in reducing the risk of thermal injury.[37]

To minimize the potential for thermal injury, it is advocated that water losses due to sweating during exercise be replaced at a rate equal to the sweat rate.[5, 19, 66, 73] Inadequate water intake can lead to premature exhaustion. During exercise, humans do not typically drink as much water as they sweat and, at best, voluntary drinking only replaces about two-thirds of the body water lost as sweat.[36]

It is common for individuals to dehydrate by 2%–6% of their body weight during exercise in the heat despite the availability of adequate amounts of fluid.[33, 35, 66, 73] In many athletic events, the volume and frequency of fluid consumption may be limited by the rules of competition (e.g., number of rest periods or time outs) or their availability (e.g., spacing of aid stations along a race course). While large volumes of ingested fluids ($\geq 1 \, l \cdot h^{-1}$) are tolerated by exercising individuals in laboratory studies, field observations indicate that most participants drink sparingly during competition. For example, it is not uncommon for elite runners to ingest less than 200 ml of fluid during distance events in a cool environment lasting more than 2 h.[13, 66] Actual rates of fluid ingestion are seldom more than 500 ml $\cdot h^{-1}$ [66,68] and most athletes allow themselves to become dehydrated by 2–3 kg of body weight in sports such as running, cycling, and the triathlon. It is clear that perception of thirst, an imperfect index of the magnitude of fluid deficit, cannot be used to provide complete restoration of water lost by sweating. As such, individuals participating in prolonged intense exercise must rely on strategies such as monitoring body weight loss and ingesting volumes of fluid during exercise at a rate equal to that lost from sweating, i.e., body weight reduction, to ensure complete fluid replacement. This can be accomplished by ingesting beverages that enhance drinking at a rate of one pint of fluid per pound of body weight reduction. While gastrointestinal discomfort has been reported by individuals who have attempted to drink at rates equal to their sweat rates, especially in excess of $1 \, l \cdot h^{-1}$, [10, 13, 52, 57, 66] this response appears to be individual and there is no clear association between the volume of ingested fluid and symptoms of gastrointestinal distress. Further, failure to maintain hydration during exercise by drinking appropriate amounts of fluid may contribute to gastrointestinal symptoms.[64, 76] Therefore, individuals should be encouraged to consume the maximal amount of fluids during exercise that can be tolerated without gastrointestinal discomfort up to a rate equal to that lost from sweating.

Enhancing palatability of an ingested fluid is one way of improving the match between fluid intake and sweat output. Water palatability is influenced by several factors including temperature and flavoring.[25, 36] While most individuals prefer cool water, the preferred water temperature is influenced by cultural and learned behaviors. The most pleasurable water temperature during recovery from exercise was 5°C,[78] although when water was ingested in large quantities, a temperature of ~15°–21°C was preferred.[9, 36] Experiments have also demonstrated that voluntary fluid intake is enhanced if the fluid is flavored[25, 36] and/or sweetened.[27] It is therefore reasonable to expect that the effect of flavoring and water temperature should increase fluid consumption during exercise, although there is insufficient evidence to support this hypothesis. In general, fluid replacement beverages that are sweetened (artificially or with sugars), flavored, and

cooled to between 15° and 21°C should stimulate fluid intake.[9,25,36,78]

The rate at which fluid and electrolyte balance will be restored is also determined by the rate at which ingested fluid empties from the stomach and is absorbed from the intestine into the blood. The rate at which fluid leaves the stomach is dependent on a complex interaction of several factors, such as volume, temperature, and composition of the ingested fluid, and exercise intensity. The most important factor influencing gastric emptying is the fluid volume in the stomach.[52, 68, 75] However, the rate of gastric emptying of water is slowed proportionately with increasing glucose concentration above 8%.[15, 38] When gastric fluid volume is maintained at 600 ml or more, most individuals can still empty more than 1000 ml $\cdot h^{-1}$ when the fluids contain a 4%–8% carbohydrate concentration.[19, 68] Therefore, to promote gastric emptying, especially with the presence of 4%–8% carbohydrate in the fluid, it is advantageous to maintain the largest volume of fluid that can be tolerated in the stomach during exercise (e.g., 400–600 ml). Mild to moderate exercise appears to have little or no effect on gastric emptying while heavy exercise at intensities greater than 80% of maximal capacity may slow gastric emptying.[12, 15] Laboratory and field studies suggest that during prolonged exercise, frequent (every 15–20 min) consumption of moderate (150 ml) to large (350 ml) volumes of fluid is possible. Despite the apparent advantage of high gastric fluid volume for promoting gastric emptying, there should be some caution associated with maintaining high gastric fluid volume. People differ in their gastric emptying rates as well as their tolerance to gastric volumes, and it has not been determined if the ability to tolerate high gastric volumes can be improved by drinking during training. It is also unclear whether complaints of gastrointestinal symptoms by athletes during competition are a function of an unfamiliarity of exercising with a full stomach or because of delays in gastric emptying.[57] It is therefore recommended that individuals learn their tolerance limits for maintaining a high gastric fluid volume for various exercise intensities and durations.

Once ingested fluid moves into the intestine, water moves out of the intestine into the blood. Intestinal absorptive capacity is generally adequate to cope with even the most extreme demands;[30] and at intensities of exercise that can be sustained for more than 30 min, there appears to be little effect of exercise on intestinal function.[84] In fact, dehydration consequent to failure to replace fluids lost during exercise reduces the rate of gastric emptying,[64, 76] supporting the rationale for early and continued drinking throughout exercise.

ELECTROLYTE AND CARBOHYDRATE REPLACEMENT DURING EXERCISE

There is little physiological basis for the presence of sodium in an oral rehydration solution for enhancing intestinal water absorption as long as sodium is sufficiently available in the gut from the previous meal or in the pancreatic secretions.[84] Inclusion of sodium (<50 mmol $\cdot$ l^{-1}) in fluid replacement drinks during exercise has not shown consistent improvements in retention of ingested fluid in the vascular compartment.[20, 23, 44, 45] A primary rationale for electrolyte supplementation with fluid replacement drinks is, therefore, to replace electrolytes lost from sweating during exercise greater than 4–5 h in duration.[3] Normal plasma sodium concentration is 140 mmol $\cdot$ l^{-1}, making sweat ($\sim$50 mmol $\cdot$ l^{-1}) hypotonic relative to plasma. At a sweat rate of 1.5 l $\cdot$ h^{-1}, a total sodium deficit of 75 mmol $\cdot$ h^{-1} could occur during exercise. Drinking water can lower elevated plasma electrolyte concentrations back toward normal and restore sweating,[85, 86] but complete restoration of the extracellular fluid compartment cannot be sustained without replacement of lost sodium.[39, 70, 89] In most cases, this can be accomplished by normal dietary intake.[63] If sodium enhances palatability, then its presence in a replacement solution may be justified because drinking can be maximized by improving taste qualities of the ingested fluid.[9, 25]

The addition of carbohydrates to a fluid replacement solution can enhance intestinal absorption of water.[30, 84] However, a primary role of ingesting carbohydrates in a fluid replacement beverage is to maintain blood glucose concentration and enhance carbohydrate oxidation during exercise that lasts longer than 1 h, especially when muscle glycogen is low.[11, 14, 17, 18, 50, 60] As a result, fatigue can be delayed by carbohydrate ingestion during exercise of duration longer than 1 h which normally causes fatigue without carbohydrate ingestion.[11] To maintain blood glucose levels during continuous moderate-to-high intensity exercise, carbohydrates should be ingested throughout exercise at a rate of 30–60 g $\cdot$ h^{-1}. These amounts of carbohydrates can be obtained while also replacing relatively large amounts of fluid if the concentration of carbohydrates is kept below 10% (g $\cdot$ 100 ml^{-1} of fluid). For example, if the desired volume of ingestion is 600–1200 ml $\cdot$ h^{-1}, then the carbohydrate requirements can be met by drinking fluids with concentrations in the range of 4%–8%.[19] With this procedure, both fluid and carbohydrate requirements can be met simultaneously during prolonged exercise. Solutions containing carbohydrate concentrations $>$10% will cause a net movement of fluid into the intestinal lumen because of their high osmolality, when such solutions are ingested during exercise. This can result in an effective loss of water from the vascular compartment and can exacerbate the effects of dehydration.[43]

Few investigators have examined the benefits of adding carbohydrates to water during exercise events lasting less than 1 h. Although preliminary data suggest a potential benefit for performance,[4, 7, 48] the mechanism is unclear. It would be premature to recommend drinking something other than water during exercise lasting less than 1 h.

Generally, the inclusion of glucose, sucrose, and other complex carbohydrates in fluid replacement solutions have equal effectiveness in increasing exogenous carbohydrate oxidation, delaying fatigue, and improving performance.[11, 16, 79, 90] However, fructose should not be the predominant carbohydrate because it is converted slowly to blood glucose—not readily oxidized[41, 42]—which does not improve performance.[8] Furthermore, fructose may cause gastrointestinal distress.[59]

FLUID REPLACEMENT AND EXERCISE PERFORMANCE

Although the impact of fluid deficits on cardiovascular function and thermoregulation is evident, the extent to which exercise performance is altered by fluid replacement remains unclear. Although some data indicate that drinking improves the ability to perform short duration athletic events (1 h) in moderate climates,[7] other data suggest that this may not be the case.[40] It is likely that the effect of fluid replacement on performance may be most noticeable during exercise of duration greater than 1 h and/or at extreme ambient environments.

The addition of a small amount of sodium to rehydration fluids has little impact on time to exhaustion during mild prolonged ($>$4 h) exercise in the heat,[73] ability to complete 6 h of moderate exercise,[5] or capacity to perform during simulated time trials.[20, 74] A sodium deficit, in combination with ingestion and retention of a large volume of fluid with little or no electrolytes, has led to low plasma sodium levels in a very few marathon or ultra-marathon athletes.[3, 67] Hyponatremia (blood sodium concentration between 117 and 128 mmol $\cdot$ l^{-1}) has been observed in ultra-endurance athletes at the end of competition and is associated with disorientation, confusion, and in most cases, grand mal seizures.[67, 69] One major rationale for inclusion of sodium in rehydration drinks is to avoid hyponatremia. To prevent development of this rare condition during prolonged ($>$4 h) exercise, electrolytes should be present in the fluid or food during and after exercise.

Maintenance of blood glucose concentrations is necessary for optimal exercise performance. To maintain blood glucose concentration during fatiguing exercise greater than 1 h (above 65% $\dot{V}o_{2max}$), carbohydrate ingestion is necessary.[11, 49] Late in prolonged exercise, ingested carbohydrates become the main source of carbohydrate energy and can delay the onset of fatigue.[17, 19, 21, 22, 51, 58] Data from field studies designed to test these concepts during athletic competition have not always demonstrated delayed onset of fatigue,[46, 47, 91] but the inability to control critical factors (such as environmental conditions, state of training, drinking volumes) make confirmation difficult. Inclusion of carbohydrates in a rehydration solution becomes more important for optimal performance as the duration of intense exercise exceeds 1 h.

CONCLUSION

The primary objective for replacing body fluid loss during exercise is to maintain normal hydration. One should consume adequate fluids during the 24-h period before an event and drink about 500 ml (about 17 ounces) of fluid about 2 h before exercise to promote adequate hydration and allow time for excretion of excess ingested water. To minimize risk of thermal injury and impairment of exercise performance during exercise, fluid replacement should attempt to equal fluid loss. At equal exercise intensity, the requirement for fluid replacement becomes greater with increased sweating during environmental thermal stress. During exercise lasting longer than 1 h, a) carbohydrates should be added to the fluid replacement solution to maintain blood glucose concentration and delay the onset of fatigue, and b) electrolytes (primarily NaCl) should be added to the fluid replacement solution to enhance palatability and reduce the probability for development of hyponatremia. During exercise, fluid and carbohydrate requirements can be met simultaneously by ingesting 600–1200 ml $\cdot$ h^{-1} of solutions containing 4%–8% carbohydrate. During exercise greater than 1 h, approximately 0.5–0.7 g of sodium per liter of water would be appropriate to replace that lost from sweating.

■ A C K N O W L E D G M E N T S ■

This pronouncement was reviewed for the American College of Sports Medicine by members-at-large, the Pronouncement Committee, and by: David L. Costill, Ph.D. (FACSM), John E. Greenleaf, Ph.D. FACSM, Scott J. Montain, Ph.D., and Timothy D. Noakes, M.D. FACSM.

■ R E F E R E N C E S ■

1. Armstrong, L.E., D.L. Costill, and W.J. Fink. Influence of diuretic-induced dehydration on competitive running performance. *Med. Sci. Sports Exerc.* 17:456–461, 1985.
2. Armstrong, L.E., R.W. Hubbard, B.H. Jones, and J.J. Daniels. Preparing Alberto Salazar for the heat of the 1984 Olympic marathon. *Physician Sportsmed.* 14:73–81, 1986.
3. Armstrong, L.E., W.C. Curtis, R.W. Hubbard, R.P. Francesconi, R. Moore, and E.W. Askew. Symptomatic hyponatremia during prolonged exercise in heat. *Med. Sci. Sports Exerc.* 25:543–549, 1993.
4. Ball, T.C., S. Headley, and P. Vanderburgh. Carbohydrate-electrolyte replacement improves sprint capacity following 50 minutes of high-intensity cycling. *Med. Sci. Sports Exerc.* 26:S196, 1994 (abstract).
5. Barr, S.I., D.L. Costill, and W.J. Fink. Fluid replacement during prolonged exercise: effects of water, saline, or no fluid. *Med. Sci. Sports Exerc.* 23:811–817, 1991.
6. Bean, W.B. and L.W. Eichna. Performance in relationship to environmental temperature. Reactions of normal young men to simulated desert environment. *Fed. Proc.* 2:144–158, 1943.
7. Below, P.R. and E.F. Coyle. Fluid and carbohydrate ingestion individually benefit intense exercise lasting one hour. *Med. Sci. Sports Exerc.* 27:200–210, 1995.
8. Bjorkman, O., K. Sahlin, L. Hagenfeldt, and J. Wahren. Influence of glucose and fructose ingestion on the capacity for long-term exercise. *Clin. Physiol.* 4:483–494, 1984.
9. Boulze, D., P. Montastruc, and M. Cabanac. Water intake, pleasure and water temperature in humans. *Physiol. Behav.* 30:97–102, 1983.
10. Brouns, F., W.H.M. Saris, and N.J. Rehrer. Abdominal complaints and gastrointestinal function during long-lasting exercise. *Int. J. Sports Med.* 8:175–189, 1987.
11. Coggan, A.R. and E.F. Coyle. Carbohydrate ingestion during prolonged exercise: effects on metabolism and performance. *Exerc. Sport Sci. Rev.* 19:1–40, 1991.
12. Costill, D.L. Gastric emptying of fluids during exercise. In: *Perspectives in Exercise Science and Sports Medicine, Vol. 3, Fluid Homeostatsis During Exercise,* C.V. Gisolfi and D.R. Lamb (Eds.). Carmel, IN: Benchmark Press, Inc., 1990, pp. 97–128.
13. Costill, D.L., W.F. Krammer, and A. Fisher. Fluid ingestion during distance running. *Arch. Environ. Health* 21:520–525, 1970.
14. Costill, D.L. and M. Hargreaves. Carbohydrate nutrition and fatigue. *Sports Med.* 13:86–92, 1992.
15. Costill, D.L. and B. Saltin. Factors limiting gastric emptying during rest and exercise. *J. Appl. Physiol.* 37:679–683, 1974.
16. Coyle, E.F. Timing and method of increased carbohydrate intake to cope with heavy training, competition and recovery. *J. Sports Sci.* 9:29–52, 1991.
17. Coyle, E.F., A.R. Coggan, M.K. Hemmert, and J.L. Ivy. Muscle glycogen utilization during prolonged strenuous exercise when fed carbohydrate. *J. Appl. Physiol.* 61:165–172, 1986.
18. Coyle, E.F., J.M. Hagberg, B.F. Hurley, W.H. Martin, A.A. Ehsani, and J.O. Holloszy. Carbohydrate feeding during prolonged strenuous exercise can delay fatigue. *J. Appl. Physiol.* 55:30–235, 1983.
19. Coyle, E.F. and S.J. Montain. Benefits of fluid replacement with carbohydrate during exercise. *Med. Sci. Sports Exerc.* 24 (Suppl. 9):S324—S330, 1992.
20. Criswell, D., K. Renshler, S.K. Powers, R. Tulley, M. Cicale, and K. Wheeler. Fluid replacement beverages and maintenance of plasma volume during exercise: role of aldosterone and vasopressin. *Eur. J. Appl. Physiol.* 65:445–51, 1992.
21. Davis, J.M., W.A. Burgess, C.A. Slentz, W.P. Bartoli, and R.R. Pate. Effects of ingesting 6% and 12% glucose/electrolyte beverages during prolonged intermittent cycling in the heat. *Eur. J. Appl. Physiol.* 57:563–569, 1988.
22. Davis, J.M., D.R. Lamb, R.R. Pate, C.A. Slentz, W.A. Burgess, and W.P. Bartoli. Carbohydrate-electrolyte drinks: effects on endurance cycling in the heat. *Am. J. Clin. Nutr.* 48:1023–1030, 1988.
23. Deuster, P.A., A. Singh, A. Hofmann, F.M. Moses, and G.C. Chrousos. Hormonal responses to ingesting water or a carbohydrate beverage during a 2 h run. *Med. Sci. Sports Exerc.* 24:72–79, 1992.
24. Eichna, L.W., W.B. Bean, W.F. Ashe, and N. Nelson. Performance in relation to environmental temperature. Reactions of normal young men to hot, humid (simulated jungle) environment. *Bull. Johns Hopkins Hosp.* 76:25–58, 1945.
25. Engell, D. and E. Hirsch. Environmental and sensory modulation of fluid intake in humans. In: *Thirst: Physiological and Psychological Aspects.* D.J. Ramsay and D.A. Booth (Eds.). Berlin: Springer-Verlag, 1990, pp. 382–402.
26. Fortney, S.M. Effect of hyperosmolality on control of blood flow and sweating. *J. Appl. Physiol.* 57:1688–1695, 1984.
27. Fortney, S.M., E.R. Nadel, C.B. Wenger, and J.R. Bove. Effect of acute alterations of blood volume on circulatory performance in humans. *J. Appl. Physiol.* 50:292–298, 1981.
28. Fortney, S.M., E.R. Nadel, C.B. Wenger, and J.R. Bove. Effect of blood volume on sweating rate and body fluids in exercising humans. *J. Appl. Physiol.* 51:1594–1600, 1981.
29. Gilsolfi, C.V. and J.R. Copping. Thermal effects of prolonged treadmill exercise in the heat. *Med. Sci. Sports* 6:108–113, 1974.
30. Gisolfi, C.V., R.W. Summers, and H.P. Schedl. Intestinal absorption of fluids during rest and exercise. In: *Perspectives in Exercise Science and Sports Medicine, Vol. 3. Fluid Homeostasis During Exercise.* C.V. Gisolfi and D.L. Lamb (Eds.). Carmel, IN: Benchmark Press, Inc., 1990, pp. 129–180.

31. Gisolfi, C.V., K.J. Spranger, R.W. Summers, H.P. Schedel, and T.L. Bleiler. Effects of cycle exercise on intestinal absorption in humans. *J. Appl. Physiol.* 71:2518–2527, 1991.

32. Gonzalez-Alonso, J., C.L. Heaps, and E.F. Coyle. Rehydration after exercise with common beverages and water. *Int. J. Sports Med.* 13:399–406, 1992.

33. Greenleaf, J.E. and F. Sargent II. Voluntary dehydration in man. *J. Appl. Physiol.* 20:719–724, 1965.

34. Greenleaf, J.E. and B.L. Castle. Exercise temperature regulation in man during hypohydration and hyperhydration. *J. Appl. Physiol.* 30:847–853, 1971.

35. Greenleaf, J.E., P.J. Brock, L.C. Keil, and J.T. Morse. Drinking and water balance during exercise and heat acclimation. *J. Appl. Physiol.* 54:414–419, 1983.

36. Hubbard, R.W., O. Maller, M.N. Sawka, R.N. Francesconi, L. Drolet, and A.J. Young. Voluntary dehydration and alliesthesia for water. *J. Appl. Physiol.* 57:868–875, 1984.

37. Hubbard, R.W. and L.E. Armstrong. The heat illness: biochemical, ultrastructural, and fluid-electrolyte considerations. In: *Human Performance Physiology and Environmental Medicine at Terrestrial Extremes.* K.B. Pandolf, M.N. Sawka, and R.R. Gonzalez (Eds.). Indianapolis: Benchmark Press, Inc., 1988, pp. 305–360.

38. Hunt, J.N. and M.T. Knox. Regulation of gastric emptying. In: *Handbook of Physiology,* Vol. IV. Washington, DC: American Physiological Society, 1969, pp. 1917–1935.

39. Lassiter, W.E. Regulation of sodium chloride distribution within the extracellular space. In: *The Regulation of Sodium and Chloride Balance.* D.W. Seldin and G. Giebisch (Eds.). New York: Raven Press, Inc., 1990, pp. 23–58.

40. Levine, L., M.S. Rose, R.P. Francesconi, P.D. Neufer, and M.N. Sawka. Fluid replacement during sustained activity in the heat: nutrient solution vs. water. *Aviat. Space Environ. Med.* 62:559–564, 1991.

41. Massicotte, D., F. Perronnet, C. Allah, C. Hillaire-Marcel, M. Ledoux, and G. Brisson. Metabolic response to [13C]glucose and [13C]fructose ingestion during exercise. *J. Appl. Physiol.* 61:1180–1184, 1986.

42. Massicotte, D., F. Perronnet, G. Brisson, K. Bakkouch, and C. Hillaire-Marcel. Oxidation of glucose polymer during exercise: comparison of glucose and fructose. *J. Appl. Physiol.* 66:179–183, 1989.

43. Maughan, R.J. Thermoregulation and fluid balance in marathon competition at low ambient temperature. *Int. J. Sports Med.* 6:15–19, 1985.

44. Maughan, R.J., C.E. Fenn, M. Gleeson, and J.B. Leiper. Metabolic and circulatory responses to the ingestion of glucose polymers and glucose-electrolyte solutions during exercise in man. *Eur. J. Appl. Physiol.* 56:356–362, 1987.

45. Maughan, R.J., C.E. Fenn, M. Gleeson, and J.B. Leiper. Effects of fluid, electrolyte, and substrate ingestion on endurance capacity. *Eur. J. Appl. Physiol.* 58:481–486, 1989.

46. Millard-Stafford, M., P.B. Sparling, L.B. Rosskopf, B.T. Hinson, and L.J. Dicarlo. Carbohydrate-electrolyte replacement during a simulated triathlon in the heat. *Med. Sci. Sports Exerc.* 22:621–628, 1990.

47. Millard-Stafford, M., P.B. Sparling, L.B. Rosskopf, and L.J. Dicarlo. Carbohydrate-electrolyte replacement improves distance running performance in the heat. *Med. Sci. Sports Exerc.* 24:934–940, 1992.

48. Millard-Stafford, M., L.B. Rosskopf, T.K. Snow, and B.T. Hinson. Pre-exercise carbohydrate-electrolyte ingestion improves one-hour running performance in the heat. *Med. Sci. Sports Exerc.* 26:S196, 1994 (abstract).

49. Mitchell, J.B., D.L. Costill, J.A. Houmard, M.G. Flynn, W.J. Fink, and J.D. Beltz. Effects of carbohydrate ingestion on gastric emptying and exercise performance. *Med Sci. Sports Exerc.* 20:110–115, 1988.

50. Mitchell, J.B., D.L. Costill, J.A. Houmard, W.J. Fink, D.D. Pascoe, and D. R. Pearson. Influence of carbohydrate dosage on exercise performance and glycogen metabolism. *J. Appl. Physiol.* 67:1843–9, 1989.

51. Mitchell, J.B., D.L. Costill, J.A. Houmard, W.J. Fink, R.A. Robergs, and J.A. Davis. Gastric emptying: influence of prolonged exercise and carbohydrate concentration. *Med Sci. Sports Exerc.* 21:269–274, 1989.

52. Mitchell, J.B. and K.W. Voss. The influence of volume of fluid ingested on gastric emptying and fluid balance during prolonged exercise. *Med. Sci. Sports Exerc.* 23:314–319, 1991.

53. Montain, S.J. and E.F. Coyle. Fluid ingestion during exercise increases skin blood flow independent of increases in blood volume. *J. Appl. Physiol.* 73:903–910, 1992.

54. Montain, S.J. and E.F. Coyle. The influence of graded dehydration on hyperthermia and cardiovascular drift during exercise. *J. Appl. Physiol.* 73:1340–1350, 1992.

55. Morimoto, T., K. Mike, H. Nose, S. Yamada, K. Hirakawa, and C. Matsubara. Changes in body fluid and its composition during heavy sweating and effect of fluid and electrolyte replacement. *Jpn. J. Biometeorol.* 18:31–39, 1981.

56. Moroff, S.V. and D.B. Bass. Effects of overhydration on man's physiological responses to work in the heat. *J. Appl. Physiol.* 20:267–270, 1965.

57. Moses, F.M. The effect of exercise on the gastrointestinal tract. *Sports Med.* 9:159–172, 1990.

58. Murray, R., D.E. Eddy, T.W. Murray, J.G. Seifert, G.L. Paul, and G.A. Halaby. The effect of fluid and carbohydrate feeding during intermittent cycling exercise. *Med. Sci. Sports Exerc.* 19:597–604, 1987.

59. Murray, R., G.L. Paul, J.G. Seifert, D.E. Eddy, and G.A. Halaby. The effects of glucose, fructose, and sucrose ingestion during exercise. *Med. Sci. Sports Exerc.* 21:275–282, 1989.

60. Murray, R., G.L. Paul, J.G. Seifert, and D.E. Eddy. Responses to varying rates of carbohydrate ingestion during exercise. *Med. Sci. Sports Exerc.* 23:713–718, 1991.

61. Nadel, E.R., S.M. Fortney, and C.B. Wenger. Effect of hydration state on circulatory and thermal regulations. *J. Appl. Physiol.* 49:715–721, 1980.

62. Nadel, E.R., C.B. Wenger, M.F. Roberts, J.A.J. Stolwijk, and E. Cafarelli. Physiological defenses against hyperthermia of exercise. *Ann. N.Y. Acad. Sci* 301:98–110, 1977.

63. National Research Council. *Recommended Dietary Allowances,* 10th Ed. Washington, DC: National Academy Press, 1989, pp. 250–255.

64. Neufer, P.D., A.J. Young, and M.N. Sawka. Gastric emptying during exercise: effects of heat stress and hypohydration. *Eur. J. Appl. Physiol.* 58:433–439, 1989.

65. Nishiyasu, T., X. Shi, G.W. Mack, and E.R. Nadel. Effect of hypovolemia on forearm vascular resistance control during exercise in the heat. *J. Appl. Physiol.* 71:1382–1386, 1991.

66. Noakes, T.D. Fluid replacement during exercise. *Exerc. Sports Sci. Rev.* 21:297–330, 1993.

67. Noakes, T.D., R.J. Norman, R.H. Buck, J. Godlonton, K. Stevenson, and D. Pittaway. The incidence of hyponatremia during prolonged ultraendurance exercise. *Med Sci. Sports Exerc.* 22:165–170, 1990.

68. Noakes, T.D., N.J. Rehrer, and R.J. Maughan. The importance of volume in regulating gastric emptying. *Med. Sci. Sports Exerc.* 23:307–313, 1991.

69. Noakes, T.D., N. Goodwin, B.L. Rayner, T. Branken, and R.K.N. Taylor. Water intoxication: a possible complication during endurance exercise. *Med Sci. Sports Exerc.* 17:370–375, 1985.

70. Nose, H., M. Morita, T. Yawata, and T. Morimoto. Recovery of blood volume and osmolality after thermal dehydration in rats. *Am. J. Physiol.* 251:R492—R498, 1986.

71. Nose, H., G.W. Mack, X. Shi, and E.R. Nadel. Role of osmolality and plasma volume during rehydration in humans. *J. Appl. Physiol.* 65:325–331, 1988.

72. Nose, H., G.W. Mack, X. Shi, and E.R. Nadel. Shift in body fluid compartments after dehydration in humans. *J. Appl. Physiol.* 65:318–324, 1988.

73. Pitts, G.C., R.E. Johnson, and F.C. Consolazio. Work in the heat as affected by intake of water, salt, and glucose. *Am. J. Physiol.* 142:253–259, 1944.

74. Powers, S.K., J. Lawler, S. Dodd, R. Tulley, G. Landry, and K. Wheeler. Fluid replacement drinks during high intensity exercise: effects on

minimizing exercise-induced disturbances in homeostasis. *Eur. J. Appl. Physiol.* 60:54–60, 1990.

75. Rehrer, N.J. The maintenance of fluid balance during exercise. *Int. J. Sports Med.* 15:122–125, 1994.

76. Rehrer, N.J., E.J. Beckers, F. Brouns, F. Ten Hoor, and W.H.M. Saris. Effects of dehydration on gastric emptying and gastrointestinal distress while running. *Med. Sci. Sports Exerc.* 22:790–795, 1990.

77. Rothstein, A., E.F. Adolph, and J.H. Wills. Voluntary dehydration. In: *Physiology of Man In the Desert*, E.F. Aldolph (Ed.). New York: Interscience, 1947, pp. 254–270.

78. Sandick, B.L., D.B. Engell, and O. Maller. Perception of water temperature and effects for humans after exercise. *Physiol. Behav.* 32:851–855, 1984.

79. Saris, W.H.M., B.H. Goodpaster, A.E. Jeukendrup, F. Brouns, D. Halliday, and A.J.M. Wagenmakers. Exogenous carbohydrate oxidation from different carbohydrate sources during exercise. *J. Appl. Physiol.* 75:2168–2172, 1993.

80. Sawka, M.N., R.G. Knowlton, and J.B. Critz. Thermal and circulatory responses to repeated bouts of prolonged running. *Med. Sci. Sports* 11:177–180, 1979.

81. Sawka, M.N., R.P. Francesconi, A.J. Young, and K.B. Pandolf. Influence of hydration level and body fluids on exercise performance in the heat. *J.A.M.A.* 252:1165–1169, 1984.

82. Sawka, M.N., A.J. Young, R.P. Francesconi, S.R. Muza, and K.B. Pandolf. Thermoregulatory and blood responses during exercise at graded hypohydration levels. *J. Appl. Physiol.* 59:1394–1401, 1985.

83. Sawka, M.N. and K.B. Pandolf. Effetcs of body water loss on physiological function and exercise performance. In: *Fluid Homeostasis during Exercise*, Vol. 3, C.V. Gilsolfi and D.R. Lamb (Eds.). Carmel, IN: Benchmark Press, Inc., 1990, pp. 1–38.

84. Schedl, H.P., R.J. Maughan, and C.V. Gisolfi. Intestinal absorption during rest and exercise: implications for formulating an oral rehydration solution (ORS). *Med. Sci. Sports Exerc.* 26:267–280, 1994.

85. Senay, L.C., Jr. Relationship of evaporative rates to serum [Na+], [K+], and osmolarity in acute heat stress. *J. Appl. Physiol.* 25:149–152, 1968.

86. Senay, L.C., Jr. Temperature regulation and hypohydration: a singular view. *J. Appl. Physiol.* 47:1–7, 1979.

87. Shapiro, Y., K.B. Pandolf, and R.F. Goldman. Predicting sweat loss response to exercise, environment, and clothing. *Eur. J. Appl. Physiol.* 48:83–96, 1982.

88. Sutton, J.R. Clinical Implications of Fluid Imbalance. In: *Perspectives in Exercise Science and Sports Medicine*, Vol. 3, *Fluid Homeostsis During Exercise*. C.V. Gisolfi and D.R. Lamb (Eds.). Carmel, IN: Benchmark Press, Inc., 1990, pp. 425–455.

89. Takamata, A., G.W. Mack, C.M. Gillen, and E.R. Nadel. Sodium appetite, thirst, and body fluid regulation in humans during rehydration without sodium replacement. *Am. J. Physiol. (Regulatory Integrative Comp. Physiol.)* 266:R1493–R1502, 1994.

90. Wagenmakers, J.M., F. Brouns, W.H.M. Saris, and D. Halliday. Oxidation rates of orally ingested carbohydrate during prolonged exercise in men. *J. Appl. Physiol.* 75:2774–2780, 1993.

91. Wells, C.L., T.A. Schrader, J.R. Stern, and G.S. Krahenbuhl. Physiological responses to a 20–mile run under three fluid replacement treatments. *Med. Sci. Sports Exerc.* 17:364–369, 1985.

92. Wyndham, C.H. Heat stroke and hyperthermia in marathon runners. *Ann. N.Y. Acad. Sci.* 301:128–138, 1977.

INDEX

Page numbers in *italics* denote figures; those followed by "t" denote tables.